Encyclopedia of
Disability and Rehabilitation

Editorial Board

Encyclopedia of
Disability and Rehabilitation

Arthur E. Dell Orto
Robert P. Marinelli

EDITORS

MACMILLAN LIBRARY REFERENCE USA

Simon & Schuster Macmillan

NEW YORK

Simon & Schuster and Prentice Hall International

LONDON   MEXICO CITY   NEW DELHI   SINGAPORE   SYDNEY   TORONTO

Macmillan Library Reference
Simon & Schuster Macmillan
866 Third Avenue
New York, NY 10022

Library of Congress Catalog Card Number: 95-24454

Printed in the United States of America

printing number
1 2 3 4 5 6 7 8 9 10

Library of Congress Cataloging-in-Publication Data
Encyclopedia of Disability and Rehabilitation / Arthur E. Dell Orto and
Robert P. Marinelli, Editors
        p.   cm.
    Includes bibliographical references and index.
    ISBN 0-02-897297-X
1. Handicapped—Rehabilitation—Encyclopedias.   I. Dell Orto, Arthur E.
II. Marinelli, Robert P.
HV1568.E53   1995   95-24454
362.4′03—dc20   CIP

This paper meets the requirements of ANSI-NISO Z39.48-1992 (Permanence of Paper).

Contents

Preface   VII

List of Articles   IX

List of Contributors   XV

Encyclopedia of Disability and Rehabilitation   1

List of Resources   775

Index   791

Editorial and Production Staff

Hélène G. Potter
Project Editor

Paul Bernabeo
Editor in Chief

William D. Drennan
Copy Editor

Ellen P. Raspitha   Helen Wallace
Proofreaders

AEIOU, Inc.
Indexer

Rose Capozzelli
Production Manager

Debra Alpern
Alison Avery
Sabrina Bowers
Jessica Brent
Jennifer Karmonick
Editorial Assistants

Gordon Macomber, President
Philip Friedman, Publisher
Elly Dickason, Associate Publisher

Preface

This volume is a reference work for people with disabilities, their families, co-workers, caregivers, and the concerned public. If the entries in this Encyclopedia have one thing in common, it is that they all view the person with a disability not individually but as part of a circle of family, friends, health care professionals, and colleagues. Each person in this large circle stands to play an active role in a rehabilitation process designed to give the person with a disability the means to live as independently as possible.

Since the passage of the Americans with Disabilities Act in 1990, persons with disabilities have not only secured more rights, they have become more empowered as well as more visible. One of the provisions of the act was to make public buildings accessible to people who use wheelchairs by installing ramps and telephones at chair height. Many city sidewalks have ramps at intersections. Theaters with live performances now routinely provide hearing devices for those who need them. However, ignorance, misconceptions, and prejudices about many disabilities on the part of both people with and without disabilities still exist.

Disability and rehabilitation challenge resources and create opportunities, often within the context of a complex and harsh reality. For the person living with a disability, the treatment and rehabilitation process is a series of demands, challenges, disappointments, and rewards. The same can be said of the primary caregiver, often a family member or significant other, whose life is equally changed by the disability of a child, sibling, spouse, parent, other relative, or friend.

Our hope is that the Encyclopedia will help in the rehabilitation process by providing relevant rehabilitation information on a vast range of disabilities—physical and mental, organic and those caused by trauma—and available rehabilitation therapies, processes, concepts, and sources of support, as well as simple explanations of terms and procedures.

Even though the primary focus of the Encyclopedia is on disability and rehabilitation, we want to emphasize that persons with disabilities share a common ground with people who are not disabled or not yet disabled. As associate editor Irving Kenneth Zola has stated, "all people are temporarily able-bodied." The dignity of a person and the potential of all people should be the core value of any rehabilitation process and a goal of health and human care systems.

The entries in the Encyclopedia, which are arranged alphabetically, deal with many areas of interest, some of which are:

- the disabilities themselves
- the rehabilitation process
- the therapies available for rehabilitation
- assistive technology
- consumer empowerment
- the workplace
- the caregivers
- psychosocial adjustment
- rehabilitation philosophy and concepts

Our understanding of the terms "disability" and "rehabilitation" was fundamental in conceiving and planning this work. "Disability" is a physical or mental impairment that substantially limits an individual's ability to perform one or more major life activities. However, disability is as much a sociopolitical and economic issue as it is a medical concept.

"Rehabilitation" is defined as the process or program designed to enable the individual with a disability to reach his or her fullest physical, psychological, and vocational potential. Throughout this work, the terms "consumers," "clients," and "patients" are used interchangeably to refer to individuals with disabilities.

Use of the Encyclopedia is facilitated by a system of cross-references that lead the reader to other entries. At the end of most entries is a section beginning with the words "See also" that lists related articles. Another type of cross-reference is the "See entry;" here we direct readers to an alternative entry under which information can be found. For example the "See entry" at the term "Empowerment" reads "See Advocacy, Civil Rights, Consumers, Philosophy of Rehabilitation."

Where appropriate, entries also include lists of organizations and foundations as resources for help or further information. Bibliographies guide the reader to other literature on a particular topic.

Many people deserve our thanks for guiding us along, from initial idea to bound book. The idea for the *Encyclopedia of Disability and Rehabilitation* was formulated by Maya De, Director of the June Holt Library at the Massachusetts Rehabilitation Commission. In 1988, under the leadership of June Holt and with the support of Commissioner Elmer Bartels, an advisory board was convened to discuss the need for such a book and to conceptualize its content and format.

In 1989 we were asked to take on the editorship of this Encyclopedia. Our twenty years of experience as editors and authors of books in the areas of disability and rehabilitation had only partially prepared us, it turned out, for the enormous task at hand. The completion of this project is a direct result of the extraordinary support and expertise of our Associate Editors, David E. Creasey, M.D., and Irving Kenneth Zola, Ph.D., the contributors, and advising editors, on the one hand, and the staff at Macmillan Reference, on the other.

None of this would have been possible without the vision, skill, and high standards of Elly Dickason, associate publisher of Macmillan Reference, who was able to keep us on course even though we sometimes wondered if we would survive the demands of the process. Elly assured us that complex challenges are solved one step at a time—much like the rehabilitation process. We would also like to thank Hélène Potter, our project editor at Macmillan, who over the past eighteen months patiently and efficiently coordinated the many tasks essential to producing the Encyclopedia and whose expertise, support, and friendship are greatly valued. We also wish to express our gratitude and appreciation to the National Rehabilitation Information Center (NARIC) for substantial assistance in locating national disability and rehabilitation resources. This federally funded library and information center has been instrumental in the development of this Encyclopedia. NARIC is funded by the U.S. Department of Education, National Institute on Disability and Rehabilitation Research (NIDRR). Finally, a special acknowledgment is due to Ken Paruti, whose administrative ability and computer skills made an overwhelming project manageable during the past six years.

A dedicatory acknowledgment is in order for Irving Kenneth Zola, friend, associate editor, colleague, disability leader, and mentor, whose untimely death in 1994 was a great loss to the disability and rehabilitation community as well as to this project. Irv embodied the best qualities of humanity by living a life that was fueled by dreams, validated by accomplishments, and fortified by respect and admiration.

ARTHUR E. DELL ORTO
ROBERT P. MARINELLI

List of Articles

A

Ability
  Richard Roessler

Accessibility
  Elmer C. Bartels

Adjustment Services
  Robert H. Couch

Adolescents, Rehabilitation of
  Richard T. Goldberg

Advocacy
  Frances G. Berko
  Robert J. Boehlert

Affirmative Action
  Frank G. Bowe

Aging
  Donna R. Falvo
  Duane A. Lundervold

Alcohol Rehabilitation
  Joseph F. Stano

Allied Health Professions
  Darlene K. Sekerak
  David E. Yoder

Alzheimer's Disease
  Linda Garand
  Kathleen C. Buckwalter

Americans with Disabilities Act
  Justin Dart
  Jane West

Amputation
  Gustav Rubin

Animals
  Bonita M. Bergin

Anxiety Disorders
  Gary B. Kaplan
  Mark S. Bauer

Aphasia
  Martha Taylor Sarno

Architectural Accessibility
  Edward Steinfeld

Art Therapy
  Deborah Farber

Arthritis
  Saralynn H. Allaire

Assessment in Rehabilitation
  Norman C. Hursh

Assistive Technology
  Bud Rizer

Attitudes
  Harold E. Yuker

Audiology
  Robert Burkard

Autism
  Barbara J. Becker

B

Back Disorders
  Malcolm H. Pope
  Antonia A. Clark

Behavior Therapy
  Robert G. Lasky

Blindness and Vision Disorders
  J. Elton Moore

Blood Disorders
  Emily E. Czapek

Burns
  Alan J. Breslau

C

Cancer Rehabilitation
  Susan J. Mellette
  Karen L. Blunk

Career Counseling
  David B. Hershenson

Caregiving
  David E. Biegel

Childhood Disabilities
  Janet Lord
  Barbara Bennett

Childhood Psychiatric Disorders
  Lisa A. Lenhart

Chronic Fatigue Syndrome
  Mario C. Battigelli

Civil Rights
  Harlan Hahn

Clinical Supervision
  James T. Herbert

Clothing
  Nora M. MacDonald

Communication Disabilities
  Louise Zingeser
  Diane Paul-Brown

Computer Applications for Visual Disabilities
  Joseph J. Lazzaro

Computers
  Dina Loebl

Consumers
  Carolyn L. Vash
  Irving Kenneth Zola

Coronary Artery Disease
  Ray W. Squires

Correctional Rehabilitation
  Vicki Dellinger Verdeyen

Credentials
  Marvin D. Kuehn

D

Dance/Movement Therapy
  Marcia B. Leventhal

Deaf-Blindness
  Marianne Riggio

Deafness and Hearing Impairment
  Douglas Watson
  Myra Taff-Watson

Deinstitutionalization
  Steven J. Taylor

Developmental Disabilities
  William E. Kiernan
  Robert L. Schalock

Disability
  Mark Nagler
  Wendy Wilson

Disability Law and Social Policy
  Kay Fletcher Schriner
  Andrew I. Batavia

Disability Management
  Donald E. Shrey

Drug Rehabilitation
  Bobby G. Greer

E

Eating Disorders
  Theodore E. Weltzin
  Elizabeth B. McCabe
  Walter H. Kaye

Economics
  David S. Salkever

Employee Assistance Programs
  Joseph E. Havranek

Endocrine Disorders
  Elliot Sternthal

Engineering, Rehabilitation
  Donald McNeal

Ergonomics
  Anil Mital

Ethics
  Henry D. Wong
  Ann T. Neulicht

Evaluation of Rehabilitation Programs
  Gregory G. Garske

F

Facilities
  Carolyn Zollar

Pat Morrissey
Karen O'Donnell

Family
Paul W. Power

Forensic Rehabilitation
Roger O. Weed

Functional Electrical Stimulation (FES)
Jeanne O'Malley Teeter

Future of Rehabilitation
John J. Benshoff
Karen E. Barrett

G

Gallaudet University
I. King Jordan

Gastrointestinal Disorders
Stephen P. Stowe

Genetic Disorders
R. Stephen Amato

Growth Disorders
Campbell P. Howard
I. David Schwartz

H

Head Injury
George Zitnay

History of Rehabilitation
Martha Lentz Walker

Homelessness
Deborah K. Padgett

Hospice
Galen Miller

Hospital, Rehabilitation
Richard P. Bonfiglio
Jan Loeffler Bergen

Housing
Ronald L. Mace

Human Immunodeficiency Virus Disease and
Acquired Immunodeficiency Syndrome
Richard P. Keeling

Human Resource Development
William G. Emener

Human Services
Paul Schmolling

I

Independent Living
Quentin W. Smith
Lex Frieden
Laurel Richards

Information Resources
Richard T. Walls
Denetta L. Dowler

International Rehabilitation
Susan R. Hammerman

J

Job Placement
David Vandergoot

K

Keller, Helen
Christopher Caiazza

Kidney Disorders
Beth Witten
Karren King

L

Labor Unions
Claude W. Whitehead

Learning Disabilities
Maurice A. Feldman

Life Care Planning
Paul M. Deutsch

Loss and Grief
Michael G. Gilewski
Elizabeth M. Zelinski

M

Management
Gopal C. Pati

Massage Therapy
Stephen K. Koepfer

Mental Retardation
Thomas L. Whitman
Cynthia L. Miller
Deirdre E. Mylod

Minorities
Sylvia Walker
Reginald Rackley

Mood Disorders
Philip G. Janicak
Anne M. Leach

Multiple Disabilities
Paul A. Alberto
Kathryn Wolff Heller

Musculoskeletal Disorders
Mark D. Klaiman
Jeanne Hicks

Music Therapy
Jean Anthony Gileno

N

Neurological Disorders
François Vingerhoets
Julien Bogousslavsky

Neurology
David C. Good

Neuromuscular Disorders
Gregory T. Carter

Normalization and Social Role Valorization
Raymond A. Lemay

Nursing, Rehabilitation
Pamela G. Watson

O

Occupational Information
Chrisann Schiro-Geist

Occupational Therapy
Mary M. Evert

Organic Mental Syndromes
David S. Geldmacher
Peter J. Whitehouse

P

Pain
Ronald J. Kulich

Pediatric Rehabilitation
Marilyn H. Lash

Personal Assistance Services
Simi Litvak

Personality Disorders
Susan J. Lewis

Pharmacology
David E. Creasey

Philosophy of Rehabilitation
Dennis R. Maki
Gerald C. Murray

Physical Therapy
Catherine Certo

Physician
Glen E. Gresham

President's Committee for the Employment of People with Disabilities
Rick Douglas

Private Sector Rehabilitation
Mary Vencill

Prosthetics and Orthotics
Dudley S. Childress
Laura Fenwick
Mark Edwards

Psychiatric Rehabilitation
Gary R. Bond

Psychiatry
David E. Creasey

Psychology
Lynda J. Katz

Psychology, Rehabilitation
Paul Leung

Psychosocial Adjustment
Donna R. Falvo

Q

Quality of Life
Ellen S. Fabian

R

Reasonable Accommodation
Gregory K. Jones
Yvonne A. Williams

Recreation
Karen C. Wenzel

Rehabilitation Center
Gregory L. Thomsen

Rehabilitation Counseling
Martha Lentz Walker

Rehabilitation Education
E. W. Stude

Religion
William Blair
Dana Davidson

Research, Rehabilitation
Donald J. Dellario

Respiratory Disease
John R. Bach

Respite Care
Gary B. Mesibov
Jemma C. Price

Rural Rehabilitation
Thomas W. Seekins

Rusk, Howard A.
Daniel Perkes

S

Schizophrenia
Susan S. Matthews
Samuel J. Keith

Self-Concept
Brenda G. Lawrence
S. G. Bennett

Self-Help
C. Kirven Weekley

Sexuality and Disability
Stanley H. Ducharme

Sickle Cell Anemia and Thalassemia (Hemoglobin-opathies)
Ruth Andrea Seeler

Social Work Practice in Rehabilitation
Allen F. Johnson

Sociology
Gary L. Albrecht

Special Education
Edna Mora Szymanski
Sarah Johnston-Rodriguez
Debra Adrian Heiss
Mary Heinrichs

Spinal Cord Injury
Michael M. Priebe
Diana H. Rintala

State–Federal Rehabilitation Program
Antonio E. Jones

Statistics
Gerry Hendershot

Stroke
Mark N. Ozer

Supported Employment
Michael D. West

Surgery
Victor L. Lewis, Jr.

Switzer, Mary
Leonard G. Perlman
James R. Burress

T

Technology and Disability
Marcia J. Scherer

Transition from School to Work
Lynda L. West

Transportation Accessibility
David M. Capozzi
Dennis J. Cannon

V

Veterans' Medical Rehabilitation in the U.S.
Department of Veterans Affairs
James L. Green

Veteran Vocational Rehabilitation in the U.S.
Department of Veterans Affairs
David T. James

Violence
Dick Sobsey

Vocational Evaluation
Paul W. Power

W

Wellness
Gary S. Skrinar
Kristy M. Hendricks

Wheelchairs
Kristjan T. Ragnarsson

Women in Rehabilitation
Charlene Poch DeLoach

Work
Susanne M. Bruyère
Joyce A. Hoying

List of Contributors

Alberto, Paul A.
Georgia State University
Multiple Disabilities

Albrecht, Gary L.
University of Illinois, Chicago
Sociology

Allaire, Saralynn H.
Boston University School of Medicine
Arthritis

Amato, R. Stephen
Greater Baltimore Medical Center
Genetic Disorders

Bach, John R.
University Hospital, Newark, NJ
Respiratory Disease

Barrett, Karen F.
Southern Illinois University
Future of Rehabilitation

Bartels, Elmer C.
Massachusetts Rehabilitation Commission, Boston, MA
Accessibility

Batavia, Andrew I.
University of Arkansas
Disability Law and Social Policy

Battigelli, Mario C.
Chapel Hill, NC
Chronic Fatigue Syndrome

Bauer, Mark S.
VA Medical Center, Providence, RI
Anxiety Disorders

Becker, Barbara J.
Marshall University
Autism

Bennett, Barbara
University of California, San Francisco
Childhood Disabilities

Bennett, S. G.
University of Nottingham, England
Self-Concept

Benshoff, John J.
Southern Illinois University
Future of Rehabilitation

Bergen, Jan Loeffler
Bryn Mawr Rehab, Malvern, PA
Hospital, Rehabilitation

Bergin, Bonita M.
Assistance Dog Institute, Rohnert Park, CA
Animals

Berko, Frances G.
New York State Office of Advocate for the Disabled
Advocacy

Biegel, David E.
Case Western Reserve University
Caregiving

Blair, William
Lifestyle Adjustment Consultants, Pinson, AL
Religion

Blunk, Karen L.
Medical College of Virginia
Cancer Rehabilitation

Boehlert, Robert J.
New York State Office of Advocate for the Disabled
Advocacy

Bogousslavsky, Julien
CHU Vaudois, Lausanne, Switzerland
Neurological Disorders

Bond, Gary R.
Indiana University/Purdue University at Indiana
Psychiatric Rehabilitation

Bonfiglio, Richard P.
Bryn Mawr Rehab, Malvern, PA
Hospital, Rehabilitation

Bowe, Frank G.
Hofstra University
Affirmative Action

Breslau, Alan J.
The Phoenix Society, Inc., Levittown, PA
Burns

Bruyère, Susanne
Cornell University
Work

Buckwalter, Kathleen
University of Iowa
Alzheimer's Disease

Burkard, Robert
State University of New York, Buffalo
Audiology

Burress, James R.
Deceased
Switzer, Mary

Caiazza, Christopher
New York, NY
Keller, Helen

Cannon, Dennis M.
U.S. Architectural Barriers and Compliance Board, Washington, DC
Transportation Accessibility

Capozzi, David M.
U.S. Architectural and Transportation Barriers Compliance Board, Washington, DC
Transportation Accessibility

Carter, Gregory T.
UC Davis Medical Center
Neuromuscular Disorders

Certo, Catherine
Boston University
Physical Therapy

Childress, Dudley S.
Northwestern University
Prosthetics and Orthotics

Clark, Antonia A.
University of Vermont, Burlington
Back Disorders

Couch, Robert H.
Auburn University
Adjustment Services

Creasey, David E.
Boston University
Pharmacology
Psychiatry

Czapek, Emily E.
Regional Comprehensive Hemophilia Center of Central and Northern Illinois
Blood Disorders

Dart, Justin
Washington, DC
Americans with Disabilities Act

Davidson, Dana
Pinson, AL
Religion

Dellario, Donald J.
Worcester State Hospital, Worcester, MA
Research

DeLoach, Charlene Poch
University of Memphis
Women in Rehabilitation

Deutsch, Paul M.
Paul Deutsch and Associates, Orlando, FL
Life Care Planning

Douglas, Rick
Department of Labor, Washington, DC
President's Committee for the Employment of
    People with Disabilities

Dowler, Denneta L.
West Virginia University
Information Resources

Ducharme, Stanley II.
Boston University Medical Center
Sexuality and Disability

Edwards, Mark
Northwestern University
Prosthetics and Orthotics

Emener, William G.
University of South Florida, Tampa
Human Resource Development

Evert, Mary M.
American Occupational Therapy Association,
    Rockville, MD
Occupational Therapy

Fabian, Ellen S.
University of Maryland
Quality of Life

Falvo, Donna R.
Southern Illinois University
Aging
Psychosocial Adjustment

Farber, Deborah
School of Visual Arts, NY
Art Therapy

Feldman, Maurice A.
Queen's University, Kingston, Ontario, Canada
Learning Disabilities

Fenwick, Laura
Northwestern University
Prosthetics and Orthotics

Frieden, Lex
ILRU Program, Houston, TX
Independent Living

Garand, Linda
College of Nursing, University of Iowa
Alzheimer's Disease

Garske, Gregory G.
University of Illinois-Urbana-Champaign
Evaluation of Rehabilitation Programs

Geldmacher, David S.
University Alzheimer Center, Cleveland, OH
Organic Mental Syndromes

Gileno, Jean Anthony
Immaculata College
Music Therapy

Gilewski, Michael J.
Cedars-Sinai Medical Center, Los Angeles, CA
Loss and Grief

Goldberg, Richard T.
Spaulding Rehabilitation Hospital, MA
Adolescents, Rehabilitation of

Good, David C.
*Bowman Gray School of Medicine,
Winston-Salem, NC*
Neurology

Gortney, Clinton
Youth for Tomorrow, Bristow, VA
Head Injury

Green, James L.
Veterans Health Administration, Washington, DC
Veterans' Medical Rehabilitation in the U.S.
Department of Veterans Affairs

Greer, Bobby G.
University of Memphis
Drug Rehabilitation

Gresham, Glen E.
State University of New York, Buffalo
Physician

Hahn, Harlan
University of Southern California, Los Angeles
Civil Rights

Hammerman, Susan R.
Rutgers University
International Rehabilitation

Havranek, Joseph
Bowling Green State University
Employee Assistance Programs

Heinrichs, Mary
University of Wisconsin/Madison
Special Education

Heiss, Debra Adrian
University of Wisconsin, White Water
Special Education

Heller, Kathryn Wolff
Georgia State University
Multiple Disabilities

Hendershot, Gerry
*U.S. Department of Health & Human Services,
Hyattsville, MD*
Statistics

Hendricks, Kristy
Simmons College
Wellness

Herbert, James T.
Pennsylvania State University
Clinical Supervision

Hershenson, David B.
University of Maryland
Career Counseling

Hicks, Jeanne
National Institutes of Health
Musculoskeletal Disorders

Howard, Campbell P.
Children's Mercy Hospital, Kansas City, MO
Growth Disorders

Hoying, Joyce A.
Cornell University, Ithaca, NY
Work

Hursh, Norman C.
Boston University
Assessment in Rehabilitation

James, David T.
Veterans Benefits Administration, Washington, DC
Veteran Vocational Rehabilitation in the U.S.
Department of Veterans Affairs

Janicak, Philip G.
University of Illinois, Chicago
Mood Disorders

Johnson, Allen F.
Auburn Family Institute, Auburn, MA
Social Work Practice in Rehabilitation

Johnston-Rodriguez, Sarah
University of Wisconsin/Madison
Special Education

Jones, Antonio E.
West Virginia Legislature
State–Federal Rehabilitation Program

Jones, Gregory K.
New York State Office for the Disabled, Albany, NY
Reasonable Accommodation

Jordan, I. King
Gallaudet University, Washington, DC
Gallaudet University

Kaplan, Gary
VA Medical Center, Providence, RI
Anxiety Disorders

Katz, Lynda J.
Landmark College
Psychology

Kaye, Walter H.
Western Psychiatric Institute, Pittsburgh, PA
Eating Disorders

Keeling, Richard P.
University of Wisconsin, Madison
Human Immunodeficiency Virus Disease and Acquired Immunodeficiency Syndrome

Keith, Samuel J.
University of New Mexico School of Medicine
Schizophrenia

Kiernan, William
Children's Hospital, Boston, MA
Developmental Disabilities

King, Karren
Missouri Kidney Program, Westwood, KS
Kidney Disorders

Klaiman, Mark D.
National Institutes of Health
Musculoskeletal Disorders

Koepfer, Stephen R.
Bayside, NY
Massage Therapy

Kuehn, Marvin D.
Emporia State University
Credentials

Kulich, Ronald J.
Tufts New England Medical Center
Pain

Lash, Marilyn
New England Medical Center, Boston, MA
Pediatric Rehabilitation

Lasky, Robert G.
Ages Health Services, Rockland, MA
Behavior Therapy

Lawrence, Brenda
University of Portsmouth, Southsea Hants, England
Self-Concept

Lazzaro, Joseph J.
Massachusetts Commission for the Blind, Boston, MA
Computer Applications for Visual Disabilities

Leach, Anne M.
University of Illinois, Chicago
Mood Disorders

Lemay, Raymond A.
Children's Aid Society, Plantagenet, Ontario, Canada
Normalization and Social Role Valorization

Lenhart, Lisa A.
Duke University Medical Center
Childhood Psychiatric Disorders

Leung, Paul
University of Illinois, Champaign
Psychology, Rehabilitation

Leventhal, Marcia B.
Dance Therapy Institute of Princeton, NJ
Dance/Movement Therapy

Lewis, Susan
Brookline, MA
Personality Disorders

Lewis, Victor L.
Chicago, IL
Surgery

Litvak, Simi
World Institute on Disability, Oakland, CA
Personal Assistance Services

Loebl, Dina
Harvard University
Computers

Lord, Janet
Children's Hospital Medical Center, Oakland, CA
Childhood Disabilities

Lundervold, Duane A.
Southern Illinois University
Aging

MacDonald, Nora M.
West Virginia University
Clothing

Mace, Ronald L.
North Carolina State University
Housing

Maki, Dennis
University of Iowa
Philosophy of Rehabilitation

Matthews, Susan
NIMH–Clinical & Treatment Research, Rockville, MD
Schizophrenia

McCabe, Elizabeth B.
University of Pittsburgh School of Medicine
Eating Disorders

McNeal, Donald
Rancho Los Amigos Medical Center, Downey, CA
Engineering, Rehabilitation

Mellette, Susan J.
Medical College of Virginia
Cancer Rehabilitation

Mesibov, Gary B.
University of North Carolina, Chapel Hill
Respite Care

Miller, Cynthia L.
University of Notre Dame
Mental Retardation

Miller, Galen
National Hospice Organization, Arlington, VA
Hospice

Mital, Anil
University of Cincinnati
Ergonomics

Moore, J. Elton
Mississippi State University
Blindness and Vision Disorders

Morrissey, Pat
American Rehabilitation Association, Reston, VA
Facilities

Murray, Gerald C.
University of Iowa
Philosophy of Rehabilitation

Mylod, Deirdre E.
University of Notre Dame
Mental Retardation

Nagler, Mark
University of Waterloo, Renison College, Waterloo, Ontario, Canada
Disability

Neulich, Ann T.
University of North Carolina, Chapel Hill
Ethics

O'Donnell, Karen
American Rehabilitation Association, Reston, VA
Facilities

Ozer, Mark N.
National Rehabilitation Hospital, Washington, DC
Stroke

Padgett, Deborah K.
New York University
Homelessness

Pati, Gopal C.
Indiana University, Northwest
Management

Paul-Brown, Diane
American Speech-Language-Hearing Association, Rockville, MD
Communication Disabilities

Perkes, Dan
New York University Medical Center
Rusk, Howard A.

Perlman, Leonard G.
Rockville, MD
Switzer, Mary

Pope, Malcolm
University of Iowa
Back Disorders

Power, Paul W.
University of Maryland, College Park
Family
Vocational Evaluation

Price, Jemma C.
University of North Carolina, Chapel Hill
Respite Care

Priebe, Michael
VA Hospital, Houston, TX
Spinal Cord Injury

Rackley, Reginald
Howard University, Washington, DC
Minorities

Ragnarsson, Kristjan T.
Mt. Sinai School of Medicine, NY
Wheelchairs

Richards, Laurel
ILRU Program, Houston, TX
Independent Living

Riggio, Marianne
Perkins School for the Blind, Watertown, MA
Deaf-Blindness

Rintala, Diana H.
Baylor College of Medicine
Spinal Cord Injury

Rizer, Bud
Maryland Rehabilitation Center, Baltimore
Assistive Technology

Roessler, Richard
University of Arkansas, Fayetteville
Ability

Rubin, Gustav
College of Podiatric Medicine, New York
Amputation

Salkever, David S.
Johns Hopkins University School of Public Health
Economics

Sarno, Martha Taylor
New York University School of Medicine
Aphasia

Schalock, Robert L.
Hastings College, Hastings, NE
Developmental Disabilities

Scherer, Marcia J.
Rochester Institute of Technology
Technology and Disability

Schiro-Geist, Chrisann
University of Illinois, Champaign
Occupational Information

Schmolling, Paul
Kingsborough Community College
Human Services

Schriner, Kay Fletcher
University of Arkansas, Fayetteville
Disability Law and Social Policy

Schwartz, I. David
Children's Mercy Hospital, Kansas City, MO
Growth Disorders

Seekins, Thomas W.
University of Montana, Missoula
Rural Rehabilitation

Seeler, Ruth Andrea
Michael Reese Hospital, Chicago
Sickle Cell Anemia and Thalassemia
(Hemoglobinopathies)

Sekerak, Darlene F.
University of North Carolina
Allied Health Professions

Shrey, Donald E.
University of Cincinnati
Disability Management

Skrinar, Gary
Boston University
Wellness

Smith, Quentin W.
ILRU Program, Houston, TX
Independent Living

Sobsey, Dick
University of Alberta, Edmonton, Canada
Violence

Squires, Ray W.
Mayo Clinic, Rochester, MN
Coronary Artery Disease

Stano, Joseph F.
Springfield College
Alcohol Rehabilitation

Steinfeld, Edward
University of New York, Buffalo
Architectural Accessibility

Sternthal, Elliot
Joslin Diabetes Center, Boston, MA
Endocrine Disorders

Stowe, Stephen P.
*Lake Morman Regional Medical Center,
Mooresville, NC*
Gastrointestinal Disorders

Stude, E. W.
California State University, Fresno
Rehabilitation Education

Szymanski, Edna Mora
University of Wisconsin, Madison
Special Education

Taff-Watson, Myra
University of Arkansas, Fayetteville
Deafness and Hearing Impairment

Taylor, Steven
Syracuse University
Deinstitutionalization

Teeter, Jeanne O'Malley
Cleveland F.E.S. Center
Functional Electrical Stimulation (FES)

Thomsen, Gregory L.
Patricia Neal Rehabilitation Center at Fort Sanders Regional Medical Center, Knoxville, TN
Rehabilitation Center

Vandergoot, David
National Center for Disability Services, Albertston, NY
Job Placement

Vash, Carolyn L.
Altadena, CA
Consumers

Vencill, Mary P.
Berkeley Planning Associates, Oakland, CA
Private Sector Rehabilitation

Verdeyen, Vicki Dellinger
Department of Justice, Annapolis Junction
Correctional Rehabilitation

Vingerhoets, François
CHU Vaudois, Lausanne, Switzerland
Neurological Disorders

Walker, Martha Lentz
Kent State University
History of Rehabilitation
Rehabilitation Counseling

Walker, Sylvia
Howard University
Minorities

Walls, Richard T.
West Virginia University
Information Resources

Watson, Douglas
University of Arkansas, Fayetteville
Deafness and Hearing Impairment

Watson, Pamela G.
Thomas Jefferson University
Nursing, Rehabilitation

Weed, Roger O.
Georgia State University, Atlanta
Forensic Rehabilitation

Weekley, C. Kirven
Baptist Rehabilitation Center, Memphis, TN
Self-Help

Weltzin, Theodore E.
University of Wisconsin School of Medicine, Madison
Eating Disorders

Wenzel, Karen C.
MS Community Resources, Denver, CO
Recreation

West, Jane
Chevy Chase, MD
Americans with Disabilities Act

West, Lynda L.
George Washington University
Transition from School to Work

West, Michael D.
Virginia Commonwealth University, Richmond
Supported Employment

Whitehead, Claude W.
Employment Related Services Associates, Hudson, FL
Labor Unions

Whitehouse, Peter
University Alzheimer Center, Cleveland, OH
Organic Mental Syndromes

Whitman, Thomas L.
University of Notre Dame
Mental Retardation

Williams, Yvonne A.
New York State Office for the Disabled, Albany, NY
Reasonable Accommodation

Wilson, Wendy
University of Waterloo, Renison College, Waterloo, Ontario, Canada
Disability

Witten, Beth
Johnson County Dialysis, Inc., Lenexa, KS
Kidney Disorders

Wong, Henry D.
University of North Carolina, Chapel Hill
Ethics

Yoder, David E.
University of North Carolina, Chapel Hill
Allied Health Professions

Yuker, Harold E.
Hofstra University
Attitudes

Zelinski, Elizabeth M.
University of Southern California
Loss and Grief

Zingeser, Louise
American Speech and Hearing Association, Rockville, MD
Communication Disabilities

Zitnay, George
Brain Injury Association, Washington, DC
Head Injury

Zola, Irving Kenneth
Brandeis University
Consumers

Zollar, Carolyn
American Rehabilitation Association, Reston, VA
Facilities

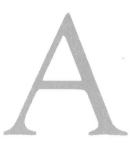

ABILITY

Indicative of a person's productive potential, "ability" refers to the individual's capacity both to learn new skills and behaviors and to perform previously learned skills and behaviors. Individual differences in abilities may or may not be limited by disabling conditions. In either case, ability is a critical construct for providers of treatment and rehabilitation services (especially rehabilitation evaluators and counselors). Measured with standardized tests and other assessment procedures, abilities provide insights into (1) the person's likelihood of success in a variety of independent living and vocational roles, and (2) the extent to which disability may have adversely affected the person's functioning.

Depending on the context in which it is used, the concept of ability may be defined narrowly or broadly. In the narrow sense, ability refers to intellectual functioning, which is composed primarily of general intelligence (g) and other constructs such as verbal, numerical, spatial, and perceptual abilities. In the field of rehabilitation, ability is used in a broader sense to refer to those capabilities required to function in both daily living and vocational roles. Each individual possesses strengths and weaknesses in abilities, and the purpose of assessment is to clarify the person's potential to perform with and without accommodation.

Useful in vocational counseling, ability measures predict the extent to which a person is capable of responding satisfactorily to a wide range of vocational training or on-the-job demands. Computer software is available that matches ability profiles of the individual with ability requirements of different jobs, thus enabling the person and the counselor or evaluator to identify feasible vocational goals for discussion during the rehabilitation-planning process (Bolton, 1987).

Ability is an important concept beyond the evaluation and counseling functions in rehabilitation. When changes in ability due to an injury or disability occur at midlife, they are often associated with termination of employment unless early rehabilitation and accommodation efforts are made. Although a variety of factors contribute to failure to return to work, two issues are particularly salient for the practice of rehabilitation. Frequently, employers will stereotype employees with disabilities as less "able" than those without disabilities (Greenwood, Fletcher-Schriner, and Johnson, 1991). In addition, employers must place greater emphasis on implementation of early rehabilitation and accommodation interventions at the workplace.

Early rehabilitation efforts instituted in the workplace are referred to as "disability management" programs. Disability management services concentrate on returning the person with a disability to the same job in the same industry and company as quickly as possible. Aspects of the disability management process include "early identification at the workplace of disability-related problems; effective management of physical symptoms; facilitation of return to work; and modification of jobs, when necessary" (Tate & Habeck, 1986).

A strong moral and economic rationale exists for disability management programs. First, a significant segment of the work force must cope with the effects of disability, and the projected number of adults with disabilities in the labor force is expected to increase with the "graying of America" (United Way Strategic Institute, 1989). Without disability management programs, many Americans with disabilities may have difficulties functioning in productive vocational roles.

An economic argument for disability management services is easily made. On an annual basis, American business commits between 3 and 6 percent of its total payroll to disability costs (Schwartz et al., 1989). The costs of disability income payments and health care services exceed $185 billion a year, and the average on-the-job injury has a total cost of $19,000 (Munrowd & Habeck, 1987; Tate, Habeck, and Galvin, 1986). Early return to work is clearly advantageous both to the employer and the employee.

The return-to-work process may also be viewed from a more positive perspective and labeled "ability management" rather than "disability management." Ability management stresses that it is to the employer's advantage to retain loyal and trained ("able") workers. Disability does not have a negative impact on all of the individual's assets. For example, the person's prior experience on the job enables him or her to continue to make good judgments about the use of personnel and resources. Moreover, the experienced worker with a disability does not need to

be retrained in the basic functions of the job, although some modifications in the way work is done may be needed. Data from an E. I. duPont corporation survey (1990) underscore the need for ability management in business: Over 90 percent of duPont employees with disabilities were rated by their supervisors as having average or above-average production and safety records.

Through such strategies as job accommodation and job restructuring, ability management services enable workers to maintain their prior positions and qualify for training and advancement opportunities. Tom Jackson and Alan Vitberg (1987) captured the philosophy of ability management in their description of career development. Career development is characterized by "real efforts of managers to encourage employees to develop their unique capabilities, to focus them in ways that are specifically related to the organization's goals, and to facilitate imagination, creativity, and entrepreneurship."

Achieving the goals of ability management or career development requires a collaborative relationship between the employer and the employee with a disability. Under the Americans with Disabilities Act, one of the employer's primary responsibilities is to review the individual's need for job modifications and provide reasonable accommodations. These accommodations, which serve to enable the person to perform the essential functions of the job without creating an undue hardship for the employer, may require additional equipment, short-term light-duty assignments, changes in schedules, or restructured job duties.

Unfortunately, the "disability" perspective on the return-to-work process is more pervasive than the "ability" (career development) perspective (Roessler & Fletcher-Schriner, 1991). Effective ability management requires a commitment on the employer's part to help returning workers identify and remove obstacles to utilization of their abilities; that is, to their career development. These obstacles may affect the worker's success in getting to and around the work site; performing certain job demands such as reaching, standing, or lifting; or mastering task demands that require cognitive and/or interpersonal skills.

In an ability management approach, the employee and the supervisor discuss these career development barriers and collaborate in devising strategies to remove them. These strategies are formulated in a career development plan, and both the supervisor and the employee participate in monitoring outcomes of the plan. The career development approach enables employees with disabilities to make maximum use of their abilities, so that they are able not only to secure and retain employment but also to advance in their careers as well.

(*See also:* ASSESSMENT IN REHABILITATION; CAREER COUNSELING; DISABILITY; DISABILITY MANAGEMENT; ECONOMICS; JOB ACCOMMODATION)

BIBLIOGRAPHY

BOLTON, BRIAN. *Occupational Report.* Fayetteville, AR, 1987.

E. I. DUPONT DE NEMOURS & COMPANY. *Equal to the Task II: 1990 duPont Survey of Employment of People with Disabilities.* Wilmington, DE, 1990.

GREENWOOD, REED; FLETCHER–SCHRINER, KAY; and JOHNSON, VIRGINIA. "Employer Concerns Regarding Workers with Disabilities and the Business-Rehabilitation Partnership: The PWI Practitioner's Perspective." *Journal of Rehabilitation* 57 (1991):21–26.

JACKSON, TOM, and VITBERG, ALAN. "Career Development, Part 2: Challenges for the Organization." *Personnel* 64 (1987):68–72.

MUNROWD, DIANE, and HABECK, ROCHELLE. *Disability Management and Rehabilitation: An Analysis of Programs, Costs and Outcomes.* East Lansing, MI, 1987.

ROESSLER, RICHARD, and FLETCHER SCHRINER, KAY. "Partnerships: The Bridge from Disability to Ability Management." *Journal of Rehabilitation* 57 (1991): 53–58.

SCHWARTZ, GAIL; WATSON, SARA; GALVIN, DON; and LIPOFF, ELISE. *The Disability Management Sourcebook.* Washington, DC, 1989.

TATE, DENISE, .and HABECK, ROCHELLE. "Disability Management and Rehabilitation in the Workplace." *Journal of Applied Rehabilitation Counseling* 17 (1986):4.

TATE, DENISE; HABECK, ROCHELLE; and GALVIN, DON. "Disability Management: Origins, Concepts, and Principles for Practice." *Journal of Applied Rehabilitation Counseling* 17 (1986):5–11.

UNITED WAY STRATEGIC INSTITUTE. *Nine Forces Reshaping America.* Alexandria, VA, 1989.

RICHARD ROESSLER

ABUSE

See VIOLENCE

ACCESSIBILITY

In ordinary conversation, the term "accessibility" is used to describe the ease of finding a location or the frequency with which a location is used. A place that is accessible is well known and frequently used. The disability community has expanded the definition of this term to mean ease of use by a person with a disability. An accessible place is one that can be readily entered and used by people with disabilities. A location without steps at the entry, and with wide doors and roomy halls and corridors, is accessible to people who use wheelchairs. A school or medical clinic is accessible to people who are deaf when a telecommunication device for the deaf (TDD) is available and the staff knows sign language. A government office is accessible to people who are blind when the hallways have no physical obstacles and people can obtain written material in braille, on an audiotape or computer diskette, or through the free services of a reader. A school is accessible to students with learning disabilities when it provides individualized education programs that meet students' learning styles and needs. Accessibility is thus a functional concept embracing architectural designs that do not impose physical barriers to mobility, modes of communication that can be understood by individuals with disabilities that affect hearing or vision, and operational methods that include people with various disabilities.

An accessible society is one in which people with disabilities can readily participate. Accessibility is a socially inclusive concept that draws its values from a belief in the basic dignity and civil rights of all individuals within a given society. This concept is premised on a civil rights foundation that holds that each individual, including those with disabilities, is entitled and obligated to participate in all of that society's activities: education, work, commerce, civic life, and government programs and services. Because so many aspects of contemporary society are based on old assumptions, patterns, and infrastructures that exclude individuals with disabilities, changes are necessary to achieve accessibility.

The importance of accessibility as a contemporary social and political issue is determined in part by the growing number of people with disabilities in modern societies. The number of individuals with severe disabilities who survive serious injuries, accidents, and illness has increased with advances in technology and modern medicine. The survival rates of American soldiers who were injured in the Vietnam War and transported by helicopter to a field hospital approached 95 percent. Adults injured on the job or in highway accidents survive their injuries with the assistance of medical technology, drugs that prevent or cure infections, and modern rehabilitation therapy. Premature infants who would have died in earlier times can live and thrive with the assistance of intensive medical intervention and follow-up treatment.

In the United States, the number of individuals with physical or mental impairments that limit one or more major life activities was estimated at 43 million in 1990 (Americans with Disabilities Act). Of this group, 34 million resided outside of institutions (National Health Interview Survey, 1989). In response to the increasing number of people with disabilities, disability policies in the United States between 1970 and 1990 began to shift away from a focus on specialized welfare programs that provided separate services for particular disability groups. A new, more comprehensive approach was aimed at making regular government services more accessible to people with disabilities and enabling them to take advantage of the same employment opportunities and use the same private sector goods and services that were available to other citizens.

Development of Accessibility Policies in the United States

In the United States, the role of government in identifying and addressing barriers to accessibility has been an important factor in promoting changes that can open up employment opportunities, government services, and commerce to people with disabilities. The federal government became involved in addressing some barriers to the employment of individuals with physical disabilities in 1920, when

a special program of vocational rehabilitation services for veterans disabled in World War I and workers injured in the course of their employment was established under the Smith-Fess Act. In the late 1960s and early 1970s, the U.S. Congress adopted laws requiring that certain measures be undertaken to improve accessibility and include individuals with disabilities in federally funded programs and facilities. Other federal and state laws were enacted to mandate changes in public and private businesses so that their services and goods would be more accessible to individuals with disabilities.

In the 1960s, citizen support for government policies to promote accessibility in the United States initially focused on transportation and architectural barriers. In a mobile modern society, transportation is the link to schools, jobs, health care, commerce, and civic events. Without accessible transportation, most individuals with severe physical disabilities cannot live or function outside an institutional environment. Traditionally, most buildings and public facilities were designed for an average adult who has average height, weight, strength, and other average physical and mental characteristics. Because of this approach to designing the environment, millions of people with disabilities who did not fit the profile of the mythical average adult experienced great difficulties in attempting to participate in ordinary activities.

American veterans with injuries who returned from World War II and found their local communities completely inaccessible led the first citizen organizations that advocated government policies to improve architectural and transportation accessibility. The Disabled American Veterans and the Paralyzed Veterans of America were a major force behind the enactment of the 1968 Architectural Barriers Act. That law required all new buildings funded by the federal government to be physically accessible. The approach taken by the 1968 law focused on new construction and alterations which had to be accessible to and usable by people with physical disabilities.

Federal accessibility policies began to converge with the enactment of Title V of the Rehabilitation Act of 1973. That law expanded federal accessibility policies by protecting "individuals with handicaps" from discrimination in all federally funded programs and services and in private employment with federal contractors. It also placed responsibility for setting accessibility standards and enforcing the Architectural Barriers Act upon the Architectural and Transportation Barriers Compliance Board.

The 1980s brought adoption of other federal policies that supported changes to make American society more accessible to people with disabilities. Among them was the Voting Accessibility for the Elderly and Handicapped Act of 1984, which required polling places in federal elections to be physically accessible to elderly voters and voters with disabilities. It also required election officials to communicate voter information in an accessible manner through the provision of large-print instructions and telecommunication devices for the deaf. In 1986 the Air Carrier Access Act was adopted to prohibit discrimination against "otherwise qualified handicapped individuals" in response to industry practices that made it impossible for many individuals with a severe disability to travel independently.

In 1988, amendments to the federal Fair Housing Act addressed the needs of individuals with severe disabilities who use wheelchairs for mobility by prohibiting disability-based discrimination in existing public and privately owned apartments. This law required landlords to make reasonable modifications to an apartment so that a tenant with a disability could occupy the premises. It also required the use of accessible or "adaptive" designs in new apartments to permit easy conversion to meet the accessibility needs of a future occupant with a severe disability.

Another federal policy that supported progress toward a more accessible society was the Technology Assistance Act of 1988. This law endorsed federal funding for projects in every state to coordinate and expand the availability of assistive technology for people with severe disabilities so that they can live independently and go to work.

A uniquely comprehensive statement of federal accessibility policy was embodied in the Americans with Disabilities Act, which became law on July 26, 1990. The law, which has been called the "Emancipation Proclamation" for people with disabilities, prohibited discrimination in employment, public accommodations, government services, and telecommunications. It required employers to make reasonable changes in the work environment so that a qualified individual with a disability could be productively employed in a public or private sector job. The law also called for modifications to ensure that people with disabilities would have equal access to all public services provided by state and local governments, including public transportation. It prohibited barriers that restrict the access of people with disabilities to restaurants, hotels, grocery stores, museums, pharmacies, and physicians' offices. It also required the establishment of a national TDD relay service, so that people with hearing impairments would have equal access to the same communications system that serves their fellow citizens. The grass-roots effort to enact this law exemplified an open democratic process in which empowered voters with disabilities and others who believe in basic civil rights for all people played a very active part.

Achieving Accessibility

In undertaking the changes needed to implement the inclusionary policies endorsed by the Americans with Disabilities Act, organizations and individuals must first recognize their own practices and attitudinal barriers that limit the full participation in society of individuals with disabilities. Section 2 of the act acknowledged the attitudinal barriers, stating, "Individuals with disabilities continually encounter various forms of discrimination, including outright intentional exclusion . . . and relegation to lesser services . . . jobs or other opportunities . . . ."

In dealing with individual situations, attitudinal barriers may be addressed on a voluntary personal basis. With the increased numbers of people with disabilities living in modern societies, more people have personal contact with a family member or friend or coworker who has a disability, and they can thus learn about the barriers to that individual's potential contributions that are imposed by inaccessibility. In a family or small social setting, the first step to barrier removal requires flexibility and a positive attitude about the potential of particular individuals with disabilities who are members of that family or group. Family members, as well as employers or leaders in community organizations who have accepted an individual with a disability, willingly make physical or operational changes in an existing situation to ensure that person's participation in family and community life or employment. The family of an individual who uses a wheelchair for mobility may build a ramp or widen the doorway to a bathroom. Employers have revised job tasks for individuals within their work force who become disabled because they know the workers and want them to continue contributing to corporate success. These accessibility measures, called "reasonable accommodations," involve changes in regular procedures or the work or business environment to permit an individual with a disability to participate or work there.

The legal mandates for government agencies and private businesses call for the adoption of a more systematic approach to making their facilities accessible to individuals with all kinds of disabilities. Eliminating barriers that keep customers with disabilities out of stores, patients out of clinics or doctors' offices, or students out of school and public recreational facilities requires analysis and planning before changes are undertaken. Accessibility standards for the federal Architectural Barriers Act required prospective compliance in the case of both new construction of and major alterations in federally funded buildings and structures.

Under the Americans with Disabilities Act, requirements for architectural accessibility were expanded to cover buildings designed or constructed by private sector businesses and organizations after 1990, with a phase-in schedule for some rules. Building owners were also required to make "readily achievable" minor modifications in existing structures so that public areas could be used by individuals with disabilities. The law also required state and local governments to review their services and operations in order to make them accessible to people with disabilities. In situations where architectural barrier removal was not feasible, the law called for governments to provide equivalent services that were readily accessible to individuals with disabilities. This could be done by modifying operations, service delivery methods, or locations and by planning for fully accessible, integrated service delivery in the future.

Independent of laws and government policies, the development of new technology has produced equipment and devices that assist individuals with disabilities at work, at home, and in community activities. An example of new technology that improves communications accessibility for people who are blind is the "talking computer," which can scan text and "read" it in a computerized voice that the user can hear. Technology has also made possible the design and manufacture of wheelchair-accessible buses and a telephone system that can be used by people who are deaf by means of a TDD and a relay system that connects TDD users with people who have standard telephones.

Future Accessibility Issues

Acceptance and support for the laws and policies that mandate changes to achieve accessibility for people with disabilities has not been unanimous. Some critics suggest that they provide special privileges to people who have disabilities. Others say that the requirements go beyond what is reasonable and will add extra expenses for businesses and government at a time when resources are limited. They question why architectural design and business practices should be changed to accommodate the needs of a minority of the population. These perspectives ignore the enormous social and economic costs of dependency. The annual cost of welfare and disability benefits paid to individuals with disabilities in the United States in 1990 was estimated at well over 60 billion dollars (National Council on Disabilities). At that time census data and employment studies indicated that two-thirds of working-age Americans with disabilities were not employed, even though more than half of them wanted to work and attributed their involuntary unemployment to inaccessible and inhospitable workplaces.

A 1982 survey of federal contractors with reasonable accommodation duties under Title V of the Rehabilitation Act demonstrated that the cost of such changes was modest when compared with the benefits of productive work. The study found that 51 percent of requested accommodations cost nothing. An economic analysis done by the Equal Employment Opportunity Commission (EEOC) in connection with the development of regulations to implement the Americans with Disabilities Act estimated that the total annual cost for reasonable accommodation in the American workplace would be $16.4 million. The EEOC anticipated that this cost would be offset by a tenfold gain in productivity reflecting wages earned by workers with disabilities, as well as decreased support payments estimated at $222 million each year. When these factors were considered the economic benefit of making workplaces accessible to workers with disabilities was obvious. Tax incentives were also enacted to assist small businesses in making workplaces and customer premises accessible so that the cost of changes needed to include individuals with disabilities as workers and consumers was reasonable for business.

Full accessibility to all opportunities, facilities, goods, and services can occur over time as new structures are built and old ones remodeled. Accessibility to workplaces and private spaces first requires attitudinal changes about the rights of individuals with disabilities to be included in all activities of a society. The features of a truly accessible society must encompass:

- environments that are truly architecturally accessible;
- workplaces, businesses, and government services that enable individuals with hearing or vision impairments to communicate freely and participate fully in all activities;
- education systems and institutions that include individuals with disabilities;
- health care that is affordable and accessible;
- housing that is affordable and accessible;
- assistive technology to enhance mobility, communications, and learning skills;
- community-based services to support and encourage individuals with disabilities living independently;
- timely disabilities benefits with incentive provisions to encourage work;
- comprehensive laws and policies that prohibit discrimination against persons with disabilities;
- law enforcement mechanisms to ensure those rights.

In 1995, existing laws and government policies endorsed accessibility in many of these areas. What is essential for a truly inclusive society is a national disability policy that encompasses all these elements, and a strong commitment from government leaders to enforce the legal rights of individuals with disabilities. Full accessibility can exist only if people with disabilities and their families, colleagues, and neighbors expect and insist on changes to bring about the inclusion of all individuals with disabilities in all activities of their communities and the larger society.

(*See also:* AMERICANS WITH DISABILITIES ACT; ARCHITECTURAL ACCESSIBILITY; ASSISTIVE TECHNOLOGY; ATTITUDES; CIVIL RIGHTS; DISABILITY LAW AND SOCIAL POLICY; REASONABLE ACCOMMODATION)

BIBLIOGRAPHY

BERKELEY PLANNING ASSOCIATES. "A Study of Accommodations Provided to Handicapped Employees by Federal Contractors." Washington, DC, 1982.

COMMITTEE ON EDUCATION AND LABOR, House Report No. 101–485 (1990).

COMMITTEE ON LABOR AND HUMAN RESOURCES. Senate Report No. 101–116 (1989):43.

EQUAL EMPLOYMENT OPPORTUNITY COMMISSION. "Equal Employment Opportunity for Individuals with Disabilities; Notice of Proposed Rulemaking, 29 CFR Part 1630," 56 Federal Register 8579, 1991.

HARRIS, LOUIS, AND ASSOCIATES. "The ICD Survey of Disabled Americans: Bringing Disabled Americans into the Mainstream." New York, 1986.

LAPLANTE, MITCHELL P. "The Demographics of Disability," *The Americans with Disabilities Act: From Policy to Practice.* New York, 1991.

NATIONAL COUNCIL ON DISABILITY. *Towards Independence: An Assessment of Federal Laws and Programs Affecting Persons with Disabilities with Legislative Recommendations.* Washington, DC, 1986.

SCOTCH, RICHARD. *From Good Will to Civil Rights: Transforming Federal Disability Policy.* Philadelphia, PA, 1989.

WEST, JANE, ed. *The Americans with Disabilities Act: From Policy to Practice.* New York, 1991.

ELMER C. BARTELS

ACCREDITATION

See CREDENTIALS

ACQUIRED IMMUNE DEFICIENCY SYNDROME (AIDS)

See HUMAN IMMUNODEFICIENCY VIRUS AND ACQUIRED IMMUNODEFICIENCY SYNDROME

ADAPTIVE TECHNOLOGY

See ASSISTIVE TECHNOLOGY

ADDICTION

See ALCOHOL REHABILITATION, DRUG REHABILITATION, PSYCHIATRIC REHABILITATION

ADJUSTMENT SERVICES

In the context of disability and rehabilitation, adjustment has been defined as a process designed to solve problems, meet individual needs, and overcome functional limitations caused by disability (Couch & Sawyer, 1992). The official definition of adjustment services is found in the glossary of the Vocational Evaluation and Work Adjustment Association (VEWAA), a professional division of the National Rehabilitation Association. This definition describes adjustment services as

> ongoing, systematic and individualized rehabilitation services designed to enable persons with disability to cope with self and situations through the acquisition of skills, behaviors, and concepts to achieve an increased, measurable functional level of personal, social, and/or vocational development (Fry & Botterbusch, 1988).

Adjustment services are generally provided by an individual known as an adjustment specialist, but other professionals may provide certain components of this treatment/training process.

The provision of adjustment services usually follows the process known as vocational evaluation in which individual rehabilitation problems, needs, and functional limitations are identified. For instance, if an individual with a disability is found to have low academic achievement, no work history, low self-esteem, and a poor attitude toward work, vocational evaluators would identify such problems and needs in the vocational evaluation process.

A period of adjustment services might then be recommended in order to meet the noted needs. For this particular individual, evaluators might recommend academic remediation. They might also recommend counseling, real work in a work setting, job readiness activities, and other procedures that would help the individual to experience success in real work assignments and mold a good work personality. Following these recommendations, the adjustment specialist and the person with the disability prepare the individual written adjustment plan (IWAP), which outlines the adjustment program appropriate for the individual.

Adjustment services are essential for anyone who has not gained the basic skills necessary to seek, obtain, and maintain employment in our society (Cull & Hardy, 1973). The general purpose of all adjustment services should be to bring about changes in any behaviors that interfere with the individual's attempt to become a functional, independent member of his or her community (Baker, 1992). George Wright (1980) divides adjustment into three categories: work, personal, and social. But all adjustment procedures are designed to assist individuals who have disabilities to work and to live happily and productively in their community. Thus, solving problems, changing behaviors, helping to meet needs, and overcoming the functional limitations of the individual constitute the role of the adjustment specialist in this rehabilitation specialty known as adjustment services.

Target Groups

Any person who has difficulty in adjusting to life's demands might benefit from adjustment services. Typically, however, individuals receiving adjustment services in rehabilitation have been excluded from many developmental activities as a consequence of their disability. Those who have lifelong disabilities that require frequent hospitalizations and absences from school may not have had after-school or part-time summer jobs and therefore did not experience the normal exposure to work common to most people. These same people may have had limited opportunities to socialize, date, engage in competitive sports, lead school organizations, play musical instruments, or drive automobiles. They may have been objects of ridicule or suffered discrimination because of their disability. Failure to participate in normal growing-up activities can lead to an absence or distorted view of the role of work in our society. It may lead to problems in relating to others and can cause personality difficulties.

For those who have developmental disabilities, learning new tasks can be slow and difficult. A person with mental retardation, for instance, might require help in learning to perform a job in the community. A job coach or trainer may work with the individual on the job, teaching him or her specific job tasks and good work habits.

Other individuals may acquire a disability later in life. An automobile, diving, or trampoline accident might result in paralysis or traumatic brain injury. Such individuals must adjust to a different life. They must relearn how to study, get around, bathe, and drive, and to care for, feed, and dress themselves. Some with spinal cord injuries must use a wheelchair. Physical strength and stamina must be redeveloped through a process known as work hardening. Newly blinded individuals must also learn how to live without sight. A program known as Adjustment to Blindness helps such persons tell time differently, use talking computers, eat, walk with a cane or guide dog, learn to read braille, use talking books, match colors in their clothing selections, and a host of other activities (American Foundation for the Blind, 1992). Adjustment to a new physical disability, therefore, is often difficult and may require the help of professionals if one is to resume a full and satisfying life.

Other disabilities that occur later in life include those associated with strokes, substance abuse, cancer, AIDS, diabetes, mental illness, amputations, and aging (Smith & Couch, 1990). Individuals with such disabilities need some form of adjustment services to help them enter or reenter the labor market so they may be self-supporting, independent, and free to live a productive and satisfying life.

Because the needs, problems, and functional limitations addressed by adjustment services are so varied, there are many different techniques used by the adjustment specialist to assist individuals with disabilities in achieving their goals. The Commission on Accreditation of Rehabilitation Facilities (1993), the independent accrediting body for rehabilitation facilities, has specified certain minimum components that adjustment programs should provide. Among these are components intended to develop physical

capacity and psychomotor skills, work-related skills, work-practice opportunities, and communication and interpersonal skills. The commission also provides standards for personal adjustment programs.

Models of Adjustment Services

Five basic models of adjustment services have been identified to help define the role and function of the adjustment specialist and illustrate the many techniques and methods that are employed in adjustment services (Couch & Sawyer, 1992).

These five models have been adopted or adapted to meet the full range of challenges presented by those with disabilities. The first is work acclimation, which uses real or simulated work to introduce the worker to the world of work. The work acclimation model has as its goal the provision of real work experience in a work setting. Such experience teaches work habits, how to get along with supervisors and fellow workers, how to meet a job's quality and quantity standards, and how to enjoy all the rewards, challenges, and demands of the world of work. The work acclimation model usually takes place in the work center of a rehabilitation facility (called a workshop, activity center, rehabilitation center, etc.), which resembles a small industrial operation or business. But it can also be used in the community on a real job in which the rehabilitation client is already employed through a supported work program. In these settings the adjustment specialist may be the work supervisor in the work center industry or the job coach/trainer providing support at the community job site.

The second adjustment service model is problem solving. The problem-solving model consists of systematically addressing real, concrete problems that interfere with the individual's rehabilitation. For instance, if one of the client's problems is the common one of transportation, it is specifically identified and its parameters explored. A statement is then formulated that outlines a goal including a solution to the specific problem (e.g., the client will arrive at work on time each day). Next, possible solutions to the problem are "brainstormed." After evaluating all the possible solutions, the most logical and practical ones are adopted. The solutions become a part of the individual written adjustment plan. The planned program is implemented, then monitored regularly to assure its success in solving the problem. In this model the adjustment specialist is a planner, problem solver, and program monitor (Barker & Barker, 1993).

The third basic approach to adjustment is the behavioral model. Borrowed from psychology, it is often referred to as behavior modification. If an individual needing adjustment has a specific problem behavior which interferes with his or her work and life, a behavior modification program is used to eliminate undesirable behaviors or shape new, more desirable behaviors. For instance, if a person is consistently tardy for work, a plan might be devised to reinforce on-time behavior by using praise, granting special privileges, or providing other desired and rewarding items or events. Quite frequently, the adjustment specialist will teach adjustment clients to use behavior modification on themselves in a process known as self-management (Magrega & Couch, 1991). When using the behavioral model, the adjustment specialist assumes the role of a behavior technician.

The education model is employed whenever the adjustment client has a knowledge or skill deficit. In such cases, adjustment specialists become teachers using special and vocational education techniques to teach such varied subjects as job readiness, activities of daily living, or specific job skills. One day adjustment specialists may be teaching an individual to cook from a wheelchair, interview for a job, or use a personal computer. The next day they may be teaching a supported employment client to make french fries at a fast-food restaurant or conducting remedial-reading classes. Adjustment specialists may also teach individuals or groups one or more of the competencies from an available curriculum, such as Donn Brolin's (1989) Life-Centered Career Education, or they may need to create their own lesson plan: to teach proper hygiene to a person with mental retardation, for example. Again, the goal is the same: teaching an individual with a disability to live and work as independently as possible in the real world.

The final adjustment model is devoted to personal growth and development. Counseling is the core activity of this model. Adjustment specialists use individual and group counseling to help individuals explore their personal situations and their values, goals, and aspirations. The interpersonal relationship between the adjustment specialist and the client is critical in the rehabilitation process. Special activities may focus on such topics as assertiveness training, goal and values clarification, problem solving, and communication. Through this process individuals with disabilities explore their feelings and options and make informed decisions about their lives, thus facilitating their personal growth development.

Adjustment Specialists in Varied Settings

As illustrated in the adjustment models, the roles of the adjustment specialist are many and varied. The adjustment specialist may at times be a work supervisor in a rehabilitation facility's work center, a job coach or trainer on site at a community job, a planner and problem solver, a behavior technician, a teacher, an adviser, or a counselor.

Studies have been conducted that describe the competencies of the adjustment specialist. Judith Early and James Bordieri (1991) identified a number of competency clusters needed by adjustment specialists. First and foremost, adjustment specialists must have a special empathy for people and their life issues. They must aspire to make positive differences in the lives of others. They must know disabilities and their effect on every aspect of an individual's life. They must be familiar with jobs and careers and know how to analyze jobs in order to identify specific job tasks. Once they become aware of the functional limitations of a specific person's disability, and analyze potential jobs for him or her, they must be able to match the individual with a suitable, desired job that he or she can handle.

The Americans with Disability Act, signed into law in 1990, prohibits discrimination against individuals with disabilities in employment and in access to government services, businesses open to the public, public transportation, and telecommunication systems. Employers must make reasonable accommodations for the qualified individual with a disability if such accommodation will permit the individual to do a particular job. This law gives added impetus to the role of the adjustment specialist.

Two-thirds of Americans with disabilities are unemployed. Many of these individuals want to work, are ready and capable, and need no adjustment services prior to employment. Rather, it is the environment—for example, physical obstacles and negative attitudes in the workplace—that must be adjusted for these capable individuals to find suitable employment. In these instances adjustment specialists, along with other rehabilitation professionals, must be educators in and advocates for changing community environments (Couch, 1992; Menchetti, 1992). They may be called upon to be rehabilitation engineers, removing architectural barriers, modifying jobs to make them accessible, and serving as consultants to employers in making job accommodations. The role and function of the adjustment specialist, therefore, is a complex one requiring many varied competencies.

Most individuals who receive adjustment services attend work-oriented rehabilitation facilities. In 1990, 1.6 million individuals were served in the nation's 5,500 work-oriented rehabilitation facilities and activity centers (McAlees, 1990). Another 86,000 were served in community-based supported-employment programs (Wehman, 1992). In addition, thousands of students with disabilities are provided education- and adjustment-type services in school-to-work transition programs in public schools.

A large majority of adjustment clients are sponsored by the State-Federal Vocational Rehabilitation Program, which has offices in all U.S. states and territories. These offices are administered nationally by the Rehabilitation Services Administration within the U. S. Department of Education. State and local mental health and mental retardation authorities may also sponsor institution- or community-based adjustment-type programs. Affiliates of the National Easter Seal Society, Goodwill Industries, Jewish Vocational Service, Catholic Charities, Salvation Army, Association of Retarded Citizens, and other charitable or government groups operate rehabilitation facilities and activity centers in which adjustment services are offered.

Thousands of adjustment clients receive services in private, specialty rehabilitation centers or hospitals, prisons, homes for the aging, and in other community-based programs. Independent living centers, operated largely by those who have disabilities, also offer certain types of adjustment services.

Actually, wherever there are people with disabilities who have problems living and working in society, one generally will find an adjustment specialist providing adjustment services nearby.

The Future of Adjustment Services

A sizable number of practicing adjustment specialists have not mastered all the needed competencies. A majority of adjustment specialists have a bachelor's degree in rehabilitation services, psychology, education, sociology, or related fields. Some have no degrees and have learned their skills on the job. Better-qualified adjustment specialists have master's degrees in rehabilitation counseling or vocational evaluation and adjustment. Continuing education of these individuals is required to supplement their educational backgrounds and experience with training in the many competencies needed to become a fully competent adjustment specialist. One of the major future challenges of adjustment services is to assure that those practicing adjustment services master the many competencies that have been identified as critical.

The profession of adjustment specialist is relatively new, and adjustment services are not well known. Yet, this specialty offers an exciting, challenging role in the family of rehabilitation professions. Most Americans with disabilities have needs, problems, and functional limitations that may require professional assistance. Many of the services described herein are essential if these individuals are to achieve their goals of full employment, independence, social integration, and access to the complete range of goods and services generally available to all Americans.

Individual adjustment services tend to be somewhat fragmented, and other professions often specialize in individual components of adjustment. Special education units for the secondary-level student with a disability are developing programs for the critical transition from school to work. Rehabilitation counselors are trained to provide a wide range of adjustment services. Occupational therapists are claiming the work hardening process that was once the exclusive domain of the work acclimation model of adjustment. Job development and placement specialists have emerged to practice the specialty of finding jobs for those with disabilities. Rehabilitation engineers are being employed to help modify jobs and consult with employers regarding job accommodations. Thus, the scope, role and function, and territorial limits of adjustment services must be better defined and delineated in the future (Sawyer, 1992). The need for adjustment-type services by people with disabilities is indisputable. The available and emerging competencies needed for such practice in a host of settings have been identified, and the standards for such practices have found their way into the professional literature and published accreditation criteria. The practice of adjustment services, therefore, is an emerging professional activity that has not yet been fully consolidated as a profession. Once the issues of training, scope and limits, and professional identity are resolved, the great potential promise of adjustment services in addressing the needs of people with disabilities will undoubtedly be fulfilled, and the goal of developing adjustment services as an accepted professional practice will be realized.

(See also: BEHAVIOR THERAPY; DEVELOPMENTAL DISABILITIES; FACILITIES; PSYCHOSOCIAL ADJUSTMENT; REHABILITATION COUNSELING; STATE–FEDERAL REHABILITATION PROGRAM; VOCATIONAL EVALUATION)

RESOURCES

Vocational Evaluation & Work Adjustment Association, 202 East Cheyenne Mountain Blvd., Suite N, Colorado Springs, CO 80906

National Rehabilitation Association, 633 South Washington St., Alexandria, VA 22314–4193

American Foundation for Blind, 15 West 16th St., New York, NY 10011

BIBLIOGRAPHY

AMERICAN FOUNDATION FOR THE BLIND. Directory of Services for Blind and Visually Impaired Persons in the United States, 23rd ed. New York, 1992.

BAKER, RICHARD J. "Determining the Goals and Techniques of Adjustment Services." Rehabilitation Counseling Bulletin 16 (1972): 29–40.

BARKER, LARRY L., and BARKER, D.A. Communication, 6th ed. Englewood Cliffs, NJ, 1993.

BROLIN, DONN E. Life-Centered Career Education: A Competency-Based Approach. Council for Exceptional Children. Reston, VA, 1989.

COMMISSION ON ACCREDITATION OF REHABILITATION FACILITIES. Standards Manual. Tucson, AZ, 1993.

COUCH, ROBERT H. "Ramps not Steps: A Study of Accessibility Preferences." Journal of Rehabilitation 58 (1992) 1:65–69.

COUCH, ROBERT H., and SAWYER, HORACE W. "Adjustment Services for Special Populations." Vocational Evaluation and Work Adjustment Bulletin 25 (1992):63–69.

CULL, JOHN G., and HARDY, RICHARD. Adjustment to Work. Springfield, IL, 1973.

EARLY, JUDITH K., and BORDIERI, JAMES E. "A National Survey of Job Tasks and Functions of Work Adjustment Specialists." In Fifth National VEWAA Forum on Issues in Vocational Assessment: The Issues Papers, Ron Fry ed. Menomonie, WI, 1991.

FRY, RON, and BOTTERBUSCH, KARL, eds. VEWAA Glossary. Menomonie, WI, 1988.

MCALEES, DANIEL C. "New Directions for Rehabilitation Facilities," Vocational Evaluation and Work Adjustment Bulletin 23 (1990):25–30.

MAGREGA, DENNIS, and COUCH, ROBERT H. "Behavior Modification for Adjustment Services: Empowerment via Self-Management." Vocational Evaluation and Work Adjustment Bulletin 24 (1991):5–9.

MENCHETTI, BRUCE M. "Transition in Adjustment." Vocational Evaluation and Work Adjustment Bulletin 25 (1992):70–74.

SAWYER, HORACE W. "Adjustment Services: Opportunities for the Future." Vocational Evaluation and Work Adjustment Bulletin 25 (1992):102–104.

SMITH, JULIA, and COUCH, ROBERT H. "Adjustment Services and Aging." Vocational Evaluation and Work Adjustment Bulletin 23 (1990):133–138.

WEHMAN, PAUL. Achievement and Challenges: A Five-Year Report on the Status of the National Supported Employment Initiative. Richmond, VA, 1992.

WRIGHT, GEORGE. Total Rehabilitation. Boston, 1980.

ROBERT HILL COUCH

ADOLESCENTS, REHABILITATION OF

The developmental tasks of adolescence are mastered with difficulty by able-bodied youth. The tasks of adolescence, when superimposed on the limitations caused by chronic physical or mental disability, are laden particularly with conflict and strife. Any rehabilitation program established for an adolescent with disability must first attend to the resolution of normative developmental tasks (Goldberg, 1981).

A developmental perspective places an adolescent with a disability within the context of his or her age; educational grade; and mental, physical, and social development. The disability may interrupt the adolescent's normal working through of developmental tasks, but it does not totally obliterate the direction and pace of adolescent development. Genetic inheritance as well as cultural, environmental, and familial factors play a large part in determining the course of adolescent development. The development of the child within the family and the varying responses of family to children with disability provide a complex set of interactions that cannot be explained by the severity of the disabling condition (Harper, 1991). Consequently there is a large number of individual differences within each group with disabilities that vary larger than the differences among groups with disabilities. Research on disabled adolescents needs to take account of these large individual differences. For example, Richard T. Goldberg and B. Delia Johnson (1978) have shown that adolescents with disabilities do not always progress through successive phases of vocational development, and that when they do, they score an average of two years below their peers in age and educational grade.

Persons with a visible disability may have greater difficulty in adjusting to their handicaps than do persons with an invisible disability. In a study comparing children with congenital heart disease with children with facial disfigurement due to facial burns, it was found that the facially burned children had greater adjustment problems in school, lowered self-esteem, less initiative, less developed vocational interests, and less specific vocational plans after high school (Goldberg, 1974). Patients with facial disfigurement had comparatively minor functional limitations compared with patients with congenital heart disease.

Problems of Coping

All adolescents have problems coping with the developmental tasks commensurate with their age and educational grade. Adolescents need to develop coping strategies for individuation and segregation from their biological families, for coming to terms with their sexual needs and sexual identity, for choice of an educational and career objective, and for learning techniques that will make them independent, self-reliant, productive members of the community.

Adolescents with a disability often have extraordinary problems and stresses that augment the usual stresses experienced by adolescents without disability. Heidi Wayment and Andrea Zetlin (1989) compared thirty adolescents with learning disabilities attending special education classes with thirty adolescents without learning disabilities attending regular classes. Both groups were asked to respond to a sentence completion test eliciting current stress in their lives. Students in regular classes developed more active coping strategies. Both groups recognized the need for individuation, independence, socialization, and autonomy; they differed on the need for academic performance. Students in special education had become hardened to the outcome of poor academic achievement. Instead of attempting to cope with this problem, they avoided it. Students in special education generally developed more passive coping strategies, characterized by dependence and lack of personal contact.

Chronic Sorrow

The parent of a child with a disability often experiences chronic sorrow. The phenomenon of chronic sorrow, first reported and described by Simon Olshansky (1962), refers to an all-encompassing psychological reaction to a child with a disability. Parents may suffer inwardly and may conceal their reaction from others. The degree to which their reaction is expressed may depend on education, gender, race, or ethnic group. A parent of a child with congenital disability may slowly accept the child's limitations or may never accept the child's demands and needs. A parent with a child with acquired disability has greater difficulty in adjusting to the child's changed mental and physical status. As the child matures into adolescence, new concerns become more pressing. The adolescent with a disability is inevitably compared with her or his nondisabled siblings or peers. Parents reluctantly give up their expectations of "normal" adult achievement and settle for less than they had planned prior to the child's birth.

The phenomenon of chronic sorrow was applied

originally to the parents of children with mental retardation. Chronic sorrow is equally applicable to parents of adolescents with a major mental disorder, life-threatening chronic illnesses, or severe physical disabilities. Parents of adolescents with schizophrenia are constantly exposed to the societal accusation that they contributed to the disorder by faulty upbringing. Moreover, the stigma of mental disorder places unusual constraints on the parent. Unlike physical disabilities, which may be visible or which may have a known viral, traumatic, or immunologic cause, major mental disorders elude the precision of genetic markers, traumas, or infective agents. Parents feel responsible and accountable for mental illnesses. The illness is concealed from neighbors and friends. Consequently the parent has less opportunity to express his or her sorrow in normal social structures, and the adolescent becomes the center of the parent's expressed emotion.

The expressions of sorrow, initial resistance, adaptation, and acceptance may be more universal than originally proposed. Minority parents of children with disabilities appear to undergo similar stages of mourning and acceptance. The most commonly expressed emotion is one of grief and sorrow (Mary, 1990).

Transition from School to Work

An American adolescent is encouraged to develop her or his vocational potential commensurate with his or her abilities, interests, and work values, in keeping with the philosophy of individual self-development. Less attention is paid to the availability of jobs in the competitive labor market. The development of a vocational interest and the completion of a vocational training program may not guarantee future occupational success. Even Ph.D. scientists in physics, mathematics, and biochemistry face a contracting labor market.

In other nations (e.g., Germany and Japan) the rehabilitation system may develop an elaborate system of vocational training in which a student is guided toward meeting the needs of the employer (Greza, 1987). In Japan, a student is taught how to integrate his or her family, social, and personal life with his or her job (Matsui, 1993). The adolescent learns how to become an active participant in the Japanese company. The emphasis of the Japanese system is not the individual development of vocational potential but fitting the individual into the structure of the company and meeting the demands of the society.

Supported Employment

Wehman and colleagues (1981, 1985, 1987, 1991) have designed, organized, and implemented a system of supported employment for individuals with severe disabilities receiving services through the vocational rehabilitation system. In this system, the amount and type of intervention correspond with the job requirements and the degree of functional limitation present in the person with a disability. Compared to the traditional vocational rehabilitation process, which evaluates the work potential of the client prior to job placement and prepares the client for the job in a vocational training institution, supported employment teaches the client all the required skills on the job site and adapts the client to the social, interpersonal, and work demands on the job site. A study of two groups of persons with developmental disabilities randomly assigned to a supported employment program and a traditional workshop program showed that the supported employment program resulted in significantly greater employment (Goldberg et al., 1990). Supported employment has been found to be cost-beneficial and cost-effective in that it enhances greater quality of life (McCaughrin et al., 1993).

Supported employment programs provide a link between school and work. The transition to competitive employment has always been difficult in the United States, where freedom of choice reigns and employer selectivity is high. Supported employment, consistent with work-study programs proposed by Secretary of Labor Robert Reich, may be favorably compared to the more rigid German and Japanese systems for preparing adolescents for the labor market.

Normalization

The concept of normalization was effective for the deinstitutionalization of persons with mental and physical disabilities in the 1960s. Recent philosophies have criticized this concept as irrelevant to the broader issues of utilization of persons with disabilities in contemporary society. Normalization has in some quarters become the rallying point for advocates of civil rights. In the United States, any suggestion that persons with disability be given special treatment in sheltered workshops or be segregated in accordance with their disability is often looked at askance. In some educational settings, the amount of time that children with disabilities spend with children without disabilities is used as a measure of their social rehabilitation. Less attention is placed on the child's educational process. James Thompson and Mary McEvoy (1992) examine the concept of normalization from the vantage point of meeting the child's needs within an integrated setting. The presumption in the United States is that children with disabilities will be integrated with those who are perceived to be able-bodied (although not necessarily nondisabled).

A useful comparison with the philosophy and method of integration in the United States may be found in the rehabilitation institutions in Germany. In Germany, children with a disability are educated in a diverse group of institutions, ranging from special schools in the local community to Berufsbildungswerk, (i.e., special occupational training centers located throughout many regions of the country). In these training centers, adolescents are given specialized training in more than six hundred occupations. The training programs combine academic preparation with specific vocational skills. After the student has completed training, normally requiring three years, the student receives a certificate indicating that he or she has met all of the requirements for the occupation. The student is positioned to gain entry into the occupation and is placed on an even scale with students from other secondary institutions. A comparison with the educational practice in the United States reveals that German students with disability are better prepared to enter the work world (Goldberg, 1989). The disadvantage is that German students have been segregated for several years from their able-bodied peers. The concept of normalization often blurs the distinction between adequately and inadequately prepared students. The transition from school to work may require imaginative techniques to make use of specialized services. The provision of special

services for adolescents with a disability may enhance rather than detract from their ability to become included in the general community.

Vocational Development

Vocational development begins at birth with parental expectations for the child and ends at death. Several studies have shown that persons with chronic physical disability can maintain their same interests and plans following a disability. Measured interests and values are stable psychological characteristics that are maintained after adolescence despite severe disability. Vocational plans are not obliterated by a severe disability. A person needs to face the realistic limitations imposed by the disability while basing any changes in occupational plans on previous capacities, interests, and work values. In counseling a person with disability, it is important to assist the person in making a modification of a predisability plan or to seek an occupation in an allied field.

Compared to a group of adolescents without disabilities, adolescents with disabilities test lower on measures of vocational development (Goldberg, 1992). Adolescents with disabilities may have unrealistic fantasies, or may deny their limitations, or may overestimate the effect of their limitations on vocational choice. Integration of adolescents with disabilities with adolescents without disabilities is a recent development in American education. The new experiences engendered by academic integration may contribute to a higher level of vocational development. The results of integration need to be measured over successive ages and grades. No study has evaluated the effect of normalization on vocational development.

Future Trends

The rehabilitation of the adolescent with a disability rests on the assumption of the completion of the developmental tasks of adolescence. The tasks of formation of a sexual identity, separation from family, independence, and transition from school to work are typically more difficult for the adolescent with disability than for the adolescent without a disability. Moreover, adolescents with disabilities have not been given opportunities to develop pro-active coping strategies.

What can be done to foster the completion of developmental tasks? In the United States, the movement toward normalization has hastened the integration of children with disabilities in public schools. Although several advantages of integration include socialization with one's age and gender peers, exploration of sexual roles, and meeting a competitive standard of normality, integration does not guarantee training opportunities, qualifications for occupations, paid employment, and adequate housing. In a free, competitive economy, all of the above goals and rehabilitation services are fragmented. Access to the labor market is earned through hard work, specific training as well as personal contacts. Students with disabilities need a variety of services after secondary school to overcome their functional limitations and the impersonality of the labor market. These services include vocational evaluation, work activity centers, transitional employment, supported employment, independent living centers, housing services, and sexual counseling. In the United States there is no agency that coordinates all rehabilitation services. Faced with the resistance of some parents of children with disabilities toward any return toward segregation and with the realities of a rapidly contracting and more technically specialized labor force, we may need to look abroad for models of integrated school and work programs in which the adolescent is fully trained and assimilated into the objectives of the general society.

(See also: CAREER COUNSELING; FAMILY; NORMALIZATION AND SOCIAL ROLE VALORIZATION; PSYCHOSOCIAL ADJUSTMENT; SPECIAL EDUCATION; SUPPORTED EMPLOYMENT; TRANSITION FROM SCHOOL TO WORK)

BIBLIOGRAPHY

GOLDBERG, RICHARD T. "Adjustment of Children with Invisible and Visible Handicaps: Congenital Heart Disease and Facial Burns." *Journal of Counseling Psychology* 21 (1974):428–432.

———. "Toward an Understanding of the Rehabilitation of the Disabled Adolescent." *Rehabilitation Literature* (1981):66–74.

———. "The Human Sciences and Clinical Methods: An Historical Perspective." *Symposium: Social Science Perspectives on Vocational Rehabilitation. Rehabilitation Literature* (1984):340–344.

———. "A Comparative Study of Vocational Development of Able-Bodied and Disabled Persons." *International Journal of Rehabilitation Research* (1989): 3–15.

GOLDBERG, RICHARD T. "Toward a Model of Vocational Development of People with Disabilities." *Rehabilitation Counseling Bulletin* 35 (1992):161–173.

GOLDBERG, RICHARD T., and JOHNSON, B. DELIA. "A Comparative Study of Five Groups of Handicapped Children in Vocational Rehabilitation." *Scandinavian Journal of Rehabilitation Medicine* 10 (1978): 215–220.

GOLDBERG, RICHARD T.; MCLEAN, MARY; LAVIGNE, R.; FRATOLILLO, J.; and SULLIVAN, F. "Transition of Persons with Developmental Disability from Extended Sheltered Employment to Competitive Employment." *Mental Retardation* 28 (1990): 299–304.

GREZA, G. "An Encouraging Half Decade: Decade of the Disabled." *Bundesarbeitsblatt* 5 (1987): 12–16.

HARPER, DENNIS C. "Paradigms for Investigating Rehabilitation and Adaptation to Childhood Disability and Chronic Illness." *Journal of Pediatric Psychology* 16 (1991):533–542.

MARY, NANCY L. "Reactions to Black, Hispanic, and White Mothers to Having a Child with Handicaps." *Mental Retardation* 28 (1990):1–5.

MATSUI, NOBUO. Personal interview. Boston, 1993.

MCCAUGHRIN, WENDY; ELLIS, WARREN; RUSCH, FRANK; and HEAL, LAIRD. "Cost-Effectiveness of Supported Employment." *Mental Retardation* 31 (1993):41–48.

OLSHANSKY, SIMON. "Chronic Sorrow: A Response to Having a Mentally Defective Child." *Social Casework* 43 (1962):190–193.

SUPER, DONALD. *The Psychology of Careers.* New York, 1957.

THOMPSON, JAMES, and MCEVOY, MARY. "Normalization, Still Relevant Today." *Journal of Autism and Developmental Disorders* 22 (1992):666–673.

WAYMENT, HEIDI, and ZETLIN, ANDREA. "Coping Responses of Adolescents with and without Learning Handicaps." *Mental Retardation* 27 (1989):311–316.

WEHMAN, PAUL. *Competitive Employment: New Horizons for Severely Disabled Individuals.* Baltimore, 1981.

WEHMAN, PAUL; HILL, MARK; HILL, JANET; BROOKE, V.; PENDLETON, P.; and BRITT, C. "Competitive Employment for Persons with Mental Retardation: A Follow-Up Six Years Later." *Mental Retardation* 23 (1985):274–281.

WEHMAN, PAUL; KREGEL, JOHN; BANKS, P. DAVID; HILL, MARK; and MOON, M. SHERRILL. "Sheltered Versus Supported Work Programs: A Second Look." *Rehabilitation Counseling Bulletin* 30 (1987):42–52.

WEHMAN, PAUL; REVELL, W. GRANT; and KREGEL, JOHN. "Supported Employment: An Alternative Model for Vocational Rehabilitation of Persons with Severe Neurologic, Psychiatric, or Physical Disability." *Archives of Physical Medicine and Rehabilitation* 72 (1991):101–108.

RICHARD T. GOLDBERG

ADVOCACY

Advocacy is an active process designed to make any social system—public, community-based, or private—more responsive to the needs of each individual served by that system. In theory, a distinction should be made between advocacy and advocacy services. The former is a specifically assigned, formal role that is separate from the service-delivery system upon which it is to have an effect, while the latter refers to functions performed by people as part of their job responsibilities within a given service delivery system that result in a change in that system. Understanding the distinction requires a brief historical review.

Before 1960, the prescribed role of rehabilitation professionals included advocacy for the total needs of the people with disabilities whom they served. However, some administrators of community-based programs for people with disabilities came to realize that some of their employees—whether clinicians, rehabilitation specialists, or even special educators—often used this "advocacy" role to avoid handling the routine aspects of their assigned jobs. For example, an employee may have found it easier and more self-satisfying to complain to supervisors about a charge's lack of adequate clothing or parental rejection than to spend hours in direct contact with the individual, who had a severe disability, teaching the person to lift a spoon to his or her mouth. Yet the latter was the primary responsibility of that employee, and its fulfillment was the basis for the agency's income.

By the late 1960s, Dr. Wolf Wolfensberger and his interpretation of the theory of normalization began to have a major impact on the way services to children and adults with developmental disabilities were viewed. In stark contrast to the ideology of institutionalization, normalization is the process of enabling people with disabilities to function equitably in natural environments within the mainstream of society. According to its proponents, normalization is achieved by focusing primarily on the environment and, when necessary, changing others' attitudes, who are in that environment, toward people with disabilities. Wolfensberger hypothesized that each person has preconceptions and/or biases toward people who have disabilities or are otherwise different. These often unconscious biases are nurtured by three factors: the structure of society, cultural diversity within the community, and individual, lifelong experience. These biases frame the experiences of the individual with disabilities from the moment that the limitations are realized; they also limit the creativity of program developers and policymakers. Too frequently, these biases are so deeply rooted in the subconscious that, when policies and programs designed to meet the needs of the general population are under consideration, it does not occur to anyone to question the appropriateness of such generic policies and programs in meeting similar needs of people with disabilities. The resultant overriding effect upon individuals with disabilities is that, from their first social experiences, they are programmed to feel personally threatened by obvious differences that exist, or are perceived to exist, between people with disabilities and others, thus creating a self-fulfilling prophecy.

Wolfensberger used the word "normalization" to denote an attitude that is expected whenever direct services or policy and program issues concerning people with disabilities are formulated and implemented. The concept of normalization has greater meaning than the sum of its major components, which are "least-restrictive environment," "advocacy," and "quality of life." Within this context, the clearly distinct, autonomous role of the advocate first emerged as a specifically assigned, structured responsibility that carried an obligation to manifest change for the betterment of the individual. In so defining the role of the advocate, normalization theory did not intend to demean the role of others who, whether through effective performance of their job functions or as volunteers, made the service delivery system more responsive to the individual's needs.

To explore this new approach to advocacy further, in 1972 the U.S. Department of Health, Education, and Welfare, the Bureau of Education of the Handicapped, and the National Institute of Mental Health jointly awarded six grants of national significance. Three of these multi-year grants established the framework for effective advocacy as still practiced. The project undertaken by the National Association for Retarded Children (NARC) focused upon measuring the effectiveness of advocacy for individual needs in bringing about changes in the way programs and services were delivered. The focus of the award to the United Cerebral Palsy Association (UCPA) was the study of the effectiveness of changing organizational structures, both governmental and private, and the award to the National Center for Law and the Handicapped was to explore the use of the courts and other legal processes for bringing about systems changes. The combined findings and recommendations of these projects contributed to the evolution of advocacy in the following ways:

1. The projects established the theoretical definition of advocacy and identified four major types—legal, systems, individual/client, and self-advocacy—which were broadly defined as follows. *Legal advocacy* was viewed as instituting or intervening in lawsuits and administrative or judicial appeal processes and effecting other systems changes through the legal process. *Systems advocacy* used deliberate and organized mechanisms to promote changes in policies and structures through which goods and services were delivered to make them more responsive to individual needs. *Individual/client advocacy* meant acting on behalf of an individual to obtain rights or benefits. *Self-advocacy* occurred when individuals made their own choices, expressed their own needs, and participated in society's decision-making processes.

2. Early objective data were compiled indicating that: (*a*) individual function, not categorical diagnosis, was most descriptive of programmatic need; (*b*) a severe communication gap existed between rehabilitation specialists and those they served; (*c*) for maximum development of potential, the options of the individual who had a disability or the parents of such an individual must be considered with regard to both what services are needed and the manner in which they are afforded; and (*d*) programs and services that separated individuals with disabilities from society's mainstream tended to reinforce dysfunction.

3. Because the indicators listed above were at such variance with concepts and processes already ingrained in the delivery systems, the projects focused upon the needed independence of the advocate. This early distinction between advocacy and advocacy services was primarily based upon potential conflicts of interest with which practitioners of the latter may be faced. For example, the employee of a service provider who insists that a given individual be afforded a service in a manner that threatens the income of the employer may jeopardize his or her continued employment.

4. The projects emphasized the need for continued funding of retraining and widespread dissemination of findings, to be modified by future experience.

Since these findings and recommendations were first promulgated in the late 1970s, experience has proved their general validity, if not gained them universal acceptance. By the early 1990s it had become clear that:

- well-planned advocacy is an effective catalyst for change;
- the overriding purpose of advocacy and advocacy services is to obtain affordable access to such rights, benefits, and appropriate services and supports as may be needed or desired by each individual with a disability;
- acceptance at any given time of concepts of service flexibility, individual choice, and inclusion, all of which find their roots in early advocacy projects, is not a predictor of universal implementation in the immediate future;
- effective advocacy techniques and orientation-specific principles are so well defined that they provide a stable foundation for future growth;

18

- the four major types of advocacy represent descriptions of initial orientations or approaches that, for successful resolution on a given issue, may be used in combination or in tandem with one another.

These four types of advocacy—legal, systems, individual/client, and self-advocacy—are discussed below.

Legal Advocacy

Legal advocacy is the use of statutorily prescribed judicial and administrative procedures to adjudicate and enforce relative rights and responsibilities. Legal advocacy with regard to disability issues can take a variety of forms and can be used to achieve a comparable variety of purposes.

In many situations, individuals with disabilities have a choice as to whether to pursue an administrative or judicial remedy. Under the New York State Human Rights Law, for example, people who feel that they have been discriminated against may file an administrative complaint with the Division of Human Rights or pursue a private right of action, but they must elect between the two remedies. In other situations, as under the nondiscrimination in employment provisions of the Americans with Disabilities Act of 1990, a complaint usually must be filed with the Equal Employment Opportunity Commission, and a "right to sue" letter must be obtained before the institution of a lawsuit. Still other statutes require exhaustion of administrative remedies as a prerequisite to a lawsuit.

Where a judicial forum and remedy are sought, a complaint may be instituted to redress a specific, individual situation, such as to request a modification of policy for a particular individual with a disability (*Board of Education of the Hendrick Hudson School District* v. *Rowley*, 1982). Where a remedy is sought for a group ("class") of people who are similarly situated, a "class action" may be instituted, as in a 1993 federal court case resulting in a decision that the city of Philadelphia was required to install curb ramps or slopes on city streets where bids for resurfacing were let after January 26, 1992 (*Kinney* v. *Pennsylvania Transportation Department*, 1993).

Administrative proceedings are often limited to a determination of rights and responsibilities relative to a specific individual. While the decision in an administrative proceeding may be applied to other individuals similarly situated, and may result in a change in a policy or procedure by a governmental entity, which is often a party to an administrative proceeding, the results of an administrative proceeding may lack the binding nature and precedential value of a judicial determination.

Where an individual has an opportunity to choose between an administrative and a judicial forum, several factors must be considered:

- Is the individual's complaint/situation unique, or could he or she benefit from joining others seeking similar remedies?
- How much time will be required for resolution of the complaint through the administrative or judicial processes?
- What level of resources will be required to pursue a judicial or administrative remedy?

A second major issue is whether the individual will represent himself or herself in a judicial or administrative proceeding or will seek the services of an attorney or other advocate. Again, several factors must be considered:

- Will an individual's decision to represent himself or herself (to appear *pro se*) advance or hinder the complaint? While individuals with disabilities are often their own best advocates, the procedural intricacies of certain administrative and most judicial proceedings may put laypeople at a disadvantage.
- What advocacy and support services are available, either to provide direct legal representation (e.g., government-funded legal service programs, *pro bono* services, etc.) or to support an individual appearing *pro se* (e.g., community-based advocacy organizations, service providers, etc.)?
- What level of resources are required to secure legal representation and professional expertise/witnesses, and what are the chances of prevailing sufficiently on the merits to be awarded both costs and attorney's fees?

In the 1980s and early 1990s, disability advocates used the various techniques of legal advocacy to achieve a number of significant victories in the field of disability rights. Institutionalized individuals were found to have a constitutional right to protection from harm and a safe environment (*Youngberg* v. *Romeo*, 1982). People whose disabilities involve contagious diseases have been protected from employment discrimination (*Arline* v. *School Board of Nassau County*, 1987). The protracted class action lawsuit commenced to ensure appropriate care for individuals placed in the Willowbrook Developmental Center, where horrendous conditions were first brought to national attention in 1972, culminated in 1993 with a permanent injunction requiring placement of all "Willowbrook Class" individuals in appropriate community or qualifying facilities (*New York State Association for Retarded Children, Benevolent Society for Retarded Children, et al.* v. *Mario Cuomo, et al.*, 1975, 1993). Equally significant but far more personalized victories have been won by individuals with disabilities, parents, and advocates who have persevered in unique and highly individualized situations.

Systems Advocacy

Systems advocacy is defined as an active process designed to make any system—public, private, or community-based—more responsive to the needs of each person served by that system. In other words, for those people it serves, the systems advocacy agency or organization (1) increases awareness of existing programs, services, and/or unmet needs; (2) identifies barriers that keep people with disabilities from accessing needed services and supports; and (3) assists in the development and implementation of strategies to eliminate identified legislative, regulatory, social, and economic obstacles that interfere with the self-determination, independence, and ability of people to contribute to their own and society's welfare. Although they may vary in terms of geographic area covered, targeted issues and populations, organizational structures, funding sources, strategies, and countless other processes, effective systems advocacy organizations usually have some internal policies and procedures in common. Such

agencies tend to function according to written statements of mission, principles, values, and goals that are periodically reevaluated and revised. While their focus is likely to be on service-delivery policies and their implementation, a concerted effort is made to obtain input from a broad spectrum of affected entities outside the advocacy organization. Unlike a multipurpose agency, which also may have a major impact upon changes in the ways that services and supports are rendered, the systems advocacy organization devotes many of its resources to networking and uniting with other groups and organizations, whether generic or disability-related, with which it shares common issues or concerns.

Principles of Systems Advocacy

Regardless of a systems advocacy organization's stated mission, targeted population, or issues of concern, its approaches are usually based upon the following principles:

1. The vast majority of the targeted population with disabilities can become independent, self-directing, and self-supporting.
2. Each member of that population is afforded the opportunity to be an equal, participating member of society.
3. Changes in policies and operations to make the delivery of services more responsive to individual needs are achieved through deliberate and organized mechanisms.
4. The individuals of primary concern are more alike than different from other people, and thus their needs are better served by agencies responsible for serving similar needs of all people rather than by separate, segregated service systems, typified by residential institutions, special education classrooms, sheltered employment settings, and special transportation systems. A primary function of the systems advocacy agency is to raise the consciousness of the generic agencies in meeting the needs of people with whom they are concerned as part of their ordinary responsibilities. It then will provide technical assistance to those agencies in determining the most effective way to meet those responsibilities.

5. Regardless of designated geographic area—national, statewide, regional, or local—when the generic agency's responsibilities are exercised on a local or regional level, linkages are made to provide technical assistance at that level.

6. Occasionally, segregated, disability-specific services and supports may be necessary, primarily on a transitional or temporary basis, to enable people to participate fully in the generic programs.

7. Given the inherent requirement that systems advocacy bring together divergent viewpoints to identify and resolve common issues, primary functions of the systems advocacy organization include (a) the fostering of interagency cooperation and coordination so that human potential can be better achieved, and (b) the development and implementation of multifaceted strategies aimed at eradicating the conscious and unconscious biases that every person is likely to hold toward people who have disabilities or are otherwise different.

8. For maximum effectiveness, the systems advocacy function must be conducted, wherever possible, through quiet negotiation rather than public debate. As a result, recognition for the effect of changes will usually go to the generic agency, and the role of the systems advocate will often go unrecognized.

Individual/Client Advocacy

Individual/client advocacy occurs when one individual or agency tries, without resorting to legal processes, to obtain rights or benefits or to satisfy unmet needs for another specific individual or group of individuals. The widespread use of such an individualized approach provides the greatest challenge in differentiating between advocacy and advocacy services. Both may exist as a creation of either statute or organizational structure. For example, the nonlegal services rendered by the states' protection and advocacy systems, mandated by federal statute, are client-oriented and independent of the delivery systems upon which they are acting. So are some community-based not-for-profit agencies, like Advocates for Children, Inc., of New York City. However, legislatively mandated case managers, whether employed by a governmental or a community-based not-for-profit agency, may perform, by definition, advocacy services as part of the assigned job responsibilities.

Self-Advocacy

Self-advocacy, usually viewed as the highest form of advocacy and the ultimate goal of all other advocacy activities, is the empowerment of people with disabilities to rely upon themselves to make their own choices, express their own needs, and be recognized as both the primary decision-maker in choices affecting their own lives and an integral part of society's decision-making processes.

To attain full potential for self-determination, self-respect, independence, and self-support, people with disabilities need training in self-advocacy skills along a developmental continuum, so that they are enabled to access not only programs, services, and supports that will appropriately meet needs arising out of their disability, but also the generic services available to all people. For the majority of the diverse social populations with disabilities, the attainment of self-advocacy proficiency is both a desirable and an achievable goal.

Self-advocacy, as an empowerment strategy, operates on two levels. On an individual level, the person who learns to speak and act on his or her own behalf opens up pathways to pursue interests and options, gains greater knowledge of his or her rights, and is better able to exercise the responsibilities attendant to ensuring that these rights are not abrogated by others. The second level involves expansion of the skills of self-determination to include uniting with others who have common interests to achieve mutual goals.

(See also: ACCESSIBILITY; AFFIRMATIVE ACTION; AMERICANS WITH DISABILITIES ACT; CONSUMERS; DISABILITY LAW AND SOCIAL POLICY; NORMALIZATION AND SOCIAL ROLE VALORIZATION)

BIBLIOGRAPHY

Arline v. School Board of Nassau County, 772 F.2d 759, 11 Cir. 1985, aff'd. 480 U.S. 273, 1987.
Board of Education of the Hendrick Hudson School District v. Rowley, 458 U.S. 176, 1982.

Kinney v. Pennsylvania Transportation Department, 2 AD Cases 444, DC EPa, 1993.

New York State Association for Retarded Children, Benevolent Society for Retarded Children, et al. v. Mario Cuomo, et al., Permanent Injunction, 72 Civ. 356, 357, EDNY, 1993; see also Consent Judgment, 393 F.Supp 715, EDNY, 1975.

NOVAK, ANGELA, and HEAL, LAIRD W., eds. *Integration of Developmentally Disabled Individuals into the Community.* Baltimore, 1980.

SCHEERENBERGER, RICHARD C. *A History of Mental Retardation: A Quarter Century of Promise.* Baltimore, 1987.

WOLFENSBERGER, WOLF. *Citizen Advocacy for the Handicapped, Impaired, and Disadvantaged: An Overview.* Department of Health, Education and Welfare Publication No. (OS) 72–42. Washington, DC, 1972.

———. *The Principle of Normalization in Human Services.* Toronto, 1972.

Youngberg v. Romeo, 457 U.S. 307, 1982.

FRANCES G. BERKO
ROBERT J. BOEHLERT

AFFECTIVE DISORDERS

See MOOD DISORDERS; PSYCHIATRIC REHABILITATION; PSYCHIATRY; PSYCHOLOGY

AFFIRMATIVE ACTION

Affirmative action in employment of individuals with disabilities means elimination of disability factors from decision making and the provision of "reasonable accommodations" as needed to assure that each protected individual receives the opportunities he or she would have received had there been no disability. It differs in one significant way from other affirmative action laws and programs: unlike the others, disability affirmative action is not based on numbers. It sets no goals, quotas, or timetables.

The disability requirements are such that a company may meet them by hiring just one person and may violate them even after hiring thousands of people with disabilities. Affirmative action with respect to people with disabilities means that each protected person receives fair treatment at every stage of the personnel process, from outreach and recruitment, through testing and hiring, including terms of employment, to eventual termination.

The rules governing Executive Order 11246 (September 24, 1965) and Title VII of the 1964 Civil Rights Act offer group protections for members of racial and ethnic minority groups and for women. They impose requirements on employers to correct for past discriminatory practices, especially if court-ordered. Goals and timetables are mandated. An individual alleging discrimination may cite numerical evidence (e.g., a paucity of class members in certain jobs) in support of a claim of discrimination. No such requirements apply in the case of disability.

Title I of the Americans with Disabilities Act (ADA) of 1990 requires virtually all American employers with fifteen or more workers to practice nondiscrimination toward qualified individuals with disabilities. Discrimination on the basis of disability is outlawed, but no correction for past discrimination is provided. The ADA Title I rules are very similar to those of sections 501, 503, and 504 in Title V of the earlier Rehabilitation Act of 1973. Those sections that cover only federal agencies and federal contractors or grant recipients were modified by the Rehabilitation Act Amendments of 1992 and remain in force despite enactment of the ADA.

Nondiscrimination on the basis of disability is a recent phenomenon in the United States. The first federal regulations, or rules, requiring such steps appeared in 1976; all Title V employment regulations were in place by 1980. The nation's employment growth between that time and the early 1990s has been most notable in the private sector "services" economy, virtually all of which is exempt from Title V, thus limiting its impact. The ADA does cover many service sector employers, but it did not take effect until mid-1992 (for employers with twenty-five or more workers) and mid-1994 (for employers with fifteen or more workers).

Accordingly, the impact of disability affirmative action laws has been limited as of the early 1990s. Of the estimated thirteen million working-age (16–64) adults with disabilities who live in American communities (i.e., are not in institutions), only some 4 million work. The unemployment rate among those who are actively seeking employment is about 14 percent, double or triple that among nondisabled working-age adults. However, a majority of working-age adults with disabilities—more than 7 million individuals—are "out of the labor force"; that is, neither working nor actively seeking employment. Two out of every three (68 percent) working-age adults with disabilities are thus not in a position to take advantage of the affirmative action provisions in Title V and in the ADA (Bowe, 1992). The Equal Employment Opportunity Commission (EEOC) received 16,000 complaints during the first eighteen months after the effective date of ADA Title I (EEOC, 1994). Protection against discrimination on the basis of disability applies to well over 650,000 American employers. However, the impact of these laws is likely to grow as more adults with disabilities seek work and thus protection.

Definitions

The definitions used in the two laws are similar. "An individual with a disability" is defined in the ADA as any person who

(A) has a physical or mental impairment which substantially limits one or more of such person's major life activities, (B) has a record of such an impairment, or (C) is regarded as having such an impairment.

The ADA and the Rehabilitation Act protect "qualified" individuals with disabilities from unjust discrimination on the basis of disability. According to the ADA, a qualified individual with a disability is one

who, with or without reasonable accommodation, can perform the essential functions of the employment position that such individual holds or desires.

The ADA limits coverage so as to exclude users of controlled substances:

[T]he term "qualified individual with a disability" shall not include any employee or applicant who is currently engaging in the illegal use of drugs, when the covered entity acts on the basis of such use.

The Rehabilitation Act has similar language.

The definition of disability is a three-part one. Individuals may qualify under any one of the three parts. Under the first, the impairment must be permanent. Broken legs and the like are not included. Additionally, the impairment must be substantial. People who use glasses or hearing aids, but who, with those aids function well on the job, are not covered. Employees who are in treatment trying to rehabilitate themselves from substance dependency and are not current abusers of controlled substances such as drugs, are protected against discrimination on the basis of disability—but they enjoy no such protection if they resume drug use.

The second part of the definition relates to a history, or record, of a disability. If an employee or applicant once was under the care of a psychiatrist for a mental disorder, once was a substance abuser, or once was disabled in another way, an employer may not use that information in any personnel or other employment decisions. People who have a "record" of an impairment are protected from discrimination on the basis of that record.

The third part of the definition protects an individual from discrimination on the basis that he or she is "regarded" as being an individual with a disability. If an employer were to take adverse action against a qualified individual because it wrongly believes him or her to be disabled, the employer would violate the rights of the employee.

"Reasonable accommodations" are required by the ADA and by sections 501, 503, and 504 when the individual has a substantial limitation. The employer is required to offer what it believes is a "reasonable" accommodation to a known limitation. The key terms here are "known" and "limitation." If the employer is aware of a permanent limitation, it should consider what reasonable accommodations might be made to that known limitation.

What is a "reasonable accommodation"? The ADA says it may include:

(A) making existing facilities used by employees readily accessible to and usable by individuals with disabilities; and (B) job restructuring . . . modified work schedules, reassignment to a vacant position, acquisition or modification of equipment or devices, appropriate adjustment or modifications of examinations, training materials or policies, the provision of qualified readers or interpreters, and other similar accommodations for individuals with disabilities.

Under Title V and the ADA, reasonable accommodations consist of adjustments in practices, modifications in building design, or the provision of special adaptive devices that help someone with a disability to do the work his or her background and training qualify him or her to perform. Accommodations are a contractual obligation; that is, they must be offered to qualified people. The two exceptions recognized by the laws are those instances in which provision of an accommodation would impose an "undue hardship" (e.g., would be very costly) or would interfere with business necessity and safety (e.g., would jeopardize the performance of work by the individual or by others in the work force). The term "reasonable" limits the employer's obligation to those changes that do not impose an "undue hardship" and do not disrupt the business or work force.

From Title V to the ADA

In section 501, Congress sought to protect the equal employment rights of people with disabilities applying for jobs at, or working in, federal agencies. Section 501 calls for "affirmative action," but what it means is "nondiscrimination" (equal employment opportunity). The section requires federal agencies to provide "reasonable accommodations" for applicants and employees with handicaps.

Administrative regulations set by the Office of Personnel Management (OPM) and the EEOC for section 501 allow federal agencies, but do not require them, to ignore personnel ceilings when hiring sign language interpreters to support deaf workers, readers for blind employees, and personal care attendants for workers with physical disabilities. While those policies help, the budgetary constraints under which most federal agencies operate limit the practical effect of these procedures. Nonetheless, federal employment of people with disabilities has improved significantly since 1973. Indeed, the federal record is strong by comparison with that of the private sector.

In section 503, Congress imposed an affirmative action obligation on private companies holding contracts with federal agencies. An example is Grumman, which makes aircraft under contract for the U.S. Department of Defense. Section 503 is administered by the U.S. Department of Labor (DoL). Coverage is limited to only some 30,000 "prime contractors" and some 85,000 subcontractors. The nation's other employers—which total some 7 million—are not covered.

Section 503 has been the subject of numerous court cases. Perhaps the most important of this body of case law is E. E. Black, Ltd. v. Marshall (1980). In Black, the issue at hand was the definition of "handicapped individual." (The term was changed to "individuals with handicaps" in the 1986 amendments to the act and then to "individuals with disabilities" in the 1992 amendments.) The case history is instructive. At the time, the Department of Labor's administrative order said that section 503 covered "every individual with an impairment which is a current bar to employment which the individual is currently capable of performing." Black, Ltd., however, contended that to be substantial, an impairment had to cause an individual difficulty in finding work across the entire spectrum of job opportunities, not just those jobs the individual was interested in or qualified to perform.

The federal district court in Hawaii decided that both were wrong, but to different degrees, siding more with DoL than with Black. In denying Black's motion for summary judgment, the court said that DoL's standard was too broad because it ignored the statutory term "substantially" and would therefore cover any person who because of an impairment is limited in employment in any way. But the court rejected Black's interpretation as well, because it would severely limit section 503's reach. The court offered a standard for use in case-by-case instances; it defined a substantial handicap as one that resulted in the individual's disqualification from jobs throughout the area to which he or she had reasonable access.

Section 504 immediately follows section 503 in the Rehabilitation Act. It applies not to contractors but to grant recipients: that is, to virtually all of the nation's 3,000 colleges and universities, its 15,000 school districts, and its many thousands of hospitals, social service agencies and facilities, and public libraries. In 1978, in the Rehabilitation Act Amendments, Congress made section 504 applicable to federal agencies as well.

Section 504 calls for "program accessibility," that

is, for all programs and activities conducted by a recipient (or by an agency) to be "accessible to and useable by" individuals with disabilities. Unlike sections 501 and 503, then, section 504 applies not only to employment but to all activities of covered entities that affect customers, students, clients, and employees.

In 1984, the U.S. Supreme Court ruled, in the *Grove City* case, that section 504's reach extended only to specific programs or activities directly benefiting from federal financial assistance, not to the entire institution as had been understood until that time. In the case of Grove City Community College in Pennsylvania, this decision meant that only the financial aid office needed to comply with section 504—not the whole college. Four years later, on March 22, 1988, Congress reversed this interpretation. The Civil Rights Restoration Act overturned the *Grove City* decision, returning the scope of coverage to programs and activities of the entire institution.

The Americans with Disabilities Act extended similar kinds of protection for individuals with disabilities to employers that receive no federal funds of any kind. The major difference in protection between the Title V employment sections and the ADA is there: More than 650,000 companies are covered by ADA Title I versus about 100,000 by Title V.

Personnel Procedures

Limitations. The laws say that employers may ask about, and be told of, any job-related limitations of the individual applicant or employee. Stated differently, the employer may ask the applicant if he or she could do the job, with or without reasonable accommodations. For example, if the individual is restricted for medical reasons from working on rotating shifts, the employer must know that to be able to assign duties and protect the safety and health of employees.

Privacy of Medical Information. However, the employer may not ask, or require applicants or employees to tell, why that limitation has been applied. Individuals with disabilities have the right to privileged and confidential treatment of medical information, including diagnostic data on disabilities.

Asking about disability prior to a job offer violates the ADA and the Title V employment sections.

Reasonable Accommodations. The only exception to the reasonable accommodations requirement discussed above relates to products or procedures that are primarily personal in use and in purpose; those are the employee's responsibility. Employers having recognized unions representing workers should discuss any proposed accommodation in advance with union representatives to assure that such adjustments do not infringe on the rights and prerogatives of other workers.

Education and Training. Qualified individuals with disabilities have a right to the same kinds of education and training they would receive if they had no limitations. They also have a right to the reasonable accommodations they need in order to take full advantage of that training. It is not acceptable to arrange for separate, segregated, or different training for such individuals if the regular training may be made available with or without reasonable accommodations.

Internal Mobility. Individuals with disabilities have the same right to transfers, promotions, and advancements as do other employees.

Universal and Standard Criteria. The ADA and the employment sections of Title V require covered employers to use only "universal and standard" criteria for personnel processes. All requirements in a job description must be job-related. There cannot be requirements that are not actually relevant to doing the job. To illustrate: it is not acceptable to say things like "writes reports" when "prepare reports" is also acceptable (it may be possible to type a report, to dictate one, to provide one orally, etc.).

Accessible Facilities. All "people use" buildings (buildings that are not used by employees or members of the general public are exempt) are to include "access" features to the extent feasible and to the extent needed by applicants and employees with disabilities. For example, at least one entrance must include wide doors and ramps, if needed; there must also be level floors, elevators, accessible restrooms, accessible common areas such as cafeterias and lobbies, and similar features. When an individual is to be assigned to work in a building, such reasonable accommodations as are necessary to make the work site accessible must be considered and, if feasible, provided. Examples might include a raised desk, an accessible restroom on that floor, and an "accessible" parking space in an employer-owned parking lot. The employer is not responsible for non-company-owned, leased, or rented facilities.

Record Keeping. Title V and the ADA require employers to keep such records as are necessary to demonstrate compliance. Thus, copies of personnel manuals, recruiting materials, and reports of reasonable accommodations made must be retained and made available to the EEOC or other authorized agencies upon request.

Adverse Action. In making demotion, layoff, termination, and other adverse-action decisions, the employer may not base its determination on disability. It is not permissible to demote, separate, or terminate an employee just because that individual has a permanent limitation due to a disability. However, if the limitation cannot be accommodated, despite the employer's best efforts, and if the limitation is such that the individual no longer can perform the job, the employee may not be qualified for the job; if that is the case, the person no longer is protected by the ADA or by the applicable section of Title V. Employers having a work force represented by a union should consult with union representatives before taking adverse action against employees with disabilities.

Complaints. Title V and the ADA require that covered employers provide a mechanism through which qualified individuals with disabilities may file internal complaints about alleged discrimination.

There is a clear private right of action under section 504 and under the ADA. EEOC rules for ADA Title I ask individuals with disabilities to first "exhaust administrative remedies," that is, wait for the EEOC to investigate the case before requesting a "right to sue letter." Section 503 does not confer a private right of action as clearly; however, EEOC rules explain that any complaint brought under section 503 will be considered a complaint under ADA, and vice versa. (See, for example, *Federal Register,* January 24, 1992.) Filing under ADA assures a private right of action following exhaustion of administrative remedies.

Employees and applicants with disabilities who believe that discrimination on the basis of disability

has occurred may file complaints with the regional office of the EEOC. The EEOC, in turn, may come into the company to investigate the complaint, or may refer the complaint to a state equal employment agency for investigation. Applicants and employees working for federal contractors also may file with the U.S. Department of Labor on the basis of section 503. As with the EEOC, the Labor Department has the right to come into the company to investigate the complaint.

After exhausting administrative remedies, qualified individuals with disabilities may have the right to go to court for relief. Under the ADA, relief may include hiring, reinstatement, promotion, back pay, front pay, reasonable accommodation, or other actions that will make an individual "whole" (the condition in which the person would have been but for the discrimination). Remedies may also include payment of attorneys' fees, expert witness fees, and court costs. Where intentional discrimination is found to have occurred, compensatory and punitive damages up to $300,000 may be awarded.

Future Impact

Although the impact of the Title V employment sections and of the ADA Title I was limited through the early 1990s, these statutes offer potentially powerful protections for individuals with disabilities. As more and more such individuals secure the education and training needed to get and keep good jobs, more will seek the protection of these statutes in their efforts to lead self-supporting lives as tax-paying citizens. The two laws provide sufficient statutory authority to enable individuals with disabilities to secure appropriate relief for any discrimination that may occur. However, the relief is available only to those to seek it. As long as millions of American adults with disabilities remain out of the labor force, such protections may as well not exist for them. Therein lies our principal challenge: to encourage tens of millions of adults with disabilities to prepare themselves for, and then seek, employment commensurate with their abilities.

(*See also:* ADVOCACY; AMERICANS WITH DISABILITIES ACT; CIVIL RIGHTS; CONSUMERS; REASONABLE ACCOMMODATIONS)

Resources

Equal Employment Opportunity Commission, 1801 L. St., NW, Washington, DC 20507

Bibliography

Bowe, Frank. *Equal Rights for Americans with Disabilities.* New York, 1992.
E.E. Black, Ltd. v. *Marshall,* 497 F.Supp 1088, 1104, D.C., Hawaii, 1980.
Equal Employment Opportunity Commission. Unpublished data on ADA Title I complaints received, October 1–December 30, 1994.

Frank Bowe

AGING

Aging, a normal process with many dimensions, is a broad concept, including changes in both the internal and external environment that occur on a continuum from conception to death. Aging encompasses not one process but many, including physical, psychological, and social processes that undergo changes throughout the life of each individual. These changes occur at varying rates within each individual and among separate individuals. Most changes resulting from the aging process are subtle, occurring in slow and at times imperceptible increments. These changes evolve over many years and gradually affect functional capacity to some degree. The duration and level of any resulting dysfunction are different for each individual and dependent on a variety of factors.

Although changes associated with aging are inevitable, increasing attention is being directed toward delaying functional decline to the extent possible for as long as possible (Brody, 1988). The aging process may influence a person's physical, psychological, and social abilities, resulting in alteration of functional capacity. Successful aging refers to balancing changes effectively in each of these areas and adapting to or modifying the environment so that maximal function and quality of life can be maintained.

As individuals reach later years, they are confronted with varying degrees of physical, psychological, and social losses. Older adults' abilities to cope

and adapt vary greatly. To be effective, interventions directed to assisting older adults regain or maintain maximal function must address not only physical changes but also include restoration of the balance among physical, psychological, social, and environmental issues within the older individual's life (Gallo, 1988). Behavior is the interactive result of these influences and the focus of rehabilitation efforts with older adults.

Defining Older Adulthood

The age at which an individual can be labeled as "old" is an arbitrary distinction, since aging is a continuing process. A variety of ways have been used to categorize individuals into different age groups and to define older adulthood. In the United States, legislative and administrative policies define "old age" in various ways. The Older Americans Act designates sixty years of age as a basis for eligibility for a variety of services (U.S Senate Special Committee on Aging, 1983). The Social Security Act defines sixty-five as the criterion for entitlement for full benefits (Atchley, 1988). Using chronological age as a basis for demarcating the onset of old age has its limitations, since chronological age alone is not always a good indicator of an individual's level of function, ability to adapt, or level of maturity.

Other means of categorizing individuals by age is according to developmental models that are based on life stages such as adolescence, middle age, or older adulthood. This approach to categorization defines age in terms of social transitions and behavior or characteristics that may be expected or that are usually observed at a particular stage of life. Changes from each life stage occur gradually, and the exact point at which an individual moves from one life stage to another is arbitrary. The life stage categorizations of age groups are general and do not account for individual differences, nor does this approach accurately reflect the individual's ability to function effectively within his or her environment (Falvo, 1991).

Another means of categorizing older age is through evaluating an individual's ability to function at varying levels. Functional definitions of aging rely on observation of individual attributes with regard to mental capacity, appearance, mobility, co-ordination, and other functional capacities. Included in the functional definition of aging is not only physical function but also psychological and social function as well as the individual's ability to adapt and cope within his or her environment. An accurate definition of the functional age of an individual must address function in each area.

Physical definitions of aging may vary depending on the context. For example, an Olympic swimmer may be considered old by age twenty-five, although by most definitions all functional capacities are still intact. Physical aging is tied to the concept of the life span—namely, maximum length of life that is possible for a certain species. Life span is genetically determined and is variable for different species. Life span is different from life expectancy, which refers to the length of time an individual may expect to survive given the current mortality rate. For humans, life span has remained relatively constant at approximately 120 years, while life expectancy over time has gradually increased (Borrow, 1992).

Physical changes take place in the human body throughout the life span. Because physical changes associated with aging are so variable, it is difficult to separate changes associated with normal aging and the pathological effects of disease. Physical changes associated with normal aging are cumulative and interact to produce consequences resulting in differing degrees of loss of physical capacity. The degree to which these losses produce severe limitation of function depends on many factors, including psychological and social changes.

Psychological function as associated with aging may be broadly defined. Two major perspectives involve mental dimensions such as perception, intelligence, and memory; the second, a more global perspective, is human development.

Psychological changes associated with aging refer to mental processes such as thinking, creativity, memory, and problem-solving; these in turn affect behavior and the individual's ability to adapt. Aging can affect psychological functions, specifically cognitive processes that are dependent on central nervous system function. However, social factors may also influence psychological functions. Many psychological changes that have an impact on ade-

quate function can be at least partially prevented or compensated for if adequate social resources are available (Geiger, 1988).

From a human development perspective, changes associated with aging involve a dynamic process in which the individual confronts continuous challenges throughout life that he or she must interpret, cope with, and adapt to. Moving through these different stages helps the individual develop personality characteristics over time, enabling him or her to form an identity, which is used to interpret experiences and assign subjective meaning to those experiences. Development is viewed as an evolving whole that does not involve discrete stages but is the result of continuous processes of development encompassing interactions among mental processes, subjective experiences, adaptive strategies, and the individual's social environment.

Aging may also be at least partially defined from a social perspective. From this perspective the social roles that individuals are expected to fulfill at different times in life are established. Most human relationships are structured to some degree by the social roles they fill. These social roles serve as a background for social interactions and determine the reactions of social groups toward an individual as well as the individual's reaction to the groups. Throughout life, individuals fill many different social roles, which change over time. Age serves to modify expectations of the individual in his or her social role. Social expectations differ, for example, for an individual who is fifteen and for one who is thirty-five. As individuals age, they engage in a process of adaptation in which they attempt to fit role demands to their individual capability and societal expectations. Social aging is used to evaluate the appropriateness of roles and expectations and to modify expectations with regard to various roles in society.

Physical, psychological, and social changes associated with aging are also modified by age norms, or what people at a given age are assumed to be capable of doing, as well as assumptions about what is appropriate behavior at any given age. A variety of factors, including gender, ethnicity, and social class, can modify not only changes in each of these areas but age norms and expectations as well.

Societal Issues in Aging

The demographics of the United States portend a significant change in the nature of the nation's population. The prolongation of life expectancy has greatly increased the proportion of older individuals within the population. In 1900 there were only three million persons, or about 4 percent of the total population, who were over age sixty-five in the United States. The average life expectancy at birth was 48.3 years for females and 46.3 years for males (Barrow, 1992). By 1983 individuals sixty-five years or older constituted about 12 percent of the population in the United States, and the life expectancy at birth was 78.3 years for females and 71.0 years for males (American Association of Retired Persons, 1990). It is projected that in the United States by the year 2000 those individuals 65 years or older will constitute 31 million, or 13 percent of the population, and it is conceivable that with increasing advancements in combating the leading causes of mortality, by the year 2030 those persons sixty-five years or older could constitute nearly 21 percent of the total population (Lewis, 1989).

Trends indicate that the number of older adults with the onset of late life disability will increase, as will the number of older adults who experience disability at a younger age (Holland & Falvo, 1990). Until the past few decades, persons with major disability did not survive to reach older adulthood (Trieschmann, 1987). With the advancement of knowledge and medical management, however, many of these individuals are surviving longer so that increasing numbers of persons with disability are now entering later years of adulthood (Smith, 1987). The large number of older adults with disability is significant (Blake, 1981). To provide comprehensive, cost-effective services to meet the complex needs of older persons with disability, a number of resources will be needed.

Statistical data indicate that older adults with disability—either those who were disabled earlier in life or those who were disabled in older age—have higher rates of unemployment and underemployment as compared to younger job applicants (Herbert & Dambrocia, 1989). The increasing number of older adults with disability who will not be effec-

tively used in the work force has significant implications for society. Not using this pool of potential workers increases the rate of unemployment and reduces the gross national product; it also fails to use the skills and experience of the older adult.

The dramatically increasing number of older adults raises tremendous health, economic, and political issues that have not been adequately addressed (Binstock, 1988). Financing and providing adequate health care for the older population, establishing an economic base for the provision of a number of social services and benefits to older adults as well as providing the economic surplus needed to finance retirement income, and establishing policies that contribute to ensuring that resources are available to meet these needs will have considerable impact on society as a whole. The dramatic increase in the older population demands attention to development of programs and services to meet the needs associated with this growth as well as to educate professionals to ensure that relevant services are provided to older adults as a group and to older adults who are physically or emotionally disabled.

Issues in Older Adulthood

While many older adults remain active with only minor limitations in function, the incidence of chronic disease and disability increases with age (Becker & Kaufman, 1988). Aging affects the kinds of illness individuals are more likely to have and the amount of associated disability (Barrow, 1992). As individuals become older their vulnerability to chronic illness and subsequent disability increases. Nearly 50 percent of persons over age seventy have at least one chronic illness that interferes to some degree with their ability to function in activities of daily living (Kemp, Brummel-Smith, and Plowman, 1989). In addition, disability from injury also increases with age. As individuals age, they increasingly incur accidental injury that is accompanied by more complications, loss of functional ability, dependency, and immobility (Kallman & Kallman, 1989).

In 1985 only about 5 percent of the older population lived in institutionalized settings (Atchley, 1988). It is projected that this percentage may nearly double by the year 2000, primarily due to the larger number of older adults who are living well into their eighth decade (Nanton & Soldo, 1985). Such an increase will place a dramatic demand on resources to support care in long-term-care facilities. Community care alternatives to institutional placement of older adults has been suggested as one method of decreasing the demand for long-term-care beds while at the same increasing the potential for older adults to remain in the community (Corthell & Fleming, 1990).

Normal changes of aging occur not only in able-bodied persons but also in individuals who have experienced disability at an earlier age. As a result, normal changes associated with aging become superimposed on other impairments related to the person's original disability (Trieschmann, 1987). Depending on the time of onset and type of disability, as individuals with disability age, body systems that have compensated for loss of function of other body systems may show increased physical decline, further impairing the residual function that the individual has intact (Issacson-Kailes, 1991).

The effects of chronic disease or disability are not the only factors that interfere with older adults' ability to reach their maximum functional capacity. Societal myths and misconceptions and negative attitudes toward aging present additional barriers that can prevent older adults from reaching their full level of function (Powel & Thorson, 1990). The effects of ageism are visible in a variety of settings but perhaps are most dramatically illustrated in employment (Atchley, 1988). Despite federal legislation prohibiting age discrimination in employment, many older adults in general experience negative biases toward hiring, training, and retention (Benedict & Ganikos, 1981).

Although some older adults welcome retirement as an opportunity to enjoy leisure or other activities they had inadequate time to pursue while working, a number of other older adults experience significant economic hardships imposed by fixed income, or rising medical costs resulting from chronic disease or disability that make gainful employment necessary (Corthell & Fleming, 1990). Economic conditions including rising inflation require income supplements for many older adults on fixed incomes if they are to maintain an adequate standard of living. Even when work is not an economic necessity for them, many older adults value the opportunity to continue to work in some capacity. The work yields more than economic rewards; it also provides social contacts and status and contributes to the individual's identity, sense of self-worth, and enhancement of self-esteem.

Older adults with disabilities experience a compounded bias with regard to work (Myers, 1987). Often they do not receive the same assistance or services needed to maintain their jobs as do younger adults, and consequently they may be forced to leave the work force even though with appropriate modifications of their job or job environment they may have been capable of continuing to function in the workplace (Herbert & Dambrocia, 1989). Older adults with the same disability tend to be occupationally disabled at a greater rate than younger adults because of the tendency to overestimate physical demands of jobs and ageism (Atchley, 1988).

Age and the number of chronic conditions present do not necessarily define older adults' ability to function independently in their environment. Physical impairment alone may not be responsible for the degree of functional limitation individuals experience that can challenge their independence (Falvo, 1991). Not all limitations experienced by older adults relate only to chronic illness or disability. While in some instances chronic illness or disability imposes functional limits that in and of themselves interfere with function, in many instances functional limitations that prevent older adults from being fully active in their environment are limits imposed by other people's perceptions of the older adults' ability to function (Atchley, 1988).

Consequences of chronic illness or disability in the older adult population include not only the functional limits of their physical condition but also potentially social limits, which can in turn lead to psychological disability such as depression. The most effective means of assessing the ability of older adults to function in their environment considers all factors that affect function rather than limiting assessment to physical function alone.

Implications for Rehabilitation

Traditionally, rehabilitation has emphasized vocational goals; consequently, older adults have not always been recipients of rehabilitation services due to perceived limits of employability. Thus, many older adults with disability have not received rehabilitation services that would enable them to increase functional capacity, maintain independence, and reduce development of complications that can affect independence. The 1978 Rehabilitation Act amendments, and specifically Title VII of that legislation, provided for comprehensive services for independent living without regard to vocational potential. The expansion of rehabilitation services to assist in meeting the needs of older adults is a logical extension of current rehabilitation practices.

The general philosophy of rehabilitation, most simply stated, is the process of restoring individuals to their highest possible level of physical, emotional, and social function. The philosophical orientation of rehabilitation is exceptionally compatible with meeting the needs of older adults. The philosophy implies a process that includes a creative and cooperative team approach, with an emphasis on learning and behavioral changes.

In addition to the basic philosophy of rehabilitation, the rehabilitationist has a knowledge of medical aspects of disability and of issues in adaptation and adjustment as well as skills to advocate for the rights of individuals with disability and to provide a comprehensive, individualized approach to dealing with the problems of the client. Such knowledge and skills provide a unique and needed background for working with the older adult (Smith, 1987).

Although many older adults remain healthy and active well into their later years, one-third of all people with functional impairments are older adults. It has been estimated that well over half of all older adults have one or more physical impairments that limit activity (Powel & Thorson, 1990). Rehabilitation services that are directed toward helping individuals adapt to disability, maintain or regain some type of gainful employment, gain or maintain function or skills that assist them to achieve their maximal level of independent living, or increase quality of life are the goals of rehabilitation practice and well suited to the needs of older adults with disability.

The process of rehabilitation includes an assessment of the individual's abilities and limitations as well as an assessment of their psychological and social resources. The number of older adults who will be experiencing functional impairment will continue to grow as the number of adults reaching older age rises and as life expectancy increases. The need for accurate and appropriate assessment, provision of services, and adaptive devices to preserve and maintain the highest level of functional capacity possible, and ongoing provision of services to assist older persons in their ability to cope and adapt to the limitations they are experiencing will continue to grow.

Rehabilitation services to older adults may be provided in a variety of contexts. Services may be directed toward helping older individuals maintain or gain employment through job restructuring, work site modification, or training. In other instances services may be directed toward providing assistance services or devices that may be needed to help the individual gain or maintain independent living within his or her own home. In some instances disability can reach the point that some type of specialized housing is needed. When this occurs, the older individual may need to move into the home of a relative, a foster care situation, or other type of specialized facility. In the event that other resources aren't available, or that the disability has a profound impact on function, the older person may be placed in an institutionalized setting (Atchley, 1988). Rehabilitation services are still appropriate in these settings to maximize function and quality of life.

Rehabilitation seeks to minimize disability through assessment of individuals' abilities, resources, and barriers that restrict them from living to their full functional capacity. Maintenance of the balance among physical, psychological, and social factors is necessary if optimal level of function is to be maintained. Dysfunction in any one area can lead to dysfunction in other areas. Specific medical diagnosis of chronic illness or disability is not as important to an individual's rehabilitation potential as is the impact of each aspect of the condition on each area of the person's daily life and daily functioning. A functional assessment approach takes into account physical, psychological, and social factors as well as environmental and economic factors that may have an impact on functional capacity.

Rehabilitation services to the older adult may include vocational considerations, or services may be directed toward maintenance or enhancement of the individual's functional capacity and consequently the degree of independence and quality of life. Environmental barriers may need to be modified to promote fuller independence, or assistive devices may be needed to increase functional capacity. In some instances services may be directed toward identifying resources or other supportive services that may contribute to the fuller independence of the older adult.

When functional capacity of the older adult becomes significantly compromised, rehabilitation may be able to offer the advocacy, resources, and innovative approaches that could make alternatives to institutionalization possible. Cost containment, particularly in the prospective payment system, requires reliance on alternatives to institutional care.

Innovative Approaches to Rehabilitation of the Older Adult

As awareness of aging and disability increases, so will the need for innovative approaches to issues and problems associated with an aging population. Traditionally a medical model that is oriented to acute or crisis care has been used in assessing individuals' needs for service and resources. The medical model focuses on specific pathological changes related to the disease or disability and treatment of symptoms. Diagnosis of a chronic illness or disability alone is not always a useful indication of the person's ability to function effectively within his or her environment, nor does it accurately identify measures that can be taken to assist individuals to adapt and adjust to regain or maintain maximum functional capacity. The functional model often used by rehabilitation and applied to the needs of older adults is a means of providing comprehensive information that can then be used to develop an effective plan for meeting the needs of the older adult.

The Seventeenth Institute on Rehabilitation Issues was convened to develop an agenda on aging in America and its implications for rehabilitation and independent living. The Institute concluded that there should be increased emphasis on education and training of rehabilitation counselors, and expansion of rehabilitation services to older adults (Corthell & Fleming, 1990). A similar recommendation was issued at the eleventh Mary E. Switzer Memorial Seminar (Myers, 1987). Recommenda-

tions from this seminar stipulated that education and training be offered to providers already in the service delivery network as well as to professional training curricula of rehabilitation practitioners and other medically related professionals to increase general knowledge of aging, discrimination, disability, and work issues. The need to train rehabilitationists about issues of aging was echoed at the fifteenth Mary E. Switzer Memorial Seminar, from which recommendations included a call for better training of rehabilitation counselors to meet the needs of older adults, and for establishment of Rehabilitation Service Administration priorities for short- and long-term training programs for rehabilitationists already working in the field (Perlman & Hansen, 1991).

Innovative approaches to helping other adults regain or maintain employment have also been addressed. Emphasis has been placed on educating employers and union representatives on the value of flexible work options that could be used by older adults as well as on promoting the value of older adults in the workplace (Perlman & Hansen, 1991). Other approaches related to development of programs to make services available to the older worker include transportation services, which would enhance their ability to obtain or maintain competitive employment, and use of functional assessment in disability determination hearings (Smith, 1987).

The role of the independent living rehabilitation movement in issues of aging has also been addressed (Corthell & Fleming, 1990). James F. Budde (1990) reports that 22 percent of the consumers of independent living rehabilitation services are older than sixty-one years of age and further suggests that with respect to older adults, the independent living concept should be expanded to include assisted living models in home settings.

Another innovative approach to meeting the needs of older adults with physical or cognitive disabilities is an adult foster care model of assisted living. Gordon Bourland and Duane Lundervold (1990) describe such a model, which is designed to provide older adults with the opportunity to engage in meaningful activities and maintain functional skills through use of assistive technology, modified environments, and skill instruction when necessary.

One approach that has been suggested as having specific utility in increasing and maintaining older individuals' functional independence longer is a behavioral one. A behavioral model as applied to the rehabilitation of older adults emphasizes individual autonomy, self-managed interventions, and direct skill acquisition to enhance more effective functioning. Behavioral models have been applied to specific functional problems such as eating disorders, incontinence, and depression as well as to social situations in which skills are taught to promote adaptation to and competence in a variety of settings. A behavioral approach combines an understanding of the effect of the social and physical environment on all levels of behavior and emphasizes function rather than diagnosis.

Research Implications for Rehabilitation

The Rehabilitation, Comprehensive Services, and Developmental Disabilities Act Amendment of 1978 established the National Institute of Handicapped Research (NIHR) and mandated that the institute conduct and coordinate research to improve the lives of all individuals with disability. Section 204 of this legislation extended the traditional research programs from issues related to working-age persons with disabilities to adults at both ends of the age spectrum, namely the very young and older adults. In 1980 the NIHR demonstrated its commitment to research on older adults with disability by requesting proposals for research and training centers with a core area in aging. Over the ensuing years research and training centers were established, and research at the centers focused on approaches to improve the functional and societal status of older adults, the effects of multidisciplinary treatment, and issues related to caregivers as well as assessment of community support systems to assist families caring for older adults with disability. Training and continuing education programs related to the rehabilitation of older adults were also developed. Although numerous studies have been conducted at the research and training centers, more are needed. Effective rehabilitation for older adults can be provided only after current rehabilitation professionals and students have been adequately trained. Working with older adults requires knowledge of their unique needs, strengths, and possible limitations as well as knowledge of the aging process and adapta-

tion to interventions. Research that assesses the effectiveness of curriculum and training materials directed toward increasing understanding of the needs and potential of older adults with disability is vital.

Research related to creative approaches to dealing with special needs of older adults with disability, as well as scientific evaluation of the effectiveness of those approaches, are also needed. Such approaches relate to environmental restructuring and behavioral approaches to a number of problems of older adults. Other research priorities may be directed toward improved methods for changing community behavior and/or attitudes toward older individuals with disability; this includes integration into programs and activities from which older persons with disability are excluded and removal of environmental or social barriers that interfere with participation. In addition, research directed toward development of advanced technology that would improve the functional ability of older adults with disability is needed. Methods to enhance development of mechanisms for increased communication and collaboration among varying agencies that could result in development of improved services to older adults should also be studied.

Integrating service, research, and training; utilizing a biopsychosocial perspective; and maximizing functional abilities are trends to consider in future rehabilitation efforts with older adults.

(*See also:* ALZHEIMER'S DISEASE; CAREGIVING; INDEPENDENT LIVING; LOSS AND GRIEF; PSYCHOSOCIAL ADJUSTMENT; STATISTICS; WELLNESS)

BIBLIOGRAPHY

AMERICAN ASSOCIATION OF RETIRED PERSONS. A *Profile of Older Americans*. Washington, DC, 1990.

ATCHLEY, ROBERT C. *Social Forces and Aging*, 5th ed. Belmont, CA, 1988.

BARROW, GEORGIA M. *Aging, the Individual, and Society*. New York, 1992.

BECKER, GAYLENE, and KAUFMAN, SHARON. "Old Age, Rehabilitation, and Research: A Review of the Issue." *The Gerontologist* 28 (1988):459–468.

BENEDICT, ROBERT C., and GANIKOS, MARY L. "Coming to Terms with Ageism in Rehabilitation." *Journal of Rehabilitation* 47 (1981):11–17.

BINSTOCK, ROBERT H. "Allocation of Resources to

Rehabilitation." In L. Gregory Pawlson and Stanley J. Brody, *Rehabilitation and Geriatric Education: Perspectives and Potential,* ed., L. Gregory Pawlson and Stanley J. Brody. McLean, VA, 1988.

BLAKE, RICH B. "Disabled Older Persons: A Demographic Analysis." *Journal of Rehabilitation* 47 (1981):19–27.

BOURLAND, GORDON, and LUNDERVOLD, DUANE. "The Caring Family Home: A Behavioral Model of Adult Foster Care." *Adult Residential Care Journal* 4 (1990):95–108.

BRODY, STANLEY, J. "Geriatrics and Rehabilitation: Common Ground and Conflicts." In *Rehabilitation and Geriatric Education: Perspective and Potential,* eds. L. Gregory Pawlson and Stanley J. Brody. McLean, VA, 1988.

BUDDE, JAMES F. "Independent Living and Rehabilitation: Concepts and Practices." In *Aging and Rehabilitation II: The State of the Practice,* eds. Stanley J. Brody and L. Gregory Pawlson. Springer, NY, 1990.

CORTHELL, DAVID W., and FLEMING, KEN. *Seventeenth Institute on Rehabilitation Issues.* Menomonie, WI, 1990.

FALVO, DONNA. *Medical and Psychosocial Aspects of Chronic Illness and Disability.* Gaithersburg, MD, 1991.

GALLO, JOSEPH J.; REICHEL, WILLIAM; and ANDERSON, LILLIAN. *Handbook of Geriatric Assessment.* Rockville, MD, 1988.

GEIGER, BRIAN F. "Cognitive Intervention in Alzheimer's Disease." *Journal of Rehabilitation* 54 (1988):21–23.

HERBERT, JAMES T., and DAMBROCIA, CYNTHIA J. "Employability of Older Persons with Disabilities: A Partnership Among Employers, Rehabilitation Counselors, and Potential Workers." *Journal of Applied Rehabilitation Counseling* 20 (1989):16–20.

HOLLAND, BEVERLY E., and FALVO, DONNA R. "Forgotten: Elderly Persons with Disability—A Consequence of Policy." *Journal of Rehabilitation* 56 (1990):32–35.

ISAACSON-KAILES, JUNE. "Aging with a Disability: Another Advocacy Priority." In *Aging, Disability, and the Nation's Productivity: A Report on the 15th Mary E. Switzer Memorial Seminar,* eds. Leonard G. Perlman and Carl E. Hansen. Reston, VA, 1991.

KALLMAN, HAROLD, and KALLMAN, SHEILA. "Accidents in the Elderly Population." In *Clinical Aspects of Aging,* ed. William Reichel. Baltimore, 1989.

KEMP, BRYAN; BRUMMEL-SMITH, K.; and PLOWMAN, VICKI J. "Geriatric Rehab Program Focuses on Research, Training, and Services." *Journal of Rehabilitation* 55 (1989):9–11.

LEWIS, KEN. "Persons with Disabilities and the Aging Factor." *Journal of Rehabilitation* 55 (1989):12–13.

MANTON, KENNETH G., and SOLDO, BETH. "Dynamics of Health Changes in the Oldest Old, New Perspectives and Evidence." *Milbank Memorial Fund Quarterly* 63 (1985):206–285.

MYERS, JANE. "Challenges for the Older Worker in the Rehabilitation Process." In *The Aging Workforce: Implications for Rehabilitation: A Report of the Eleventh Mary E. Switzer Memorial Seminar,* eds. Leonard G. Perlman and Gary F. Austin. Alexandria, VA, 1987.

PERLMAN, LEONARD G., and HANSEN, CARL E. *Aging, Disability, and the Nation's Productivity: A Report on the 15th Mary E. Switzer Memorial Seminar.* Reston, VA, 1991.

POWEL, CHUCK, and THORSON, JAMES A. *Rural Elderly and Their Needs: Understanding, Developing, and Using a Needs Assessment.* Kansas City, MO, 1990.

SMITH, MAE. "Aging and Employment." In *The Aging Workforce: Implications for Rehabilitation: A Report of the Eleventh Mary E. Switzer Memorial Seminar,* eds. Leonard G. Perlman and Gary F. Austin. Alexandria, VA, 1987.

TRIESCHMANN, ROBERTA B. *Aging with a Disability.* New York, 1987.

SENATE SPECIAL COMMITTEE ON AGING. *Developments in Aging: 1982.* Washington, DC, 1983.

DONNA R. FALVO
DUANE A. LUNDERVOLD

ALCOHOL REHABILITATION

According to Glen Evans, Robert O'Brien, and Morris Chafetz (1991), alcoholism is defined as a "chronic disorder associated with excessive consumption of alcohol over a period of time." There is much room for interpretation in this definition. What is excessive consumption? Over what period of time does the drinking need to take place? Although there is room for discussion in the points raised above, there is a consensus among health care professionals that alcoholism and alcohol abuse have a significant effect on American society. One cannot consider the impact of alcoholism without considering the physical, psychological, social, legal, and economic effects that alcohol has on the person and on society as a whole.

No one definition of alcoholism is satisfactory. As a disabling condition, alcoholism affects each person individually. One person with the diagnosis of alcoholism may have substantial physical health problems as a result of drinking, while another may have minimal physical complaints. Another person with alcoholism may have lost several jobs as a result of drinking, while another has been on one job for years with no absenteeism. Alcoholism manifests itself in a unique manner for each individual who acquires this disease. The American Psychiatric Association (1994) publishes a list of diagnostic criteria; however, the health care professional must also understand how alcoholism affects that person in a unique way.

Since alcohol use has been present since the onset of human existence, one can also assume that alcohol abuse has been present for just as long. Mark Keller, as cited in William J. Filstead, Jean J. Rossi, and Mark Keller (1976), suggests "that the first plant man cultivated deliberately was the grapevine." The discovery of fermentation may have been by chance, but it has been developed ever since, and alcohol has been part of cultures across the planet. The use or nonuse of alcohol is an important component of culture; alcohol has been an important part of American culture since its inception.

The prevalence of drinking problems in American society is sizable. According to the American Psychiatric Association (1994), a U.S. national sample of noninstitutionalized adults (ages 15–54) studied in 1990–1991 using DSM-III-R criteria reported that around 14 percent had alcohol dependence at some time in their lives, with about 7 percent having had dependence in the past year. Fourteen percent of adults would make persons with alcohol problems the largest group of persons with a disability in American society and the subsequent cost upon society to be enormous.

Physical, Psychological, Social, Legal, and Economic Factors

Alcohol abuse and dependence problems have a holistic effect on the individual. Every aspect of the person's life is affected. Because alcohol problems are both progressive and chronic, the individual often does not see the effects that his or her drinking

has on that person's life until many years have elapsed, if ever. Progression refers not only to the fact that the person will need to drink more over time to achieve the desired effect, it also means that the effects of continued drinking over several years will have a cumulative impact on every aspect of that person's life. Chronic means that this disease is characterized by periods of exacerbation and remission but that the disease can continue unabated until death unless the person stops drinking.

Physically, the person with alcohol abuse or dependence may experience many problems. According to James Wright and others as cited in Glen Evans, Robert O'Brien, and Morris Chafetz (1991), these include cardiac disease, neurological disorders, hypertension, gastrointestinal disorders, and peripheral vascular disorders. The presence of these disorders does not constitute a diagnosis of alcohol abuse or dependence, but the health care provider should be aware of the correlation between these physical disorders and alcohol abuse and dependence.

Psychologically, according to the American Psychiatric Association (1994), "Alcohol dependence and abuse are often associated with dependence on, or abuse of other substances, including cannabis, cocaine, heroin, amphetamines, various sedatives and hypnotics, and nicotine. Alcohol may be used to alleviate the unwanted effects of these other substances or to substitute for them. Symptoms of depression, anxiety, and insomnia frequently accompany alcohol dependence and sometimes precede it." According to Wright and others as cited in Glen Evans, Robert O'Brien, and Morris Chafetz (1991), the diagnosis of mental illness occurs in 27.7 percent of male abusers and 52.8 percent of female abusers. An individualized approach must be taken to ascertain the effects of other psychological disorders on the alcohol-dependent person. Dual diagnosis will complicate treatment and rehabilitation efforts.

Social, legal, and economic factors related to alcoholism are numerous. Social relationships are often strained or broken. The alcoholic's behavior is the cause of difficult family dynamics that often result in codependency. Persons who live with an active alcoholic may suffer from the perceived loss of human potential as a result of these conditions. The alcoholic also interfaces with the legal system at a much higher rate than the average adult. The reasons are numerous. The primary reason is that of driving under the influence of alcohol, the cause of approximately 25,000 deaths each year. In addition, since alcohol is a disinhibiting drug and the ability to make good judgments is impaired while under its influence, many persons may become involved in criminal behavior when drinking. Finally, there is a relationship between alcohol use and spousal and child abuse. All of these factors will result in the heavy drinker or alcoholic coming into contact with the legal system.

Economically the alcoholic costs society $108 billion in lost production per year. This cost results from both the increased use of medical and social services as a result of the alcoholism, and lost production in the workplace by alcoholic employees. According to Henrick Harwood, Patricia Kristiansen, and J. Valley Rachal, as cited in *Alcohol and Health* (U.S. Department of Health and Human Services, 1990), the economic cost of alcohol abuse and dependence was projected to be $150 billion in 1995.

Major Societal Problems Arising from Alcohol Abuse

The social consequences of alcohol abuse and alcoholism are multitudinous. Motor vehicle crashes as a result of alcohol abuse or alcoholism number in the hundreds of thousands annually. Alcoholics are also much more likely to be involved in falls when inebriated. In addition to the risk of death, alcoholics may suffer serious medical consequences as a result of falls, including head trauma. Fires and burns occur more frequently for alcoholics than among the general adult population. Fires resulting from "careless disposal of smoking materials" often occur when the alcoholic passes out with a lit cigarette in his or her mouth. Drowning also occurs more frequently to persons who have been drinking. According to Jonathan Howland and Ralph Hingson, as cited in *Alcohol and Health* (U.S. Department of Health and Human Services, 1990), victims who have been exposed to alcohol account for approximately 38 percent of drowning deaths.

Suicide is another considerable risk factor associated with alcohol use. According to Judy Roizen, James Colliver, and Henry Malin, as cited in *Alcohol and Health* (U.S. Department of Health and Human Services, 1990), research indicates that 20 to 36 percent of suicide victims have a history of alcohol abuse or were drinking shortly before their suicide. There is also a link between trauma and alcohol abuse. This link may be shown through the increased use of emergency medical services among alcohol abusers. Finally, there are links among crime, alcohol abuse, and family violence. Prison populations have a high incidence of persons with alcoholic problems, and, as mentioned above, there is also increasing evidence of a link between alcohol abuse and both spousal and child abuse.

Etiology, Diagnosis, Prevention, and Treatment

The origins of alcohol abuse and alcoholism are found in a complex set of variables. No one set of variables can be said to be the reason why one person develops a problem with alcohol. One can best understand the development of a problem with alcohol as a process that takes place over a number of years. There is evidence that both genetic and environmental factors are part of the development of alcoholism in a particular individual. The interaction of genetic and environmental factors is most likely the most accurate way to understand the acquisition of the disease of alcoholism. Because each person's life, and his or her perception of it, is unique, the best way to understand the etiology of alcoholism is that a variety of factors were involved for the development of alcoholism in a person.

The diagnosis of alcoholism is a complex task that should be undertaken only by appropriate trained health care providers. Classifications of alcohol-use disorders have evolved gradually; both the World Health Organization and the American Psychiatric Association have played prominent roles (U.S. Department of Health and Human Services, 1990). Diagnostic systems are based on using multiple diagnostic criteria that are holistic in nature. Only by understanding the person's life, and the role that alcohol plays in that life, is an accurate diagnosis possible. Diagnosis is best accomplished through a combination of interviewing, psychological screening tests such as the Michigan Alcoholism Screening Test, and medical evaluation.

Prevention of alcohol abuse problems is based on the premise that if one never starts abusing alcohol, then one will never have a problem with it. Since the early 1970s there has been considerable effort in the prevention field. The sooner one starts prevention efforts the better, but prevention programs can be effective for every age group. Persons are never too young to be exposed to prevention efforts. Both government and the private sector have supplied the impetus for prevention efforts. They have been successful from the preschool level through the college-age adult population. The premises behind prevention are that the knowledge base about alcohol use and its effects can be developed; that attitudes toward alcohol use can be challenged and explored; that positive decision-making and coping skills can be taught; and that positive, healthy behaviors will result. Examples of prevention programs include Drug Awareness Resistance Education (DARE) and the federal government's Fund for the Improvement of Post-Secondary Education (FIPSE) program.

Treatment of persons with alcohol abuse and dependence issues takes many forms. In considering treatment for the individual patient, the first thing that must be taken into consideration is management of alcohol dependence. Alcohol is a depressant drug, and in most cases patients who have a long-term pattern of heavy drinking must be medically withdrawn from alcohol. This is accomplished in detoxification centers; thousands of public and private centers exist throughout the country. The reason for withdrawal under medical supervision is that patients may experience a variety of severe complications if they withdraw on their own. Neurological effects, cardiovascular effects, seizures, and distorted perceptions may occur during withdrawal. The medical staff of a detoxification center is trained to deal with medical problems such as these and to determine when patients need to be transferred to a general medical facility because of the severity of complications.

Once detoxification has occurred, the patient or client must be evaluated for further treatment. Some withdrawal symptoms may persist for several weeks, and the client needs to be supported medically and psychologically to deal with these issues. An evaluation must be made on treatment setting and intensity. A wide range of options exist. Some patients may still be experiencing significant medical complications from alcoholism and need to be admitted to a twenty-eight-day inpatient program where further medical treatment can occur under the auspices of a counseling regimen. Other clients benefit from further inpatient treatment that is primarily psychological and supportive in nature. Still other patients need a supportive living environment, and they are accepted into halfway houses for an extended time.

Finally, other clients will leave a detoxification center and return to their home and begin a period of outpatient counseling at a local alcoholism treatment center. The types of clients who are mentioned above will eventually be referred to outpatient counseling centers. Alcoholics Anonymous (AA) is a major force in the treatment and rehabilitation of the person disabled by the effects of alcohol. At every step of the process the client is exposed to AA meetings and AA members. In inpatient facilities, including detoxification centers, AA members put on nightly meetings. Treatment centers where patients are allowed off the grounds generally require client participation in a certain number of AA meetings per week. Thousands of AA meetings take place every day in this country, literally around the clock. Large U.S. cities have over a hundred meetings a week or more.

Individual and group counseling may continue for an extended time. In addition, as self-awareness develops and sobriety continues, other issues may surface in the patient's life. Referral for family and marital therapy, sex therapy, social skills training, and other specialized psychological services may be warranted. The goal for the client who is alcoholic is abstinence, and the patient must learn to live sober in a world where other people drink.

A controversy that exists in the alcohol abuse field is whether a person with a history of abusing alcohol can control his or her drinking. Many clients wish to return to appropriate drinking. Appropriate drinking can be defined as being able to drink without loss of control in any given situation or over an extended period of time. The evidence concerning the ability to control drinking is scant. While it may be argued that an occasional person may return to appropriate drinking, for the overwhelming majority of clients who abuse alcohol the only realistic solution is complete abstinence. The fact that this debate exists is evidence of the prominent role that alcohol maintains in this society.

Treatment and Rehabilitation Implications for Those Clients Who Have Alcoholism as a Primary Versus Secondary Diagnosis

Many of the clients seen by alcoholism treatment agencies have a primary diagnosis of alcohol dependence or alcoholism. This means that the foremost issue in their lives is their alcoholism. Medical complications and family, social, legal, and economic problems result from their alcoholism. For example; a client reports a history of job losses. Previous employers have told the client that drinking during business hours and poor job performance will result in termination. One could deduct that the employment history problems are secondary to the primary problem: the client's alcoholism. If the client did not have a drinking problem, one could reason that there may not have been employment problems.

However, due to the way that denial and other defenses are used by alcoholics, they would not see things in the way that was just stated. He or she would argue that the lousy job or unreasonable supervisor was the reason for the job loss. An alcoholic might say, "You'd drink, too, if you had my job." The alcoholic would believe that a better job, one where she or he was left alone, would be the cure. Three or six or ten jobs later the alcoholic would still be using this line of reasoning. When the general public sees this happening to someone, they shake their heads and say, "Can't they see what they are doing to themselves?" The answer to this question is no. Alcoholism is a progressive disease, and over a period of years the use of alcohol affects an alcoholic's thinking processes. Alcoholics cannot see themselves as they are; they use the psychological defenses of denial, distortion, deletion, and generalization to hide from the reality of their own lives. They no longer have a choice of whether they can drink; they are physically and psychologically addicted to ethyl alcohol in its various forms. They cannot not drink.

Other clients will come into treatment centers, and the determination is eventually made that al-

though they have a problem with alcohol, it is secondary to another diagnosis. For example, a client with a primary diagnosis of schizophrenia also uses alcohol to excess. The person is using the alcohol to help blunt hallucinations that he or she is experiencing. Treating the alcoholic without treating the schizophrenia would result in a client who still has a significant mental health issue. Even if this could be accomplished in the short term, the patient may revert to alcohol because the hallucinations would still be there if left untreated.

Regardless of whether alcohol dependence is the primary or secondary diagnosis, a holistic approach must be adopted if the client is to return to health. In both cases the use of alcohol must stop completely. One cannot know the true health status, both physical and mental, of the individual until all drinking has ceased. In the case of alcoholism as the primary diagnosis, one cannot determine all the health services needed until sobriety is attained. In the case of alcoholism as the secondary diagnosis, the use of alcohol may obscure the total health of the client, and this cannot be evaluated until there is sobriety. In both of these cases the patient may not ever drink safely again; abstinence must be part of the treatment plan.

Major Roles and Functions of Professionals

Allied health professionals from a variety of fields work together in providing care and treatment to persons with the diagnosis of alcoholism. Regardless of their occupational specialty and education, individuals need to be trained to work in the addictions field; often a master's degree or more education is required to become certified and licensed. Physicians in several specialties regularly provide health services to clients with a diagnosis of alcoholism. The medical specialty of addictionology addresses the problem of alcoholism. Psychologists provide counseling and allied services to clients. Rehabilitation counselors and other mental health professionals are often trained to work with people with the diagnosis of alcoholism. These counselors are specially trained to understand how alcoholism relates to disability and can influence the treatment and rehabilitation process.

Social workers often work with alcoholics in a variety of settings. Some social work programs have a specialization in addictions. Occupational therapists can specialize in the psychosocial aspects of alcoholism and work with clients in a variety of settings. Nurse practitioners and registered nurses provide diverse services in many health care settings. Finally, recreation therapists are employed by many alcoholism treatment agencies.

An increasing number of states require alcoholism counselors to be certified. The requirements for certification vary from state to state; interested persons should contact the division of alcoholism in their state department of health. The existence of a certification movement is evidence of the continued growth of the field of alcoholism counseling.

Role and Functions of Professional, Consumer, and Governmental Organizations

Professional organizations have as their goals the advocacy of continued research and professional practice in the betterment of the human condition. Organizations such as the American Psychiatric Association, the American Psychological Association, the American Counseling Association, and the National Rehabilitation Association are examples of such groups. In addition, the National Association of Alcoholism and Drug Abuse counselors is evidence of a professional organization whose total focus is on the training of alcoholism counseling professionals.

The major consumer group, in that it is made up of alcoholics, is Alcoholics Anonymous. AA was founded in 1935 by Bill Wilson and Dr. Bob Smith. Since its origins in Akron, Ohio, AA has spread across the globe. AA has helped millions of men and women achieve sobriety. There are thousands of daily meetings in every locale in the United States. AA meetings in any area can be found by looking up Alcoholics Anonymous in the telephone book, calling the number, and asking where the meetings are for the day. For nonalcoholics some of the meetings are designated "open" meetings. Some persons do not like the emphasis on spirituality in AA. Rational Recovery was started in the early 1980s; there is an emphasis on personal empowerment without a spiritual component. Religion has also played an important part in recovery for many people. Persons should be encouraged to explore that aspect of their life if they feel it can help.

Government at all levels is an important partner in providing treatment and rehabilitation services to alcoholics. State and federal governments fund alcoholism programs. Through the grant process they fund research into every aspect of alcoholism and its treatment, from basic science to staff training. Each state has a division of alcoholism, and the federal government funds both the National Institute of Alcohol Abuse and Alcoholism (NIAAA) and the National Institute of Drug Abuse (NIDA).

A View of the Future

Until at least the first few years of the twenty-first century the public will see progress on several fronts with regard to the treatment and rehabilitation of persons with alcohol dependence. First, research into basic science will continue to reach a further understanding into the biochemical and physiological nature of alcohol dependence, including possible genetic links of the disease. Second, prevention efforts at all levels will continue to grow; the results of prevention efforts indicate that they are working. Third, treatment programs will continue to grow, but the emphasis will be less on inpatient treatment and more on partial hospitalization and outpatient programming. Finally, the self-help movement, as exemplified by Alcoholics Anonymous, will continue to expand; it has been very successful. The disease of alcoholism may never be eradicated, but with continued progress, allied health professionals will continue to have better treatment techniques and skills to help individuals with this illness.

(*See also;* DRUG REHABILITATION; ECONOMICS; MOOD DISORDERS; ORGANIC MENTAL DISORDERS; PSYCHIATRIC REHABILITATION; WELLNESS)

RESOURCES

A.A. World Services, Inc., 475 Riverside Dr., New York, NY 10163

Al-Anon Family Group Headquarters, P.O. Box 862, Midtown Station, New York, NY 10018–0862

Alcohol, Drug Abuse, and Mental Health Administration, Department of Health and Human Services, 5600 Fishers Lane, Room 6c15, Rockville, MD 20857

Hazelden Foundation, Inc., Pleasant Valley Road, P.O. Box 176, Center City, MN 55012–1076

National Association of State Alcohol and Drug Abuse Directors, 918 F St., NW, Suite 400, Washington, DC 20004

National Clearinghouse for Drug Abuse Information, Department of Health and Human Services, 5600 Fishers Lane, Room 10a53, P.O. Box 2345, Rockville, MD 20857

National Council on Alcoholism and Drug Dependence, 12 West 21st St., 7th Floor, New York, NY 10010

National Institute on Alcohol Abuse and Alcoholism, Department of Health and Human Services, P.O. Box 2345, 5600 Fishers Lane, Rockville, MD 20857

Office of National Drug Control Policy, Executive Office of the President, Washington, DC 20500

Office of Substance Abuse Prevention, P.O. Box 2345, 5600 Fishers Lane, Rockville, MD 20857

BIBLIOGRAPHY

ALCOHOLICS ANONYMOUS. *Twelve Steps and Twelve Traditions.* New York, 1953.

———. *Alcoholics Anonymous,* 3rd ed. New York, 1976.

AMERICAN PSYCHIATRIC ASSOCIATION. *Diagnostic and Statistical Manual of Mental Disorders,* 4th ed., rev. Washington, DC, 1994.

BEATTIE, MELODY. *Codependent No More.* Center City, MN, 1987.

CAPUZZI, DAVE, and GROSS, DOUGLAS R. *Youth at Risk: A Resource for Counselors, Teachers, and Parents.* Alexandria, VA, 1989.

DUPONT, ROBERT L., ed. *Stopping Alcohol and Other Drug Use Before It Starts: The Future of Prevention.* Rockville, MD, 1989.

EVANS, GLEN; O'BRIEN, ROBERT; and CHAFETZ, MORRIS. *The Encyclopedia of Alcoholism,* 2nd ed. New York, 1991.

FILSTEAD, WILLIAM J.; ROSSI, JEAN J.; and KELLER, MARK. *Alcohol and Alcohol Problems: New Thinking and New Directions.* Cambridge, MA, 1976.

LUDWIG, ARNOLD M. *Understanding the Alcoholic's Mind.* New York, 1988.

U.S. DEPARTMENT OF HEALTH AND HUMAN SERVICES. *Alcohol and Health.* Rockville, MD, 1990.

JOSEPH F. STANO

ALLIED HEALTH PROFESSIONS

Occupational therapists, physical therapists, speech and language pathologists and audiologists, and rehabilitation counselors make up the core of rehabilitation professionals from allied health fields. Although more than 100 disciplines are recognized by the U.S. Bureau of Health Professions, these four activities are traditionally recognized as the most prominent in rehabilitation. These professions share a common goal of prevention of injury or disease and the restoration of function or the prevention of progressively increasing dysfunction. The breadth of knowledge and skill of these professionals makes them ideally suited to respond to the variety of needs of individuals with disabilities. Allied health professionals contribute to the recovery of infants, young children, adolescents, adults, and elderly individuals experiencing physical, emotional, mental, genetic, or developmental conditions that might result in disability.

Participating as members of the interdisciplinary rehabilitation team, these professionals seek to assist the client in regaining or attaining physical and social skills, environmental adaptations, and economic opportunities to live and work as independently and productively as possible. Although these services may be delivered in isolation, rehabilitation professionals most frequently work collaboratively with each other and the client as a rehabilitation team. This interdisciplinary team, including the client and family, is collectively responsible for evaluation, goal-setting, service planning, assessing progress, and revising the service plan. All activities and decisions of the team are patient-focused and depend, to whatever extent possible, on the patient's acceptance of responsibility for his or her own program. Allied health professionals in rehabilitation base their services on theories of normal development over the life span, the dynamic interaction of biological and environmental systems, full inclusion of individuals with disabilities in society, and the integration of clinical and scientific knowledge. The rehabilitation process evolves in consultation with the client's family and physician who may also be supported by psychologists, social workers, respiratory therapists, or recreation therapists.

Each discipline represented on the rehabilitation team provides both overlapping and unique contributions to the rehabilitation process. This promotes cooperation and collaboration, continuity of service, and multiple perspectives on the same problem to assist the individual in meeting his or her rehabilitation needs. All four disciplines are concerned about the functional abilities of the individual, with the goal of returning him or her to an independent and productive lifestyle.

Occupational therapy is grounded in the notion of "curing by doing" (Hopke, 1990). The occupational therapist evaluates the individual's ability to perform routine activities at home, at work, and for recreation. The occupational therapist then helps that individual relearn routine activities or finds new ways to accomplish an activity. For example, an individual who has lost the use of an arm may need to learn how to dress, eat, drive, and play tennis with one hand. Occupational therapists are especially interested in using purposeful activity and occupation, with or without assistive devices, as a way of rehabilitating the individual. Even though its inception was in the psychiatric field, occupational therapy has developed an equally important role in rehabilitation of individuals with physical disabilities. Therapists in this field are especially adept at evaluating and treating problems associated with sensory loss or dysfunction.

Physical therapists are also concerned with returning the individual to his or her level of function before disease or injury. The physical therapist, however, is more likely to view functional activity as an outcome or goal of therapy than as a mechanism for treatment. Physical therapists attempt to identify components of movement that are interfering with successful and productive movement and to remediate the problem as a means to improve function. All functional movement is dependent on a dynamic interaction of variables, including posture, balance, muscle strength, endurance, coordination, joint mobility, flexibility, pain, and heart and lung function. The physical therapist evaluates each of these components of movement in the context of the environment in which the individual is asked to perform and considers the impact of modification in each of the components on function. Assistive devices, including crutches, walkers, artificial limbs, and electrical stimulation devices, may be used to compensate for the loss of a component or ability or to facilitate the reeducation of lost abilities. Heat, cold, ultrasound, electrical stimulation, and other physical agents may be used as adjuncts to movement techniques and exercise to reduce pain and promote tissue healing.

Rehabilitation counselors use counseling, planning, and case management expertise to assist individuals with disabilities to regain their best level of autonomy, independence in living, and return to purposeful activity. They assist their clients in solving life problems and in training for and locating work that is suitable to their physical and mental abilities, interests, and aptitudes. Rehabilitation counselors identify barriers to medical, psychological, personal, social, and vocational adjustment. They determine the extent of disability and, with the individual, develop a plan of services to overcome handicaps to employment or independent living. Services may include counseling to assist individuals and their families with emotional and psychological adjustment to disability, academic or vocational training, vocational counseling, job analysis, job modification, or reasonable accommodation and job placement.

Speech and language pathologists are essential for the rehabilitation of persons with developmental handicaps, genetic disorders, cerebral palsy or other neuromotor disorders, severe head injuries, stroke, or physical impairments such as cleft lip or palate. Speech and language pathologists and audiologists are concerned about the recovery or compensation for loss of the ability to articulate words, organize language, and understand and communicate language. They treat problems of articulation and problems of information processing and language acquisition and understanding. Speech and language pathologists assist individuals in learning or regaining communication skills, as well as compensating by using communication strategies such as sign language and computerized voice output communication devices. Audiologists are concerned with identifying and rehabilitating persons with hearing disorders; this may include the prescription of assistive hearing devices. Because speech and hearing are so closely interrelated, a therapist competent in one must have a familiarity with the other to determine if the individual's difficulties are associated with the inability to hear or the inability to understand and speak, or both.

Professionals in the disciplines of allied health require highly technical training and considerable skill in problem-solving and interpersonal relations. Professional education for these disciplines typically is at the master's level, and graduates must pass a national examination to meet requirements for state licensure or certification. Some of these professions are supported by licensed assistants with two-year degrees who are specifically trained to assist in the rehabilitation process.

(*See also:* ART THERAPY; ASSISTIVE TECHNOLOGY; AUDIOLOGY; DANCE/MOVEMENT THERAPY; MASSAGE THERAPY; MUSIC THERAPY; NURSING, REHABILITATION; OCCUPATIONAL THERAPY; PHYSICAL THERAPY; RECREATION; REHABILITATION COUNSELING; SPECIAL EDUCATION)

RESOURCES

American Occupational Therapy Association, 1383 Piccard Drive, P.O. Box 1725, Rockville, MD 20849–1725

American Physical Therapy Association, 1111 North Fairfax Street, Alexandria, VA 22314–1488

American Speech/Language and Hearing Association, 10801 Rockville Pike, Rockville, MD 20852–32879

BIBLIOGRAPHY

FAHERTY, KATHLEEN. *North Carolina Health Careers '92.* Chapel Hill, NC, 1992.

HOPKE, WILLIAM E. *The Encyclopedia of Careers and Vocational Guidance,* Vol. 2. Chicago, 1990.

DARLENE K. SEKERAK
DAVID E. YODER

ALZHEIMER'S DISEASE

Alzheimer's disease (AD) was first described in 1906 as a progressive dementing disorder associated neuropathologically with senile plaques and neurofibrillary tangles that lead to loss of mental functions and functional abilities. More than seventy conditions cause dementia (Blass, 1982; Katzman, 1986). AD is the most prevalent form of dementia, accounting for approximately 50 to 60 percent of diagnosed cases. AD is commonly found in the elderly population, but it has been diagnosed in people as young as thirty years old. Many times a distinction is made between presenile dementia of the Alzheimer's type (onset before age sixty-five) and senile dementia of the Alzheimer's type (onset after age sixty-five), even though they do not differ pathologically. Epidemiologically, AD is described as a unitary disorder regardless of age of onset.

Etiology

The severity of symptoms exhibited by a person with AD is closely related to the extent of lesions to the brain. Under microscopic examination, the brain of an individual with AD has an increased number and abnormal distribution of senile plaques and neurofibrillary tangles throughout the cerebral cortex, granulovacuolar degenerations (mostly confined to the hippocampus and subiculum), and a reduction in the number of cortical neurons. Neurochemically, AD specifically affects the cholinergic neurotransmitters in the brain. The cholinergic system (which produces acetylcholine) is involved in the brain's capacity to learn and remember (Drachman & Leavitt, 1974).

There are a number of theories set forth to explain the cause of AD, including environmental factors, genetic factors, and immunologic factors. Environmental factors that have been associated with onset of AD include head trauma, exposure to heavy metals (such as aluminum, manganese, and silicon), and viruses or other infectious agents. There is growing genetic evidence that chromosomes 14 and 21 are linked to early-onset AD, and a normal cholesterol-carrying protein produced by a gene on chromosome 19 (apolipoprotein E or APOE) has been strongly associated with late-onset AD. Because AD is associated with neuritic plaques (concentrated in the hippocampus and neocortex of the brain) and neurofibrillary tangles (often found in the neocortex, hippocampus, substantia innominata, hypothalamus, and brainstem reticular formation), defects in the immune system have been suspected as a possible etiology. Defects in the immune system may be an independent cause of AD, or may interact with other proposed causative agents (i.e., toxins, infections, or genetic factors). Despite exciting breakthroughs, research aimed at identifying a single cause of AD has led to incomplete explanations. This may be because Alzheimer's disease is really a final common pathway for disorders with several etiologies.

Characteristics

People afflicted with AD experience a decline in intellectual capacity, including memory, language, the ability to conceptualize and perform tasks, mood, concentration, cooperation, as well as thought processes, perceptions, and reasoning. Memory losses are progressive and affect both recent and remote memory. Language and ability to speak deteriorate; early word-finding difficulties eventually progress to loss of all meaningful verbal abilities. Mood changes may be characterized by emotional instability or by blunted and/or exaggerated emotional responses. Expressions of anxiety, fear, sadness, and anger are seen in many people with AD. These mood changes have been related to both physiologic responses in the brain as well as to the reactions to the disease process (Cohen, Kennedy, and Eisdorfer, 1984).

A four-stage model provides a useful framework for describing the progressive decline in functioning associated with AD (Reisberg, 1983). These stages include the forgetful phase, the confused phase, the dementia phase, and the end phase. Persons with dementia progress through these phases (stages) at different rates. Highly learned skills are generally retained as the disease progresses (e.g., a homemaker may retain the ability to cook long into the disease).

The forgetful phase is characterized by subjective cognitive deficits that do not interfere with daily functioning. In the first phase, mood changes are usually anxiety and/or depression, and the cognitive loss is forgetfulness. Persons are often aware of their forgetfulness and are able to compensate for it by using reminder lists, calendars, etc.

The confused phase is characterized by more severe impairments in functioning. In this phase, individuals tend to experience profound recent memory deficits, are increasingly disoriented to their surroundings, and may not be able to concentrate. Language deficits may appear; word recall becomes noticeably impaired. The individual demonstrates increasing difficulty with money management, legal decisions, transportation, home maintenance, meal preparation, and housekeeping.

The dementia phase is characterized by severe cognitive deficits. The individual begins to withdraw from family and friends, stress-related behaviors are common (e.g., insomnia, pacing, wandering, confusion, and agitation), communication becomes more difficult, the ability to reason and to recognize others becomes impaired, and the individual is unable to plan for safety. Eventually the individual becomes totally dependent on a caregiver, needing help with activities of daily living such as eating, bathing, dressing, and toileting. It is most often during this phase that families are forced to consider nursing home placement of the person with AD.

In the end, or terminal phase of AD, the individual is no longer able to walk and has little purposeful activity. Recognition of the environment or other individuals is generally lost, although the person may experience moments of lucidity. Eventually the afflicted individual forgets how to eat, chew, and swallow, which leads to malnutrition and weight loss. Problems associated with immobility, such as skin breakdown, urinary tract infections, muscle contractures, and pneumonia are common in the end phase of AD. As the individual becomes increasingly vegetative, death follows, usually from pneumonia or other complications of the disorder.

The progression of AD varies, with length of onset from diagnosis to death from one to twenty years (average, eight to ten years). The loss of cognitive functioning is variable and unpredictable. Death results from the physical deterioration that accompanies the profound cognitive changes, not from the brain pathology itself.

Diagnosis

Microscopic examination of the brain is necessary to differentiate AD from other types of dementias precisely. The insidious onset, slow progression, and clinical features of AD do not distinguish it from dementia due to many other causes (e.g., Pick's disease, multi-infarct dementia, and Parkinson's disease). The diagnosis of AD can be made with better than 85 percent accuracy by conducting a thorough family history as well as psychological, physical, and neurological examinations. Occasionally, high-technology scans such as MRI, CAT, and SPECT will be used to help distinguish Alzheimer's disease from dementia due to other causes. However, examination of brain tissue at death is the only means confirming a diagnosis of AD.

Impact of Alzheimer's Disease on the Individual, Family, and Society

The effects of AD are felt throughout the health care and social service delivery systems of the United States. While AD is not an inevitable consequence of aging, the prevalence of AD increases dramatically with each decade of life after age sixty-five. As society as a whole ages, AD and the associated burden of care that is placed on families and society at large have emerged as important health care issues. The human and financial costs of AD are devastating. The economic cost of AD is difficult to gauge precisely, as the indirect costs (e.g., lost productivity incurred by family caregivers) are indisputably great. AD devastates the lives of spouses and family members, who must watch the mental deterioration of a loved one while carrying the burden of care over a prolonged time. As the prevalence of AD continues to increase (AD is projected to affect more than 5 million Americans by the year 2040), and the cost of caring for an afflicted individual soars, there is increased recognition of the need for both science policy and public policy to respond to long-term needs of both afflicted persons and their caregivers (U.S. Department of Health and Human Services, 1991). The unpredictable and changing needs of AD patients and their families place a burden on the already fragmented social support and health care networks at the community level. Without a coherent and well-funded national long-term-care policy, AD threatens to overwhelm the disjointed collection of public and private mechanisms that attempt to provide and pay for health care delivery to older and chronically disabled persons in our society.

Prevention and Treatment of Alzheimer's Disease

Specialized training programs must be provided for the wide variety of care providers required throughout the continuum of care for a person with AD.

Since there is no single known cause or cure for AD, treatment strategies are aimed at maximizing remaining brain function and preventing excess disability in the affected person. It is postulated that persons with AD have diminished ability to tolerate both internal and external stressors, such as television, caffeine, pain, and fatigue. Stress is believed to produce excess disability, which can be controlled by interventions (Hall & Buckwalter, 1987).

Medication management may be indicated for the treatment of cognitive and affective (mood) symptoms that are distressing to the affected person. Judicious use of psychotropic medication may be needed for symptomatic relief of anxiety, insomnia, and/or anorexia associated with depression, delusions, or hallucinations. Many times, medications used to treat the distressing symptoms at one stage in the disease process will no longer be of therapeutic benefit in subsequent stages. Therefore it is recommended that psychotropic medications be periodically discontinued so that their therapeutic benefit may be reevaluated.

Brief psychotherapy can be beneficial for the management of cognitive and affective symptoms associated with early AD. Psychotherapy fosters the use of adaptive coping skills and completing the developmental tasks of the older adult. Although persons with AD are not candidates for insight-oriented psychotherapy, they often can benefit from supportive and solution-focused techniques that are used to modify stress-producing behaviors, promote ventilation of feelings, and reinforce use of adaptive coping strategies. In addition, family members can often benefit from individual, group, and/or family therapy aimed at helping them understand and cope with the enormous emotional, physical, and financial burdens associated with caregiving.

Environmental manipulation is one of the most effective treatment strategies for the management of behavioral problems associated with AD. Activities should be modified based on the individual's stress response. A predictable routine is of paramount importance for the person who experiences increasing memory deficits. The daily routine should be simplified and adhered to whenever possible. Scheduled rest periods, elimination of caffeine, and breaking up daily activities into small steps can be very helpful in modifying stress.

In the early stages, the person with AD may use memory aids (e.g., calendars, lists, signs, and pictures) to help cope with memory loss. Socialization activities and levels of stimulation may need modification. It is important to evaluate continuously the affected person's response to environmental noise and large group activities (church, shopping, and family gatherings), and to remove the individual from these settings or activities when signs of stress are evident. As the disease progresses and the person is less able to communicate, nonverbal communication such as use of gestures and signs is more heavily relied on. Comfort, distraction, and removal of noxious stimuli are helpful when the person with AD experiences false sensations or beliefs (e.g., hallucinations or delusions). It is important to avoid arguing with such individuals, since their perceptions, no matter how bizarre, are real to them, and their ability to reason logically is usually diminished.

In the end stage of AD, palliative care is needed. Complications of immobility (e.g., muscle contractures and decubitus ulcers) must be prevented whenever possible. For example, frequent repositioning and range-of-motion exercises are essential to avoid complications for the person who no longer moves voluntarily. It also may be necessary to puree food and stroke the individual's neck to stimulate the swallowing response when he or she is no longer able to swallow.

All interventions must be systematically evaluated to determine effectiveness when caring for a person who has AD. Desired outcomes are measured primarily by the affected person's behavioral responses. There are no "cookbook" treatment strategies for this disease; rather, each intervention must be modified based on individual behavioral responses on a twenty-four-hour continuum and over an unpredictable and changing clinical course. It is important to remember that abilities will vary from one day to the next in persons with AD. They may remember how to eat with utensils on one day and forget how to do so the next. A decreased incidence of stress-related behaviors (wandering, pacing, aggression, refusal to participate, and inappropriate social behaviors) is one important indication that treatment strategies are successful. Health care providers are well advised to solicit the input of knowledgeable family members

on an ongoing basis regarding the effectiveness of various medical and nonmedical approaches.

Professional Care of Individuals with Alzheimer's Disease

The family or primary caregivers are the foundation for planning care for a person with AD. The more caregivers learn about the disease and its management, the better able they are to provide quality care and to enter into the complex and dynamic care planning process.

Care of the person with AD is multidisciplinary and involves both formal and informal providers. AD is a highly complex disease with a variety of behavioral manifestations that require expertise from several disciplines (neurologists, nurses, social workers, physicians, activity therapists, physical therapists, occupational therapists, and rehabilitation therapists). The treatment team involved in the care of individuals with AD intervenes to maintain personal integrity, promote desired social and environmental conditions, and to assist individuals to function optimally in both home and institutional environments. To do this, care planning must consider various ways to sustain the strengths of the affected person, not only as an individual but also in relationship to family and community/institutional settings.

When a person with AD is asked to carry out even a relatively simple task, such as eating, the care provider must be willing to demonstrate and supervise the task. Oftentimes the person with AD forgets the appropriate use of items, and "cues" must frequently be given, such as showing the person that a toothbrush is to be used in the mouth rather than on the hair. Thus repeated cuing and demonstrations, one step or one command at a time, can help to diminish inappropriate task performance and maintain the demented individual's level of self-esteem.

Rehabilitation planning should consider various ways to sustain the cognitive and functional levels of a person who has AD by maximizing opportunities to use remaining strengths (e.g., laying out clothes for the person who can no longer decide appropriate clothing), supporting rather than challenging remaining functions (e.g., not asking the person to achieve beyond his or her abilities), and anticipating future problems and designing interventions to prevent or ameliorate them (e.g., removing the distributor cap from the car when the person with AD insists on driving and it is no longer safe for him or her to do so). Many times assistive devices such as large-handled spoons or cups will enable the person with AD to continue to eat independently. Similarly, provision of clothing with Velcro fasteners, rather than tiny buttons, will promote the individual's ability to accomplish activities of daily living such as dressing and toileting.

Health care professionals must also continuously assess the environment for cues that may be misleading and potentially dangerous for persons with both cognitive and perceptual impairments. For example, light glare off highly polished floors may resemble pools of water over which the person with AD may try to jump. Hallways, bathrooms, and other high-traffic areas should also be assessed for excessive clutter that the person with AD may trip over. Unending spaces that invite visually cued wanderers to "pace" continuously should be broken up with chairs or culturally appropriate artwork and other wall decorations that command their attention and interest. Alzheimer's disease and many other degenerative neurological disorders are often accompanied by gait changes that impair ambulation and that lead to falls, hip fracture, and other adverse outcomes. Therefore it is essential that therapists evaluate the need of persons with AD to use assistive ambulation devices such as walkers or quad canes, in an ongoing effort to prevent falls, especially in a population prone to wandering and elopement from safe environments. In addition, occupational, rehabilitation, activity and physical therapists should consult with formal and informal caregivers regarding environmental simplification, use of assistive devices, and effective alternatives to restraints.

Given the wide range of challenges associated with providing care to a person with AD, special efforts are needed to develop information and referral services, coordinate care, and to offer personal and professional support to informal caregivers. Health, social service, case management, respite, foster care, and nutritional and transportation services differ considerably from one locale to another and may not even be available in some rural set-

tings. Moreover, even when services are available, they may be means-tested (accessible only to those of certain income range) or age-tested (available only to persons under or over a particular age). The local Alzheimer's Disease and Related Disorders Association chapter is a general screening agency for determining which local services can best meet the needs of AD victims and their families. If no local chapter has been established, see the Resources section for organizations that provide information related to specific services offered nationwide.

(*See also:* AGING; CAREGIVING; FAMILY; LOSS AND GRIEF; ORGANIC MENTAL SYNDROMES; QUALITY OF LIFE; RESPITE CARE)

RESOURCES

Alzheimer's Association, 919 North Michigan Ave., Suite 1000, Chicago, IL 60611

American Association of Retired Persons, 1909 K St., NW, Washington, DC 20049

Children of Aging Parents (CAPS), 2761 Trenton Rd, Levittown, PA 19056

National Association of Area Agencies on Aging, 600 Maryland Ave., SW, S. 208, Washington, DC 20024

National Association for Home Care, 519 C St., NE, Stanton Park, Washington, DC 20002

The National Council on the Aging, Inc., P.O. Box 7227, Ben Franklin Station, Washington, DC 20044

BIBLIOGRAPHY

BLASS, JOHN P. "Dementia." *Medical Clinics of North America* 66 (1982):1143–1160.

COHEN, DONNA; KENNEDY, JOHN G.; and EISDORFER, CARL. "Phases of Change in the Patient with Alzheimer's Dementia: A Conceptual Dimension for Defining Health Care Management." *Journal of American Geriatric Society* 32 (1984):11–15.

DRACHMAN, DAVID A., and LEAVITT, JANET. "Human Memory and the Cholinergic System: Relation to Aging." *Archives of Neurology* 30 (1974):113–121.

HALL, GERI R., and BUCKWALTER, KATHLEEN C. "Progressively Lowered Stress Threshold: A Conceptual Model for Case of Adults with Alzheimer's Disease." *Archives of Psychiatric Nursing* 6 (1987):399–406.

KATZMAN, ROBERT. "Alzheimer's Disease." *New England Journal of Medicine* 314 (1986):964–973.

REISBERG, BARRY. *Alzheimer's Disease: The Standard Reference.* New York, 1983.

U.S. DEPARTMENT OF HEALTH AND HUMAN SERVICES. *Third Report of the Advisory Panel on Alzheimer's Disease.* Washington, DC, 1991.

LINDA GARAND
KATHLEEN C. BUCKWALTER

AMERICANS WITH DISABILITIES ACT

The Americans with Disabilities Act (ADA) is landmark civil rights legislation. Signed into law on July 26, 1990, the ADA prohibits discrimination against people with disabilities in virtually every aspect of society—from employment, to telecommunications, to movie theaters, to banks, to subways. It marks a revolutionary turning point in public policy for people with disabilities—away from the role of the federal government as caretaker for people with disabilities through the provision of special programs and services, and toward the federal government as empowerer of people with disabilities, supporting and facilitating the exercising of individual rights and full participation in the mainstream of societal life. The ADA calls for the re-creation of society over time, so that all aspects of public life are accessible to and inclusive of people with disabilities—mental, physical, and sensory.

Philosophy of the ADA

Historically, people with disabilities have been physically segregated and socially isolated from the mainstream of society. They have routinely experienced discrimination and purposeful unequal treatment based on stereotypic assumptions that do not reflect their abilities to participate in and contribute to society. The results have been significant social, vocational, economic, and educational disadvantages and political powerlessness. The ADA acknowledges that it is not so much the disability per se that makes life difficult for a person with a disability, but rather the way society responds to that individual.

The ADA seeks to change the status of people with disabilities by requiring a more enlightened attitude toward them. It rejects the long-standing and outmoded view of people with disabilities as helpless and pitiful and the primary role of the government as a charitable one—to take care of them through provision of special programs and services. The ADA affirms the view of people with disabilities as full citizens who rightfully assert their claims to equal access and full participation, and the role of the government as one of facilitating and supporting such assertions.

The ADA affirms that disability is a natural part of the human experience. It rejects the notion that disability is somehow an experience separate and different from the experience of being human. The ADA is often described as the emancipation proclamation for people with disabilities, comparable in significance to the Civil Rights Act of 1964 for African Americans.

Legislative Roots of the ADA

The notion of providing comprehensive civil rights protection for people with disabilities through federal legislation emerged soon after the enactment of the Civil Rights Act of 1964, which prohibits discrimination on the basis of race, color, religion, or national origin. The 1977 White House Conference on Handicapped Individuals called for the inclusion of people with disabilities in the Civil Rights Act of 1964. In the 1970s and the 1980s a number of amendments were introduced in Congress to do just that; however, none of them received serious consideration (Burgdorf, 1990).

While no comprehensive antidiscrimination legislation was enacted until the ADA in 1990, numerous federal laws were passed that covered various aspects of nondiscrimination. These served as the policy and political building blocks for the ADA. They include the following:

- The Architectural Barriers Act of 1968 mandated that all buildings constructed, altered, or financed by the federal government after 1969 be accessible to and usable by persons with physical disabilities.
- Sections 501, 503, and 504 of the Rehabilitation Act of 1973 prohibit discrimination in any

program or activity receiving federal funds, in executive agencies and the U.S. Postal Service, and require affirmative-action plans for hiring and advancement of people with disabilities in the federal government and by contractors with the federal government. Section 504 was the major building block for the ADA. It was amended in 1988, along with other civil rights statutes, by the Civil Rights Restoration Act. A provision in the amendment clarified that people with HIV and AIDS were protected by Section 504. This became a key policy clarification when questions about HIV and AIDS emerged during the debate over the ADA. The disability community gained important lobbying skills and toned its political muscles on this legislation in preparation for the ADA (West, 1992).

- The Education for All Handicapped Children Act of 1975, renamed in 1990 the Individuals with Disabilities Education Act, entitles all children with disabilities to a free appropriate public education, to take place in an integrated setting to the maximum extent appropriate.
- The Developmental Disabilities Assistance and Bill of Rights Act of 1975 authorizes state developmental disabilities councils to coordinate and fund services for people with significant long-term disabilities. Enacted largely in response to substandard and abusive situations in institutions for people with mental retardation, the legislation includes a bill of rights for people with developmental disabilities. The act also authorizes protection and advocacy systems in every state, intended to advocate for the rights of people with disabilities and provide them with legal representation.
- The Voting Accessibility for the Elderly and Handicapped Act, enacted in 1984, requires registration and polling places for federal elections to be accessible to people with disabilities.
- The Air Carrier Access Act of 1986 prohibits discrimination by air carriers against people with disabilities.
- The Fair Housing Act Amendments of 1988 added people with disabilities as a group protected from discrimination in housing. This was the first extension of antidiscrimination cover-

age into the private sector, thus setting a precedent for the ADA.

The Critical Role of Advocacy

The ADA was generated by advocacy from the disability community—both those within government and those outside government. The law is a crowning achievement for the independent-living movement and the disability rights philosophy—both of which are at the heart of advocacy in the disability community. The independent-living movement finds its modern roots in the early 1970s in California, when a number of individuals with disabilities came together with the unifying belief that people with disabilities themselves can find the solutions to their problems. The movement has since grown considerably, so that there are now federally supported independent living centers throughout the country (Heumann, 1993). National disability rights leaders from both major political parties find their roots in this movement. For example, Judith Heumann, who was one of the early organizers of the Berkeley, California, Center for Independent Living and who is often considered the mother of independent living, was a lead spokesperson for the ADA and was appointed by President Clinton in 1993 as assistant secretary for the Office of Special Education and Rehabilitative Programs in the U.S. Department of Education. Lex Frieden, the executive director of the National Council on Disability under President Reagan when the ADA was initially drafted, was a founder of Independent Living Research Utilization in Texas.

One of the goals of the independent living movement has been for people with disabilities to establish control over their own lives. One way this has been accomplished is through the establishment of organizations that are controlled and run by people with disabilities. Many of these organizations were at the forefront during the development of the ADA, such as the Disability Rights Education and Defense Fund and the World Institute on Disability.

After two decades of limited progress with limited civil rights protection, disability rights leaders concluded that comprehensive federal protection was needed. Without such protection the message of total equality would not be transmitted. Justin Dart, who is often called the father of the disability rights movement, led the way in transforming a fragmented community into a united, powerful grassroots lobby.

Legislative History of the ADA

The ADA was initially proposed and drafted by a small, independent federal agency, the National Council on Disability (NCD) (then the National Council on the Handicapped), which was comprised of individuals appointed by President Reagan and confirmed by the U.S. Senate. Members of the Council are people with disabilities, family members of people with disabilities, or professionals working with people with disabilities. Under the leadership of Sandra Parrino, NCD chair; Justin Dart, NCD vice chair; Lex Frieden, NCD executive director; and Robert Burgdorf, civil rights attorney, the ADA became the flagship recommendation in a 1986 landmark report to the President and Congress, *Toward Independence*.

The legislation was first introduced in April 1988 by then senator Lowell Weicker, ranking member and former chair of the Senate Subcommittee on Disability Policy. A key reason for introduction at that time was to gain support from both parties during an election year and build congressional support. Both goals were accomplished, as several members of Congress signed on as cosponsors and both presidential candidates endorsed the concept of the legislation. Congress adjourned at the end of 1988 without legislative action on the bill.

During this period advocates worked all over the country to build support for the ADA. Justin Dart visited each state four to twenty times, meeting with individuals in groups of three to six thousand to promote the ADA. He developed a network of more than a thousand disability community leaders and generated thousands of messages to members of Congress. He chaired the ADA-focused Congressional Task Force on the Rights and Empowerment of Americans with Disabilities, presiding over a total of sixty-three public forums in every state.

Disability leaders worked with leaders in the business community, Congress, and the Administration to draft an improved bill for introduction in the 101st Congress. Bob Silverstein, staff director of the Sub-

committee on Disability Policy, played a central role in drafting this legislation, which was introduced by Senator Tom Harkin, chair of the subcommittee, in 1989. Congressman Tony Coehlo introduced the legislation in the House of Representatives.

Disability interest groups in Washington, DC, were actively organizing and developing legislative strategy to ensure enactment of the legislation within the 101st Congress (1989–1990). Organized under the umbrella of the Consortium for Citizens with Disabilities (CCD), the interest groups had grown to number more than a hundred. Led by veteran advocate Pat Wright of the Disability Rights Education and Defense Fund, the CCD met one to three times a week to develop legislative strategies and examine negotiations. CCD chair Paul Marchand of the Association for Retarded Citizens and activist Liz Savage of the Epilepsy Foundation of America worked tirelessly to mobilize grassroots networks across the country to send Congress messages about the need for the ADA.

Dialogue and advocacy—especially through the efforts of presidential counsel Boyden Gray and Equal Employment Opportunity Commission chair and disability rights attorney Evan Kemp—led to the August 1989 endorsement of the Senate version of the ADA by President Bush. After months of inspired negotiation led by Senators Harkin, Kennedy, Hatch, and Dole; by Representatives Hoyer, Bartlett, Mineta, Brooks, and others; by Bob Silverstein and other congressional staffers; and, of course, by Pat Wright, the ADA was passed by Congress on July 13, 1990. The final votes in support of the ADA were overwhelming: 377–28 in the House and 91–6 in the Senate. However, this was misleading, as there was considerable opposition by some powerful organizations, including the National Federation of Independent Business and the U.S. Chamber of Commerce.

There were a number of efforts to weaken the ADA during the legislative process, including exempting people with mental illness and AIDS from protection. The disability community determined that amendments of this nature would legalize discrimination for generations to come and that the ADA would be withdrawn before such amendments would be accepted. Advocates were firm in their conviction that the law had to declare the unequivocal equality of people with disabilities.

This view prevailed, and on July 26, 1990, President Bush signed the ADA into law. More than three thousand members of the disability community gathered on the South Lawn of the White House for this event. "Let the shameful wall of exclusion finally come tumbling down," President Bush said as he signed the bill into law.

Legal Requirements of the ADA

The legal requirements of the antidiscrimination mandate of the ADA are drawn from two sources. The substantive requirements are based on Section 504 of the Rehabilitation Act of 1973. The procedural requirements are drawn from Title VII of the Civil Rights Act of 1964.

Antidiscrimination. The overarching substantive requirement of the ADA is the prohibition of discrimination. Antidiscrimination requirements for people with disabilities may be considered to have two central aspects. The first, which is shared by other minority groups and women, is that of not being treated in a prejudicial manner because of an individual, and often immutable, characteristic that has no bearing on the individual's skills or capabilities. For example, being an African American has no bearing on an individual's ability to be a physician. In this situation, the intention of the antidiscrimination mandate is to ensure that the characteristic in question is not used to limit or foreclose opportunities or individual choices.

The second aspect of antidiscrimination requires paying particular attention to the individual characteristic (e.g., race, sex, age, or religion) to use the interaction between the individual and society to ameliorate or end the limitation or exclusion to equal access. This second aspect of antidiscrimination applies when the societal structure prevents equal access. If the disability per se limits equal access, the antidiscrimination mandate will likely not apply. For example, an individual who is blind would not likely be qualified to drive a bus no matter what societal barriers are removed. The inherent lack of vision likely prevents the act of driving. This distinction must be considered with caution, however. Technology and creativity have enabled people with disabilities to perform in ways that were previously thought impossible. For example, with the help of computers, people who are blind can read, and people who lack speech can talk. Limited thinking about the capacities of people with disabilities has resulted in significant restraint on their achievements and exclusion of their participation. The goal of the ADA is to eliminate such thinking and the resultant limitation it yields (Feldblum, 1993; West, 1991a). However, an individual who uses a wheelchair may be qualified to be an attorney if law schools are architecturally accessible, dorm rooms are built to accommodate wheelchairs, accessible transportation to law school is available, the bar exam is offered in an accessible location, and law firms do not discriminate in hiring and are in accessible locations.

This second aspect of antidiscrimination, which requires paying particular attention to the characteristic in question, is especially important for people with disabilities, but is also relevant for other minority groups. While it requires the provision of accommodations and the removal of structural barriers for people with disabilities, it also requires employers to allow people of different religions to practice their faiths by having religious holidays from work that may not be the traditional holidays. This second aspect of antidiscrimination may require what has been called "legitimate permanent differential treatment necessary to achieve and maintain equal access" (Longmore, 1987, p. 363).

In terms of the first aspect of antidiscrimination, the traditional prohibition applies. People with disabilities may not be excluded or otherwise discriminated against on the basis of their disability. In terms of the second aspect of discrimination, the covered entity assumes an affirmative obligation to remove architectural and communication barriers; modify policies, practices, and procedures; provide reasonable accommodation in the workplace; and provide auxiliary aids and services in places of public accommodation. This requirement has been referred to as the "accommodation imperative," requiring the removal of barriers that are "any aspects of the social or physical environment that prohibit meaningful involvement by persons with disabilities" (West, 1991a). Both of these types of prohibitions are described in greater detail in the various sections of the law (see below).

Who Is Considered a Person with a Disability? The definition of who is protected by the ADA antidiscrimination mandate is a functional one. It is parallel to the definition of who is protected by Section 504 of the Rehabilitation Act of 1973. Disability is defined as "(A) a physical or mental impairment that substantially limits one or more of the major life activities of such individual; (B) a record of such an impairment; or (C) being regarded as having such an impairment."

The functional definition is a critical aspect of the ADA. A list of specific conditions, diseases, and impairments would be virtually impossible to compile and would need routine updating. The functional definition allows application of the criteria to the individual in question and encompasses new disabilities and/or illnesses when they emerge.

The Department of Justice regulations implementing the ADA further delineate what is meant by a physical or mental impairment and provide a list of examples of conditions covered. The list includes visual, speech, and hearing impairments; diseases and conditions such as cancer; diabetes; epilepsy; heart disease; emotional illness; mental retardation; emotional illness; and HIV disease, both symptomatic and nonsymptomatic.

The second aspect of the definition—a person with a record of an impairment—includes people who had an impairment or condition but who no longer have it, and people misclassified as having such an impairment. The first category would include people who have recovered from cancer or mental illness. The second category would include people who have been misclassified as having mental retardation, learning disability, or mental illness.

The third aspect of the definition—those regarded as having an impairment—covers individuals who are treated by others as if they have an impairment that substantially limits a major life activity, when that is not the case. For example, if an individual has slightly high blood pressure that does not substantially limit a major activity and an employer refuses to hire him or her for a high-pressure job, believing he or she could not manage it because of the high blood pressure, this individual would be protected by the ADA because the employer perceived him or her to be someone with a disability.

Employment. The ADA prohibits employers from discriminating against qualified people with disabilities in hiring, firing, promotions, recruitment, and any conditions of employment. The employer may not limit, segregate, or classify applicants or employees on the basis of disability in a way that adversely affects the opportunities or status of the individual. Employers must provide reasonable accommodations to the known physical or mental limitations of an applicant or employee unless the provision or such accommodation would impose an undue burden. Reasonable accommodations include making modifications to the physical layout of a job facility, restructuring a job, establishing a part-time or modified work schedule, reassigning to a vacant job, acquiring equipment or devices, and providing readers and interpreters for people with vision and hearing impairments. A "qualified" applicant or employee is one who meets the skill, experience, education, and other job-related requirements and who can perform essential functions of the job with or without reasonable accommodation. An undue burden is a significant difficulty or expense. The law sets forth factors to be considered in determining if a particular accommodation is an undue burden. These include the cost, the resources available to the employer, and the impact of the accommodation on the employer and the business.

Employers covered by the law were phased in over time. As of July 26, 1994, all of the phase-ins were complete. At that time employers with fifteen or more employees were covered by the ADA.

The remedies available under Title VII of the Civil Rights Act of 1964 are also available under the Employment Title of the ADA. The Equal Employment Opportunity Commission (EEOC) provides administrative enforcement of the act, and when those remedies are exhausted, there is a right to sue in federal court for injunctive and monetary relief in the form of back pay. Compensatory and punitive damages can be awarded, subject to monetary ceilings that are determined by the number of employees of the employer.

State and Local Government. Otherwise qualified people with disabilities must have meaningful access to programs, services, and activities of nonfederal governmental agencies. Government activities such as meetings of state legislatures, town meetings, meetings of school boards, and licensure and registration activities must be accessible. Administration of benefits programs such as social services must be conducted in an accessible, nondiscriminatory manner.

Programs provided by governmental entities must be accessible to people with disabilities in the most integrated setting appropriate to the needs of the individual. While separate programs can be provided to individuals with disabilities, individuals with disabilities cannot be required to participate in such programs and cannot be denied participation in the generic program (e.g., a recreation program). If auxiliary aids and services are needed by the individual with a disability to participate, the governmental entity must provide them. Examples of auxiliary aids and services include provision of assistive listening devices for people who are hearing impaired and readers for people who are blind. If provision of such aids and services requires a fundamental alteration of the program or an undue burden, such provision is required only to the point where it becomes a fundamental alteration or undue burden.

Architectural access to existing government buildings is required when program access without architectural modifications cannot be achieved. New construction and alterations must be readily accessible to and usable by people with disabilities. Technical standards for accessibility, known as Uniform Federal Accessibility Standards (UFAS) and Americans with Disabilities Act Accessibility Guidelines (ADAAG), must be followed.

Employees of nonfederal governmental entities are covered by the employment provisions of the ADA.

Enforcement remedies under Section 505 of the Rehabilitation Act apply to state and local government requirements. These include damages and injunctive relief. The Department of Justice (DOJ) enforces these provisions of the law.

Transportation.   Discrimination is prohibited in the provision of both publicly and privately funded transportation. All newly purchased public buses must have lifts and be accessible to people with disabilities. Retrofitting is not required. Supplementary paratransit services must be provided to individuals who, because of the significance of their disabilities, are unable to use accessible fixed-route public transpoation systems. If provision of paratransit ser-

vices becomes an undue burden, it must be provided only to the undue burden level.

All new rail vehicles and stations must be accessible. Existing rail systems had to have one accessible car per train by 1995. Key rail stations had to be accessible by 1993. Time limit extensions of up to thirty years are available from the Department of Transportation (DOT) if extraordinarily expensive structural changes are required.

Van services, hotel shuttle buses, taxis, limousines, and other private transportation systems are also covered by various antidiscrimination provisions of the ADA.

The DOT administers the transportation requirements of the ADA.

Public Accommodations.   Public accommodations includes the broad range of private entities that affect commerce, such as banks, restaurants, doctors' offices, hotels, zoos, stadiums, stores, and educational institutions. This section of the act has been described as the most expansive section of the law (Parmet, 1993), extending the antidiscrimination mandate fully into the private sector. Virtually all businesses are covered by the ADA, no matter how small.

The ADA prohibits the use of eligibility criteria that screen out or tend to screen out individuals with disabilities unless such criteria are necessary for the operation of the business. For example, it would be a violation of the ADA for a dry cleaner to have a policy refusing to serve deaf people. In addition, reasonable modifications to policies, practices, and procedures are required unless such modifications would fundamentally alter the nature of the business. For example, a store might be required to modify a "no pets" rule to allow guide dogs to accompany people who are blind.

Architectural and communications barriers must be removed if such removal is "readily achievable," meaning accomplishable without much difficulty or expense. An example would be placing a portable ramp over one step at the entrance to a bank.

Businesses are required to provide auxiliary aids and services to persons with disabilities as long as such provision is not an undue burden on the business. Provision of these auxiliary aids and services is a flexible requirement, with the goal being effective participation. For example, a doctor's office might be required to provide an interpreter for a patient who is deaf. However, communicating through writing notes may well suffice.

All new construction and alterations must be accessible.

The DOJ enforces the public accommodations title of the ADA. Enforcement remedies available include private suits, injunctive relief, attorneys' fees, and court costs. The attorney general only may seek monetary damages and civil penalties in pattern or practice cases or suits.

Telecommunications. Telephone relay services must be provided in every state and nationwide. Relay services enable persons who are deaf, hard of hearing, or speech-impaired to use nonvoice telecommunications devices and a communications assistant to relay messages to a speaking person over the telephone. Thus speaking and nonspeaking persons can communicate in an effective and timely manner. This provision seeks to end the isolation experienced by many deaf or hard-of-hearing persons who were often unable to use the telephone because of its inaccessibility. It is administered by the Federal Communications Commission (FCC).

Early Implementation of the ADA

The DOJ is the lead agency in implementing and enforcing the ADA. In addition to its enforcement responsibilities, the DOJ coordinates efforts of other federal agencies involved in implementation and enforcement.

The four key government agencies with ADA responsibilities (DOJ, EEOC, FCC, and DOT) issued implementing regulations for the ADA shortly after the law's enactment. In the early 1990s the EEOC and the DOJ funded technical assistance efforts to facilitate implementation, including a contract to the Disability Rights Education and Defense Fund to train people with disabilities about their rights under the law. The National Institute on Disability and Rehabilitation Research (NIDRR), a division of the U.S. Department of Education, has established ADA technical assistance centers in each region of the country. Private foundations, under the leadership of the Dole Foundation in Washington, DC, have established the Funding Partnership for People with Disabilities, which has pooled resources

of more than fifteen foundations to support projects that promote implementation of the law.

(*See also*: ACCESSIBILITY; ADVOCACY; AFFIRMATIVE ACTION; ARCHITECTURAL ACCESSIBILITY; CIVIL RIGHTS; CONSUMERS; DISABILITY LAW AND SOCIAL POLICY; HISTORY OF REHABILITATION; INDEPENDENT LIVING; REASONABLE ACCOMMODATION; TRANSPORTATION ACCESSIBILITY)

RESOURCES

ADA Materials Development Project Relating to Employment, Cornell University, 106 ILR Extension, Ithaca, NY 14853–3901

Disability Rights Education and Defense Fund, 2212 Sixth St., Berkeley, CA 94710

National Council on Disability, 1331 F St., NW, Suite 1050, Washington, DC 20004–1107

World Institute on Disability (WID), 510 16th St., Suite 100, Oakland, CA 94612

BIBLIOGRAPHY

BURGDORF, ROBERT L. "History." *The Americans with Disabilities Act: A Practical and Legal Guide to Impact, Enforcement, and Compliance.* Washington, DC, 1990.

DART, JUSTIN. "ADA. Landmark Declaration of Equality." In *Worklife: A Special Issue*, ed. Dick Dietl. Washington, DC, 1990.

———. "Introduction: The ADA: A Promise to Be Kept." In *Implementing the Americans with Disabilities Act: Rights and Responsibilities of All Americans*, eds. Larry Gostin and Henry Beyer. Baltimore, 1993.

FELDBLUM, CHAI. "Antidiscrimination Requirements of the ADA." In *Implementing the Americans with Disabilities Act: Rights and Responsibilities of All Americans*, eds. Larry Gostin and Henry Beyer. Baltimore, 1993.

GOSTIN, LARRY, and BEYER, HENRY, eds. *Implementing the Americans with Disabilities Act: Rights and Responsibilities of All Americans.* Baltimore, MD, 1993.

HEUMANN, JUDITH. "Building Our Own Boats." In *Implementing the Americans with Disabilities Act: Rights and Responsibilities of All Americans*, eds. Larry Gostin and Henry Beyer. Baltimore, 1993.

LONGMORE, PAUL K. "Uncovering the Hidden History of People with Disabilities." *Reviews in American History*, Sept. 1987.

NATIONAL COUNCIL ON THE HANDICAPPED. *Toward Independence.* Washington, DC, 1986.

PARMET, WENDY E. "Title III Public Accommodations." In *Implementing the ADA: Rights and Responsibilities of All Americans,* eds. Larry Gostin and Henry Beyer. Baltimore, 1993.

PRESIDENT'S COMMITTEE ON EMPLOYMENT OF PEOPLE WITH DISABILITIES. *Worklife ADA Special Issue.* Washington, DC, 1990.

Temple Law Review. The Americans with Disabilities Act Symposium: A View from the Inside. Philadelphia, 1991.

WEST, JANE. "The Social and Policy Context." In *The Americans with Disabilities Act: From Policy to Practice,* ed. Jane West. New York, 1991a.

———. *Moving Toward the Mainstream: Disability Rights Policy and Politics in the 100th Congress.* Washington, DC, 1992.

———, ed. *The Americans with Disabilities Act: From Policy to Practice.* New York, 1991b.

JUSTIN DART
JANE WEST

AMPUTATION

Of the approximately 50,000 amputations that are done each year in the United States (Staats, 1985), some 85 percent are of the lower extremity, and the great majority of these are the result of vascular deficiency (Medhat, 1983). Most of the persons with lower-extremity amputations have diabetes, with small artery occlusion. Large-vessel blockage secondary to arteriosclerosis is another major cause of amputations of the lower limbs. Most upper-extremity amputations are the result of accidents, if, indeed, injuries caused by shell fragments or bullets can be considered accidental. Other causes will be discussed below.

Classification of the types of upper- and lower-limb amputation is most often related to the length of the residual limb (stump). The terms "stump" and "residual limb" will be used interchangeably. The amputation level is a major factor defining basic prosthetic components. Variants within each component category should be selected by a knowledgeable clinic team, comprised, at the minimum, of a surgeon, a prosthetist, and a physical therapist. The team must consider the person's vocational needs, avocation, and the environment in which the prosthesis will have to function, as well as the person's physiological age, the purpose for which the pros-

thesis will be used, and, not least, the patient's wishes.

Types of Amputation

The following classification is a simplified version and, within each gross level of amputation, prosthetic requirements will vary with the length of the residual limb, as, for example, in the cases of the below-knee and above-knee prostheses; and, in the case of the partial foot amputation, the portion of the foot retained will dictate the prosthetic components.

Lower-Limb Amputations

1. Partial foot
2. Total foot (Syme)
3. Below-knee
4. Knee disarticulation
5. Above-knee
6. Hip disarticulation
7. Hemipelvectomy
8. Transcorporectomy (through the lower trunk)
9. Multiple limbs

Upper-Limb Amputations

1. Partial hand
2. Total hand
3. Wrist disarticulation
4. Below-elbow
5. Elbow disarticulation
6. Above-elbow
7. Shoulder
8. Shoulder girdle
9. Multiple limbs

Etiology of Amputations

The causes of amputation are, in most instances, trauma, disease, or genetic abnormality. In the physiologically elderly group, diabetic neurovascular disease and arteriosclerosis are the most prominent factors leading to lower-extremity gangrene and amputation. Younger, more physiologically active individuals will most often sustain amputations as a result of trauma, such as industrial or farm accidents, or from war-incurred wounds due to shell fragments, antipersonnel mines, booby traps, or bullets.

In the very young, amputation may occasionally be the result of elective surgery advised to rehabilitate children with genetically caused abnormalities, some of which were secondarily induced by the mother's ingestion of drugs such as thalidomide in the past (Jentschura, Marquardt, & Rudel, 1967). When a limb cannot be reconstructed to become functionally useful, partial amputation may be indicated, as for example, for unilateral lower-limb hypertrophy. Extreme care must be taken to avoid amputating functioning elements as in many cases of phocomelia (foreshortened upper extremities).

At any age amputation may result from infection such as uncontrolled osteomyelitis or gas gangrene, malignancy, frostbite, or even snakebite.

Children have been unfortunate victims of lawn mower accidents with partial loss of a foot, or even loss of a lower limb.

Prevention

Prevention of amputation of vascularly impaired lower limbs with major artery blockage is based on surgical bypass revacularization. Appropriate attention to the care of the feet is extremely important (Lee et al., 1988), particularly for the person with diabetes for whom bypass surgery may not be clinically feasible because the problem in such cases is usually small vessel occlusion, although both types of vascular deficiency, of varying degree, may be present.

Absence of sensation may also be found in the feet of persons with diabetes as a consequence of nerve involvement frequently associated with this disease. The feet must be visually inspected frequently for areas of irritation and potential breakdown of the skin. Sources of irritation must be removed. One must not wait until blisters have formed; simple reddening is an adequate warning sign. Individuals who have this problem must be especially careful to inspect the feet several times a day, cleanse the feet daily, and dry them thoroughly.

Foot callosities should be treated by a podiatrist on a regular basis. Dense callosities may cause subcutaneous trauma, hemorrhage, tissue breakdown, infection, and eventually osteomyelitis, leading to amputation.

Treatment and Rehabilitation

When an amputation is elective, there is an opportunity to help the person requiring amputation to face the impact of the severe, emotionally depressing effect of the anticipated loss of a limb. Under ideal circumstances socially and occupationally adjusted persons with amputations should be invited to the patient's bedside to counsel the patient and demonstrate that the person's world will not end with limb ablation. An example of an organization of rehabilitated persons who have had amputations and who are prepared to provide such counsel is Chapter 76 of the Disabled American Veterans, National Amputation Foundation (Kaminsky, 1992).

Besides emotional preparation, physical therapy of a person with below-knee or higher-level amputation should be instituted, aimed particularly at improvement of the abdominal and contralateral extremity musculature as well as that of the other uninvolved extremities. The need to avoid deformities caused by habitually maintaining a comfortable position, such as a bent knee, is important.

Immediate fitting, popular in recent years, has been superseded to a large degree by postop fitting with a cast, and delayed ambulation. Both immediate fitting and rigid postop casting of a residual limb will decrease hospital time. It is essential that the surgeon make every effort to save the knee and provide the patient with a below-knee amputation where possible (Rubin, 1972a). A physiologically elderly person with an above-knee amputation and cardiac or pulmonary impairment may not be capable of ambulation, whereas such a person with a below-knee amputation is very likely to walk (McCullough et al., 1971).

When a person with a lower-limb amputation has been rehabilitated to the extent of being able to stand and make forward progress with parallel bars solely on the intact extremity, the prosthetist should fabricate a temporary prosthesis. A permanent prosthesis is indicated when adequate stump shrinkage has occurred. This will take about six weeks to three months in most instances and is a matter of clinic team judgment. When the residual limb shrinks sufficiently under the influence of nightly bandaging with an elastic bandage, such as an Ace bandage, and daily use of a temporary prosthesis, a permanent prosthesis may be prescribed.

Prescription of Prosthesis

Prior to prescription, cardiopulmonary clearance from an internist, particularly for a person in poor physical condition (physiologically elderly), is advisable. Clearance is most important for the person with an above-knee amputation, who must expend a great deal of energy while walking. The energy expenditure experienced by the person with the unilateral above-knee amputation walking on level ground, at the same speed as a person without such an amputation, has been reported to be from 25 percent (McCullough et al, 1971) to 100 percent greater (Gordon, 1958) than that of a person with both limbs intact.

Lower-Limb Amputation

1. Partial Foot Amputation. There is disagreement about the functional usefulness of short partial-foot amputations. When such amputations can be done to avoid deformity of the stump and achieve weight-bearing on the heel pad, ambulation may be anticipated.

Posterior foot amputations (hind-foot amputations) are best fitted with the patellar-tendon-bearing (PTB) orthosis (Rubin, 1972b). This will partially unweight the heel by accepting weight-bearing in a socket resembling that of the below-knee prosthesis (see below).

2. Syme Amputation. When the Syme amputation has been meticulously performed it provides the person with a lower-limb amputation with an excellent stump capable of accepting partial weight-bearing within a Syme prosthesis (Harris, 1961). Incorrectly designed Syme stumps (Rubin, 1981) make fitting with a prosthesis difficult; and if the heel pad has shifted or is hypermobile, the tolerance of the stump for weight-bearing is limited.

3. Below-Knee Amputation. It is extremely important that every effort be made to save the knee (Rubin, 1972a). Almost all persons with below-knee amputations can be rehabilitated, whereas most above-knee amputation patients who are physiologically in poor physical condition, regardless of age, will not be able to become independent ambulators.

There is essentially no controversy about the below-knee prosthetic prescription. Most patients with below-knee amputations are prescribed a total-contact PTB (patellar-tendon-bearing) prosthesis with soft socket insert, supracondylar suspension, endoskeletal or exoskeletal shank, and an energy-storing foot.

4. Through-Knee Amputation. This is a partially end-bearing amputation, utilizing a socket that provides supracondylar suspension, a four-bar linkage knee, and an energy-storing foot. Depending on the activity of the individual, a swing-phase hydraulic element (see below) may be added to the four-bar linkage knee component. The four-bar linkage has the advantage of ease of swing, stability, and cosmesis because it does not extend the limb during sitting: The knee component folds behind the knee.

A variant of this is the bent-knee prosthesis, which is designed to accommodate a below-knee amputation stump that cannot be straightened out.

5. Above-Knee Amputation. When the internal medicine specialist has provided clearance of cardiopulmonary adequacy, a prosthesis should be prescribed. The pre-World War II plug fit socket has been replaced by the two-socket designs currently in use.

6. Hip Disarticulation Amputation. The Canadian hip disarticulation prosthesis is universally accepted. A low-resistance, fluid-controlled knee will provide a more physiologic function than a single-axis, alignment-stabilized knee. Weight support is on the ischial tuberosity.

7. Hemipelvectomy Amputation. A bucket socket is required to encompass the soft tissues of the trunk. The components are those of the Canadian hip disarticulation prosthesis. A certain amount of pistoning on walking is unavoidable in the absence of bone support because the socket is fabricated around the soft tissues of the trunk. For the knee component a low-resistance, fluid-controlled knee is the first choice, and, with appropriate alignment stabilization, a single axis knee, the second choice. Elderly persons are unlikely to ambulate with either a hip disarticulation or hemipelvectomy prosthesis.

8. Transcorporectomy. When this procedure is indicated, the entire pelvis and lower limbs are removed, almost always because of a malignancy. The patient is fitted with a body socket of plastic laminate mounted on a platform that allows the patient to be erect in a modified wheelchair with seat sufficiently lowered so that the wheel rims can be reached and manipulated. Cosmetic artificial limbs are usually refused by the patients.

9. Multiple-Limb Amputation. Each limb is individually fitted in accordance with established principles. The elderly bilateral person with an AK (above knee) amputation is unlikely to walk and should be prepared to accept a wheelchair.

Upper Extremity Amputation

1. Partial Hand Amputation. In the absence of a thumb, it is most important to restore opposition, and a rigid thumbpost that has no sensation may be fabricated but is rarely worthwhile. Cosmetic fingers and gloves may also be used when appearance rather than function is of prime importance for individuals in direct public relations. Surgically, transportation of the index to the thumb position, or first-toe transplantations, have both been successful. It is important to retain sensation if possible, and these surgical procedures do so. The choice is the patient's.

2. Total Hand Amputation. If wrist function is retained, a functional prosthesis such as that designed by Gustav Rubin employs a useful concept (Rubin, 1972c). An artificial hand with fingers is provided, with linkage to the wrist stump, and powered by the wrist in such manner that dorsiflexion of the wrist stump achieves opposition of the fingers (index and middle) to the thumb, and volarflexion opens the hand—that is, separates the fingers.

3. Wrist Disarticulation. A forearm socket of plastic laminate designed to accommodate the broad distal stump of the wrist disarticulation uses a thin wrist fitting to avoid length discrepancy when the hook or hand terminal device is attached. The terminal device may be manipulated by a shoulder harness and cable system or myoelectric components.

4. Below-Elbow Amputation. Here again there is a choice between myoelectric and cable control via a shoulder harness. The patient's occupation and avocation as well as the patient's wishes should be factors in making a choice; for example, a farmer, who would not only be a hard user but also might live in an isolated area far from a prosthetic shop, should not be provided with a delicate myoelectric mechanism.

The socket will usually be of a double-wall configuration, with the inner wall conforming to the stump and the outer serving to restore limb length and provide cosmesis (Sears, 1991). Terminal devices are various but basically of a hook or hand type. Functional electric hands and electric hooks are available. Functional or cosmetic terminal devices may also be selected for cable-driven prostheses. Since the artificial hook or hand has no sensation, and since no *acceptable* method of transferring sensation has been developed, visual clues are needed. The hook is less bulky than the hand, and such clues are more readily visible when the hook is used.

The Krukenberg procedure splits the forearm into a two-pronged fork useful for the patient with visual impairment with bilateral upper limb amputation, who is thereby provided with sensory feedback in the absence of visual clues. This operation separates the radius and ulna but retains the pronator teres muscle to provide a pinch function, enabling the person with this type of operation to hold objects between the radius and the ulna and to feel such objects.

5. Elbow Disarticulation. Since there is no socket space for a prosthetic elbow, this level requires outside rigid joints at the elbow. The hook or hand terminal device is controlled by a shoulder harness and dual control cable. The dual control accomplishes elbow flexion, elbow locking, and terminal device operation utilizing shoulder and stump motion to pull the cable.

6. Above-Elbow Amputation. The socket of plastic laminate is suspended from the shoulder harness (Figures 1 and 2). A turntable elbow permitting manual rotation is used as well as the dual control system.

An excellent electrical system is a hybrid, using a Boston electric elbow and a cable-controlled hand. An even more sophisticated, although very expensive, system is the Utah arm, which employs myoelectric signals to operate both the elbow and the terminal device. Forearm rotation capability may also be added.

7. Shoulder Disarticulation. Excursion amplifiers such as levers or pulleys can be used within the cable systems to increase power and operate the elbow and terminal devices, but these are rarely acceptable for long-term function since they are inadequate. Myoelectric controls or hybrid systems are more practical for this level of amputation. When myoelectric controls are not possible, switch electric controls may be used: A small pull on a switch incorporated in the harness will operate the device. The switch is employed when the muscle contraction does not transmit sufficient microvoltage to the skin surface to operate the unit myoelectrically.

8. Shoulder Girdle Amputation. Some switch-controlled electrical components can provide function, but it is the author's impression that persons with this amputation are best served, if unilateral

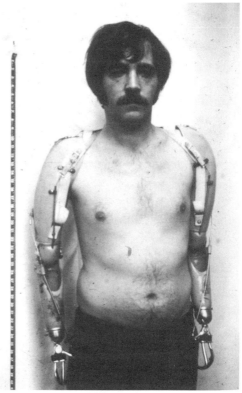

Figure 2. Patient with bilateral above-elbow amputation fitted with "conventional," i.e., body-powered (shoulder and stump movement) cable controls. (Photo courtesy of Gustav Rubin)

and if the opposite extremity functions well, by providing them with a cosmetic plastic laminate shoulder cap to fill out their clothes.

Additional Aspects of Rehabilitation

Muscle power of the stump, the contralateral limb, and the trunk should be developed. Where possible, a preoperative exercise program should be instituted and the support of friends and family enlisted. The patient, when in bed, should never put pillows behind the stump. Flexion contractures, deformities due to soft tissue, may develop. For the same reason, the patient should spend at least four hours of twenty-four lying prone, and should avoid spending long periods in a wheelchair with knee and hip flexed.

A temporary limb or a cast should be applied as early as feasible postop, even before the incision is

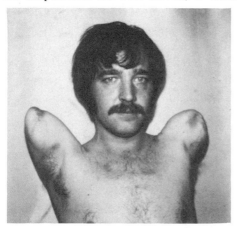

Figure 1. Bilateral above-elbow amputee. (Photo courtesy of Gustav Rubin)

healed, but weight-bearing should be delayed for the vascularly impaired person with an amputation until healing has occurred. The popularity of immediate fitting has waned in recent years. An experienced team must be constantly available if immediate fitting is employed. A loose socket must be replaced without delay.

As shrinking and stump maturation progress, the socket will become loose, and additional stump socks will be necessary to provide a more adequate fit. When fifteen ply of stump socks have been added, a new socket will be needed, since that amount of padding of the stump will eliminate the possibility of conformity of the stump with the socket.

Touchdown on the prosthetic foot should be taught in such a manner that only thirty to thirty-five pounds of weight are initially applied. A bathroom scale may be used to estimate weight pressure, or a weight-sensitive device may be incorporated in the endoskeletal unit. Walking is limited at first and will gradually be increased by the therapist, followed by progression from a walker, to crutches, to a cane. The achievement of ambulation without any support should be rapid for the below-knee amputee.

The above-knee amputee should follow similar procedures, but progress will be slower. Parallel bars are necessary in the beginning stages. The physiologically able person with bilateral lower extremity amputation will usually start the rehabilitation process on the tilt table and proceed to parallel bars, a walker, crutches, and hopefully a cane. Persons with amputation must be taught a technique of falling and arising after falling.

Most persons with bilateral-lower-limb amputations will, at times, be wheelchair-dependent, and transfer techniques should be taught. The wheelchair must have removable armrests, enabling the patient to use a transfer board. The doorways of the home should be wide enough for a wheelchair, and the hallways adequate for turnaround. Handrails can be strategically placed in the bath and toilet areas. A shower chair is useful, and ramps must be installed where possible to access the outside.

Appropriate gait must be taught, particularly in the case of the patient with above-knee amputation, using sophisticated knee components such as the Swing-N-Stance (SNS) Mauch knee, which is a hydraulic unit with special stance phase stability char-

acteristics as well as a swing phase (Kegel & Byers, 1977).

Once the person with an amputation has been taught to walk stairs and curbs, he or she will be ready for the outside world. All of these functions should be accomplished under physical therapy supervision. Later the patient can be taught to drive a car with appropriate modifications for the level of amputation.

Rehabilitation of the person with an upper limb amputation requires strengthening of the other limbs and the abdominal muscles, as well as specific training in the use of a prosthesis. The therapist should have a set of wood blocks of various configurations, and the patient should be taught to manipulate them, then taught to hold a telephone, use a filing system type if necessary, and also to drive an automobile with the proper accessories.

Most persons with amputations can be provided with prostheses that will enable them to participate in sports such as swimming, skiing, fishing, and golf. Prostheses may be modified to allow them to participate in almost all avocations (Figures 3 and 4).

Although children fall into a different category, methods are not too different. Fitting should be accomplished as early as the crawling stage for the patient with below-knee amputation and as soon as the child with an above-knee amputation can stand on his or her intact limb with assistance. The knee of the AK prosthesis should be locked until the child demonstrates balance and security before teaching the AK prosthesis user a heel-and-toe gait on a single-axis knee.

An upper-extremity padded terminal device with grasp capability may be provided for the infant to aid in teaching the sensation of grasp; when the child reaches about one year (Sauter, 1972), a functional prosthesis with a conventional child-size hook terminal device should be fitted. It is important to teach the child independent personal care such as dressing, body hygiene, and toileting (Jentschura et al., 1967).

Children require frequent adjustments to accommodate for growth, and endoskeletal modular systems will simplify this problem. In a thorough discussion of the treatment and prosthetic fitting of the child with an amputation, emphasis is placed on

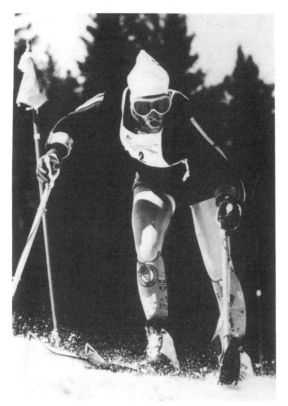

Figure 3. Most persons with amputations can be provided with prostheses that enable them to practice sports such as skiing. (Photo courtesy of the Veterans Administration)

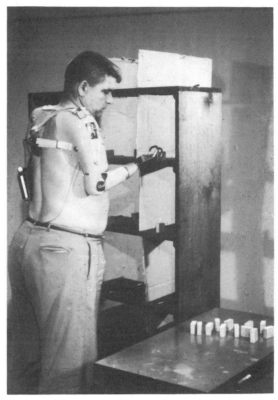

Figure 4. Prostheses can be designed to allow patients to participate in almost all avocations. Here, a patient with bilateral shoulder disarticulation was fitted with electrically controlled artificial limbs. (Photo courtesy of the Veterans Administration)

the need for early fitting and the speed with which children learn to use their prostheses (Jentschura, Marquardt, & Rudel, 1967). Physical therapy and occupational therapy, are, in the case of children as well as adults, primarily directed at generalized muscle development and teaching the use of the prosthesis as well as other means of coping with absence of the limb.

For the child with an amputation, balance must be taught, and the child must learn to sit, manage stairs, fall, and arise after falling. A trunk harness attached to a walker will help to teach balance. G. Jentschur et al., (1967) advise therapists to teach children with high bilateral amputations to use their feet and toes to do things that cannot be done with upper-limb prostheses.

The child with high bilateral upper-limb amputations can, as is the case with the adult as well, benefit from fitting with an electric elbow and body-powered terminal device.

Future Developments

A final report has been submitted for a computer-aided socket design and computer-aided manufacture of a below-knee socket (Houston et al., 1992). The usefulness of this system will await wide future application. If this approach is found to be worthwhile, socket techniques for other levels of amputation will be anticipated.

A hydraulic ankle and a hydraulic hip unit will eventually reach the consumer (Rubin & Wilson, 1981) but has not to date.

Direct skeletal attachment of a prosthesis is still awaiting successful application—even at this writing—for long-term use (Peizer, 1983). An untethered, ambulatory, vertical trunk support system will aid in unweighting individuals who have borderline ambulation capability. This would be useful as an interim training device.

Persistent research into the etiology and effective treatment of phantom pain and phantom sensation should yield results in the near future. Recent research suggests that phantom sensation has a central rather than a peripheral origin; investigation into the treatment of phantom pain continues but has not yet been resolved.

Upper-limb sensory feedback systems, including the use of transducers and implanted nerve stimulators, have not yet reached a clinically useful stage of development. Research continues but a practical application remains elusive.

(See also: CHILDREN; PEDIATRIC REHABILITATION; PHYSICAL THERAPY; PROSTHETICS AND ORTHOTICS; PSYCHOSOCIAL ADJUSTMENT; SURGERY; WHEELCHAIRS)

RESOURCES

Child Amputee Prosthetics Project (CAPP), 3160 Geneva St., Los Angeles, CA 90020

Institute for Rehabilitation Medicine, New York University Medical Center, 550 First Ave., New York, NY 10016

International Center for the Disabled, 340 East 24th St., New York, NY 10010

National Amputation Foundation, 73 Church St., Malverne, NY 11565

Ontario Crippled Children's Center, Toronto, Ont. M5R3B4, Canada

Prosthetics Research Center, Northwestern University, 345 E. Superior St., Chicago, IL 60611

Rehabilitation Research and Development Service, 103 South Gay St., 5th Floor, Baltimore, MD 21202-4051

U.S. Department of Veterans' Affairs, 810 Vermont Ave., Washington, DC 20420

War Amputees of Canada, National Headquarters, 2827 Riverside Dr., Ottawa, Ont. R1V0C4, Canada

World Rehabilitation Fund, Inc., 386 Park Ave. South, New York, NY 10001

BIBLIOGRAPHY

BONGARD, O., and KRAHENBUHL, B. "Predicting Amputation in Severe Ischemia." *The Journal of Bone and Joint Surgery* 70B (1988):465–467.

GORDON, E. E. "Energy Costs of Activities in Health and Disease." *Archives of Internal Medicine* 101 (1958):702–713.

HARRIS, R. I. "The History and Development of Syme's Amputation." *Artificial Limbs* 6 (1961):4–28.

HOUSTON, V. L.; BURGESS, E. M.; CHILDRESS, D.; LEHNEIS, H. R., "Automated Fabrication of Mobility Aids (AFMA): Below-Knee CASD-CAM Testing and Evaluation Program Results." *Journal of Rehabilitation Research and Development* 29 (1992): 78–124.

JENTSCHURA, G.; MARQUARDT, E.; and RUDEL, E. M. *"Malformations and Amputations of the Upper Extremity."* New York, 1967.

KAMINSKY, SOL. Personal communication, 1992.

McCULLOUGH, N. C. III; SHEA, J. D.; WARREN, W. D.; and SARMIENTO, A. "The Dysvascular Amputee: Surgery and Rehabilitation." In *Current Problems in Surgery.* Chicago, 1971.

MEDHAT, MOHAMMAD A. "Rehabilitation of Vascular Amputees." *Orthopaedic Review* XII (1983):51–52.

PEIZER, EDWARD. "Research Trends in Upper Limb Prosthetics." *Orthopaedic Review* XII (1983):219–258.

RUBIN, GUSTAV. "The Below-Knee Amputation Prosthesis." *Bulletin of the American College of Surgeons,* March, 1972a.

———. "The Patellar-Tendon-Bearing (PTB) Orthosis." *Bulletin of the Hospital for Joint Diseases* XXXIII (1972b):155–173.

———. "A Wrist-Driven Hand Prosthesis." *Bulletin of Prosthetic Research* 10 (1972c):40–46.

———. "Prosthetic Fitting Problems of the Quasi-Syme Amputation." *Clinical Orthopedics and Related Research,* October (1981):233–241.

———. "S-N-S Knees and the Bilateral A-K Amputee." *Clinical Prosthetics and Orthotics* 7 (1983): 1–2.

RUBIN, GUSTAV; COHEN, ELLEN; and RZONCA, EDWARD C. "Prostheses and Orthoses for the Foot and Ankle." In *The High-Risk Foot in Diabetes Mellitus,* ed. Robert G. Frykberg. New York, 1991.

RUBIN, GUSTAV, and WILSON, A. BENNETT. "Research Trends in Lower Limb Prosthetics." In *Atlas of Limb Prosthetics.* St. Louis, 1981.

SAUTER, WILLIAM F. "Prostheses for the Child Amputee." In *The Orthopedic Clinics of North America* 3 (1972):483–494.

SEARS, HAROLD H. "Approaches to the Prescription of Body-Powered and Myoelectric Prostheses." In *Physical Medicine and Rehabilitation Clinics of North America,* ed. Lawrence W. Friedmann. Philadelphia, 1991.

STAATS, TIMOTHY B. "Advanced Prosthetic Techniques for Below-Knee Amputation." *Orthopaedics* 8 (1985):249–258.

GUSTAV RUBIN

AMYOTROPIC LATERAL SCLEROSIS (ALS)

See NEUROLOGY; NEUROMUSCULAR DISORDERS

ANIMALS

Animals have played a significant role in the lives of people for thousands of years. They have provided us with food, shelter, clothing, transportation, protection, and entertainment. Domestication of certain species of animals provided partnerships that made those pursuits more easily attainable—and in the case of the dog, that partnership may have existed for as long as 15,000 years.

Dogs, horses, donkeys, burros, goats, and even the cat served humans in capacities that stretched the limits of animal servitude into areas of partnership and mutual dependency. With the role of the domesticated animal in human activities minimized by modern technology in the form of cars, trucks, tractors, doorbells, and sentry alarms, a subtle shift has occurred. These animals are now moving into service for individuals who are physically, emotionally, or developmentally limited.

That many of these "new" service roles existed in times past but were inadequately documented can be surmised from a review of the roles animals still serve in developing countries, which rely on methods used by their forefathers, and their fathers before.

Donkeys and burros in Nepal, India, and other Asian countries still carry those who cannot walk or wares of those who cannot lift to a vendor's street corner shop. Dogs alert individuals with hearing impairments to the presence of visitors, predators, and other unusual events. Cats sit contentedly on the laps of those with physical or mental limitations.

In Asian countries use of animals is an integral part of culture and daily life. Europeans and Americans are just now rediscovering their value. Recognizing that the versatility of animals often surpasses the capabilities of machines and other innovations, we are rapidly evolving and refining animal roles in ways that benefit people with disabilities.

Assistance Dogs

Guide Dogs. The best known of all assistance dogs, they continue a sixty-year tradition of bringing mobility to blind and visually limited persons. The primary job of guide dogs is to prevent the individual from injury by bumping into a low-hanging tree branch or unwittingly stepping off a curb. Thus these dogs are trained to think of themselves as larger than their own two-foot-high, one-foot-wide selves—to incorporate the person's bulk into their senses and guide them around all that might affect the two, as if one being. They are also taught that curbs and other uneven terrain are reasons to pause, allowing the individual with the visual limitation to adjust his or her footing accordingly. They do not, as is so often rumored, take the person here or there, unless the path is so often threaded that it is a patterned pathway. Rather, the visually limited or blind individual counts his or her steps to each locale, and is totally in charge of the dog's activities and direction.

Hearing Dogs. These dogs are formally trained to alert their deaf or hearing-impaired master to such sounds as the doorbell, the telephone ring, an alarm clock, a kitchen timer, and even a baby's cry. Often a Border Collie rescued from the pound is ideal for the job. These small dogs race from sound to person to sound again, leading their master to the sound's source in exchange for a treat or a word of thanks. Trained almost completely by incentive techniques, these usually small, enthusiastic dogs have a high sensitivity to sound, a lot of energy, and a strong drive for treats or play rewards.

Service Dogs. Working with individuals whose physical limitations are other than hearing or visual limitations, service dogs serve the broadest range of disabilities in the assistance dog field. Primary service areas include individuals with cerebral palsy, muscular dystrophy, spina bifida, paraplegia, quadriplegia, multiple sclerosis, or amputeeism. Trained to do tasks that their masters cannot manage themselves, these dogs turn lights on and off, open doors, pull wheelchairs, retrieve dropped or needed items, and wear a backpack to keep items within reach of those with hand or arm limitations. Opening a refrigerator door, retrieving a cold drink, and closing the door are not uncommon tasks for one of these highly trained canine companions. Other commands can be taught, specialized to individual needs.

Of equal importance to its work performance is the importance of the dog's role as a social icebreaker. So frequently ignored or avoided by the nondisabled public, some individuals with physical disabilities find themselves socially isolated—that is, until they get a service dog; then their social life changes. So, for that matter, does their own personal life—now partnered with a canine companion whose unconditional love accompanies them through life.

Social/Therapy Dogs. These dogs function similarly to service dogs except that there is by definition a third party who facilitates the interactions with the individual whose disability prevents him or her from being able to have or directly manage a dog. These dogs work in schools for children with disabilities, or in families with a developmentally disabled child or other family member. Such dogs may be someone's personal pet trained to go with him or her on visitations to local nursing homes, hospitals, or other institutions. Or they may have been program-trained, together with a family member, to be placed to live with and work for one specific individual. In either case, the third-party handler guides the interactions and caretakes the dog. Social dogs are primarily activity-oriented. Their involvement with patients and staff is guided by the handler's knowledge and innovation. The work of a therapy dog is generally directed by a physician or therapist who writes the dog into the treatment plan for an individual. The handler then is committed to follow that plan.

The Americans with Disabilities Act provides for public access rights for assistance dogs and their disabled partners. This regulation includes dogs and other animals specifically trained to perform tasks for the benefit of an individual with a disability and has no limitations such as certification or other forms of identification. This well may change over time if abuses or other significant problems arise, creating public safety or etiquette issues that come to the attention of legislators.

Other Assistance Animals

This category covers quite an assortment.

Monkeys. These animals are trained to serve people with quadriplegia in more refined and specific ways than the service dog is able. Individuals with spinal cord injuries that limit movement to their head and neck, and in some cases minimal movement of hands and arms, may have a monkey attendant and friend. Trained to do everyday chores such as transferring drinks or sandwiches from a refrigerator to a feeding tray, placing books on a reading stand, or putting cassettes into a VCR by following a beam of light the individual with disability directs from a mouth-operated laser pointer, these amazing simian aides work with a great degree of reliability. If and when it is necessary to correct an inappropriate monkey behavior, an aversive high-frequency sound is used. As with assistance dog users, persons with quadriplegia who have monkey helpmates find their affectionate, responsive, and entertaining ways a welcome addition to an often unstimulating environment. Social implications are also reported. People with quadriplegia who acquire a monkey aide feel that overnight they have become a minicelebrity in their neighborhood, because the monkey's presence facilitates discussion and social interaction.

Horses and Therapeutic Horseback Riding. Hippotherapy has become not only a means of entertainment for individuals with disabilities but also a viable physical and psychological therapy. Sitting astride a horse as the animal moves often stimulates those parts of the rider's body that do not function normally. For individuals with cerebral palsy or other neuromuscular disorders, an arm or a leg may feel like it requires a ton of energy to move, due to the tautness of the nerves and muscles. Yet the rhythm and stride of a horse beneath them allow for a relaxation and neuromuscular flow that may free the body of those physical counterweights. Also, the body on a horse experiences a movement not unlike that of an able-bodied walk because the horse's motions so closely resemble a person's. Thus those who cannot force their body parts to function can still get the benefits of that bodily movement, reducing potential for muscular atrophy. And certainly there is a greater incentive to ride than to sit home and exercise.

Rabbits, Llamas, Goats, Cats, Snakes, Lizards. Domesticated or nondomesticated, these animals provide social or therapeutic help to individuals who are confined, institutionalized, or in any way deprived of the companionship of animals in much the same way as the social/therapy dogs mentioned earlier. Carefully screened and trained, these animals are taken by volunteers to visit schools, hospitals, nursing homes, prisons, rehabilitation centers, and hospices to share the love and uniqueness of their special pet with others in need. Stimulated by the uniqueness or the familiarity of a visiting animal, elderly individuals who have lost a reason for communicating may resume that precious exchange. Others who hold hands and arms to themselves, reach out again. Still others cry, laugh, or both in response to the invitation to be involved in a world with love to share.

Perspectives

New and expanded roles for assistance dogs are developing at a rapid rate. A seizure-alert dog is being developed to accompany people with epilepsy and either stay nearby or bring help when a seizure is being experienced. Some dogs appear to alert their owners to the onset of a seizure, which allows that person time to position himself or herself safely prior to the seizure. For the thousands of individuals with uncontrollable epilepsy, this use of a dog could be a solution to what has been an unresolvable problem: confinement to the safety of their homes since seizures remain unpredictable.

With dogs' intense desire to be a viable part of our lives, we are limited only by the extent of our knowledge about the dog. A consortium of universities and institutes is being formed to concentrate studies on the dog and thus gain the knowledge that will open the field of dogs assisting persons with disabilities even more. We know that the dog's brain, for all its small size, has wondrous capabilities. Teaching the animal motor skills that allow the dog to open and close refrigerator doors, turn on and off light switches, and pull wheelchairs is only the tip of the iceberg. And as we add more to our knowl-

edge about teaching methods, such as trial-and-error learning, mimicking (observational learning), synchronized learning (dogs responding to the same stimuli), modeling (positioning the dog's body in different postures), reflex training (causing the dog to move based on application of a technique that causes a reflex), operant conditioning (reinforcing something the dog did), and insight learning (the broad spectrum of accumulation and application of knowledge that cannot be traced to one of the above), we will undoubtedly discover a capability that the dog has offered us were we only smart enough to recognize it. And once again we will achieve a breakthrough in the dog's ability to serve humans in general, and individuals with disabilities in particular.

Ironically, while the working role of animals in modern society has diminished in recent history, their role in the lives of people with disabilities has expanded. Social and psychological benefits have been documented in scientific studies. The versatility of these animals' movements, coupled with their intelligence and desire to cooperate, have made available solutions no machine is yet able to provide. And their genuine interest in working for and sharing with people has endeared them to us all.

(*See also:* ASSISTIVE TECHNOLOGY; BLINDNESS AND VISUAL DISORDERS; DEAFNESS AND HEARING DISORDERS; SPINAL CORD INJURY)

RESOURCES

Guide Dog Programs
Guide Dog Foundation for the Blind, Inc., 371 Jericho Turnpike, Smithtown, NY 11787
Guide Dogs of America, 13445 Glenoaks Blvd., Sylmar, CA 91342

Hearing Dog Programs
Companion Dogs for the Deaf & Hearing Impaired, 4200 E. Britton Rd, Oklahoma City, OK 73131
National Hearing Dog Center, 116 Main St., Athol, MA 01331

Service Dog Programs
Assistance Dog Institute, P.O. Box 2334, Rohnert Park, CA 94927
Assistance Dogs of America, 85 Morse Rd., Columbus, OH 43214
Independence Dogs, Inc., 146 State Line Rd, Chaddsford, PA 19317

Social/Therapy Dog Programs

Delta Society Pet Partners, 321 Burnett Ave. S., Renton, WA 98055

People Animal Linking System, 716 Channel Lane, Climax, NC 27233

Therapy Dogs, Inc., 639 33rd St., Richmond, CA 94804

Other Assistance Animals

North American Riding for the Handicapped Association, P.O. Box 33150, Denver, CO 80233

Helping Hands—Simian Aides for the Disabled, 1505 Commonwealth Ave., Boston, MA 02135

BIBLIOGRAPHY

BERGIN, BONITA. "Companion Animals for the Handicapped." In *The Loving Bond: Companion Animals in the Helping Professions*, Saratoga, CA, 1987.

COPESTAKES, VESTA. "Canine Companions." *Abilities: Canada's Journal of the Disabled*, Fall 1988, pp. 8–9.

COWLEY, GEOFFREY. "The Wisdom of Animals." *Newsweek*, May 23, 1988, pp. 52–59.

COX, LOIS M. "Born to Do." *Dog Fancy*, Sept. 1984, pp. 42–45.

CUSACK, ODEAN, and SMITH, ELAINE. *Pets and the Elderly*. New York, 1984.

FINCHER, JACK. "All You Have to Do Is Tell Them What You Want." *Smithsonian*, Jan. 1992, pp. 80–87.

HAMPTON, JANIS E. "Opening New Doors for the Handicapped." *Pure-Bred Dogs/American Kennel Gazette*, June 1983, pp. 35–38.

HART, LYNETTE; HART, BENJAMIN; and BERGIN, BONITA. "Socializing Effects of Service Dogs for People with Disabilities." *Journal of the Delta Society* 2 (1985): 64–65.

"Helping Hand." *Picture Week*, Oct. 20, 1986, pp. 30–35.

HENDERSON, BRUCE B. "A Dog for Kris." *Reader's Digest*, July 1986, pp. 127–131.

HIRSHEY, GERRI. "Retrieving Independence for the Handicapped." *Family Circle*, Feb. 14, 1984, p. 10.

"Independence Dogs." *Petsmart News*, July 1993, p. 16.

KELLEY, BARBARA BAILEY. "Teaching Dogs New Tricks." *San Francisco Examiner*, June 29, 1986, pp. 4–6.

KELMAN, JUDITH. "Safe in Mother's Arms." *Redbook*, July 1990, pp. 112–114.

MADER, BONNIE; HART, LYNETTE; and BERGIN, BONITA. "Social Acknowledgments for Children with Disabilities: Effects of Service Dogs." *Child Development* 60 (1989): 1529–1534.

MASON, JAN. "A Boy and His Dog." *Life*, Nov. 1986, pp. 51–55.

MEADOWS, GRAHAM. *Animal Friends*. Auckland, New Zealand, 1991.

MOWRY, RANDOLPH; CARNAHAN, SAMMYE; and WATSON, DOUGLAS. *A National Study on the Training, Selection and Placement of Hearing Dogs*. University of Arkansas, 1994.

"North Bay Based Assistance Animals." *North Bay Pets*, Feb. 1992, pp. 4–5.

OSIECZANEK, CINDI. *Hearing Dog Recipient Manual*. Denver, 1984.

OGDEN, PAUL. *Chelsea: The Story of a Signal Dog*. Boston, 1992.

O'NEILL, CATHERINE. "Dogs Giving a Hand." In *Dogs on Duty*. Washington, DC, 1988.

REAGAN, RONALD. "Reflections of a Self-Made American." *Success*, Nov. 1986, p. 36.

RUCKERT, JANET. *The Four Footed Therapist*. Berkeley, CA 1987.

SMITH, ELIZABETH SIMPSON. *A Service Dog Goes to School*. New York, 1988.

TONG, DAVE. "Canine Companions for Independence." *People Animals Environment: Bulletin of the Delta Society*, Fall 1985, pp. 23–24.

WARZECHA, MARY. "A Special Educator." *Dog Fancy*, Jan. 1992, pp. 24–26.

WHITE, BETTY with WATSON, THOMAS J. *Pet Love*. New York, 1983.

BONITA M. BERGIN

ANOREXIA NERVOSA

See EATING DISORDERS

ANXIETY DISORDERS

Anxiety is a universally experienced, unpleasant sensation of tension, worry, or fearful anticipation often associated with multiple somatic symptoms. For most, it occurs transiently during stressful situations that are novel, demanding, or conflictual. Anxiety syndromes that are experienced with great intensity and chronicity, and that cause impairments in occupational and interpersonal function, are considered anxiety disorders. Anxiety disorders are commonly occurring psychiatric syndromes with incidences estimated in the general population of between 5 and 20 percent. The onset of these disorders usually occurs in the late teens and early twenties, and the course of illness is either continuous or intermittent. Anxiety disorders are often associated with substance abuse, depression, occupational instability, and relationship problems.

Types of Anxiety Disorders

Individuals with panic disorder (PD) experience recurrent attacks, which are unanticipated episodes of intense fear that last for minutes or hours and are accompanied by physical symptoms such as shortness of breath, palpitations, chest pain, dizziness, shaking, and sweating, among others. PD patients describe their panic attacks as the most distressing and frightening experiences of their lives. They often believe that the attacks are a medical problem, such as a heart attack or stroke, and use medical services with great frequency. PD is diagnosed if an individual has recurrent, and unexpected panic attacks, as defined by the *Diagnostic and Statistical Manual for Mental Disorder* (*DSM-IV*). The lifetime prevalence of PD is 2 percent, while that of infrequent panic attacks may be as high as 10 percent. Individuals with panic disorder often have coexisting agoraphobia. This condition is a fear of being in situations from which escape might be difficult or embarrassing (e.g., being a passenger in a car or subway train). As a result of this fear, they avoid such situations or bear them with intense anxiety; people with extensive agoraphobia can be completely housebound.

Generalized anxiety disorder (GAD) is defined as a persistent condition of excessive anxiety with about two or more life circumstances lasting longer than six months. It is associated with physical symptoms that include fatigue, palpitations, dry mouth, dizziness, diarrhea, insomnia, edginess, irritability, and poor concentration, among others. Patients in their forties report an average of more than twenty years of symptoms and say that even after they are successfully treated, their symptoms recur once medication is stopped.

Simple phobias are conditions in which there are excessive and irrational fears of objects (e.g., animals) and situations (e.g., heights). Social phobia is a fear of humiliation in certain social situations (e.g., performing in public, using public lavatories, eating or drinking in public). Exposure to the phobic situation provokes an immediate anxiety response, and the affected person avoids these situations or endures them with intense discomfort. The prevalence rate for simple phobia is at least 7 percent, but those having it rarely receive psychiatric attention because their symptoms do not cause as widespread dysfunction as social phobia. Social phobia is more disabling than simple phobias because its victims have difficulty functioning in many important interpersonal, public, and work situations.

Obsessive-compulsive disorder (OCD) is an often chronic and debilitating condition consisting of recurrent obsessive thoughts and compulsive actions. Obsessions are intrusive ideas that the person attempts to ignore or neutralize using compulsive actions, that is, intentional behaviors performed excessively according to certain rules (e.g., hand washing, which relieves the anxiety of contamination fears). The lifetime prevalence rate is estimated at 2 to 3 percent, and patients fall into four major symptom clusters: washers, checkers, ruminators, and pathological slow-movers.

Post-traumatic stress disorder (PTSD) develops in some individuals who experience traumatic events. The traumas are considered outside the range of usual human experience, and include crime, physical or sexual abuse, natural disasters, medical stress, combat experience, and others. The traumatic event is reexperienced as daytime recollections, distressing dreams, or sudden sensations that the event is recurring (flashbacks). There is persistent avoidance of thoughts, activities, or feelings associated with the trauma. Feelings of detachment, loss of interest, and heightened arousal may develop, and this syndrome may be chronic and severe.

Treatment and Rehabilitation

Treatment and rehabilitation for those with anxiety disorders usually entails the use of both medication and psychotherapy. The initial goal is to resolve or minimize the symptoms within days or weeks of initiating treatment. In the subsequent few months, and sometimes years, the goal is to help patients overcome their phobic avoidances, restore self-esteem, minimize adverse effects from medications, and facilitate return to their previous lifestyle. Pharmacotherapy and psychotherapy should be discontinued only after a prolonged period of improved functioning.

Benzodiazepines and tricyclic antidepressants (TCAs) have anxiety-relieving and antipanic effects and have been used extensively in the treatment of anxiety disorders. However, benzodiazepines have the disadvantage of causing physiological dependence with long-term use, while tricyclics cause multiple side effects. Relatively newer serotonergic agents such as buspirone, clomipramine, and fluoxetine (and possibly sertraline and paroxetine) appear to be useful in the treatment of GAD, OCD, and PD. These are nonaddictive, unlike benzodiazepines, and have fewer side effects than TCAs. However, further studies are necessary to determine their usefulness in treating anxiety disorders. Benzodiazepines and antidepressants have been only partially effective in the treatment of PTSD.

Psychotherapeutic approaches are an important component of treatment of all anxiety disorders. For the transiently anxious patient, a supportive, problem-solving approach is usually sufficient. If anxiety symptoms are very intense, however, short-term use of benzodiazepines may be necessary. For patients with anxiety disorders, behavioral interventions such as relaxation, exposure, and desensitization techniques are effective. Recognition and reframing of cognitive distortions are helpful therapeutic techniques in the hypersensitive anxious patient. Longer-term treatments such as psychodynamically oriented psychotherapy or psychoanalysis have been found clinically useful in the case of generalized anxiety symptoms.

Aggressive treatment of anxiety disorders is essential because they can cause impairment. For example, panic disorder equals or exceeds major depressive disorder in terms of social dysfunction, marital stress, medical services utilization, financial dependence, alcohol abuse, and even suicide attempts. Unfortunately, the treatments for anxiety disorders are themselves associated with significant adverse effects, especially in elderly people or those with medical impairments.

In summary, anxiety disorders are distinct and usually chronic psychiatric conditions that can be associated with significant distress, disability, and social and occupational disability. An integrated approach, including psychotherapy and pharmacotherapy, can minimize this distress, restore self-esteem, and help the patient return to a normal lifestyle.

(*See also:* PHARMACOLOGY; PSYCHIATRIC REHABILITATION; PSYCHIATRY; PSYCHOLOGY)

RESOURCES

Anxiety Disorders Association of America, 6000 Executive Blvd., Suite 513, Rockville, MD 20852–3801 [All anxiety disorders]

Council on Anxiety Disorders, P.O. Box 17011, Winston-Salem, NC 27116 [All anxiety disorders]

Information Resources and Inquiries Branch, National Institute of Mental Health (Room 7C-02), 5600 Fishers Lane, Rockville, MD 20857 [All anxiety and other mental health disorders]

Obsessive-Compulsive Foundation, P.O. Box 70, Milford, CT 06460 [Obsessive-compulsive disorder]

National Center for Post-Traumatic Stress Disorder, Department of Veterans Affairs Medical Center, White River Junction, VT 05009 [Combat-related post-traumatic stress disorder]

BIBLIOGRAPHY

AMERICAN PSYCHIATRIC ASSOCIATION. *Diagnostic and Statistical Manual of Mental Disorders*, 4th ed., rev. Washington, DC, 1994.

FEIGHNER, JOHN P. "Impact of Anxiety Therapy on Patients' Quality of Life." *American Journal of Medicine* 82 [supplement 5a] (1987):14–19.

MARKOWITZ, JEFFREY S.; WEISSMAN, MYRNA M.; OUELETTE, ROBERT; LISH, JENNIFER D.; and KLERMAN, GERALD L. "Quality of Life in Panic Disorder." *Archives of General Psychiatry* 46 (1989):984–992.

RAPOPORT, JUDITH. *The Boy Who Couldn't Stop Washing: The Experiences and Treatment of Obsessive-Compulsive Disorder*. New York, 1989.

RICKELS, KARL, and SCHWEIZER, EDWARD E. "Current Pharmacotherapy of Anxiety and Panic." In *Psychopharmacology: The Third Generation of Progress*, ed. H.Y. Meltzer. New York, 1987.

SOLOMON, SUSAN D.; GERRITY, ELLEN T.; and MUFF, ALYSON. "Efficacy of Treatments for Posttraumatic Stress Disorder: An Empirical Review." *Journal of the American Medical Association* 268 (1992):633–638.

ZINBARG, RICHARD E.; BARLOW, DAVID H.; BROWN,

Timothy A.; and Hertz, Robert M. "Cognitive-Behavioral Approaches to the Nature and Treatment of Anxiety Disorders." *Annual Review of Psychology* 43 (1992):235–267.

Gary B. Kaplan
Mark S. Bauer

APHASIA

The term "aphasia" refers to an acquired disorder caused by damage to the brain that affects an individual's communication skills. The most common symptom of aphasia is an impairment in the ability to express oneself when speaking. Individuals who have acquired aphasia usually also have difficulty in reading, writing, and understanding speech.

Aphasia occurs when the brain centers that control communication and that generally are in the left hemisphere in most individuals are damaged. The most frequent cause of aphasia is stroke. Approximately one-third of those who have sustained severe head injuries acquire aphasia. Brain tumors can also cause aphasia.

Temporary aphasia, called *transient aphasia*, refers to a communication disorder that lasts for only a few hours or days. More than half of those who initially show symptoms of aphasia recover completely during the first few days.

The diagnosis of aphasia depends on establishing the presence of certain linguistic symptoms in an individual with a confirmed brain lesion, using standardized tests of aphasia. The degree of aphasia severity may range from mild to severe and differs from person to person with respect to impairment. When aphasia is severe, individuals may be totally unable to express themselves using speech, writing, or gesture and also may have difficulty comprehending speech and/or reading. When deficits are severe in all communication skills, the condition is referred to as global aphasia. In some instances, aphasia symptoms may be so mild that they may barely be perceptible. For example, the only apparent symptom may consist of the person having a greater than average amount of difficulty finding words in a conversation when the topic is unfamiliar.

Aphasia is sometimes described in terms of whether the primary difficulty is in the expression (speaking) or the reception (understanding) of language. The symptoms of aphasia, however, are rarely purely expressive or receptive, and it has been found to be more useful to identify types of aphasia by referring to the observed fluency of speech. Fluency refers to the "flow" of speech, the uninterrupted phrases and sentences generally used by normal speakers to communicate their thoughts and feelings. Aphasia can be designated as either fluent or nonfluent.

Nonfluent aphasia is generally characterized by an effortful, hesitant, telegraphic style of speech marked by pauses. A person with nonfluent aphasia tends to use more nouns and verbs than prepositions and articles. Speech is slow, and sentences are frequently incomplete. In severe nonfluent aphasia the individual is generally restricted to using a small single-word vocabulary. The same reduction in vocabulary and grammatical skills when speaking is usually evident in writing as well. The understanding of speech may be relatively spared in nonfluent aphasia. Individuals with nonfluent aphasia often have an associated paralysis or weakness of the right arm and leg.

Fluent aphasia is usually characterized by a normal rate of speech without the pauses and hesitations typical of nonfluent aphasia. Although the person with fluent aphasia may speak in full sentences, there is sometimes an obvious reduction in the ability to retrieve specific nouns. The person may, therefore, tend to "talk around" a point—for example, for the word "pencil" the person may say "the thing you write with," substitute a word that is similar (i.e. brother for sister), or use a nonsense word. Most individuals with fluent aphasia also have difficulty understanding speech. Unlike those with nonfluent aphasia, people with fluent aphasia do not ordinarily have weakness of the right arm and leg.

It is estimated that more than 1.5 million persons in the United States have acquired aphasia. Although aphasia is more common in persons over age fifty, it may occur in individuals of any age, gender, race, nationality, or vocation. Intelligence and education are not determining factors.

Speech-language pathologists are the professionals qualified to manage individuals with acquired aphasia. Certain speech-language pathologists have special interest and expertise in the diagnosis and treatment of aphasia. More often than not, the individual speech-language pathologist with specialized experience in aphasia works in a hospital or rehabilitation center but may also be in private practice.

The rehabilitation of aphasia is a long process in which improvement can be noted over months and years. Unfortunately, medical insurance reimbursement for aphasia treatment is generally limited to a small number of sessions over a short period. As a result, the onset of aphasia in an otherwise normal language user often has a strong negative impact on the quality of life of the individual, his or her family, and/or significant other. The degree of grief over the loss of function and the isolation experienced by the majority of people with aphasia do not always correlate with the degree of severity—that is, a mildly impaired individual may find living with aphasia more difficult than someone with severe aphasia. Depression is a common reaction to aphasia. In the same vein, there is great variability among patients with regard to their ability to circumvent their aphasia impairment. The ability to communicate in everyday situations, called functional communication, is not necessarily commensurate with task performance on language tests. Given the dependence of contemporary Western society on communication in all aspects of life, returning to employment and community reintegration are especially difficult for individuals with aphasia. As a result, many are dependent on others to carry out personal, everyday activities (e.g., banking).

The American Speech-Language-Hearing Association (ASHA), 10801 Rockville Pike, Rockville, MD 20852, tel. (301) 897–5700, is the professional association that establishes standards of clinical practice in speech-language pathology. Fully qualified speech-language pathologists have a master's degree from an accredited university graduate training program, meet ASHA's specific educational and experiential requirements, and hold the Certificate of Clinical Competence (CCC/SLP). In most states licensure is required for the practice of speech-language pathology.

(*See also*: COMMUNICATIONS DISABILITIES; HEAD INJURY; PSYCHOSOCIAL ADJUSTMENT; STROKE)

RESOURCE

The National Aphasia Association (NAA)(P.O. Box 1887, Murray Hill Station, New York, NY 10156–0611) is the only national organization dedicated exclusively to advocating for the aphasia community and developing a support group network (aphasia community groups). The NAA is also committed to increasing public awareness of aphasia by distributing informational materials, publishing a quarterly newsletter, and sponsoring the National Aphasia Awareness Week annually. The organization also maintains an 800 number (1-800-922-4NAA) and a directory of Aphasia Community Groups (ACG).

BIBLIOGRAPHY

EWING, SUSAN A., and PFALZGRAF, BETH. *Pathways: Moving Beyond Stroke and Aphasia. What Is Aphasia?* Detroit, 1990.

LAFOND, DENISE; JOANETTE, YVES; PONZIO, JACQUES; DEGIOVANI, RENÉ; and SARNO, MARTHA TAYLOR. *Living with Aphasia: Psychological Issues.* San Diego, 1993.

SARNO, JOHN E.; SARNO, MARTHA TAYLOR; and DEGRABA, THOMAS J. *Stroke: The Condition and the Patient.* New York, 1994.

MARTHA TAYLOR SARNO

ARCHITECTURAL ACCESSIBILITY

Architectural accessibility refers to the support provided by the built environment to compensate for limited functional abilities. Access to the built environment is of critical importance to an individual with a disability. Rehabilitation may help develop a certain level of function; however, an inaccessible environment can counter the effects of treatment. Moreover, through restricting action, it can cause a decline in function. Without a relatively accessible environment, it is extremely difficult, if not impossible, for many people with disabilities to live independently. Even if they can manage, an inaccessible environment limits quality of life and opportunities. Barriers, in effect, create spatial segregation, which is strongly associated with the oppression of minorities. It is no wonder, then, that achieving full access to the community is a major goal of the disability rights movement.

Key Concepts

Architectural barriers are the features of buildings that limit access and use by people with disabilities. The most obvious examples are stairs at entrances, doors that are too narrow, and bathrooms that are unusable for people confined to wheelchairs. However, there are also barriers that affect people who have other mobility impairments, low stamina, and disabilities affecting the senses, communications, and intellectual functions.

Architectural barriers limit function and independence directly. They also have a psychosocial impact. Barriers can be viewed as a message from society at large about the place of people with disabilities. They are territorial markers defining the boundaries of "the disabled world." The presence of barriers limits the opportunities of people to develop competence. Limited access to a city, for example, effectively precludes obtaining knowledge about its resources. This lack of knowledge, in turn, makes it even more difficult to use those resources. Finally, barriers can be viewed as arbitrary limitations on equal opportunity. For example, even if an individual with a disability is highly capable of performing the required skills of a job, the presence of architectural barriers precludes that individual from taking it. The building is, in effect, an agent of discrimination.

Given the serious impacts of architectural barriers, the quest to achieve a barrier-free society became an early goal of the disability rights movement. The concept of "barrier-free design" emerged in the late 1950s and early 1960s. Barrier-free design conceptualized the idea of independence in architectural terms. It means full use and access to buildings for people with a wide range of disabilities. It can be viewed as one of many strategies for overcoming the limitations of a disability, along with prosthetics and assistive technology. While the latter are also attempts to improve competence, barrier-free design is directed at a broad class of people rather than at individuals.

Designing an accessible environment for a known individual or group starts with identifying the specific abilities of the client. Then an appropriate environment is designed that fits those abilities. However, the design of buildings and products for users who are not known presents a problem. Without standardization, an individual might encounter a wide variety in the level of accessibility of various buildings. Early experience with barrier-free design demonstrated the need for establishing a generally accepted minimum level of accessibility. Eventually, detailed regulations, called "accessibility codes," evolved that define a level of accessibility intended to accommodate a broad range of people.

There is a real difference between the design of a public building or a speculative apartment building and the design of a workplace and an individual home for a person with disabilities. Workplace and home modifications are concerned with meeting specific needs of known individuals. In some cases, this may mean going far beyond the minimum requirements of accessibility codes. In other cases, not all the code issues need to be addressed since an individual has only a limited number of disabilities, not all those addressed by codes. However, the design of workplace and home modifications requires a more in-depth understanding of disability as well as a more detailed analysis of the person's interactions with the environment. They often involve the use of both assistive technology and barrier-free design. It is often hard to draw a clear boundary between the two.

By the mid-seventies there had been enough experience with barrier-free design to allow other ideas to emerge to extend the concept. In the design of housing, it became clear that a single design feature was often needed to accommodate people with a wide range of needs. For example, the choice of height to install a countertop can become a compromise between the needs of those who stand and those who sit in a wheelchair. Even among wheelchair users, there is a wide range of comfortable heights, depending on the seat height of the wheelchair, the design of the armrests, and the stature of the individual. Households often include both people with and people without disabilities. Thus, a countertop that adjusts in height was identified as a more appropriate solution than a compromise height. This concept of "adaptability" has been applied extensively in the design of housing, but it is also appropriate for other applications, such as public bathrooms or work environments. Adaptable environments also acknowledge that use of the environment changes over time. An office or apartment may be used by a person in a wheelchair for several years. The next occupant may not have any disability or may have a hearing impairment. Adaptable features accommodate differences in needs, help to avoid compromises that satisfy no one, and mitigate conflicts between the needs of different people.

Barrier-free design has been viewed primarily as design "for people with disabilities." Special provisions allow people with disabilities to gain access. Like many assistive devices, barrier-free design features are simply alternative products for people with disabilities. A new term, "universal design," is now used to refer to design for all people as opposed to special design for those with disabilities. Although this sounds like a semantic distinction, there are fundamental differences. In the case of barrier-free design one can have accessibility without equality. An entrance to a building that has a ramp around the side, or even a separate doorway, is an example. Universal design transcends code requirements. The basic idea is that accessibility and usability, defined in the broadest sense, should be a major goal of good design in general.

Universal design also embraces a concern for aesthetics. The roots of barrier-free design were in the design of health care facilities—specifically, chronic care hospitals. Thus, many products used to achieve accessibility have an appearance that is associated with such settings. For example, because they associate disability with medical problems, architects often select grab bars that look institutional and belong in a hospital. But when designing a decorative balcony railing, they will select a more attractive, less institutional product but not necessarily one that is easy to grasp. Taking the universal design perspective, both grab bar and railing would be designed for everyone to use. Aesthetics and function for everyone would be considered an integral part of the basic design problem. There would be no difference in the way each design decision was treated.

Factors Leading to Increases in Accessibility

The concept of rehabilitation and the creation of rehabilitation centers as specialized health care settings shifted the focus of medical care. The patient was no longer a passive participant in treatment; the goal now was for individuals with disabilities to achieve independence in activities of daily living. This type of medicine required a different environment. It made no sense to design a health care facility in which a patient couldn't maintain the skills learned in rehabilitation therapy sessions. It became clear that a different approach to the design of doors, bathrooms, corridors, and other features of health care facilities was necessary to support rehabilitation. Likewise, it did not make sense to invest in resources to help a person live independently and hold a job if the buildings in which those activities took place were inaccessible. Rehabilitation professionals had come to realize that general community settings must also be accessible to ensure employment and independence.

Advances in medical and rehabilitation technology after World War II, along with the development of the lightweight folding wheelchair, made it possible for paraplegics and hemiplegics to have much greater mobility in the community and use automobiles on their own. Later, the development of the electric wheelchair equipped with sophisticated control systems put mobility in the community within the reach of people with very severe limitations. We are experiencing the rapid development of microprocessor-controlled equipment, portable power systems, and sophisticated communications technology. Text telephones allow people with hearing and communication disabilities to use the telephone system with a keyboard. Environmental control units (ECUs) allow people who cannot use their hands and arms to access automated devices for operating equipment.

Soldiers disabled in World War II stood a much higher chance of surviving than had those disabled in previous military confrontations. Upon returning to the United States and undergoing rehabilitation, they found many barriers in the way of living a normal life. The GI Bill allowed veterans to return to school with government benefits. The first organized attempt to make a college campus accessible was a program at the University of Illinois in Champaign-Urbana designed to provide college education for veterans with disabilities. That university became a testing ground for the idea of accessible architecture as it sought to integrate a large number of people with disabilities into its campus population. Prior to this effort, very few people with severe disabilities had attended universities. Veterans' groups such as the Paralyzed Veterans of America launched important advocacy efforts to ensure that the country lived up to its moral responsibility to returning soldiers. This activity continued in the aftermath of the Korean War and later the Vietnam War.

In the late 1940s and early 1950s, the polio epidemic swept through the United States. Polio, like war, struck people of all economic and social classes. World War II and Korean War veterans, together with the survivors of the polio epidemic, were a large and articulate grass-roots constituency for disability rights and accessibility in particular. As these groups passed through the stages of childhood, early adulthood, and child rearing, they and their families demanded accessibility to allow them to fulfill their expectations of independence and equal opportunity.

The movement to end segregation of racial minorities was a model for disability rights activists. The concepts of front-door access, mainstreamed education, and integrated housing opportunities have direct parallels in accessible design. From the beginning of the disability rights movement, architectural barriers have been a target of activism. The symbolic impact of eliminating barriers has clearly contributed to the emphasis that the movement places on achieving accessibility. Polling places, civic buildings, recreation facilities, and the public streets have to be accessible if people with a disability are to have equal opportunity and the same quality of life that is available to the rest of the population. Making them accessible is concrete evidence that there is progress toward those goals.

The theory of normalization was developed in northern Europe as a way to improve the quality of life of people with developmental disabilities. This theory maintains that institutional environments perpetuate and reinforce perceptions of difference and devalued status of their inhabitants. Integrating people with severe disabilities into community settings and giving them the opportunity to live a life that is as culturally normative as possible will reduce difference, change perceptions, and improve their social status. Normalization as implemented in the United States led to the rapid deinstitutionalization of people with disabilities and the need to find appropriate and accessible living environments for them in the community as well as to provide them with access to general community facilities.

The changing demographics of the nation are another important factor that has led to increased public awareness of the need for architectural accessibility. Due to improved medical technology, increasing numbers of people with disabilities have survived disease, accidents, injuries from war, and genetic disorders. In addition, the extension of the life span has greatly increased the proportion of the population who have some degree of limited mobility. Armed with statistics demonstrating that at least 10 percent of the population has some limitation in a major life activity, proponents of accessibility have been able to argue successfully for their goals.

Codes and Standards

Perhaps one of the most powerful forces for improving accessibility has been the development of building standards and codes requiring it. The original accessibility standard was the American National Standards Institute's (ANSI) A117.1 (1961). This document, originally titled *Making Buildings and Facilities Accessible to the Physically Handicapped,* was intended as a voluntary standard. After its adoption, it became clear that a voluntary standard alone would not lead to large-scale removal of architectural barriers. The President's Committee for the Employment of People with Disabilities and the National Easter Seal Society, which sponsored the development of the ANSI standard, led a campaign to adopt a federal law requiring accessibility to federally funded projects. This campaign resulted in the Architectural Barriers Act of 1968. States throughout the nation developed similar laws modeled on the federal legislation. While initially these laws covered only buildings built with public funds, they soon were extended to encompass a wide range of publicly used buildings.

Although the laws were on the books, compliance

was sporadic. In response the advocacy community began to work toward more effective enforcement and more extensive coverage. Many stages established special commissions or boards who were given the responsibility of implementing the state statutes. These groups included people with disabilities themselves as representatives because building code officials at that time knew very little about accessibility.

The federal Rehabilitation Act of 1973 built on the experience of state organizations. It created the U.S. Architectural and Transportation Barriers Compliance Board and made that agency responsible for the coordination of federal efforts in the area of accessibility. Sections 503 and 504 of the act instituted the concept of "program accessibility," meaning that covered entities had to modify their facilities in order to ensure that architectural barriers would not result in discrimination. The law did not require that every building and every space be accessible, only that enough accessibility would be present to eliminate discrimination.

Other laws enacted in the 1970s, such as the Urban Mass Transportation Act and the Education for All Handicapped Children Act, extended the mandate for accessibility. The combined effect of these laws and companion state legislation was to institutionalize the concept of accessible design as part of building code compliance and public programs. Although the Architectural Barriers Act had applied only to new construction, the new laws meant that existing buildings had to be modified to meet the mandates of program accessibility, job accommodation, and mainstreamed education.

The Rehabilitation Act and the Architectural Barriers Act covered only federally assisted housing. Many of the state laws also covered state-supported housing programs. Some states extended their barrier-free design regulations to cover all multifamily rental housing. The majority of housing in the United States, however, was not covered. In 1988 the federal Fair Housing Act Amendments applied the concept of adaptable housing to all new multifamily construction, including privately owned condominiums.

The Americans with Disabilities Act of 1990 (ADA) created provisions that have approached near-universal coverage. Title I of the ADA requires reasonable accommodations in workplaces. Title II reaffirms the program accessibility concept in the Rehabilitation Act with tougher sanctions and more extensive implementation procedures. Title III of the act requires reasonable accommodations in publicly used facilities. The ADA was a major milestone because it was the first time that a federal law mandated access to existing facilities neither constructed nor operated with government funds. The ADA's provisions for existing buildings are much less stringent than those for new construction, and, in cases of undue hardship or technical nonfeasibility, accessibility can be avoided. Yet Title III is still an acknowledgment that inaccessibility amounts to discrimination that is not acceptable in American society.

Professional Roles

Architects, landscape architects, and other design professionals, such as interior designers and industrial designers, have the responsibility to ensure that the environments and products they design are usable by people with disabilities. At a minimum, all their work must comply with accessibility regulations where applicable. Some design professionals have decided to specialize in accessible design. They act as consultants to other architects or building owners and help them meet accessibility laws and regulations. They practice universal design or design home and office modifications for individuals. They also teach accessible design to professionals in training and to practitioners through continuing education programs.

There are many other professionals involved in the creation of accessible communities. Rehabilitation therapists, particularly occupational therapists, do evaluations of individual needs, recommend products, and design modifications for their clients. Because they are not qualified to design structural changes for buildings, nor are they usually knowledgeable about construction practices and aesthetics, on complex or large projects they work with professional designers in a team approach or as consultants. Rehabilitation engineers design and construct assistive technology. They are often involved in the design of home and office modifications for individual clients.

Many consumer advocates have become proficient in identifying architectural barriers and recommending solutions. Some are heavily involved in the development of improved-accessibility codes. Independent living centers (ILCs) often take a lead role in community education and advocacy activities. They complete "accessibility audits," or surveys of barriers in facilities. A few ILCs even offer home modification services. These may involve home evaluations and recommendations, design of modifications, and construction.

Local and state building code officials and other government officials are playing an increasingly active role in the accessibility field. They are becoming more knowledgeable about accessibility issues, although usually only from the standpoint of laws and regulations. Federal and state agencies now have officials who administer accessibility regulations and arrange financing for home and office modifications or large-scale building renovation programs. A comparable role in the private sector is played by facility managers, who complete accessibility audits, plan renovation programs, develop funding priorities, and identify needs in their organizations.

The Future

Deinstitutionalization has resulted in increased recognition of the many unmet needs of people with multiple disabilities, particularly those with developmental disabilities. Technology is becoming available that will allow more attention to be devoted to the needs of people with communication and respiratory disabilities, among others. Disability policy is putting greater emphasis on independent living. Coupled with the graying of the population and the lack of sufficient funding to build new accessible, affordable housing, this means that more attention is being paid to home modifications. There is a growing awareness that environmental sensitivity should be considered a disability and addressed by limitations on the use of certain building materials and by improvements in ventilation systems. The ADA mandate to make existing buildings accessible is becoming a major focus of accessible architecture. In particular, there is increasing pressure for steady improvements to be made in the level of accessibility through facilities management. This will include providing a greater level of adaptability, ensuring fire safety for people with disabilities, and identify-

ing ways to make historic structures more accessible without destroying their historic value.

(*See also:* ACCESSIBILITY; ADVOCACY; AMERICANS WITH DISABILITIES ACT; CIVIL RIGHTS; DISABILITY LAW AND SOCIAL POLICY; HOUSING; INDEPENDENT LIVING; TRANSPORTATION ACCESSIBILITY; WHEELCHAIRS)

BIBLIOGRAPHY

BEDNAR, MICHAEL, ed. *Barrier Free Environments.* New York, 1977.

BOSTROM, JAMES; MACE, RONALD; and LONG, MARIA. *Adaptable Housing.* Washington, DC, 1987.

DEJONG, GERBEN, and LIFCHEZ, RAY. "Physical Disability and Public Policy." *Scientific American* 6 (1983).

MACE, RONALD. *Universal Design: Housing for the Lifespan of All People.* Washington, DC, 1988.

STEINFELD, EDWARD, ed. *Access to the Built Environment: A Review of Literature.* Washington, DC, 1979.

EDWARD STEINFELD

ART THERAPY

Art therapy is a method of treatment in which the unique blending of art and therapeutic practice is used as a vehicle for exploring individual problems and potentials. Through the use of therapeutic art experiences, emotional, motor, and cognitive abilities can be enhanced. Art therapists use the healing power of the creative process as a way of both reconciling emotional difficulties and facilitating self-knowledge, communication, and personal development.

Artistic expression has been an essential element within societies throughout history, beginning with drawings on the walls of caves. The desire to create is universal. Psychiatrists in the late 1800s discovered that individuals suffering from mental illnesses were compelled to create paintings and drawings (on walls, floors, lavatory paper, scraps) as a way of coping with their illness, and studied these productions in an effort to understand the artists and their suffering. The use of art for both diagnosis and treatment by art therapists was a natural outgrowth of this work.

Art is a unique reflection of the artist and can thus be a window through which we can view an individual's unconscious processes. It is a powerful form of communication, a special language for expressing emotions. Visual art can offer a portrait of the artist and his or her reality, from which it is possible to step back to attain perspective. Art can be viewed at a later date as a way of documenting progress over time. Another unique advantage of art as therapy is the natural spatial aspect of visual expression, which can portray many facets of experience simultaneously. Artistic creation can be enjoyable as well as function as a mirror of one's thoughts and feelings. Art production involves human emotion, and the creative process can yield cathartic emotional responses (Nadeau, 1993). Therapeutic art experiences offer an avenue to give one's inner self some form of artistic expression. Art therapists believe that the process of artistic creation is often more important than the product. One of the intrinsic benefits of the creative process is to help facilitate honest personal expression.

In art therapy, the therapist must build a partnership or therapeutic alliance with the patient. Only through the formation of a trusting relationship, in which the therapist conveys respect for the unique experience of the patient, can the patient feel free to express conflicts freely. Through this process the patient can mobilize his or her own inner resources and give them form in outer reality (Adamson, 1984). The art that results from giving aesthetic form to the specific event or emotions that disrupted one's life is a powerful vehicle for change and reparation within the safety of the therapeutic relationship.

Numerous studies have indicated the value of art therapy as a significant mode of treatment and as a way of changing behaviors, reinforcing learning, and improving the lives of persons with disabilities. Painting, collage, and claywork, for example, can enhance the functioning of children who are emotionally disturbed by increasing emotional expression without inhibition, enhancing nonverbal expression, augmenting appropriate venting of feelings, and providing a vehicle for expression of wishful thinking (Mills, 1990).

Art as therapy is distinguishing itself in the treatment of elders with mental retardation through the use of drawing, sculpture, and painting, by exploring the developmental components of aging, and by providing age-appropriate leisure activities. Participants exhibit significant positive changes in socialization, autonomous functioning, and self-expression (Harlan, 1990).

Art therapy has made significant inroads in the treatment of sexual abuse and trauma by helping individuals access previously repressed memories (Consoli, 1991). Drawing and painting have been successfully used with children with learning disabilities to improve eye-hand coordination. Art therapy can also be used to modify behavior in students who have learning disabilities with attention deficits, hyperactivity, and to facilitate task completion (Miller, 1986). Language development has been shown to be enhanced significantly through a unique blending of art therapy and language curriculum for children with hearing impairments (Green & Hasselbring, 1981).

Art therapists treat a multitude of populations in a variety of settings, including people with physical disabilities, those who are chemically dependent and their families, and persons with psychiatric illness. They also work with people in prisons, those living with catastrophic illness, older persons, and people who are developmentally delayed. Art therapists are employed in rehabilitation centers, schools for normal and exceptional students, mental health settings, medical centers, correctional facilities, private practice, and in other settings.

Many of the methodologies used by art therapists have proved beneficial for use with those persons with a disability by helping them attain increased control and understanding of their bodies and emotions. One significant result is that they are better able to explore their own creative expression. The challenge to art therapists is to enhance self-knowledge and morale and augment motor ability as well as the quality of physical and mental health of their patients. Art therapy can help individuals change their conception of their disability so as not to be consumed by it through acceptance of the limitations of their illness and the possibilities inherent despite it.

The American Art Therapy Association (AATA) was established in 1969 and represents a membership of almost 5,000 professionals and students. The AATA considers entry level into the profession at the postgraduate level. Art therapists have graduated from a master's program that includes approximately 1,000 hours of supervised internship experience. Art therapists registered by the AATA are designated ATR (Art Therapist Registered) to assure the general public that the individual providing art therapy services has met certain standards and conditions as developed by AATA. The American Art Therapy Association will soon require certification (through qualifying examination) for all art therapists to enhance professionalism in the field. The AATA has thirty-four affiliate chapters throughout the United States.

"Art therapists have rigorous training in the therapeutic use of art as well as the behavioral sciences, visual symbol production and are skilled in methods of intervention. Intensive supervision of clinical work is also a requirement." (AATA, 1990).

The field of art therapy is rapidly expanding. There has been a significant increase in the number of art therapists as well as the range of settings in which they are employed. New contexts will yield changes in the practice of art therapy. This innovative field offers a valuable contribution to the care of people living with mental and physical disabilities. Art therapists are attuned to an inner language of imagery, and through this unusual framework may help give rise to a new comprehension of human functioning.

(*See also:* MUSIC THERAPY; RECREATION)

RESOURCE

The American Art Therapy Association, Inc., 1202 Allanson Rd, Mundelein, IL 60060

BIBLIOGRAPHY

ADAMSON, EDWARD. *Art As Healing.* London: 1984.

AMERICAN ART THERAPY ASSOCIATION. *Education Requirement Bylaws.* 1990.

ANDERSON, FRANCES E. "A Critical Analysis of the Published Research Literature in Arts for the Handicapped: 1971–1981, with Special Attention to the Visual Arts." *Art Therapy* 1 (1983):26–39.

CONSOLI, JIM. *Psychimagery: Healing the Child Within.* 1991.

GREEN, J. C. and HASSELBRING. "The Acquisition of Language Concepts by Hearing Impaired Children Through Selected Aspects of an Experimental Core Art Curriculum." *Studies in Art Education* 22 (1981):32–37.

HARLAN, JANE E. "The Use of Art Therapy for Older Adults with Developmental Disabilities–Special Issue: Activities with Developmentally Disabled Elders and Older Adults": *Activities Adaptation and Aging* 15 (1990):67–77.

JOHNSON, DAVID READE. "On Being One and Many." *The Arts in Psychotherapy* 18 (1991):1–5.

LIEBMAN, MARIAN. *Art Therapy for Groups.* Cambridge, MA 1984.

MILLER, MARGARET G. "Art–A Creative Teaching Tool." Academic Therapy 22 (1986):53–56.

MILLS, ANNE. "Art therapy on a Residential Treatment for Troubled Children." *Journal of Child and Youth Care* 6 (1990):49–59.

NADEAU, ROBERTA. "Using the Visual Arts to Expand Personal Creativity." In *Using the Creative Arts in Therapy,* ed. B. Warren. New York, 1993.

NAUMBURG, MARGARET. *An Introduction to Art Therapy.* New York, 1973.

RUBIN, JUDITH AARON. "Art Therapy Today." *Art Education* (1990):8.

WADESON, HARRIET. *Art Psychotherapy.* New York, 1980.

———. *The Dynamics of Art Psychotherapy.* New York, 1987.

WARREN, BERNIE, ed. *Using the Creative Arts in Therapy.* New York, 1993.

DEBORAH FARBER

ARTHRITIS

The term arthritis means inflammation of a joint and is used to describe a large collection of disorders in which such inflammation is merely one component. Rheumatic disorders is a more appropriate name because joint involvement may be relatively non-inflammatory or a minor component. Three major types of rheumatic disorders are described in this entry: osteoarthritis, diffuse connective tissue disorders, including rheumatoid arthritis, and spondyloarthropathies, such as ankylosing spondylitis.

Osteoarthritis

Also referred to as degenerative joint disease, osteoarthritis (OA) is the most common rheumatic disorder, being nearly universal among elderly people. It is a relatively noninflammatory disorder that affects a limited number of joints. Typical sites of osteoarthritis are the distal and proximal interphalangeal finger joints; carpometacarpal joints of the thumbs, neck and lower back, hips, knees, and first metatarsophalangeal toe joints. Ankle, wrist, elbow, and shoulder involvement is rare, although the elbow and shoulder are often affected by bursitis and tendinitis, similar degenerative processes.

Osteoarthritis is characterized by progressive thinning of the cartilage that lines the ends of bones at joints, by enlargement of the margins of bones at the joints (spur formation), and by hardening of the bones. In the distal interphalangeal finger joints, bony enlargement takes the form of nodes called Heberden's nodes.

Although OA is found most often in older individuals (by age sixty-five, 75% of the population has OA of the hands determinable by X ray), additional risk factors determine which joints are affected, when, and the degree of effect; these factors appear to vary for different joints. Repetitive use in occupational activities, injuries, obesity, and female gender are risk factors for OA of the knees. Hip involvement is more common in men and may result primarily from inherited factors. The association of OA with sports activities may be related more to injury than use. Heredity is another major risk factor and can take the form of genetic predisposition; rates of joint deformities in a population; characteristics of bones, such as osteoporosis; and the tendency to deposit crystals in degenerated cartilage. Heberden's nodes are most often found in successive generations of women in certain families.

Diagnosis is based on symptoms of joint pain and stiffness and on X-ray findings. Typical X-ray changes indicating definite OA include moderate-to-large osteophytes (spurs) and joint space narrowing. The aims of treatment are to relieve pain and maintain joint motion. Acetaminophen drugs, such as Tylenol, are prescribed to reduce pain and promote joint movement. In highly inflammatory phases of OA, nonsteroidal anti-inflammatory drugs, such as aspirin, Motrin, Naprosyn, and so forth, may be used, as acetaminophen has no anti-inflammatory properties.

Range-of-motion and muscle-strengthening exercises are important to maintain joint motion and position. Affected joints should not be stressed by impact-loading activities, such as running, or repetitive tasks. Thirty-minute periods of fitness walking, however, do not have negative effects on knee OA. Joint-replacement surgery often becomes necessary for severe OA of the knees or hips. These surgeries tend to be highly successful, especially for pain relief.

While OA accounts for a large amount of disability on a societal level because of its frequent occurrence, the level of severity per individual is often mild. Many people in whom OA shows on an X ray have no symptoms. About 10 percent of the population with OA, usually those with hip or knee involvement, have severe disability. Preventive measures include weight reduction, avoidance of repeated injury to joints, and redesigning occupational tasks.

Diffuse Connective Tissue Disorders

Diffuse connective tissue disorders, also called autoimmune disorders, are chronic diseases characterized by inflammation, spontaneous flare and remission, and autoimmune phenomena. The etiology of these disorders, which include rheumatoid arthritis, juvenile rheumatoid arthritis, lupus erythematosus, and others, is unknown. A degree of genetic influence is often evident. Higher rates in females indicate hormonal influences, although these are not understood. Environmental factors, including common infectious agents, may also be involved. Diagnosis is based on a combination of symptoms, history, examination, and laboratory test findings. Positive autoantibody tests (rheumatoid factor and antinuclear antibodies) are commonly, but not universally, found. In addition, autoantibodies may be found in combination with other illnesses or in people with no illness. Misdiagnosis is common. Treatment tends to be nonspecific. No preventive measures are known.

Rheumatoid Arthritis (RA). Rheumatoid arthritis is the next most common rheumatic disorder after OA, affecting up to 1 percent of the population. People of any age may be affected although the onset is most common in the fourth through sixth decades of life. The disorder is systemic (affects the whole body), but its primary effect is on joints with synovial linings. Many joints tend to be affected in a symmetric pattern.

The distribution of RA varies throughout the world, being more common in some native American tribal groups and less common among rural black South Africans. The disorder usually goes away during pregnancy, presenting further evidence of hormonal influences.

Symptoms include fatigue and malaise; prolonged morning stiffness; signs of inflammation in joints, that is, redness, swelling, warmth, and pain; and low-grade fever and weight loss. Symptoms must be present for at least six weeks for the diagnosis to be confirmed. Joint motion is restricted by both pain and swelling. Involvement of the heart, lungs, lymph glands, blood, peripheral nervous system, eyes, and small-to-medium blood vessels (vasculitis and arteritis) may also be found. These latter effects are generally not severe; the major exception is Felty's syndrome, which can cause extremely low white-blood counts and anemia. Subcutaneous nodules located around joints, and occasionally in the lungs, and skin ulcers are evidence of vasculitis.

Laboratory findings include positive rheumatoid factor, found in about 75 percent of patients, and, less commonly, antinuclear antibody tests. The sedimentation rate is generally elevated, and a mild anemia is often present. The latter is an anemia of chronic disease rather than iron deficiency. Typical X-ray changes, which may take months or years to develop, consist of cartilage thinning, erosion of bone in the area of joints, and osteoporosis.

The objectives of treatment are to reduce joint destruction, relieve inflammation, and maintain function. The first objective may be achieved through the use of antirheumatic drugs, primarily methotrexate, gold salts, sulfasalazine, penicillamine, and antimalarials. Methotrexate is the most effective of these drugs, and early use is advocated. All these drugs have anti-inflammatory actions and relieve symptoms. They are frequently used in combination with high doses of nonsteroidal anti-inflammatory drugs; patients with mild disease may be treated with only the latter drugs.

As corticosteroids are potent anti-inflammatory and possibly antirheumatic drugs, they may be used, especially for short-term relief. The oral form, prednisone, is used for generalized effect but because serious side effects are likely when taken in high dosages (greater than ten milligrams per day) for long periods of time, use is limited as much as possible. Injectable forms are used for acutely inflamed joints. Although RA is painful, the use of narcotic drugs is usually limited to short-term treatment of extreme flares. Acetaminophen also provides extra pain relief for less acute flares.

Other treatments besides medications are important. Generalized acute flares respond to bed rest. Individual inflamed joints may be rested by the use of splints and treated with ice. Passive range-of-motion exercises should be done during acute flares to maintain joint motion.

During more stable phases, active range-of-motion and muscle-strengthening exercises are needed. While repetitive, stressful joint use increases inflammation, modified fitness-walking programs (limited to twenty-minute periods) and swimming do not exacerbate disease and help to maintain aerobic conditioning. Energy-conservation techniques help to manage fatigue. Adaptive-aid use increases independence. Wrist splints that leave the fingers free provide support while facilitating function. When mobility aids are needed, platform crutches or walkers put less stress on upper-extremity joints. Flexible orthotics help relieve foot problems; running or tennis shoes provide stability and cushioning. Joint replacement and other orthopedic surgery often become necessary.

Disability as an outcome of RA is more prominent than early death, but studies suggest that survivorship is decreased by 50 percent, a rate similar to Hodgkin's disease, diabetes, and stroke. A moderate level of disability occurs most often. Disease onset is typically gradual; the largest functional decline occurs within the first two years, followed by slow decline thereafter. Disease onset and course are variable, however. Onset variations include acute and interrupted onset. About 10 percent of individuals have mild disease and another 10 to 15 percent severe disease that does not yield to treatment; the latter individuals experience severe disability.

Juvenile Rheumatoid Arthritis (JRA). The term JRA is used to describe chronic inflammatory joint diseases in children, although for the most part these diseases differ from adult rheumatoid arthritis. There are three subtypes: systemic-onset JRA; polyarticular (many joints) JRA; and pauciarticular (few joints) JRA. Systemic-onset JRA is characterized by general symptoms such as spiking fever; rash; enlarged lymph glands, liver, and spleen; and heart or lung effusions. Usually, a chronic arthritis affecting many joints develops within weeks or months. Pauciarticular JRA affects the eyes in 10 to 50 percent of children and can lead to blindness. In older boys pauciarticular JRA may be similar to ankylosing spondylitis or other spondyloarthropathies. The three JRA subtypes are also differentiated by the proportions of boys and girls affected, ages affected, and presence or absence of rheumatoid factors and antinuclear antibodies. Altogether, JRA is uncommon, the prevalence of active disease being estimated at 0.06 percent.

Diagnosis and treatment are similar to that of adult rheumatoid arthritis. As arthritis in children can affect the growth of bones, JRA can affect overall height as well as the growth of specific bones, creating limb-length discrepancies and disproportionately small jaws. Periodic eye evaluation is needed for up to ten years after the onset of pauciarticular JRA.

Remission after several years of JRA is common, especially in children who are rheumatoid-factor negative. A subset of children with polyarticular JRA—older girls who are rheumatoid-factor positive—tend to have a disease similar to adult rheumatoid arthritis and often experience severe disability.

Lupus Erythematosus. There are two forms of lupus erythematosus: discoid lupus, which primarily affects only the skin, and systemic lupus (SLE), which has diffuse effects and is more severe. Systemic lupus is highly variable in presentation because it can involve many body systems; each individual has a unique set of affected systems. Systems most commonly involved are the joints, skin, and blood. The arthritis that accompanies lupus is generally not as severe as rheumatoid arthritis. A "butterfly" rash across the cheeks is characteristic of SLE but occurs in a minority of patients; other types of skin lesions occur also. Other systems commonly affected are the kidneys, heart, lungs, blood vessels, lymph glands, stomach and intestines, and central nervous system.

The prevalence of SLE is estimated at 0.05 percent; it is more common among African Americans and possibly Asians. The occurrence of lupuslike syndromes as side effects from certain drugs suggests environmental factors. People of all ages may be affected, but onset is most common in the childbearing years. The disease may flare during pregnancy, and the fetus may be affected.

Antinuclear antibody tests are most often positive in lupus. Other blood abnormalities can include anemia, either the mild anemia of chronic disease or a more severe form, as well as low white-blood counts and low platelet counts.

Corticosteroid drugs are used for the more severe effects of lupus. High doses of prednisone may be required for long periods of time, producing additional disability. Other medical treatment depends on the systems involved. General measures for disease flares include increased rest and reduction of stress. Energy-conservation measures are most important in that fatigue is an especially prominent feature.

The prognosis is variable, but some level of disability and/or early death is frequent. Seventy percent of individuals with SLE live for twenty years or more. Kidney and cardiovascular involvement most commonly lead to early death. Hospitalization for disease flares is required, on average, every two years. Kidney involvement may require dialysis and transplantation. Cognitive deficits, psychosis, and seizures may result from central nervous system involvement.

Other Diffuse Connective Tissue Disorders. Two other diffuse connective tissue disorders each have a prevalence of approximately 0.01 percent. Scleroderma means "hard skin"; the term is used to describe two probably separate disorders, localized scleroderma and systemic sclerosis. Localized scleroderma affects limited areas of the skin and underlying tissues. Mild disability due to limb impairment and disfigurement may result. Systemic sclerosis is a more serious disorder; in addition to skin hardening, the disorder affects the internal organs and can result in early death.

Polymyositis and dermatomyositis are similar disorders that consist primarily of inflammation of the skeletal muscles; heart, gastrointestinal, and lung involvement is also common. Dermatomyositis also affects the skin. Polymyositis, especially, may be associated with cancer.

Spondyloarthropathies

This term is used to describe a group of related disorders that include ankylosing spondylitis (AS), Reiter's syndrome, psoriatic arthritis (affecting 7 percent of people with psoriasis), arthritis associated with inflammatory bowel disease, and reactive arthritis. These disorders primarily involve the sacroiliac and lower weight-bearing joints; when present, hand involvement classically affects the distal interphalangeal joints. Joint inflammation occurs at sites of ligamentous insertion into bone rather than the synovial lining of joints. Besides joints, the eyes, heart, lung, and skin may be involved.

Heredity and, in some cases, environmental factors play important etiological roles in these disorders. Ninety percent of individuals with AS and Reiter's syndrome are positive for the gene HLA-B27, as are smaller proportions with the other disorders. Both Reiter's syndrome and reactive arthritis occur after either an intestinal infection or, in the case of Reiter's, a genitourinary infection. Autoantibodies are not found in these disorders. Gender proportions in general are equal, although men may have more severe disease.

Diagnosis is based on symptoms, history, physical examination, and X-ray findings. Laboratory test abnormalities can include a mildly increased sedimentation rate and other mild, nonspecific findings.

The aims of treatment are to reduce joint destruction and inflammation. Medications include nonsteroidal anti-inflammatory drugs, methotrexate, and sulfasalazine. Range-of-motion and muscle-strengthening exercises are important, as is maintenance of good posture. Smokers are urged to stop due to the possibilities of lung disease and/or compression from spinal deformity.

The prognoses for these disorders are variable. Mild-to-moderate levels of disability occur in most cases, but severe illness can result (rarely) in early death. Prevention of Reiter's syndrome and reactive arthritis is by avoidance of dysentery and of urinary urethral infection (by the use of condoms).

Impacts of Rheumatic Disorders

Physical impacts may include loss of function, pain, fatigue, appearance changes, and early death. The functional loss initially and universally experienced is in the area of recreational activities. Varying degrees of impairment in mobility, activities of daily living, social activities, and roles occur also. The degree of disability caused by rheumatic disorders—contrary to more fixed impairments—may vary from day to day due to flare and remission characteristics. Another difference between rheumatic and more fixed impairments is that in rheumatic disorders activities may be done once or twice—although not repetitively.

Pain, along with stiffness and fatigue, is a hallmark of rheumatic disorders. During acute flares, pain may be severe, but chronic aching is more usual. Treatment usually reduces pain significantly, enabling the individual to resume active living, but it is not eliminated totally. Although frustrating, this enables the individual to recognize that the illness is present and take appropriate action. Despite the fact that pain is ongoing, most individuals are able to adjust and do not develop the so-called chronic-pain syndrome. Like pain, fatigue is often a sign of disease activity and is increased in times of flare. Because of fatigue, six-hour workdays may be best, although hard to arrange.

The most common appearance change is impaired movement. Severe joint deformities occur most often in rheumatoid arthritis, while hair loss and skin rashes frequently affect people with systemic lupus erythematosus. Those who take large amounts of corticosteroids typically gain substantial weight. The effect of scleroderma on the face is a pinched appearance. Kyphosis (abnormal spine curvature that produces a hunched back) is common in ankylosing spondylitis.

Psychological impacts include the need to adjust to the losses of free and comfortable movement, function, and appearance changes and the possibility of early death. Mild-to-moderate depression is common for one to two years after diagnosis. The level of depression is usually that of mood alteration, but clinical depression may exist in up to 20 percent of patients. Because of varying courses and flare and remission characteristics, the adjustment process may be interrupted and renewed in times of major declines in function or hospitalization. Like many individuals with adult-onset disorders, people with rheumatic disorders may not identify with the disability community and thus not avail themselves of needed services.

Loss of mobility and illness often reduce participation in community social affairs. Spouses frequently suffer nearly as much as patients, and their needs may not be recognized. Family recreational activities may be curtailed or the affected individual left out. Divorce may be instigated by disease onset but is not statistically more common than in the general population. Remarriage, however, is less likely, resulting in a lack of social support for many patients. Role shifting between spouses occurs frequently. Children may need to participate more in household work. Although these effects are generally not harmful, overburdening may occur.

Arthritis (rheumatic diseases generally) is the second leading cause of work disability in the United States. After ten years of disease, the rate of work disability in rheumatoid arthritis is 50 percent. Individuals in jobs with high physical demands (including repetitive-motion requirements) and low autonomy over work hours and job procedures become work-disabled earlier. Surprisingly little use is made of state-federal vocational rehabilitation services. Loss of income is the largest economic cost for individuals with rheumatic disorders. In most cases outpatient care is the highest medical cost. The cost of joint replacement surgery, however, is substantial.

Rehabilitation Considerations

A team approach is beneficial though frequently not provided because many patients receive care in private physicians' offices. Besides physicians, important team members include physical therapists, occupational therapists, nurses, podiatrists, social workers, rehabilitation counselors, nutritionists, and psychologists.

Appropriate exercises are an important treatment component; routine daily-living activities are not sufficient, and most exercise programs for the general public are too stressful. Exercises should be prescribed by a physical therapist with rheumatology experience.

Patient education requires special consideration in the case of rheumatic disorders. Information provided when needed and desired over time meets the needs of adults with chronic disorders better than complete information provided at the time of diagnosis. Educational programs designed specifically for people with rheumatic disorders, such as the Self-Help Program sponsored by the Arthritis Foundation, have been found to increase individuals' feelings of self-efficacy with respect to control of symptoms. The group sharing that occurs at these programs is also beneficial.

A family approach is especially important, considering that women, who often have a central role in families, are commonly affected. Rheumatic disorders often affect sexual relationships because of pain, fatigue, and inability to assume positions; also, spouses may fear causing pain.

Future Developments

Greater prevention of osteoarthritis is expected through the identification of risk factors and reduction of occupational and sports hazards. Due to breakthroughs in the ability to detect change in joints, new treatments will be forthcoming. Further advances are expected in the treatment and prevention of connective tissue disorders from research specific to these disorders as well as from research on other immunological disorders such as AIDS and cancer.

Consumer and Professional Organizations

The main consumer organization is the Arthritis Foundation, which provides services such as information and referral, Self-Help and other educational programs, water and land exercise programs, support groups, camping and other programs for children, and peer counseling, primarily through local chapter offices. Other consumer organizations include the Lupus Foundation and the Scleroderma Federation. The main professional organization is the American College of Rheumatology (ACR) whose membership is composed of rheumatologists. The Association of Rheumatology Health Professionals is a division of ACR; its members are nurses, physical and occupational therapists, social workers, and the like.

(*See also:* BACK DISORDERS; FAMILY; MUSCULOSKELETAL DISORDERS; OCCUPATIONAL THERAPY; PAIN; PHYSICAL THERAPY; PSYCHOSOCIAL ADJUSTMENT)

RESOURCES

Arthritis Foundation, 1314 Spring St., NW, Atlanta, GA 30309

Lupus Foundation of America, 4 Research Place, Suite 180, Rockville, MD 20850

BIBLIOGRAPHY

ALLAIRE, SARALYNN H. "How a Chronically Ill Mother Manages." *American Journal of Nursing* 88 (1988): 46–49.

———. "Employment and Household Work Disability in Women with Rheumatoid Arthritis." *Journal of Applied Rehabilitation Counseling* 23 (1992):44–51.

ARTHRITIS FOUNDATION. *Guide to Independent Living.* Atlanta, 1988.

FELSON, DAVID T. "Osteoarthritis." *Rheumatic Disease Clinics of North America* 16 (1990):499–511.

HARKCOM, THOMAS M.; LAMPMAN, RICHARD M.; BANWELL, BARBARA F.; and CASTOR, C. WILLIAM. "Therapeutic Value of Graded Exercise Training in Rheumatoid Arthritis." *Arthritis and Rheumatism* 28 (1985):32–39.

HARRIS, JENNIFER A.; NEWCOMB, ANDREW F.; and GEWANTER, HARRY L. "Psychosocial Effects of Juvenile Rheumatic Disease: The Family and Peer Systems as a Context for Coping." *Arthritis Care and Research* 4 (1991):123–130.

STAPLETON, BARBARA. "Keep Moving: Exercise and Arthritis." In *Joint Movement* 2 (1990):1–3 (available from the Arthritis Foundation).

KOVAR, PAMELA A.; ALLEGRANTE, JOHN P.; MacKENZIE, C. RONALD; PETERSON, MARGARET G.; GUTIN, BERNARD; and CHARLSON, MARY E. "Supervised Fitness Walking in Patients with Osteoarthritis of the Knee." *Annals of Internal Medicine* 116 (1992):529–534.

KUSHNER, IRVING, and DAWSON, NEAL V. "Changing Perspectives in the Treatment of Rheumatoid Arthritis." *Journal of Rheumatology* 19 (1992):1831–1833.

LAWRENCE, REVA C.; HOCHBERG, MARC C.; KELSEY, JENNIFER L.; McDUFFIE, FREDERIC C.; MEDSGER, THOMAS A.; FELTS, WILLIAM R.; and SHULMAN, LAWRENCE E. "Estimates of the Prevalence of Selected Arthritic and Musculoskeletal Diseases in the United States." *Journal of Rheumatology* 16 (1989):427–441.

LORIG, KATE. "Arthritis Patient Education." In *Rheumatic Diseases: Rehabilitation and Management,* ed. Gail K. Riggs and Eric P. Gall. Boston, 1984.

LORIG, KATE, and FRIES, JAMES F. *The Arthritis Helpbook.* Reading, MA, 1991.

ROGERS, MALCOLM; PARTRIDGE, ALISON; and LIANG, MATHEW. "Psychological Care of Adults with Rheumatoid Arthritis." *Annals of Internal Medicine* 96 (1982):344–348.

SCHUMACHER, H. RALPH; KLIPPEL, JOHN H.; and ROBINSON, DWIGHT R., eds. *Primer on the Rheumatic Diseases.* Arthritis Foundation, Atlanta, 1988.

SARALYNN H. ALLAIRE

ARTIFICIAL LIMB

See AMPUTATION; ENGINEERING, REHABILITATION; PROSTHETICS AND ORTHOTICS

ASSESSMENT IN REHABILITATION

Individuals with a disability are confronted with complex issues, multiple needs, and a seemingly overwhelming assortment of bureaucratic resources. They have immediate and long-term concerns about medical and health care needs, ability to provide personal and economic support for their family, a variety of legal issues, and are often overwhelmed by the disability experience itself. They question their employment potential and career options, how to access educational and training resources, how to overcome learning and other difficulties, and/or how to avail themselves of benefits available under the various entitlement programs.

Assessment represents the first step in helping a person with a disability to understand rehabilitation options and to develop his or her realistic potential. By definition, rehabilitation assessment is a comprehensive and interdisciplinary evaluation of the individual's physical, emotional, cognitive, behavioral, and sensory abilities in relation to the functional demands of the environments in which a person is expected to participate. Information is obtained from medical, vocational, educational, and psychological evaluations that form the basis for the creation of an individualized rehabilitation plan that is developed between a rehabilitation professional and the consumer. As a comprehensive process, assessment focuses on a person's ability to function in the family, on the job, at school, in independent living situations, and in the community.

For the rehabilitation professional, assessment provides the foundation for subsequent rehabilitation interventions and program planning, and a documented course of action leading to desired rehabilitation outcomes. Rehabilitation assessment recommendations serve the consumer, case manager, and service agency as a program evaluation tool to determine whether goals are being met in a timely and cost-efficient manner.

Current Issues

The role, function, and practice of assessment are influenced and shaped by advances and trends in the rehabilitation field. Many of the more significant factors include the following:

- Medical advances. Medicine has become more accurate and effective in diagnosing and treating individuals who experience severe and chronic injury and disability, including traumatic head injury, cardiac impairment, psychiatric disability, and AIDS. Individuals who previously may not have survived traumatic or chronic injury now turn to rehabilitation for accurate evaluation and planning to improve their quality of life. The challenge for assessment is to develop or adapt assessment procedures that respond to the unique needs of these individuals.
- Rehabilitation advances. Rehabilitation has developed an expanded range of services for individuals with disabilities, including supported employment in integrated work settings, supported education, assistive technology, work hardening and ergonomic interventions, and independent living centers. Services are also expanded to individuals with more severe disabilities, with an emphasis on inclusion and integration in work, classroom, and community settings. Disability legislation such as the Americans with Disabilities Act (ADA) has created greater access to public transportation, community services, and employment opportunities. Rather than limited to state vocational rehabilitation agencies or rehabilitation workshops, rehabilitation services are now found in schools,

in hospitals, and in industrial settings. These advances mean that the evaluator has multiple services to consider when developing a rehabilitation plan with the individual.
- Technology advances. Advances in medical and rehabilitation assessment tests and procedures allow for more accurate measurement of an individual's impairment. The application of computers in assessment provides immediate interpretation of assessment results and the capacity to manipulate large databases to assist in diagnosis and decision-making. In addition, evaluators have access to computer information networks, making resources easier to identify (e.g., assistive technology devices).

Another example of technological advances in rehabilitation is the use of assistive and augmentative devices that allow individuals to participate independently in community, job, home, and school.
- Ecological assessment trends. Rehabilitation models and practice are shifting from a focus on disability and impairment of the person to a model that considers the person within the context of his or her environment. This "ecological paradigm" recognizes that a person's behavior and performance can best be understood as interaction between the person's skills and abilities and the supports or characteristics that may or may not be present in the environment. This means that assessment must be "environment-specific" and must consider the aids, resources, and environmental characteristics that support an individual's performance.
- Eligibility determination. Rather than requiring individuals to have potential for employment to be eligible for rehabilitation, legislation, policies, and regulations stress a presumption of eligibility, an emphasis on inclusion in rehabilitation. Assessment functions less in a "gatekeeper" role and more as a process to identify the appropriate person-service-outcome match.
- Self-determination trends. Persons who seek rehabilitation services, including assessment, play a more collaborative role in the rehabilitation process. The person is viewed as having the right and the responsibility to participate in the decision-making and planning that will affect

his or her life. Assessment is a service that is not provided *to* the person but that is done *with* the person.

Objectives of Assessment in Rehabilitation

Assessment in rehabilitation has a broader and more dynamic function than traditional assessment approaches that emphasize strengths and limitations of the person to determine eligibility for services, or readiness for school, work, or community placement. Objectives of rehabilitation assessment reflect the range and diversity of assessment procedures and the potential of assessment to impact directly on the person with a disability and the structure of subsequent rehabilitation services. The following objectives identify the descriptive or diagnostic role as well as the dynamic or instrumental role of assessment in rehabilitation.

1. Diagnostic objectives. A primary objective of assessment is to identify the strengths and abilities of the person, and to clarify the impact of the impairment on the person's ability to function in different situations or settings. In addition, rehabilitation assessment describes the contextual elements of the school, work, family, social, and community environment that may be modified to facilitate successful independent functioning.

   Rehabilitation assessment is often required to determine the existence of a disability, to develop a functional disability rating, or medical impairment rating. Predictions about duration of disability or inability to perform are incorporated into disability determinations and impairment ratings for determining eligibility for programs and benefits under Social Security programs (SSI, SSDI), workers' compensation, or vocational rehabilitation.

2. Adjustment to disability. Identification of the person's present adjustment to his or her disability must be an initial focus of assessment. The person's adjustment reflects his or her readiness for rehabilitation planning, need for immediate counseling, and the level of assessment that will follow.

3. Individualized rehabilitation plan. An objective of assessment is the development of an individu-

alized rehabilitation plan leading to achievement of realistic functional outcomes. The Individual Written Rehabilitation Plan (IWRP) is a collaborative effort between counselor and client to synthesize assessment results, to identify functional outcomes and the services needed to reach identified goals, to establish time frames for services and goals attainment, and to clarify responsibilities of individuals involved. Rehabilitation assessment is also used in formal plans called Individualized Education Plans (IEP) in education, and Individualized Service Plans (ISP) in mental health.

4. Identification of accommodations, supports, and resources. An objective of assessment is the identification of accommodations and supports that can be utilized in the person's vocational, educational, home, or community environment to promote independence and performance. Assessment functions to identify how present environmental characteristics could be modified, or how natural cues, supports, or resources could be used to increase the individual's functioning.

5. Facilitation of a counseling relationship. Rehabilitation assessment encourages development of counseling and other facilitative relationships by increasing the individual's awareness and understanding of his or her disability and its impact on living, learning, and working. The objective of assessment is to engage the individual in a goal-directed counseling process to resolve issues that may range from the person's adjustment to his or her disability and commitment to rehabilitation, to career planning directions, to family reactions to the disability experience, or to decision-making and independence within the rehabilitation process.

6. Empowerment and self-determination. An objective of the assessment process is to empower the individual to take ownership of his or her rehabilitation plan. Assessment is a decision-making process. Effective assessment results in the individual taking increasing responsibility for the decisions that affect his or her life.

Rehabilitation assessment is more than a process to identify disability factors, establish a diagnosis, or determine readiness for rehabilitation. Assessment is also an educational process, assisting the individual to understand his or her disability as it relates to different environmentally specific demands, requirements, and opportunities. Assessment is also an individualized process, taking part in the environs and under the conditions that approximate what the individual is expected to experience in the future. Assessment is an instrumental process that aggressively seeks to empower the individual through presenting opportunities for choice, decision-making, and self-determination. Assessment is also a dynamic service applied throughout the rehabilitation process, using a variety of tests, procedures, and perspectives to integrate information with counseling, case management, and other service activities.

Methodology Issues in Assessment

Assessment in rehabilitation uses a variety of tests, tools, and procedures to acquire information and engage the individual in rehabilitation planning. Because of the critical nature of the decisions that are made by and about the person, methodological questions are frequently raised by both the individual and rehabilitation professionals. Of concern is how confident one can be that results are an accurate description of the individual and his or her potential. The following sections review several methodological issues that respond to this question.

Criterion Issues. To interpret assessment results, there must be a means of comparing a person's performance or status against objective criteria. The majority of tests in rehabilitation and education use a norm-referenced comparison method. Individual performance on a test is compared to the performance of a group of similar individuals on the same test (Anastasi, 1987). The assumption in norm-referenced testing is that the individual being tested is similar to the sample on which the test was normed. The adequacy of the norm group for persons with a disability is often questioned, as most norm groups do not have a representative sample of individuals with disabilities (Power, 1991). The adequacy of the norm group is further questioned as individuals from minority and culturally diverse groups are increasingly involved in rehabilitation and assessment (Hursh, 1995). The rehabilitation professional should look for tests that use norm

groups that are current, well described, sufficient in size, and that relate to questions being asked by the consumer and professionals.

Norm-referenced tests use statistical procedures to compare performance with a related sample. In contrast, criterion-referenced tests compare the individual's performance with the ability, behavior, or knowledge requirements of a particular skill area. Interpretations are linked to performance criteria rather than to performance characteristics of a relative norm group. The criterion-referenced test asks, "Does Bill assemble brake systems correctly?" or "How many safety rules is Sally able to identify correctly?" Criterion-referenced tests allow interpretation of the person's present and needed level of skill and behavior and are particularly useful in rehabilitation planning.

Test Validation Issues. Validity is a psychometric standard used to evaluate the characteristics and usefulness of a test or assessment activity. Basically, the validity of a test is defined in terms of the extent to which a test measures what it is designed to measure (Anastasi, 1987; Cronbach, 1990). However, it is important to understand that evaluation of the validity of a test should not be based on a statistical correlation coefficient alone. Test validation is specific to the population sample as well as to the intent of the test or instrument (Power, 1991). A test may be useful (valid) in answering questions about a person who is representative of one population but not about an individual from another population sample. Paul Power (1991) highlights the importance of the last point in noting that validation of tests on individuals with a disability is a rare occasion. Understanding all the factors that contribute to the validity of a specific instrument allows the evaluator to interpret the results with a greater degree of confidence.

Several methods are used to validate a test, depending on the questions being asked. These include content, construct, predictive, and concurrent validity. Resources that discuss test development and validation procedures in more depth are by Anne Anastasi (1987) and Lee Cronbach (1990).

Validity is not only an important psychometric characteristic but also a critical applied function, often central to decisions that are made about a person's life. This consideration was highlighted by the Americans with Disabilities Act (ADA) guidelines related to employment testing. The ADA requires that assessment procedures used in hiring, selection, and promotion do not discriminate against a person because of his or her disability. This means that (1) assessment procedures must not influence the individual's performance because of his or her disability (e.g., using a written test for a person with dyslexia) and (2) that the assessment procedure must be a valid measure of the abilities needed to perform the essential functions of the job for which he or she is being considered. Validating assessment procedures against the demands and requirements of a job increase the likelihood that decisions will be based on an accurate description of the individual's ability to perform.

Assessment Stages

From the beginning, assessment is an individualized process that considers the person's needs, goals, and planning options. The evaluator helps the individual to understand the purpose of assessment activity, the individual's responsibilities during assessment, and his or her role in understanding its results, establishing rehabilitation goals and selecting services to achieve identified goals in a timely manner.

Assessment occurs in three basic stages. The goal of the first stage is to identify rehabilitation needs in relation to the person's work, education, social, community, or independent living areas. This stage functions to identify whether an agency or program is able to provide the kinds of services the person desires and to ascertain that the services are consistent with the individual's goals. It is also important at this stage to clarify the individual's readiness to participate in rehabilitation planning and readiness to establish realistic rehabilitation goals (Cohen et al., 1989). A person may present himself or herself at the request of a significant other but have little personal investment in rehabilitation. Another person may fear loss of benefits, or experience other secondary gains from disability and not desire a change in disability status. Others may have great dissatisfaction with their present situation but not have the personal supports to consider change.

The second stage in assessment involves developing and implementing a rehabilitation assessment plan that is responsive to the individual's identified needs. The assessment plan is structured to examine the individual's strengths and abilities in the context of the requirements, supports, resources, and characteristics of a specific environment. It is important to recognize that individuals require different levels of assessment, depending on their rehabilitation goals. One individual may have a clear understanding of his or her independent living needs and may need assistance only in identifying sources for financial assistance, or modifications of a living area to achieve independence. Another individual may require more comprehensive assessment and planning to identify medical, vocational, educational, and supported living services due to a traumatic head injury. During this stage, the evaluator assists the individual to understand the meaning of the assessment results, integrate multidisciplinary testing into an understandable format, and use the information to gain a more realistic understanding of his or her rehabilitation potential and possible alternatives.

During the third stage of assessment, the evaluator works with the individual to develop a rehabilitation plan. The evaluator functions to confirm the person's understanding of the assessment results and how the results contribute to defining a goal, and to identify and select appropriate services. In addition, ongoing evaluation activity is planned to check the individual's progress or implement specialized assessments. For example, an ergonomic evaluation may be planned at the time of job placement for a person with spinal cord problems to identify needed workstation adaptations.

Multidisciplinary Assessment Approaches

Assessment is a decision-making process that utilizes professionals from many disciplines to respond to the complex needs of the individual. Essential characteristics of specific approaches are identified in the following sections.

Medical Assessment. The focus of medical assessment is on identifying the impairment status of the individual and how the injury or disability affects the individual's functioning. Typically, the primary medical person in rehabilitation is a physiatrist, although with different disabilities a psychiatrist, psychologist, cardiologist, neurologist, or other specialist may be involved. Medical evaluations for qualified workers with a disability have assumed greater importance under the ADA. Assessment in employment decisions is used to establish whether there is a disability and to what extent the disability may represent a direct threat to the health or safety of the individual or coworkers. Medical findings that are used to demonstrate the existence of a disability and to make decisions regarding employability must be related to the person's ability to perform the essential function of a job. It is the responsibility of the physician to use information from a job analysis and, when appropriate, information from a work capacity evaluation.

Resources that discuss rehabilitation medical assessments include Walter Stolov and Michael Clowers (1981); Donna Falvo (1991); Myron G. Eisenberg et al. (1993); Steven J. Scheer (1991).

School-based Assessment. The role of evaluation for students with special needs has largely been diagnostic in focus and, less frequently, academically based. As a result of legislation (Individuals with Disabilities Education Act, Carl D. Perkins Act) emphasizing school-to-work transition, vocational-academic integration, and tech-prep curricula models, schools have an increased interest in functional assessment that facilitates planning and implementing transition to community, postsecondary education, and work. Assessment uses both school and community-based sites to explore a student's interests, develop an understanding of functional strengths, orient curriculum instruction around functional needs, and plan for placements after public school (Hursh & Kerns, 1989). Assessment activity is developmental in function, responding to the student's needs, interests, experiences, and goals as he or she transitions through middle school and high school to the community. Rehabilitation counselors, psychologists, speech therapists, occupational therapists, and learning specialists are used to assess students and support teachers.

Neuropsychological Assessment. Neuropsychological evaluation provides information on the relationship between how the brain functions and functional behaviors, usually in terms of the individual's cognitive, psychomotor, and perceptual processing skills. This evaluation is useful in the treatment and rehabilitation of individuals with head injury, learning disabilities, or when central nervous system involvement is suspected. Typically the evaluation is performed by a skilled neuropsychologist and consists of medical, academic, and work history review, individual and family interviews, and psychological and neuropsychological assessment. Although a wide battery of tests may be used, there is usually reliance on one of two neuropsychological test batteries: the Halstead-Reitan, a widely utilized and thoroughly validated battery, and the Luria-Nebraska, a more recent battery based on the pioneering work of Russian psychologist A. Luria. In addition, the McCarron-Dial Work Evaluation System is a neuropsychologically based battery that yields results reflecting the individual's work potential and suggested vocational placement levels.

The neuropsychologist should be able to discuss the vocational implications of a range of cognitive findings, including (Boll & Bryant, 1988; Uomoto, 1991):

- general neuropsychological functioning;
- sensory-motor integrity;
- attention and concentration;
- verbal and spatial memory;
- language and communication skills;
- complex problem-solving and abstract ideas processing

The primary goal of the neuropsychological evaluation is to understand the individual's ability to perform everyday activities, to perform job tasks, and to sustain effort on a task.

Ergonomic Evaluation. Ergonomics is the process of evaluating and adapting the motions, movements, body mechanics, and effort required in the use of tools, machines, and equipment within a specific work setting. Although ergonomics was developed to respond to work site characteristics, the principles can also be applied to the individual's home and living requirements. Ergonomic evaluation is both a prevention and a rehabilitation service that aims at eliminating or minimizing injuries, strains, sprains, and fatigue as well as maximizing safety, efficiency, comfort, and productivity (Mital, 1995; Mital, Nicholson, and Ayoub, 1993). As a prevention intervention, an ergonomic evaluation may identify work site repetitive force and stress factors contributing to cumulative trauma disorders and repetitive motion disorders such as carpal tunnel disorders or low back pain. As a rehabilitation process, the work station may be redesigned to fit the desk, telephone, computer, and filing system for someone with low vision. Ergonomic evaluation results may make recommendations about tool redesign, equipment modification, or organization of the workplace layout.

Functional Behavior Assessment. Assessment recognizes the benefits of observing and responding to the individual in actual environments in which he or she is expected to function, either at work, school, or home. Functional assessment uses observation and behavior rating forms in a criterion-referenced approach to assessment. Observations document the person and his or her skills as well as the characteristics of the environment that may support or prompt the behavior. In a behavior analysis approach, the evaluator considers the individual's behaviors and the means by which environmental supports, cues, or resources may be used to prompt and maintain performance. A benefit of this approach is that evaluation information can be applied to the site immediately to determine how it may impact on the person's activity. The focus of functional behavior assessment may range from cooking, budgeting, and personal hygiene to transportation, use of the community library, applied functional academics, and both avocational and vocational skills.

Useful checklists and behavior rating scales include the *Independent Living Behavior Checklist* (Walls, Zane, and Thvedt, 1979) and the *Functional Assessment Inventory* (Crewe & Athelstan, 1984).

Future Considerations

Disability legislation in the United States promotes access and opportunity in all aspects of society for more than 43 million people with disabilities. Advances in medical and rehabilitation practice improve the quality of life for an increasing number of individuals, including the older person with a disability, individuals with AIDS, adolescents with autism, minority and multicultural individuals with disabilities, and individuals who develop cumulative trauma disorders. The challenge for assessment is to develop methods and approaches that are responsive to the unique needs of an expanding population

base, to use developing technologies that promote effective and efficient assessment, and to access the expanding range of rehabilitation services. Assessment in rehabilitation, including each multidisciplinary specialization, must be conceptualized to contribute as an ongoing support to counseling, case management, placement, support, and maintenance interventions.

(*See also:* ASSISTIVE TECHNOLOGY; BEHAVIOR THERAPY; ERGONOMICS; EVALUATION OF REHABILITATION PROGRAMS; PSYCHOLOGY; PSYCHOSOCIAL ADJUSTMENT; REHABILITATION COUNSELING; VOCATIONAL EVALUATION)

BIBLIOGRAPHY

ANASTASI, ANNE. *Psychological Testing*, 6th ed. New York, 1987.

BOLL, THOMAS, and BRYANT, BRENDA K., eds. *Clinical Neuropsychology and Brain Function: Research, Measurement, and Practice.* Washington, DC, 1988.

COHEN, MIKAL; FARKAS, MARIANNE; COHEN, BARRY; and UNGER, KAREN. *Setting an Overall Rehabilitation Goal: Assessing Readiness.* Boston, 1989.

CREWE, NANCY M., and ATHELSTAN, GARY T. *Functional Assessment Inventory Manual.* Menomonie, WI, 1984.

CRONBACH, LEE. *Essentials of Psychological Testing*, 5th ed. New York, 1990.

EISENBERG, MYRON G.; GLUECKANF, ROBERT L.; and ZARETSKY, HERBERT H., eds. *Medical Aspects of Disability: A Handbook for the Rehabilitation Professional.* New York, 1993.

FALVO, DONNA F. *Medical and Psychosocial Aspects of Chronic Illness and Disability.* Gaithersburg, MD, 1991.

HURSH, NORMAN C. "Essential Skills in Industrial Rehabilitation and Disability Management: Implications for Rehabilitation Counselor Education." In *Principles and Practices of Disability Management*, eds. Donald E. Shrey and Michel Lacerte. Winter Park, FL, 1995.

HURSH, NORMAN C., and KERNS, ALLEN F. *Vocational Evaluation in Special Education.* Austin, TX, 1989.

MITAL, ANIL. "Ergonomics, Injury Prevention, and Disability Management." In *Principles and Practices of Disability Management*, eds. Donald E. Shrey and Michel Lacerte. Winter Park, FL, 1995.

MITAL, ANIL; NICHOLSON, ANDREW; and AYOUB, MOH. *A Guide to Manual Materials Handling.* Bristol, PA, 1993.

POWER, PAUL. *A Guide to Vocational Assessment*, 2nd ed. Austin, TX, 1991.

SCHEER, STEVEN J., ed. *Medical Perspectives in Vocational Assessment of Impaired Workers.* Gaithersburg, MD, 1991.

STOLOV, WALTER, and CLOWERS, MICHAEL. *Handbook of Severe Disabilities.* Washington, DC, 1981.

UOMOTO, JAY M. *The Neuropsychological Evaluation in Vocational Planning.* Orlando, FL, 1991.

WALLS, RICHARD; ZANE, T.; and THVEDT, J. *Independent Living Behavior Checklist.* Dunbar, WV, 1979.

NORMAN C. HURSH

ASSISTIVE TECHNOLOGY

Assistive technology, or "AT," has many definitions, usually dictated by the environment in which the technology is being applied. Due to the proliferation of many new types of affordable commercially available technologies, and a rapidly expanding interest in the phenomenon of applying these technologies to persons with special needs, occupationally related or population-based definitions have been formulated. For example, the rehabilitation profession has traditionally referenced the provision of technologically based services as rehabilitation engineering. Occupational therapy may use the description of compensatory devices, emphasizing the fact that the assistance is being provided to an area of function that is impaired.

Perhaps the most inclusive definition of AT is found in the Technology Related Assistance for Individuals with Disabilities Act of 1988, and is as follows:

"Assistive technology device: Any item, piece of equipment, or product system, whether acquired commercially off the shelf, modified, or customized, that is used to increase, maintain, or improve functional capabilities of individuals with disabilities.

"Assistive technology service: Any service that directly assists an individual with a disability in the selection, acquisition, or use of an assistive technology device."

This law provides examples of this definition, including:

A. the evaluation of the needs of an individual with a disability, including a functional evaluation of the individual's customary environment;

B. purchasing, leasing, or otherwise providing for the acquisition of assistive technology devices by individuals with disabilities;

C. selecting, designing, fitting, customizing, adapting, applying, maintaining, repairing, or replacing of assistive technology devices;

D. coordinating and using other therapies, interventions, or services with assistive technology devices, such as those associated with existing education and rehabilitation plans and programs;

E. training or technical assistance for an individual with disabilities, or, where appropriate, the family of an individual with disabilities; and

F. training or technical assistance for professionals (including individuals providing education and rehabilitation services), employers, or other individuals who provide services to, employ, or are otherwise substantially involved in the major life functions of individuals with disabilities.

The term "assistive technology" is often used in conjunction with "adaptive technology" or "special education and rehabilitation technology." While these terms may have similar connotations, assistive technology is more far-reaching and, as is described above, involves both the process and the product of the provided assistance.

It is necessary to distinguish between "mainstream technology" and "assistive technology." It is quite possible that these two terms could represent the same definition. The term "technology" is often synonymous with the most recent developments in a particular field, such as computers, electronics, or medicine. A typical user of technology is looking to accomplish a specific task or tasks. Technology may also be synonymous with "improvement" or "progress" and, as such, may connote an improved way of performing tasks. For example, use of a word processing program with spell checking, grammar correction, and outline functions on a microcomputer is certainly an improvement over use of a manual typewriter. This is particularly evident in the area of editing, whereby final perfect copies are not generated on paper until all attributes of the project are perfect, including grammar and spelling. The person using the computer-based word processor is certainly benefiting from this technology, spending less time on a project, and being more efficient with his or her other resources. This word processor is not necessarily functioning as assistive technology for the user, since the user may indeed have other options available, including use of a manual typewriter, use of paper and pen, or the ability to dictate the project for someone else to generate on paper. If, however, the user of the word processor has a severe physical disability, and accesses the computer by a modified keyboard, or perhaps through an eye-gaze tracking system, then the word processor is a crucial component of the overall assistive technology system. The technology, the word processor, was not created specifically for use by persons with disabilities, but rather for the larger population of people without disabilities who need to complete printed documents quickly and accurately. It becomes assistive technology only when it is applied to the specialized needs of a person with a disability who may have no alternative way of efficiently completing the task at hand.

Fundamentals

Many of the newest specialized assistive technology devices and processes can be directly attributed to advancements in the mainstream of technology. This might include such items as infrared remote control systems, voice-activated appliances, and even fax machines. While each of these technologies serves the general population, there are specific unintended applications that can address specific needs of an individual with a disability. The infrared remote control system can be used by a person with a mobility impairment who wishes to control electronic components within his or her home. This could include television, security systems, or an entertainment system. Voice-activated appliances, while developed to enable the mainstream of society to control specific devices through the most commonly used interface, the voice, can nonetheless also be used by individuals with disabilities that prevent them from operating devices that require fine motor control. Finally, the popular fax machine, the fast and convenient method for sending copies of information anywhere in the world, allows persons with many types of disabilities to send and receive printed information without having to leave their home, or their home work station.

Other types of assistive technology are designed, fabricated, and integrated into specialized areas from the moment of inception. This is true since there are many needs of persons with disabilities that simply cannot be addressed by available, off-the-shelf, mainstream devices. Many popular types of assistive technology devices and processes, while not products designed for the mainstream, are derived from portions of technologies or processes used in the mainstream and are adapted to serve the needs of a particular group with a disability. An example would be the newer and stronger lightweight materials that can be used to construct wheelchairs or even artificial limbs. Specialists in the field of assistive technology have available to them an unending source of potential resources to use during the problem-solving process, as many new mainstream technologies hold unintended applications for persons with disabilities.

Assistive technology has been described as both a process and a product. In general, an assistive device can be synonymous with the word "tool," as a tool is functional only in the hands of a skilled user. As a further expansion on the analogy with tools, assistive technology solutions are often as volatile as tools. It is possible that several different tools may provide the same desired results, but there are other instances where the most efficient tool is the only one that can actually complete the job. Knowing, therefore, that assistive technology allows for the same degree of volatility, it is possible that a solution that is less than the best can be chosen for an individual and be deemed effective. Because of the variability that can exist among possible solutions, it is crucial that a method of measuring impact be in place.

Assistive technology runs the spectrum from low tech to high tech. "Low" and "high" are not necessarily synonymous with "inexpensive" and "costly," respectively. Likewise, they are not the same as "traditional" and "advanced." These descriptors may be more akin to "simple" and "complex." A solution can be simple but still be expensive. Likewise, a solution can be complex but can be very inexpensive to secure. Regardless of which descriptive category holds the appropriate solution, assistive technology can range from the horizontal handle that is attached to a round doorknob to allow for operation by a person with poor hand dexterity or strength, to a computer system controlled by speech activation that allows the user to complete educational assignments, control the telephone, the environment, and that person's wheelchair. In both instances, the technology functions in an assistive mode to allow the individual to complete a task independently. In these particular examples, there are numerous other differences among the solutions, including the cost, the amount of time involved in the problem-solving process, the immediacy of the impact of the solution, and the type of professionals involved. While these differences do exist, it is not possible to weigh the benefits of the outcome. If applied to the same case, a person with a severe physical disability would now be capable of entering a room where he or she could then access an adaptive computer system.

Legislation

The issues involved in the provision of AT, while launched by the simple availability of many new forms of low-cost and effective technologies, have also been greatly influenced by key legislation. The 1986 Amendments to the Rehabilitation Act of 1973 provide for the first time a definition of rehabilitation engineering, to include a range of services and devices that can supplement and enhance individual functions. States were required to describe their plan on how rehabilitation technology services would be provided to assist an increasing number of individuals with disabilities. The Rehabilitation Act Amendments of 1992 contain much more specific expectations regarding the provision of rehabilitation technology to eligible individuals. Congress elected to use the term "rehabilitation technology" to reflect all activities previously incorporated under the term "rehabilitation engineering," and clarified that the term includes assistive technology devices and assistive technology services (Senate Report 102-357, p. 17). Furthermore, Congress specified that "in terms of rehabilitation technology, the Individualized Written Rehabilitation Plan (IWRP) should provide for regular and periodic assessments to ensure that a match exists between the supports, the technology, and the current and changing needs of the individual who will be using the technology, as well as other people involved in the provision of services who require the information" (Senate Report 102-357, p. 39).

Further significance was granted the subject of assistive technology with the passage of the Technology-Related Assistance Act for Persons with Disabilities in 1988. This federal mandate provided financial assistance to states on a competitive grant basis, to plan and implement a consumer-responsive system of technology services for individuals of all ages with disability. Technology services and devices were defined in a broad context to stimulate creative problem-solving, interagency coordination, and professional consumer collaboration. Unlike already existing public programs, this federal initiative represented the first time Congress targeted new public resources exclusively to expand access to assistive technology.

The Americans with Disabilities Act (ADA), signed into law by President Bush on July 26, 1990, protects more than 43 million Americans with disabilities from discrimination in employment, public services, transportation, public accommodations, and telecommunications. Each title of the act specifically references assistive technology equipment or devices as means to achieve access and equal opportunity. In Titles I and III, the purchase or modification of equipment and devices is included within the definition of "reasonable accommodation." However, the removal of architectural, physical, or communication barriers, through "reasonable accommodation," is not an absolute civil right. Title IV of the ADA expands access rights to the important area of telecommunications. Telephone services offered to the public in every state must include interstate and intrastate telecommunications relay services so that these services provide individuals with speech and hearing impairments access to communications equivalent to those provided to individuals able to use voice telephone systems.

In a policy letter from the Office of Special Education Programs on August 10, 1990, the Office of Special Education Programs director, Dr. Judy Schrag, clarified the rights of children with disabilities to access assistive technology. This policy letter states clearly and unequivocally that assistive technology services and devices may be considered special education, related services, or supplementary aids and services to enable a student with a disability to remain in the regular education classroom. Assistive technology needs must be considered when developing a child's individualized education program (IEP).

The Individuals with Disabilities Education Act (IDEA) for the first time includes definitions of assistive technology devices and services identical to those included in the TECH Act.

Measurement of Outcome

Measuring the impact of assistive technology is often a difficult task. Methods of reporting impact vary tremendously, but most rely on subjective reporting from the end user in terms of general satisfaction with the device or the process. Despite increasing emphasis on assistive technology for persons with disabilities, including legislation and consumer demands, and despite documentation of some highly effective outcomes in specific case study situations, there is not a large volume of data available supporting objective outcomes on a widespread basis. Lack of supportive data can be interpreted in one of two ways. First, it could be assumed that the widespread application of assistive technology is not effective to the point of being measurable. Second, it could be assumed that the results of assistive technology applications are conjectured—that is, that the provision of any type of device or service, regardless of the degree of improvement demonstrated in outcome, is, in and of itself, a successful application.

Assistive technology can have a major impact on the lives of people with disabilities, enabling them to capitalize on their abilities and minimize the effect of their disabilities. Assistive technology does not necessarily eliminate the disability, but it can act as an intermediary to allow the person with a disability to increase his or her functioning, independence, and ability to utilize fully the capabilities that are limited or not affected by specific disability. Assistive technology should be considered in all aspects of the lives of a person with a disability. Traditionally, professionals involved in an individual case will address the issues pertinent to that professional, the facility they represent, the profession they represent, the funding source they represent, or the type of agency they represent. As such, the problems identified and for which solutions are found may be quite focused. For instance, a specialist in vocational rehabilitation may identify assistive technology that can enable a person with a disability to perform more independently on the job. Whatever the limiting factors of the disability, they will be present not only on the job but also in school, in the home, and in places of public access. It is important that the needs of individuals with disabilities be considered in light of all of the environments in which they will come in contact. Assistive technologies can be chosen that will be functional across environments, but there are cases where the need specified in one environment, perhaps as part of an independent living solution, would not have an impact or play a role in any other environment.

Nearly all professional organizations responsible for providing services to persons with disabilities have a personal investment in assistive technology. By simply lessening the impact of one's disability, a professional is able to increase that person's independence and promote success in whatever type of program involved.

Sources of Assistive Technology

Provision of assistive technology is a very individualized process, and care should be taken not to prescribe solutions based on single factors, such as diagnosis or age of the targeted user. Factors which should be considered in the prescription of assistive technology generally include: (1) characteristics of the person (user); (2) characteristics of the environment; and (3) characteristics of the task to be performed. While some forms of assistive technology are generic in application for the given individual—for instance, a magnification lens that can be used in multiple environments for many different types of print—others are much more specific, such as the automatic page turner that will be used for a specific type of document (looseleaf binder paper) and involve a specific task (looking up phone numbers or other types of corresponding codes).

Assistive technology is appropriate for nearly all types of disabilities, ranging from physical disabilities that limit mobility or manipulation of one's environment, to sensory disabilities that result in a need for alternative modalities of information and communication. Individuals with specific learning disabilities can be aided through appropriate applications of assistive technology that, while not removing the impairment to the learning process, can enable the person to perform the same tasks as the population without learning impairment. A simple example of such a concept would be use of a calculator or a cash register to perform math functions required on a job but for which an individual with a learning disability would experience difficulties.

The proliferation of assistive technologies may solve one problem for persons with disabilities, but it can create another. Competing solutions, products, devices, or processes can make decision-making difficult and complex. A wide range of professionals can be involved in the provision of assistive technology services. There is tremendous opportunity for conflicts in the prescription process.

Historically, assistive technology may have been more the domain of occupational therapists, physical therapists, and rehabilitation engineers. The multiplicity of today's technology, ranging from simple low-tech devices to very complex microcomputer systems and related peripherals, has resulted in the diversification of individual professionals involved in this process. Colleges and universities have created programs and degrees in the area of assistive technology, with some programs focusing on special education while others specialize in rehabilitation applications of technology. In terms of service delivery mechanism, legislation has focused much attention on state vocational rehabilitation agencies and local school systems to act as central points for assistive technology services. As a result, a popular model of service delivery during the early 1990s was a centralized model, where a team of professionals collaborate on individual cases. Such teams include occupational therapists, physical therapists, speech and language specialists, rehabilitation technologists, special education teachers and resource personnel, significant others, and the person in need of the assistive technology. As a team operating from a centralized facility, it is possible to respond in a time-efficient manner to identified needs by designating resources, devices, or processes that can be used on a trial basis. Such a model eliminates, or significantly reduces, the time between evaluation and the actual fitting of the assistive technology.

In summary, assistive technology is a product and a process, with the common denominator of im-proving the functioning of persons with disabilities by decreasing their dependence in the completion of vital tasks. The application of assistive technology can benefit the user personally, educationally, vocationally, or in all three areas. The provision of assistive technology is a dynamic process, as emerging technologies provide new resources for application and as improvement experienced through the use of initial assistive technology leads to a need for additional technology to continue the growth process.

(See also: AMERICANS WITH DISABILITIES ACT; COMPUTER APPLICATIONS FOR VISUAL DISABILITIES; COMPUTERS; ERGONOMICS; OCCUPATIONAL THERAPY; REASONABLE ACCOMMODATION; REHABILITATION ENGINEERING; SPECIAL EDUCATION; TECHNOLOGY AND DISABILITY; WORK)

RESOURCES

ABLEDATA Database Program, Macro International, 8455 Colesville Rd, Suite 935, Silver Spring, MD 20910–3319

American Foundation for the Blind, National Technology Center, 15 West 16th St., New York, NY 10011

Apple Computer, Inc., Worldwide Disability Solutions Group, Mail Stop 38DS, 1 Infinite Loop, Cupertino, CA 95014

Applications of Technology to the Rehabilitation of Children with Orthopedic Disabilities, Rancho Los Amigos Medical Center, 7503 Bonita St., Bonita Hall, Downey, CA 90242

Association for Retarded Citizens (ARC) of the United States, Bioengineering Program, 2501 Ave. J, Arlington, TX 76011

AT&T Accessible Communications Products Center (ACPC), 14250 Clayton Rd, Ballwin, MO 63011

Cerebral Palsy Center, Griggs-Midway Building, 1821 University Ave., St. Paul, MN 55104

Electronic Industries Association, Assistive Devices Division (EIA/ADD), 1901 Pennsylvania Ave., NW, Washington, DC 20006

ERIC Clearinghouse on Handicapped and Gifted Children, c/o The Council for Exceptional Children (CEC), 1920 Association Drive, Reston, VA 22091

Health Resource Center, National Clearinghouse on Postsecondary Education for Handicapped Individuals, One Dupont Circle NW, Suite 800, Washington, DC 20036-1193

IBM National Support Center for Persons with Disabilities, P.O. Box 2150, Atlanta, GA 30055 and 2500 Windy Ridge Parkway, Marietta, GA 30067

Library of Congress, National Library Service for the Blind and Physically Handicapped, Washington, DC 20542

BIBLIOGRAPHY

BORDEN, PETER A. *Meeting the Needs of Employees with Disabilities.* Lexington, MA, 1993.

COOK, ALBERT M., and HUSSEY, SUSAN M. *Assistive Technologies: Principles and Practice.* St. Louis, MO, 1995.

CORTHELL, DAVID W., and THAYER, TED. *Rehabilitation Technologies.* Little Rock, AR, 1986.

COSTON, CAROLINE A. *Planning and Implementing Augmentative Communication Service Delivery. Proceedings of the National Planners' Conference on Assistive Device Service Delivery.* Washington, DC, 1988.

ENDERS, ALEXANDRIA, and HALL, MARIAN. *Assistive Technology Sourcebook.* Washington, DC, 1990.

FATHERLY, SARAH; FORD, KELLEY; and VANDERHEIDEN, GREGG C., eds. *Trace Resourcebook: Assistive Technologies for Communication, Control and Computer Access.* Madison, WI, 1993.

LAZZARO, JOSEPH J. *Adaptive Technologies for Learning and Work Environments.* Chicago, 1993.

MANN, WILLIAM C., and LANE, JOSEPH P. *Assistive Technology for Persons with Disabilities: The Role of Occupational Therapy.* Rockville, MD, 1991.

PERLMAN, LEONARD G., and AUSTIN, GARY F. *Technology and Rehabilitation of Disabled Persons in the Information Age.* Alexandria, VA, 1984.

STEEL, RICHARD D., ed. "Augmentative and Alternative Communication." In *Presentations at the RESNA 12th Annual Conference & USSAAC First National Conference, New Orleans, LA.* Washington, DC, 1989.

TOBIAS, JIM, and WOODS, DIANE E., eds. *Volunteer Rehabilitation Technology: International Perspectives and Possibilities.* New York, 1988.

BUD RIZER

ATTENDANT CARE

See PERSONAL ASSISTANCE SERVICES

ATTENTION DEFICIT DISORDERS

See CHILDHOOD PSYCHIATRIC DISORDERS; LEARNING DISABILITIES

ATTITUDES

Attitudes toward people with disabilities influence the ways that others interact with them. Attitudes toward people with disabilities are quite different from attitudes toward the disabilities themselves. People often have positive attitudes toward those who are blind, but negative attitudes toward blindness and a fear of becoming blind.

Positive attitudes toward people with disabilities usually result in warm feelings and positive behavior and interactions. Negative attitudes usually result in bias and discrimination. Negative societal attitudes result in the erection of barriers that prevent people with disabilities from participating in society. Such barriers can restrict participation in education, employment, housing, transportation, and social and leisure time activities. These barriers and discriminatory behavior can be reduced or eliminated through legislation. Although laws may not change attitudes, they do affect behaviors, which often, over time, have an effect on attitudes.

Positive and negative attitudes toward people with disabilities are relatively obvious and easily described, but ambivalent attitudes are more complex (Katz, Hass, and Bailey, 1988). On the one hand there are negative feelings such as aversion, dislike, or hostility; on the other hand there can be feelings of liking, sympathy, or compassion. This is demonstrated in the attitudes of some members of families that include children with disabilities. There may be positive attitudes of love, compassion, and caring as well as negative attitudes of rejection or resentment. As a consequence of this ambivalence, overt verbalized expressions of attitudes toward people with disabilities are often positive, while negative feelings of rejection tend not to be expressed in public.

Attitudes toward people with disabilities are influenced by several types of variables. One set of variables relates to the perceived characteristics of the person with a disability. These perceptions are influenced by the amount and content of information the perceiver has about such people, which in turn is influenced by the amount and type of contact that person has had with them. Contact is a function of role and status variables. Important role relationships of people with and without disabilities include parent, rehabilitator, teacher, and friend. In addition, attitudes can be influenced by the personal characteristics of the individual without disabilities and the attitudinal norms prevalent in the environment.

The extent of the relationship between attitudes and behavior depends to a large degree on how each variable is measured. The correlation is highest if it involves a specific behavior and the attitudes toward that specific behavior. The relationship tends to be low to moderate when both measures are general rather than specific. It is usually very low when it involves a general measure; that is, overall attitudes toward people with disabilities, and a specific behavior such as willingness to teach retarded children (Ajzen & Fishbein, 1977).

Characteristics That Influence Attitudes

Attitudes toward people with disabilities are a function of their perceived characteristics and the way these characteristics are evaluated. Both disability-related and general characteristics of the person with the disability are influential. The perception and evaluation of characteristics often changes as a result of extended contact between the perceiver and the person with the disability.

Those who believe that people with disabilities are different, incompetent, inferior, and/or have negative characteristics tend to have negative attitudes. Many studies have shown this to be true both for people in general and for groups such as teachers (Hannah, 1988) and hospital and treatment personnel (Rabkin, 1972; Wills, 1978). In addition, people who believe that disability is a major characteristic of individuals with disabilities tend to exhibit negative biases (Wright, 1988). In contrast, believing that such individuals can be competent, that they are similar to people without disabilities, and that special skills or training are not necessary for interacting with or teaching them tends to be associated with positive attitudes.

Initial attitudes toward individuals with disabilities often are influenced by disability-related characteristics, such as the type of disability and its severity, visibility, origin, and prognosis. In later interaction the disability characteristics, like other external characteristics of an individual, become less

important, while personal characteristics and behavior become more so.

In initial impressions and reactions to disability labels, some disabilities are evaluated more positively than others. People with disabilities such as asthma, diabetes, and heart disease are acceptable in most situations. Those with disabilities such as cerebral palsy, mental illness, and mental retardation are often avoided. But many disabilities are acceptable in some role relationships and not in others; that is, the degree of acceptance tends to vary according to whether an interaction is educational, employment-related, treatment-related, or social. Blind people, for instance, tend to be acceptable socially but are often considered unemployable.

If people with disabilities have a positive attitude toward their disability (as reflected in self-acceptance and disability acknowledgment), this often has a positive effect on the attitudes of others toward them. When most of the non-disability-related attitudes of individuals with disabilities are similar to those of the people with whom they are interacting, this, too can result in positive attitudes. In addition, people with disabilities who have good social skills are generally positively evaluated by others.

Labels sometimes influence the way people are perceived, although the conditions under which labels have either positive or negative influences on attitudes have not been determined. Labels probably have the most influence on people who have little information about or contact with people with disabilities because such people tend to have stereotyped perceptions based on the label.

Information and Contact

Although the amount and content of information about people with disabilities can affect attitudes, few studies have investigated the specific types of information that have positive or negative effects (Shaver et al., 1989). Information about disabilities probably has little effect, whereas information about people with disabilities can have positive or negative effects, depending on the content of the information and whether it results in stereotyping or individuation. Often information doesn't change attitudes. Mass media presentations probably influence attitudes only when they provide pertinent new information. Like labels, they primarily influence people with minimal prior information about people with disabilities.

The effect of contact with people who are perceived as disabled depends on variables such as the characteristics of both the person with the disability and the person without a disability, the role relationship between the two, and the types of interactions that occur. The data indicate that for contact to result in positive attitudes, the person with the disability should be perceived as competent, likable, able to communicate successfully, and accepting of his or her disability (Yuker, 1988). In addition, for positive attitudes to result, the person without disability should be free of negative beliefs; that is, such beliefs as that the most important characteristic of a person with a disability is the disability or that people with disabilities are different, incompetent, inferior, and/or have other negative characteristics.

Interaction that is personal, rewarding, and characterized by cooperation, intimacy, and equal status (e.g., friendship) usually provides positive information and tends to result in positive attitudes (Yuker, 1988). Interaction that spotlights either the disability (e.g., in medical or rehabilitation settings) or negative behavioral or personal characteristics often results in negative attitudes (Wright, 1988; Yuker & Block, 1986).

It often has been asserted that information and contact together are more effective in bringing about attitude change than either variable by itself. Such assertions ignore the fact that contact provides information. Unfortunately, the type of information provided by contact seems never to have been studied systematically, even though such research could help explain the varying effects of contact on attitudes.

Attitudes of Various Groups

The attitudes of group members are influenced by the kinds of individual characteristics discussed above, most particularly by the amount and type of contact and information they have about people with disabilities. Group attitudes are also influenced by the status and role relationships of the interacting

individuals and the ways in which they enact their roles. These variables help to account for the differences between the attitudes that are "typical" of family members, friends, neighbors, teachers, rehabilitation personnel, employers, and others. The following evaluations of the attitudes of various groups are simply summary descriptions of presumably typical attitudes. In real life there are often large differences in the attitudes of members of the same group as a consequence of different past experiences.

Friends. The attitudes of people who are close friends of one or more people with disabilities are usually more positive than those of any other group. There are various degrees of friendship. While a casual acquaintanceship may increase rather than dispel prejudice, a sustained relationship tends to lessen prejudice (Allport, 1954). Friendship is strongly influenced by similar views regarding favorite activities, likes, dislikes, values, and so forth.

Family Members. Attitudes of family members often are ambivalent. These attitudes are influenced by the ways in which the characteristics of the individual with the disability affect the other family members, evoking either positive reactions such as love and empathy or negative reactions such as annoyance, anger, and even disgust. Factors such as the disabled person's responsiveness, need for care, intelligence, and general ability level have been shown to be important. Some family members are concerned about their ability to provide adequate care and supervision, and they worry about the future of the individual with the disability.

Teachers. The effects of occupational contact (e.g., the contact of people working in fields such as education or health) are complex. Differences among occupations arise because different personal attributes are valued in different role relationships. The attitudes of teachers, for example, are influenced by characteristics of the child that influence his or her teachability and classroom behavior, such as academic performance, compliance, and misbehavior. Positive attitudes tend to be held by regular and special education teachers who have had positive contact with children with disabilities, teachers who believe they are competent to relate to and teach such children, and teachers who believe they have support personnel available.

Health Workers. The attitudes of many people in medical and rehabilitation occupations toward individuals who are sick or disabled often are negative (see the literature reviews by Wills, 1978; Wright, 1988; Yuker & Block, 1986). Many people in these occupations make personal attributions that blame and devalue their clients and tend to emphasize negative rather than positive characteristics. People in these occupations tend to value clients who exhibit characteristics such as manageability, treatability, likability, and rehabilitation motivation.

Employers and Coworkers. The attitudes of employers reflect the effects of information and contact. Employers who have experience with employees with disabilities usually have positive attitudes, particularly toward those with the types of disabilities that are familiar to them. The data indicate that employers seek and value characteristics such as job skills, dependability, and social skills and are willing to employ people with disabilities perceived as having these characteristics. Although their perceptions may be negatively influenced by their preconceptions about the characteristics of people with disabilities, the preconceptions can be changed by experience with employees who are disabled. The attitudes of fellow workers reflect their perceptions of the working behavior of people with disabilities as well as their prior information and contact. Their attitudes are positive toward fellow workers with disabilities who are competent, cooperative, and friendly.

Children. Studies of the attitudes of children without disabilities show they are strongly influenced by the type and amount of interaction they have had with children with disabilities. This depends, in part, on the location and status of the children with disabilities within a school. Obviously, if there are no students with disabilities in the school, there is no interaction. If such students spend all or most of their time in segregated classrooms, there is minimal interaction, particularly if they come to school in separate buses. If the students with disabilities spend some or all of their time in integrated classes, the effects are usually positive. The type and amount of interaction, and the resulting attitudes of the children, also are influenced by the attitudes of teachers and the way that classroom activities are structured. Mainstreaming often results in positive attitudes. However, there seldom is a carryover of these attitudes from one setting to another. Friendships at school often are not reflected in out-of-school activities.

Based on their review of sociometric research, Macmillan and Morrison (1984) concluded that acceptance of children with disabilities is related to their personal characteristics and behavior more than to their disability characteristics. Children tend to like peers who exhibit athletic or game skills, are easy to get along with, show academic competence, and do not misbehave. The situation is also important. Children with disabilities may be accepted in play situations where specific physical skills are valued more than academic abilities. The attitudes of children usually are influenced by those of their teachers, peers, and parents.

Neighbors. Finally, the attitudes of neighbors toward people with disabilities appear to be primarily influenced by characteristics such as friendliness, social skills, and lack of aggressive behavior. Physical proximity and accessibility can promote either positive or negative attitudes, depending on other variables. A significant social issue exists with respect to the attitudes of neighbors toward community homes for people with various types of disabilities. The data indicate that there is often initial community opposition, which may take the form of zoning changes or licensing requirements, court actions, petitions, and even firebombings. The extent of opposition varies with the type of disability and the personal characteristics of the neighbors. The most opposition is shown to drug addicts, followed by alcoholics, with less opposition shown to mentally retarded, terminally ill, physically handicapped, and elderly people. The opposition usually dies out after the facility has been established.

Norms. Although attitudes are largely a function of the variables of contact, information, and role characteristics, they are also influenced by attitudinal norms prevalent in the local and national environments. The attitudes of significant others—people one listens to and whose opinions one respects—provide information that may significantly influence one's own attitudes. Each of the groups discussed above provides a set of norms for its members. If there is convergence among the norms of several groups of significant others, they can be particularly influential.

In addition to the norms of local groups such as these, larger societal norms as reflected in laws, regulations, and statements by public figures also can be quite influential. The increasingly positive acceptance of people with disabilities in the United States can undoubtedly be attributed in part to the passage of nondiscrimination laws and laws guaranteeing equal treatment in education and employment. These laws have also resulted in additional opportunities for equal status contact, which frequently leads to positive attitudes.

Nondisabled Persons

The relationship between the individual characteristics of people without disabilities and their attitudes toward people with them has been extensively studied. Many variables that have been examined yielded low correlations with attitudes. Thus, variables such as the following often are minor influences on attitudes toward people with disabilities. Relatively more important is past experience as reflected in variables such as information and contact.

Demographic Variables. Several demographic characteristics of people without disabilities, including age and socioeconomic status, have low correlations with their attitudes toward people with disabilities. On the other hand, characteristics such as occupation, gender, education, and national and cultural values can influence attitudes. Occupation was discussed above. In the past, more studies reported that in the United States women had more positive attitudes than men, but the gender difference seems to be diminishing. Years of education yield a moderately low average correlation of about .20 (Yuker & Block, 1986).

Personality Variables. The psychological and personality characteristics of people without disabilities mostly show very low correlations to attitude toward people with disabilities. For about fifty different personality variables, the highest average correlations are about .20, indicating only 4 percent explained variance (Yuker & Block, 1986).

National and Cultural Values. These can be important influences on attitudes toward people with disabilities, although there are large individual differences within cultures. There are national differences based on gender—in some countries (e.g., Greece and Israel) men have more positive attitudes than women—and attitudes toward people disabled in war are more positive than attitudes toward those disabled in other ways. Differences in attitudes among religions have been documented based on their views of the origin of the disabilities (e.g., as a punishment for sins). Overall, the United States is probably the country that is most accepting of disabilities although there are differences among its various cultural and ethnic groups.

Attitude Measurement and Attitude Measures

Attitudes can be measured by attitude scales, interviews, adjective checklists, semantic differential scales, social distance scales, and sociometric measures. Attitude scales are often preferred to other types of measures. Between 1959 and 1964 some important scales for measuring attitudes toward people with disabilities were developed that were still being used in the early 1990s. They include the Attitudes Toward Disabled Persons scale (ATDP), the Disability Factor scales (DFS-G), and the Opinions about Mental Illness scale (OMI). Each of these scales is both reliable and valid and has been used in many studies since its development. New instruments, including multivariate scales, have also been developed.

Many instruments are described and reproduced in a book by Antonak and Livneh (1988). It includes scales for measuring general attitudes toward people with disabilities, people with mental illness, mental retardation, and mainstreaming, as well as scales for measuring attitudes toward blindness, deafness, and epilepsy. The description of each scale includes data pertaining to its administration, scoring, reliability, and validity. In addition, copies of most scales are supplied. There are also recommendations, the most important of which are that researchers should refine or update previous measures rather than create new ones and that multidimensional scales should be used. Some people (e.g., Soder, 1990), however, are critical of all measurement procedures in use.

Attitude Change

Like most salient attitudes, those toward people with disabilities are hard to change. Although there have been hundreds of studies of attempts to change attitudes toward people with disabilities, most have been unsuccessful. They have yielded small to moderate effect sizes. A comprehensive meta analysis of 273 studies by Shaver et al. (1989) yielded an average effect size of .37 (small to moderate), and 23 percent of the studies had negative effects on attitudes. Much of the research was of poor quality. The conclusion of Shaver et al. was disappointing: The data failed to indicate which procedures are most effective. There is a need for better-designed research studies and for replication of single studies that seem to be effective in modifying attitudes.

(*See also:* ACCESSIBILITY; CONSUMERS; PSYCHOSOCIAL ADJUSTMENT; SELF-CONCEPT)

BIBLIOGRAPHY

AJZEN, I., and FISHBEIN, M. "Attitude-Behavior Relations: A Theoretical Analysis and Review of Empirical Research." *Psychological Bulletin* 84 (1977):888–918.

ALLPORT, G. W. *The Nature of Prejudice.* Reading, MA, 1954.

ANTONAK, R. F., and LIVNEH, H. *The Measurement of Attitudes Toward People with Disabilities.* Springfield, IL, 1988.

HANNAH, MARY ELIZABETH. "Teacher Attitudes Toward Children with Disabilities: An Ecological Analysis." In *Attitudes Toward Persons with Disabilities,* ed. Harold E. Yuker. New York, 1988.

HORNE, M. D. *Attitudes Toward Handicapped Students: Professional, Peer and Parent Reactions.* Hillsdale, NJ, 1985.

KATZ, I.; HASS, R. G.; and BAILEY, J. "Attitudinal Ambivalence and Behavior Toward People with Disabilities." In *Attitudes Toward Persons with Disabilities,* ed. Harold E. Yuker. New York, 1988.

MACMILLAN, D. L., and MORRISON, G. M. "Sociometric Research in Special Education." *Attitude and Attitude Change in Special Education: Theory and Practice,* ed. R. L. Jones. Reston, VA, 1984.

RABKIN, J. G. "Opinions about Mental Illness: A Review of the Literature." *Psychological Bulletin* 77 (1972):153–171.

SHAVER, J. P.; CURTIS, C. K.; JESUNATHADAS, J.; and STRONG, C. J. "The Modification of Attitudes Toward Persons with Disabilities: Is There a Best Way?" *International Journal of Special Education* 4 (1989):33–57.

SODER, M. "Prejudice or Ambivalence? Attitudes Toward Persons with Disabilities." *Disability, Handicap, and Society* 5 (1990):227–241.

WILLS, T. A. "Perceptions of Clients by Professional Helpers." *Psychological Bulletin* 85 (1978):968–1000.

WRIGHT, B. A. "Attitudes and the Fundamental Negative Bias: Conditions and Corrections." In *Attitudes toward Persons with Disabilities,* ed. Harold E. Yuker. New York, 1988.

YUKER, H. E. "The Effects of Contact on Attitudes Toward Disabled Persons: Some Empirical Generalizations." In *Attitudes Toward Persons with Disabilities,* ed. Harold E. Yuker. New York, 1988.

YUKER, H. E., and BLOCK, J. R. *Research with the Attitude Toward Disabled Persons Scales: 1960–1985.* Hempstead, NY, 1986.

HAROLD E. YUKER

AUDIOLOGY

Audiology is a health-related profession concerned with the diagnosis, remediation, and prevention of hearing impairment. A practitioner in the field of audiology is referred to as an audiologist.

In the United States an audiologist must be certified by the American Speech-Language and Hearing Association (ASHA). This certification is recognized by the award of a certificate of clinical competence in audiology (CCC-A). Certification is awarded once the applicant has received a master's degree (or equivalent) in audiology, passed a national certification examination, and completed a clinical fellowship year (CFY). Academic requirements for certification include courses in the anatomy and physiology of the speech and hearing mechanism, the perception of sound, auditory pathology, auditory habilitation/rehabilitation, and hearing testing. Graduate students of audiology must engage in a clinical practicum to develop their clinical skills via supervised experience.

The responsibilities of an audiologist fall into three categories: diagnosis, remediation, and prevention. Diagnosis involves the identification of hearing impairment and site-of-lesion testing. Identification of hearing impairment requires quantification of the magnitude of hearing loss, which is recorded on an audiogram. To obtain an audiogram, the audiologist places earphones on a person's ears and asks him or her to indicate when he or she is able to hear a tone presented to one of the ears. The level at which a tone is just barely audible is called a hearing threshold. The audiogram plots hearing thresholds for each ear across several tone frequencies (pitch levels). In this way a person's hearing is classified as ranging from within normal limits ("normal hearing") to profoundly impaired ("deaf"). Also of interest is the pattern of hearing loss. For example, a person might have an equal amount of hearing loss across frequencies, which would be called a "flat" hearing loss, or more of a loss in the high frequencies (high pitches), which is termed a high-frequency hearing loss. The magnitude and pattern of hearing loss can provide clues to the etiology of the hearing loss, in addition to giving information about the person's receptive auditory abilities. However, the audiogram provides only information about the sound levels necessary for tones to become audible; it does not address the clarity of the signal. Speech discrimination tests use speech stimuli to determine how well the person can understand speech. Since humans have a highly developed linguistic system, and the auditory channel is the most common mode of speech reception in everyday communicative situations, the speech discrimination test gives a measure of an individual's speech reception abilities.

Site-of-lesion testing seeks an answer to the question, "Where in the auditory pathway is the abnormality?" Traditionally abnormalities are divided into three categories: (1) outer and middle ear ("conductive"); (2) inner ear ("sensory"); and (3) eighth nerve or central nervous system ("retrocochlear"). A battery of tests is available to identify the site of lesion. Pure tone testing as recorded on an audiogram is useful for this purpose as are speech discrimination tests. There are a number of tests which, unlike audiograms and speech discrimination tests, do not require behavioral responses. Acoustic impedance tests involve the measurement of sound reflected off the eardrum. In people with conductive loss due to fluid in the middle ear (e.g., children with a middle-ear infection), more sound bounces off the eardrum than in people with no middle-ear

fluid. Electrical responses from the brain can be recorded with electrodes taped to the scalp. One of these responses is called the brainstem auditory evoked response (BAER). The BAER is useful in separating cochlear (sensory) hearing loss from disorders of the eighth nerve and brainstem. This test is also popular for threshold testing of people who cannot or will not cooperate behaviorally (e.g., human infants).

The next concern of the audiologist is remediation of auditory impairment. To this end, the audiologist may fit a hearing-impaired person with a hearing aid. The first step in doing so is to perform an evaluation to identify the optimal hearing aid characteristics and to determine which ear to fit and whether the person would benefit from hearing aids in both ears. The person will then be oriented to the hearing aid and provided with strategies to optimize the use of the hearing aid under various environmental conditions. The audiologist may provide speech-reading (sometimes called "lipreading") training to aid the individual in combining information from the auditory and visual systems. One form of remediation for people who are deaf is a cochlear implant. This involves the surgical implantation of a device that stimulates the inner ear electrically. Alternatively, deaf people may be fitted with a vibrotactile aid, which translates acoustic signals into vibrations that are used to stimulate the skin mechanically. The audiologist is often involved in both the hearing testing and training of those who are fitted with a cochlear implant or a vibrotactile aid.

The third area of audiologist responsibility is the prevention of hearing loss. For example, an audiologist may develop a hearing conservation program in a noisy industrial setting. In such a case the audiologist might measure the noise levels in the work setting, perform periodic hearing tests of the people who are working there, and institute measures to minimize the effects of such a work setting on hearing. These measures might include the use of hearing protectors by workers at risk for hearing loss because of noise exposure, rotation of workers between noisy and quiet work environments, and sound isolation of noisy machinery.

Audiologists work in a variety of settings, including school systems, university clinics, hospitals, industry, government agencies, and private practice.

They also interact with a variety of medical and allied health personnel, including otorhinolaryngologists (ear-nose-throat doctors), neurologists, pediatricians, neonatologists, speech pathologists, rehabilitation counselors, physical therapists, occupational therapists, primary- and secondary-level teachers, and hearing aid dealers.

(*See also:* COMMUNICATION DISABILITIES; DEAFNESS AND HEARING IMPAIRMENTS)

RESOURCE

American Speech-Language and Hearing Association (ASHA), 10801 Rockville Pike, Rockville, MD 20852

BIBLIOGRAPHY

BESS, FRED, and HUMES, LARRY. *Audiology: The Fundamentals.* Baltimore, MD, 1990.

KATZ, JACK. *Handbook of Clinical Audiology,* 3rd ed. Baltimore, MD, 1985.

MARTIN, FREDERICK. *Introduction to Audiology,* 3rd ed. Englewood Cliffs, NJ, 1986.

NEWBY HAYES, and POPELKA, GERALD. *Audiology,* 3rd ed. Englewood Cliffs, NJ, 1985.

ROBERT BURKARD

AUTISM

Autism is a lifelong disability resulting from a neurological disorder of the brain. Autism occurs in approximately 15 out of every 10,000 persons and is three times more common in males than females. The syndrome was first described by Leo Kanner in 1943. Autism was originally considered to be an emotional and mental disorder resulting from poor parenting, but in 1964 Bernard Rimland introduced a neurologically based theory of autism, which was subsequently supported by medical research. The approach to treatment has since accordingly changed from psychotherapy to behavioral and medical intervention.

Researchers have found no single cause of autism. Rather, autism results from multiple neurological impairments associated with the brain's processing of information. Several areas of the brain, including the cerebellum and the brainstem, may be directly involved. Neurochemical studies suggest that abnormal functioning of serotonin, a neurotransmitter, may play a role in causing the symptoms of autism. Some forms of autism have a genetic component.

The criteria for a diagnosis of autism are still being debated, but most authorities agree that autism always becomes apparent before an individual reaches thirty-six months of age. In some cases symptoms are apparent from birth. There are no known medical tests available that clearly result in a diagnosis of autism. Autism is diagnosed by its behavioral symptoms. Behavioral symptoms vary from person to person, but all people with autism display mild to severe deficits in communication and social behaviors. Researchers have estimated that 50 percent of all persons with autism are nonverbal. Those individuals with autism who are verbal, however, have problems related to the content and form of their speech. They also have difficulty sustaining conversation. Other characteristic behaviors include excessive rocking and spinning of the body, repetitive behaviors, insistence on following structured routines, and persistent preoccupation with the parts of objects or with a few particular objects. People with autism may appear to be unaware of the presence of other people. In the severe form of autism, individuals may injure themselves or show other aggressive and bizarre behaviors. The absence of imaginative play is highly characteristic of autism in children, and lack of empathy characterizes autism in adults.

Sensory and cognitive abilities may also be affected. Some people with autism may be unable to tolerate a light touch, though they tolerate deep pressure. Many individuals with autism have difficulty processing auditory information and may be extremely sensitive to certain sounds (Grandin & Scariano, 1986; Stehli, 1991). The extent of cognitive deficits in people with autism is difficult to measure, particularly when there are communication deficits that interfere with testing. It has been estimated that 70 to 90 percent of people with autism have cognitive ability levels that fall within the range of mental retardation (Romancsyk, Lockshin, and Harrison, 1991). "Savant," or exceptional skills, such as those exhibited by the character Raymond in the 1990 movie "Rain Man," are found only in a small percentage of people with autism.

Because the etiology of this syndrome is unclear, there are no known ways to prevent or cure it. There are, however, treatments available that reduce symptoms. The most commonly used treatment for autism is behavior therapy, derived from the principles and techniques of applied behavioral research (i.e., positive reinforcement, shaping, and modeling). Pharmacological treatments (typically neuroleptics, tricyclic antiobsessional antidepressants, and opiate antagonists) have been used for the treatment of behavioral symptoms. Such drug therapy, however, may have no effect on some people with autism and may have adverse effects on others. Vitamin therapy has been shown in a number of studies to be helpful for some individuals with autism (Rimland, 1987).

For all people with autism, training in communication and social skills is essential. Communication training strives to teach functional language. Some nonverbal people with autism have been taught to communicate through alternative methods such as sign language and picture boards. Computers have been used to augment expressive communication through visual screen display, synthesized voice output, and/or printed messages. Social skills training entails the analysis of complex social behaviors, breaking them into small steps that may be taught separately and in sequence. The use of role modeling with feedback, repeated practice, and peer-mediated strategies have also been proven effective with this population.

Behavioral treatment is also employed to decrease undesirable behaviors. Such treatment depends on the identification of the function or purpose of the behavior. While in some cases such behavior seems to be driven by a neurologically based compulsion (Geyde, 1992), in other cases undesirable behaviors may be caused by the inability to communicate a need for attention, a particular object, or escape. Treatment plans address the purpose of the behavior and incorporate the training of alternative appropriate behaviors to achieve that purpose (Carr & Durand, 1986).

Treatment must take into consideration the special characteristics of autism. People with autism often exhibit the need for sameness; thus, a structured, consistent environment and the use of daily schedules are often very helpful. Giving short, consistent, clear instructions, as well as providing visual cues, has also been beneficial. Environmental factors such as noise levels should be considered because many people with autism are hypersensitive to sounds.

The prognosis of autism depends on several factors. Indicators for a positive prognosis include speech before the age of five and an intelligence quotient of 50 or above. Early intervention is often critical to favorable progress. Parental involvement in early intervention programs is known to facilitate learning and overall treatment effects. Total recovery from autism has been reported in only a few individuals.

Since autistic symptoms differ considerably in severity, the prognosis for independence in adulthood varies. Group homes throughout the country provide residential programs that may be, at least to some degree, suitable for the special needs of this population. The degree to which an individual with autism requires supervised support depends on the severity of the behavioral symptoms. Vocational habilitation focuses on the individual's strengths. Some people with autism have highly developed skills in mechanics, rote memory, music, or art. Whereas such individuals may be gainfully employed in situations that utilize these and other skills, they usually need some level of behavioral support.

In addition to those mentioned above, treatments and methods that have been used include facilitated communication, auditory integration training, and sensory integration. Researchers continue to study the efficacy of these treatments. As medical and educational research expands, additional information concerning the exact nature of this syndrome should shed more light on new, effective treatments.

(*See also:* BEHAVIOR THERAPY; CHILDHOOD PSYCHIATRIC DISORDERS; DEVELOPMENTAL DISABILITY; PHARMACOLOGY)

RESOURCES

Autism Research Institute, 4182 Adams Ave., San Diego, CA 92216

Autism Society of America, 7910 Woodmont Ave., Suite 650, Bethesda, MD 20814–3015

BIBLIOGRAPHY

BERKELL, DIANNE E., ed. *Autism: Identification, Education, and Treatment,* Hillsdale, NJ, 1992.

CARR, EDWARD G., and DURAND, MARK. "The Social-Communicative Basis of Severe Behavior Problems in Children." In *Theoretical Issues in Behavior Therapy*, eds. Steven Reiss and Richard Bootzin. New York, 1986.

GEDYE, ARCEE. "Anatomy of Self-Injurious, Stereotypic, and Aggression Movements: Evidence for Involuntary Explanation." *Journal of Clinical Psychology* 48 (1992):766–778

GRANDIN, TEMPLE, and SCARIANO, MARGARET. *Emergence: Labeled Autistic.* Novato, CA, 1986.

POWERS, MICHAEL D., ed. *Children with Autism: A Parent's Guide.* New York, 1989.

RIMLAND, BERNARD. *Infantile Autism: The Syndrome and Its Implications for a Neural Theory of Behavior.* New York, 1964.

———. "Megavitamin B$_6$ and Magnesium in the Treatment of Autistic Children and Adults." In *Neurobiological Issues in Autism*, eds. Eric Schopler and Gary Mesibov. New York, 1987.

ROMANCZYK, RAYMOND G.; LOCKSHIN, STEPHANIE; and HARRISON, KELLY. "Schizophrenia and Autism." In *Psychopathology in the Mentally Retarded*, 2nd ed., eds. Johnny L. Matson and Rowland Barrett. San Antonio, 1991.

STEHLI, ANNABEL. *The Sound of a Miracle: A Child's Triumph Over Autism.* New York, 1991.

BARBARA J. BECKER

AUTOIMMUNE DISORDERS

See ARTHRITIS; HUMAN IMMUNODEFICIENCY VIRUS DISEASE AND ACQUIRED IMMUNODEFICIENCY SYNDROME

B

BACK DISORDERS

Musculoskeletal disorders include some of the most disabling and costly health problems in our society, and low back disorders are, by far, the most common and the most costly. Back and spine impairments, excluding those of the spinal cord, rank in frequency second only to impairments of hearing and sight. Twenty-five percent of all disabling injuries involve the back or spine, and such disabilities affect more than 4 million Americans.

Back injuries, which represent 32 percent of compensable injuries, account for 42 percent of compensable costs. Estimates of the costs associated with disabling back conditions vary from $16 billion to $56 billion a year, depending on how they are computed. Total medical costs, combined with indirect costs, including compensation payments, might be as high as $100 billion a year (Frymoyer, 1991).

About 80 percent of adults experience impairing back pain at some time in their lives, and most people recover within four to six weeks. However, about 10 percent develop chronic back pain, and nearly 50 percent of those with chronic back pain

become disabled. Since most people do recover from back problems rather quickly, immediate medical treatment and long-term treatments are usually not warranted. Those who become disabled by chronic pain, however, often have trouble finding relief.

Although many pain-producing back conditions have been identified, back disorders elude precise diagnosis about 70 percent of the time. Damage to spinal structures and degenerative conditions of the spine, such as herniated disks, spinal stenosis, facet arthropathy, and segmental instability, probably cause much low back pain. Since the spine bears much of the body's weight, it must be able to stay rigid, but it must also be flexible, allowing one to bend and twist. The spine has three primary components: vertebrae, the bony structures that interlock with one another; disks, the softer structures that rest between each pair of vertebrae; and ligaments, which absorb shock and protect other structures from damage. Over time, disks wear out; this is part of the normal aging process. Sometimes disks are damaged prematurely or exposed to conditions that accelerate normal degenerative processes, leading to disk herniation. However, the most common

105

diagnoses for acute low back pain are nonspecific; for example, lumbosacral strain and sprain.

The duration of disability has been directly related to the likelihood of successful treatment and rehabilitation. Only about 20 percent of those whose disability persists for a year or more eventually return to work, and those whose disability persists for two years or more rarely ever work again. Research shows that chronic back disability is not simply a physical condition but a far more complex phenomenon that involves social, occupational, and psychological factors, and thus it is not surprising that traditional medical treatments often fail.

Treatment approaches encompass a range of therapeutic components that address the complex nature of chronic disability. Pain centers offer a range of services, including behavior modification, spinal injection therapy, manipulation, and acupuncture. The usual approach involves modifying behavior associated with pain through counseling, education, and stress management. Although participants report improved functioning and reduced medication use, long-term pain reductions and cost savings have not been well documented. Work-hardening programs, first developed for those with occupational disabilities, involve activities that simulate work tasks with a goal of returning to work. These programs, designed primarily for those who have jobs to which they can return, usually include physical and occupational therapy and some psychological counseling. Return-to-work rates, ranging from 50 to 80 percent, reflect variations in patient population and program content. Functional restoration programs that include behavioral support have gained a reputation for unprecedented return-to-work rates and for increases in activity levels. With a primary aim of functional improvement, these programs usually involve an integrated team of physicians, physical and occupational therapists, psychologists, and exercise instructors.

The high costs of back disorders, although borne by society as a whole, are most keenly felt by employers. Most back injuries are associated with work, and they represent the second most common cause of work absence. The highest rates of back injuries occur in occupations that require heavy manual labor, repeated lifting, long-term exposure to vehicle vibration, and static positions, especially in awk-ward or unsupported postures. Disabling low back injuries and chronic back pain reports are most common among workers in agriculture, aviation, construction, health care (nurse's aides, orderlies, attendants), mining, transportation, and warehousing. But office workers who sit for most of the workday also report high levels of back discomfort and fatigue, which may predispose them to injury.

The factors that account for high injury rates in the occupations listed above are well known. Like other musculoskeletal injuries, back injuries can be caused by direct trauma, a single overexertion, or repetitive or chronic loading. Direct trauma usually results from an accident such as a fall or a blow to the back. Overexertion associated with manual handling of materials accounts for two-thirds of back injuries in industry, and the cumulative effects of repetitive lifting, particularly in forward-flexed and/or twisted postures, also place workers at high risk for back pain.

Occupational low back pain has been associated with sedentary work, which is increasingly common in business and industry. Three-quarters of all workers sit for prolonged periods on the job. People with low back pain often report an intolerance for sitting, and pain severity is inversely related to the opportunities to change posture while seated. Even those without a history of back pain report discomfort with prolonged static sitting. Also, prolonged immobility can have deleterious effects on the spine that make back injuries more likely. Static sitting reduces the movement of nutrient-rich fluids through the intervertebral disks, which reduces their shock-absorbing capacity. Good seating should allow a worker to maintain a relaxed, but supported, posture and should allow for freedom of active motion over the course of the day.

Vibration has also been identified as a significant risk factor for low back pain. Both epidemiological and laboratory research suggest a relationship between long-term vehicle vibration (both vertical and horizontal) and disk herniation. A structure that vibrates at its resonant frequency is more likely to fail, and whole-body-vibration studies have established that the seated human has a resonant frequency close to those produced by cars and trucks, buses, trains, tractors, and heavy construction and mining equipment. A vehicle driver may be at even higher risk for mechanical disk damage when unloading the vehicle after driving, since back muscles fatigue with vibration.

Efforts to prevent low back pain in the workplace have become increasingly important because diagnostic and therapeutic approaches have proven inadequate to curb the soaring incidence and cost of this problem. Most methods can be classified as primary, secondary, or tertiary prevention strategies. Primary prevention strategies include preplacement testing of workers, training workers in safe and effective performance of job tasks, ergonomic job design or job modification, and employee fitness programs. Secondary prevention strategies aim to identify those who have experienced an injury and to intervene appropriately and early enough to prevent disability. Such interventions may take many forms, such as treatment, education, ergonomic counseling, and job accommodation and modification. Tertiary prevention strategies include treatment and rehabilitation programs to minimize the consequences of injury, reduce the duration of chronicity or disability, restore function, and return people to work.

Several sources of information are available for those with chronic or disabling back pain. The National Chronic Pain Outreach Association maintains a computerized registry of chronic pain support groups in the United States and provides referral services to support groups and to pain management specialists and clinics. The Back Pain Association of America offers education and support to people with back disorders as well as to their family members and health care providers. The Vermont Rehabilitation Engineering Research Center for Low Back Pain, a research center funded by the National Institute on Disability and Rehabilitation Research, offers brochures, fact sheets, toll-free telephone and electronic information services, and referrals to research and rehabilitation programs. Newsletters for employers, as well as occupational health and rehabilitation personnel, include *The Back Letter* and *Spine Letter*, both of which provide timely articles based on recent research. *Back to Back*, the newsletter of the Back Association of Canada, addresses the concerns of people with back pain.

(*See also*: DISABILITY MANAGEMENT; ECONOMICS; ERGONOMICS; MUSCULOSKELETAL DISORDERS; PAIN; WORK)

RESOURCES

Back Association of Canada, 83 Cottingham St., Toronto, Ontario M4V 1B9

Back Pain Association of America, P.O. Box 135, Pasadena, MD 21122–01351

The Back Letter, 1351 Titan Way, Brea, CA 92621–3787

National Chronic Pain Outreach Association, Inc., 7979 Old Georgetown Rd, Suite 100, Bethesda, MD 20814–2429

Spine Letter, 12107 Insurance Way, Hagerstown, MD 21740

Vermont Rehabilitation Engineering Research Center for Low Back Pain, 1 South Prospect St., Burlington, VT 05401

BIBLIOGRAPHY

BIGOS, STANLEY J., and ANDARY, MICHAEL T. "Practitioner's Guide to Industrial Back Problems." *Neurosurgery Clinics of North America* 2 (1991):863–875.

BIGOS, STANLEY J., and BATTIÉ, MICHÈLE C. "Acute Care to Prevent Back Disability: Ten Years of Progress." *Clinical Orthopaedics and Related Research* 221 (1987):121–130.

BUCKLE, PETER, and STUBBS, DAVID. "The Contribution of Ergonomics to the Rehabilitation of Back Pain Patients." *Journal of Social and Occupational Medicine* 39 (1989):56–60.

CHAFFIN, DONALD B. "Manual Materials Handling and the Biomechanical Basis for Prevention of Low Back Pain in Industry—An Overview." *American Industrial Hygiene Association Journal* 48(1987):989–996.

CHAFFIN, DONALD B., and ANDERSSON, GUNNAR B. J. *Occupational Biomechanics.* New York, 1984.

DEYO, RICHARD A. "Nonsurgical Care of Low Back Pain." *Neurosurgery Clinics of North America* 2 (1991):851–862.

———. "The Role of the Primary Care Physician in Reducing Work Absenteeism and Costs Due to Back Pain. *Occupational Medicine—State of the Art Reviews* 3 (1988):17–30.

FRYMOYER, JOHN W., ed. *The Adult Spine.* New York, 1991.

FRYMOYER, JOHN W., and CATS-BARIL, WILLIAM L. "An Overview of the Incidences and Costs of Low Back Pain." *Orthopaedic Clinics of North America* 22 (1991):263–271.

FRYMOYER, JOHN W., and MOONEY, VERT. "Current Concepts Review: Occupational Low Back Pain."

Journal of Bone and Joint Surgery 68A (1986):469–474.

Haag, Annette B. "Ergonomic Standards, Guidelines, and Strategies for Prevention of Back Injury." *Occupational Medicine—State of the Art Reviews* 7 (1992):155–165.

Himmelstein, Jay S., and Andersson, Gunnar B. J. "Low Back Pain: Risk Evaluation and Preplacement Screening." *Occupational Medicine—State of the Art Reviews* 3 (1988):255–269.

Jensen, Roger C. "Epidemiology of Work-Related Back Pain: Topics in Acute Care and Trauma." *Rehabilitation* 2 (1988):1–15.

Kelsey, Jennifer L., and Golden, Anne L. "Occupational and Workplace Factors Associated with Low Back Pain." *Occupational Medicine—State of the Art Reviews* 3 (1988):7–16.

Nachemson, Alf L. "Newest Knowledge of Low Back Pain: A Critical Look." *Clinical Orthopaedics and Related Research* 279 (1992):8–20.

Pope, Malcolm H.; Andersson, Gunnar B. J.; Frymoyer, John W.; and Chaffin, Donald B. *Occupational Low Back Pain: Assessment, Treatment, and Prevention.* St. Louis, 1991.

Snook, Stover H. "Approaches to the Control of Back Pain in Industry: Job Design, Job Placement, and Education/Training." *Occupational Medicine—State of the Art Reviews* 3 (1988):45–59.

Snook, Stover H., and Webster, Barbara S. "The Cost of Disability." *Clinical Orthopaedics and Related Research* 221 (1987):77–84.

Waddell, Gordon. "A New Clinical Model for the Treatment of Low Back Pain." *Spine* 12 (1987):632–644.

Malcolm H. Pope
Antonia A. Clark

BARRIERS

See ACCESSIBILITY; AFFIRMATIVE ACTION; ATTITUDES

BEHAVIORAL DISORDERS

See AUTISM; CHILDHOOD PSYCHIATRIC DISORDERS

BEHAVIOR THERAPY

The years since the mid-1950s have witnessed tremendous growth and development in the fields of health care and rehabilitation. Medical breakthroughs continue to be commonplace, with advances on many fronts reported regularly in scientific journals, newspapers and magazines, and in television documentaries and news features. Less common is the increasing knowledge base from scientific investigations, showing the importance of psychological, behavioral, and social influences on health care and well-being. Many health care and rehabilitation specialties have emerged to examine the prevention and treatment of health-related problems from non-biological perspectives. Behavior therapy is one of the most prominent systems of treatment and rehabilitation for many kinds of health care difficulties.

The purposes of this entry are to (1) provide a brief overview of behavior therapy and its related specializations; (2) present various behavior therapy applications used in health care and rehabilitation; and (3) examine issues concerning the future of behavioral therapy in health care and rehabilitation.

What Is Behavior Therapy?

Behavior therapy began in the late 1950s as a learning-based response to the prevailing disease-oriented model of psychodynamic psychotherapy (Dollard & Miller, 1950; Eysenck, 1959; Lazarus, 1958; Skinner, 1953; Wolpe, 1958). There were also significant historical forerunners to the development of behavior therapy, including Pavlov, Watson, Hull, Thorndike, and Skinner, in the areas of learning and conditioning of animal and human behavior. Proponents of behavior therapy reject traditional beliefs that inferred motives, needs, or drives explain behavior. Rather, the emphasis for behavior is placed on situational and environmental conditions that influence behavior. Also, in behavior therapy, the majority of behaviors are considered learned or changeable through learning procedures. There are many comprehensive reviews of the history of behavior therapy, learning theories relating to behavior therapy foundations, and numerous strategies and techniques derived from an equally large number of behavior therapy research studies. Given the availability of such reviews, and limitations regarding the focus of this entry (i.e., behavior therapy applied to health care and rehabilitation), readers interested in more extensive aspects of behavior therapy are encouraged to consult other sources (e.g., Franks & Barbrack, 1991; Hersen & Bellack, 1985; Jacobs, 1993; Kazdin, 1989). Also, there are extensive reports of the efficacy of behavior therapy in the mental health field, including patients with chronic mental illness (Curran et al., 1985; Monti, Corriveau, and Curran, 1982; Paul & Lentz, 1977), marital dysfunction (Epstein, 1982; Jacobson, 1983; Margolin & Fernandez, 1985), and stress and anxiety (Beck, 1984; Woolfolk & Lehrer, 1985).

Behavior therapy does not lend itself to an easy and precise definition. The Association for the Advancement of Behavior Therapy regards behavior therapy as focusing largely on the use of research-related principles derived from experimental and serial psychology, with an emphasis on measuring the effectiveness of treatment interventions (Franks & Wilson, 1975). This definition has two key aspects: (1) Behavior therapy techniques are based on techniques derived from research in experimental and social psychology; and (2) it emphasizes empirical evaluation of its effectiveness. Behavior therapy is also evolving into a variety of specializations, especially in the areas of health care and rehabilitation.

Two specialization fields emphasizing the relationship of contemporary behavior therapy with health care and rehabilitation are behavioral medicine and health psychology. Both are concerned with behavior therapy principles and practices for promoting health and well-being of adults and children.

Behavioral medicine is the interdisciplinary field concerned with the development and integration of behavioral and biomedical science, knowledge, and techniques relevant to health and illness and the application of this knowledge and these techniques to prevention, diagnosis, treatment, and rehabilitation (Schwartz & Weiss, 1978). Behavioral medicine has emerged since the mid-1960s in response to many empirical studies showing that lifestyle and behavior and psychological factors affect health and illness. Such a belief originated in the earliest of recorded Eastern and Western civilizations and provided the foundations for scientific inquiry that continues to validate the relationship that multiple influences have on personal health and recovery from illness and disability. Health psychology is a specialty area within the broader field of psychology

and emphasizes a biopsychosocial model of health care. This model contends that health and illness are best understood not only in terms of biological factors but also psychological and social factors (Gentry, 1984; Rodin & Stone, 1987; Stone, 1987; White, 1988).

The specific application of principles relating to behavioral medicine and health psychology includes behavior analysis, cognitive behavior modification, and cognitive therapy. There is a large variety of specific techniques and treatment strategies associated with each of these contemporary behavior therapy treatment approaches. Behavior analysis may be regarded as a form of treatment that (1) focuses on techniques of learning and functional skill development; (2) uses treatment strategies designed to meet the unique needs of the individual; and (3) emphasizes discrete measures to evaluate functional change and treatment outcome (Jacobs, 1993). Behavior analysis emphasizes the use of operant procedures to understand the antecedents and consequences of behavior and ways to change and improve targeted behaviors.

Cognitive behavior modification emphasizes the role of a person's subjective perception of events, interpretations and attributions of one's own behavior, thought patterns, self-statements, and cognitive strategies (Mahoney, 1974; Wilson & O'Leary, 1980). Cognitive-behavior therapy approaches include several major tenets, such as:

1. The human organism responds primarily to cognitive representations of its environments rather than the environments per se.
2. Most human learning is cognitively mediated.
3. Thoughts, feelings, and behaviors are causally interrelated.
4. Expectancies, attributions, self-talk, and other cognitive activities are central to producing, predicting, and understanding psychopathological behavior.
5. Cognitive processes can be cast into testable formulations that are integrated with other behavioral paradigms.
6. The task of the cognitive-behavior therapist is to act as a diagnostician, educator, and consultant who assesses maladaptive cognitive processes and works with the client to design learning experi-

ences that may remediate dysfunctional cognitions and the behavioral and affective patterns with which they correlate (Kendall, Vitousek, and Kane, 1991).

Cognitive therapy describes a comprehensive treatment approach developed by Aaron T. Beck (1976), although related approaches to cognitive therapy have also emerged. According to Michael E. Thase (1986), Beck's view on dysfunctional behavior is:

1. Certain psychopathological states are either caused and/or maintained by rather automatic distorted and dysfunctional patterns of thinking.
2. Cognitive distortions reflect unrealistic and frequently negative views of self, world, and future (the cognitive triad).
3. Dysfunctional cognitions may appear illogical to others but are consistent with the patient's personal views of reality.
4. Clinically troublesome cognitive distortions are often triggered by adverse life events, yet are maintained by fixed perceptual rules or schemata.
5. Schemata provide the basis for organizing, categorizing, evaluating, and judging new experiences and recollections of past events.
6. Schemata often develop early in life and are shaped by relevant experiences.

A large variety of cognitive therapy techniques have been developed to help reduce and eliminate dysfunctional thoughts often leading to many different kinds of problems in living (McMullin, 1986).

Behavior Therapy Applications Used in Health Care and Rehabilitation

Numerous applications of behavior therapy in health care and rehabilitation are found in the corresponding specialties of behavioral medicine and health psychology, often emphasizing behavior analysis, cognitive-behavior modification, and cognitive therapy. Behavior therapy and related specializations have been found effective in reducing problems in living associated with many health care and rehabilitation problems, including the treatment of chronic headaches (Blanchard, 1992), cancer (Anderson, 1992), AIDS and HIV (Kelly & Murphy, 1993),

insomnia, coronary heart disease (Smith & Leon, 1992), and rheumatoid arthritis (Young, 1992). The following clinical applications of behavior therapy are representative of contemporary behavior therapy practices in health care and rehabilitation.

Chronic Pain. One of the first uses of a behavioral approach for chronic pain was based on operant conditioning principles (Fordyce, 1976). The focus of this approach was on the modification of various maladaptive pain-related behaviors (e.g., excessive time spent in bed, excessive reliance on pain medications), using reinforcement procedures aimed to change environmental conditions influencing such behaviors. Dennis Turk, Donald Meichenbaum, and Myles Genest (1983) argued for use of a cognitive-behavioral approach to managing pain behaviors by including cognitive and affective aspects in the treatment of chronic pain conditions. In this way, chronic pain patients were taught about the relationship of chronic pain to cognitive, behavioral, and affective components of pain to help them restructure and manage their pain experiences. Their cognitive-behavioral approach also encouraged the development of skills such as relaxation skills and various coping skills to manage chronic pain better.

There have been many advances in the use of cognitive-behavioral approaches to chronic pain. Cognitive variables have been shown increasingly to be a critical aspect relating to the maintenance of chronic pain. Studies have shown that individuals experiencing chronic pain who view themselves as more capable to control their pain report greater pain tolerance and increased physical performance when compared with those who do not feel able to control their pain (Bandura et al., 1987). Behavioral treatment of patients with chronic pain has also been shown effective in several studies. In one such study patients with chronic pain receiving a treatment package of relaxation training, exercise, activity pacing, and cognitive therapy, were compared with patients in a waiting-list control condition (Philips, 1987). Patients receiving the treatment package showed significant favorable changes in mood, affective reactions to pain, medication intake, and exercise capability. The waiting-list control group showed no such changes over the duration of the study. Also, patients receiving the treatment package not only maintained their improvement over a twelve-month follow-up but actually improved on most outcome measures.

In a review of behavioral and cognitive-behavioral approaches to chronic pain, a variety of studies have shown the efficacy of behaviorally oriented treatment programs (Keefe, Dunsmore, and Burnett, 1992). The majority of outcome studies cited used control groups when assessing behavioral treatments. Future research directions in the use of behavioral approaches to chronic pain were noted in the areas of assessment of chronic pain and treatment. Regarding assessment, a need was recognized to find quantifiable biomedical data relating to pain. It has been suggested from previous research relating to assessment that being able to assess both psychosocial and biomedical data may be useful in suggesting treatment interventions and in the prediction of treatment outcome (Turk & Rudy, 1987). Most research relating to chronic pain has focused on chronic low back pain, given that pain clinics see a majority of such patients, and studies are heavily reliant on using such samples due to availability. Future research directions were also suggested for chronic pain relating to cancer, arthritis, sickle cell disease, and other conditions.

Brain Injury. Brain injury rehabilitation has grown in scope and numbers since the mid-1970s. Numerous brain injury rehabilitation programs exist throughout the United States, and an equally growing number of rehabilitation practitioners are specializing in head injury rehabilitation. The fastest growing specialization for psychologists has been neuropsychology, evidenced by increasing numbers of (1) opportunities for pre- and postdoctoral training in clinical neuropsychology; (2) professional associations for neuropsychologists; and (3) neuropsychologists becoming members of these professional organizations. Training in neuropsychology has historically emphasized diagnostic evaluations aimed at understanding the impact of traumatic brain injury and other brain insults (e.g., stroke, brain lesions) on cognitive behavioral functioning. Neuropsychologists continue to be challenged to produce neuropsychological evaluations aimed at understanding the impact of brain injury. However, such evaluations have increasingly been seen as secondary to the importance of changing aberrant behaviors frequently shown by persons who are brain-injured.

Behavioral change is frequent following severe and traumatic brain injury. It is not uncommon for individuals with brain injury in postacute rehabilitation programs to experience behavioral problems, including:

1. increased physical and verbal aggressiveness toward staff and other residents;
2. sexual disinhibition;
3. reduced capacity for insight;
4. impaired awareness, alertness, and arousal;
5. reduced motivation for rehabilitation;
6. obsessional disorders;
7. denial;
8. depression (Rosenthal, 1987; Wood, 1987).

These and related behavioral problems are not typically responsive to traditional psychiatric care or medications. Brain injury rehabilitation has increasingly encouraged the use of behavioral strategies aimed at reducing and eliminating maladaptive behaviors and increasing adaptive and functional behaviors. Behavior therapy has been the treatment of choice for improving the functional capabilities of individuals with brain injury.

It is likely that behavior therapy will continue to play a significant role in the rehabilitation of individuals with brain injury, given the many documented successes of this approach. A large variety of journal articles and texts have been written pertaining to behavioral brain injury rehabilitation (e.g., Ewert et al., 1989; Levin & Grossman, 1978; Malec, 1984; Wood, 1987).

Obesity. Many Americans experience problems with their weight, with 24 percent of men and 27 percent of women being obese, using a criterion of being 20 percent or more above desirable weight (Kuczmarski, 1992). Obesity contributes to coronary heart disease, hypertension, diabetes, cancer, and other diseases (Manson et al., 1990; Pi-Sunyer, 1991). Obesity is a complex problem that is associated with high-fat diets, reduced physical activity, genetics (Price, 1987; Stunkard et al., 1990), and a wide variety of behavioral and psychosocial factors (Rodin, 1992; Wadden & Stunkard, 1985). Behavior therapy is one of the key components of most comprehensive weight control strategies.

Behavior therapy in the treatment of obesity usually includes (1) identifying eating or related lifestyle behaviors to be modified; (2) setting specific behavioral goals; (3) modifying determinants of the behavior to be changed; and (4) reinforcing the desired behavior. Such interventions have been shown to be effective, although given the complexity of factors associated with obesity, additional treatment interventions are usually encouraged to assure successful weight loss and maintenance (Jeffery, 1987).

Stress. Stress may be defined as a particular relationship between the person and the environment that is appraised by the person as taxing or exceeding his or her resources and endangering his or her well-being (Lazarus & Folkman, 1984). Hans Selye (1956) examined physiological responses to stress, finding that when individuals experience stress, the nervous and endocrine systems are activated to increase the awareness of threat to well-being. This complex stress activation process also reduces the efficiency of the body's immune system, thus making the individual more vulnerable to disease and illness. Individuals suffering greater stress than they are able to cope with successfully are at greater risk of experiencing physical, emotional, cognitive, interpersonal, or behavioral disorders (Lasky, 1994).

Behavior therapy is a treatment of choice for a variety of stress-related disorders. Generalized anxiety is a common stress response that has been responsive to relaxation training, including progressive relaxation, biofeedback training, and visualization procedures (Benson, 1975). Stress is often mediated by cognitive factors, shown by individuals using cognitive distortions and cognitive errors that increase the stress response. For example, a person may worry that he will lose his job, thinking that his superiors are out to get him or focusing excessively on the potential loss of employment and its implications. This situation may contribute to muscular tension, emotional distress, and behavioral problems, including alcohol and drug use, to alleviate distressful symptoms. Cognitive therapy is often a helpful intervention in such cases, with the focus on identifying and changing faulty thinking styles of cognition contributing to maladaptive thinking and behavior (Beck, 1976, 1984; Beck & Emery, 1979).

The stress of work is also an increasing concern, given that the workplace is experiencing significant change and the realization that change is related strongly to worker stress (National Institute for Oc-

cupational Safety and Health, 1988; Price, 1992). Occupational stress and its consequences are being given increasing attention due to documented costs affecting worker health and well-being (e.g., Fitzgerald, 1992) and the financial impact on business and industry (National Safety Council, 1991). Behavior therapy and related responses to workplace stress have focused on organizational change (McClennan, 1992), strategies and tactics for preventing stress in the workplace (Sauter, Murphy, and Hurrell, 1990), and early psychological intervention when workplace stress is detected (Balzer & Kocher, 1993).

The Future of Behavior Therapy in Health Care and Rehabilitation

American health care and rehabilitation have changed remarkably since the mid-1970s, and will likely continue to change dramatically in the years ahead. The relationship of emotional, behavioral, psychological, social, environmental, and interpersonal influences on health and rehabilitation is gaining increasing support. More succinctly, such a relationship, often referred to as a biopsychosocial paradigm, represents the impact of such factors on personal health and well-being. There is increasing research support for the influence of lifestyle on health and well-being. Lifestyle patterns have been found to play a significant role in deaths related to cardiovascular disease, cancer, and strokes (Matarazzo, 1984). Also, it has been estimated that up to 50 percent of all mortalities from the ten leading causes of death in the United States can be attributed to behavioral or lifestyle patterns (U.S. Department of Health and Human Services, 1985). This recognition has led to increasing use of behavioral therapy interventions to reduce health risk factors such as cigarette smoking, alcohol and drug abuse, cardiovascular diseases, and stress.

Behavior therapy is becoming recognized as a treatment of choice for many medical and psychosocial illnesses, given research support for its use and reduced cost when compared with other psychological therapies (e.g., psychoanalysis, psychodynamic psychotherapy). There have been increasing demands for the delivery of quality services with proven effectiveness and at low cost. This charge, usually from managed care insurers, has been responded to by behavior therapy, especially given the importance of behavior therapy research regarding the efficacy of behavioral treatment approaches within a relatively brief time. Research used in behavior therapy has traditionally focused not only on the study of large groups but also of single subject designs. Behavior therapists typically seek to use documented empirical research findings to support selected treatment interventions. Such practices help to assure that treatment outcome will be favorable and timely. This direction is the mandate and direction of the managed care industry that is likely to continue. Current and future research on the effectiveness of behavior therapy—and related treatment approaches in health care and rehabilitation—aims to determine which specific treatments are best for what identified problems, and under what specific conditions. Given the many documented research findings supporting the efficacy of clinical behavior therapy, it is likely that it will continue to grow in influence and effectiveness in the treatment of problems relating to health care and rehabilitation.

(*See also:* EATING DISORDERS; HEAD INJURY; PAIN, PSYCHOLOGY; PSYCHOSOCIAL ADJUSTMENT; REHABILITATION PSYCHOLOGY; WELLNESS)

BIBLIOGRAPHY

ANDERSON, B. L. "Psychological Interventions for Cancer Patients to Enhance the Quality of Life." *Journal of Consulting and Clinical Psychology* 60 (1992):552–568.

BALZER, D., and KOCHER, B. "Early Psychological Intervention Limits Chronic Claims Costs." *Work Injury Mangement* 2 (1993):1–4.

BANDURA, ALBERT; O'LEARY, A.; TAYLOR, C. B.; GAUTHIER, J.; and GOSSARD, D. "Perceived Self-Efficacy and Pain Control: Opioid and Non-Opioid Mechanisms." *Journal of Personality and Social Psychology* 35 (1987):563–571.

BECK, AARON T. *Cognitive Therapy and the Emotional Disorders.* New York, 1976.

———. "Cognitive Approaches to Stress." In *Principles and Practices of Stress Management,* eds. R. L. Woolfolk and P. M. Lehrer. New York, 1984.

BECK, AARON T., and EMERY, GARY. *Cognitive Therapy of Anxiety and Phobic Disorders.* Philadelphia, 1979.

BENSON, HERBERT. *The Relaxation Response.* New York, 1975.

BLANCHARD, EDWARD B. "Psychological Treatment of Benign Headache Disorders." *Journal of Consulting and Clinical Psychology* 60 (1992):537–551.

CURRAN, JAMES P.; SUTTON, ROBERT G.; FARAONE, STEPHEN V.; and GUENETTE, SIMONE. "Inpatient Approaches." In *Handbook of Clinical Behavior Therapy with Adults,* eds. Michel Hersen and Alan S. Bellak. New York, 1985.

DOLLARD, JOHN, and MILLER, NEAL D. *Personality and Psychotherapy.* New York, 1950.

EWERT, J.; LEVIN, H. S.; WATSON, M. G.; and KALINSKY, Z. "Procedural Memory During Posttraumatic Amnesia in Survivors of Closed Head Injury: Implications for Rehabilitation." *Archives of Neurology* 46 (1989):911–916.

EYSENCK, HANS J. "Learning Theory and Behavior Therapy." *Journal of Mental Science* 105 (1959): 61–75.

FITZGERALD, TERENCE E. "Psychosocial Aspects of Work-Related Musculoskeletal Disability." In *Stress and Well-Being at Work,* eds. James C. Quick, Lawrence R. Murphy, and John J. Hurrell. Washington, DC, 1992.

FORDYCE, WILBERT. *Behavioral Methods for Chronic Pain and Illness.* St. Louis, 1976.

FRANKS, CYRIL M., and BARBRACK, CHRISTOPHER R. "Behavior Therapy with Adults: An Integrative Perspective for the Nineties." In *The Clinical Psychology Handbook,* 2nd ed., eds. Michel Hersen, Alan E. Kazdin, and Alan Bellack. New York, 1991.

FRANKS, CYRIL M., and WILSON, TERENCE, eds. *Annual Review of Behavior Therapy: Theory and Practice,* Vols. 1–7. New York, 1973–1979.

GENTRY, W. D. "Behavioral Medicine: A New Research Paradigm. In *Handbook of Behavioral Medicine,* ed. W. D. Gentry. New York, 1984.

HERSEN, MICHEL, and BELLACK, ALAN S. *Handbook of Clinical Behavior Therapy with Adults.* New York, 1985.

JACOBSON, NEIL S. "Clinical Innovations in Behavioral Marital Therapy." In *Advances in Clinical Behavior Therapy,* eds. K. Craig and D. McMahon. New York, 1983.

JEFFERY, R. W. "Behavioral Treatment of Obesity." *Annals of Behavioral Medicine* 9 (1987):20–24.

KAZDIN, ALAN E. "Behavior Therapy: Evolution and Expansion." *The Counseling Psychologist* 7 (1978): 34–37.

———. *Behavior Modification in Applied Settings,* 4th ed. Pacific Grove, CA, 1989.

KEEFE, FRANCIS J.; DUNSMORE, J.; and BURNETT, R. "Behavioral and Cognitive Behavioral Approaches to Chronic Pain: Recent Advances and Future Directions." *Journal of Consulting and Clinical Psychology* 60 (1992):528–536.

KELLY, J. A., and MURPHY, D. A. "Psychological Interventions with AIDS and HIV: Prevention and Treatment." *Journal of Consulting and Clinical Psychology* 60 (1993):576–585.

KENDALL, P. C.; VITOUSEK, K. B.; and KANE, M. "Thought and Action in Psychotherapy: Cognitive-Behavioral Approaches." In *The Clinical Psychology Handbook*, 2nd ed., eds. Michel Hersen, Alan E. Kazdin, and Alan Bellack. New York, 1991.

LASKY, ROBERT G. "A National Strategy for the Prevention of Psychological Disorders." In *Proposed National Strategies for the Prevention of Leading Work-Related Diseases and Injuries*, Part 2. Cincinnati, OH, 1988.

————. *Accident Facts.* Chicago, 1991.

————. "Occupational Stress: A Disability Management Perspective." In *Principles and Practices of Disability Management in Industry*, ed. D. Shrey and M. Lacerte. Winter Park, FL, 1994.

LAZARUS, ARNOLD A. "New Methods of Psychotherapy: A Case Study." *South Africa Medical Journal* 32 (1958):660–663.

LAZARUS, RICHARD, and FOLKMAN, SUSAN. *Stress, Appraisal, and Coping.* New York, 1984.

MACLENNAN, BERYCE W. "Stressor Reduction: An Organizational Alternative to Individual Stress Management." In *Stress and Well-Being at Work*, eds. J. Quick, L. Murphy and J. Hurrell. Washington, DC, 1992.

MATARAZZO, JOSEPH D. "Behavioral Health: An Overview." In *Behavioral Health: A Handbook of Health Enhancement and Disease Prevention*, eds. J. D. Matarazzo, N. E. Miller, S. M. Weiss, and J. A. Herd. New York, 1984.

MCMULLIN, RIAN E. *Handbook of Cognitive Therapy Techniques.* New York, 1986.

PAUL, GORDON L. and LENTZ, R. J. *Psychosocial Treatment of Chronic Mental Patients: Milieu versus Social Learning Programs.* Cambridge, MA, 1977.

PHILIPS, H. CLARE. "The Effects of Behavioral Treatment on Chronic Pain." *Behavior Research and Therapy* 25 (1987):365–377.

PI-SUNYER, F. X. "Health Implications of Obesity." *American Journal of Clinical Nutrition* 53 (1991):1595S–1603S.

PRICE, R. A. "Genetics of Human Obesity." *Annals of Behavioral Medicine* 9 (1987):9–14.

PRICE, R. H. "Employee Stress Levels." In *Employee Burnout: Causes and Cures.* Minneapolis, MN, 1992.

RODIN, JUDITH. *Body Traps.* New York, 1992.

RODIN, JUDITH, and STONE, GEORGE C. "Historical Highlights in the Emergence of the Field." In *Health Psychology: A Discipline and a Profession*, eds. G. C. Stone, S. M. Weiss, J. D. Matarazzo, N. E. Miller, J. Rodin, C. D. Belar, M. J. Follick, and J. E. Singer. Chicago, 1987.

ROSENTHAL, MITCHELL. "Traumatic Head Injury: Neurobehavioral Consequences." In *Rehabilitation Psychology Desk Reference*, ed. B. Caplan. Rockville, MD, 1987.

SAUNDERS, R. W. "Systematic Desensitization in the Treatment of Child Abuse." *American Journal of Psychiatry* 135 (1978):483–484.

SAUTER, STEVEN L.; MURPHY, LAWRENCE R.; and HURRELL, JOSEPH J. "Prevention of Work-Related Psychological Disorders: A National Strategy Proposed by the National Institute for Occupational Safety and Health." *American Psychologist* 45 (1990):1146–1158.

SCHWARTZ GARY E., and WEISS, STEVEN M. "Yale Conference on Behavioral Medicine: A Proposed Definition and Statement of Goals." *Journal of Behavioral Medicine* 1 (1978):3–12.

SELYE, HANS. *The Stress of Life.* New York, 1956.

SHAH, M., and JEFFERY, R. W. "Is Obesity Due to Overeating and Inactivity, or to a Defective Metabolic Rate? A Review." *Annals of Behavioral Medicine* 13 (1991):73–81.

SKINNER, B. F. *Science and Human Behavior.* New York, 1953.

————. *About Behaviorism.* New York, 1974.

SMITH, T. W., and LEON, A. S. *Coronary Heart Disease: A Behavioral Perspective.* Champaign, IL, 1992.

STONE, GEORGE C. "The Scope of Health Psychology." In *Health Psychology: A Discipline and a Profession*, eds. G. C. Stone, S. M. Weiss, J. D. Matarazzo, N. E. Miller, J. Rodin, C. D. Belar, M. J. Follick, and J. E. Singer. Chicago, 1987.

THASE, MICHAEL E. "Cognitive Therapy." In *Dictionary of Behavior Therapy Techniques*, eds. Alan S. Bellack and Michel Hersen. New York, 1986.

TURK, DENNIS C.; MEICHENBAUM, D.; and GENEST, M. *Pain and Behavioral Medicine: A Cognitive-Behavioral Perspective.* New York, 1983.

TURK, DENNIS C., and RUDY, THOMAS E. "Towards a Comprehensive Assessment of Chronic Pain Patients." *Behavior Research and Therapy* 25 (1987): 237–249.

114

U.S. DEPARTMENT OF HEALTH AND HUMAN SERVICES. *Health: United States 1985.* Washington, DC, 1985.

WADDEN, THOMAS A., and STUNKARD, ALBERT J. "Social and Psychological Consequences of Obesity." *Annals of Internal Medicine* 103 (1985):1062–1067.

WHITE, N. F. "Medical and Graduate Education in Behavioral Medicine and the Evolution of Health Care." *Annals of Behavioral Medicine* 10 (1988): 23–29.

WILSON, TERENCE G., and O'LEARY, K. DANIEL. *Principles of Behavior Therapy.* Englewood Cliffs, NJ, 1980.

WOLPE, JOSEPH. *Psychotherapy by Reciprocal Inhibition.* Stanford, CA, 1958.

WOOD, ROBERT. *Brain Injury Rehabilitation: A Neurobehavioral Approach.* London, 1987.

WOOLFOLK, R. L., and LEHRER, P. M. "Stress and Generalized Anxiety." In *Handbook of Clinical Behavior Therapy with Adults,* ed. M. Hersen and A. S. Bellak. New York, 1985.

YOUNG, L. D. "Psychological Factors in Rheumatoid Arthritis." *Journal of Consulting and Clinical Psychology* 60 (1992):619 627.

ROBERT G. LASKY

BIOENGINEERING

See ENGINEERING; REHABILITATION

BIPOLAR DISORDER

See MOOD DISORDERS

BIRTH DEFECTS

See DEVELOPMENTAL DISABILITIES; GENETIC DISORDERS; GROWTH DISORDERS

BLINDNESS AND VISION DISORDERS

This article focuses on significant vision disorders and provides a basic explanation of the structures of the eye, an overview of the eye-care service-delivery system, and an introductory framework for discussing the visual process.

The Visual System

The eye is a small but complex organ, about one inch in diameter, in which images are formed as specialized nerve cells respond to light and generate electrical signals that are carried to the visual areas of the brain (Bailey & Hall, 1990). The eye has a tough outer coat formed by the sclera and the cornea (Figure 1). The sclera, which can be seen as the white part of the eye, forms most of the back of the eye's outer coat. The transparent cornea forms a clear, curved coat in front of the eye and serves as protection and a window through which light rays enter. Behind the cornea is the iris, the colored part of the eye, which is shaped like a flat disk with a hole in the center. The hole or aperture is called the pupil. This iris contains blood vessels, pigments, and muscle fibers that act to vary the size of the pupil. Immediately behind the iris is the crystalline lens of the eye, whose front and back surfaces are both curved. The eye's ability to focus results from changes in the shape of the lens. Fibers from the edge of the lens connect to the ciliary body, a circle of muscle tissue located directly behind the iris. Ciliary muscle action changes the tension of the lens, thus controlling its shape and focus.

On the inside surface of the sclera is a layer of blood vessels called the choroid. On top of the choroid is the third and innermost layer of the eye, the retina, a special tissue that contains approximately 100 million specialized nerve cells, called rods and

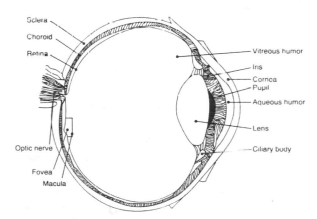

Figure 1. The parts of the eye

SOURCE: *Visual Impairment: An Overview,* the American Foundation for the Blind

115

cones, that respond to light. Rods and cones relay signals to nerve cells of the retina, which in turn generate electrical messages that are sent to the brain along the optic nerve. At the center of the retina is the macula, a specialized region used for looking at fine details and differentiating colors. The fovea, which is the central portion of the macula, responds to fine visual acuity requirements.

The space between the retina and the back of the crystalline lens is filled with a clear, jellylike material called the vitreous humor. In front of the lens, between the iris and the cornea, is a watery fluid called the aqueous humor. On the outside of the eye, attached to the sclera, are various muscles responsible for controlling movements of the eye.

For all practical purposes, the eye works very much like a camera. The cornea and lens focus an image on the surface of the retina and, just as a film in a camera does, each small region of the retina reacts according to the light falling on it. The image that is projected to the retina is an upside-down image. Through the complex activity in the brain in which electrical signals pass along the optical nerve, we eventually "see" an image that is a correct representation of the world around us (Bailey & Hall, 1990).

Visual Functions

Visual function refers to one's ability to obtain impressions through the eyes of the shape, size, distance, motion, color, or other characteristics of objects. The major visual functions are (1) acuity, far and near; (2) depth perception; (3) field of vision; (4) accommodation; and (5) color vision. While all of these are important, visual acuity plays the most vital role in occupational success.

Visual acuity has been defined as the measurement of the amount of detail an individual sees in relation to the amount of detail someone with normal vision sees (Sardegna & Paul, 1991). Visual acuity refers to normal distance vision, which is usually recorded as 20/20. The eye chart customarily used for the visual acuity test is called the Snellen Chart or Snellen System. "20/20" is the "normal" distance vision. While there are a number of systems for vision notation, distance (far) vision is usually noted in the "20" system. Here the numerator denotes the distance at which the examination is conducted, 20 feet. The denominator denotes that the vision is "normal" for 20 feet. In the metric system, normal distance acuity would be 6/6, the examination being conducted at 6 meters, which is approximately 20 feet. If the individual is evaluated at 20 feet, but the smallest letter he or she can see is the size that normally could be seen at 40 feet, then the vision would be recorded as 20/40; in the metric system, it would be 6/12. Many people see better than 20/20; for example, a person with a visual acuity of 20/15 sees at 20 feet what people with normal vision see only at 15 feet. The 20/40 letter on the eye chart is twice the size of the 20/20, the 20/80 is four times the size of the 20/20, and so on. The usual range of visual acuity is from 20/15 to 20/200. A measurement of 20/200 means that the individual is able to see only the largest letter on the chart, the big *E*. The term "count fingers" refers to the vision of an individual who cannot see the big *E* but who can count the number of fingers the examiner holds up. "Hand motion" is the term used to describe the vision of someone who cannot see the separate fingers but who can discern some movement when the hand is waved. Light perception (LP) describes the vision of a person who can perceive only light or its absence. No light perception (NLP) refers to the vision of someone who is unable to discern any light at all. Near acuity refers to the clarity of vision at 20 inches or less; most near acuity measures are taken at 14 inches.

The remaining visual functions are also important and can be crucial to the successful performance of certain occupations. Depth perception or three-dimensional vision refers to the ability to judge distance and space relationships so as to see the objects where and as they actually are. Field of vision refers to the area that can be seen up and down or to the right or left while the eyes are fixed on a given point. Accommodation refers to the adjustment of the lens of the eye to bring an object into sharp focus. This function is especially important when one is doing near-point work at varying distances from the eye. Color vision refers to the ability to identify and distinguish colors.

Most countries and many states have created their own definition of blindness. The term "blindness" may have a variety of meanings, but it is most often thought to mean some type of anatomic and functional disturbance of the sense of vision of sufficient magnitude to cause total loss of light perception. Visual impairment (Hoover & Bledsoe, 1981) refers to any deviation from the generally accepted norm that effects central visual function, peripheral visual function, binocular visual function, or color perception. The deviation may be anatomic or functional, partial or total, and temporary, reversible, progressive, or permanent.

"Legal blindness" is a term used by a wide variety of government agencies, including the Internal Revenue Service and the Social Security Administration, to determine whether an individual is eligible for federal or state benefits. Legal blindness is generally determined by measuring visual acuity (how much detail one sees at a specific distance) and visual field (the area of vision). A person is generally classified as legally blind if the visual acuity of the better eye, with best correction, is 20/200 or less. One may also be described as legally blind if the visual field of the better eye, even with 20/20 vision, is limited to 20 degrees or less. An individual with loss in the visual field may experience peripheral or central acuity-vision loss.

People who are legally blind should not necessarily be considered totally blind. The term includes a wide range of visual abilities, and two individuals with 20/200 visual acuity or 20-degree visual fields may have vastly different vision levels. It is estimated that over 75 percent of the legally blind individuals in the United States have some remaining vision. These individuals are often able to use their remaining vision to work, read, travel, and continue their daily routines by using adaptive devices or by developing accommodating body or head movements. Since most legally blind people have some residual vision, a misconception exists about what people who are blind can actually see. Therefore, many agencies that serve individuals who are blind suggest that the word "blind" be used to describe only those with no usable vision and the phrases "low vision" or "visually impaired" be used to describe people who have some remaining usable vision. A person with a visual acuity measurement of 20/50 or less and visual field of 20 to 40 degrees or less in the better eye, with correction, is generally considered to have low vision (Sardegna & Paul, 1991), although the definition varies widely.

The visual impairment generally denoted by the term "blindness" varies according to at least four variables: (1) the degree of sight retained; (2) the age at onset of blindness; (3) the time lapsed since the onset of blindness; and (4) the cause and the kind of onset (i.e., sudden or slowly developing). The degree of sight retained may range from none in total blindness to a considerable amount of sight (e.g., 20/100 Snellen Distance Vision, which is equivalent to a loss of 80 percent, according to the ophthalmological definition). Individuals vary dramatically in their ability to make functional use of whatever sight they have, and thus degree of sight retained is a very important variable to be considered. The age at onset of blindness is also very important because those who are congenitally blind or become blind when younger than about five years of age do not retain a workable visual imagery. Those who become blind later in life must adjust to the demands of the world of the seeing, which they have known and can more or less clearly remember. They also tend to know what they have lost and thus have to cope with the emotional effects of the loss, which vary according to their personalities. The time elapsed since the onset of blindness is also an important factor because it must be considered in judging the adjustment of the individual and also in providing educational or rehabilitative assistance. The person who has lived with blindness for a long time is obviously in a different position than one who has just become blind. The cause and kind of onset of blindness are related factors because the cause of blindness determines whether the onset was slowly developing or sudden. The former can put the person in a prolonged state of insecurity and uncertainty, while sudden onset causes a shock from which the individual recovers according to his or her ego strength and environmental support. The cause of blindness also tends to indicate whether an individual's general health is affected, as in such systemic diseases as diabetes or tuberculosis, or whether the pathological process is confined only to the eyes.

Eye-Care Service-Delivery System

A wide variety of medical and nonmedical services are needed by people who are blind or severely visually impaired. A number of professionals may be involved in the care of an individual with a vision impairment. These include the ophthalmologist who is a physician (M.D.) specializing in the total care of the eyes including (but not limited to) the evaluation of the health of the eyes and the visual system, diagnosis, medical interventions with drugs, noninvasive treatments, surgery, and the prescription of optical corrections. The optometrist is a doctor of optometry (O.D.) who provides a wide variety of services including diagnosis of visual conditions, prescription of optical corrections, and other noninvasive procedures (e.g., patching an amblyopic [lazy] eye). Optometrists are trained primarily to diagnose and treat refractive efforts and perceptual dysfunction (Michelson, 1980). Optometrists' roles and responsibilities vary according to the licensing and regulating legislation in the state in which their practice is located. An optician is a professional who fills the optical prescriptions of ophthalmologists and optometrists. The optician grinds lenses and produces different types of spectacle corrections (e.g., glasses, bifocals, contact lenses, etc.). The ocularist constructs and fits a cosmetically pleasing device when an individual is in need of a prosthesis for a missing eye. The ocularist becomes a member of the rehabilitation team when an individual has had an eye removed (enucleation) due to trauma or disease or when there has been a congenital condition for which an absent (anopthalmic) eye or a small (micropthalmic) eye needs to be corrected. Low vision specialists usually work in low vision clinics or in private practice providing low vision care. They assist ophthalmologists or optometrists in the instruction of people who receive optical devices, and they may also deliver other services for which they are qualified (e.g., rehabilitation teaching or orientation and mobility). Other professionals who are actively involved in serving individuals who are blind or severely visually impaired include rehabilitation counselors, rehabilitation engineers, ophthalmic nurses, rehabilitation teachers, and orientation and mobility specialists.

Demographics

Visual impairment is the most frequently reported chronic health problem in the United States (LaPlante, 1988). Blindness and severe visual impairment are prevalent throughout the world. According to the World Health Organization (1980), an estimated 30 million to 40 million people in the world are blind. Prevent Blindness America (1992) estimates that there are approximately 900,000 legally blind people over the age of forty in the United States and more than 11.4 million people who have a severe vision impairment that precludes reading normal newsprint. Blacks have a higher rate of blindness than whites, but much of this difference may be due to poor access to appropriate eye care services. Worldwide, the most common causes of blindness are cataract, trachoma, onchocerciasis, xerophthalmia, injuries, glaucoma, macular disease, optic nerve atrophy, diabetic retinopathy, and retinitis pigmentosa. Much of the blindness throughout the world is preventable through nutritional, therapeutic, and sanitation-improvement programs.

The four leading causes of blindness in the United States are macular degeneration, glaucoma, cataract, and diabetic retinopathy (Prevent Blindness America, 1994). Macular degeneration results from changes in the back of the eye that cause blurred vision or loss of the center of vision. In glaucoma, increased intraocular tension causes atrophy of the optic nerve. Cataract is a condition in which the lens of the eye becomes opaque, resulting in progressive loss of vision. In diabetic retinopathy, high blood-sugar levels lead to blood vessel changes inside the eye, resulting in blurring, cloudiness, blind spots, and, sometimes, total loss of vision.

Different groups in the population are affected differently by these diseases. For example, whites tend to have more macular degeneration than blacks, whereas blacks are blinded from glaucoma more frequently than whites. Also, the incidence of visual impairment increases with age. It has been estimated that more than 70 percent of the visually impaired people in the United States are over age sixty-five (Bailey & Hall, 1990). In this population, age-related maculopathy, glaucoma, senile cataracts, and diabetic retinopathy are the most frequent causes of blindness. Retinal degeneration, a condition characterized by tunnel vision, difficulty with night vision, and difficulty with close work because of damage to the part of the eye that picks up visual images and sends them to the brain, is another common cause of vision loss among those over sixty-five.

Among new cases of blindness, the four major causes are, in order of prevalence, age-related maculopathy, glaucoma, diabetic retinopathy, and senile cataract. These disorders and diseases are responsible for nearly half of all new cases of blindness (Sardegna & Paul, 1991).

Responding to Vision Loss

Within the visually impaired population, there is a wide variety of visual characteristics and rehabilitation needs. These include a loss of visual acuity, which may range from slight to profound; visual-field loss, which may be predominantly peripheral or predominantly central, with severity ranging from slight to profound; and other vision problems, such as night blindness, color blindness, decreased contrast sensitivity, sensitivity to glare, or prolonged recovery from the effects of glare. The extent of the impairment created by the vision loss depends not only on the nature and extent of the loss, and when it occurs (i.e., adventitious vs. congenital blindness), but also on the needs, aspirations, attitudes, and physical abilities of the individual involved. Some of the more significant functional impairments resulting from vision loss include diminished ability to read, recognize faces and facial expressions, or perform visually guided motor tasks, as well as an inability to be aware of the important features of one's immediate environment and move freely within it.

Vision loss affects virtually every aspect of a person's life. Individuals who have experienced vision loss often fear that they will lose their jobs and/or their ability to support themselves. Many fear that they will be unable to take care of themselves or that they will become the object of pity (Resources for Rehabilitation, 1990). Vision loss often threatens an individual's independence, and there is often concomitant diminishment of self-esteem. When self-esteem is reduced or diminished, people are often reluctant to accept assistance offered by others, including services from rehabilitation counselors.

Individuals with vision loss often need time to adjust psychologically before they are able to begin the rehabilitation process (Resources for Rehabilitation, 1990). The amount of time needed before they accept their vision loss and are able to benefit from rehabilitation services depends on the individual and may be a matter of days, months, or even years. In most cases individuals who are visually impaired and who are slow to accept their condition and prognosis will benefit from discussing their situation with a professional counselor or with others who have gone through similar experiences. The professional rehabilitation counselor can be crucial in determining the individual's response to blindness or severe visual impairment.

Employment and Vision Loss

Work is an activity of central importance in the lives of millions of Americans. Holding a job provides the means to support oneself and one's family, to engage in a regular, predictable daily routine, and to experience the satisfaction of accomplishment and increased self-esteem. People who are blind or severely visually impaired are no different from sighted persons in ascribing value to being contributing members of society. Rehabilitation professionals such as those mentioned earlier are the essential link in the total rehabilitation process and, as such, must be prepared to take on an array of responsibilities in training people who are blind for gainful employment.

People who are blind or severely visually impaired make up a large and growing segment of the disabled population in the United States. Employers have expressed concern about their ability to accommodate workers who are blind or severely visually impaired under the requirements of the Americans with Disabilities Act (ADA). They will need the help of skilled rehabilitation professionals and others in order to deal with the new challenges presented by the ADA. Given the proper training and adaptive equipment, people who are blind or visually impaired would be able to hold the vast majority of jobs in this country.

(See also: COMPUTER APPLICATIONS FOR VISUAL DISABILITIES; KELLER, HELEN; PSYCHOSOCIAL ADJUSTMENT)

RESOURCES

American Academy of Ophthalmology, P.O. Box 7424, San Francisco, CA 94120–7424

American Council of the Blind, 1155 15th St., NW, Suite 720, Washington, DC 20202

American Foundation for the Blind, Eleven Penn Plaza, New York, NY 10001

American Optometric Association, 243 North Lindbergh Blvd., St. Louis, MO 63141

American Printing House for the Blind, P.O. Box 6085, Louisville, KY 40206

Association for Education and Rehabilitation of the Blind and Visually Impaired, 206 N. Washington St., Suite 320, Alexandria, VA 22314

Blinded Veterans Association, 477 H St., NW, Washington, DC 20001–2694

Canadian National Institute for the Blind, 1931 Bayview Ave., Toronto, Ont. M4G 4C8

Job Accommodation Network (JAN), 918 Chestnut Ridge Rd, Suite 1, P.O. Box 6080, Morgantown, WV 26506–6080

Library of Congress—National Library Service for the Blind and Physically Handicapped, 1291 Taylor St., NW, Washington, DC 20542

National Council of Private Agencies for the Blind, Carroll Center, 770 Centre St., Newton, MA 02158

National Council of State Agencies for the Blind, 1213 29th St., NW, Washington, DC 20007

National Eye Institute, Building 31, Room 6A03, Bethesda, MD 20892

National Federation of the Blind, 1800 Johnson St., Baltimore, MD 21230

National Industries for the Blind, 524 Hamburg Turnpike, Wayne, NJ 07472

Prevent Blindness America, 500 East Remington Rd., Schaumburg, IL 60173

Rehabilitation Research and Training Center on Blindness and Low Vision, P.O. Drawer 6189, Mississippi State, MS 39762

Smith-Kettlewell Eye Research Institute, Rehabilitation Engineering Center, 2232 Webster St., San Francisco, CA 94115

BIBLIOGRAPHY

BAILEY, IAN L., and HALL, AMANDA. *Visual Impairment—An Overview.* New York, 1990.

HOOVER, RICHARD E., and BLEDSOE, C. WARREN. "Blindness and Visual Impairment." In *Handbook of Severe Disability,* eds. Walter Stolov and Michael R. Clowers. Washington, DC, 1981.

LAPLANTE, MITCHELL P. *Data on Disability from the National Health Interview Survey, 1983–85 (An InfoUse Report).* Washington, DC, 1988.

MICHELSON, PAUL. *Insight into Eyesight.* Chicago, 1980.

PREVENT BLINDNESS AMERICA. *Vision Problems in the U.S.—Blindness and Visual Impairment.* Schaumburg, IL, 1994.

RESOURCES FOR REHABILITATION. *Rehabilitation Resource Manual—Vision.* Lexington, MA, 1990.

SARDEGNA, JILL, and PAUL, T. OTIS. *The Encyclopedia of Blindness and Vision Impairment.* New York, 1991.

WORLD HEALTH ORGANIZATION. "International Classification of Impairments, Disabilities, and Handicaps." Geneva, 1980.

J. ELTON MOORE

BLOOD DISORDERS

Blood can be divided into two major components: cellular and fluid. The cellular component consists of white blood cells (WBCs) that fight infection, red blood cells (RBCs) that carry oxygen, and platelets that help stop bleeding. The most common white blood cell disorders are the leukemias. The leukemias represent the abnormal growth of one of the types of white blood cells. The common red blood cell disorders are due to an abnormality of hemoglobin, the substance in the red blood cell that carries oxygen. In sickle-cell anemia, the structure of hemoglobin is abnormal, whereas in thalassemia, the production of hemoglobin is disrupted. Increased numbers of RBCs occur in polycythemia vera and can lead to blood vessel occlusion and stroke. Platelet disorders may be either quantitative (abnormal number) or qualitative (abnormal function). A markedly elevated platelet count is seen in thrombocytosis. This can result in abnormal bleeding and/or excessive clotting (thrombosis). If either occurs in the brain, a stroke can result. Chronic idiopathic thrombocytopenia (ITP) causes low platelets. This condition is manifested by easy bruising and internal bleeding into organs such as the brain; joint bleeding is rare. Qualitative platelet disorders are usually mild. Severe disorders (Glanzmann's thrombasthenia, Bernard-Soulier syndrome) are rare; any disability is secondary to internal bleeding.

The fluid part of blood, plasma, contains a variety of substances such as salts and proteins. One group of proteins is the clotting factors, which interact with platelets to form a blood clot. When a blood vessel is injured, the platelets stick to the vessel wall and form a "plug." The "platelet plug" is most effective in small blood vessels and stops bleeding for about four hours; hence the name "temporary clot formation." Vessel injury also results in activation of clotting factors. This occurs sequentially, with the activated form of one factor activating the next factor in line. The end result is a fibrin mesh, which traps blood cells and seals the hole in the vessel; this constitutes a blood clot. Clotting factors are now named in order of discovery, from I to XIII. Another protein, the von Willebrand Factor, is not part of the "clotting cascade" but is necessary for platelets to stick to blood vessels and for Factor VIII to circulate in the blood. Von Willebrand's disease (formerly referred to as pseudohemophilia) is the most common hereditary bleeding disorder, occurring in 1 to 3 percent of the general population, but it is usually mild and does not result in disability.

Although an inherited deficiency has been described for all of the numbered clotting factors, Factor VIII and Factor IX deficiencies are the most common. The lack of either Factor VIII or Factor IX results in the hereditary bleeding disorder known as hemophilia. Factor VIII and Factor IX deficiencies result in the same medical problems and will be discussed together.

There are approximately 20,000 individuals with hemophilia in the United States. Factor VIII deficiency (Hemophilia A) occurs in approximately 1 in 7,500 boys; Factor IX deficiency (Hemophilia B or Christmas Disease) occurs one-fifth as frequently. The gene for hemophilia is on the X chromosome, one of the sex chromosomes. Therefore, only males are affected; females are carriers (Miller, 1992). In many individuals it is now possible to find the exact gene defect that resulted in their hemophilia. Women with a history of hemophilia in the family can then be told with more than 98 percent accuracy if they carry a hemophilia gene. Prenatal diagnosis of hemophilia is also possible.

Individuals with hemophilia have normal platelets. They do not have problems with small vessel or superficial bleeding such as skinned knees, razor nicks, and blood drawing. Their major bleeding is internal (Hilgartner & Pochedly, 1989). Bleeding into joints and muscles is most common and, if not treated promptly, eventually leads to severe crippling and disability. Bleeding into internal organs is less common but has the potential for more serious immediate consequences. Bleeding into the brain is the most feared, because death or severe mental and/or physical impairment often result.

Hemophilia is classified as mild, moderate, and severe, depending on the baseline Factor VIII or IX level (see Table 1). All persons with hemophilia will bleed with surgery or major trauma. Persons with mild disease may not experience any other bleeding problems and often are not diagnosed until adolescence or adulthood. People with moderate hemophilia bleed with minor trauma and occasionally bleed spontaneously (with no history of injury). The person with severe hemophilia often bleeds weekly; most bleeding episodes occur spontaneously.

Table 1. Classification of Hemophilia A and B

Factor Level (Normal >50%)	Severity	Symptoms
<1%	Severe	Spontaneous bleeding
1%–5%	Moderate	Bleeding with trauma
>5%	Mild	Bleeding with major trauma/surgery

Bleeding into the brain is the most serious type of bleeding. Other than blood borne viruses, it is the major cause of death in individuals with hemophilia. Bleeding into joints and muscles is the most frequent type of bleeding and the most common cause of disability.

Treatment of Hemophilia

Chronic illness affects all aspects of an individual's life: physical, mental, social, vocational, and economic. Thus the treatment of a chronic disease cannot be undertaken in a "medical vacuum." Hemophilia treatment has served as a model for comprehensive multidisciplinary care in the United States since the mid 1970s. Comprehensive hemophilia treatment centers are located throughout the country. The core comprehensive care team consists of a physician knowledgeable in the medical treatment of individuals with congenital bleeding disorders, a nurse coordinator whose role includes extensive patient education, a physical therapist, and a psychosocial counselor. Extended team members readily available for a referral include an orthopedist, a dentist, a genetics counselor, a nutritionist, and HIV and hepatitis specialists. Increasingly, case management and reimbursement responsibilities also are incorporated into the jobs of core team members (Standards and Criteria for the Treatment of Individuals with Congenital Bleeding Disorders, 1994).

Bleeding episodes are conventionally treated as they occur (on-demand therapy) by infusing the missing clotting factor ("factor" or "concentrate"), either Factor VIII or Factor IX, into the individual's vein. Once in the blood, Factor VIII and IX last only a short time. For an individual with severe Hemophilia A to have any Factor VIII measurable in the blood, that person would need to get an infusion every second or third day. Most parents learn to infuse their child by the time he is five or six years old. Many children learn self-infusion when they are nine to twelve years old. Infusions can be done virtually anywhere—at home, in school, on airplanes, while camping—and take only a few minutes. In addition to the convenience this provides, it also gives the individual and his family some control over the disease.

Even with the best on-demand treatment, some individuals with hemophilia develop joint damage. Although this often does not restrict activity during childhood, such joint abnormalities form the basis of arthritis in later years. In an attempt to minimize and/or prevent arthritis and to allow individuals with hemophilia to have a normal lifestyle, physicians are increasingly advocating routine factor infusion two or three times weekly. Such routine administration of factor concentrates to prevent rather than to treat bleeding is called prophylaxis. When prophylaxis is begun before the onset of joint damage, it is referred to as primary prophylaxis. When instituted to prevent rebleeding in and allow aggressive rehabilitation of specific joint(s), it is known as secondary prophylaxis. Treatment regimens for both primary and secondary prophylaxis vary greatly. In Sweden, high-dose primary prophylaxis (5,900 U factor VIII/IX kilogram/year) has been routinely practiced in all children with severe hemophilia since 1981, beginning at one to two years of age. Patients have had virtually no joint bleeds and, to date, have normal joints clinically and by X ray (Nilsson, Berntorp, Ljung et al, 1994). Individuals treated with lower dose prophylaxis prior to 1980 have had an average of 2.6 joint bleeds/year for those ages thirteen to twenty, and approximately 5 bleeds/year for those over age twenty. Depending when prophylaxis was initiated, they have shown only mild joint defects or minor orthopedic problems that have not interfered with education or work. In the Netherlands, where intermediate dose prophylaxis (1,753 U/kg/yr) is begun around age four after some joint bleeds have occurred, the number of joint bleeds/year has been reduced from approximately twenty to five to eight. Clinically, patients have done well, but 35 percent have minor damage, which will probably result in arthritis in later years (van den Berg, Nieuwenhuis, Karel et al, 1994). In a United States study of fourteen boys placed on secondary prophylaxis, all children demonstrated clinical improvement, including a marked reduction in the number of joint bleeds. In spite of the decreased bleeding, however, in nine that had follow-up X rays, X-ray abnormalities did not regress in any and progressed in two of fifteen evaluable joints (Manco-Johnson, Nuss, Geraghty et al, 1994).

Problems associated with routine prophylaxis include difficulty in assessing veins, family and financial stress, and, theoretically, the possibility of an increased incidence of inhibitor information (see below). In young children, it is usually necessary to place a small, indwelling, plastic tube, known as a central line, into a larger vein; clotting factor is infused through the end of the tube or into a port buried under the skin. Such lines may become infected; this in turn can lead to blood poisoning. The Swedish center reports very few problems with line infections (Ljung, Lindgren, Tengborn et al, 1994). In the United States study by Manco-Johnson and coworkers, six of fourteen boys, all under seven years of age, required central lines. Three experienced one or more line infections (Manco-Johnson, Nuss, Geraghty et al., 1994). In addition to the medical problems posed, line infections usually necessitate hospitalization, adding to overall medical costs. In the same study, prophylaxis was discontinued in four of fourteen boys because of financial limitations. Seven of fourteen boys received fewer doses than prescribed because of financial limitations and fear of exceeding lifetime insurance caps. Neither the Swedish study nor the American study demonstrated an increased incidence of inhibitor formation.

One of the problems in both choosing and comparing prophylactic regimens is deciding which individuals are at the greatest risk of recurrent joint bleeds before such bleeds and resulting damage have occurred. Clinicians have repeatedly observed that there exists a subgroup of individuals with hemophilia in whom a relatively low number of bleeds occurs independent of product usage. In a large international study individuals with hemophilia were followed annually, both clinically and with joint X rays, for five years. Fifty percent of patients receiving relatively little factor (less than 500U/kg/yr) and entering the study with normal joints, still had normal joints five years later (Aledort, 1992). Although prophylaxis offers the ability to greatly minimize, if not eliminate, joint bleeds in individuals with hemophilia, it is no different than any other medical treatment in that the risks as well as the benefits must be taken into consideration. These should be discussed on an individual basis so that the patient and his family can make an informed decision.

Bleeding into joints results in an increase in the number of cells (hypertrophy) of the joint lining (synovium). These synovial cells produce chemicals which destroy the smooth joint surface (cartilage), eventually leading to painful arthritis. If a joint bleed is not treated early, the pain results in disuse. The disuse, even for only a few days, results in weakened muscles and tight tendons (contracture). Muscles stabilize the joint; when they are weak, joint bleeds occur more frequently. Therefore, evaluation by a physical therapist is essential (Gilbert & Greene, 1990). Ideally, this occurs routinely so that small problems will be caught and rectified. For children, normal activity, including sports, is the easiest way to maintain or build muscle strength. Today most hemophilia treaters restrict only contact sports such as football, wrestling, and boxing (*Hemophilia and Sports*, 1992). The grade school child can participate in regular gym and recess. In high school, highly competitive intervarsity sports where head trauma is likely should be avoided, but other sports should be encouraged.

To achieve the concentration of relatively pure Factor VIII or IX needed, blood from up to 20,000 donors is pooled. This pooling resulted in more than 90 percent of persons with severe hemophilia being infected with the HIV (AIDS) virus in the early

1980s. Almost 100 percent were also infected with hepatitis C. Those persons not immunized with hepatitis B vaccine were also infected with hepatitis B virus. Factor concentrates derived from human blood are now treated to kill viruses. There has been no case of HIV virus transmitted by treated concentrate since January 1986. Since the 1980s, transmission of hepatitis has occurred rarely, if at all.

In December 1992, the first lab-made genetically engineered (recombinant) Factor VIII was licensed. As production of recombinant Factor VIII increases, it should become more widely available.

Other than transmission of bloodborne viruses, the major complication of hemophilia treatment is the development of antibodies or inhibitors of Factor VIII or IX. Inhibitors are produced by the body and neutralize ("soak up") clotting factor as soon as it enters the blood. If the inhibitor is high enough, a measurable Factor VIII or Factor IX level cannot be achieved, no matter how much factor is given, and bleeding continues. Several other concentrates that cause clotting can be given to these individuals to stop bleeding; they are effective in approximately 75 percent of individuals. In many individuals, daily infusions of factor will greatly lower or eradicate the inhibitor so that Factor VIII or IX concentrates are again effective (immune tolerance). Treatment of individuals with hemophilia who have developed an inhibitor is complex and should be undertaken only under the supervision of a hemophilia specialist.

The individual with hemophilia should receive the same dental care as any individual. Unfortunately, the combined fears of patient and dentist often result in severe neglect, a "dental cripple." Cleaning and superficial infiltrative anesthesia require no special precautions. One dose of factor is usually given before block anesthesia in the event a blood vessel is entered. One dose of factor is also given before dental extractions. These can usually be managed thereafter with an oral medication (Amicar or tranexamic acid) until the extraction site is healed in seven to ten days.

Rehabilitation

A joint into which acute hemorrhage occurs repeatedly over several months is known as a target joint. As mentioned above, inflammation of the joint lining (synovium) from bleeding leads to progressive destruction of the smooth joint surface (cartilage) and, eventually, to arthritis. Therefore, target joint bleeds are treated more aggressively in an attempt to decrease synovial inflammation, break the bleeding cycle and reduce joint damage. Medical therapy in the form of some type of routine infusions, such as every-other-day prophylaxis, is attempted first. Physical therapy and regular exercise should be stressed throughout because strong muscles will provide joint support and decrease the number of bleeding episodes. Passive range of motion exercises require prior infusion of factor concentrate. If aggressive medical therapy is not successful, consideration should be given to removing much of the synovium surgically to reduce the number of bleeding episodes and decrease the number of destructive chemicals produced. With modern technology this can be done through a few very small incisions (arthroscopic synovectomy). Factor concentrates must be given during surgery and rehabilitation to prevent bleeding. Alternatively, a radioactive material that causes the synovium to scar and thus shrink can be injected into the joint space (radionucleotide synovectomy). This has been done for over ten years in Venezuela with good results. The theoretical possibility of causing cancer by administering a radioisotope does not appear to be a real problem.

Treatment of arthritic pain is difficult because most arthritis medicine interferes with platelet function and can cause increased bleeding. Aspirin interferes with the platelet function for up to ten days and should never be used. Nonsteroidal anti-inflammatory drugs (e.g. ibuprofen, naproxen) can be used in select, compliant patients if carefully monitored by a hemophilia specialist.

For the individual with severe debilitating pain secondary to advanced arthritis, joint replacements provide relief from pain and more normal stance and gait, thus reducing stress on other muscles and joints. Hip and knee replacements are the most common. Pain and quality of life rather than age should be the important indicators for the timing of joint replacements.

Although bleeding can be well controlled with the infusion of clotting factors, the complexity of clotting assays and the coordination of surgery and rehabilitation with factor dosages require specific ex-

pertise and should be undertaken at a hemophilia center. Bracing can sometimes delay surgery and should be considered in high-risk individuals.

Functional Limitations and Handicaps

Bleeding into the brain is the most serious complication of a bleeding disorder. This is analogous to stroke and should be rehabilitated in the same manner. Clotting factor concentrates are given for at least six weeks to prevent rebleeding. Joint damage with accompanying muscle damage and tendon shortening are the most common forms of disability. Knees, ankles, and elbows are the most commonly affected. Before clotting factor became available, most people with severe hemophilia were using wheelchairs by young adulthood. With prompt infusion of clotting factor when bleeding occurs and aggressive physical therapy to strengthen muscles and increase range of motion of joints, this extent of crippling should no longer happen. Even with optimal on-demand therapy, however, some arthritis still occurs, making walking long distances, climbing stairs, and standing for long periods difficult. Heavy lifting is problematic if elbows are involved. The above exclude some types of employment. In addition, jobs associated with frequent mild trauma, such as construction work, will result in frequent bleeding episodes and are therefore not practical. The most important limitation to employment today is the high cost of clotting factor. Employers' insurance rates invariably increase greatly, making it difficult for small businesses to employ individuals with hemophilia.

Psychosocial Issues

The combination of a hereditary disease occurring in males and the resulting restriction excluding them from major contact sports is a setup for psychosocial problems. Mothers often feel severely guilty for having "done this" to their child. Fathers are resentful that their son cannot play football. These reactions are combined with the fear that the child will bleed to death from the slightest injury. Each developmental stage produces new challenges. Ongoing psychosocial assessment and support are essential if one wishes to have individuals who are mentally as well as physically healthy. Parents and children must be taught to achieve the balance between being over-protective and restricting most physical activities and avoiding high-risk behaviors, such as tackle football. During high school, vocational counseling is important to channel abilities into occupations that are not associated with frequent trauma and that do not unduly stress joints.

Economic Issues

A normal life expectancy is projected for a child born with hemophilia. With early aggressive therapy, arthritis should be minimized. The licensing of recombinant ("man-made") factor VIII is a major breakthrough in terms of both safety and potential supply. One of the major challenges is how to pay for therapy. Clotting factor is extremely expensive. The estimated cost for an adult with no complications is $60,000 per year for clotting factor alone. Insurance policies vary greatly in what the insurer will pay as well as in lifetime caps. Some states have programs that will serve as a "payer of last resort" for clotting factor. Unfortunately, an increasing number of families have to resort to public aid to cope with medical bills. This is both demoralizing for the individual who usually wants to work, and wasteful, as tax dollars are subsidizing a family who could be earning and paying taxes.

Consumer and Government Organizations

In the mid-1970s, the U.S. government established a network of comprehensive hemophilia centers across the country. These centers offer multidisciplinary care with strong emphasis on early intervention and have been shown to be cost-effective (Smith, Levine, and Directors, 1984). The National Hemophilia Foundation (NHF) has set standards of hemophilia care (*Standards and Criteria,* 1994) and has a directory of hemophilia treatment centers and facilities (*Directory of Hemophilia Treatment Centers,* 1991). It also has a variety of educational materials, an information resource center (HANDI), and sponsors peer-driven support networks for men and women affected by bleeding disorders. Local chapters likewise provide education and are knowledgeable about resources in their area. Some provide services such as camp, case management, and counseling as well.

Future Research

For the child born with hemophilia, the future looks bright. The goal is no longer preventing death and disability; it is preventing arthritis. As mentioned in the section dealing with treatment, more physicians are recommending routine infusions of factor concentrates two or three times weekly to prevent bleeding episodes, rather than treating them after they occur. The development of very small infusion pumps concurrent with purer, more concentrated and less expensive factor concentrates, should permit continuous rather than intermittent infusions of Factors VIII and IX. This should not only provide more consistent factor levels, but reduce the total amount of factor necessary to maintain a measurable (greater than 1%) factor level.

Finally, a "cure" for hemophilia through gene therapy is a real possibility. Gene therapy will not change the individual's own genes. Rather, a normal gene for Factor VIII or IX production is inserted into such cells as muscle and liver taken from the person with hemophilia. These cells are grown in the laboratory and put back into the individual's body (e.g., muscle cells can be placed under the skin). The cells, now containing the normal Factor VIII or IX gene, produce clotting factor, which they release into the circulation. Although normal factor levels will not be achieved, enough factor will be produced to turn a person with severe hemophilia into one with mild disease, requiring factor for surgery and major trauma only.

(*See also:* ARTHRITIS; CANCER REHABILITATION; HUMAN IMMUNODEFICIENCY VIRUS DISEASE AND ACQUIRED IMMUNODEFICIENCY SYNDROME; SICKLE CELL ANEMIA AND THALASSEMIA [HEMOGLOBINOPATHIES]; STROKE)

RESOURCES

Hemophilia and AIDS/HIV Network for the Dissemination of Information (HANDI), 110 Greene St., Suite 406, New York, NY 10012

The National Hemophilia Foundation (NHF), The SoHo Building, 110 Greene St., Suite 303, New York, NY 10012

BIBLIOGRAPHY

ALEDORT, LOUIE M. "Orthopedic Outcome Study." In *Abstract Book, XX International Congress of the World Federation of Hemophilia.* Athens, Greece, 1992.

GILBERT, MARUIN S. "Prophylaxis: Musculoskeletal Evaluation." *Seminars in Hematology* 30 (1993):3–6.

GILBERT, MARUIN S., and GREENE, WALTER B. *Musculoskeletal Problems in Hemophilia*, New York, 1990.

HILGARTNER, MARGARET W., and POCHEDLY, CARL, eds. *Hemophilia in the Child and Adult*, 3rd ed. New York, 1989.

KELLY, LORAN A. *Raising a Child with Hemophilia.* New York, 1991.

LJUNG, ROLF; LINDGREN, ANN–CHRISTINE; TENGBORN, LILIAN; and PETRINI, PIA. "The Feasibility of Long Term Venous Access in Children with Hemophilia." *Seminars in Hematology* 31 (1994):16–18.

MANCO-JOHNSON, MARILYN J.; NUSS, RACHELLE; GERAGHTY, SUE; and FINK, SHARON. "A Prophylactic Program in the United States: Experience and Issues." *Seminars in Hematology* 31 (1994):10–12.

MILLER, CONNIE. *Inheritance of Hemophilia.* New York, 1992.

NATIONAL HEMOPHILIA FOUNDATION. *Standards and Criteria for the Care of Persons with Congenital Bleeding Disorders.* New York, 1994.

———. *Hemophilia and Sports.* New York, 1992.

NILSSON, INGA MARIE; BERNTORP, ERIC; LJUNG, ROLF et al. "Prophylactic Therapy of Severe Hemophilia A and B Can Prevent Joint Disability." *Seminars in Hematology* 31 (1994):5–9.

PETTERSON, HOLGER. "Can Joint Disease Be Quantified?" *Seminars in Hematology* 31 (1994):1–4.

———. "Radiographic Scores and Implications." *Seminars in Hematology* 30 (1993):7–11.

SMITH, PETER S.; LEVINE, PETER H.; and the Directors of Eleven Participating Hemophilia Centers. "The Benefits of Comprehensive Care of Hemophilia: A Five-Year Study of Outcomes." *American Journal of Public Health* 74 (1984):616–617.

VAN DEN BERG, H. MARIJKE; NIEUWENHUIS, H. KAREL; MAUSER-BUNSCHOTEN, EVELINE P., and ROOSENDAAL, GORIS. "Hemophilic Prophylaxis in the Netherlands." *Seminars in Hematology* 31 (1994):13–15.

EMILY E. CZAPEK

BODY IMAGE

See SELF-CONCEPT; PSYCHOSOCIAL ADJUSTMENT

BONE DISEASES

See MUSCULOSKELETAL DISORDERS

BRACES

See PROSTHETICS AND ORTHOTICS

BRAIN INJURY

See HEAD INJURY

BULIMIA NERVOSA

See EATING DISORDERS

BURNS

One of the most devastating traumas in human experience is severe burn injury. Two million Americans suffer burn injury each year, the highest rate of all industrialized nations. Annually, over 7,000 die from fire and burn injuries, a rate of about 3 per 100,000. About 70,000 are hospitalized with burn injuries (National Commission on Fire Prevention and Control, 1977), half of whom are treated in one of the 170 hospitals that have specialized burn treatment centers (Burn Care Resources in North America, 1993). More than one-third of deaths and injuries from burns are to children; burns are the second leading cause of death of children aged one to four and the third leading cause of death of all under the age of nineteen. The elderly, persons with disabilities, and those with psychopathology and diseases, such as epilepsy or diabetes, are also highly prone to injury and death from burns. Twenty to 40 percent of burn patients have a previous psychiatric history (Tucker, 1986), dementia, mental retardation, and epilepsy being the most common conditions (Antebi, 1993).

Types of Burns

There are five basic types of burns:

1. thermal burns, which result from flame, hot surfaces, or explosion;
2. scalds, which result from hot liquids and steam;

3. chemical burns, caused by both acids and bases, and other chemical oxidizing agents;

4. electrical burns, generally caused by high-voltage electricity and lightning;

5. radiation burns, the most common type of burn, which usually result from sunburn and are considered minor although they can be serious and can even result in death. (Other sources of radiation are radioactive chemicals and waves of the spectrum such as X rays.)

Although most major burns appear as large burns on the body's surface, electrical burns may not appear as large but may be considerably more serious. Electrical burns may enter the body at one small point and come out at another (sometimes explosively) without appearing too traumatic, but the path through the body between these two points may coagulate the blood, completely cutting off the supply. Amputation of one or more limbs may be required, and death may ensue.

Two factors involving burns determine the nature of the injury and the possible course of recovery: depth of burn and size of burn. At one time, depth of burn was described by the medical profession, and still is by laypeople, in terms of degree. First degree is the least serious and is generally just a reddening of the skin, usually from sunburn. Although a first-degree burn may be uncomfortable, it is self-healing and normally requires no medical treatment.

Second-degree burns result in the destruction of the outer layer of the skin, called the epidermis, which generally heals by itself. Second-degree burns can, under certain conditions, progress to third-degree burns unless proper precautions are taken. Second-degree burns can be very painful, are pink to red in color that blanches when pressed, and can be marked by blistering. The skin beneath the blister will have a moist appearance. Blisters should be retained as long as possible to maintain a sterile environment.

In the case of third-degree burns, all of the skin has been destroyed, and since no skin cells remain, it cannot regenerate by itself and usually requires surgery unless the burned area is small. The skin will be firm and leathery, with colors of white, black, and brown. It does not blanch when pressed. Although considered to be painless because the sensory

nerves in the area have been destroyed, most burn survivors suggest that these are painful burns as well.

Fourth-degree burns involve not only all the skin layers, but also the organs, muscles, and/or bones beneath the skin. These are obviously the most serious.

Burn care professionals tend to not use degree to describe depth of burn but refer instead to partial-thickness burns for second-degree burns (first-degree burns are not usually considered in that they are of little medical consequence), full-thickness burns for third-degree burns, and deep full-thickness burns for fourth-degree burns (Figure 1, p. 128).

In addition to the depth of the burn, the percent of the total body surface area (TBSA) that is burned is of considerable importance in determining treatment and outcome. Assessing the extent of the burn is usually done according to the "Rule of Nines" (Figure 2, p. 129). On a diagram of the full front and rear of the adult human body, the entire head and neck and each arm are assigned a value of 9 percent, the front torso, back torso, and each leg are assigned 18 percent, and the perineum, 1 percent (totaling 100%). The diagrams are shaded by the physician to match the patient's burn topography. Solid shading indicates full-thickness burns; hatched shading, partial-thickness burns. A technique has also evolved that uses computer modeling on a screen display of a three-dimensional mannequin. Because the ratio of body parts varies from infancy to age fifteen and above (an infant's head, for example, represents a significantly larger percentage of the total body surface than an adult's), corrections must be factored in. This is usually done according to a Lund and Browder Chart, which is a table of age versus percent of surface for each external body component. Several other diagrams and nomograms are also used for this purpose.

First Aid

Over the millennia that humankind has suffered burn injury, a panoply of suggested remedies has proliferated. Few of these have proved helpful, and most are actually harmful. The recommended treatment for burns is as follows.

1. Stop the burning process. Remove the victim from the heat source. Stop, drop, and roll to

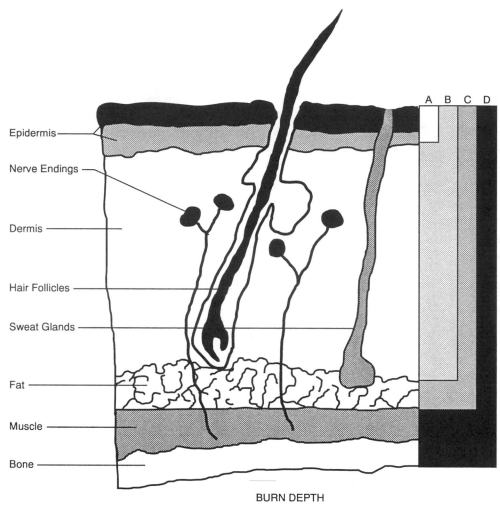

Epidermis
Nerve Endings
Dermis
Hair Follicles
Sweat Glands
Fat
Muscle
Bone

A B C D

BURN DEPTH
A. First Degree (Superficial)
B. Second Degree (Partial Thickness)
C. Third Degree (Full Thickness)
D. Fourth Degree (Deep Full Thickness)

Figure 1. Burn Depth
SOURCE: Alan J. Breslau

smother the flames, cutting off the oxygen needed for combustion.

2. Quickly remove any clothing that could retain the heat and cause even deeper burning. Be careful not to remove any clothing sticking to the skin.

3. Cool the burn with tap water. Do not use ice, which may cause further skin damage. Do not cool too large a body area because this might cause hypothermia, a dangerous lowering of the body temperature and a life-threatening condition. Do not apply butter, petroleum jelly, or other ointments. These may hold in the heat and cause problems in removal at a hospital.

4. For large burns, cover the victim with a clean, dry cloth to prevent shock and retain normal body heat. Calm the victim until help arrives.

5. Do not break any blisters that form; these help to maintain a sterile field and reduce pain.

6. For burns of the head, hands, feet, and perineum, or if the victim is an infant, child, or sick or elderly person, seek medical help at once. Help should also be obtained if a third-degree burn is suspected or if swelling or infection de-

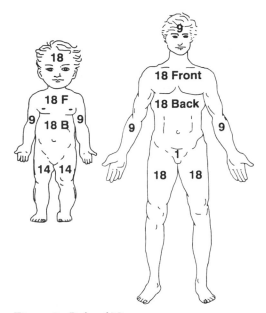

Figure 2. Rule of Nines

SOURCE: Alan J. Breslau

the dermis, or corium. It is packed with a wide variety of cells and nerves that perform many different functions: Ruffini's corpuscles sense heat in one temperature range; Krause's end bulbs sense it in another range; Meissner's corpuscle is sensitive to a light touch; the Pacinian to a heavy one. The skin plays a role in the production of vitamin D, actually a hormone, and is involved in a number of biochemical functions, many of which may be lost as the result of a severe burn, creating problems that go beyond those involving the skin as a barrier to the outside world (Schmeck, 1988).

Melanocytes produce the pigment melanin, which gives the skin its shades of color and helps to protect us from harmful ultraviolet light. The number of melanocytes is fairly constant; variations in their production of melanin make one skin light and another skin dark. Carotenes, which Orientals have in abundance, add a yellowish component. Hemoglobin adds a pinkish tinge to very fair-skinned individuals. Eccrine sweat glands help to cool the body via evaporation, and the sebaceous glands lubricate the skin around the hair follicles. The skin is also the organ through which we are recognized and evaluated. It mirrors our age, ethnicity, health, and emotions.

The lowest level of the skin is called subcutaneous tissue. This layer helps to protect the body against heat and cold, and against physical shock.

velops. Burns may be more serious than they first appear. Inhalation of combustion gases, fumes, and hot air can cause life-endangering damage to the airways, even if the actual burns are limited in extent. Immediate medical help is necessary.

The Skin

The skin is an organ of the body. In fact, it is the largest organ. It serves many functions. It prevents us from dissolving into our surroundings. It is porous but at the same time leakproof in order to retain vital fluids that constantly circulate through our bodies. We are encrusted with dead skin cells that take about fourteen days to reach the body's surface and then survive there, for perhaps an equal amount of time, before sloughing off. Yet the skin is a hotbed of chemical and disease-fighting activity.

The skin is composed of three layers, and in some parts of the body, four layers. The epidermis, or outer layer, is composed of flattened cells called keratinocytes that fill with keratin (the principal constituent of the skin, hair, nails, horny tissues, and tooth enamel) as they move to the skin surface. No matter how supple and healthy the skin looks, it is covered with dead cells. Beneath this thin crust is

Emergency Treatment

Approximately 170 hospitals in the United States have specialized departments for the treatment of burns. Most burn patients, however, are treated in hospitals that lack this special expertise. In many areas of the country, victims with large burns may be evacuated from the accident scene by specially equipped aircraft, helicopter or fix-wing (essentially, flying ambulances), directly to a burn center for treatment. If burn victims are first taken to a local hospital to be given emergency treatment, they are stabilized before being sent on to a burn center.

A burn is defined as major if the TBSA involved is greater than 10 percent; if the age of the victim is below six or greater than thirty-five; if the burn involves the face, hands, feet, perineum, or joints or is circumferential; if there is concurrent injury (fracture), electrical injury, or chemical injury; if there is suspicion of child abuse/neglect; if the patient/family cannot manage aftercare; or if there is a medical history of chronic/severe illness (diabetes, etc.).

After burn assessment and treatment of other concurrent life-threatening conditions that may take precedence (breathing problems, bleeding, shock, head and spinal injuries, fractures, soft-tissue damage, and foreign bodies that may have entered the body in the case of an explosion or accident), replacement of fluids lost to the oozing of the wounds and the dumping of fluid from the blood vessels into the interstitial tissues (which results in life-threatening thickening of the blood) must be initiated as soon as possible. These fluids are dripped through an intravenous catheter at prescribed rates directly into the bloodstream. The urinary output is collected and measured in order to ensure a proper balance.

Treatment of the Burn

Major burns should be treated in a specialized burn treatment center, where the entire medical team is dedicated only to that purpose. The team may consist of burn surgeons, plastic and reconstructive surgeons, physicians, psychiatrists, psychologists, burn nurses, physical therapists, occupational therapists, recreational therapists, social workers, dietitians, and an entire cadre of other support services. Each team member performs a special service.

After smoke inhalation, the leading cause of burn death in the hospital is infection. All bodies are covered with bacteria that can contaminate the burn wound, and the accident itself may be another source. At one time many burn survivors succumbed to massive infection, but with the development of topical antibiotics, this cause of mortality has been reduced tremendously. (Systemic antibiotics are not used to fight wound infection because blood circulation to the wound itself is compromised, preventing the antibiotic from reaching the site.)

The scabs that form over the burn wound, called eschar, are a breeding ground for bacteria and have to be removed. This is done by picking them off, or removing them when they adhere to the gauze dressings placed over them, in a process called debride-

ment (pronounced *dee BREED ment*). This is probably the most painful part of burn treatment and the most difficult for the patient. Sometimes this procedure is performed in large stainless-steel bathtubs called Hubbard tanks or by using hand showers with the patient suspended over the tank.

Traditionally there has been a reluctance to administer sufficient narcotic pain medication to the burn patient undergoing treatment for fear that the patient might become addicted and that lung function might be impaired. This is rarely the case, but the fears still persist. Thus, the pain of treatment is often much worse than the pain from the burn itself. Theoretically, full-thickness burns should not be painful because all of the sensory nerves in the skin have been destroyed. Burn survivors do not confirm this lack of pain, however (U.S. Department of Health and Human Services, 1992).

Alternatives to pain medication are sometimes used. These include distraction therapy, such as counting backward from one hundred, deep breathing, listening to music, and sometimes hypnosis. Patients have been known to resort to self-hypnosis in order to overcome the excruciating pain (Breslau, 1977). Self-administered analgesia, in which the patient uses a medication pump and decides how much of the total allotted dosage to administer, is also finding wide use.

If the burn wound is circumferential—that is, if it runs completely around a limb or the torso—it can act as a natural tourniquet and trap the body fluids in the restricted compartment, causing severe swelling and endangering the limb. Then it becomes necessary, as an emergency treatment, to make deep incisions parallel to the axis of the limb in order to relieve the pressure.

At one time, the survivor of a massive burn could expect to be hospitalized for treatment and reconstructive surgery for many months and years, sometimes decades. With newer techniques, hospitalization time has been reduced to days and weeks. The general rule for acute care is one day of hospitalization for each percentage of burn. The need for debridement has also been considerably reduced and sometimes eliminated by a technique that involves early incision and grafting. In this process, the eschar is excised, sometimes along with unburned tissue, within days of the accident and the area covered immediately with a skin graft (explained below). This not only stops the pain and reduces the chance of infection but imposes the functional and cosmetic outcome as well. The procedure is performed in the operating room with the patient under anesthesia.

Since third- and fourth-degree burns do not heal by themselves because all of the skin cells have been destroyed, it is necessary to cover them with skin from another part of the patient's own body. (Skin from others—except a genetically identical twin—will be rejected by the body's immune system when it recognizes that a foreign material has been attached.) This process is called a skin graft. The place on the patient's body where the skin has been harvested to cover the wound is called the donor site. Sometimes the full thickness of skin is excised from the donor site to repair certain burn wounds, and the donor site is closed by suturing the margins together. The full-thickness skin removed from the donor site cannot be too large. For large areas of coverage, only a split thickness of donor-site skin is harvested, using an instrument called a dermatome. This shaves off a precisely controlled thickness of skin, usually the epidermis with a small amount of dermis attached. The donor site will heal naturally within ten days to two weeks and may be harvested again and again, in rare cases as many as twenty-nine times.

For burns of 50 percent of body surface area or less, there is theoretically sufficient donor skin available (the other 50%) to cover the burn. For larger burns, however, there would not be sufficient skin for full coverage. Many techniques have been developed for covering larger and larger burn wounds so that even patients with burn wounds greater than 90 percent are surviving. This has been accomplished in a number of ways. A small wound heals from the margins toward the center. There is a limit to the amount of coverage that will result from this lateral growth in a reasonable period of time, and leaving the wound open is too risky. One early technique used to increase coverage of the donor skin so that it could close a larger wound was to cut the donor skin into postage-stamp-sized pieces, spread them out over the wound, and allow the gaps between "stamps" to grow in. This was a tedious and difficult procedure, and retention of the stamps in place until they "took" was not always effective. A series of devices, called skin meshers, overcomes some of the shortcomings of the postage-stamp grafts. The harvested donor skin is passed through a device that incises it with parallel dotted lines spaced closely together so that the skin can be stretched anywhere from one and a half to nine times its original size. The small triangular openings in the mesh grow inward, closing the openings with new skin. The healed product has the appearance of chicken skin and smooths out somewhat as the new skin matures.

But even nine-to-one expansion of the donor skin may not be sufficient to provide full coverage of the massively burned patient. Other techniques must be used. Even if the patient has remaining skin only the size of a thumbnail, it can be harvested (biopsied) and reduced to clusters of only a few cells each. These are "seeded" onto a nutrient medium in a large number of special glass dishes. In about three weeks each dish contains a patch of skin about two inches square. After several manipulations, these are lifted off onto a Vaseline-covered gauze, frozen, and returned to the patient. The process is called cultured epithelial autograft.

While this is taking place, the patient is usually covered with a temporary skin, such as pigskin (heterograft or xenograft), which is the closest skin to human skin, cadaver skin (allograft or homograft), or a synthetic skin covering. Because burn injury suppresses the immune response somewhat, these foreign coverings are not rejected as quickly as they normally would be in a healthy patient. When the patient's cultured skin is returned, the foreign skin is excised and replaced with the autograft patches.

Unfortunately, the autograft is extremely thin, perhaps only a half-dozen cells deep, and does not offer sufficient protection. It was found that if only the epidermis (or outer) layer of the cadaver skin has been excised, leaving behind the much thicker dermis layer, the body's immune system will not recognize it as a foreign substance. (Apparently, the cells that signal the immune system are contained only in the epidermis.) Thus, the resulting combination of homograft dermis and autograft epidermis will provide sufficient coverage and protection to extremely large burns.

Synthetic skins, reconstituted from biologic materials, are being developed and have been clinically tested successfully for permanent use. These can be stored and used by any patient as a permanent skin covering without rejection, with excellent cosmetic and functional results.

Because of increased metabolism, the number of calories a burn survivor needs, even to maintain his or her initial weight, is about double the normal—as many as 5,000 to 6,000 calories a day. The need for the patient to consume excessive amounts of food (called hyperalimentation) is difficult at the early stages, as there is generally a loss of appetite. In such cases, a tube is passed through the patient's nose down into the stomach, and a nutritious high-calorie fluid is slowly pumped into the patient, sometimes twenty-four hours a day. If this is not possible, intravenous feeding is used to feed nutrients directly into the bloodstream.

Physical Rehabilitation

Once all of the patient's wounds have been covered with skin, and sometimes even before this has been completed, the patient begins a regimen of physical and occupational rehabilitation, the aim of which is to return the patient to the full range of motion. The patient also is trained in ways to overcome any disabilities or limitations imposed by his or her new condition. This can be a painful and stressful period. Joints sometimes fuse when kept inactive for prolonged periods; muscle mass may be lost due to atrophy; and the injury may have damaged muscles, tendons, nerves, and bones. Yet in most cases, recovery usually is quite successful.

Burn scars typically have a ropelike appearance and are hypertrophic; that is, they often heal above the surface of the surrounding skin because of the nodular formation of collagen fibers (Robberson & Maxwell 1990). A proliferation of capillaries may leave them deeper in color. Keloid scars are benign tumors that are sharply elevated and ever growing due to excessive collagen formation. Surgical removal is usually ineffective in that there is a high rate of recurrence. They generally cause no harm except that they may produce contractures (shortening of tissue).

Contractures of burn scars and grafted areas are a continuing source of problems for the survivor, and further remedial surgery is necessary to eliminate this tightening of the skin, especially over joint areas. Surgical procedures called releases and Z-plasties, as well as further grafting, help to reduce these contractures.

Itching is another major scourge of the burn survivor. The healing wounds itch severely as new nerves are being formed, and few techniques provide satisfactory alleviation. After about six months, the itching generally ceases.

One technique used to smooth out the raised scars, contractures, and discoloration, and to reduce itching, is the use of pressure garments. These are custom-made stretch-fabric garments, carefully measured and constructed to apply an even pressure to all of the scarred areas. They must be worn twenty-three hours a day for periods ranging from six months to two years until the scars have matured and no further benefit can be expected. Masks for facial burns, made of either fabric or hard clear plastic, are also used, although these sometimes create embarrassing situations for adult burn survivors in banks and convenience stores.

Psychosocial Rehabilitation

In spite of all the pain and suffering, the physical and financial loss, the feelings of guilt, and perhaps the loss of loved ones that a burn survivor undergoes, it is almost universally agreed that the most difficult part of the experience is the staring of the public at the disfigurement. Burn injury results in a completely new physical appearance. The survivor and the family must go through the stages of grief that one undergoes when someone dies—denial and isolation, anger, bargaining, depression, acceptance (Kübler-Ross, 1975). The former self no longer exists. A new person has been born physically, mentally, and emotionally. For many, this can be a difficult transition.

The patient's feelings and moods may change from day to day, and even during the course of a single day, as he or she adapts to the new realities. Family members also experience great difficulty in coping with the many problems and guilt associated with the trauma. They, too, must develop coping mechanisms and strategies that vary with the different stages of the healing process and are dependent on many factors. Psychological and emotional support are also important for them; their problems tend to be neglected and all attention directed toward the burn patient.

Burn survivors often go through hallucinations, nightmares, and insomnia in the first days and weeks after the accident. These phenomena generally cease after discharge from the hospital but may persist from time to time. Flashbacks to the trauma and other indicators of post-traumatic stress disorder (PTSD) are quite common after burn injury.

Even if the patient receives psychological and psychiatric counseling, being out in public may still be difficult. Psychosocial peer-support groups are available to help burn survivors make the transition.

Marriage relationships are sometimes strained by the many changes—physical, psychological, and emotional—that result from severe burn injury. There may also be difficulties in obtaining or retaining employment as a result of any consequent disfigurement and/or disability. Hospital social workers and psychologists are often available to offer assistance in these areas.

The pressure to attain stereotypical beauty is tremendous. To suddenly become disfigured may be overwhelming to many survivors. Since we cannot prevent the public from staring at someone whose appearance is outside the parameters of "normal," the survivor must learn to cope with this. People are genetically programmed to study anyone or anything that could be a potential threat to their genetic heritage in order to protect themselves. We cannot, and should not, expect them not to look. One technique that has proven effective is for people who are disfigured to speak to the person studying them and explain why they look different, thus allaying any fears.

People who are able to conceal their scars, and tend to do so, may suffer emotionally even more than the obviously disfigured survivor. Those whose faces or hands are disfigured usually come to terms with their condition in time and with counseling, while those with hidden disfigurements are always fearful that their anomalies will be seen and constantly focus on their problem without ever coming to terms with it. This is particularly a syndrome of female children who have been burned and whose parents encourage them to conceal their scars so as not to be ridiculed by peers (Breslau, 1992). This is counterproductive. People must not be ashamed of their scars. They must learn to accept their new body image; once they do that, others will as well.

(*See also:* LOSS AND GRIEF; PAIN; PSYCHOSOCIAL ADJUSTMENT; SURGERY)

RESOURCE

The Phoenix Society for Burn Survivors, Inc., 11 Rust Hill Rd, Levittown, PA 19056

BIBLIOGRAPHY

AMERICAN BURN ASSOCIATION. *Burn Care Resources in North America, 1993–1994.*

ANTEBI, DANIEL. "The Psychiatrist on the Burn Unit." *Burns* 19 (1993):43–46.

BRESLAU, ALAN J. *The Time of My Death.* New York, 1977.

———. "Establishing a World-wide Burn Support Network." *ANZBA Bulletin* (Australian and New Zealand Burn Association) 8 (1992):24–26.

KÜBLER-ROSS, E. *On Death and Dying.* New York, 1975.

NATIONAL COMMISSION ON FIRE PREVENTION AND CONTROL. *America Burning.* Washington, DC 1977.

ROBBERSON, STACY, and MAXWELL, GAIL. *You and Your Family: A Pictorial Book for Burn Patients and Their Families.* Oklahoma City, 1960.

TUCKER, P. "The Burn Victim: A Review of Psychosocial Issues." *Australia and New Zealand Journal of Psychiatry* 20 (1986):413.

U.S. DEPARTMENT OF HEALTH AND HUMAN SERVICES. Agency for Health Care Policy and Research, Clinical Practice Guideline. *Acute Pain Management: Operative or Medical Procedures and Trauma.* March 1992.

ALAN J. BRESLAU

C

CANCER REHABILITATION

"Cancer" is a term applied to a variety of diseases in which some cells in the body have lost their normal regulatory control over growth and can invade other body tissues and spread distantly. More than one million people will be diagnosed with cancer each year, and it is estimated that more than 8 million people are living with cancer in the United States (Cancer Facts & Figures, 1994). The etiology of cancer is multifactorial, but some cancers are associated with tobacco use, alcohol use, or a genetic predisposition.

The treatment of cancer involves surgery; chemotherapy; radiation therapy; hormonal manipulation of the tumor; and immune therapy, attempting to improve the body's normal immune defenses that attack cancer cells. These treatments may be given in combination or singly in an attempt to cure or lessen symptoms of the disease.

Earlier diagnosis and advances in treatments have led to improved survival and many cures. Accordingly, cancer is now regarded more as a chronic illness than an acutely terminal disease. Because of this, there has been an interest in the rehabilitation and assessment of quality of life of the person with cancer. Cancer rehabilitation, as an area of research at the National Cancer Institute, accelerated in the 1970s in response to the National Cancer Act.

Once cancer is diagnosed, it inevitably changes the life of the individual physically, psychologically, and socially. Cancer, as well as its treatment, is associated with a wide variety of disabilities. Cancer rehabilitation involves a coordinated multidisciplinary care approach to the patient in an effort to overcome any physical, psychosocial, or vocational disabilities by preserving or optimizing function and independence.

The cancer rehabilitation and continuing care team involves professionals from multiple fields, including physicians, nurses, physical therapists, occupational therapists, psychologists, speech pathologists, social workers, counselors, clergy, and nutritionists. The team discusses the unique needs and goals of each patient and how best to deal with them. Ideally the rehabilitation team is consulted early after the diagnosis, assisting the patient through and after therapy.

Rehabilitation needs of the patient with cancer

are determined by the type of cancer, and the extent to which normal function has been affected as well as the availability and effectiveness of rehabilitation measures. Lung cancer, for example, is the leading cancer in terms of deaths; and the incidence is high in both sexes. However, the majority of these patients do not live long enough to benefit from major rehabilitative measures, since the five-year survival rate is only 13 percent. Conversely, cancer of the colon and the rectum accounts for approximately 150,000 new cases each year in the United States, but the five-year survival rate is nearly 60 percent, and is almost 90 percent for people with early diagnosis. Except for patients who require a colostomy (an opening of the bowel through the skin of the abdomen), the rehabilitation needs of patients with colon cancer are limited. The need for colostomies has been continually decreasing due to better surgical techniques and, sometimes, the use of radiation therapy and chemotherapy. Colostomy patients can receive instruction in the care of the colostomy from specially trained nurses called enterostomal therapists. Also, organizations such as the United Ostomy Association and the American Cancer Society can offer assistance in education as well as recommend support groups that may be available.

Cancers of the genitourinary system are frequently associated with sexual dysfunction. Prostate cancer is a very common cancer developing in one in ten men by age eight-five. With advances in surgical treatment, potency can frequently be preserved or penile prostheses can be placed to regain sexual function. Sexual dysfunction is also common in women who have undergone treatment for one of the gynecological cancers. The use of lubricants or hormonal replacements, when appropriate, can alleviate vaginal dryness. Ongoing patient and family counseling may also be required. The cancers with unique rehabilitation needs or in which there have been marked advances in rehabilitation include cancers of the head and neck, breast, and the extremities. These are considered in more detail.

Cancers of the Head and Neck

Cancers originating in the mouth, throat, larynx, and sinuses account for only about 8 percent of all cancers in men and 4 percent in women in the United States (Cancer Facts & Figures, 1994). Nevertheless, cancers of the head and neck are among the most disabling. Patients may present with an unresolving sore throat, ear pain, change in voice, or difficulty swallowing. The diagnosis is made by biopsying the abnormal area or an unhealing ulcer.

The primary treatment is usually surgical removal, which may result in major defects and loss of function, depending on the site and size of the cancer. Radiation therapy may be utilized alone in early cancers of the vocal cords, thereby preserving speech. Also, combinations of radiation therapy and chemotherapy are increasingly being used in an attempt to eliminate or reduce the extent of the surgery. However, a sizable number of people later require salvage surgery.

Surgery for cancer of the sinus may involve removal of the cheekbone, eye, and roof of the mouth. An upper dental plate can be fashioned to close the defect in the roof of the mouth. External prostheses may be constructed of synthetic materials such as methylmethacrylate to match the opposite side of the face and can be attached with skin adhesives or anchored to the bone. Prosthetic noses and ears may also be constructed when needed. Reconstructive surgery requires large flaps of skin and muscle to be transferred from another part of the body, such as tissue from the front of the chest up to the head and neck area. Free tissue transfers from more distant areas can be done using microvascular surgical techniques to reestablish the blood supply.

When the larynx is surgically removed because of cancer, normal speech is lost. Air now enters the lungs through an opening or stoma in the neck. Patients who have undergone this procedure can learn to speak again by using air vibrating in the upper esophagus and throat. This is known as esophageal speech. To do this, air is swallowed and then released under the control of the patient to produce speech. Another approach, devised by Mark Singer and Eric Blom (1980), is the creation of an opening between the trachea and the esophagus to supply the air in the esophagus. This opening, or tracheoesophageal fistula, is maintained by a small silicone device with a one-way valve to prevent food from getting into the lungs. Still another manner in which speech can be achieved is by use of a battery-powered vibratory device that produces a tone that can be converted to speech by lip and tongue movements. This device, called an electrolarynx, is usually held to the neck while speaking. Speech pathologists are involved in retraining the patient to speak. Peer assistance and support are provided to patients by clubs such as Lost Chord or New Voice, which are sponsored by the American Cancer Society, and the International Association of Laryngectomees. National and international meetings and training sessions are held for persons with a laryngectomy and their family members.

A significant number of people who have had removal of the larynx are able to return to their previous jobs, depending on the requirements of their occupation. Because of the stoma, the patient with laryngectomy cannot hold his or her breath without using a finger to close the opening. Therefore, heavy lifting cannot be done, since the breath is usually held during the initiation of the lift. Also, occupations in which the person is exposed to dust, chemical fumes, or in which water may get into the stoma are not advised.

Treatment for cancer of the tongue may involve removal of all or part of the tongue. This usually results in difficulty swallowing as well as in speech. Since speech usually requires the tongue to touch the roof of the mouth, a thick upper dental plate can be made to decrease this space. Swallowing problems can be alleviated or improved by instruction from a speech pathologist or occupational therapist in the types or consistency of foods that are easier to swallow. It may be necessary to use a long-handled spoon or a short feeding tube to deliver the food to the throat, where it can be swallowed. Many patients with cancer of the head and neck region also undergo removal of the lymph nodes in the neck to further evaluate the extent of the cancer. A common aftereffect of this procedure is drooping of the shoulder due to loss of function of some of the shoulder muscles. This may prevent the patient from resuming his or her normal occupation if the work involves manual labor.

Radiation therapy to the head and neck may result in disability due to stiffening of the tissues that were in the radiation field, and damage to the salivary and/or lacrimal glands. This can cause varying degrees of neck and lip stiffness to the point where the person has limited neck movement or difficulty

eating. Exercises during and after treatment may help to prevent this complication. Eye and mouth dryness can be improved by use of artificial tears and saliva.

Breast Cancer

Breast cancer is a major problem in our society. In the United States it affects about one in nine women at some time during their life. Early diagnosis is now being achieved through use of screening mammography or X-ray examination of the breasts. A cancer may be detected in this manner even before it can be felt on physical exam. Treatment formerly involved having a radical mastectomy, which consisted of complete removal of the breast as well as the muscles of the chest wall. This procedure always causes some disability. However, radical mastectomies are now rarely performed. Currently, treatment options include either removal of the breast, sparing the chest wall muscles (modified radical mastectomy), or removal of only the tumor (lumpectomy), followed by radiation therapy. In addition, the woman undergoes removal of the lymph nodes or "glands" under the arm to further assess her risk of recurrence of the cancer. Depending on the woman's risk of recurrent disease, she may undergo additional treatment with chemotherapy or hormonal therapy.

When radiation or chemotherapy is given, the treatment may extend over weeks for radiation or over months for chemotherapy. During such therapies the woman may experience a wide range of side effects, with some of the most common being fatigue, nausea, loss of appetite, and hair loss. However, the majority of patients are able to work or do their normal activities, with only minor allowances for appointments during therapy.

The loss of a breast may not be considered a disability for most occupations but may affect the person's arm mobility and ability to lift heavy objects. In addition, a person's self-image, ability to dress as desired, or engage in athletics may be affected after a mastectomy, despite the availability of a prosthesis that is made to match the other breast.

Many women elect to have breast reconstruction, either at the time of surgery or at a later date. There are several options for reconstruction of the breast. The surgery may involve transplanting skin and muscle from the back of the chest, from the lower abdominal wall, or as a free tissue transfer. For example, tissue from the posterior hip area may be transferred up to the breast area, using microsurgical techniques to reestablish the blood supply.

Another option that has found much favor is reconstruction of the breast by inserting a prosthetic breast filled with either silicone or a saline-filled gel under the skin. The tissues overlying the breast area must often be stretched to accommodate a prosthesis that matches the opposite breast in size and shape. This can be accomplished by weekly injections of saline into the prosthesis to stretch the overlying tissue gently and gradually until the desired size is obtained. There has been concern about the safety of silicone prostheses, in particular regarding their possible relationship to some connective tissue disorders. In 1992, the Food and Drug Administration removed silicone-filled breast implants from general use, and further testing continued. Sherine E. Gabriel and a team of colleagues conducted a large and well designed study of women with breast implants and found no evidence of increased risk of connective tissue diseases or cancer (1994). The study showed a slightly greater risk of joint stiffness in patients who had breast prosthesis surgery because of cancer, but the reason is still not known. Further work in this area may help clarify this issue.

After breast surgery, patients need to be instructed in exercises that will return the arm on the affected side to its full range of motion. Occasionally patients may require instructions in alternate ways of accomplishing certain daily tasks, by modification of their current way of performing the task or by use of assistive devices.

Swelling of the arm on the side of the original breast cancer may occur at any time after surgery when the woman has had the lymph nodes under the arm removed or radiated. This condition, known as lymphedema, may be mild or so severe as to be disabling. Prevention of lymphedema includes protection of the arm on the affected side from cuts, sunburn, or other trauma. Infections can develop more easily and may lead to chronic swelling or worsening of the preexisting lymphedema. Occupations in which trauma to the arm and hand are likely to occur need to be avoided or modified to protect the arm from injury or infection. Sometimes just wearing protective gloves will alleviate the potential problem. Treatment of lymphedema may include elevation of the arm; massage; or use of pneumatic compression devices, but their effectiveness is limited.

Spread, or metastasis, of breast cancer to other areas of the body occurs in a significant number of women in spite of effective local treatment and even follow-up or adjuvant chemotherapy. Spread is most often to the bones or the lungs, but many body organs may be affected. Women may live for a number of years even with widespread cancer, which often can be controlled with chemotherapy or hormone treatments. Many of these women continue with their usual work or other activities. Metastasis to the bone may produce pain and may result in spontaneous fractures, particularly of the hip or the spine. Radiation therapy often is a useful form of treatment for these patients.

Of the multiple community organizations with an interest in research in breast cancer and in the breast cancer patient, the Reach to Recovery Program of the American Cancer Society is one of the best known. This organization has now expanded its program to include services to breast cancer patients at any stage of the disease.

Cancers of the Musculoskeletal System

A decrease in a cancer patient's mobility or even the capacity to walk is a common finding. There are multiple reasons why this may occur in a cancer patient. Severe generalized weakness is a common complaint and can be related to the cancer as well as its treatment. Generalized weakness can lead to decreased activity. Also, some lung cancers produce substances that cause muscular weakness. The condition of these people can be evaluated by physical and occupational therapists, and individualized treatment can be initiated using strengthening exercises, braces, walkers, and when necessary wheelchairs to optimize their function and independence.

Cancers can also directly affect mobility and the ability to walk by invading the bone, spinal cord, or brain. Limb-sparing treatment, avoiding amputation, is now possible for up to 90 percent of cancers that start in the muscles or soft tissues of the extremities, according to Walter Lawrence and colleagues (1987). Limb-sparing surgery is also possible for many cancers arising in the bone. Treatment usually involves chemotherapy and radiation along with surgery. The surgery involves excision of the cancerous bone and replacement with other bone or either ceramic or metallic replacement. With new expandable, adjustable metallic replacements, the limb can be lengthened as a child grows.

Vocational Rehabilitation

The financial costs of cancer in this country are enormous. Cancer costs exceed $100 billion a year (Cancer Facts & Figures, 1994). Besides the direct medical costs incurred due to cancer and its treatment, there is the indirect cost to our society in the form of disability and death. This nation is deprived of millions of years of lost productivity and billions of dollars in lost revenue annually.

Returning individuals to their precancer functional lifestyle is the ultimate goal of cancer rehabilitation. However, the scope of the problem of vocational rehabilitation is immense. Patients must contend with negative employer and coworker attitudes and concerns about possible frequent absences, job performance, and the company's health insurance costs.

There is a widespread perception that individuals with cancer suffer discrimination in the workplace solely as a result of the diagnosis of cancer. The extent to which this occurs in patients without impaired function is not known. The Rehabilitation Act of 1973, as amended, specifically mentions cancer and includes wording that covers the "perception" of disability as well as actual disability (Scotch, 1984). Similar provisions are included in the 1990 Americans with Disabilities Act (ADA). In the first year of the ADA more than 12,000 complaints were filed from July 1992 to July 1993, but only 2.7 percent were brought by individuals with cancer. The first case brought to court by the federal Equal Employment Opportunity Commission (EEOC) involved a patient with terminal, inoperable brain cancer. The patient was awarded more than $500,000 on the basis that he had been successfully carrying out his job responsibilities at the time he was fired.

Patients with cancer may not seek to return to work after treatment due to the misconception that work may worsen their condition. Also, patients do not always realize that they are medically able to return to work. However, the majority of cancer survivors hold gainful employment. According to Vincent Mor (1987), 77 percent of cancer survivors who were employed prior to the diagnosis of cancer were still employed one year later. Of the 23 percent no longer employed, the majority had had lung cancer or were blue-collar workers.

Insurance problems are also frequently encountered by cancer patients. In particular, it is very difficult for anyone who has had a cancer diagnosis to obtain or change health or life insurance. Individuals also may feel trapped in their current job due to insurance benefits and the possibility of not being able to obtain new insurance if they leave.

Out-of-pocket expenses encountered by patients with cancer and their families can be staggering. Nonreimbursable out-of-pocket expenses can be 25 to 50 percent of the patient's or family's income (Houts et al., 1984; Lansky et al., 1979).

Continued education and communication among patients, physicians, employers, and insurance companies can work to alleviate the misconceptions, clarify the problems faced by the patient returning to work, and assist patients through their therapy and follow-up.

(*See also:* DISABILITY MANAGEMENT; PROSTHETICS AND ORTHOTICS; PSYCHOSOCIAL ADJUSTMENT; QUALITY OF LIFE; SURGERY)

RESOURCES

The American Cancer Society, 1599 Clifton Rd, NE, Atlanta, GA 30329
  The following programs can be reached by writing to the American Cancer Society
    —International Association of Laryngectomees
    —Look Good . . . Feel Better
    —Lost Chord
    —New Voice
    —Reach to Recovery
Equal Employment Opportunity Commission, 1801 L. St., NW, Washington, DC 20507
National Cancer Institute, Office of Cancer Communications, 31 Center Drive, Mail Stop Code 2580, Bethesda, MD 20892

United Ostomy Association, 36 Executive Park, Suite 120, Irvine, CA 92714

International Association of Enterostomal Therapy, 2081 Business Center Drive, Suite 290, Irvine, CA 92715

The Canadian Cancer Society, 2 Carlton St., Suite 710, Toronto, Ont. M5B 2J2

National Cancer Institute of Canada, 10 Alcorn Ave., Suite 200, Toronto, Ont. M4V 381

Canadian Association for Enterostomal Therapy, 158 Cameron Crescent, Pointe Claire, PQ, H9R 4E1

BIBLIOGRAPHY

AMERICAN CANCER SOCIETY. *Cancer Facts & Figures.* Atlanta, 1994.

GABRIEL, SHERINE E.; O'FALLON, W. MICHAEL; KURLAND, LEAONARD T.; et al. "Risk of Connective-Tissue Diseases and Other Disorders After Breast Implantation." *New England Journal of Medicine* 330,24(1994):1697–1702.

HOUTS, PETER S.; LIPTON, ALLEN; HARVEY, HAROLD A.; et al. "Nonmedical Costs to Patients and Their Families Associated with Outpatient Chemotherapy." *Cancer* 53(1984):2388–2392.

LANSKY, SHIRLEY B.; CAIRNS, NANCY U.; CLARK, GARY M.; ET AL. "Childhood Cancer: Nonmedical Costs of the Illness." *Cancer* 43(1979):403–408.

LAWRENCE, WALTER; DONEGAN, WILLIAM L.; NATARAJAN, NACHIMUTH; et al. "Adult Soft Tissue Sarcomas: A Pattern of Care Survey of the American College of Surgeons." *Annals of Surgery* 205,4(1987):349–359.

MOR, VINCENT. "Work Loss, Insurance Coverage, and Financial Burden Among Cancer Patients." *American Cancer Society: Proceedings of the Workshop on Employment, Insurance and the Patients with Cancer—1987* (1987):5–10.

SCOTCH, RICHARD K. *From Goodwill to Civil Rights: Transforming Federal Disability Policy.* Philadelphia, 1984.

SINGER, MARK I. and BLOM, ERIC D. "An Endoscopic Technique for Restoration of the Voice after Laryngology." *Annals of Otology, Rhinology, and Laryngology* 89 (1980):529–533.

SUSAN J. MELLETTE
KAREN L. BLUNK

CARDIOVASCULAR DISORDERS

See CORONARY ARTERY DISEASE; STROKE

CAREER COUNSELING

Career counseling is a recognized counseling specialty in its own right, and so a number of definitions of the field have been proposed in its growing body of literature. Two particularly comprehensive, albeit differently oriented, definitions will be provided here. A 1991 position paper of the major professional organization in the field, the National Career Development Association (NCDA), stated, "Career counseling is defined as counseling individuals or groups of individuals about occupations, careers, life/career roles and responsibilities, career decision making, career planning, leisure planning, career pathing, and other career development activities (e.g., resume preparation, interviewing and job search techniques), together with the issues or conflicts that individuals confront regarding their careers." This definition places its heaviest emphasis on the first word of "career counseling." Another definition, which instead places greater emphasis on the second word, is by Linda Brooks and Duane Brown (1986): "Career counseling is an interpersonal process designed to assist individuals with career development problems. Career development is that process of choosing, entering, adjusting to, and advancing in an occupation. It is a lifelong psychological process that interacts dynamically with other life roles. Career problems include, but are not limited to, career indecision and undecidedness, work performance, stress and adjustment, incongruence of the person and work environment, and inadequate or unsatisfactory integration of life roles with other life roles (e.g., parent, friend, citizen)."

Here the term "career counseling" will be used to refer to the kinds of corrective interventions indicated in these two definitions, but several other aspects of vocational behavior, including career development, work adjustment, and career programming, will also be defined and discussed.

For the first fifty-three years of its existence, U.S. federal legislation authorizing programs for the rehabilitation of persons with disabilities preceded the word "rehabilitation" with the modifier "vocational," and even since that modifier was removed in 1973, return to work has remained one of the two stated goals of the state-federal rehabilitation program (along with independent living). Moreover, return to work has undisputedly always been the principal goal of insurance rehabilitation and of disability management programs in industry. During the half century that rehabilitation was known as vocational rehabilitation, what is now called career counseling was known first as "vocational guidance" and later changed to "vocational counseling" to reflect the ascendance of a less directive approach to the helping process. The goal of both vocational counseling and vocational rehabilitation was to help the client (in the former case, school leavers, immigrants, or able-bodied unemployed persons; in the latter case, persons with disabilities) to choose and obtain an appropriate line of work. Over time, just as rehabilitation broadened its mission, the field of vocational counseling broadened its conceptualization of its function from offering ad hoc assistance with a single, one-time choice to viewing work behavior as a lifelong developmental process in which any single career decision must be placed within the context of that process. This change led the field to change its name to career counseling. This change in perspective should have closed any conceptual gap between career counseling and rehabilitation because now a personal history of disability, whether congenital or acquired, becomes just one idiosyncratic aspect of a person's career development.

Therefore, at least theoretically, career counseling for persons with disabilities should not differ from career counseling for any other client. In practice, however, this is less than totally true, primarily because the person with a disability presents unique issues that were not presented by the nondisabled population on whom career counseling approaches were developed. Samuel H. Osipow (1976) summarized some of these issues as follows: (1) the person with a disability is more frequently forced to take whatever job he or she can get, rather than being free to follow a preferred career development plan; (2) for many persons with mental disabilities, the capacity for personal choice and the decision-making process may be impaired; (3) severe disability may override otherwise dominant personal characteristics in determining career behavior; (4) realistically, options for persons with many disabilities may be quite limited; (5) the disability may have arrested or slowed the person's career development process; and (6) for persons with disabilities, career development is often continuously stressful

rather than stressful just at choice points. Consequently, we must continue to treat the career development and career counseling of persons with disabilities as a special instance rather than just another example of a general principle. Accordingly, this entry will first consider career counseling processes in general and then their specific applications in rehabilitation.

Components of Career Intervention

Three basic components of career intervention have developed largely independently of each other. These components, presented in the sequence in which they emerged as systematic activities, are career counseling, career development, and career programming. Although there were some attempts in the 1880s to develop a system of vocational guidance based on phrenology (the study of the bumps on a person's skull as an indication of mental faculties and character), the first systematic, scientific approach to career counseling is credited to Frank Parsons (1854–1908), a law professor and social activist who in the year of his death founded the first documented career counseling program, the Vocation Bureau, in Boston, Massachusetts. Its stated purpose was "to aid young people in choosing an occupation, preparing themselves for it, finding an opening in it, and building up a career of efficiency and success. And to help any, young and old, who seek counsel as to opportunities and resources for the betterment of their condition and the means of increasing their economic efficiency" (Parsons's statement in *The Arena*, July 1908, quoted in Davis, 1969). Thus the initial statement of purpose by the visionary founder of the field incorporated the words "career" and "counsel." In Parsons's book, *Choosing a Vocation*, published posthumously in 1909, he outlined the factors involved in the choice of a vocation as "(1) a clear understanding of yourself, your aptitudes, abilities, interests, ambitions, resources, limitations, and their causes; (2) a knowledge of the requirements and conditions of success, advantages and disadvantages, compensation, opportunities, and prospects in different lines of work; (3) true reasoning on the relations of these two groups of facts." Since that time the field of career counseling has been attempting to implement and build upon Parsons's statement. For the first half of the twentieth century the field focused on developing objective measures by which a person could gain that "clear understanding of [themselves and their] aptitudes, abilities, interests, ambitions, resources, limitations," and vocational guidance consisted of administering and interpreting these measures to clients. Since the middle 1960s, the approach of matching personality types with characteristics of occupations has been best represented by the work of John L. Holland (1985) and his widely used instrument, the Self-Directed Search.

Just before World War II, in part influenced by European psychotherapists who emigrated to America to escape Nazi persecution, the field of counseling took on a strong orientation toward human development. This orientation found its way into the career field primarily through the work of Donald E. Super, who in 1953 published "a theory of vocational development" in the *American Psychologist*. This theory contained ten propositions, among them that people differed in abilities, interests, and personalities in ways that qualify them for a number of occupations; that vocational development involves the development and implementation of a self-concept through a continuous process of choice, adjustment, and compromise; that this developmental process follows a defined pattern of successive stages; and that satisfaction involves finding work that provides adequate outlets for one's abilities, interests, and personality. Thus a shift in focus was introduced, from Parsons's attention to the single event of choosing a vocation to a new conception of vocational development as an ongoing, lifelong process. This movement resulted in the creation of two new elements within the field of careers: one, a new field of theory and research in career development, closely related to the general field of human development; and the other, an alternative approach to career counseling that placed its emphasis on examining career issues as life-span issues of personal growth and development rather than on the single, focused issue of vocational choice that Parsons and his following espoused. The approach of Parsons and his followers became known as the trait-and-factor approach, and the newer alternative became known as the developmental approach.

Subsequently, a third major approach, the information-processing approach, arose out of two sources. One source was the use of occupational information in arriving at a career choice, and the other source was the developing area of cognitive psychology, with its interest in how people take in, store, and use information to make decisions. Since the choice of an occupation generally involves deciding on something that one has never before fully experienced, information about possible options is extremely important. Donald Zytowski (1972) has shown that occupational information existed as early as the year 1468. Modern examples of occupation information include the U.S. Department of Labor's *Dictionary of Occupational Titles* and *Occupational Outlook Handbook*, brochures put out by commercial sources, and computerized systems such as CHOICES, DISCOVER, and SIGI. Interest in the area of human information processing was largely stimulated by the invention of the computer. The application of this approach to career counseling is best exemplified by John D. Krumboltz's statement in the book *Social Learning and Career Decision Making* (1979). In this approach, career counseling focuses on assisting clients in how to develop their information-seeking, processing, and decision-making skills and to apply these skills to resolving their career issues.

Finally, a fourth school of thought holds that career development is primarily determined by one's cultural or socioeconomic background or even by sheer accident, such as being in the right place at the right time. As these views place control largely outside the individual, they offer relatively little that is applicable in career counseling beyond an awareness that these factors may be operating.

Since the late 1980s, attempts have been made in the literature to define a general process of career counseling that incorporates insights from all major schools of thought. Elizabeth B. Yost and M. Anne Corbishley (1987) have listed the steps in career counseling as (1) initial assessment to determine feasibility for career counseling; (2) exploring the client's values, interests, abilities, and experiences; (3) synthesizing the findings in step 2 to arrive at general career goals; (4) generating a list of possible alternatives congruent with those goals; (5) obtaining occupational information about these options; (6) making a choice among these options, based on all the information at hand; (7) making plans to reach that goal; and (8) implementing those plans. This sequence of steps is applicable to career counseling regardless of whether the counselor's theoretical orientation is trait and factor, developmental, or information processing.

The third component of career intervention is known as career programming. It is obvious that while just about everyone goes through career development, relatively few people seek career counseling. As that is the case, educators and career counseling professionals came to recognize the need to facilitate the career development process for the majority of people who did not seek help. Thus programs to instruct people in the selection and pursuit of career goals have been developed in schools, colleges, community agencies, government departments, and business and industry. In business and industry, career programs are often company-specific, focusing on how to attain optimal career pathing within that setting. As with career counseling, career programming may follow a trait-and-factor, developmental, or information-processing orientation, depending on the orientation of the person who designs the program.

Thus the career field may be thought of as a three-by-three matrix. On one side are three relatively distinct areas: (1) the basic science of career development as a specific area of human development; (2) career counseling as a generic helping process with clearly defined steps; and (3) career programming as programs of learning and activities designed to facilitate career development. Along the other dimensions of the matrix are the three principal theoretical orientations: (1) trait and factor; (2) developmental; and (3) information processing. Any and all of these orientations can be applied in any of the three areas indicated above.

Application to Persons with Disabilities

As was noted earlier, the life experiences of many persons with disabilities render invalid many of the assumptions on which normative career development theory and career counseling practice are based. Therefore the need was recognized for an approach to career behavior that was applicable to persons with disabilities. This need has been addressed by the construction of several theories of work adjustment. These theories were developed and empirically tested specifically on persons with disabilities. Working since the middle 1960s, Rene V. Dawis and Lloyd H. Lofquist (1984) developed the Minnesota Theory of Work Adjustment, which follows a trait-and factor orientation. This approach seeks to match a client's needs and values with specific reinforcers that different occupations offer and to match the client's abilities with the specific demands of different occupations. The closer the match between needs and reinforcers, the more likely the person will be satisfied with the job; the closer the match between abilities and demands, the more likely the person will perform satisfactorily on the job. The greater the job satisfaction of the individual and the more satisfactory his or her performance, the better the work adjustment and the longer the person is likely to remain on that job (i.e., not quit or be fired). The theory has good empirical support.

Working during the same time period, David B. Hershenson (1981) constructed a theory of work adjustment that follows a developmental orientation. According to this theory, which also has received empirical support, three work-related domains develop successively within the person. First, during the preschool years, the domain of work personality develops. This domain includes the person's self-concept as a worker and the person's system of work motivation. Next to develop, during the school years, is the domain of work competencies, which includes work habits, physical and mental skills applicable to jobs, and work-related interpersonal skills. Finally, as the person begins to prepare to leave school and enter the world of work, the domain of work goals develops. These three domains—work personality, work competencies, and work goals—interactively affect each other and remain in dynamic balance over the course of the person's career. The output of this dynamic balance is work adjustment, which includes the elements of satisfaction and task performance (as does the Minnesota theory) and of work-role behavior (e.g., promptness, appropriate dress, accepting supervision).

While there has been no information-processing theory developed specifically for persons with disabilities, there have been a number of computerized career counseling programs for rehabilitation clients.

These programs include information on disability-related functional limitations among the factors used in arriving at career options that the program suggests to the client.

Several major rehabilitation approaches are highly relevant to career counseling. One of these is the increased attention being given to assisting students with disabilities to make the transition from school to work; another is supported employment, which provides ongoing, work-related supportive services that permit persons with severe disabilities to engage in competitive employment. A third major approach is job accommodation, in which job tasks and job sites are modified to make them accessible to workers with disabilities.

Finally, in career counseling persons with disabilities, it is important to distinguish those whose onset of disability was precareer (e.g., congenital or in early childhood) from those whose onset of disability was after the person had entered upon a career. Richard T. Goldberg (1992) concluded that past research has shown that people with acquired disabilities tend to choose occupations consistent with their predisability plans, while people with precareer disabilities tend to choose occupations consistent with their parents' aspirations and social class.

While different theories of career development/work adjustment and career programming have been created for persons with disabilities, no model of career counseling specific to persons with disabilities has been proposed. The general model suggested by Yost and Corbishley and outlined above should adequately apply to persons with disabilities. Naturally, for different individuals with different disabilities, some steps may require more time or specialized methods of implementation.

Career Professionals and Professional Associations

The professional concerned with general career counseling, who may or may not work with persons with disabilities, is the National Certified Career Counselor (NCCC). To obtain this credential from the National Board for Certified Counselors, the person must possess a master's degree in counseling, have several years of supervised experience doing ca-

reer counseling, and pass both general counseling and specialty career counseling national examinations. To maintain the certification, the career counselor must take continuing education in the field and abide by the professional code of ethics.

A related professional who definitely does counsel clients with disabilities, but may or may not deal with career issues, is the Certified Rehabilitation Counselor (CRC). A third career professional is the school counselor, who works with rehabilitation or career counselors to promote a smooth school-to-work transition for students with disabilities. School counselors also have master's degrees and are certified by the same board as career counselors, following a parallel process. Two other professional groups that work with persons with disabilities on career issues are vocational evaluators, who assess the current and potential vocational functioning of clients and suggest interventions needed to improve vocational functioning, and employment counselors, who work to place persons with or without disabilities in appropriate jobs.

Two other career assistance occupations that have no specific educational requirements are those of the job developer, who tries to create jobs in competitive employment for persons with disabilities, and the job coach, who provides various types of assistance in instances of supported employment.

There are two principal professional organizations to which many of these professionals belong: the American Counseling Association (ACA), which has divisions for career counselors, school counselors, employment counselors, and rehabilitation counselors, and the National Rehabilitation Association (NRA), which also has a division for rehabilitation counselors as well as divisions for vocational evaluators and job developers. As their organizational names imply, the ACA is primarily concerned with counseling fields, while the NRA is primarily active in rehabilitation fields; thus rehabilitation counselors have a place in both organizations.

The Future of Career Counseling with Persons with Disabilities

The subfields of career development theory and research, career counseling, and career programming are likely to move closer together so that theory will more directly guide practice, and practice will more directly shape theory. Moreover, career counseling and career programming should become better integrated, making both activities more effective and more efficient. The pressures for increased productivity in the workplace that exist in the broader society should hasten these changes. These trends should lead to improved integration among theories of work adjustment and career counseling and career programming for persons with disabilities.

The greatest long-term impact on the careers of persons with disabilities will probably result from the passage of the Americans with Disabilities Act (1990), which requires equal access and equal employment opportunity for individuals with disabilities. This should have a major effect on career options for persons formerly excluded because of disabilities. Over a long period of time, this may invalidate some of the points Osipow (cited earlier) made about the restrictive career development of persons with disabilities so that it will eventually become possible to apply the concept of career development to persons with disabilities for whom that concept has not been applicable.

Two other related factors that should have an impact on the career development and career counseling of persons with disabilities are projected changes in the economy and job market and in the nature of work and the work force. The study *Workforce 2000*, by William B. Johnston and Arnold E. Packer (1987), predicted that the proportion of women and minorities in the work force will continue to grow and that the demand for skilled workers will increase while the demand for unskilled workers will decrease. This development will help the prospects of some persons with disabilities, particularly if they obtain the skills that are in high demand and short supply. For many others, however, with marginal skills and impaired capacities to develop high-level skills, there are few promising signs other than an expansion of supported employment programs and programs that seek to foster the employment of persons with disabilities in the private sector, such as the federally supported Projects with Industry.

Clearly, the need to develop more relevant theories of career development and more effective methods of career counseling and career programming for persons with disabilities will continue to occupy career professionals for a long time.

(*See also:* DISABILITY MANAGEMENT; JOB PLACEMENT; SPECIAL EDUCATION; TRANSITION FROM SCHOOL TO WORK; VOCATIONAL EVALUATION; WORK)

RESOURCES

American Counseling Association, 5999 Stevenson Ave., Alexandria, VA 22304

National Career Development Association (at the same address)

BIBLIOGRAPHY

BROOKS, LINDA, and BROWN, DUANE. "Career Counseling for Adults: Implications for Mental Health Counselors." In *Foundations of Mental Health Counseling*, eds. Artis J. Palmo and William J. Weikel. Springfield, IL, 1986.

DAVIS, HOWARD V. *Frank Parsons: Prophet, Innovator, Counselor*. Carbondale, IL, 1969.

DAWIS, RENE V., and LOFQUIST, LLOYD H. *A Psychological Theory of Work Adjustment*. Minneapolis, 1984.

GOLDBERG, RICHARD T. "Toward a Model of Vocational Development of People with Disabilities." *Rehabilitation Counseling Bulletin* 35 (1992):161–173.

HERSHENSON, DAVID B. "Work Adjustment, Disability, and the Three R's of Vocational Rehabilitation: A Conceptual Model." *Rehabilitation Counseling Bulletin* 25 (1981):91–97.

HOLLAND, JOHN L. *Making Vocational Choices: A Theory of Vocational Personalities and Work Environment*, 2nd ed. Englewood Cliffs, NJ, 1985.

JOHNSTON, WILLIAM B., and PACKER, ARNOLD E. *Workforce 2000: Work and Workers for the 21st Century*. Indianapolis, 1987.

KRUMBOLTZ, JOHN D. "A Social Learning Theory of Career Decision Making." In *Social Learning and Career Decision Making*, eds. Anita M. Mitchell, G. Brian Jones, and John D. Krumboltz. Cranston, RI, 1979.

NATIONAL CAREER DEVELOPMENT ASSOCIATION (NCDA). Position paper approved by the Board of Directors. Alexandria, VA, Jan. 11, 1991.

OSIPOW, SAMUEL H. "Vocational Development Problems of the Handicapped." In *Contemporary Vocational Rehabilitation*, eds. Herbert Rusalem and David Malikin, New York, 1976.

PARSONS, FRANK. *Choosing a Vocation*. Boston, 1909.

SUPER, DONALD E. "A Theory of Vocational Development." *American Psychologist* 8 (1953):185–190.

U.S. DEPARTMENT OF LABOR. *Dictionary of Occupational Titles*, 4th ed. Washington, DC, 1991.

———. Bureau of Labor Statistics. *Occupational Outlook Handbook*, 1994–95 ed., Washington, DC, 1994.

YOST, ELIZABETH B., and CORBISHLEY, M. ANNE. *Career Counseling: A Psychological Approach.* San Francisco, 1987.

ZYTOWSKI, DONALD G. "Four Hundred Years Before Parsons." *Personnel and Guidance Journal* 50 (1972):443–450.

DAVID B. HERSHENSON

CAREGIVING

Caregiving has become such a ubiquitous term that its meaning is often taken for granted. The provision of assistance and support by one family member to another is a regular and usual part of family interactions, and is in fact a normative and pervasive activity. Thus caregiving due to chronic illness and disability represents something that, in principle, is not very different from traditional tasks and activities rendered to family members. The difference, in real terms, however, is that caregiving in this situation represents the increment of extraordinary care that goes beyond the bounds of normal or usual care. The provision of care to a family member who has a chronic illness implies a significant expenditure of time and energy over potentially long periods of time, involves tasks that may be unpleasant and uncomfortable, is likely to be nonsymmetrical (the caregiver often gives more than he or she receives in return from the care recipient), and is often a role that had not been anticipated. Actual caregiving role tasks vary considerably with the type and stage of illness. Thus caregiving is illness- and disability-related (Biegel, Sales, and Schulz, 1991).

The roles and functions of family caregivers vary by type and stage of illness and include both direct and indirect activities. Direct activities can include provision of personal care tasks, helping with bathing, grooming, dressing, or toileting; health care tasks, such as catheter care, giving injections, or monitoring medications; and checking and monitor-

ing, such as continuous supervision, regular checking, or telephone monitoring. Indirect tasks include care management such as locating services, coordinating service use, monitoring services, or advocacy; and households tasks such as cooking, cleaning, shopping, money management, transportation of the family member to medical appointments, or day care programs (Noelker & Bass, 1994).

The provision of care by family members to other family members who become dependent due to the physical and/or mental effects of chronic illness is not a new phenomenon. In fact, families in the United States, as well as in other parts of the world, have always provided care to their dependent members. However, there is growing recognition among service providers and researchers that caregiving will become a more salient public policy issue in the future because of a number of recent (and anticipated) demographic, economic, and social changes. Key changes include the following:

- Life expectancy and aging of the population have increased dramatically during this century.
- Shifts in the epidemiology of disease from acute to chronic diseases and also a decrease in accidental deaths have resulted in an increase in the number of persons in the population with functional activity and mobility limitations.
- Death rates for heart disease and stroke have decreased and five-year cancer survival rates have increased.
- The number of multigenerational families has increased, resulting in a growing number of elderly caregivers.
- Family structures are changing due to declining fertility rates and increase in the divorce rate. The result is that the average woman now spends eighteen years of her life helping an elderly parent, as compared to seventeen years of her adult life caring for a dependent child.
- Greater numbers of women, the traditional caregivers, are in the labor force. The combination of working and providing care for children, disabled adults, or the elderly can be particularly difficult.
- Changes in health-care reimbursement and medical technology have increased responsibilities for family caregivers.

Research on the effects of caregiving shows very clearly that caregiving is not without costs to the caregiver. Many families report caregiving to be an emotional, physical, and at times, financial burden. Significant caregiving problems identified by researchers include the following (Kahana, Biegel, and Wykle, 1994):

1. coping with increased needs of the dependent family member caused by physical and/or mental illnesses;
2. coping with disruptive behaviors, especially those associated with cognitive disorders or mental illness such as dementia or schizophrenia;
3. restrictions on social and leisure activities;
4. infringement of privacy;
5. disruption of household and work routines;
6. conflicting multiple role demands;
7. lack of support and assistance from other family members;
8. disruption of family roles and relationships;
9. lack of sufficient assistance from human service agencies and agency professionals.

Caregiving can have positive aspects for the caregiver as well. For example, parents caring for adults with schizophrenia report that the caregiving experiences aided their personal growth and increased their understanding of family problems (Bulger, Wandersman, and Goldman, 1993). Adult children who are caregivers to elderly parents report that they find caregiving gratifying because they can "pay back" the care the parent provided to them when they were young. In addition, caregivers report that being a caregiver helps them gain inner strength or learn new skills.

A variety of services have been developed for caregivers that are designed to reduce the burden that caregivers often experience and to provide supportive assistance to enable families to continue their caregiving roles. These services can be categorized into support groups, educational interventions, and clinical/direct services.

Support groups are designed to provide caregivers with emotional support, informational support, and enhancement of coping skills. These groups are either professionally led, typically for a set number of sessions, or peer-led and usually of an ongoing nature. There is a strong emphasis on sharing of feelings, experiences, and coping strategies among group members. Support groups are designed to:

1. reduce emotional isolation, anxiety, and fear in families and allow them to develop supportive networks;
2. provide a safe atmosphere for expressing negative emotions;
3. give and receive advice and support from others in the same situation;
4. address gaps in knowledge and provide information and techniques useful for the caregiving role;
5. develop needed coping skills and learn from others how to cope more effectively.

Educational interventions emphasize the provision by professionals of information and/or skills, usually in a group format, to enable caregivers to meet their needs better. They can be divided into three types: cognitive information only, cognitive information plus self-enhancement and/or behavioral management skills, and self-enhancement and/or behavioral management skills only. In cognitive information only interventions, information is provided on such topics as the nature of the disease and/or physical disability, issues of medication management, management of patient behaviors, and available community resources for patients and caregivers. Educational interventions incorporating emphases on skills may include patient management skills, stress management skills, and such social skills as the enhancement of assertive behaviors and social network building skills.

Clinical or direct service interventions vary considerably more than either support group or educational interventions. Such interventions can be broadly categorized into six different types: counseling/therapy, respite care, behavioral/cognitive stimulation, hospice care, day hospital care, and general psychosocial interventions. Even within these classifications, direct service interventions vary considerably. Thus counseling/therapy interventions can include caregivers only, or both patients and caregivers only, or both patients and caregivers, with interventions lasting from one month to two years or more. Similarly, respite care can include in-home as well as out-of-home care.

Despite the extensive literature in caregiving, which increased by more than 200 percent from 1988 to 1993, many limitations in the extant literature must be addressed by future research. For example, we know relatively little about the ways in which the caregiving experience is similar or different across illnesses; many studies of caregivers have been based on nonrepresentative samples, often clinical populations, and have used cross-sectional rather than longitudinal designs; the range of caregiving variables that have been examined is often fairly narrow; the process and context of caregiving, especially the relationship of family caregivers to broader social systems in society, have not been fully examined; and we have little empirical knowledge concerning barriers to the use of caregiver services or of the effectiveness of services that are utilized (Biegel, Sales, and Schulz, 1991; Burton & Sorensen, 1993; Kahana, Biegel, and Wykle, 1994; Pearlin et al., 1990). Thus there are significant opportunities for further conceptual and methodological work in this field.

(See also: AGING; FAMILY; HOSPICE; RESPITE CARE)

RESOURCES

Alzheimer's Association, 919 N. Michigan Ave., No. 1000, Chicago, IL 60611

Older Women's League, 666 11 St., NW, Suite 700, Washington, DC 20001

Well Spouse Foundation, P.O. Box 801, New York, NY 10023

BIBLIOGRAPHY

BIEGEL, DAVID E.; SALES, ESTHER; and SCHULZ, RICHARD. *Family Caregiving in Chronic Illness: Alzheimer's Disease, Cancer, Heart Disease, Mental Illness and Stroke.* Newbury Park, CA, 1991.

BULGER, MICHAEL W.; WANDERSMAN, ABRAHAM; and GOLDMAN, CHARLES R. "Burdens and Gratifications of Caregiving: Appraisal of Parental Care of Adults with Schizophrenia." *American Journal of Orthopsychiatry* 63 (1993):225–265.

BURTON, LINDA M., and SORENSEN, SILVIA. "Temporal Context and the Caregiver Role: Perspectives from Ethnographic Studies of Multigenerational African-American Families." In *Caregiving Systems: Informal and Formal Helpers,* eds. S. H. Zarith, L. I. Pearlin, and J. W. Schaie. Hillsdale, NJ, 1993.

COULTON, CLAUDIA. "Prospective Payment Requires Increased Attention to Quality of Post-hospital Care." *Social Work in Health Care* 13 (1988):19–31.

KAHANA, EVA; BIEGEL, DAVID E.; and WYKLE, MAY L., eds. *Family Caregiving Across the Life Span.* Newbury Park, CA, 1994.

NOELKER, LINDA S., and BASS, DAVID M. "Relationship Between the Frail Elderly's Informal and Formal Helpers." In *Family Caregiving Across the Life Span.* eds. E. Kahana, D. Biegel, and M. Wykle. Newbury Park, CA, 1994.

PEARLIN, LEONARD I.; MULLAN, JOSEPH T.; SEMPLE, SHIRLEY J.; and SKAFF, MARILYN M. "Caregiving and the Stress Process: An Overview of Concepts and Their Measures." *The Gerontologist* 30 (1990):583–591.

DAVID E. BIEGEL

CARPAL TUNNEL SYNDROME

See ARTHRITIS; MUSCULOSKELETAL DISORDERS

CEREBRAL PALSY

See CHILDHOOD DISABILITIES; DEVELOPMENTAL DISABILITIES; MENTAL RETARDATION

CEREBROVASCULAR DISEASE

See ORGANIC MENTAL SYNDROMES; STROKE

CERTIFICATION

See CREDENTIALS

CHARACTER DISORDERS

See PERSONALITY DISORDERS

CHILDHOOD DISABILITIES

Treating childhood disability requires both an understanding of the concept of disability and an awareness of the natural changes in skill levels and roles that occur during normal child development. Thus, when applied to children, the concept of disability as "any restriction or lack . . . of ability to perform an activity in the manner or within the range considered normal for a human being" (World Health Organization, 1980), must incorporate a set of norms that are appropriate for the child's age. Behavior that is normal at one age may become a significant disability when the child grows older and the expected normal range changes. For example, inability to walk is considered normal during infancy but becomes a significant disability by age two. By adolescence it can lead to the even more serious handicap of social isolation.

Identification and Evaluation

The most common mechanism for early identification of disability in the United States is based on the medical model, with a parent or physician initiating concern about a child's development. The initial screening is done by the child's physician, with a routine physical examination identifying motor control or other difficulties. For the child who is not suspected of having any abnormality, routine vision and hearing tests are usually done at the prekindergarten physical examination (about age five), thus delaying diagnosis of sensory deficits in some cases. Formal developmental screening tests (Table 1) are designed to identify abnormal development while minimizing referrals of developmentally normal children. Abnormal screening results do not diagnose developmental delay, but they can help identify children who need further evaluation.

Relying on parents and the medical system to initiate evaluation for potential childhood disability is effective for many—particularly those with medically oriented problems—but can lead to underidentification among some families. Identification and referral by the public schools is now mandated under the Education for All Handicapped Children Act of 1975 and its 1986 and 1990 amendments, but identification through this approach tends to occur after three to five years of age.

Early identification of all children with disabilities is ideal, as it promotes referral for evaluation and treatment during the critical infant and toddler years. Unfortunately, while early developmental screening of entire populations is occasionally done

Table 1. Common standardized assessment instruments

Screening Tests

Denver Developmental Screening Test—II (DDST-II)
Denver Prescreening Developmental Questionnaire (PDQ)
Alpern Boll Developmental Profile II
Early Language Milestone Scale (ELM)
Peabody Picture Vocabulary Test
Receptive-Expressive Emergent Language
Miller Assessment of Preschoolers (MAP)

Developmental Evaluation

Bayley Scales of Infant Development
Griffiths Mental Developmental Scale
Fagan Test of Infant Intelligence
Mullen Scales of Early Learning

General Intelligence

Stanford-Binet Intelligence Scale
Wechsler Preschool and Primary Scale of Intelligence
Wechsler Intelligence Scale for Children: Revised
McCarthy Scales of Children's Abilities
Kaufman Assessment Battery for Children

Adaptive Behavior

Vineland Adaptive Behavior Scale
American Association of Mental Deficiency (AAMD) Adaptive Behavior Scale
Pediatric Evaluation of Disability Inventory (PEDI)
Functional Independence Measure for Children (WeeFIM)

Motor Performance

Peabody Developmental Motor Scales
Erhardt Developmental Prehension Assessment
Bruininks-Oserestsky Test of Motor Proficiency
Motor Assessment of Infants (MAI)
Jebsen Test of Hand Function

Language

The Rosetti Infant Toddler Language Scale
Preschool Language Scale
Test of Problem Solving
The Word Test
Clinical Evaluation of Language Fundamental—Revised
Goldman Fristoe Test of Articulation

for research purposes, the cost is prohibitive for general use. A less expensive approach is to provide special surveillance for children and families who demonstrate particular medical, physical, situational, or psychosocial risk factors that are commonly associated with developmental disabilities. Children with medical problems, such as low birth weight, prematurity, or neonatal seizures, and children born to mothers with drug abuse problems, children whose mothers do not receive prenatal care, or to families who lack permanent housing are considered at high risk for developmental disabilities, thus justifying the expense of developmental surveillance. Because this approach bypasses otherwise "normal" children with developmental problems, however, such screening programs have tended to include increasing numbers of factors that place children "at risk," thereby requiring screening of larger and larger numbers of children and undermining the cost-control component of the concept.

Once a child with a possible disability has been identified, the exact nature of the problem must be evaluated. Evaluation procedures rely heavily on a comprehensive, multidisciplinary approach, including the expertise of physicians, teachers, audiologists, speech pathologists, physical therapists, occupational therapists, social workers, and psychologists. For very young children, the evaluation should focus on the strengths and weaknesses of both the family and the child because of the family's crucial role in promoting long-term development and ultimate independence. Not every child requires evaluation by every type of practitioner, but all relevant ones should be included. About 30 percent of children with handicaps are affected by more than one condition. In such cases, professionals from multiple disciplines must collaborate to prioritize treatment goals.

Evaluation includes a medical examination, with emphasis on the neurological, musculoskeletal, vision, and hearing systems. Behavior—either directly observed or reported by an adult familiar with the child—is noted, and then standardized testing is done. Numerous test instruments exist, many of them designed for specific populations or purposes. A partial listing of common instruments is provided in Table 1.

Standardized cognitive testing of young children with disabilities is filled with pitfalls. First, assessment of any very young child is complicated by the limited repertoire of possible behaviors and by the difficulty in obtaining the child's cooperation. At best, testing of infant intelligence—which has traditionally relied on eliciting age-appropriate language, social, or motor behaviors—has been useful only for identification of developmental or neurological deficits that might benefit from intervention. It has not been useful in predicting long-term functioning or later intelligence (Honzik, 1983).

Significant physical disability further limits the number of behaviors available as test responses, making test selection and interpretation even more complicated for children with disabilities than it is for the children without disabilities. Thus traditional test instruments may not be helpful for evaluating children with specific sensory or motor impairments. In an effort to obtain better information about infant intelligence as well as to provide motor-free cognitive testing of children with physical impairments, researchers have suggested a "perceptual-cognitive" approach to early assessment. This technique relies on the infant or young child's ability to attend, remember, and recognize differences in repeatedly presented visual and auditory stimuli. By using response measures such as changes in heart rate, visual fixation, and smiling rather than gross motor behavior, the technique offers promise in providing cognitive assessment of even children with severe physical disabilities (Kearsley, 1982; Zelazo, 1979).

Description

Typical childhood disabilities can be divided into three categories, based on the way they are typically identified: (1) disabilities that are evident at or shortly after delivery; (2) developmental disabilities that, although they may stem from impairments present at birth, become evident only over time; and (3) disabilities with their onset later in childhood. Disabilities can further be divided into those involving physical limitations, those involving cognitive deficits, and combinations of the two.

Disabilities Evident at or Shortly After Birth. This category includes birth defects such as musculoskeletal anomalies, congenital brain malformations, or chromosomal abnormalities. Musculoskeletal defects, which are generally obvious at delivery, can range in severity from the trivial (extra digits on the hands or feet) to the profound (congenital absence of multiple limbs). Clubfeet, joint contractures (arthrogryposis), and a variety of hand anomalies all fit in this category (Warkany, 1971). Myelomeningocele, the most common of the major disabling birth defects (spina bifida), consists of abnormal intrauterine development of the lower portion of the spinal cord, with resulting partial or complete lower extremity paralysis and an inability to develop bowel and bladder control. In about 80 percent of cases the spinal cord anomaly is associated with inadequate drainage of cerebrospinal spinal fluid (CSF) from the center of the brain. Untreated, this condition, called hydrocephalus, can lead to severe brain damage and even death. Treatment generally consists of surgical placement of a tube to drain excess CSF from the brain to the abdominal cavity. Other brain malformations may not be immediately obvious at delivery but are commonly diagnosed in early infancy, either because the head size is abnormal at birth or because the rate of head growth is abnormal. Poor sucking ability or neonatal seizures may also prompt medical evaluation.

Chromosomal anomalies are also commonly diagnosed shortly after birth. Down syndrome, caused by the presence of forty-seven instead of forty-six chromosomes, is the most common and most readily identifiable chromosome abnormality. More than fifty clinical signs are associated with it, including epicanthal folds in the eyes, flat nasal bridge, and a small head. Affected children may also have specific health problems such as poor resistance to infection, hearing loss, gastrointestinal problems, and heart defects. Mental retardation is a prominent component of Down syndrome, although there are wide variations in mental ability, behavior, and developmental progress (Cicchetti & Beeghly, 1990).

Among conditions evident at delivery, prematurity deserves special consideration. While the fact of a premature birth is obvious at delivery, whether a child will ultimately demonstrate a disability may remain uncertain for some time. Major neurological deficits (blindness, deafness, severe cerebral palsy, or mental retardation) may become apparent early, but subtle learning disabilities or visual-motor inte-

gration abnormalities may not be diagnosable until children reach school age (Nickel, Bennett, and Lamson, 1982; Sagail et al., 1990). As technologically sophisticated medical care has improved survival rates for ever-smaller premature infants, the potential for high rates of resulting long-term disability has become an increasing concern.

Developmental Disabilities. Physical or cognitive impairments may be present at birth and yet require months to years before becoming evident. This process of "unmasking" occurs as normal developmental changes fail to materialize, creating a gradually increasing level of concern among parents, physicians, caretakers, and/or teachers.

Cognitive dysfunction is the most common of the developmental disabilities. It encompasses a continuum of problems, from profound mental retardation to mild learning difficulties or attentional problems. In the Education for All Handicapped Children Act of 1975, mental retardation is defined as "significantly subaverage general intellectual functioning existing concurrently with deficits in adaptive behavior and manifested during the developmental period that adversely affects a child's education performance." "General intellectual functioning" refers to an IQ score of 70 or below, while "adaptive behavior" refers to adjustment to everyday life. Mental retardation itself is not a disease, although there are numerous biological risk factors associated with it and, when of profound degree, it can be associated with reduced life expectancy. The reported prevalence of mental retardation increases from the preschool years through late adolescence, although this probably reflects increasing identification of affected individuals rather than any age-specific increase in "true" prevalence (Kiely, 1987). The 1975 act defines learning disabilities as "disorder(s) in one or more of the basic psychological processes involved in understanding or . . . using . . . language, which many manifest . . . in an imperfect ability to listen, think, speak, read, write, spell, or to do math calculation." Depending on the definition used, 10 to 30 percent of the population has some degree of learning disability (Levine, 1987).

Evaluation of very young children for visual or hearing deficits remains a substantial challenge. Whether congenital or acquired, vision or hearing deficits often go undiagnosed until preschool or even

151

later (Drews et al., 1992). Delay in diagnosis is largely due to the difficulty inherent in testing very young children. Early visual testing relies on careful observation of infant preferences in visual focus. A normal infant will preferentially focus on a human face. The child's head and eye movements will try to follow the face as it moves across his or her line of vision. More sophisticated testing includes presentation of standardized stripes or patterns to stimulate visual focus (Nelson et al., 1984). Infant hearing tests include careful observation of behaviors such as blinking, head turning, or startle reactions in response to standardized sounds. Tests that monitor brain waves in response to visual or auditory stimuli (visual or auditory evoked potentials) are available but require sophisticated equipment and trained personnel (Grimes, 1985; Nelson et al., 1984).

Untreated, vision or hearing deficits can have serious developmental consequences. Both blind and deaf children have a high incidence of mental retardation, delay in motor development, and emotional difficulties (Fraiberg, Smith, and Adelson, 1969; Grimes, 1985). Since the earliest bond between mother and child is visual—the infant's focus on the mother's face—a child who is blind from early infancy may suffer from disrupted maternal-infant bonding. In addition, without the ability to observe the surrounding world, an infant is placed at considerable disadvantage in his or her attempts to learn about that world. Lacking normal visual stimuli that prompt the infant to reach, grasp, creep, and ultimately walk, overall development may be severely impaired (Elonen & Zwarenstey, 1964). Early or congenital deafness presents a different set of developmental obstacles. While initial emotional bonding may be unimpeded, the child is denied opportunity for early language acquisition and communication with other people. Delay in language comprehension or production is commonly the first sign of a hearing deficit, and any child with abnormal language development should undergo detailed audiometry as soon as the problem is noted (Coplan, 1985).

Cerebral palsy (CP), which affects 1.5 to 5.0 children per 1,000 live births, is the most common developmental disability affecting the musculoskeletal system (Lord, 1984; Nelson & Ellenberg, 1978). It is an inconsistently defined syndrome of abnormal motor control stemming from nonprogressive malfunction of the central nervous system. The cause or causes of cerebral palsy are not well understood. Difficulties with labor or delivery may cause brain damage that ultimately leads to CP in some cases. However, many children with obstetrical difficulties develop normal motor control, while others with normal birth histories ultimately demonstrate motor control problems (Freeman et al., 1985). Although severe CP sometimes is diagnosed during early infancy, mild to moderate cases commonly remain undiagnosed until one to two years of age. Initial concern usually focuses on a child's failure to acquire developmental milestones, such as sitting, creeping, or walking, on schedule. Examination typically reveals involuntary movement, stiff, "spastic" muscles, and/or persistence of immature reflex and movement patterns. Since different clinical syndromes can include abnormal motor development, evaluation by a pediatric neurologist or physiatrist is necessary to assure accurate diagnosis (Lord, 1984).

Developmental problems of children with cerebral palsy include limited mobility and self-care skills. Because these children exhibit developmental patterns that are different from those of children without disabilities, parenting is complicated by a lack of information regarding what parents can reasonably expect of their child. Associated disabilities, particularly mental retardation, exert an independent, major effect on ultimate functional capabilities (Cohen & Kohn, 1979; Molnar & Taft, 1977).

Childhood-Onset Disabilities. Medical illness and trauma are both major causes of childhood-onset disabilities. Severe childhood injuries include burns, injuries requiring amputations, brain damage resulting from near-drowning episodes, penetrating injuries to the head or abdomen, long bone fractures, blunt abdominal trauma, and closed head injuries. A combination of head and extracranial injury can also occur.

Severe head injury (HI) with associated brain damage is one of the most common traumatic causes of long-term childhood disability. Long-term sequelae to severe HI include posttraumatic seizures, impaired motor function, intellectual and memory deficits, language disorders, and personality change. HI carries a higher risk of long-term disability than extracranial injury (ECI), with combinations of the two carrying the highest risk of disability as well as the highest mortality rate. Accidents involving motor vehicles are the most common cause of ECI, serious HI, and combination injuries. While automobile seat belts do reduce both the mortality rate and the extent of injuries among passengers, pedestrian and bicycle-related automobile accidents also account for a significant fraction of serious injuries. Among infants under one year of age, nonaccidental trauma (child abuse) is also a significant cause.

Medical illnesses can create long-term disability in two separate ways. In the first, an acute illness, although followed by complete resolution, may leave permanent, residual damage. Vascular injury or tumor may force limb amputations, and central nervous system infections may cause permanent brain damage. The second mechanism involves chronic illnesses that may be disabling by their nature and severity. Cystic fibrosis, severe asthma, diabetes, and childhood arthritis all fit in this category.

Treatment

As in any rehabilitation program, the hallmarks of pediatric rehabilitation include individual assessment, concrete goal-setting, and a multidisciplinary approach to treatment structured to facilitate maximum independence. Pediatric rehabilitation differs from adult rehabilitation in its focus on the child's developmental stage at the time of intervention and on its long-term perspective in relation to normal growth and development. Goals shift through the growing years, demanding repeated interventions, each time with a new set of goals reflecting the child's new developmental stage. Thus at age four occupational therapy may focus on independence in dressing and bathing, whereas at age fourteen the same child might receive occupational therapy to focus on kitchen and homemaking skills. Since the majority of children with disabilities never have known any other state, they rarely understand their own long-term treatment goals (Selekman, 1991).

Rehabilitation programs can go on in a variety of places, including at home, in a hospital, at a therapy center, or in school. In practice they are frequently carried out simultaneously in several different locations. A child may receive special education in consultation with an occupational therapist at school and go to a therapy center several times a week for motor control and ambulation training with a physical therapist. That same child may also be hospitalized for orthopedic surgery, followed by intensive physical therapy during the hospitalization. The home, too, provides a major arena for rehabilitation. Daily routines can provide innumerable opportunities to learn and practice motor control and self-care skills. Particularly for infants and very young children, physical and occupational therapists may spend considerable time training parents in handling, positioning, and specific interventions with their child (Eigsti, Aretz, and Shannon, 1990).

Parents, physicians, physical and occupational therapists, speech pathologists, teachers, psychologists, and rehabilitation engineers each offer a unique contribution toward a child's rehabilitation. While the specific members of each rehabilitation team will vary based on the child's needs, the concept of team functioning—with consensus regarding goals and frequent communication among team members—remains.

Parents

Ultimately, parents affect rehabilitation outcome far more than any professional can. The parents' psychological and emotional approach to their child can be a powerful motivator toward independence or a major discouraging influence. A family that accepts their child's disability and insists on maximum functioning, typically in mainstream environments, provides the child with both motivation and self-confidence necessary for ultimate independence (Crothers & Paine, 1959). Commonly, parents do not know where to begin to obtain resources for their child. A partial listing of national organizations that address the needs of children with disabilities appears at the end of this entry.

Physicians

Pediatricians, pediatric physiatrists, child developmentalists, orthopedic surgeons, neurosurgeons, ophthalmologists, otolaryngologists, and urologists all participate in caring for children with disabilities. Generally, one individual—either a developmental pediatrician or a pediatric physiatrist—takes on the role of "team leader," assuming responsibility for coordination of services and long-term medical surveillance. The team leader prescribes rehabilitation services and equipment as needed and then monitors the child several times a year, with an awareness that normal growth can lead to medical complications such as joint contractures, scoliosis (curvature of the spine) or skin breakdown, while ongoing intellectual development mandates ongoing revision of rehabilitation goals (Noll, Molnar, and Badell, 1989).

Physical Therapists

Physical therapists focus on muscle control, strength, posture, and walking. Their goals are to develop maximum physical capacity and to prevent musculoskeletal deformities. Treatment of infants and young children consists of promoting normal movement and teaching parents effective ways of handling and positioning their child. As children get older, play activities can be used during treatment sessions. The ultimate goal is functional independence. If independent walking is excessively difficult or unrealistic, a physical therapist may teach wheelchair or other compensatory skills (Eigsti, Aretz, and Shannon, 1990).

Occupational Therapists

Occupational therapists are concerned with the capacity of the child with disability to participate in the normal roles expected of children their age (family member, playmate, student). Training in hand use and daily living skills such as dressing or feeding, as well as environmental adaptations such as special seating, built-up handles for utensils, or bathroom modifications, all can promote functional independence. The occupational therapist may also consult with a child's classroom teacher so that skills learned during occupational therapy sessions can be promoted during general classroom time (Royeen & Gorga, 1990).

Speech Pathologists

A speech pathologist is a specialist in human communication, including comprehension, verbal expression, and nonverbal interaction. Since the same mouth and tongue movements initially used for sucking, swallowing, and chewing are ultimately refined to produce speech, speech pathologists commonly work with feeding disorders among infants and very young children. Often occupational therapists share in this task. As children grow older, the focus shifts to language comprehension and expression. The speech pathologist may recommend special evaluations for hearing and cognition. They may also consult with classroom teachers. Training in language production may include motor control training, signing, or the use of special equipment. Augmentative communication refers to equipment ranging from boards or books that display pictures of common items, to sophisticated computers with voice synthesizers (Cohen, 1985; Gardner & Workinger, 1990).

Rehabilitation Nurses

Rehabilitation nurses support overall programs by concentrating on family education and support. Nurses train families in routine care, particularly care of the bowels and bladder. They also teach families how to prevent medical complications such as skin breakdown or contractures.

Rehabilitation Engineers

Specialized equipment for children with disabilities promotes function by bypassing the child's impairment and providing alternate means of accomplishing a task. Devices range from hearing aides to artificial limbs to voice synthesizers to electric wheelchairs. The hallmark of rehabilitation engineering is its individualized focus and its ultimate goal of promoting independent function and development. While some equipment is available ready-made, much of it requires custom fitting, and is, therefore, quite expensive. Families often have difficulty obtaining funding for more sophisticated (and expensive) equipment items. A number of new materials and techniques have been developed to facilitate custom fitting and fabrication. Rehabilitation engineers typically consult with physicians and physical and occupational therapists who know the child well before developing a specific item of equipment (Milner et al., 1990; Motloch, 1974).

Psychologists

Clinical psychologists participate in rehabilitation programs in two distinct ways. First, they assist in assessing intellectual potential by identifying cognitive strengths and weaknesses. This commonly requires standardized testing, scoring, and interpretation. In addition, psychologists can help both parents and children with their emotional reactions to the child's disability and help them find more effective coping strategies for everyday problems. For parents this involves resolution of anger, guilt, and the chronic grieving that often accompanies parenting a child with a disability. Children, particularly adolescents, may suffer from inadequate social skills and poor self-esteem. Mildly involved children seem to be at greater risk for emotional suffering than the more severely involved (Crothers & Paine, 1959).

Teachers

Under the Education for All Handicapped Children Act of 1975, public schools must provide "free and appropriate" education for all children, regardless of disability. Federal regulations also mandate that children receive education in the "least restrictive environment" appropriate. Thus, although special education teachers bear considerable responsibility for education and educationally related services, children are often placed in mainstream classes for a large fraction of their school experience (*Special Education Rights and Responsibilities*, 1992). Mainstream placement has the advantage of requiring children to learn appropriate social skills.

Legal Resources

In 1973 Congress passed the Vocational Rehabilitation Act, which has been called the "first civil rights law protecting the rights of the handicapped." This legislation provides that no person with a handicap shall, solely by reason of his or her handicap, be excluded from participation in, denied benefits of, or be subject to discrimination under any program receiving federal financial assistance. The law stresses the basic human right to full participation in society for individuals with handicaps. Section 504 of this legislation requires that public buildings be physically accessible to persons with handicaps. The

Rehabilitation Act was written primarily for adults, although the law applies equally to children.

To address the specific needs of children, Congress passed the Education for All Handicapped Children Act of 1975, which requires public schools to provide free and appropriate public education for all children, regardless of handicap. Public schools must identify, diagnose, educate, and provide educationally related services to all children with handicaps between five and eighteen years of age. To be eligible for services, a child must have an identifiable condition that may interfere with his or her educational process, thus requiring special educational services.

Other components of this law include the following:

1. Each child must be evaluated by an interdisciplinary team, which will design the individual educational plan (IEP).

2. Each child must be educated in the least restrictive environment appropriate.

3. Related services such as transportation, speech and language services, and counseling must be provided by the school when considered necessary by the IEP team.

4. Parents must be involved in decisions regarding their child's education. If disagreements arise, parents and children have a right to a due process hearing (Community Alliance for Special Education, 1992).

For children under school age, the 1986 and 1990 amendments to the Education for All Handicapped Children Act of 1975 provide that children from three to five years of age with disabilities also receive education followed by coordinated, multidisciplinary interagency care. Program eligibility requires a significant difference between a child's age and current level of functioning or a high risk of developmental delay. Risk factors include medical or social characteristics of the child or family. Commonly, children need more than one risk factor to qualify for services. For these young children, the family participates in the evaluation, assessment, and planning process and must ultimately approve of the individualized family service plan (IFSP) that is developed.

155

Two other legal areas affect children with disabilities: the "baby Doe" regulations, which mandate medical care for children with disabilities; and the Social Security System, which may provide disability income and eligibility for Medicaid to children with disabilities.

The baby Doe regulations provide protection from medical neglect under laws regarding child abuse and neglect. The only situations in which treatment may be withheld include those in which children are permanently comatose or terminally ill, or in situations where treatment would not be curative or would be inhumane. When questions or disagreements regarding ongoing care of children with multiple severe problems arise, hospital ethics teams can meet with physicians and parents to assist in decision-making (Barnett, 1990).

The Supplemental Security Income (SSI) program under Social Security is a need-based disability program for both adults and children that provides monthly cash benefits and, in most states, automatic Medicaid eligibility. To qualify for benefits, a child must live in a family that has limited income and resources, be a U.S. citizen or legal resident, and have a severe disability. For purposes of SSI eligibility, disability is defined as a physical or mental impairment of "comparable severity" to one that would prevent an adult from engaging in "substantial gainful activity" (Perrin & Stein, 1991).

In 1990 the U.S. Supreme Court, in *Sullivan* v. *Zebley* (110 S. Ct. 885 [1990]), mandated a change in the guidelines for determination of "disability" in children. Accordingly, SSI regulations were revised to make it easier for children to qualify, and the Social Security Administration implemented an evaluation process for children that is comparable to the one used for adults. The Social Security Administration then began considering not only medical conditions but also the effect a condition might have on the child's ability to develop in an age-appropriate manner and to perform age-appropriate activities (Matthews, 1991).

Conclusion

Pediatric rehabilitation addresses the entire spectrum of childhood disability. Programs can be coordinated by a pediatrician, pediatric physiatrist, pediatric neurologist, developmentalist, otolaryngologist, or ophthalmologist, and the members of the rehabilitation team vary according to individual needs. The concept of a multidisciplinary approach to promote maximum independence remains in all programs, however, with the ultimate goals of comfort, function, and life satisfaction.

(*See also:* ASSISTIVE TECHNOLOGY; AUTISM; CHILDHOOD PSYCHIATRIC DISORDERS; DEVELOPMENTAL DISABILITIES; DISABILITY; FAMILY; HEAD INJURY; LEARNING DISABILITIES; MULTIPLE DISABILITIES; MUSCULOSKELETAL DISORDERS; PEDIATRIC REHABILITATION; PSYCHOSOCIAL ADJUSTMENT; SPECIAL EDUCATION)

RESOURCES

American Foundation for the Blind, 15 West 16th St., New York, NY 10011

Association for Children and Adults with Learning Disabilities, 4156 Library Rd, Pittsburgh, PA 15234

Association for Retarded Citizens (ARC), 500 East Border St., Arlington, TX 76010

Exceptional Parent, 209 Harvard St., Suite 303, Brookline, MA 02146

March of Dimes Birth Defects Foundation, 1275 Mamaroneck Ave., White Plains, NY 10605

Muscular Dystrophy Association, 3300 East Sunrise Drive, Tucson, AZ 85718

National Down Syndrome Society, 666 Broadway, New York, NY 10012

National Easter Seal Society, 230 West Monroe St., Chicago, IL 60606

National Head Injury Foundation (NHIF), 1776 Massachusetts Ave., NW, Suite 100, Washington, DC 20036

National Information Center on Deafness, Gallaudet University, 800 Florida Ave., NE, Washington, DC 20002

National Organization for Rare Disorders, P.O. Box 8923, New Fairfield, CT 06812

Spina Bifida Association of America, 4590 MacArthur Blvd., Washington, DC 20007–4226

United Cerebral Palsy Association, 1522 K St., NW, Suite 1112, Washington, DC 20005

BIBLIOGRAPHY

BARNETT, TERRY J: "Baby Doe: Nothing to Fear but Fear Itself." *Journal of Perinatology* 10 (1990):307–311.

CICCHETTI, DANTE, and BEEGHLY, LEONARD, eds.

Children with Down's Syndrome: A Developmental Perspective. Cambridge, Eng., 1990.

COHEN, CAROL. A. "Augmentative Communication: A Perspective for Pediatricians." *Pediatric Annals* 14 (1985):232–240.

COHEN, PETER, and KOHN, JEAN, G. "Follow-up Study of Patients with Cerebral Palsy." *Western Journal of Medicine* 130 (1979):6–11.

COMMUNITY ALLIANCE FOR SPECIAL EDUCATION (CASE). *Special Education Rights and Responsibilities.* 3rd ed. San Francisco, 1992.

COPLAN, JAMES. "Evaluation of the Child with Delayed Speech or Language." *Pediatric Annals* 14 (1985):203–208.

CROTHERS, BRONSON, and PAINE, RICHMOND S. *The Natural History of Cerebral Palsy.* Cambridge, MA, 1959.

DREWS, CAROLYN D.; YEARGIN-ALLSOPP, MARSHALYN; MURPHY, CATHERINE C.; and DESOUFLE, PIERRE. "Legal Blindness Among 10-Year-Old Children in Metropolitan Atlanta: Prevalence, 1985 to 1987." *American Journal of Public Health* 82 (1992): 1377–1379.

EIGSTI, HEIDI; ARETZ, MARYBETH; and SHANNON, LOU. "Pediatric Physical Therapy in a Rehabilitation Setting." *Pediatrician* 17 (1990):267–277.

ELONEN, ANNA S., and ZWARENSTEY, SARAH B. "Appraisal of Developmental Lag in Certain Blind Children." *Journal of Pediatrics* 65 (1964):599–610.

FRAIBERG, SELMA; SMITH, MARGUERITE; and ADELSON, EDNA. "An Educational Program for Blind Infants." *Journal of Special Education* 3 (1969):121–139.

FREEMAN, JOHN M.; AVERY, GORDON; BRANN, ALFRED W.; GILLES, FLOYD H., HOBEL, CALVIN J., HOLMES, LEWIS E., MOORE, ROBERT Y.; MOSER, HUGO; ROSEN, MORTIMER; SUSSER, MERVYN; and FINK, LESLIE. "National Institute of Health Report on Causes of Mental Retardation and Cerebral Palsy." *Pediatrics* 76 (1985):457–458.

GARDNER, JUDY., and WORKINGER, MARILYN SEIF. "The Changing Role of the Speech-Language Pathologist in Pediatric Rehabilitation/Habilitation." *Pediatrician* 17 (1990):283–286.

GRIMES, CHARLES T. "Audiologic Evaluation in Infancy and Childhood." *Pediatric Annals* 14 (1985): 211–219.

HONZIK, MARJORIE P. "Value and Limitation of Infant Tests: An Overview." In *Origins of Intelligence Infancy and Early Childhood,* ed. Michael Lewis. New York, 1983.

KEARSLEY, RICHARD B. "Cognitive Assessment of the Handicapped Infant: The Need for an Alternative Approach." *American Journal of Orthopsychiatry* 51 (1981):43–54.

KIELY, MICHELE. "The Prevalence of Mental Retardation." *Epidemiologic Reviews* 9 (1987):194–218.

LEVINE, MELVIN D. "Developmental Variations and Dysfunctions in the School Child." In *Developmental Behavioral Pediatrics,* eds. M. Levine, W. Carey, and A. Crocker. 2nd ed. Philadelphia, 1987.

LORD, JANET. "Cerebral Palsy: A Clinical Approach." *Archives of Physical Medicine and Rehabilitation* 65 (1985):542–548.

MATTHEWS, MARTHA. Many More Infants Eligible for SSI Under *Zebley* Regulations. *Youth Law News* (Sept.–Oct. 1991):14–17.

MILNER, M.; NAUMANN, S.; LITEROWICH, M.; RYAN, MARTIN S.; SAUTER, W. F.; SHEIN, G. F.; and VERBURG, G. "Rehabilitation Engineering in Pediatrics." *Pediatrician* 17 (1990):287–296.

MOLNAR, GABRIELLA E., and TAFT, LAURENCE T. "Pediatric Rehabilitation, Part I: Cerebral Palsy and Spinal Cord Injuries." *Current Problems in Pediatrics* 7 (1977):6–46.

MOTLOCH, WALLACE M. "Human Needs and Orthotic Goals for Spina Bifida Patients." Presented at the Conference on Mobility Acts for Spina Bifida Patients. Toronto, 1974.

NELSON, KARIN B., and ELLENBERG, JONAS H. "Epidemiology of Cerebral Palsy." *Advances in Neurology* 19 (1978):421–435.

NELSON, LEONARD B.; RUBIN, STEPHEN E.; WAGNER, RUDOLPH S.; and BRETON, MICHAEL E. "Developmental Aspects in the Assessment of Visual Function in Young Children." *Pediatrics* 73 (1984):375–381.

NICKEL, ROBERT E.; BENNETT, FORREST C.; and LAMSON, FRED N. "School Performance of Children with Birth Weights of 1,000 g or Less." *American Journal of Diseases of Children* 136 (1982):105–110.

NOLL, STEPHEN F.; MOLNAR, GABRIELLA E.; and BADELL, ANGELES; BINDER, HELGA; DYKSTRA, DENNIS D.; EASTON, JESSIE K. M.; MATTHEWS, DENNIS J.; and PERRIN, JANE C. "Pediatric Rehabilitation. 1. General Principles and Special Considerations." *Archives of Physical Medicine and Rehabilitation* 70 (1989):162–165.

PERRIN, JAMES M., and STEIN, RUTH E. K. "Reinterpreting Disability: Changes in Supplemental Security Income for Children." *Pediatrics* 88 (1991): 1047–1051.

RIVERA, FREDERICK P.; THOMPSON, ROBERT S.; THOMPSON, DIANE C.; and CALONGE, NED. "Injuries to Children and Adolescents: Impact on Physical Health." *Pediatrics* 88 (1991):783–788.

ROYEEN, CHARLOTTE B., and GORGA, DELIA. "Occupational Therapy in Pediatric Rehabilitation." *Pediatrician* 17 (1990):278–282.

SAGAIL, SAROJ; SZATMARI, PETER; ROSENBAUM, PETER; CAMPBELL, DUGAL; and KING, SUZANNE. "Intellectual and Functional Status at School Entry of Children Who Weighed 1000 Grams or Less at Birth: A Regional Perspective of Births in the 1980s." *Journal of Pediatrics* 116 (1990):409–416.

SELEKMAN, JANICE. "Pediatric Rehabilitation: From Concepts to Practice." *Pediatric Nursing* 17 (1991):11–14.

WARKANY, JOSEF. *Congenital Malformations Notes and Comments.* Chicago, 1971.

WORLD HEALTH ORGANIZATION. *International Classification of Impairments, Disabilities, and Handicaps: A Manual of Classification Relating to the Consequences of Disease.* Twenty-ninth World Health Assembly, 1976. Geneva, Switzerland, 1980.

ZELAZO, PHILIP R. "Reactivity to Perceptual-Cognitive Events: Application for Infant Assessment." In *Infants at Risk: Assessment of Cognitive Functioning,* eds. R. B. Kearsley and I. E. Sigel. Hillsdale, NJ, 1979.

JANET LORD
BARBARA BENNETT

CHILDHOOD PSYCHIATRIC DISORDERS

The rehabilitation, or treatment, of childhood psychiatric disorders is an area undergoing continual refinement as more information regarding treatment outcome and efficacy is gathered. Before 1986 there were few treatment options for children diagnosed with a mental illness, and the regimens available were designed to focus on distress in general rather than targeting the specific difficulties that a child was exhibiting. The primary mode of intervention for children was play therapy, which tended to be nondirective in approach (Axeline, 1947) and did not target specific behavioral symptoms. Given the trend in mental health settings to favor short-term treatment regimens, as well as outcome data regarding treatment efficacy, there is now an emphasis on implementing differential treatment programs based on the symptomatology exhibited by the child. As rehabilitation effects depend on diagnosis, this entry will begin by reviewing the history of diagnosis for childhood psychiatric disorders. This will be followed by a review of the various diagnostic categories, and the treatment modalities found to be effective for alleviating the difficulties noted within each diagnostic category. Special emphasis will be placed on disruptive behavior disorders (i.e., conduct disorders and attention disorders).

Diagnosis of childhood psychiatric disorders was initially poorly conceptualized, with little differentiation between disorders or symptom patterns. The earliest diagnostic system, the *Diagnostic and Statistical Manual of Mental Disorders* (DSM-I), enumerated only two categories for childhood mental disorders (American Psychiatric Association, 1952), testimony to the fact that psychiatric disorders in childhood had not yet been closely examined. Subsequent to the original version of this taxonomic system, a broader and more comprehensive manual for the diagnosis of mental disorders was established, with the *Diagnostic and Statistical Manual of Mental Disorders,* 4th ed. (DSM-IV) (American Psychiatric Association, 1994) listing forty possible diagnoses subsumed within ten major diagnostic categories for disorders that are usually first diagnosed in infancy, childhood, or adolescence. Additionally, it is suggested that children can receive diagnoses classified within the adult sections of the manual if the criteria, or the modified criteria, are met. This expanded nosologic system has resulted from extensive research within the field of child psychiatry, and is based on behavioral criteria rather than theoretical viewpoints with little empirical validity. A diagnostic system based on symptom patterns allows for greater consistency in diagnosis, as well as for better communication among clinicians and researchers (Kazdin, 1987a). Although many advances have been made in the classification of childhood psychiatric disorders, this is an area that continues to be in the formative stages, and descriptions of the disorders will be altered as new data emerge. An important issue to be addressed in future diagnostic classification systems is how discrete various disorders are from one another, versus how much overlap exists between different diagnostic categories; this issue is related to comorbidity and dual diagnoses, as well as clarity of symptom patterns. Although the DSM-IV offers the clearest depiction of childhood mental illness, it has been difficult to establish a reliable and valid diagnostic system, as psychiatric illness in children tends to be less stable and to have more global behavioral effects than mental illness in adults (Rutter & Tuma, 1988). Determination of the appropriate diagnosis is essential for treatment effectiveness, which suggests that the less reliable the diagnostic system, the less efficacious will be the treatment. Thus the outcome for rehabilitation attempts can only be as effective as the diagnostic system in use. To improve positive outcome, it is essential to establish a reliable and valid taxonomic system.

One of the difficulties encountered in the establishment of a reliable diagnostic system is the fact that, for children, psychiatric symptomatology may change form as the child matures; an additional difficulty in diagnosis is that certain behaviors may be considered problematic at one age but may be normative at a different developmental period. Some behavioral symptoms may be resolved in the absence of intervention when exhibited at a particular developmental period or when fairly mild in form, but these same behaviors may be an indicator of more serious difficulties when expressed at a different developmental stage. For example, some oppositional behavior and temper tantrums during early childhood (i.e., two to three years of age) are normative, while oppositional behavior and temper tantrums later in childhood (i.e., nine to ten years old) are nonnormative and may be indicative of difficulties that can worsen (develop into a conduct disorder). To make an accurate diagnosis, the clinician needs to be aware of the normal developmental progression in behavior and the patterns of behavior that are to be expected at each developmental stage (Greenspan, 1981). In addition to being aware of normal developmental behavioral patterns, the clinician should be cognizant of the patterns of abnormal behavior development and the indicators that portend a worsening at a later time. There have been efforts to understand better the risk and resilience factors related to various diagnostic categories, which may assist clinicians in recognizing the warning signals in children's behavioral symptoms. Risk factors are those variables that contribute to the prediction of a particular negative outcome, while resilience factors are those variables that act to offset the development of later difficulties. For example,

poor academic performance (Loeber, 1990) and inconsistent discipline (Frick et al., 1992) are risk factors for later conduct disorders, while advanced social problem solving or social cognitive skills protect (or operate as a resilience factor) against the development of conduct problems (Downey & Walker, 1989).

In establishing a diagnosis for a child, the assessment process should involve an evaluation of the child's emotional and behavioral symptoms, as well as an evaluation of the child's environment. Evaluating children in the context within which they reside is essential, as children continue to be dependent on contextual or environmental factors, and their level of functioning will be affected by these factors. Obtaining an accurate account of a child's functioning involves assessing the child in multiple domains, including the areas of family/parents, scholastic, peer, general and cultural environment. Parental functioning is an important consideration, given the impact that parents have on children. Included in an assessment of parental functioning would be: an evaluation of psychopathology, parental discipline techniques, emotional and physical availability for the child, any relevant stressors, and resources available to the parents (i.e., financial, family, friends). The child's scholastic functioning should also be evaluated, which would involve an assessment of the child's academic performance (achievement level), the child's academic potential (ability level), behavioral functioning in the classroom, and peer relations at school. Environmental considerations include neighborhood resources (i.e., recreation centers, peer availability), violence/criminal activity in the neighborhood, and peer/family support available to the child in his or her living environment. Cultural factors should be taken into consideration, which would involve an examination of the prevailing norms within the child's community. Gathering data on the child's functioning in these various settings would allow the diagnostician to make a better informed decision regarding the appropriate diagnosis for a child, which would then have an impact on the treatment of choice.

As noted above, the most comprehensive diagnostic system to date is the DSM-IV (American Psychiatric Association, 1994). Included within this structure are a number of categories for disorders that are first diagnosed in infancy, childhood, or adolescence; the primary categories include developmental disorders, attention-deficit and disruptive behavior disorders, feeding/eating disorders, elimination disorders, and other disorders. The DSM-IV employs a categorical approach to diagnosis, which consists of evaluating current symptomatology and ascertaining whether a child meets the criteria for a particular diagnostic category. An alternative approach to diagnosis involves a dimensional rating, in which the child is evaluated on a number of dimensions and a profile of behavioral and emotional symptoms is established (Kazdin, 1987a). This approach is more consistent with the multiple domain analysis proposed above. The categorical approach can suggest to the clinician potential treatment regimens for the particular symptomatology, while a dimensional approach offers a broader and more comprehensive view of the child. The value inherent in the two evaluation techniques suggests that applying a combination of the two approaches would be most beneficial for the clinician when assessing a child (Rutter & Tuma, 1988).

Attention-Deficit and Disruptive Behavior Disorders

The attention-deficit and disruptive behavior disorders classification includes behavioral symptom patterns that are referred to as "externalizing" (Achenbach & Edelbrook, 1983). Externalizing behaviors are those marked by a lack of impulse control that have an impact on others in the environment (i.e., aggression, disruptiveness) and that are asocial or antisocial in nature. Children who exhibit externalizing behaviors tend to be problematic for others in their surroundings, and thus these children tend to be referred for intervention. Approximately 60 percent to 80 percent of all children referred to mental health settings exhibit externalizing behaviors (Stroul, 1993), reinforcing the idea that externalizing behavioral symptom patterns represent the most common motivation for pursuing intervention.

Attention-Deficit Hyperactivity Disorder. Attention-deficit hyperactivity disorder (ADHD) is one of the most common childhood psychiatric disorders, with referrals generated by teachers and by parents. The core symptoms of this disorder include difficulty

sustaining attention, easy distractibility, excessive activity, and impulsive behavior. Translated into behavioral terms, a child may exhibit difficulty following directions, difficulty attending in class or structured activities, being easily distracted by extraneous stimuli, speaking or acting out of turn, leaving tasks uncompleted, difficulty remaining still or seated, and engaging in activities without considering the consequences. There are three different types of ADHD listed in the DSM-IV: inattentive, hyperactive, and combined. ADHD-inattentive is characterized primarily by difficulty sustaining attention and the concomitant behavioral symptoms; ADHD-hyperactive is characterized primarily by excessive activity and restlessness; and ADHD-combined is characterized by both attentional difficulties and excessive activity. Symptoms of ADHD tend to be situation-specific, indicating that a child will not necessarily exhibit behavioral symptoms in all situations, but the symptoms may be more or less severe depending on the specific situation (American Psychiatric Association, 1994). For example, a child who has no siblings may be more distractible and overactive in the classroom than at home, given the greater stimulation at school. In contrast, a child may exhibit fewer difficulties in the classroom if the teacher has structured the class's activities and has clearly established rules, expectations, and consequences for the children; however, the child may have more difficulty maintaining appropriate behavior at home if there are fewer external controls over his or her behavior. For this reason, it is advantageous for the clinician to assess the child in multiple domains and to have different respondents regarding the child's behavior.

In terms of etiology, several hypotheses have been examined, including the proposals that artificial food additives lead to hyperactivity (Feingold, 1975), that children with ADHD may have suffered minimal brain damage at an early age (Ross & Ross, 1976), and that there is a genetic basis to this disorder (Morrison & Stewart, 1973). Although different theories continue to be developed regarding the etiology of ADHD, the most support has been found for theories focusing on a biological predisposition and genetic influence. Russell A. Barkley (1988) reported that paternal ADHD behavior patterns were found in 25 percent of children with

ADHD, suggesting that there is some degree of genetic heritability to this disorder. The concordance rates for temperamental factors associated with ADHD (i.e., overactivity) are lower in fraternal (dizygotic) twins than the concordance rates for these factors in identical (monozygotic) twins, again suggesting that there is a genetic etiological component to ADHD (Buss & Plomin, 1975).

The form of treatment that has consistently received the most empirical support is the use of stimulant medication, primarily methylphenidate (Ritalin) (Gadow, 1992). Indeed, it has been remarked that no other form of intervention is effective for the treatment of ADHD behavioral patterns (Ross & Ross, 1976). Despite this sentiment, behavioral treatment regimens have been used with some success (Barkley, 1988); behavioral approaches are not necessarily less effective in terms of treating ADHD, but it takes longer to observe positive treatment effects (Wells, 1994), and medication may affect different behavioral patterns or symptoms. The benefits for considering alternatives to medication rehabilitation techniques are that behavioral approaches are more generalizable, as the child will be able to use the strategies taught in different settings, and the child may assume greater responsibility for behavioral control. Furthermore, children who show a poor response to Ritalin may be able to benefit from behavioral or cognitive behavioral approaches.

Ritalin has been found to be effective in terms of reducing the attentional difficulties and the behavioral overactivity associated with ADHD according to parental reports, teacher reports, and other measures of attention (Barkley, et al., 1988); 80 percent of children with diagnosed ADHD exhibited some improvement in symptomatology following the introduction of methylphenidate. Children's response to medication, however, depends on the initial level of behavioral disturbance, as those who exhibit the highest rates of inattentive and distractible behaviors benefit the most from medication (Murray, 1987). This latter phenomenon is known as "rate dependency" and refers to the idea that medication response depends on the initial rate or level of behavioral disturbance. In terms of long-term improvement, there is evidence that children who received medication for a longer period of time have a better outcome (Satterfield, Hoppe, and Schell, 1982), although not all children will show continued benefit from medication administration and not all children will experience a worsening in symptomatology following medication withdrawal (Sleator, Neumann, and Sprague, 1974).

The second broad category of intervention for children with ADHD, behavioral treatment regimens, is of two varieties: parent training, and contingency management techniques. Parent training involves having parents provide greater external structure, such that the child may be better able to maintain attention and concentration, as well as rewarding the child when attention has been maintained. The first organized parent training manuals were formulated in the 1970s and 1980s (Wells, 1994) and were based on research findings that revealed a strong relationship between family dysfunction or parenting styles and poor outcome in adulthood (Schachar & Wachsmuth, 1991). The focus on parent training grew out of research in which excessively harsh, aversive, or inconsistent parenting styles were found to be associated with aggressive and disruptive behavioral patterns in children (Kazdin, 1985). Several studies have examined the effectiveness of parent training in comparison to medication treatment, with the general outcomes indicating that parent training is effective in reducing some of the ADHD symptomatology but does not have a significant independent contribution when combined with medication (Horn et al., 1991). In other words, medication treatment in isolation produces the same level of improvement as medication in conjunction with parent training. One caveat to these findings, as pointed out by Karen Wells (1994), is that the research designs have not included an assessment of behavior in the home, which would likely be affected most strongly by parent training intervention. Furthermore, most research examines proximal treatment outcome rather than examining outcome at later time points, which may not offer a valid assessment of the efficacy of parent training or behavioral treatment, as these approaches do not affect behavior as quickly as medication. In terms of the specific strategies used in parent training, Philip C. Kendall and Lauren Braswell (1985) developed a structured program that involves rewarding children for displaying less distractibility, greater control over motoric restlessness, and greater attentional capacity; another component of this treatment protocol is the use of self-instructional training, which is designed to assist children with developing conscious control over behavior by changing the thought patterns used in various situations. This treatment approach has demonstrated some limited effectiveness in reducing the symptomatology associated with ADHD. The most judicious plan appears to be providing pharmacological intervention in conjunction with parent training or self-instruction training to achieve the most positive treatment outcome.

Conduct Disorders

There are two primary diagnoses within this general category: oppositional defiant disorder (ODD) and conduct disorder (CD). Both diagnostic categories involve an unwillingness to adhere to societal norms or expectations, with conduct disorder involving a more serious violation of these norms. Children with oppositional defiant disorder or conduct disorder tend to display verbally or physically aggressive behaviors, which has been found to be a poor prognostic indicator. Research has shown that aggression tends to be one of the most persistent and stable behavior patterns in children (Olweus, 1979), and may be related to a variety of other negative outcomes, including substance use, delinquency, and more severe psychopathology (Coie et al., 1992). For these reasons, it is essential that clinicians adequately assess aggressive symptomatology and related behavioral patterns, to provide treatment that can offset the development of later difficulties. The vast majority of children diagnosed with CD met the criteria for ODD at an earlier age, suggesting the possibility of a developmental progression from one disorder (ODD) to the other (CD); however, there is not a direct one-to-one correspondence between these two disorders, as some children with ODD never develop CD (Loeber, Lahey, and Thomas, 1991). Some authors have speculated that ODD is a milder version of CD (Werry, Reeves, and Elkind, 1987), with these disorders having different anchor points along a disruptive-behavior continuum. Rolf Loeber (1990) diagrammed a developmental continuum for disruptive behaviors that suggested that although these behaviors are manifested differently at

different developmental periods, there is great continuity over time in the expression of some form of disruptive behavioral symptoms—the form of the behavior changes and worsens over time, but the presence of the behavioral symptoms is consistent. One suggestion has been that the phenotypic expression of the disorder may change over time but the underlying genetic influence remains the same (Simonoff, McGuffin, and Gottesman, 1994); these authors further posit that the environmental influence on the exhibition of conduct-disordered behaviors decreases over time, with the genetic influence becoming more prominent as children become older. In sum, the symptomatology associated with ODD may be, but is not necessarily, an early stage in the development of CD.

The criteria listed in the DSM-IV for oppositional defiant disorder include difficulty controlling one's temper, arguing with others, noncompliance with adult requests, engaging in deliberately annoying behaviors, being easily annoyed by others, blaming others (not assuming responsibility for own behavior), and displaying anger or vindictiveness. These symptoms are generally present before age eight, with this disorder being somewhat more common in males than females (American Psychiatric Association, 1994). These symptoms are always observed in the child's home environment, and may or may not be present at school or in other environments, as a child may have better control over these behaviors in some situations than in others; this is similar to the situation specificity noted in ADHD symptomatology. Relationship disturbances or dysfunction are common between family members and children with ODD symptomatology, such that this behavioral pattern is always evident at home. Clinicians may want to solicit information from parents and/or teachers to have a clearer picture of the child's behavior patterns in multiple settings; often the oppositional behaviors are not observed in the office at the time of initial assessment, and the clinician benefits from obtaining information from multiple sources.

The DSM-IV indicates that behavioral symptoms such as stealing (with or without direct confrontation of the victim), breaking and entering, running away from home overnight, truancy, lying, setting fires, vandalism, engaging in physical altercations or cruelty with other people, cruelty to animals, and using a weapon in a fight are indicators of conduct disorder. There are four broad categories within which these characteristics are classified, including aggression to people and animals, destruction of property, deceitfulness/theft, and serious violations of rules. This classification system allows the clinician to pinpoint the area or areas of greatest concern for a child, which can have implications for the treatment regimen. In addition to the general symptom categories, there are two primary types of conduct disorder: childhood onset and/or adolescent onset. Childhood onset conduct disorder has a poorer prognosis, as the child exhibits the more severe behavioral disturbance at an earlier age; there is evidence that early age of onset is related to more serious and chronic behavioral disturbances in adulthood (Loeber & Dishion, 1983).

In terms of etiological factors for conduct disordered behaviors, David P. Farrington (1991) indicated that there are six primary categories into which these factors can be classified: socioeconomic deprivation and associated features of such deprivation, parenting styles, family history of conduct-disordered behaviors, poor academic achievement, hyperactivity or impulsivity, and early childhood oppositional behaviors. Each of these factors may have an independent contribution to the development of conduct-disordered behavior, with the greater number of factors representing greater risk for the development of a behavioral disturbance. Each of these factors can be considered to be a risk factor or marker for the development of conduct-disordered behavior; thus the greater number of risk factors present, the greater likelihood that conduct disorder will develop. Ronald J. Prinz and Gloria E. Miller (1991) discussed the need for the clinician to maintain cultural sensitivity when assessing children for aggressive or disruptive behaviors, as in some contexts aggression is both normative and adaptive. For children who live in violent neighborhoods, aggression may be necessary in terms of survival and peer support. In this case, the clinician may be doing the child a disservice by focusing on a reduction in the level of aggression the child exhibits, at least in certain environments. A more sensitive approach may be to assist the child in recognizing the contexts within which aggression is acceptable and those in which it is not; in other words, assisting the child with discrimination training rather than eliminating the aggression altogether. Another option suggested by Prinz and Miller (1991) is to recruit a mentor from within the child's community to assist the child in developing additional coping skills and to reduce reliance on aggression as a coping skill.

In terms of the rehabilitation of children with a conduct disorder, it is important to assess the areas of functioning that have been adversely affected. Kenneth A. Dodge (1993) suggested that multiple factors are associated with the development and maintenance of conduct disorders; treatment will have long-lasting effects and be truly beneficial only if all areas affected are targeted and if all etiological factors are addressed. The areas that should be included in a thorough assessment are reminiscent of those listed above and include family functioning and patterns of familial interaction, the child's cognitive ability and academic achievement level, the child's peer group and interpersonal relationship skills, and broader community or neighborhood factors (i.e., availability of extracurricular activities in the neighborhood, level of violence, and a positive support system readily available to the child). If a multifaceted treatment approach is not used, the clinician may observe some changes in behavior, but these changes are not likely to be maintained, as other forces will be operating to counteract the positive effects of the treatment. There is some validity to the idea that the clinician treating a child with conduct disorder should use multiple treatment approaches and target as many areas of functioning as possible, as there have been no empirical studies that have effectively isolated the curative factors in the rehabilitation of conduct disorders (Dodge, 1993).

James K. Luiselli (1991) related that the DSM system does not guide the clinician in assessing the different areas of functioning, given the categorical nature of this system; thus he provided an outline of various control variables that may be operative in the maintenance of conduct disorders, as well as the different treatment approaches that can be used to deal effectively with each of the identified control variables. The variables he indicated to be of importance in the development and maintenance of conduct disorders include desire for adult attention, desire for peer attention, desire to avoid or escape from certain demands, poor social skills, and poor cognitive ability with associated academic difficulty. The belief is that children with conduct-disordered behaviors experience difficulties cross-situationally, with a variety of etiological factors contributing to the development and maintenance of the behavioral disturbances. Isolating behaviors in only one situation or focusing on only one of the etiological factors will lead to negative treatment outcome in that the forces maintaining the negative behavioral patterns will be stronger than the factors maintaining treatment gains. A thorough assessment is essential before implementing any rehabilitation plan.

Rehabilitation of conduct-disordered behavior can be accomplished in a variety of ways, including group treatment, individual treatment, family therapy, pharmacotherapy, and parent training. The primary goal of each rehabilitative approach is to increase the child's level of compliance and to decrease the oppositionality. Individual treatment regimens have not been found to be as effective in working with conduct-disordered youth, and a multimodal treatment regimen is the treatment of choice for children with a disruptive behavior disorder (Lochman, 1992). There have been more than 200 treatment regimens proposed for the rehabilitation of conduct disorders (Kazdin, 1993), but only two types of treatment have demonstrated effectiveness: parental management training and problem-solving skills training. Problem-solving skills training involves instructing children in the art of problem-solving. Kenneth A. Dodge and colleagues (1986) delineated a series of five steps involved in the problem-solving process, including the encoding of stimuli in social situations, interpretation of the stimuli encountered, alternative solution generation, consequence identification and evaluation, and behavioral enactment. Children with conduct-disordered or aggressive behaviors have been found to be deficient at each step in this problem-solving process (Dodge et al., 1986; Lochman et al., 1991). Therefore, problem-solving skills training consists of training children in the requisite skills associated with each step in this problem-solving process. Group therapy is the most widely used method for training children in problem-solving because this modality allows for role-playing and the concomitant improvement in social skills,

peer versus adult feedback, and interpersonal stimulation that allows the opportunity to focus on misinterpretations (Rose & Edelson, 1987).

Alan E. Kazdin (1987b) developed a cognitive-behavioral treatment regimen for teaching problem-solving skills to conduct-disordered youth, with a focus on improving the accuracy of interpretations of social stimuli and increasing the number of solutions in a child's repertoire. Research on this treatment protocol indicated that problem-solving training is more effective than relationship therapy in terms of reducing the severity of conduct-disordered behaviors, but this reduction is not great enough to warrant classification of the treated children into the normative range (Kazdin et al., 1987). A second problem-solving skills training protocol is that developed by John E. Lochman and colleagues (1987). This manual describes a structured program for implementation in a school setting and is designed to improve perspective-taking skills (or gain better understanding of other people's perspectives), increase awareness of the physiological signals associated with anger, improve problem-solving skills, and increase awareness of alternative strategies to use in conflictual situations. This program has received empirical support in decreasing the level of aggression exhibited by children, based on parent reports (Lochman et al., 1984), reducing the level of off-task behavior in the classroom (Lochman & Lampron, 1988), increasing self-esteem, and reducing substance use three years later (Lochman, 1992).

Parent management training is the second form of treatment that has been shown to have positive effects on conduct-disordered behaviors in children and adolescents. Parents are trained in procedures to use with their child at home, with this training based on the idea that negative behavior patterns are maintained in the home by dysfunctional or maladaptive parent-child interactions (Kazdin, 1993). The basic goal of parent training is to assist parents in gaining more control over their child's behavior by improving parental monitoring of the child's behavior; altering the contingencies operating to maintain the negative behavior; and developing greater consistency in the rules, expectations, and consequences in the home. Parent training has been found to be useful for reducing the level of problematic behaviors in conduct-disordered children, with the posttreatment behavioral functioning falling within the normative range (Forehand & Long, 1988). For this treatment modality to be effective, the parents need to be willing to participate in the parental training process and therefore must exhibit relatively high levels of motivation to work in therapy. Referring back to the risk factors noted above, if several risk factors are present, it is less likely that parents will become or stay involved in parent training sessions and less likely that positive gains will be made if they do complete the parent training program (Dumas & Wahler, 1983; Webster-Stratton, 1985). Alan E. Kazdin, Todd C. Siegel, and Debra Bass (1992) found that combining problem-solving skills training with parent management training was more effective than either treatment choice in isolation; this is consistent with the recommendation made above that a multimodal treatment package will be the most beneficial in reducing the level of conduct-disordered behaviors that a child exhibits.

Medication has been suggested to have some benefit for reducing the level of aggression that children and adolescents exhibit, although few controlled studies have examined the efficacy of pharmacotherapy for conduct-disordered behavior. Neuroleptic medications have been tried with aggressive children, with some demonstrated effectiveness based on behavior rating scales (Greenhill et al., 1985). Lithium has been proposed to be effective in reducing aggression in children with conduct-disordered behaviors (Campbell et al., 1984; DeLong & Aldershof, 1987). Additionally, there has been the suggestion that seizure medications or anticonvulsants reduce aggression in some children and adolescents (reviewed by Evans, Clay, and Gualtieri, 1987). For children who experience explosive or impulsive aggression and who are not responding to other forms of treatment, antidepressants may be an option for clinicians to consider, although the evidence of potential efficacy of this treatment choice is based on a small sample (Zubieta & Alessi, 1992). In general, the use of medication for the treatment of aggression appears to be most useful if the aggression occurs explosively or in a rageful manner (Campbell, Gonzalez, and Silva, 1992). However, the use of medication for the treatment of aggressive behavioral patterns should be done cautiously, as there are few well-controlled studies examining the efficacy of

medications in comparison to other forms of treatment for untreated children.

Some question regarding the efficacy of the judicial system for the rehabilitation of conduct-disordered behavior has been raised. Joan McCord (1985) found that males who were processed through the court system between ages seven and seventeen were less likely to be repeat offenders or to be convicted of a more serious crime at a later date; this indicates that there may be some value to punishing children for engaging in antisocial or delinquent activities. However, there is also some concern with the labeling of children and the associated stigmatization, as well as a caution that an increase in delinquent activity may follow a court appearance (Farrington, Osborn, and West, 1978). Thus, for some children, becoming involved in the judicial system may serve as a deterrent for later criminal activity and therefore function as a rehabilitative factor, while for other children the process of being convicted of a crime may intensify the exhibition of conduct-disordered behavior due to the child labeling himself or herself as a "delinquent," or to a desensitization to the threat of court proceedings. It may be useful to identify the factors associated with the different response patterns, and to respond to different children in different ways to maximize the rehabilitation efforts.

Internalizing Disorders

In contrast to externalizing behavioral disturbances, internalizing disorders are characterized by symptoms that tend to be more problematic for the child than for the people in his or her surroundings. For this reason, internalizing symptoms can be overlooked by others in the child's environment, particularly if the symptoms are mild or if the child does not acknowledge the internal distress. The symptoms associated with internalizing disorders include fearfulness, withdrawal, worries or anxieties, and depression. One of the hallmarks of internalizing disorders is the exhibition of overcontrolled behaviors, compared to the undercontrolled behaviors associated with externalizing disorders. The DSM-IV enumerates the following psychiatric disorders that would be classified as internalizing disorders in children: separation anxiety disorder, major depression, dysthymic disorder, specific phobias, obsessive-compulsive disorder, posttraumatic stress disorder, and generalized anxiety disorder. Of these, only separation anxiety disorder is a disorder restricted to use with children. Each of these disorders can have an adverse impact on the child's scholastic, social, and familial functioning and as such may interfere with the normal developmental processes. In terms of specific symptomatology, separation anxiety disorder, specific phobias, obsessive-compulsive disorder, and generalized anxiety disorder all have symptoms of anxiety, which can include excessive and unrealistic fear or worry associated with a particular stimulus (i.e., object or situation); avoidance of the feared stimulus; and physiological arousal in the presence of, or in anticipation of, the feared stimulus. Generalized anxiety disorder interferes with the child's functioning to a greater extent than the other disorders, as the fears are more general and pervasive, and the child will experience a need to avoid many different stimuli. The prevalence rate for anxiety disorders in children is 2.5 percent (Offord, 1985). Major depression and dysthymic disorder are both characterized by feelings of worthlessness, depression, hopelessness, withdrawal, and some disturbance of sleep and appetite. Dysthymic disorder is a milder version of major depression and tends to be more commonly observed in children and adolescents, with the prevalence for major depression being 1.1 percent and the prevalence for milder depressive episodes being 9.7 percent (Offord, 1985).

Fewer data are available related to etiological factors for internalizing disorders, but the information that has been obtained indicates that there is a higher prevalence of internalizing disorders in children who have hostile, withdrawn fathers (Katz & Gottman, 1993), deficient or absent communication patterns with the mother (Burge & Hammen, 1991), and depressive symptomatology in the mother (Hammen, Burge, and Stansbury, 1990). Children are more likely to develop depressive symptomatology if there is positive history for an affective (depressive) disorder in the family (Rutter, 1986), suggesting that there may be a genetic component to the development of this disorder. Few studies, however, have examined the etiology of depression in children, or identified the factors associated with greater risk for developing this disorder.

The different forms of treatment proposed for the amelioration of internalizing symptomatology tend to be classified as either individual therapy approaches or pharmacotherapy. Systematic desensitization is one of the more common approaches for assisting children with overcoming phobic or fearful behaviors (King, Hamilton, and Ollendick, 1988). This procedure is generally implemented in individual therapy sessions and involves exposing the child to the feared stimulus either *in vivo* or via imagery, while the child is relaxed. Use of a live model or of relaxation exercises can facilitate the process of systematic desensitization (Ollendick & Cerney, 1981). If a child exhibits generalized anxiety, the clinician may want to consider use of a multicomponent treatment program, which could involve relaxation, cognitive restructuring, and rewards for nonanxious behaviors (Strauss, 1988). Philip C. Kendall and colleagues (1992) devised a cognitive-behavioral treatment program that has been found to be effective in reducing anxious symptomatology, with this program focusing on increasing children's cognitive and behavioral control over the reaction to feared situations and feared stimuli. The more pervasive the symptomatology, the more likely it will be necessary to use a treatment package that incorporates different components in order to increase the likelihood of positive treatment outcome. In terms of targeting depressive symptomatology, cognitive-behavioral and relaxation techniques have been found to be useful for reducing the level of depression (Reynolds & Coats, 1986); thus similar treatment options are effective for the different forms of internalizing distress.

Pharmacological intervention has been proposed to affect internalizing difficulties in children and adolescents. Reduction in anxious symptomatology was noted following introduction of antianxiety medication for children with avoidant and generalized anxiety (Simeon & Ferguson, 1987), and for children with chronic illnesses (Pfefferbaum et al., 1987). An antidepressant was found to be effective in reducing symptomatology related to school phobia in one study (Gittelman-Klein & Klein, 1971), but these results were not supported in a subsequent controlled study (Bernstein, Garfinkel, and Borchardt, 1990). The use of antidepressant medication to reduce depressive symptomatology has been called into question, with the results of several double blind studies indicating that medication is no more effective than a placebo (Geller et al., 1990). Neal D. Ryan (1992) has further expanded on this topic and has suggested that the effectiveness of antidepressant medication in children has not been empirically established, and that medications in isolation do not resolve the associated features of depression (i.e., distorted or negative thought patterns) (Kazdin, 1990). It appears wise to use these medications judiciously and only in cases where a child is not responding to other forms of treatment. The same general rule applies to the use of antianxiety agents in children, with the treatment of choice being cognitive-behavioral intervention supplemented by medication only if the child is not responding to other forms of therapy (Kutcher et al., 1992).

Comorbidity

Comorbidity refers to the presence of multiple psychiatric diagnoses rather than one diagnosis. There is some evidence, based on prevalence estimates, that approximately one-third (Hogan et al., 1989) to one-half (Martinez & Smith, 1993) of children are reported to have symptoms related to more than one DSM-IV diagnosis. Comorbidity can occur at one point in time (cross-sectional) or at different points in time (longitudinal), and can occur within or between the broad categories of internalizing and externalizing behavioral disorders. Several hypotheses have been generated to explain the presence of comorbid disorders in children. These include the possibility that particular disorders operate as precursors for the development of other disorders, that two comorbid disorders arise from similar etiological components, that the presence of one disorder operates as a risk factor for the development of a different disorder, and that the two disorders actually represent subtypes of a more heterogeneous diagnostic category (Biederman, Newcorn, and Sprich, 1991). Given that the presence of comorbid disorders would have implications for rehabilitation efforts and prognosis, it is important for the clinician to complete a thorough assessment, including a systematic evaluation of each disorder, to develop a rehabilitation plan most effectively. John E. Clarkin and Philip C. Kendall (1992) discussed treatment considerations for comorbid disorders and suggested that if both disorders occur at the same time, it is advantageous to treat both symptom patterns either sequentially or simultaneously. There is also the possibility that one disorder may be the precursor for the development of a later disorder, and as such there may be a causal relationship; if this is the case, then the rehabilitation of the initial disorder should offset the development of the later disorder. Unfortunately, the data available on the course and etiology of many childhood psychiatric disorders do not allow clinicians to make an accurate determination of the future course of symptomatology; thus a focus on intervention rather than prevention prevails.

Approximately one-fourth (August & Garfinkel, 1993) to one-third (Keller et al., 1992) of children with one externalizing disorder meet criteria for another externalizing disorder. These estimates refer to comorbidity among ADHD, ODD, and CD, and suggest that there is some overlap among the undercontrolled behaviors associated with these three disorders. In terms of treatment recommendations and prognosis, Rolf Loeber and Benjamin B. Lahey (1989) indicated that children who are comorbid for two externalizing disorders tend to exhibit more severe behavioral disturbances within each diagnostic category than children with only one diagnosis, and comorbidity for two externalizing disorders is associated with greater risk for the development of antisocial behavior in adulthood. Thus it is difficult to ascertain whether the poorer prognosis for children comorbid within the externalizing category is due to the greater severity of behavioral disturbance or to the presence of two disorders. When externalizing comorbidity is observed, the clinician may want to recommend a more intensive, comprehensive rehabilitation plan in an attempt to reduce the likelihood of the unfolding of more severe difficulties at a later time.

Comorbidity within the internalizing category has been empirically examined to a lesser extent, but the available evidence suggests that the comorbidity rates are similar to those seen within the externalizing disorders, with approximately one-fourth (Puig-Antich & Rabinovich, 1986) to one-third (Strauss et al., 1988a) of children with one internalizing disorder meeting the criteria for a second internalizing disorder. Cyd C. Strauss and colleagues (1988b) indicated that there are age differences in the disorders that will be observed in comorbid children, with younger children tending to receive both separation anxiety and overanxious diagnoses, and older children receiving both overanxious and depressive diagnoses.

There can also be overlap in the expression of internalizing and externalizing symptomatology, and some children receive diagnoses within both categories. As many as 40 percent of children diagnosed with ADHD also meet criteria for an anxiety disorder, with children comorbid for these two types of disorders tending to exhibit less severe ADHD symptomatology (Pliszka, 1992). Comorbidity has been observed between ADHD and depressive disorders at a "higher than expected rate," although no prevalence estimates were provided regarding the rate of occurrence (August & Garfinkel, 1993). There is a high degree of comorbidity between substance use, an undercontrolled behavior, and conduct disorder, with approximately 75 percent of adolescents who meet criteria for conduct disorder also meeting criteria for moderate substance use (Greenbaum et al., 1991). A high degree of comorbidity was also found between substance use and depression, with approximately 25 percent of adolescents with a depressive disorder also meeting criteria for moderate substance use (Greenbaum et al., 1991). For adolescents, substance use history should be assessed thoroughly, given these rates, particularly if the child meets criteria for a conduct disorder. Children with mixed internalizing-externalizing disorders have been found to improve more in the absence of treatment than children with an externalizing disorder in isolation, suggesting that the internalizing disorder may operate at least partially as a resilience factor for children comorbid for these disorder types (Rutter, 1976). One possible explanation for this finding is that children who experience some anxiety are more likely to experience anxiety when engaging in undercontrolled behaviors (i.e., oppositional behavior), and this anxiety may then operate as an inhibitory mechanism at a later time. This issue raises the possibility that the identification of comorbid symptomatology patterns may allow for more accurate prediction of treatment outcome, prognosis, and relapse rates, as well as the possibility that different intervention techniques may be recommended for comorbid difficulties than would be suggested for children with a single diagnosis.

(*See also:* ADOLESCENTS, REHABILITATION OF; ANXIETY DISORDERS; AUTISM; BEHAVIOR THERAPY; CAREGIVING; EATING DISORDERS; FAMILY; LEARNING DISABILITIES; MOOD DISORDERS; PEDIATRIC REHABILITATION; PHARMACOLOGY; PSYCHIATRIC REHABILITATION; RESPITE CARE)

RESOURCES

National Alliance for the Mentally Ill (NAMI), 2101 Wilson Blvd., Suite 302, Arlington, VA 22201

National Mental Health Association (NMHA), 1021 Prince St., Alexandria, VA 22314

BIBLIOGRAPHY

ACHENBACH, THOMAS M., and EDELBROOK, CRAIG S. *Manual for the Child Behavior Checklist and Revised Child Behavior Profile.* Burlington, VT, 1983.

AMERICAN PSYCHIATRIC ASSOCIATION. *Diagnostic and Statistical Manual of Mental Disorders* (DSM-I). Washington, DC, 1952.

———. *Diagnostic and Statistical Manual of Mental Disorders,* 4th ed. (DSM-IV). Washington, DC, 1994.

AUGUST, GERALD J., and GARFINKEL, BARRY D. "The Nosology of Attention-Deficit Hyperactivity Disorder." *Journal of the American Academy of Child and Adolescent Psychiatry* 32 (1993):155–165.

AXELINE, VIRGINIA M. *Play Therapy.* New York, 1947.

BARKLEY, RUSSELL A. "Attention Deficit Hyperactivity Disorder: A Workshop Manual for Clinicians." Cleveland, 1988.

BARKLEY, RUSSELL A.; FISCHER, MARIELLEN; NEWBY, ROBERT F.; and BREEN, MICHAEL J. "Development of Multimethod Clinical Protocol for Assessing Stimulant Drug Response in Children with Attention Deficit Disorder." *Journal of Clinical Child Psychology* 17 (1988):14–24.

BERNSTEIN, GAIL A.; GARFINKEL, BARRY D.; and BORCHARDT, CARRIE M. "Comparative Studies of Pharmacotherapy for School Refusal." *Journal of the American Academy of Child and Adolescent Psychiatry* 29 (1990):773–781.

BIEDERMAN, JOSEPH; NEWCORN, JEFFREY; and SPRICH, SUSAN. "Comorbidity of Attention Deficit Hyperactivity Disorder with Conduct, Depressive, Anxiety, and Other Disorders." *American Journal of Psychiatry* 148 (1991):564–575.

BURGE, DORLI, and HAMMEN, CONSTANCE. "Maternal Communication: Predictors of Outcome at Follow-up in a Sample of Children at High and Low Risk for Depression." *Journal of Abnormal Psychology* 100 (1991):174–180.

BUSS, ARNOLD H., and PLOMIN, ROBERT. *A Temperament Theory of Personality Development*. New York, 1975.

CAMPBELL, MAGDA; GONZALEZ, NILDA M.; and SILVA, RAUL R. "The Pharmacologic Treatment of Conduct Disorders and Rage Outbursts." *Pediatric Psychopharmacology* 15 (1992):69–85.

CAMPBELL, MAGDA; SMALL, ARTHUR M.; GREEN, WAYNE H.; JENNINGS, S. J.; PERRY, RICHARD; BENNETT, WILLIAM G.; and ANDERSON, LOWELL. "Behavioural Efficacy of Haloperidol and Lithium Carbonate: A Comparison in Hospitalized Aggressive Children with Conduct Disorder." *Archives of General Psychiatry* 120 (1984):650–656.

CLARKIN, JOHN F., and KENDALL, PHILIP C. "Comorbidity and Treatment Planning: Summary and Future Directions." *Journal of Consulting and Clinical Psychology* 60 (1992):904–908.

COIE, JOHN D.; LOCHMAN, JOHN E.; TERRY, R.; and HYMAN, CLAIRE. "Predicting Early Adolescent Disorder from Childhood Aggression and Peer Rejection." *Journal of Consulting and Clinical Psychology* 60 (1992):783–792.

DODGE, KENNETH A. "The Future of Research on the Treatment of Conduct Disorder." *Development and Psychopathology* 5 (1993):311–319.

DODGE, KENNETH A.; PETTIT, GREGORY S.; McCLASKEY, CYNTHIA L.; and BROWN, MELISSA M. "Social Competence in Children." *Monographs of the Society for Research in Child Development* 51 (1986).

DOWNEY, GERALDINE, and WALKER, ELAINE. "Social Cognition and Adjustment in Children at Risk for Psychopathology." *Developmental Psychology* 25 (1989):835–845.

DUMAS, J. E., and WAHLER, R. G. "Predictors of Treatment Outcome in Parent Training: Mother Insularity and Socioeconomic Disadvantage." *Behavioral Assessment* 5 (1983):301–313.

EVANS, RANDALL W.; CLAY, THOMAS H.; and GUALTIERI, C. THOMAS. "Carbamazepine in Pediatric Psychiatry." *Journal of the American Academy of Child and Adolescent Psychiatry* 26 (1987):2–8.

FARRINGTON, DAVID P. "Childhood Aggression and Adult Violence: Early Precursors and Later-Life Outcomes." In *The Development and Treatment of Childhood Aggression*, eds. D. J. Pepler and K. H. Rubin. Hillsdale, NJ, 1991.

FARRINGTON, DAVID P.; OSBORN, S. G.; and WEST, DONALD J. "The Persistence of Labelling Effects." *British Journal of Criminology* 21 (1978):277–284.

FEINGOLD, BEN F. "Hyperkinesis and Learning Disabilities Linked to Artificial Food Flavors and Colors." *American Journal of Nursing* 75 (1975):797–803.

FOREHAND, REX, and LONG, NICHOLAS. "Outpatient Treatment of the Acting-Out Child: Procedures, Long-Term Follow-up Data, and Clinical Problems." *Advances in Behavior Research and Therapy* 10 (1988):129–177.

FRICK, PAUL J.; LAHEY, BENJAMIN B.; LOEBER, ROLF L.; STOUTHAMER-LOEBER, MAGDA; CHRIST, MARY ANNE; and HANSON, KELLY. "Familial Risk Factors to Oppositional Defiant Disorder and Conduct Disorder: Parental Psychopathology and Maternal Parenting." *Journal of Consulting and Clinical Psychology* 60 (1992):49–55.

GADOW, KENNETH D. "Pediatric Psychopharmacology: A Review of Recent Research." *Journal of Child Psychology and Psychiatry and Allied Disciplines* 33 (1992): 153–195.

GELLER, BARBARA; COOPER, THOMAS B.; GRAHAM, DONNA L.; MARSTELLER, FREDERICK A.; and BRYANT, DEBRA M. "Double-Blind Placebo-Controlled Study of Nortriptyline in Depressed Adolescents Using a 'Fixed Plasma Level' Design." *Psychopharmacology Bulletin* 26 (1990):85–90.

GITTELMAN-KLEIN, RACHEL, and KLEIN, DAVID F. "Controlled Imipramine Treatment of School Phobia." *Archives of General Psychiatry* 25 (1971): 204–207.

GREENBAUM, PAUL E.; PRANGE, MARK E.; FRIEDMAN, ROBERT M.; and SILVER, STARR E. "Substance Abuse Prevalence and Comorbidity with other Psychiatric Disorders Among Adolescents with Severe Emotional Disturbances." *Journal of the American Academy of Child and Adolescent Psychiatry* 30 (1991):575–583.

GREENHILL, LAURENCE L.; SOLOMON, MARDI; PLEAK, RICHARD; and AMBROSINI, PAUL. "Molindone Hydrochloride Treatment of Hospitalized Children with Conduct Disorder." *Journal of Clinical Psychiatry* 46 (1985):20–25.

GREENSPAN, STANLEY I. *The Clinical Interview of the Child*. New York, 1981.

HAMMEN, CONSTANCE; BURGE, DORLI; and STANSBURY, KATHY. "Relationship of Mother and Child Variables to Child Outcomes in High Risk Sample: A Causal Modeling Analysis." *Developmental Psychology* 26 (1990):24–30.

HOGAN, ANNE E.; QUAY, HERBERT C.; VAUGHN,

SHARON; and SHAPIRO, STEVEN K. "Revised Behavior Problem Checklist: Stability, Prevalence, and Incidence of Behavior Problems in Kindergarten and First Grade Children." *Psychological Assessment* 1 (1989):103–111.

KATZ, LYNN F., and GOTTMAN, JOHN M. "Patterns of Marital Conflict Predict Children's Internalizing and Externalizing Behaviors." *Developmental Psychology* 29 (1993):940–950.

KAZDIN, ALAN E. *Treatment of Antisocial Behavior in Children and Adolescents.* Homewood, IL, 1985.

———. *Conduct Disorders in Childhood and Adolescence.* Newbury Park, CA, 1987a.

———. "Treatment of Antisocial Behavior in Children: Current Status and Future Directions." *Psychological Bulletin* 102 (1987b):187–203.

———. "Childhood Depression." *Journal of Child Psychology and Psychiatry and Allied Disciplines* 31 (1990): 121–160.

———. "Treatment of Conduct Disorder: Progress and Directions in Psychotherapy Research." *Development and Psychopathology* 3 (1993):277–310.

KAZDIN, ALAN E.; ESVELDT-DAWSON, KAREN; FRENCH, NANCY H.; and UNIS, ALAN S. "Problem-Solving Skills Training and Relationship Therapy in the Treatment of Antisocial Behavior." *Journal of Consulting and Clinical Psychology* 55 (1987):76–85.

KAZDIN, ALAN E.; SIEGEL, TODD C.; and BASS, DEBRA. "Cognitive Problem-Solving Skills Training and Parent Management Training in the Treatment of Antisocial Behavior in Children." *Journal of Consulting and Clinical Psychology* 60 (1992):733–747.

KELLER, MARTIN B.; LAVORI, PHILIP W.; BEARDSLEE, WILLIAM R.; WUNDER, JOANNE; SCHWARTZ, CARL; ROTH, JOAN; and BIEDERMAN, JOSEPH. "The Disruptive Behavioral Disorders in Children and Adolescents: Comorbidity and Clinical Course." *Journal of the American Academy of Child and Adolescent Psychiatry* 31 (1992):204–209.

KENDALL, PHILIP C., and BRASWELL, LAUREN. *Cognitive-Behavioral Therapy for Impulsive Children.* New York, 1985.

KENDALL, PHILIP C.; CHANSKY, TAMAR E.; and KANE, MARTHA. *Anxiety Disorder in Youth: Cognitive-Behavioral Interventions.* New York, 1992.

KING, NEVILLE J.; HAMILTON, DAVID H.; and OLLENDICK, THOMAS H. *Children's Phobias: A Behavioral Perspective.* New York, 1988.

KUTCHER, STAN P.; REITER, SHARON; GARDNER, DAVID M.; and KLEIN, RACHEL G. "The Pharmacotherapy of Anxiety Disorders in Children and Ad-

olescents." *Pediatric Psychopharmacology* 15 (1992): 41–67.

LOCHMAN, JOHN E. "Cognitive-Behavioral Interventions with Aggressive Boys: Three-Year Follow-up and Preventive Effects." *Journal of Consulting and Clinical Psychology* 60 (1992):426–432.

LOCHMAN, JOHN E.; BURCH, PETER R.; CURRY, JOHN F.; and LAMPRON, LOUISE B. "Treatment and Generalization Effects of Cognitive Behavioral and Goal-Setting Interventions with Aggressive Boys." *Journal of Consulting and Clinical Psychology* 52 (1984):915–916.

LOCHMAN, JOHN E., and LAMPRON, LOUISE B. "Cognitive-Behavioral Interventions for Aggressive Boys: Seven-Month Follow-up Effects." *Journal of Child and Adolescent Psychotherapy* 5 (1988):15–23.

LOCHMAN, JOHN E.; LAMPRON, LOUISE B.; GEMMER, THOMAS V.; and HARRIS, STEVE R. "Anger Coping Interventions for Aggressive Children: Guide to Implementation in School Settings." In *Innovations in Clinical Practice: A Source Book,* eds. P. A. Keller and S. R. Heyman. Sarasota, FL, 1987.

LOCHMAN, JOHN E.; MEYER, BRIAN L.; RABINER, DAVID L.; and WHITE, KAREN J. "Parameters Influencing Social Problem-Solving of Aggressive Children." In *Advances in Behavioral Assessment of Children and Families,* ed. R. Prinz. Greenwich, CT, 1991.

LOEBER, ROLF. "Development and Risk Factors of Juvenile Antisocial Behavior and Delinquency." *Clinical Psychology Review* 10 (1990):1–41.

LOEBER, ROLF, and DISHION, THOMAS J. "Early Predictors of Male Delinquency: A Review." *Psychological Bulletin* 94 (1983):68–99.

LOEBER, ROLF, and LAHEY, BENJAMIN B. "Recommendations for Research on Disruptive Behavior Disorders of Childhood and Adolescence." In *Advances in Clinical Psychology,* eds. Benjamin B. Lahey and Alan E. Kazdin. New York, 1989.

LOEBER, ROLF; LAHEY, BENJAMIN B.; and THOMAS, CHRISTOPHER. "Diagnostic Conundrum of Oppositional Defiant Disorder and Conduct Disorder." *Journal of Abnormal Psychology* 100 (1991):379–390.

LUISELLI, JAMES K. "Assessment-Derived Treatment of Children's Disruptive Behavior Disorders." *Behavior Modification* 15 (1991):294–309.

MCCORD, JOAN. "Deterrence and the Light Touch of the Law." In *Reactions to Crime: The Police, Courts, and Prisons,* eds. D. P. Farrington and J. Gunn. Chichester, Eng., 1985.

MORRISON, JAMES R., and STEWART, MARK A. "Evidence for a Polygenetic Inheritance in the Hyperactive Child Syndrome." *American Journal of Psychiatry* 130 (1973):791–792.

MURRAY, JOHN B. "Psychophysiological Effects of Methylphenidate (Ritalin)." *Psychological Reports* 61 (1987):315–336.

OFFORD, DAVID R. "Child Psychiatric Disorders: Prevalence and Perspectives." *Psychiatric Clinics of North America* 8 (1985):637–652.

OLLENDICK, THOMAS H., and CERNEY, J. A. *Clinical Behavior Therapy with Children.* New York, 1981.

OLWEUS, D. "Stability of Aggressive Behavior Patterns in Males: A Review." *Psychological Bulletin* 86 (1979):852–875.

PFEFFERBAUM, BETTY; OVERALL, JOHN E.; BOREN, HALLIE A.; FRANKEL, LAWRENCE S.; SULLIVAN, M. P.; and JOHNSON, K. "Alprazolam in the Treatment of Anticipatory and Acute Situational Anxiety in Children with Cancer." *Journal of the American Academy of Child and Adolescent Psychiatry* 26 (1987):532–535.

PLISZKA, STEVEN R. "Comorbidity of Attention-Deficit Hyperactivity Disorder and Overanxious Disorder." *Journal of the American Academy of Child and Adolescent Psychiatry* 31 (1992):197–203.

PRINZ, RONALD J., and MILLER, GLORIA E. "Issues in Understanding and Treating Childhood Conduct Problems in Disadvantaged Populations." *Journal of Clinical Child Psychology* 20 (1991):379–385.

PUIG-ANTICH, JOAQUIN, and RABINOVICH, HARRIS. "Relationship Between Affective and Anxiety Disorders in Childhood." In *Anxiety Disorders of Childhood*, ed. Rachel Gittelman. New York, 1986.

REYNOLDS, WILLIAM M., and COATS, KEVIN I. "A Comparison of Cognitive-Behavioral Therapy and Relaxation Training for the Treatment of Depression in Adolescents." *Journal of Consulting and Clinical Psychology* 54 (1986):653–660.

ROSE, STEVEN D., and EDELSON, J. L. *Working with Children and Adolescents in Groups.* San Francisco, 1987.

ROSS, DAVID, and ROSS, SUSAN. *Hyperactivity.* New York, 1976.

RUTTER, MICHAEL L. *Helping Troubled Children.* New York, 1976.

———. "Child Psychiatry: The Interface Between Clinical and Developmental Research." *Psychological Medicine* 16 (1986):151–169.

RUTTER, MICHAEL L., and TUMA, A. HUSSAIN. "Diagnosis and Classification: Some Outstanding Issues." In *Assessment and Diagnosis in Child Psychopathology*, eds. Michael L. Rutter, A. Hussain Tuma, and I. S. Lann. New York, 1988.

RYAN, NEAL D. "The Pharmacologic Treatment of Child and Adolescent Depression." *Psychiatric Clinics of North America* 15 (1992):29–40.

SATTERFIELD, JAMES; HOPPE, CHRISTIANE M.; and SCHELL, ANNE M. "A Prospective Study of Delinquency in 100 Adolescent Boys with Attention Deficit Disorder and 88 Normal Adolescent Boys." *American Journal of Psychiatry* 139 (1982):795–798.

SCHACHAR, RUSSELL J., and WACHSMUTH, R. "Family Dysfunction and Psychosocial Adversity: Comparison of Attention Deficit Disorder, Conduct Disorder, Normal and Clinical Controls." *Canadian Journal of Behavioural Science* 23 (1991):332–348.

SIMEON, JOVAN G., and FERGUSON, H. BRUCE. "Alprazolam Effects in Children with Anxiety Disorders." *American Journal of Psychiatry* 32 (1987):570–574.

SIMONOFF, EMILY; McGUFFIN, PETER; and GOTTESMAN, IRVING I. "Genetic Influences on Normal and Abnormal Development." In *Child and Adolescent Psychiatry*, 3rd ed., M. Rutter, E. Taylor, and L. Hersou, eds. Oxford, 1994.

SLEATOR, ESTHER; VON-NEWMANN, ALICE; and SPRAGUE, ROBERT L. "Hyperactive Children: A Continuous Long-Term Placebo Controlled Follow-up." *Journal of the American Medical Association* 229 (1974):316–317.

STRAUSS, CYD C. "Behavioral Assessment and Treatment of Overanxious Disorder in Children and Adolescents." *Behavior Modification* 12 (1988):234–251.

STRAUSS, CYD C.; LAST, CYNTHIA G.; HERSEN, MICHAEL; and KAZDIN, ALAN E. "Association Between Anxiety and Depression in Children and Adolescents with Anxiety Disorder." *Journal of Abnormal Child Psychology* 16 (1988a):57–68.

STRAUSS, CYD C.; LEASE, CYNTHIA A.; LAST, CYNTHIA G.; and FRANCIS, GRETA. "Overanxious Disorder: An Examination of Developmental Differences." *Journal of Abnormal Child Psychology* 16 (1988b):433–443.

STROUL, BETH. *Systems of Care for Children and Adolescents with Severe Emotional Disturbances: What Are the Results?* Washington, DC, 1993.

WEBSTER-STRATTON, CAROLYN. "Predictors of Treatment Outcome in Parent Training for Conduct Disordered Children." *Behavior Therapy* 16 (1985):223–243.

WELLS, KAREN. "Parent Training Studies of ADHD Children." Unpublished manuscript, Duke University Medical Center, 1994.

WERRY, JOHN S.; REEVES, JAN C.; and ELKIND, GAIL

S. "Attention Deficit, Conduct, Oppositional, and Anxiety Disorders in Children: I. A Review of Research on Differentiating Characteristics." *Journal of the American Academy of Child and Adolescent Psychiatry* 26 (1987):133–143.

ZUBIETA, JON K., and ALESSI, NORMAN E. "Acute and Chronic Administration of Trazodone in the Treatment of Disruptive Behavior Disorders in Children." *Journal of Clinical Psychopharmacology* 12 (1992):346–351.

LISA A. LENHART

CHROMOSOME DISORDERS

See GENETIC DISORDERS

CHRONIC FATIGUE SYNDROME

Fatigue is a common fact of human life, frequently observed in health as well as in disease states, reflecting the body response to a multitude of experiences. Hence, the biological meaning of persisting fatigue is diverse and complex, often remaining elusive in its causes. The particular entity of persisting fatigue, occurring in the absence of recognizable primary causes, has received popular and medical attention in the late 1980s and early 1990s under the term of chronic fatigue syndrome (CFS). This clinical entity is a poorly understood disease characterized by persisting and debilitating fatigue accompanying the neuromuscular and neuropsychological clinical picture. The large variety of descriptive reports generated by this syndrome has suggested the formulation of a conventional definition, proposed under the auspices of the Center for Disease Control (CDC; Table 1). Severe fatigue, as part of conventionally defined CFS, is characteristically unresponsive to rest and is associated often with malaise, a feverish feeling, headache, sore throat, and painful joints, among other symptoms. Enlarged and/or painful lymph nodes are often noted. In contrast with these disabling findings, a remarkable absence of positive laboratory information is equally characteristic.

Chronic fatigue syndrome as defined by the CDC panel (Holmes et al., 1988) is an operational concept, agreed on by a committee of experts for the purpose of gathering information on and gaining understanding of this syndrome (complex of symptoms and signs). In this concept, there is not a definite cause. CFS as defined in this way must be distinguished from the whole range of effects of acute and chronic diseases such as chronic anemia; malignancies; infections; and cardiovascular, respiratory, metabolic, endocrine, neurological, and kidney disorders. It is the exclusion of these identifiable causes that allows the appropriate use of the CFS term.

Causes

The early reports on CFS related this disorder to the cryptic process of certain infections, particularly viral ones. In this connection, mononucleosis and its causative agent, the Epstein-Barr virus, have attracted vigorous attention and study. As of the early 1990s, however, the verification of a viral infection in the conventional picture of CFS remains unconfirmed. Similarly, yeast infection, particularly candidiasis, proposed as a causative factor of certain forms of CFS, has not been adequately documented. Psychological factors such as depression often accompany this syndrome and may even precede it in the perception of the patient. It cannot be readily concluded, however, that the mere presence of the emotional disorder explains the cause of this syndrome.

Because the large majority of CFS cases do not present significant or characteristic laboratory abnormalities, a laboratory verification of the syndrome is not available at the present time. It remains that a case is identified only on the basis of its correspondence with the diagnostic criteria listed in Table 1.

In general, chronic fatigue is a common experience. Several surveys in the United States and abroad suggest a frequency ranging from 14 to 25 percent of the general population (Shafran, 1991). Among certain categories of patients, chronic fatigue reaches even higher prevalence rates. This is particularly noted among individuals affected with psychiatric disorders, where rates of 50 to 80 percent

Table 1. Diagnostic definition of Chronic Fatigue Syndrome (CFS)

I. Major Criteria (all of A must be present and none of B)

    A. Persistent or recurring fatigue, of disabling intensity
        1. Fatigue persisting after rest; readily occurring fatigability
        2. Recognized onset (i.e., no previous history)
        3. Disabling effects resulting in marked limitation of usual activities
        4. Duration of at least 6 months (or greater)
    B. Exclusions
        1. Concurrent physical or psychiatric illness
        2. Drug use or abuse
        3. Nutritional factors (weight or diet abnormalities)

II. Minor Criteria (at least 6 of the 10 symptom criteria and 2 or more of the physical criteria; or 8 or more of the 10 symptom criteria)

    A. Symptom criteria
        1. Fever, mild
        2. Sore throat
        3. Enlarged or painful lymph nodes
        4. Muscular weakness, generalized
        5. Muscular ache
        6. Headache
        7. Aching joints
        8. Neuropsychologic disorders
        9. Sleep disorder
    B. Physical criteria (Objective)
        1. Low-grade fever
        2. Pharyngitis
        3. Enlarged or tender lymph nodes

SOURCE: CDC Criteria, 1988

are not unusual (Price et al., 1992). Conventionally defined CFS, however, is a much less common entity, perhaps even rare (estimated at 7.4 cases per 100,000).

Treatment

Options for successful treatment of CFS are admittedly limited. Clinical management of these cases includes cognitive behavior measures, controlled and increasing physical activity, analgesics and anti-inflammatory drugs, and, in appropriate cases, antidepressants. Attempts to use infection-suppressing medications or immunologically active devices have yielded uncertain and contradictory results. The general consensus calls for determined efforts toward the identification of correctable causes (e.g., meta-

bolic or endocrine disorders) before embarking on a treatment program fraught with many uncertainties.

It should be recognized that the adverse impact of fatigue in general, including chronic fatigue associated with the CFS clinical picture, may antagonize significantly the process of an applied rehabilitation program and return to work potential. This fact requires vigorous attention focused on developing the most positive motivation and outlook in the client under treatment. Here again any prescription for rest and inactivity must be tempered with an equal emphasis on exercise and diversified activities implemented through a judicious and persuasive care program. It is only in this context that deficiencies in muscular function and in attitude may be effectively ameliorated if not entirely corrected. Counteracting the penalizing influence of fatigue remains an arduous task calling for the best clinical resources of the care provider.

(*See also:* PSYCHOSOCIAL ADJUSTMENT)

RESOURCES

Center for Disease Control and Prevention, U.S. Public Health Service, Division of Viral and Rickettsial Diseases, 1600 Clifton Rd, NE, Building CDC 6, Room 110, Atlanta, GA 30333

Chronic Fatigue and Immune Dysfunction Syndrome Association, P.O. Box 220398, Charlotte, NC 28222–0398

Chronic Fatigue Syndrome Society, P.O. Box 230108, Portland, OR 97223

National CFS Association, 3521 Broadway, Suite 222, Kansas City, MO 64111

National Institute of Allergy and Infectious Diseases, Office of Communications, NIH Building 31, Room 7A50, 9000 Rockville Pike, Bethesda, MD 20892

Office of Special Education and Rehabilitation Services, Dissemination and Information Utilization Office, 3420 Mary E. Switzer Building, 330 C St., SW, Washington, DC 20202

BIBLIOGRAPHY

FEIDEN, KARYN. *Hope and Help for Chronic Fatigue Syndrome.* New York, 1990.

HOLMES, GARY P.; KAPLAN, JONATHAN E.; GANTZ, NELSON M.; KOMAROFF, ANTHONY L.; SCHONBERGER, LAWRENCE B.; STRAUS, STEPHEN E.; JONES, JAMES F.; DUBOIS, RICHARD E.; CUNNINGHAM-RUNDLES, CHARLOTTE; PAHWA, SAVITA; TOSATO, GIOVANNA; ZEGANS, LEONARD S.; PURTILO, DAVID T.; BROWN, NATHANIEL; SCHOOLEY, ROBERT T.; and BRUS, IRENA. "Chronic Fatigue Syndrome: A Working Case Definition." *Annals of Internal Medicine* 108 (1988):387–389.

PRICE, RUMI K.; NORTH, CAROL S.; WESSELY, SIMON; and FRASER, VICTORIA J. "Estimating the Prevalence of Chronic Fatigue Syndrome and Associated Symptoms in the Community." *Public Health Reports* 107 (1992):514–522.

SHAFAN, STEPHEN D. "The Chronic Fatigue Syndrome." *American Journal of Medicine* 90 (1991): 730–739.

MARIO C. BATTIGELLI

CHRONIC OBSTRUCTIVE PULMONARY DISEASE (COPD)

See RESPIRATORY DISEASE

CIVIL RIGHTS

The application of the concept of civil rights is emerging as a primary means of improving the lives of citizens with disabilities. While there is no commonly accepted formal definition of this concept, civil rights usually refer to the legal status of minority groups that evolved during the seventeenth and eighteenth centuries from the belief in the natural rights of man. This philosophy was reflected in the fundamental values of equality, freedom, and justice embodied in the Declaration of Independence, the U.S. Constitution, and subsequent laws. The use of the concept of legal rights in promoting the employment of people with disabilities has resulted from the increasing realization that discrimination is a major barrier to their participation in the work force. To demonstrate the existence of discrimination, litigants often must prove in court the disparate treatment of individuals who are similarly situated. Discrimination is the unequal treatment of equal persons. Recognition of the civil rights of people with disabilities, therefore, implies that they are inherently similar to the people without disabilities; hence they are entitled to equal opportunities under the law.

Although persons with disabilities long have been considered a minority group by researchers (e.g., Barker et al., 1953), the adoption of laws that prohibit discrimination against such individuals in the 1970s and 1980s was based on the growing acceptance of the "minority group" model (Gliedman & Roth, 1980; Hahn, 1982), which challenged the traditional "functional limitations" paradigm for the study of disability (Hahn, 1985). The minority group model is based on a sociopolitical definition of disability as a product of the interaction between the individual and the environment. This perspective avoids the common fallacy of perceiving disability as the final stage of a progression from pathology to impairment to functional limitation (Pope & Tarlov, 1991). In fact, in some versions of this definition, the dimension of performance or functioning is even removed, and the mere appearance of a disability as disclosed by visibility or labeling is considered sufficient to evoke discriminatory responses. Thus disability is socially or culturally constructed, and the basic source of the problems encountered by people with disabilities is ascribed to a disabling environment instead of to their personal defects or deficiencies.

The realization that the fundamental source of an individual's disability is external rather than internal could remove the burden of shame or inferiority from persons with disabilities. The resulting heightened self-esteem could in turn promote a positive sense of social identity to sustain a continuing struggle for equal rights. As a result, increased research has been devoted to historical and cultural circumstances in which favorable rather than negative connotations have been attached to the perceptible signs of a disability (Hahn, 1988a).

In addition, the minority group paradigm is founded on three major postulates: (1) that prevalent public attitudes form the principal environmental barriers confronting citizens with disabilities; (2) that all facets of the social or physical environment are molded by public policy; and (3) that public policy is a reflection of pervasive social attitudes or values. The isolation of attitudes as the fundamental source of discrimination against citizens with disabilities indicates that concepts and precedents developed in prior civil rights movements by African Americans, women, and other disadvantaged groups can be applied to another minority, people with disabilities. Perhaps to a greater extent than comparable sentiments about other groups, however, biases against people with disabilities are deeply ingrained in the architectural as well as the attitudinal environment.

These postulates also frame the logic for assessing the unequal treatment of people with disabilities as a consequence of a definite though barely perceptible intent, instead of mere happenstance or coincidence. Public attitudes are regarded as primarily responsible for the fact that the social status of citizens with disabilities reflects the discrimination and

deprivation inflicted on other minorities. The unemployment rate among adults with disabilities is approximately two-thirds, the highest level in almost all industrialized countries in the world (Hahn, 1984). In the United States, persons with disabilities also exhibit high rates of welfare dependency, and three-fifths of them live below the poverty line (Bowe, 1978). Many have attended separate schools, and they have been compelled to face a rigid pattern of segregation in transportation, housing, and public accommodations. Finally, attitudinal aversion to individuals with disabilities has been traced to "existential" anxiety, which seems related to the functional limitations paradigm, and to "aesthetic" anxiety, which is most closely associated with the minority group model. From the latter perspective, for instance, discrimination frequently results from perceptions of an obvious disability that yield unfavorable evaluations in a job interview or from questions on employment applications that are used to screen out potential employees on the basis of disability. In fact, the minority group model implies that it is stigma that may be a greater source of employment and other forms of discrimination against people with disabilities than functional impairments.

Historical Background

The major federal statutes designed to combat discrimination against persons with disabilities include section 504 of the Rehabilitation Act of 1973, the Civil Rights Restoration Act of 1988, and the Americans with Disabilities Act (ADA) of 1990. In 1975 Congress also sought to create a system of legal advocacy and appeals to protect the civil rights of children with disabilities by enacting the Developmental Disabilities Assistance and Bill of Rights Act and P.L. 94-142, the Individuals with Disabilities Education Act. Perhaps in part due to a general feeling of paternalism toward individuals with disabilities, these antidiscrimination measures have never been effectively enforced or administered (Percy, 1989). Congress has consistently failed to appropriate the funds necessary to implement P.L. 94-142 (Levine & Wexler, 1981; Lipsky & Gartner, 1989). Section 504 was added to the Rehabilitation

Act of 1973 only at the last moment by congressional staffers who copied the language of the provision from an earlier civil rights statute (Scotch, 1984). More important, the administrative regulations to enforce this section were not signed until 1977 after widespread sit-ins at the Department of Health, Education, and Welfare, which marked the birth of the modern disability rights movement.

In the subsequent decade, the leaders of this movement intervened in many issues, including appeals to prevent efforts to terminate the lives of adults as well as infants with disabilities in so-called Baby Doe and right-to-die cases. In actions that seemed reminiscent of the struggle over public buses in the civil rights movement of the 1960s, ADAPT (which was then an acronym for Americans Disabled for Accessible Public Transportation) staged a series of demonstrations at the annual meetings of the American Public Transit Association to protest the organization's refusal to support accessible public vehicles for passengers with disabilities. The guarantee of equal access to public accommodations and transportation, even after a twenty-year delay, was eventually included in the Americans with Disabilities Act. The ADA was adopted largely as the result of efforts by activists—without the support of a powerful national organization, professional lobbyists, contributions from political action committees, or a cohesive electoral constituency. After the passage of the ADA, ADAPT and other groups of activists turned their attention to the establishment of a national program for attendant services, health care reform, and the reduction of "disincentives" to employment in social welfare programs. Some leaders sought to develop theoretical perspectives based on personal experience with disability in the social sciences, the arts, and the humanities, as well as in professional fields such as law, health care, social work, education, architecture, gerontology, and engineering, through organizations such as the Society for Disability Studies. Many persons with disabilities also attempted to strengthen antidiscrimination laws at the state and local level.

In general, legislative bodies seemingly have been more responsive to the positions of the disability rights movement than the courts. By failing to examine the advantages conferred on people without disabilities by the existing environment, which was designed almost exclusively to fit their needs, judges have apparently confused the meaning of equal treatment with that of special treatment. In *Southeastern Community College* v. *Davis* (1979), the U.S. Supreme Court upheld the exclusion of a hearing impaired student from a nursing curriculum under Section 504 on the grounds that the accommodation of her needs would fundamentally change the nature of the program. What the justices neglected to understand was that, by confining instructional methods to verbal rather than visual modes of communication, the school was in effect granting special treatment to students who lacked a hearing impairment. In *Grove City College* v. *Bell* (1984), the Supreme Court also interpreted the statutory requirement of nondiscrimination in activities receiving federal assistance narrowly, to refer to specific programs, rather than broadly, to include the environmental context within which people with disabilities must operate. As a result, Congress was compelled to pass the Civil Rights Restoration Act to reassert its true legislative intent.

Other Supreme Court decisions have restricted both the statutory and the constitutional basis of claims by people with disabilities for equal rights. In *Alexander* v. *Choate* (1985), the Court rejected the use of Section 504 to invalidate a Tennessee ban on hospitalization with Medicaid support that would have an adverse effect on persons with disabilities. Although the justices implied that an analysis of disparate treatment could be applied in some circumstances involving bias against persons with disabilities, they declined to accept evidence of a prejudicial or disparate intent to discriminate against this minority.

Similar perspectives appeared to shape the Court's conclusion in the controversy about whether persons with disabilities should be considered a "suspect class" within the meaning of the "equal protection" clause of the Fourteenth Amendment to the U.S. Constitution. In *San Antonio Independent School District* v. *Rodriguez* (1973), the Court had defined a "suspect class," which requires the "strict scrutiny" of laws that treat them differently than the dominant majority, as a group "saddled with disabilities, or subjected to such a history of purposeful unequal treatment, relegated to such a position of political powerlessness as to command extraordinary protection from the majoritarian political process." Yet, in an opinion permeated by greater concern about the competence of persons with mental retardation than about the stigma they have endured, the Court, in *City of Cleburne* v. *Cleburne Living Center* (1985), refused to apply the literal meaning of its own words to this group, and these people were not regarded as a "suspect class." Instead, the justices relied on the relatively flimsy standard of "reasonableness" to declare unconstitutional a municipal ordinance forbidding group homes in residential neighborhoods. Since most civil rights advocates are reluctant to pursue litigation that would require them to draw invidious distinctions between mental retardation and other forms of disability, legal interest has shifted from constitutional arguments to the statutory interpretation of the Americans with Disabilities Act.

Perhaps the most critical provisions of the ADA are the requirements that employers provide "reasonable accommodation" for workers with disabilities unless doing so would impose an "undue hardship" on the firm. Furthermore, as a basis for interpreting "reasonable accommodation," it has been proposed that judges adopt a standard of equality of environmental adaptations requiring an analysis of the advantages, ordinarily taken for granted, that are bestowed on employees without disabilities by the existing environment. To cite only one example, furnishing chairs for people without disabilities might be considered equivalent to building ramps for persons who use wheelchairs. The objective of equal environmental adaptations is to achieve parity in the opportunities available to all personnel.

Future Outlook

The growing emphasis on equality and freedom for citizens with disabilities has illuminated critical questions about the link between efforts to improve the status of this minority group through both the delivery of social services and the provision of civil rights. Both strategies, of course, fundamentally seek to empower people with disabilities. Jane West (1991) has suggested, "The ADA is an orienting framework that can be used to construct a comprehensive service-delivery system." Yet to fulfill this goal, service providers need to enter into a new kind of cooperative and equal relationship with clients. At a minimum, the educational curricula for rehabilitation and other health professionals must be revised to include material on historic values that support basic principles of civil rights, political influences that have shaped disability policy, and diverse theoretical approaches to the study of disability as well as the lived experience of members of this minority group. They also need to realize that, for their clients, having a disability may offer both an unusual chance to become involved in a historic movement to extend the concept of civil rights and a different perspective that can provide a unique opportunity to explore aspects of life in human habitats that are ordinarily taken for granted. This different perspective constitutes a valuable creative capacity that might contribute economic or social rewards; such creativity can also become a meaningful source of empowerment. Women and men with disabilities can acquire purpose and meaning in their lives by playing a role in expanding the concept of civil rights in the future.

Many people with disabilities still have not gained equal rights in numerous areas of their lives. Persons who use wheelchairs, for example, are denied freedom of movement in their own neighborhoods by the absence of curb cuts at many corners and by omnipresent steps that prevent them even from visiting the homes of their friends. Similarly, anyone with a vision or hearing impairment who must rely exclusively on printed or verbal modes of communication cannot be said to enjoy unrestricted freedom of speech. Arbitrary work schedules might result in employment discrimination against people who endure the periodic intervals of exacerbation and remission of chronic arthritis, which is the main "cause" of limitations on major life activities in the United States (Pope & Tarlov, 1991). The bodily contortions required to enter a motor vehicle or use a hotel bathtub may deprive an aging person with low back pain of equal opportunities at work or in public accommodations. Every facet of the built environment has been designed for *someone*; the problem is that they have been adapted exclusively to suit the demands of the able-bodied majority in a manner that precludes people with disabilities from exercising their rights as citizens of a democratic society. More significantly, these environmental barriers often are a thinly veiled means of avoiding deeper emotions about the "other," including even those with seemingly minor impairments, who evoke either an annoying sense of uneasiness and discomfort or a troubling anxiety about the physical appearance and attractiveness of the observer. As a result, an estimated 36 million to 50 million people with discernible impairments might be expected to benefit from efforts by the disability rights movement to promote a firm definition of equal rights for persons with disabilities.

There are many ways in which people without disabilities can support these endeavors. An especially crucial role for rehabilitation professionals might entail programs to monitor enforcement of the ADA both to assist in filing complaints against recalcitrant employers and to publicize businesses that compile favorable records of compliance. Civil suits against firms that engage in particularly egregious practices of discrimination also could have a salutary remedial effect. Perhaps the most significant results of the continual pursuit of equal rights for citizens with disabilities, however, might be realized through the educational benefits of teaching all people to appreciate human differences and to value the rich diversity of a heterogeneous society.

(See also: ACCESSIBILITY; AMERICANS WITH DISABILITIES ACT; ARCHITECTURAL ACCESSIBILITY; CONSUMERS; DISABILITY LAW AND SOCIAL POLICY; HISTORY OF REHABILITATION; REASONABLE ACCOMMODATION)

RESOURCE

Disability Rights Education and Defense Fund (DREDF), 2212 Sixth St., Berkeley, CA 94710

BIBLIOGRAPHY

Alexander v. Choate, 469 U.S. 287 (1985).

BARKER, ROGER G.; WRIGHT, BEATRICE A.; MEYERSON, LEE; and GONICK, MOLLY R. *Adjustments to Physical Handicap and Illness: A Survey of the Social Psychology of Physical and Disability.* New York, 1953.

BOWE, FRANK. *Handicapping America: Barriers to Disabled People.* New York, 1978.

City of Cleburne v. Cleburne Living Center, 473 U.S. 432 (1985).

GLIEDMAN, JOHN, and ROTH, WILLIAM. *The Unexpected Minority: Handicapped Children in America.* New York, 1980.

Grove City College v. Bell, 465 U.S. 555 (1984).

HAHN, HARLAN. "Disability and Rehabilitation Policy: Is Paternalistic Neglect Really Benign?" *Public Administration Review* 43 (1982):385–389.

———. *The Issue of Equality: European Perceptions of Employment Policy for Disabled Persons.* New York, 1984.

———. "Changing Perceptions of Disability and the Future of Rehabilitation." In *Societal Influences in Rehabilitation Planning: A Blueprint for the Twenty-first Century,* eds. Leonard G. Perlman and Gary F. Austin. Alexandria, VA, 1985.

———. "Public Policy and Disabled Infants: A Socio-Political Perspective." *Issues in Law and Medicine* 3 (1987b):3–27.

———. "Can Disability Be Beautiful?" *Social Policy* 18 (1988):26–32.

———. "Theories and Values: Ethics and Contrasting Perspectives on Disability." In *The Psychological and Social Impact of Disability,* 3rd ed., eds. Robert P. Marinelli and Arthur E. Dell Orto. New York, 1991b.

LEVINE, ERWIN L., and WEXLER, ELIZABETH M. *P.L. 94-142: An Act of Congress.* New York, 1981.

LIPSKY, DOROTHY KERZNER, and GARTNER, ALAN, eds. *Beyond Separate Education: Quality Education for All.* Baltimore, MD, 1989.

PERCY, STEPHEN L. *Disability, Civil Rights, and Public Policy: The Politics of Implementation.* Tuscaloosa, AL, 1989.

POPE, ANDREW M., and TARLOV, ALVIN R., eds. *Disability in America: Toward a National Agenda for Prevention.* Washington, DC, 1991.

San Antonio Independent School District v. Rodriguez, 411 U.S. 1 (1973).

SCOTCH, RICHARD K. *From Good Will to Civil Rights: Transforming Federal Disability Policy.* Philadelphia, 1984.

Southeastern Community College v. Davis, 442 U.S. 397 (1979).

WEST, JANE. "The Social and Policy Context of the Act." In *The Americans with Disabilities Act: From Policy to Practice,* ed. Jane West. New York, 1991.

HARLAN HAHN

CLINICAL SUPERVISION

Administrative and clinical supervision of personnel represents a critical aspect in assuring that effective rehabilitation services are provided to persons with disabilities. Administrative supervision generally refers to those activities that increase efficiency of agency services including planning, organizing, and evaluating personnel, clients, nonhuman resources, and the work environment (Haimann & Hilgert, 1977). Activities within this domain include fiscal and production management, program planning and evaluation, public relations, marketing, labor relations, purchasing, and research (Matkin et al., 1982). In contrast, clinical supervision addresses professional management of direct service personnel to develop supervisees' personal/professional growth (Emener, 1978). In clinical supervision, the important "meta-question" for the supervisor is: "What change does the supervisor need to make so that the supervisee can facilitate subsequent client change?" (Williams, 1988).

Although clinical supervision has been touted as an element crucial to professional skill development (Bernard & Goodyear, 1992), it is a process that has been generally ignored in the rehabilitation literature. Of the available information, a prevailing theme outlines why supervision is important to professional competence and/or suggests how to facilitate the supervision process. These writings can be found in general (Butts & Witmer, 1992) and psychiatric nursing (Hughes, 1985), occupational (Booy & Lawson, 1986), physical (Scully & Shepard, 1983), and recreational therapy (Austin, 1986), rehabilitation counseling (Atkins, 1981), psychology (Worthington & Roehlke, 1979), medicine (Gjerde & Coble, 1982), social work (Eisikovits & Guttman, 1983), speech pathology (Anderson, 1988), and multidisciplinary treatment approaches within comprehensive rehabilitation settings (Stutts, 1991). They indicate that although supervision is a pervasive topic that cuts across rehabilitation and related disciplines, at the same time very little is known with respect to the conduct of supervision. This status has resulted in a very fragmented picture, and as a consequence, supervision research and practice have not advanced within the various rehabilitation professions. This entry examines existing supervision literature among rehabilitation disciplines to identify what aspects constitute effective supervision; outlines the goals, methods, and processes found in effective clinical supervision within generic and discipline-specific domains; and

identifies current controversies within the supervision field.

Definition, Goals, and Methods of Clinical Supervision

Janine M. Bernard and Rodney K. Goodyear (1992) developed a definition of clinical supervision that seems applicable to all rehabilitation professionals. According to these authors, supervision involves a relationship between a senior and a junior member within the same profession whereby the senior member evaluates the professional functioning of the junior member, monitors the quality of services provided to clients he or she interacts with, and serves as a gatekeeper for those persons seeking to enter the profession. Within this definition, a number of clinical supervision goals have been chronicled in the literature, including enhancing client treatment (Gruver & Austin, 1990); expanding therapist knowledge; assisting in developing clinical proficiency, autonomy, and self-esteem as a professional (Platt-Koch, 1986); promoting self-awareness and motivation of clinician behavior and developing personal endowments (Hughes, 1985); enhancing greater sensitivity of oneself and client behavior and integrating theory with clinical process (Critchley, 1987); generating positive attitudes about self and work (Graham, 1981); facilitating program effectiveness (Jaffe & Epstein, 1992); and/or developing therapeutic competence in another person (Loganbill, Hardy, and Delworth, 1982). To accomplish these goals, clinical supervisors use a variety of methods such as case review, audiotapes and videotapes of client/supervisee interaction, live observation of supervisor, supervisee or other supervisees performing clinical duties, or supervisor and supervisee simultaneously providing clinical services to clients.

Although each method can be used in either individual or group supervision settings, individual supervision has been the prevailing method among counseling professionals (Bernard & Goodyear, 1992). Despite clinical reports that group supervision offers greater input from several sources, which enhances learning (Sansbury, 1982), reduces trainee dependence (Getzel & Salmon, 1985), and offers opportunities for supervisees to challenge and support one another (Kadushin, 1992), there is little research to support its efficacy over individual supervision (Holloway & Johnston, 1985).

Several articles have provided specific suggestions when using such supervision methods to facilitate clinical competence. For example, Carol Loganbill and Cal D. Stoltenberg (1983) suggest that case review methods would be more productive in conveying information and problem-solving if a structured format were used. This format could include client demographic information; presenting problems and previous interventions to address problems; client interpersonal style; environmental stressors and support; behavioral, cognitive, and emotional client factors; counselor perception of client problems; and treatment plan. Although medically trained personnel such as nurses and physical and occupational therapists might focus on these as well as physical functioning parameters, the primary intent of case review is to assist supervisees in developing an action plan based on relevant client information. The case review method, although a primary method in delivering supervision (Herbert & Ward, 1989), has been criticized because trainee self-reports tend to be unreliable due to forgetting information (Stoltenberg & Delworth, 1987) or conscious attempts to present oneself in the most favorable light (Borders & Leddick, 1987). Further, without systematic supervisor input, supervisee self-perception and behavior will not change (Worthington, 1987). As a result, discrepancies occur between supervisee and supervisor concerning client problems, motivation for treatment, and prognosis (Biggs, 1988).

To obtain a more accurate indication of supervisee and client interaction, use of audio and video recordings has become a popular method to allow supervisors to highlight segments that were most and least productive, identify potential problem areas or confusing segments, and focus on supervisee/client dynamics (Bernard & Goodyear, 1992). Use of videotape over audiotape in clinical supervision may depend on a number of considerations such as costs to purchase and maintain equipment, client or supervisee preference, or confidentiality issues. For supervisors who rely on audiotaping, David Hurt and Robert Mattox (1990) suggest using a dual-cassette recorder so that the supervisor can listen to the su-

pervisee/client session and, when appropriate, insert supervisory comments on the second tape when needed. In this way the supervisee maintains the original recorded session on one tape plus the recorded session with supervisor comments on the other tape.

Videotaping or audiotaping requires additional time for both supervisee and supervisor. Although these methods are believed to enhance professional competency, it is surprising to find little empirical study as to whether such technology actually aids in supervisee development. Instead, the literature simply indicates that these methods are helpful. An exception was a study by Phillip B. Palmer, Jill N. Henry, and David A. Rohe (1985), who examined physical therapy students' accuracy and quality of self-evaluations of manual muscle testing and goniometry skills. It was found that videotaped feedback did not enhance self-assessment when evaluation immediately followed performance of a skill. The authors concluded that using less costly and time-consuming procedures may be better in providing supervisee feedback. It should be noted that this study did not evaluate supervisor-supervisee interaction. As a result, self-assessment even with videotape may not be as effective when supervisor input is absent. Similarly, research by Susan Bazyk and John Jezwrowsk (1989) found that occupational therapy students prefer live instruction over videotape because of the interaction benefits.

Another strategy to enhance clinical competence is to use role-playing, which provides opportunities for supervisees to experience client issues as well as clarify supervisee thoughts or feelings about the helping process (Byrd, Lesnik, and Byrd, 1981). To facilitate clinical insight, Anthony J. Williams (1988) advocates that supervisees visualize client qualities that exist symbolically or verbally and consider various client roles. DiAnne Borders (1991) also uses role playing, but within a group supervision context. In her structured group approach, Borders assigns various supervisees different alter egos that may exist for both client and clinician. The supervisor's role is to serve as moderator and process commentator of any group dynamics that may arise.

In contrast to delayed supervision models that use audiotape, role playing, or structured group interaction, live observation offers supervisors an opportunity to observe supervisee/client interaction directly. Similarly, live supervision also allows for observation plus an opportunity for supervisors to intervene during supervisee/client interaction. This model enables the supervisor to communicate and thus influence supervisee behavior. Supervisory interaction may occur using "bug in the ear," *in vivo* supervision in the presence of client or clients, telephone, consultation breaks, and written message formats (Bernard & Goodyear, 1992). Live supervision techniques have been touted as offering great potential for increasing counselor trainee professional growth, reducing anxiety, enhancing learning and accountability, and maximizing the value of supervision (Reynolds & McWhirter, 1984). Despite these perceived benefits, such approaches are often avoided in preprofessional (Herbert & Ward, 1989) and professional rehabilitation counseling practice (English, Oberle, and Byrne, 1979). With respect to preprofessional training of rehabilitation counselors, there seems to be strong opposition to live supervision among practica supervisees by both supervisors (Herbert & Ward, 1989) and supervisees (Herbert, Hemlick, and Ward, 1991). This opposition rests in the belief that such methods increase supervisee anxiety and interfere with the supervisee-client relationship. With the exception of the family therapy literature (McKenzie et al., 1986; Roberts, 1983), it is not known whether these same perceptions exist in preprofessional training of allied rehabilitation health professionals. Unlike counselor training, however, live supervision seems to be a primary method in occupational therapy (American Occupational Therapy Association, 1991), physical therapy (American Physical Therapy Association, 1993), as well as in the nursing profession (Butterworth & Faugier, 1992; Jaffe & Epstein, 1992).

All of the aforementioned methods in ascertaining clinical competence have relied on supervisor and supervisee perceptions. Other information sources, however, such as peers and rehabilitation clients, may prove valuable in evaluating clinical competence. For instance, Barney E. Dale and Andrew A. McDonald (1982) contend that while supervisors have intimate knowledge of clinician performance, the authority and power associated with this position can interfere with the supervision process. One method to reduce the negative effects would be to use other information sources, such as rehabilitation clients and other colleagues, to evaluate clinical competence. Client appraisal has the benefit of being the least expensive in terms of staff time and resources, but this process may also be biased because of client preferences that may not be germane to required job tasks. By contrast, colleague input or peer supervision has the benefit that people who provide clinical input also know the job requirements of the person being evaluated. Additional benefits described in the literature suggest that peer supervision improves accountability, maintains ethical behavior and conduct, provides a forum for reexamination of familiar experiences (Schreiber & Frank, 1983), and reduces isolation and professional burnout (Bernard & Goodyear, 1992). If the peer supervision method is adopted, Pamela Schreiber and Elaine Frank say that peers should come not only from a variety of theoretical orientations and areas of expertise but should have similar years of clinical experience and educational training. Peer supervision then promotes professional development and can prove an effective supervision method in cases where traditional supervisory dyads are often unavailable or inappropriate for experienced clinicians (Bernard & Goodyear, 1992). Given the complexities of work environments; professionals' roles and functions; and diversity of clientele, staff, and supervisors, perhaps the best appraisal system to evaluate clinical competence requires a variety of supervision methods (Dale & McDonald, 1982).

Supervision Assessment. Assessment of the supervision process often involves using some combination of standardized/unstandardized, formal/informal methods to provide supervisory feedback. Examples of these instruments can be found in counseling (Efstation, Patton, and Kardash, 1990; Lanning, 1986; Worthington & Roehlke, 1979), occupational therapy (Brown et al., 1989), speech-language pathology (Sleight, 1990), and nursing professions (Kent & Larson, 1983; Stalker et al., 1986). Typically these assessments measure supervisee clinical competence and professional attitudes and behaviors as evaluated by the supervisor. Whether rating scales, competency-based questionnaires, or narrative formats are used to assess the supervision process, a major problem with many of these assessment instruments is that they have little psychometric support. In most cases, assessment instruments used in rehabilitation supervision have not undergone serious empirical validation as to what they purport to measure or how consistently they measure the supervision domains of interest. In addition, as with any rating scales, there is the question of evaluator bias. In the absence of other sources of input, reliance on a single measure to evaluate supervisee performance might be seriously questioned.

Another important assessment theme concerns whether supervisee evaluation of the supervision process should be undertaken. Most supervision assessment instruments are from the supervisor perspective. To what extent supervisees reciprocate evaluation of their supervisors concerning the nature of supervision is, in large part, left to the discretion of the supervisor. It would seem that if supervisors are concerned with improving the supervisory process, it is incumbent that some form of analysis occur without fear of recrimination by the supervisor. Such assessment must, however, recognize the obvious power differential in supervision. After all, the supervisor may assign the grade, recommend whether continuation in one's professional program is warranted, or provide an assessment that will determine merit salary increase or promotion.

Characteristics of Effective Supervision. The literature on performance appraisal suggests that in many instances evaluation can be an emotionally charged, ineffective experience (Dale & McDonald, 1982). To facilitate clinical supervision, Chris Graham (1981) outlines a five-step process that could be applied to the supervision process regardless of professional discipline.

The first step includes an orientation where supervisor and supervisee understand the essential criteria against which performance is to be evaluated and recognize the anxiety associated with conducting an appraisal. Observation, the next step, requires active assessment of the behavior to be observed and under what situations. Observations may require using a variety of recording methods, such as outcome, event, interval, or time-sampling (cf. Miller, 1980).

Next, supervisor and self-evaluation are used to heighten self-understanding, insight, and behavior change needed to develop clinical competence. It is critical during this stage that appraisal from both

perspectives be conducted; otherwise supervision is severely compromised. The fourth step involves a final evaluation conference to review accomplishment and improvement needs. Chris Graham contends that "Motivation is often considered the primary function of a supervisor and yet the hardest to accomplish" (p. 175). This summary review is intended to enhance supervisee motivation.

The fifth and final step, individual development plan, parallels the same kind of plans that rehabilitation professionals implement when working with people with disabilities. This plan is intended to outline specific objectives to improve competency as well as to outline contingencies for accomplishment. The plan outlines target dates, expected outcomes, contingencies, monitoring procedures, and resources. For performance appraisals to be effective, both supervisee and supervisor must be involved in setting mutually agreed-upon supervisory goals, and the supervisor must be perceived as being helpful and willing to provide solutions to job problems (Burke & Wilcox, 1963). If these guidelines are not followed, it is likely that performance appraisal will remain an anxiety-laden experience that does not contribute to improving clinical competence. It is also important to recognize that, as supervisors, rehabilitation personnel must serve as models for their supervisees. Such modeling represents the most important influence on professional development of those being supervised (Stephens & Emener, 1988).

Nancy Webb (1983) proposes a number of guidelines that she believes constitute competent clinical supervision. Although her article was directed toward social work supervisors, these guidelines seem applicable to all clinical supervisors. Accordingly, effective supervisors are people who encourage maximum input from supervisee regarding the content of supervision; respect supervisee judgment concerning priority issues and topics for supervision; encourage supervisee self-evaluation; reinforce learning progress; encourage thoughtful case planning; promote consideration of alternative strategies; expect and welcome questions; avoid giving ready answers; tolerate some silence; permit and encourage disagreement; periodically ask for feedback; promote synthesis and integration of learning; stress commitment to lifelong learning and development; respect supervisee input regarding his or her own learning needs; and recognize and support the supervisee's commitment to professional values. Webb describes applications and accompanying rationale for each goal that may be of interest to readers who desire further information.

Supervision Within Various Rehabilitation Professions

A review of generic counseling and psychology literature suggests that effective supervisors are characterized by counselor-facilitator roles (James, 1973); teacher, therapist, and consultant roles (Bernard, 1979); or scholar/teacher, teacher, master therapist, consultant, evaluator, and therapist roles (Hess, 1980). Although these roles will vary according to one's supervisory style and counseling orientation (Williams, 1988), they are all designed to assist supervisees to explore and understand client problems, make clinical judgments, and develop treatment plans (Biggs, 1988) so that trainees become effective counselors (Worthington & Roehlke, 1979).

Rehabilitation Counseling Personnel. Within the rehabilitation counselor literature a number of qualities have been outlined that characterize effective supervisors, including those who encourage independent thought (Bozarth & Emener, 1981); demonstrate qualities such as concern for others, decisiveness, efficiency, flexibility, leadership, and personal honesty (English, Oberle, and Byrne, 1979); appreciate and embody qualities of a high-functioning counselor and continually improve his or her knowledge, skills, and expertise in helping counselors learn and grow (Emener, 1978); and/or serve as a technical expert and trainer (Luck, 1978). Further empirical support for these guidelines was identified by William English, Judson Oberle, and Andrew Byrne (1979), who found that rehabilitation counselors indicated the five highest rated characteristics necessary to be a successful supervisor were personal honesty, flexibility, concern for others, concern for state regulations, and decisiveness. Almost ten years later, Carolyn Tucker and colleagues (1988) found similar results when they asked what characteristics constituted effective supervision. Supervisor qualities that were most important to supervisees were availability for guidance and

direction; knowledge of policies, procedures, and regulations; demonstration of good decision-making/problem-solving skills; responsibility and dependability; having good listening skills, high ethical standards, and a sense of fairness; and relating well to others and building a cooperative team. Even though these characteristics are important in evaluating effective rehabilitation supervision, what is not known is whether supervisors actually demonstrate such behaviors, knowledge, or skills. Earlier research by William English and colleagues indicates that "first-line" vocational rehabilitation supervisors do a poor job in counselor consultation and counselor evaluation. In fact, the large majority of state vocational rehabilitation counselors rate the quality of supervisors' case consultation in job placement and development, time management, personal adjustment, and vocational counseling as being "poor" or "fair." Perhaps if effective supervision can be instituted within the state vocational rehabilitation program, it may reduce the number of counselors who quit, are fired, or are counseled out of the agency. Staff turnover rates in excess of 11 percent in state rehabilitation agencies and 22 percent in private nonprofit rehabilitation facilities have been partially attributed to perceptual differences between supervisor and counselor (Crimando, Hansen, and Riggar, 1986; Crimando, Riggar, and Hansen, 1986). Although state agency supervisors express a clear need for inservice training that addresses supervision skills of vocational rehabilitation counselors (Markin et al., 1982), many rehabilitation counselor educators believe that the only viable way to provide rehabilitation counselor supervisors with all of the administrative and clinical training necessary to be effective supervisors is through long-term education (Beardsley, Riggar, and Hafer, 1984; English et al., 1979).

Other Vocational Rehabilitation Personnel. A review of the professional journals associated with job placement, vocational evaluation, work adjustment, and vocational rehabilitation reveals that clinical supervision is a topic that has not been addressed. Although no direct references could be found in the professional literature, there have been related references with respect to administration priority needs of vocational rehabilitation personnel (Botterbusch, 1988), training needs of job coaches (Johnson,

Kelley, and Wilson, 1990), rehabilitation facility production staff (Smith & Bordieri, 1988), and vocational evaluators (Sankovsky, Brolin, and Coffey, 1977). These surveys reveal that vocational evaluators could benefit from further training and supervision in multicultural aspects, learning styles, vocational evaluation of persons with severe disabilities (Eldredge, Fried, and Grissom, 1991), report writing (Bordieri & Crimando, 1990), community resources, job market information, and improving client interpersonal relations (Sankovsky, Brolin, and Coffey, 1977). Training needs for rehabilitation facility staff reveal that further skill development is needed in job coaching, transitional employment, and supported work (Botterbusch, 1988). Production staff who work in rehabilitation facilities report that training in quality control, safety/first aid, client motivation and program planning, behavior modification, and communication skills represent the most important inservice training needs (Smith & Bordieri, 1988). Finally, deficits in applied behavior analysis, interagency coordination, and job replacement were noted regarding training needs for job coaches (Johnson, Kelley, and Wilson, 1990).

These training needs may offer insight as to potential problem areas for professionals who supervise these personnel. Although there are certainly unique aspects for various vocational rehabilitation personnel, research by Michael J. Leahy, Pamela B. Shapson, and George N. Wright (1987) and by Michael J. Leahy and George N. Wright (1988) found significant overlap with respect to competency areas shared by rehabilitation counselors, vocational evaluators, and job placement specialists. In fact, Leahy and Wright found that 90 percent of professional competency areas were shared by rehabilitation counselors and placement specialists, while 50 percent of competencies were similarly shared between counselors and vocational evaluators. Their study revealed that vocational counseling, assessment planning and interpretation, personal adjustment counseling, case management, and job analysis were competencies that these three professional groups shared. Rehabilitation counselors and job placement specialists also indicated that job placement, consultation, group and behavioral techniques, and professional and community involvement were important competency areas. Although

this review provides an indication of the variety of training needs, it does not provide any information concerning supervisory practices. For now, supervisors who practice in these areas are not afforded information to assist them in providing effective supervision. At best they must rely on information found in the rehabilitation counseling and generic counseling literature and apply such to their own practice.

Medically Related Personnel. Butterworth and Faugier (1992) report that clinical supervision of psychiatric or general nursing is a topic that has received very little attention. According to these authors, what literature is available is more related to implementing professional standards than how to facilitate clinical supervision and, in instances where clinical supervision is provided, it is generally viewed as a negative experience, the primary reason being that supervision interaction has been traditionally associated with disciplinary dealings between nursing managers and their staff. Given these circumstances, clinical supervision is perceived as an "emerging idea" in nursing. Further, it also appears that clinical supervision will not evolve until it is clear which nursing professional is assigned clinical supervision duties—that is, the head nurse, clinical specialist, or other nurse practitioner (Wallace & Corey, 1983). Although the job title of clinical specialist may infer designation of clinical supervision, the problems associated with this title include role ambiguity, lack of administrative support and authority to carry out clinical functions, and resistance from staff nurses (Harrell & McCulloch, 1986). Until nurses view supervisors in a less authoritarian way and consider clinical supervision as a critical task to assure professional development and quality patient care, it is not likely that clinical supervision will evolve (Hill, 1989).

With regard to preprofessional nursing training, Mary Haack (1988) reported that students experience increased stress and burnout as clinical training proceeds. Perhaps, as Phyllis Brust (1986) contends, a number of predisposing factors contribute to stress, such as not knowing clinical supervisor expectations or not receiving appropriate and timely feedback regarding clinical performance. Similar trends have also been reported in occupational and physical therapy preprofessional training. In fact, a major

184

complaint of clinical training has to do with unsatisfactory supervisory relationships (Christie, Joyce, & Moeller, 1985; Walish, Schuit, & Olson, 1986). Unfortunately, supervisors continue to receive little formal training in how to conduct effective clinical supervision (Yuen, 1990).

Development of clinical competencies among preprofessional students depends on educational training models. Within medically related professions, students are exposed to concurrent (portions of university-based and clinical work occur simultaneously), nonconcurrent (full-time education followed by full-time clinical work), or combination models (interspersing concurrent and nonconcurrent patterns throughout the curriculum). Although such preprofessional training varies within each discipline and across educational institutions and training facilities, each model presents unique challenges when providing clinical supervision. A study by Jane Walish, Dale Schuit, and Ronald Olson (1986) that investigated a concurrent training model found that physical therapy students reported greater skill development and confidence in supervisory and professional interactions at the end of the clinical training period. On the negative side, students also reported greater frustration at being unable to assist certain patients at the end of the initial clinical training period as opposed to when they first began training. This study supports the belief that before the initial clinical assignment, student trainees are concerned most about interactions with their clinical supervisor. Because of this perception, clinical supervisors need to be sensitive to which behaviors are most helpful in facilitating clinical competence. A subsequent study by Robert Jarski, Kornelia Kulig, and Ronald Olson (1990) revealed that effective teaching behaviors as perceived by physical therapy supervisees were characterized by interactions that encouraged feedback, discussion, and answering supervisee concerns. Interpersonal behaviors including approachability, enthusiasm, and sensitivity to patient needs were also important. In contrast, the most negative supervisor behaviors were those that students perceived as threatening (e.g., questioning supervisee in an intimidating manner or correcting supervisee in front of patient) and not fulfilling supervisory obligations (e.g., failing to adhere to schedule, unavailability for consultation). The authors concluded that facilitating a positive learning relationship was more a function of supervisor interpersonal relationships than technical knowledge. The importance of supervisors who provide a supportive learning environment, as shown in this study as well as others (e.g., Burnett and colleagues, 1986; Walish, Schuit, and Olson, 1986), will have a significant impact on emerging professionals' attitudes toward lifelong learning (Deusinger, Sindelar, and Stritter, 1986).

Recreation/Leisure Personnel. The literature concerning clinical supervision as applicable to therapeutic recreation is quite sparse. Bonita Gruver and David Austin (1990) found only one article with respect to supervision and concluded that therapeutic recreation was "far behind other health professions in developing a practice of clinical supervision." Their national survey of therapeutic recreation curricula revealed that although most faculty believed it was essential to provide undergraduates and graduates with integrated clinical supervision instruction, fewer than one half of university programs had incorporated this area into their curriculum.

Controversies Within Supervision Practice

A fundamental controversy concerns the question "Why has there been a noticeable lack of information concerning the practice of clinical supervision?" As noted in this entry, most supervision articles could be described as opinion or observations from the field as to how to conduct supervision. There is an obvious lack of empirical study. However, rehabilitation professionals have started to inquire about the nature and conduct of supervision within their respective fields. As a result, clinical supervisors have to rely on the information found in the counseling supervision literature and apply this knowledge to their own profession. To what extent such information pertains to medically oriented professions such as nursing and occupational, physical, and speech therapy remains unknown. If the situation in these professions parallels that indicated in the rehabilitation counseling supervision literature, then clinical supervision is the most important component of preprofessional training (Scofield & Scofield, 1978), which serves as the critical transition to employment (Atkins, 1981). Despite this perceived importance, there is an obvious void among rhetoric, research, and practice (Herbert & Ward, 1990).

In answering the aforementioned question, the lack of empirical work seems attributable to several influences. First, professionals may subscribe to the myth that "If one is a good clinician, then one will also be a good supervisor." This myth, as noted by Patricia McCarthy and colleagues (1988), fails to recognize that supervision constitutes a set of knowledge and skills that are unique and not similar to those required as a practitioner. Second, as noted by McCarthy and colleagues, the limited supervision research does not provide any clear theoretical base that addresses how supervision skills are acquired. In addition, there is a perception that supervision training is not necessary and, as a result, does not represent a high priority in professional training programs. This criticism seems particularly applicable to master's degree programs that are designed to train practitioners but fail to realize that these individuals eventually go on to assume supervisory positions. Given that most rehabilitation administrators and clinical supervisors are secured from the practitioner ranks with little or no management training and experience (Matkin et al., 1982; Stephens & Emener, 1988), this predicament results in supervisors who are not prepared to deliver clinical supervision. For those who would argue that on-the-job experience as a supervisor is an acceptable substitute for formal training and professional development, this position, by some accounts, is fallacious (Stephens & Emener, 1988). Third, preservice training at the bachelor's or master's level is already inundated with course content and clinical training requirements, and many educators are not receptive to any additional requirements (Patterson & Pankowski, 1988). As such, educators assigned to work in preservice programs are more concerned with developing practitioner skills and not management or clinical supervision skills. Even though recommendations for more preservice education in supervision have been called for (Riggar et al., 1988), it seems that the preferred method of field supervisors is to provide post-employment training (Hutchinson, Luck, and Hardy, 1978; Matkin et al., 1982; Menz & Bordieri, 1987). Once offered, it

is incumbent upon supervisors to participate in such training. Otherwise, as James Stephens and William Emener (1988) admonish, supervisors who do not model involvement in learning activities should not be surprised when subordinates show similar disinterest in professional development activities.

These three proposed influences have resulted in rehabilitation professions continuing to provide supervision without serious inquiry as to the nature and process of supervision. As both role and function, supervision has remained unchecked, and therefore there is little empirical evidence that guides practice. If rehabilitation supervision is to advance as a field, then professionals must undertake scientific inquiry and initiate dialogue that will have an effect on practice. Some initial questions that may facilitate dialogue could include the following: What supervision methods and procedures are used in delivering clinical supervision to beginning, advanced, and experienced professionals? Which of these methods are most effective given supervisor and supervisee developmental levels? What is the impact of supervisor/supervisee characteristics such as age, ethnicity, gender, and developmental level on supervision effectiveness? What constructs should be applied in assessing the impact of supervision? What instruments exist to measure supervision impact, and how appropriate are they across disciplines? How should university-based supervision facilitate field-based supervision? In what ways are both training environments similar, and where differences occur, how do these affect supervisee performance? What criteria are used to determine who is qualified to supervise? How can the costs of providing on-site supervision become more cost-effective? How do we train supervisors to achieve minimal competency to supervise? What, if any, considerations should be made in assigning supervisees to supervisors? How has supervision been applied in a harmful manner, and what steps are necessary to prevent such? How should supervisees be prepared to address unethical or unprofessional supervision? How should supervision be addressed within respective professional ethical codes of conduct and accreditation procedures?

Although such questions may, in themselves, not be considered controversial, the answers that follow these questions may lead to controversial dialogue within rehabilitation professions. To date, there has been very limited discussion to guide professional theory and practice of clinical supervision within the rehabilitation process. For the most part, what is known about clinical supervision is confined to pre-professional experience. Information to facilitate supervision of more experienced clinicians is almost nonexistent despite the reality that such professionals provide rehabilitation services. For now, clinical supervision remains much more an art than a science. Although this assessment is not necessarily a negative one, it offers rehabilitation personnel tremendous opportunity to engage in dialogue as to how to facilitate clinical supervision and to assess its impact on supervisee performance and ultimately client service delivery.

(*See also:* ALLIED HEALTH PROFESSIONS; CREDENTIALS)

BIBLIOGRAPHY

AMERICAN OCCUPATIONAL THERAPY ASSOCIATION. "Essentials and Guidelines for an Accredited Educational Program for the Occupational Therapist." *American Journal of Occupational Therapy* 45 (1991):1077–1092.

AMERICAN PHYSICAL THERAPY ASSOCIATION. *Clinical Education Guidelines and Self-Assessments.* Alexandria, VA (1993).

ANDERSON, JEAN. *The Supervisory Process in Speech-Language Pathology and Audiology.* Boston, MA (1988).

ATKINS, BOBBIE J. "Clinical Practice in Master's Level Rehabilitation Counselor Education." *Counselor Education and Supervision* 21 (1981):169–175.

AUSTIN, DAVID R. "Clinical Supervision in Therapeutic Recreation." *Journal of Expanding Horizons in Therapeutic Recreation* 1 (1986):7–13.

BAZYK, SUSAN, and JEZWROWSK, JOHN. "Videotaped versus Live Instruction in Demonstrating Evaluation Skills to Occupational Therapy Students." *American Journal of Occupational Therapy* 43 (1989):465–468.

BEARDSLEY, MARK; RIGGAR, TED F.; and HAFER, MARILYN. "Rehabilitation Supervision: A Case for Counselor Training." *The Clinical Supervisor* 2 (1984):55–63.

BERNARD, JANINE. "Supervision Training: A Discrimination Model." *Counselor Education and Supervision* 19 (1979):60–68.

BERNARD, JANINE M., and GOODYEAR, RODNEY K. *Fundamentals of Clinical Supervision.* Needham Heights, MA, 1992.

BIGGS, DONALD A. "The Case Presentation Approach in Clinical Supervision." *Counselor Education and Supervision* 27 (1988):240–248.

BOOY, M. J., and LAWSON, A. "Bridging the Gap in Clinical Supervision." *Occupational Therapy,* December (1986):382–384.

BORDERS, L. DIANNE. "A Systematic Approach to Peer Group Supervision." *Journal of Counseling and Development* 69 (1991):248–252.

BORDERS, L. DIANNE, and LEDDICK, GEORGE R. *Handbook of Counseling Supervision.* Alexandria, VA, 1987.

BORDIERI, JAMES E., and CRIMANDO, WILLIAM. "Evaluating Vocational Evaluation Reports: Preliminary Findings on the Development of a Critique Form." *Vocational Evaluation and Work Adjustment Bulletin* 23 (1990):79–83.

BOTTERBUSCH, KARL F. "A Survey of Needs in Six Rehabilitation Services Administration Priority Areas in Vocational Rehabilitation Facilities." *Vocational Evaluation and Work Adjustment Bulletin* 21 (1988):15–24.

BOZARTH, JEROME D., and EMENER, WILLIAM G. "A Person-Centered Approach to Administration and Supervision in Rehabilitation." *Rehabilitation Counseling Bulletin* 24 (1981):299–303.

BROWN, SUZANNE; STREETER, LYNN A. C.; STOFFEL, VIRGINIA C.; and MCPHERSON, JAMES J. "Development of a Level I Fieldwork Evaluation." *American Journal of Occupational Therapy* 43 (1989):677–682.

BRUST, PHYLLIS L. "Student Burnout: The Clinical Instructor Can Spot It and Manage It." *Clinical Management in Physical Therapy* 6 (1986):18–21.

BURKE, RONALD J., and WILCOX, DOUGLAS S. "Characteristics of Effective Employee Performance Review and Development Interviews." *Personnel Psychology* 22 (1969):291–305.

BURNETT, CAROLYN N.; MAHONEY, PATRICK J.; CHIDLEY, MARJORIE J.; and PIERSON, FRANK M. "Problem-Solving Approach to Clinical Education." *Physical Therapy* 66 (1986):1730–1733.

BUTTERWORTH, TONY, and FAUGIER, JEAN. *Clinical Supervision and Mentorship in Nursing.* London, Eng., 1992.

BUTTS, BETTY J., and WITMER, DOROTHY M. "New Graduates: What Does My Manager Expect?" *Nursing Management* 23 (1992):46–48.

BYRD, E. KEITH; LESNIK, MICHAEL J.; and BYRD, DIANNE P. "A Role Play Model for Teaching Supervision in Rehabilitation Settings." *Journal of Rehabilitation Administration* 5 (1981):137–141.

CHRISTIE, BARBARA A.; JOYCE, PEGGY C.; and MOELLER, PATRICIA L. "Fieldwork Experience, Part I: Impact on Practice Preference." *American Journal of Occupational Therapy* 39 (1985):671–674.

CRIMANDO, WILLIAM; HANSEN, GERI; and RIGGAR, TED F. "Employee Turnover: The Scope of a State DVR Personnel Problem." *Journal of Rehabilitation Administration* 10 (1986):125–128.

CRIMANDO, WILLIAM; RIGGAR, TED F.; and HANSEN, GERI. "Personnel Turnover: The Plague of Rehabilitation Facilities." *Journal of Applied Rehabilitation Counseling* 17 (1986):17–20.

CRITCHLEY, DEANE L. "Clinical Supervision as a Learning Tool for the Therapist in Milieu Settings." *Journal of Psychosocial Nursing* 25 (1987):18–22.

DALE, BARNEY E., and McDONALD, ANDREW A., SR. "Toward a Comprehensive Philosophy of Personnel Performance Appraisal in Rehabilitation Facilities." *Journal of Rehabilitation Administration* 6 (1982): 80–88.

DEUSINGER, SUSAN S.; SINDELAR, BETTY; and STRITTER, FRANK, T. "Assessment Center: A Model for Professional Development and Evaluation." *Physical Therapy* 66 (1986):1119–1123.

EFSTATION, JAMES F.; PATTON, MICHAEL J.; and KARDASH, CAROLANNE M. "Measuring the Working Alliance in Counselor Supervision." *Journal of Counseling Psychology* 37 (1990):322–329.

EISIKOVITS, ZVI, and GUTTMAN, EDNA. "Toward a Practice Theory of Learning Through Experience in Social Work Supervision." *The Clinical Supervisor* 1 (1983):51–63.

ELDREDGE, GARTH M.; FRIED, JULIET H.; and GRISSOM, JULIE K. "Vocational Evaluator Training Needs: Food for Thought." *Vocational Evaluation and Work Adjustment Bulletin* 24 (1991):11–13.

EMENER, WILLIAM G. "Clinical Supervision in Rehabilitation Settings." *Journal of Rehabilitation Administration* 2 (1978):44–53.

ENGLISH, WILLIAM R.; OBERLE, JUDSON B.; and BYRNE, ANDREW R. "Rehabilitation Counselor Supervision: A National Perspective" [Special Issue]. *Rehabilitation Counseling Bulletin* 22 (1979):7–123.

GETZEL, G. S., and SALMON, R. "Group Supervision: An Organizational Approach." *The Clinical Supervisor* 3 (1985):27–43.

GJERDE, CRAIG L., and COBLE, ROLLO J. "Resident and Faculty Perceptions of Effective Clinical Teaching in Family Practice." *Journal of Family Practice* 14 (1982):323–327.

GRAHAM, CHRIS S. "The Supervisor's Role in the Performance Appraisal Process." *Journal of Rehabilitation Administration* 5 (1981):170–178.

GRUVER, BONITA M., and AUSTIN, DAVID R. "The Instructional Status of Clinical Supervision in Therapeutic Recreation Curricula." *Therapeutic Recreation Journal* 24 (1990):18–24.

HAACK, MARY R. "Stress and Impairment Among Nursing Students." *Research in Nursing and Health* 11 (1988):125–134.

HAIMANN, T., and HILGERT, R. L. *Supervision: Concepts and Practice of Management,* 2nd ed. Cincinnati, 1977.

HARRELL, JOANNE S., and McCULLOCH, SALLY D. "The Role of the Clinical Nurse Specialist: Problems and Solutions." *Journal of Nursing Administration* 16 (1986):44–48.

HERBERT, JAMES T.; HEMLICK, LISA M.; and WARD, THOMAS J. "Supervisee Perception of Rehabilitation Counseling Practica." *Rehabilitation Education* 5 (1991):121–129.

HERBERT, JAMES T., and WARD, THOMAS J. "Rehabilitation Counselor Supervision: A National Survey of NCRE Graduate Training Practica." *Rehabilitation Education* 3 (1989):163–175.

———. "Supervisory Styles Among Rehabilitation Counseling Practica Supervisors." *Rehabilitation Education* 4 (1990):203–212.

HESS, ALLEN K. "Training Models and the Nature of Psychotherapy Supervision." In *Psychotherapy Supervision: Theory, Research and Practice,* ed. A. K. Hess. New York, 1980.

HILL, J. "Supervision in the Caring Professions: A Literature Review." *Community Psychiatric Nursing Journal* 9 (1989):9–15.

HOLLOWAY, ELIZABETH L., and JOHNSTON, REBECCA. "Group Supervision: Widely Practiced, but Poorly Understood." *Counselor Education and Supervision* 24 (1985):332–340.

HUGHES, CYRILLA M. "Supervising Clinical Practice in Psychosocial Nursing." *Journal of Psychosocial Nursing* 23 (1985):27–32.

HURT, DAVID J., and MATTOX, ROBERT J. "Supervision Feedback Using a Dual-Cassette Recorder." *The Clinical Supervisor* 8 (1990):169–172.

HUTCHINSON, J.; LUCK, RICHARD; and HARDY, R. "Training Needs of a Group of Vocational Rehabilitation Administrators." *Journal of Rehabilitation Administration* 2 (1978):156–159; 178.

JAFFE, EVELYN G., and EPSTEIN, CYNTHIA F. *Occupational Therapy Consultation: Theory; Principles; and Practice.* St. Louis, MO, 1992.

JAMES, D. T. "The Supervisor as Counselor-Facilitator." *Journal of Rehabilitation* 39 (1973):18–20, 43.

JARSKI, ROBERT W.; KULIG, KORNELIA; and OLSON, RONALD E. "Clinical Teaching in Physical Therapy: Student and Teacher Perceptions." *Physical Therapy* 70 (1990):173–178.

JOHNSON, KURT L.; KELLEY, SUSAN D. M.; and WILSON, LISA M. "Training Needs of Job Coaches." *Journal of Job Placement* 6 (1990):28–31.

KADUSHIN, ALFRED. *Supervision in Social Work,* 3rd ed. New York, 1992.

KENT, LINDA A., and LARSON, ELAINE. "Evaluating the Effectiveness of Primary Nursing Practice." *Journal of Nursing Administration* 13 (1983):34–41.

LANNING, WAYNE. "Development of the Supervisor Emphasis Rating Form." *Counselor Education and Supervision* 25 (1986):191–196.

LEAHY, MICHAEL J., and WRIGHT, GEORGE N. "Professional Competencies of the Vocational Evaluator." *Vocational Evaluation and Work Adjustment Bulletin* 21 (1988):127–132.

LEAHY, MICHAEL J.; SHAPSON, PAMELA R.; and WRIGHT, GEORGE N. "Rehabilitation Practitioner Competencies by Role and Setting." *Rehabilitation Counseling Bulletin* 31 (1987):119–130.

LOGANBILL, CAROL; HARDY, EMILY; and DELWORTH, URSULA. "Supervision: A Conceptual Model." *The Counseling Psychologist* 10 (1982):3–42.

LOGANBILL, CAROL, and STOLTENBERG, CAL D. "The Case Conceptualization Format: A Training Device for Practicum." *Counselor Education and Supervision* 22 (1983):237–238.

LUCK, RICHARD S. "Rehabilitation Supervisor: Technical Expert and Trainer." *Journal of Rehabilitation Administration* 2 (1978):66, 72.

MATKIN, RALPH E.; SAWYER, HORACE W.; LORENZ, JEROME R.; and RUBIN, STANFORD E. "Rehabilitation Administrators and Supervisors: Their Work Assignments, Training Needs, and Suggestions for Preparation." *Journal of Rehabilitation Administration* 6 (1982):170–183.

MCCARTHY, PATRICIA; DEBELL, CAMILLE; KANUHA, VALLI; and MCLEOD, JEFFREY. "Myths of Supervision: Identifying the Gaps Between Theory and Practice." *Counselor Education and Supervision* 28 (1988):22–28.

MCKENZIE, PAUL; ATKINSON, BRENT; QUINN, WILLIAM; and HEATH, ANTHONY. "Training and Supervision in Marriage and Family Therapy: A National Survey." *American Journal of Family Therapy* 14 (1986):293–303.

MENZ, FREDERICK E., and BORDIERI, JAMES E. "Training Experiences and Perceptions of Rehabilitation Facility Administrators." *Journal of Rehabilitation Administration* 11 (1987):60–67.

MILLER, L. K. *Principles of Everyday Behavior Analysis.* Monterey, CA, 1980.

PALMER, PHILIP B.; HENRY, JILL N.; and ROHE, DAVID A. "Effect of Videotape Replay on the Quality and Accuracy of Student Self-Evaluation." *Physical Therapy* 65 (1985):497–501.

PATTERSON, JEANNE B., and PANKOWSKI, JOSEPH. "Preparing the Consumer of Rehabilitation Administration, Management, and Supervision: Preservice, Inservice, and Continuing Education Issues." *Journal of Rehabilitation Administration* 12 (1988):117–121.

PLATT-KOCH, LOIS M. "Clinical Supervision for Psychiatric Nurses." *Journal of Psychosocial Nursing* 26 (1986):7–15.

REYNOLDS, EMILY, and MCWHIRTER, J. JEFFRIES. "Cotherapy from the Trainee's Standpoint: Suggestions for Supervision." *Counselor Education and Supervision* 12 (1984):205–213.

RIGGAR, TED F.; CRIMANDO, WILLIAM; BORDIERI, JAMES; and PHILLIPS, J. STUART. "Rehabilitation Administration Preservice Education: Preparing the Professional Rehabilitation Administrator, Manager and Supervisor." *Journal of Rehabilitation Administration* 12 (1988):93–102.

ROBERTS, JAMES. "Two Models of Live Supervision: Collaborative Team and Supervisor Guided." *Journal of Strategic and Systemic Therapies* 2 (1983):40–50.

SANKOVSKY, RAY; BROLIN, JAMES; and COFFEY, DARRELL. "Vocational Evaluators Identify Training Needs: Report of a National Survey." *Vocational Evaluation and Work Adjustment Bulletin* 10(1977):15–19.

SANSBURY, DAVID L. "Developmental Supervision from a Skill Perspective." *The Counseling Psychologist* 10 (1982):53–57.

SCHREIBER, PAMELA, and FRANK, ELAINE. "The Use of a Peer Supervision Group by Social Work Clinicians." *The Clinical Supervisor* 1 (1983):29–36.

SCOFIELD, MICHAEL E., and SCOFIELD, B. J. "Ethical Concerns in Clinical Practice Supervision." *Journal of Applied Rehabilitation Counseling* 9 (1978):27–29.

SCULLY, ROSEMARY M., and SHEPARD, KATHERINE F. "Clinical Teaching in Physical Therapy Education: An Ethnographic Study." *Physical Therapy* 63 (1983):349–358.

SLEIGHT, CHRISTINE C. "Off-Campus Supervisor Self-

Evaluation." *The Clinical Supervisor* 8 (1990): 163–173.

SMITH, CHRISTOPHER A., and BORDIERI, JAMES E. "The Provision of Training and Perceived Training Needs of Rehabilitation Facility Production Staff." *Journal of Rehabilitation Administration* 12 (1988): 67–71.

STALKER, MARTHA Z.; KORNBLITH, ALICE B.; LEWIS, PATRICIA M.; and PARKER, ROGER. "Measurement Technology Application in Performance Appraisal." *Journal of Nursing Administration* 16 (1986): 12–17.

STEPHENS, JAMES E., and EMENER, WILLIAM G. "Preparing the Professional Rehabilitation Administrator, Manager and Supervisor: In-Service and Continuing Education Issues and Approaches." *Journal of Rehabilitation Administration* 12 (1988):106–114.

STOLTENBERG, CAL D., and DELWORTH, URSULA. *Supervising Counselors and Therapists.* San Francisco, CA, 1987.

STUTTS, MICHAEL L. "Supervision in Comprehensive Rehabilitation Settings: The Terrain and the Traveler." *The Clinical Supervisor* 9 (1991):33–57.

TUCKER, CAROLYN M.; MCNEILL, PAULINE; ABRAMS, JULIE M.; and BROWN, JAMES G. "Characteristics Important to an Effective Supervisor: Perceptions of Vocational Rehabilitation Staff." *Journal of Rehabilitation Administration* 12 (1988):40–43.

WALISH, JANE F.; OLSON, RONALD E.; and SCHUIT, DALE. "Effects of Concurrent Clinical Education Assignment on Student Concerns." *Physical Therapy* 66 (1986):233–236.

WALISH, JANE F.; SCHUIT, DALE; and OLSON, RONALD E. "Preaffiliation and Postaffiliation Concerns Expressed by Physical Therapy Students." *Physical Therapy* 66 (1986):691–696.

WALLACE, MARY A., and COREY, LINDA J. "The Clinical Specialist as Manager: Myth versus Realities." *Journal of Nursing Administration* 13 (1983):13–15.

WEBB, NANCY B. "Developing Competent Clinical Practitioners: A Model with Guidelines for Supervisors." *The Clinical Supervisor* 1 (1983):41–51.

WILLIAMS, ANTHONY J. "Action Methods in Supervision." *The Clinical Supervisor* 6 (1988):13–27.

WORTHINGTON, EVERETT L., JR. "Changes in Supervision as Counselors and Supervisors Gain Experience: A Review." *Professional Psychology Research and Practice* 18 (1987):189–208.

WORTHINGTON, EVERETT L., JR., and ROEHLKE, HELEN J. "Effective Supervision as Perceived by Beginning Counselors-in-Training." *Journal of Counseling Psychology* 26 (1979):64–73.

YUEN, HON KUENG. "Fieldwork Students Under Stress." *American Journal of Occupational Therapy* 44 (1990):80–81.

JAMES T. HERBERT

CLOTHING

Physical attractiveness affects the perception people have of one another. If a person is perceived to be physically attractive, positive responses are generated. In addition, people who are well groomed and attractively dressed create a positive impression when interacting with others. Clothing can play a part in this process for people with physical or mental disabilities by being both attractive and functional.

Appearance is the image presented to others in social situations and encompasses both the body and clothing. Body variables include body forms (size, shape, and deviations from the norm), body expressions (skin color, hair color and texture, eye color and shape, etc.), and body motions (gait, use of limbs, use of assistive devices, etc.). Variables related to clothing include both physical and symbolic aspects. The physical value of clothing includes protection, freedom of movement, independence in dressing, thermal comfort, and comfort of garment structure. The symbolic value of clothing includes both psychological and sociological aspects. Clothing can be used to indicate a person's values and beliefs, self-esteem and self-worth, adherence to fashion, group affiliation, and status or rank. Therefore clothing portrays what a person thinks about himself or herself and is used as a means of communicating.

Appearance, cost, care, and situational factors such as work, school, and social environments need to be considered when selecting clothing. Cost includes the price of the item in relation to the benefit of the item to the consumer over time. A consumer may be willing to pay more for a classic garment that can be worn for a number of years. Care considerations involve ease of care (the amount of time, energy, and cost required for garment upkeep) and performance (how long the item will last).

Situational factors affect clothing selection decisions; for example, comfort may be a higher priority for active-wear clothing, while fashion may be more important for social encounters. Effective clothing selection and coordination can generate positive responses in both work and social situations. When an individual is physically attractive and appropriately dressed, an employer is more likely to hire that person. Also, a person is judged to be a more competent, sociable, and desirable coworker if he or she is attractively dressed.

Specific clothing designs should be selected that flatter the figure to produce a look that portrays the current fashion. If a person deviates from the current ideal, he or she should emphasize positive attributes. Clothing can be used to draw attention to certain parts of the body by manipulating the proportions of an outfit and emphasizing a selected body part.

Clothing can be designed or adapted to meet the needs of people with physical or mental disabilities. It is important to evaluate the person's functional limitations. Impaired movement may be the limiting factor and often is associated with the use of assistive devices. For example, if a person uses a wheelchair for mobility, his or her body configuration is that of a seated figure. Standard clothing is designed for the body in a standing position; therefore clothing must be redesigned to accommodate the seated figure. Fitting problems occur for men and women and for upper torso and lower torso garments. Upper torso garments need to allow for the slight forward curve of the spine when seated, which elongates the back length and shortens the front length from neck to waist. Garments also need to allow room for shoulder movement; jacket length needs to be shortened to hip level.

Lower torso garments should reflect the contours of an angled figure rather than a straight figure. Standard pants, worn by a person who is seated, have extra fabric in the lap area, not enough fabric at the back waist area or front hemline, and the pockets are difficult to reach. Pants for the seated figure can be cut with a high back and low front waistline, a hemline that is longer in the front than in the back, and pockets placed on the thigh, or in some cases the calf area. Double pockets and pleated pockets with zippered or Velcro closures contribute to a more functional garment. Skirts for the seated figure also require the same waistline and hemline adjustments and should be cut to allow extra fullness in the knee area. This can be achieved by designing a fitted skirt with a horizontal seamline above the knee with pleats, gathers, or flare in the lower part of the skirt to allow for controlled fit through the hipline and for modest coverage of the knees.

Sources of clothing acquisition include standard ready-to-wear, functional ready-to-wear, adapted ready-to-wear, and custom-designed. Functionally designed ready-to-wear clothing can be purchased primarily through mail order. Many of the companies are small, although larger retailers have entered this market. Sears, Roebuck and Company caters to the older consumer in their *HealthCare* catalog. The J. C. Penney *Easy Dressing Fashions and More* catalog features apparel with Velcro fasteners for women and men with dexterity problems. A line of clothing for people who use wheelchairs is carried by Avenues Unlimited and features garments ranging from sportswear to business attire.

Occupational therapists (OTs) and physical therapists (PTs) are interested in the physical needs of persons with disabilities, including clothing. OTs in particular are concerned with teaching activities of daily living that include dressing techniques, clothing comfort, and safety, with an emphasis on independence in dressing. Textiles and clothing educators are concerned with both the creative and functional aspects of clothing for persons with disabilities. Their students are trained to work in apparel design or fashion merchandising and have a working knowledge of the needs of this market segment. Both textile and clothing educators and cooperative extension personnel at the state or county level serve as sources of information about adaptive clothing and resources for functional, fashionable clothing.

The future of this area looks bright because of the passage of the Americans with Disabilities Act (1990). Solutions to many functional design problems were developed in the mid-1950s; however, many potential consumers still are unaware that functional, fashionable clothing designs exist. Because of this limited awareness, consumer demand has not been overwhelming, so many manufacturers and retailers have not entered this market. Consumers and rehabilitation personnel alike need to encourage manufacturers and retailers to meet the needs of this large consumer group. At the retail level, stores will be made more accessible, management will hire some people with disabilities, sales associates will be trained to work with consumers with disabilities, and there will be an increase in the use of people with disabilities in fashion promotions.

(*See also:* INDEPENDENT LIVING; PSYCHOSOCIAL ADJUSTMENT; QUALITY OF LIFE)

RESOURCES

Avenues Unlimited. 1199–15 Avenida Acaso, Camarillo, CA 93012. Catalog of clothing, accessories, and some equipment for people who use a wheelchair.

Easy Dressing Fashions and More. J. C. Penney Company, Inc., 11800 W. Burleigh St., Wauwatosa, WI 53222. Catalog of clothing and equipment for women and men with functional limitations; available at catalog counters of J. C. Penney retail stores.

Health Care. Sears Healthcare, P.O. Box 19009, Provo, UT 84605–9009. Catalog of health care products, including clothing, for people with special needs; available at catalog counters of Sears retail stores.

International Textile and Apparel Association. P.O. Box 1360, Monument, CO 80132–1360. A global organization of textile and apparel scholars.

Special Clothes for Special Children. P.O. Box 4220, Alexandria, VA 22303. Catalog of clothing and accessories for children with disabilities.

BIBLIOGRAPHY

QUINN, M. DELORES, and CHASE, RENEE WEISS. *Simplicity's Design Without Limits: Designing and Sewing for Special Needs.* New York, 1990.

TATE, SHARON LEE, and EDWARDS, MONA SHAFER. *The Fashion Handbook: A Guide to Your Visual Image*, 2nd ed. New York, 1991.

NORA M. MACDONALD

COMMUNICATION DISABILITIES

Communication is the essence of human life. Although other animals use simple signaling systems, human communication is a complex, rich system of symbols for encoding, transmitting, receiving, and understanding information from other people and the environment. Communication is central to human activities and basic to our capacity to establish relationships, interact, learn, and work. The ability to communicate effectively is often taken for granted, but a communication disability can affect every aspect of a person's life.

More than 3 million Americans have communication disabilities—disabilities of hearing, language, and/or speech processes that reduce the ability to receive and/or process a symbol system, represent concepts or symbol systems, and/or transmit and use symbol systems. A communication disability may be a primary handicapping condition in and of itself, or may be secondary to other handicapping conditions. One person may have a hearing loss; another may develop a speech and language disability after a stroke. A person may have more than one communication disability, and there may be a dependent relationship between or among them such as that between early hearing loss and speech articulation errors.

Communication disabilities affect individuals of all ages and all socioeconomic and ethnic groups. They may be congenital, manifest themselves in early development, or be acquired at any time. Severity may range from mild and barely noticeable to extremely severe. The causes of communication disabilities are varied.

The impact of communication disabilities must not be underestimated. In terms of financial toll they are estimated to cost our nation at least $30 billion a year for medical care, lost productivity, and special education. Less easy to quantify is the impact of communication disabilities on the individual, family, and community. Many communication disabilities in children affect their ability to learn basic life skills, including acquiring academic knowledge and a trade or profession. This limitation of potential burdens the child, and the family and society as well. Further, these children may experience negative reactions from both peers and adults, which may further reduce self-esteem and limit social and emotional development. Communication disabilities that manifest early may persist into adulthood, carrying lifelong implications. According to the Department of Education's National Institute on

Disability and Rehabilitation Research, speech disability ranks among the five most prevalent chronic conditions that limit activity for persons under age eighteen years.

In adults, acquired communication disabilities may lead to loss of the ability to work, which affects both financial status and self-esteem. Home and family life are often disrupted, as are social interactions and the ability to enjoy leisure pursuits. Adults with communication disabilities may feel isolated and become depressed. General health may suffer through an inability to indicate pain or other medical symptoms. Personal safety may be compromised by the inability to hear environmental sounds or express necessary information easily.

Because some communication disabilities are not immediately visible, they have not always received adequate or timely attention from the public, employers, or regulatory agencies. Many people with communication disabilities have limited work opportunities and access to public accommodations (such as hotels or entertainment). The Americans with Disabilities Act of 1990 provides important protection and opportunities for people with disabilities, including communication disabilities. The law prohibits discrimination against people with disabilities in all employment practices, and secures the right of access to public accommodations and telecommunication systems.

Human communication may take many forms—oral and written language, sign, gesture, facial expression, and body posture. Adequate use of each mode relies on many structural, physiological, psychological, environmental, and/or sociological factors. Vital to healthy communication are integrity of the basic structures for communication (auditory system; oral motor apparatus; and, for sign and gesture, vision and limb function) and intact operation of the central and peripheral nervous systems, including cognitive, psychological, motor, and sensory components. General health, too, is important; many diseases affect communication competence.

Communication takes place in a physical and social context and thus is vulnerable to the effects of the surrounding environment. Communication requires a physical setting in which sound or visual information may be exchanged readily. Speaker and listener cultural background and biases, communication intentions, mind-set, and attention come into play in any exchange. These factors may play a role in the development of a communication disability and may significantly affect the degree to which the disability imposes a handicap on the individual's life.

Communication disabilities may be classified as (1) a hearing disability involving altered auditory sensitivity, acuity, function, processing, and/or damage to the integrity of the physiological auditory system; (2) a speech disability involving articulation, voice, or fluency; or (3) a language disability involving the form, content, or function of language.

Hearing disabilities, which are diagnosed and treated by audiologists, are discussed here only in the context of their effects on speech and language disabilities; deafness and hearing loss are discussed in a separate entry.

Speech Disabilities

Articulation Disabilities. Articulation disabilities—difficulties producing correct speech sounds—affect how a message sounds to the listener and whether it is intelligible (understandable). Articulation disabilities may involve distortion of a sound, substitution of one sound for another ("wabbit" for "rabbit"), omission of a sound ("treet" for "street"), or a combination of these errors. Diagnosis of an articulation disability in a child is made in reference to normative information for the child's age group because all children pronounce speech sounds with some errors as they develop speech. A poor overall level of intelligibility is another factor in diagnosing an articulation disability. These disabilities are common, affecting an estimated 5 percent of school-age children. Children with hearing loss don't perceive a clear model of the speech signal so speech sound development may be poor or nonexistent, depending on the degree of hearing loss and the training the child receives. Similarly, articulation problems are more common in children with recurrent middle ear infections. Articulation problems are frequent in structural abnormalities such as cleft palate or lip, or neurological problems such as cerebral palsy. The vast majority of articulation problems in children result from slow development with no known physical cause.

In adults, articulation disabilities may result from structural damage to the speech production mechanism from neurological disorders, injuries, tumors, or surgery. The extent and location of the damage determine the type and severity of speech disturbance. Many adults can achieve a reasonable degree of intelligibility even with considerable structural damage to the articulators. Impairment of nervous system functioning may occur after stroke or infection, or as the result of degenerative disease such as amyotrophic lateral sclerosis or multiple sclerosis. Speech disturbance caused by neurological damage is called dysarthria or apraxia. Dysarthria symptoms include speech rate disturbances; distortions or omissions of sounds; slurring of speech; inadequate loudness of speech; voice problems; and weakness, incoordination, or paralysis of the muscles involved in articulation. Apraxia is characterized by variable, inconsistent articulatory errors, typically substitutions of sounds that are not attributable to muscular weakness, incoordination, or paralysis but rather to a deficit in motor planning.

Voice Disabilities. Voice refers to the production of sound by the vocal folds of the larynx and alteration of this basic tone by different shapes of the oral and nasal cavities. Voice is the sound source for speech and many other sounds involved in communication, such as singing, laughing, and crying. Full command of voice allows expression of messages, emotional state, intent, and reactions to the environment. A voice is judged adequate when it is perceived as appropriate for the speaker's age, sex, and physical characteristics, and when it does not interfere with or distract from communication. Judgments of perceived voice pitch, quality, and loudness contribute to the overall impression of adequacy.

Voice disabilities can involve inappropriate pitch (too high or too low), unchanging pitch, or breaks in pitch. The pitch may seem inappropriate for an individual, such as an adult male with an excessively high-pitched voice. Difficulties in loudness may be noted, including excessively or insufficiently loud voice. Voice quality disabilities refer to harshness, hoarseness, breathiness, hypernasality, or hyponasality. Mild voice disabilities may not be noticed because society tolerates a broad range of voice behaviors within normal limits. However, a moderate to severe voice disability may interfere with communication and disrupt daily functioning. Further, some noticeable voice disabilities indicate a serious health condition, such as cancer of the larynx, and warrant a full medical evaluation.

Voice disabilities from a structural change to the larynx may be temporary, as in laryngitis with a cold, or more persistent, as in vocal fold swelling, growths (polyps, nodules, tumors), or trauma. Neurological problems such as stroke or Parkinson's disease may affect control of the voice. One or both vocal cords may be paralyzed after surgery; depending on the degree of paralysis, the result may be a voice disability or a life-threatening condition that blocks the airway. Spasmodic dysphonia is a movement disability of the vocal folds that causes a severely strained, strangled-sounding voice. Functional voice problems generally occur through mislearning, as when a child habitually speaks in a loud voice; this in turn may lead to structural changes in the larynx.

Fluency Disabilities. Stuttering is a disability in the fluency of speech and affects rate and rhythm of the flow of verbal expression. Children with normal speech commonly have periods of disfluent speech; only 4 percent have true stuttering that lasts longer than six months. Disfluent speech is marked by hesitations, repetitions, blocks, and prolongations of sounds, syllables, words, and phrases ("p-p-p-p-uppy"; "sssssun"; "----bat"). Fluent periods may be mixed with disfluent periods. Stuttering may also be situational for some individuals who are fluent at times, but disfluent at others, particularly when under pressure. Disfluent speech may be accompanied by secondary behaviors used as attempts to escape the stuttering, such as eye blinking, interjection of filler words ("um," "well"), or facial or bodily contortions.

The cause of stuttering is unknown, but it is thought to have a neurological basis and involves incoordination in executing the speech production functions of respiration, voice, and articulation. Its impact may be severe. Some people with stuttering may be disfluent on every word and choose to avoid speaking in many communication situations. Even when stuttering is less severe, frustration at the inability to control speech may lead to problems in self-esteem, social relationships, and employment.

Language Disabilities. Language disabilities may occur in the form, content, or use of language, alone, or in any combination. These difficulties may be noted in understanding or expressing language in any mode—spoken, written, or gestural. A disability in language form may affect phonology—the selection and ordering of sounds; morphology—the structure and construction of words; or syntax—the ordering and combination of words to create sentences. Language content disabilities affect the semantic (meaning) system of words and sentences. Language use (pragmatic) disabilities involve errors in selecting language that is appropriate to the listener or the environmental and social context, with errors in using language to express the speaker's intent (request, demand, persuade), in comprehension of humor, or in nonverbal body language.

Children and adults may have language disabilities in any area of language form, content, and/or use. In children these disabilities may be developmental, starting in early stages of language acquisition. A child may be slow to begin to talk or have a limited, slowly expanding vocabulary. Other language disabilities may be indicated by difficulties putting words together correctly in sentences ("I chair sit"), improper use of markers for tenses or plurals ("I goed there," "the boys hits"), selection of a semantically incorrect word ("catch" for "throw"), or failure to use language in accord with the social or environmental context (only using commands in place of requests, statements, etc.). In children, a language disability may be the only presenting difficulty or may be found with other developmental problems, including mental retardation, autism, attentional deficits, or learning disabilities. In deaf children, sign language develops at a rate similar to that of spoken language in hearing children. If deaf children are exposed only to oral language, their ability to read lips, understand oral language, and express themselves through oral language may be limited. Children may also acquire a language disability through head injury, infection, or tumor. Acquired disabilities may affect any aspect of language, but the resulting pattern may differ from developmental language disabilities because a language foundation has already been established.

In adults, language disabilities may result from brain damage from stroke, infection, trauma, or diseases such as Alzheimer's. All types of language disabilities may be noted, though the nature of the problem can be related to the extent and location of the damage in the brain. In general, the left side of the brain is responsible for language form and content function, and damage to this part of the brain may result in aphasia, affecting phonological, morphological, syntactic, semantic, and/or pragmatic abilities. Aphasia may primarily affect language expression or reception, or both. The affected individual may speak rapidly and fluently but with empty or incorrect content; or slowly and disfluently with good content but impaired sentence structure. If the right side of the brain is damaged, semantics may be affected to some degree, language use disabilities are common, and comprehension may be reduced in difficult listening situations.

Among all aphasic symptoms, word-finding deficits are most common. Extent of recovery from aphasia in adults depends on treatment; the nature and extent of the damage; the individual's age, level of education, and motivation; and family or community support. Some individuals regain a level of function close to that before brain damage; others continue to have severe disabilities.

Treatment of Communication Disabilities. Speech-language pathologists are the health and education professionals responsible for the diagnosis and treatment of speech and language disabilities and related conditions such as swallowing disorders, accent reduction, and myofunctional (muscle use) disorders such as tongue thrust. They also counsel individuals and families affected by these disabilities, work in prevention, and conduct research on communication disabilities. Speech-language pathologists hold master's or doctoral degrees and have earned the Certificate of Clinical Competence from the American Speech-Language-Hearing Association (ASHA). To be certified by ASHA, speech-language pathologists must complete a rigorous program of academic study, clinical practicum, and supervised clinical fellowship, and pass a national examination. Additionally, most states require licensure for speech-language pathologists. They work in schools, clinics, hospitals, rehabilitation facilities, private practice, or collaboratively with other health professionals, such as physicians, physical and occupational therapists, and psychologists.

To help people with communication disabilities, the speech-language pathologist must first assess communication status through administration of standardized diagnostic tests, examination of the functioning of oral structures, and analysis of conversational speech, combined with systematic observation and information from the client and family. All diagnostic evaluations must be made with full awareness of the individual's cultural and ethnic background because a speech or language difference or an accent attributable to background is not a communication disability. Early intervention is critical, particularly for children. Despite a tendency to ignore communication problems in children under the assumption that they'll "grow out of it," this frequently does not happen, and in general, the later the intervention, the greater the long-term effects of a communication disability.

Once all data are collected from the evaluation, a diagnosis of a communication disability may be made and an individual treatment plan formulated. Treatment techniques vary greatly, depending on the nature and severity of the difficulty and the age of the client. They may involve practice of speech sound patterns that are incorrectly produced in an articulation disability, or elicitation of language forms that present difficulties in a person with aphasia. For voice or fluency disabilities, speech-language pathologists teach clients techniques to enhance vocal production or increase fluency. If a client/patient cannot communicate verbally, an alternative or augmentative form of communication, such as a communication board, sign language, or computer system may be used. For children and adults, speech-language treatment is often conducted in the most natural context possible. In all cases, the goal of speech-language treatment is to optimize communication abilities.

Research in communication disabilities is aimed at determining their causes, specific characteristics, better diagnostic techniques, more efficacious treatments, and prevention strategies.

Prevention of Communication Disabilities. Many communication disabilities are preventable; progression may be arrested through appropriate intervention. "Healthy People 2000," a national initiative of the U.S. Department of Health and Human Services, is designed to improve the health of all Americans through a coordinated, comprehensive emphasis on prevention. As part of this initiative, communication disabilities are important targets for intensive preventive efforts and research. Some health factors that may affect the risk of communication disabilities are genetic abnormalities; birth defects; low birth weight; maternal exposure to drugs, alcohol, and/or tobacco; immunization; middle ear infection; accidental injury; chronic conditions such as high blood pressure; diseases associated with aging such as Parkinson's disease; dementia; and HIV infection and AIDS, among others. Promoting general wellness strategies is a major goal of *Healthy People 2000*; the guidelines for good nutrition, good health care, good physical and mental health practices, lobbying for seat-belt and helmet use and other vehicle safety devices, and teaching effective caregiver-child interactions all directly affect communication abilities.

Organizations Involved in Communication Disabilities. The American Speech-Language-Hearing Association is the scientific, professional, and credentialing association for more than 75,000 speech-language pathologists, audiologists, and speech, language, and hearing scientists. ASHA's major programs and activities are directed toward ensuring that the best professional services possible are available to persons with communication disabilities. This task is accomplished through ASHA's credentialing program; continuing education and in-service programs for professionals; information, education, and referral services for consumers; and legislative and regulatory efforts to ensure rights and opportunities for people with communication disabilities.

Consumer and health organizations also serve the needs of people with communication disabilities by providing self-help and peer support. Groups such as the American Cancer Society, the American Heart Association, the Alzheimer's Disease and Related Disabilities Association, the National Easter Seal Society, the National Head Injury Foundation, and groups for specific communication disabilities are excellent resources for local support groups.

Many states have regulatory boards that control licensing and practice issues for speech-language pathologists. At the federal level, the Department of Health and Human Services, especially through work funded at the National Institute on Deafness and Other Communication Disabilities (part of the National Institutes of Health) and the departments of Education and Justice, have agendas concerned with the needs of persons with communication disabilities.

(*See also:* APHASIA; AUDIOLOGY; DEAFNESS AND HEARING IMPAIRMENTS; STROKE)

RESOURCE

American Speech-Language-Hearing Association, 10801 Rockville Pike, Rockville, MD 20852

BIBLIOGRAPHY

COSTELLO, JANIS M., and HOLLAND, AUDREY L., eds. *Handbook of Speech and Language Disorders.* San Diego, CA, 1986.

HEGDE, MAHABALAGIRI N. *Introduction to Communication Disorders.* Austin, TX, 1991.

KENT, RAYMOND D. *Reference Manual for Communicative Science and Disorder.* Austin, TX, 1994.

LASS, NORMAN J.; MCREYNOLDS, LEIGA V.; NORTHERN, JERRY L.; and YODER, DAVID E., eds. *Handbook of Speech-Language Pathology and Audiology.* Toronto, Canada, 1988.

NICOLOSI, LUCILLE; HARRYMAN, ELIZABETH; and KRESHECK, JANET. *Terminology of Communication Disorders: Speech-Language-Hearing.* Baltimore, MD, 1989.

SHAMES, GEORGE H., and WIIG, ELISABETH H., eds. *Human Communication Disorders: An Introduction.* Columbus, OH, 1982.

LOUISE ZINGESER
DIANE PAUL-BROWN

COMMUNITY LIVING

See DEINSTITUTIONALIZATION; HOUSING; INDEPENDENT LIVING

COMPUTER APPLICATIONS FOR PERSONS WITH VISUAL IMPAIRMENTS

The personal computer (PC) has led to independence for persons with vision impairments because standard computers can often be adapted with speech, Braille, and magnification systems. Adapted personal computers permit individuals with vision impairments to function independently at home,

school, and work. Large amounts of information can be accessed using personal computers such as on-line information data banks, local area networks, and compact-disk-based storage systems. This entry focuses on computer-based speech, Braille, magnification, and optical character recognition systems intended for use by persons who are blind and visually impaired. We shall use the term "adaptive technology" to indicate any device that permits individuals with disabilities to utilize personal computers independently.

The term "visual impairment" is used in this entry to indicate individuals who have a significant vision loss or a serious restriction in their visual field. Obviously, a significant loss of vision can create barriers in accessing unmodified personal computers. We shall discuss these barriers briefly in the next section.

For persons with vision impairments, the chief barrier to personal computer access revolves around the video display screen. Based on the television cathode ray tube, the standard computer screen uses illuminated alphanumeric characters to display processed information to the user and is thus largely inaccessible to persons with vision impairments. To adapt the personal computer to permit persons with vision impairments access, computer monitor output must be converted to an alternative format, or the existing character set must be enlarged. A number of assistive technologies designed to interface with personal computer platforms can perform these adaptive functions. These technologies include speech synthesis and magnification systems as well as Braille printers and displays. We shall discuss these individual technologies in upcoming sections of this entry.

Personal Computers

The electronics industry of the twentieth century has led to the development of sophisticated computing machines. In 1951 Univac, the first commercial digital computer, was a commercial success. During the 1960s and 1970s computer platforms greatly diminished in size and cost with the trend toward less expensive and more powerful computer hardware. Since the early 1980s personal computers have become an integral part of many homes, offices, schools, and public institutions. Because of their small size, modest cost, and compatibility with various forms of adaptive technology, personal computers are also increasing the quality of life for numerous persons with disabilities.

Personal computers are a combination of hardware and software. The hardware is the physical body or structure of the computer, while the software consists of the instructions and commands that drive the hardware. As do their larger mainframe and mini counterparts, personal computer hardware consists of several fundamental components, including a central processing unit, keyboard, video monitor, and storage systems.

The central processing unit is the engine that drives the system and is also referred to as a microprocessor. The keyboard allows the user to enter information into the computer and is based on the familiar typewriter-style keyboard. The monitor is the output device and displays processed information to the user in text or graphics characters. Personal computers also have storage devices to record data and other information permanently. Personal computers use disk drives to make permanent copies of information and are based on magnetic recording media.

For persons with vision impairments, the monitor presents the greatest barrier to equal access to the computer system. The goal is to bypass the video monitor or enhance the output into an accessible format. Adaptive technology can consist of hardware, software, or a combination of both. Within most personal computers are expansion slots that enable circuit cards to be installed to provide additional capability. Also, the bulk of personal computers have interface ports to connect external devices to the system. Many adaptive devices are circuit cards that plug into most personal computers or attach via interface ports. In the next sections we shall explore speech synthesis systems, magnification systems, Braille systems, and optical character recognition (OCR) systems.

Speech Synthesis Systems

Speech synthesis systems can be used by persons with a wide range of visual disabilities, no matter how much vision they happen to possess. Speech synthesizers translate the printed word into the spoken word and can automatically translate computer-generated text into speech output. Speech synthesizers are dedicated computers with the task of translating text into speech. Speech synthesis systems enable persons with vision impairments to access personal computer systems independently by "verbalizing the keyboard" and by verbalizing information displayed on the videoscreen. The bulk of speech synthesis systems consists of both hardware and software. The hardware can either be installed inside the computer system or installed externally via an input/output port. Both internal and external speech synthesizers require software to drive them.

The software that controls a speech synthesizer is known as a screen reader. Screen reading software permits the user to verbalize text in any desired unit, such as letter by letter, word by word, line by line, or in larger units, such as page by page. Screen readers can verbalize both text and graphics and can be used in conjunction with word processing, database, spreadsheet, telecommunications, and other applications software. The user can define verbal windows to be spoken when select function keys are struck, allowing any region of the video display to be read aloud on command.

Speech synthesis systems can verbalize both text and graphics-based operating systems and applications software packages. Examples include the MS DOS Operating System, Microsoft Windows, IBM's OS/2, Apple Macintosh, and Apple IIGS. Speech synthesis systems can be used with word processing software, allowing blind users to hear their keystrokes aloud and to verbalize text displayed on the videoscreen. These systems can also be used to operate spreadsheet software, permitting users to conduct financial management independently. Database software can also be accessed using speech synthesis systems that allow electronic records to be entered, stored, recalled, and printed. On-line data banks can be accessed using personal computers equipped with speech synthesis systems.

Screen Magnification Systems

Magnification systems can enlarge computer text and graphics as well as printed materials. Magnification systems create larger images on the retina, thus making objects easier to perceive. Magnification systems enable users with limited but still functional vision to operate personal computers and other devices independently. Many personal computer platforms can be adapted to generate enlarged text and graphics by adding magnification software or magnification hardware.

Magnification software can enlarge text and graphics from 1.5X to 16X, depending on the specific software program. Enlargement programs are loaded into memory and can enlarge the output from most commercial software such as word processors, databases, speadsheets, terminal emulators, and other software. The typical magnification software program allows the user to alter the size of the screen images on command for both text and graphics. Magnification software uses standard graphics video circuit cards to generate enlarged images. Since the bulk of modern personal computers can generate graphics as part of their standard operating procedure, many brands of personal computers can run magnification software programs.

If a given computer does not have the required video hardware to function with a software-based magnification program, then a hardware-based magnification processor circuit board can be added to the computer. Hardware-based magnification processors consist of graphics-based video circuit cards that are plugged into the computer. The hardware-based enlargement processor circuit card thus replaces the existing video circuit card, which is removed from the computer altogether. A graphics monitor is then interfaced to the magnification processor circuit card. A pointing device known as a mouse is also attached, permitting the user to control the system and select objects from screen-based menus. Magnification processor circuit cards also come packaged with software to drive the system, allowing the user to increase or decrease size of text and graphics displayed on the videoscreen or to change colors to a more comfortable viewing scheme. Magnification processors can also accept input from an external video camera to enable users to display printed text on the computer monitor in a split-screen format. For example, the user can dedicate half of the screen to a printed book and the other half of the screen to a word processor, database, or other software application.

Closed-Circuit Television Systems

Closed-circuit television systems (CCTV) are used as reading machines by persons with low vision. CCTV systems can be linked with hardware-based magnification processors allowing the user to split the video screen and view both printed material and computer-generated information. These systems consist of four basic components. The first component is a videocamera, which is used to focus on the desired reading material. The next component is a monitor screen, which can be in either color or black-and-white. The monitor can be used with magnification software to enlarge computer-generated text. The next two components consist of a monitor stand and a reading table. The monitor stand permits the camera to reside beneath the monitor, allowing the monitor to be positioned at a comfortable viewing angle. The reading table allows the user to place a book or other printed material under the camera. The reading table can move in any four of the compass directions, allowing any portion of the text to be focused under the camera. The videocamera output is routed to the video monitor, permitting the user to view the reading material in a bright, bold image. CCTV systems can magnify text from about 2X to about 60X magnification. These systems can be used for both text and graphics. Most CCTV systems also can display an inverse image, allowing users to read in either black-on-white or white-on-black backgrounds. CCTV systems are used at home, school, and on the job to accomplish a myriad of reading tasks for users with limited but still usable vision.

Braille Output Systems

Braille has been in use by persons with vision impairments since 1829. Braille consists of a raised-dot alphabet, which is read tactually. Personal computers can be adapted to generate Braille output by adding a Braille printer and Braille translation software to the system. Computers can generate Grade I and Grade II Braille. (Grade I Braille consists of the standard alphabet, punctuation, and mathematics symbols; Grade II Braille also includes hundreds of contractions and special symbols to conserve space on the Braille page.) There are two basic types of Braille output systems for personal computers: Braille printers and refreshable Braille displays.

Braille printers connect to the computer system much in the same manner as a standard ink printer. Braille printers can emboss at speeds from 20 to 200 characters per second, depending on the requirements of the end user. Braille printers require software packages known as Braille translators to print contracted (Grade II) Braille. Braille translation software translates standard word processing files into files suitable for embossing on a Braille printer. Refreshable Braille displays attach to personal computers and provide paperless Braille output, allowing the user to feel a line of mechanical Braille dots. The mechanical dots pop up and down under computer control and change as the user moves the cursor around the screen.

Optical Character Recognition Systems

Optical character recognition systems, working in conjunction with personal computers, can read printed material and translate the printed material into spoken, enlarged, or Braille format. Optical character recognition systems connect to personal computers and thus can scan a document directly into computer memory, enabling the user to access the scanned information with either speech synthesis, magnification, or Braille output systems. Optical scanning systems use pattern matching to convert printed text into computer-readable code (ASCII), which can be converted to speech, enlarged text, or Braille by most adaptive equipment. (These computerized reading machines also have practical applications for persons with learning disabilities, permitting the printed word to be spoken aloud, which may be a more appropriate environment for some individuals.)

There are two basic types of reading machines for blind persons: stand-alone reading machines and computer-based reading systems. The stand-alone variety contain their own scanner, imbedded computer, and software, as well as a speech output device. These systems can be carried from one site to another. Computer-based reading machines are peripherals and attach to personal computers using an interface card. Computer-based reading systems also require software to operate; this software is loaded

onto the host PC. Computer-based scanners thus use the processing power of a personal computer to accomplish reading tasks but also require the host PC to have some form of speech output system connected to provide voice output.

CD-ROM Information Systems

Compact disk-Read only memory (CD-ROM) systems represent a highly efficient data storage technology, permitting personal computers to become a library of information. The typical CD-ROM can hold hundreds of megabytes of information and can contain more than a gigabyte using data compression techniques. The data can consist of text, graphics, sound, or animation. CD-ROM systems are being incorporated into PCs by many personal computer manufacturers as standard equipment, and numerous companies manufacture drives that can be installed in most computer systems. For persons with vision impairments, the CD-ROM represents an available library of information that can be accessed using speech, Braille, or magnification technology. CD-ROM discs are being used for publishing encyclopedias, book collections, databases, dictionaries, magazines, and other technical and reference works. CD-ROM systems are also used to publish software packages containing executable programs and documentation on a single disc.

Local Area Networks

A computer network consists of a number of stand-alone computers linked into a system that can easily share files and data. The trend toward computer networking is a positive one for persons with vision impairments. Local area networks (LANs) consist of groups of personal computers that have been linked together to share information and files across an office or across the world. Using a local area network, persons with vision impairments can access information using either speech, Braille, or magnification technology.

Many local area networks contain an electronic mail server, allowing members of the network to send and receive messages. Electronic mail (e-mail) is an empowering mainstream technology for persons with disabilities in that electronic mail messages can be read using adaptive hardware and software. Adaptive software can also be stored and accessed on a local area network, permitting users with disabilities to use speech, Braille, or magnification software on their desktop computer.

On-Line Services

On-line services consist of large centralized computer systems containing information readily accessible via telephone dial-up. On-line services can be accessed using a personal computer, telephone, and modem. A modem is a device that translates computer signals into telephone signals and back again, permitting the two-way exchange of information across telephone lines. Private and commercial on-line data banks have created an environment wherein persons with vision impairments can gain rapid access to information. A computer equipped with a modem and the appropriate adaptive technology can be used to access most on-line data banks for sending and receiving information.

On-line services not only contain stored information of many types but also allow the user to communicate with others on the system. Most on-line services offer electronic mail to their subscribers, permitting near-instant worldwide communication. Message bases are another feature of on-line services, allowing subscribers to share information on a wide variety of subjects. Live chatting is also offered by many on-line services, permitting individuals to talk with one another in real time, with each subscriber typing messages back and forth using their keyboards and video displays. If a subscriber utilizes a personal computer with adaptive hardware and/or software, both electronic mail and live chatting can be accessed.

Future Technology

The future of the adaptive technology market is one of increased products and services. As personal computers continue to develop into less expensive and more powerful machines, future adaptive systems are being created in parallel to interface with these computer platforms. Also, the trend toward miniaturization is leading to a new generation of adaptive devices that can be carried or worn on the body. This trend is promising, leading to portable devices that can be used in multiple environments such as at home, at school, and on the job. Federal and state legislation is also causing technology to grow and develop. The Americans with Disabilities Act (1990) is increasing the demand for assistive technology.

Major computer manufacturers are developing adaptive equipment for persons with vision impairments and offer speech synthesis, magnification, Braille, optical scanning systems, and adaptive training materials.

(*See also:* ASSISTIVE TECHNOLOGY; BLINDNESS AND VISION DISORDERS; COMPUTERS; REHABILITATION ENGINEERING; TECHNOLOGY AND DISABILITY)

RESOURCES

Apple Computer, Worldwide Disability Solutions, Mail Stop 38DS, 1 Infinite Loop, Cupertino, CA 95014

IBM Special Needs Systems, 1000 NW 51 St., Boca Raton, FL 33432

Perkins School for the Blind, 175 North Beacon St., Watertown, MA 02172

Syntha-Voice Computers, Inc., 304-800 Queenston Road, Stoney Creek, Ont. L8G 1A7

BIBLIOGRAPHY

LAZZARO, JOSEPH J. "Adaptive Computing." *Byte Magazine,* May 1994.
———. "Computers for the Disabled." *Byte Magazine,* June 1993.
———. *Adaptive Technologies for Learning and Work Environments.* Chicago, 1993.
McCORMICK, JOHN. *Computers and the Americans with Disabilities Act.* New York, 1993.

JOSEPH J. LAZZARO

COMPUTERS

Our era is referred to as the age of information processing, the age of computer technology. Computers are integrated into our lives and have become a critical part of our daily activities. They are used to regulate air traffic; to control heating systems; to enhance communication around the world; and for banking, accounting, writing, and playing games.

The impact of computer technology is far more meaningful to people with disabilities. In addition to using computers as people without disabilities do, people with disabilities use computers to compensate for loss of sensory-motor and cognitive skills, enabling them to perform tasks they could not do without the computer.

People with severe physical limitations who cannot hold a pen or write with a typewriter can write with an adapted word processor just by generating a single consistent movement such as moving a hand, elbow, chin, or tongue. In addition, people who are homebound can gain meaningful employment by operating the computer from home while being connected to their workplace via modem. In schools, computers assist students in the communication and learning process.

In essence, for people with disabilities, the computer can mean the difference between isolation and communication, between unemployment and employment, and between dependent and independent living.

In 1982, the personal computer was introduced to the rehabilitation and special education field. The real impact of the computer on the lives of people with disabilities has yet to come. With the Americans with Disabilities Act (ADA) regulations in place, more people with disabilities will be employed and educated in the mainstream. The versatility and flexibility of computer technology increase the gamut of vocational, educational, and recreational opportunities for people with various impairments. Thus more and more computers will be used by more people. This situation will force computer manufacturers to fine-tune computer technology to meet the various needs of people with disabilities.

Human-Computer Interface

Most of the personal computer software programs were designed to work in conjunction with a standard keyboard as an input device and a screen as an output device. People who have sensory motor disabilities that prevent them from using the keyboard and the screen cannot reap the benefits of software. Some adaptations in computer access (input and output devices) may have to be made to enable people with physical disabilities to use standard software.

Theoretically, any device that can generate an electronic pulse can serve as an input or output de-

vice. This flexibility makes computers very adaptable for users with various disabilities. Those who cannot manipulate a keyboard because of limited fine motor control can use an enlarged keyboard or, if necessary, a single switch to input the information into the computer.

Each access device places cognitive and physical demands on the users. For example, in order to operate a keyboard, the user must have eye-hand coordination and fine motor dexterity (sensory-motor abilities) in addition to being able to discriminate among the letters and understand the meaning of the letters (cognitive abilities). The cognitive demands of the device on the user must be taken into consideration when interfacing input and output devices with the user.

Accessing Computers (Input Devices)

Based on the user's needs, adaptations to the access device can be minor, low-tech adaptations (such as tilting the keyboard) or major, high-tech adaptations (such as using a voice recognition system). Adaptations depend on the severity of the sensory motor impairment and the cognitive ability of the user. The rule of thumb is that the more physically challenged a person is, the more advanced the technological adaptations need to be.

Low-Tech Adaptations of Standard Keyboard. For people who cannot position their hands in a functional typing position, there are several low-tech support systems. These systems are designed either to support the arms or to adapt the keyboard to the user's abilities. For the arms, there are armrests and slings that hold the hand in a typing position. For the keyboard, mounting clamps are available to hold the keyboard in a position other than horizontal.

For people who have limited hand dexterity, there are several low-tech adaptations such as Keyguard, which is a flat board with holes that correspond to the keys of the keyboard fence. Each key is thus "fenced in," preventing an inadvertent pressing of the wrong key. Pointers are long sticks, usually a foot or more long, that enable the user to poke at an individual key via a headband, mitten, or mouthpiece, often through a keyguard. For one-hand keyboard users, key latches will hold down a key such as the shift key to free the hand for typing. A key latch can be a physical add-on device or a software program.

Alternative Keyboard. For people who have difficulty accessing the standard keyboard, other keyboards are available. Alternative keyboards are designed to compensate for deficit in range of motion or fine motor skills and vary in shape and size. Some examples are the MINI Keyboard from TASH and the Magic Wand Keyboard from In Touch Systems; they are small keyboards that enable the user with a limited range of motion to access the computer.

For users with limited fine motor skills, expanded keyboards can be a valuable alternative. The surfaces of these keyboards are membrane panels with touch-sensitive areas. These areas can be programmed to represent any combination of keys. Examples of membrane keyboards are IntelliKeys from IntelliTools and the PowerPad from Dunamis. Most of the alternative keyboards need a keyboard emulator to interface with a computer. A keyboard emulator is a program that enables an alternative keyboard to communicate with the computer. These programs can be ingrained into the hardware (such as Ke:nx and Adaptive Firmware Card, both from Don Johnston Developmental Equipment) or come in the form of software (such as BEST Switch Interface from BEST, Inc., a partial keyboard emulator that allows switches to function as a key or string of keys).

On-Screen Keyboards. For users who have very limited control of their extremities and cannot physically activate a keyboard or an alternative physical keyboard, an on-screen keyboard can be a viable option. A replica of the keyboard is displayed on the screen. A user selects a key by placing the cursor on it. The cursor is activated by either a mouse, which moves the cursor to the desired key, or a switch. When using a switch, the computer moves the cursor from one letter to another, and the user activates a switch to stop the cursor on the desired key. This process is called scanning. On-screen keyboards include EZ Keys from Word+, FreeWheel Head Pointing System from Pointer Systems, Inc., and HandiWare from Microsystems Software, Inc.

Most on-screen keyboards have other utility files that increase the speed of accessing the computer and thus productivity. Such utilities include word prediction, which prompts the computer to suggest a word based on the first few letters the user has typed, and abbreviation expansion, which prompts the computer to retrieve a preset phrase or paragraph just by typing a few letters.

The input devices for an on-screen keyboard are usually a switch, mouse, mouse emulator, and eye gaze (see the section on nonkeyboard input devices below). The choice of the input device depends on the severity of sensory motor disability and cost.

Nonkeyboard Input Devices. Switches are input devices that enable people with severe, multiple handicaps to access an electronic device with only a single movement. Users who have very limited control of their extremities and cannot physically activate a keyboard can access computers with a switch. The type of switch chosen depends on the nature of movement the user is capable of producing in a controlled and consistent manner and for a reasonable time. This movement can be generated by a hand, thumb, foot, toe, mouth, tongue, eyebrow, and even by the user's respiratory system.

Many switches are available, ranging from simple low technology to sophisticated high technology. There are simple push switches that are activated by pressure generated by any body part, thumb switches that can be pressed with the thumb, and sip and puff switches that are activated by blowing air into a tube. These types of switches are sold by TASH and Toys for Special Children.

Other, more sophisticated switches include a sound input switch that is activated by users' vocalization (Toys for Special Children), an electromyographic switch that is applied to the skin and activated by muscle contraction (Prentke Romich), and a photoelectric beam switch that is activated whenever a light beam is interrupted by a body part (Toys for Special Children).

With a keyboard emulator, switches can access most of the standard "off the shelf" software. They are used as pointers for on-screen keyboards. There are also programs designed specifically for use with a single switch. These programs are designed mostly for children with cognitive delays; for cause-and-effect training; and for training for scanning skills used for other functions, such as communication, environmental control, and mobility.

A mouse is a pointing system. The user glides the

mouse on a flat surface (table), which results in the cursor moving in the direction that the mouse is moving. When the cursor is on the desired symbol on the screen, the user presses a button mounted on the mouse to edit that symbol. More and more off-the-shelf programs are designed for use with a mouse. People who have difficulty activating a mouse must use a mouse emulator such as Head-Master from Prentke Romich. This emulator is positioned on a headband. By moving the head, the user can move the cursor on the screen as it would be activated by a mouse. The user presses a switch that performs the same action as a button on a mouse. In addition, there are mouse emulators that provide alternative selection schemes for cursor control. Examples of mouse emulators include Don Johnston Developmental Equipment's Ke:nx, IntelliTools' IntelliKeys, and TASH, Inc.'s, mouse emulator.

Joysticks are traditionally designed to activate games. Some software uses the joystick to simulate a pencil in conjunction with drawing programs. Although joysticks are common input devices for games, they are in essence quite difficult to activate. A variety of joystick emulators are available, such as KY Enterprises' Mouth Operated Joystick and Prentke Romich's JS-4 Joystick.

A touch screen is a transparent touch-sensitive membrane that is either a tablet mounted on the screen or built into the screen. The screen displays information that shows through the touch screen. The user can change the presentation on the screen by touching the screen in assigned places. This device is a natural way of selecting stimuli that eliminates the potentially difficult task of manipulating a keyboard or other input device. A touch screen that is built into the monitor is produced by IBM, and a touch screen that is a tablet mounted on the screen is EDMARK's Touch Window.

Voice recognition: Also at the high-tech end of the adaptation spectrum is the voice recognition system, an input device that translates the human voice into digitized symbols. These symbols are then translated into words, which are displayed on the screen. The computer can recognize any language or sound as long as the user produces consistent sounds for a given word. The computer has to be trained to recognize the user's voice and to correlate it with the corresponding symbols. DragonDictate is a speech recognition system for IBM computers that has 25,000 preprogrammed words and space for another 5,000 words. The user trains the computer to recognize his or her own pronunciation of these words and thus eliminates the use of hands and extremities to access the computer.

Optical character recognition is a device that scans a hard-copy document and transforms and stores the information into a computer file. The Kurzweil reading machine is a combination of a scanner and a voice synthesizer. In this case, the hard copy can be read by the computer and translated into a synthetic voice. This machine enables people who are blind to "read" books independently that were not originally written in Braille.

The Eyegaze computer system is a high-tech input device that allows the user to access a computer by eye movement only. The system comes with a camera which tracks the eye movement of the user and spots the location that the user gazes at on the on-screen keyboard.

Accessing Computers (Output Devices)

Screen Displays. The most common computer output devices are videoscreens. Like a TV, the image on a desk-top computer's monitor is generated through a picture tube called a cathode-ray tube (CRT). The image is composed of many dots, called pixels. The more pixels there are per square inch, the higher the picture resolution, and the better the representation of the image. The newer generations of computer monitors have better resolution.

Notebook computers are small, laptop-size units that have built-in flat-panel displays called LCD (liquid crystal displays). These displays do not emit light and can be read only from a certain angle. LCD screens consume less electricity, are less bulky, and weigh less. With current technology, images on LCD screens are not as crisp as on CRT monitors.

Screens come in a variety of sizes, resolutions, and color capacities. The large variety of screens enables the user to use a screen that meets his or her individual needs. People with a small degree of eyesight deterioration can purchase a large monitor with high resolution. People with a higher degree of visual loss can adjust the screen with low-tech adaptations such as screen magnification sheets. The magnifying "sheet" is placed on any computer screen and magnifies the text two to four times the original size. Mechanical devices are also available which enlarge the text sixteen times the original size.

Software programs designed to produce the same effect without any physical adaptation are also available in the market. These include HandiVIEW, produced by Microsystems Software, Inc., which is a computer software that magnifies each line of text eight times the original size. This software can be used with off-the-shelf programs such as word processors. Some new-generation screen enlargement programs are able to enlarge graphics, window, and menu bars. Voice output systems act as screen readers, enabling people who are totally blind to "see" the screen.

Printer. Printers are available that can print Braille for visually impaired people. The computer has to have a software program that translates computer commands into Braille.

Voice Output. Technology adds voice to the computer output capabilities. Voices output is a supplement to or a replacement of the visual output. This capability can provide innumerable benefits to people with disabilities, particularly to blind or mute people. For children with various learning disabilities, a speaking computer that reinforces the visual presentation enhances the learning experience.

Computers can generate three types of voice output: (1) text-to-speech synthesis; (2) digitized speech; and (3) linear predictive coding.

A text-to-speech synthesis system enables any text being input into a computer to generate a computer-voice output. The quality of the sound output is a synthetic, robotics voice, but the advantage is that the system uses minimal memory.

Digitized speech records real sounds (e.g., a person's words, or music) and translates the sounds into digitized information that a computer can process, store, and play back. The quality of the sound output is a replication of the recorded sound; however, this recording system uses a large amount of memory.

Linear predictive coding contains elements of both digitized and text-to-speech synthesis. It records real human speech, translates the sounds into digital data, stores the speech, and generates a computer-voice output with a high quality that resembles the human voice.

Music synthesizers also fall under the category of voice output. The computer is able to generate sound that imitates most of the musical instruments or an entire orchestra. Music is input into the computer through a pianolike keyboard or through the computer keyboard.

Computer Application in Rehabilitation

The unlimited combination of computer technology input devices, output devices, and software programs, and the computer's ability to store and retrieve an enormous amount of information, make computers viable tools in all facets of life. In addition to enabling people with disabilities to operate off-the-shelf programs such as word processors, spreadsheets, graphics software, communication software, and games as able-bodied people do, the computer also can compensate for specific sensory-motor losses.

A computer equipped with a voice synthesizer can "read" back to a blind person as he or she is typing, thus giving that person immediate feedback on the quality of the writing. Formatting codes, menus, and prompts may also be spoken, allowing visually impaired users to write independently on a computer. A voice synthesizer also allows a mute person to communicate vocally with a hearing person via the computer. The person types the information into the computer, and the computer speaks for him or her. People who are blind, deaf, and physically impaired to the extent that they cannot type information into the computer, can operate the computer via a single switch activated by a single movement.

The computer enables people who have severe physical limitations to control their environment by pushing just one key. They can operate radios, microwaves, and open doors from the convenience of their beds. With the assistance of a computer, people with severe disabilities can cook their own meals and gain more independence in their daily living.

Computers are also used for assessment and remediation of the cognitive and perceptual skills of children (COLORS & SHAPES from BEST) and brain-damaged adults (ThinkAble from IBM). These programs enable the therapist to assess the cognitive deficits of clients and to tailor programs to meet their specific needs. The capacity of computers to generate sound and creative graphics makes it an especially powerful tool for children. Computers are utilized in schools to augment the learning process and focus on remediating specific learning skills.

Computers have revolutionized the workplace, particularly for people with various disabilities, because they have opened the door to many opportunities. Because most office functions are computerized and people with disabilities can easily gain access to computers, these persons can now participate in the work force, performing tasks they could not do before the widespread use of computers. The employer is also required by law to provide access to the computer and arrange the work station to meet the needs of people with disabilities. Computers are also used to assess and remediate vocational skills.

Computers have enhanced the lives of people with various disabilities and enabled them to function more independently in their home, in educational settings, and in the workplace. We are only at the beginning of the computer revolution.

(See also: AMERICANS WITH DISABILITIES ACT; ASSISTIVE TECHNOLOGY; COMPUTERS FOR PERSONS WITH VISUAL IMPAIRMENTS; QUALITY OF LIFE; REHABILITATION ENGINEERING)

RESOURCES

ABLEDATA, 8455 Colesville Rd, Silver Spring, MD 20910–3319

Apple Computer, Worldwide Disability Solutions, Mail Stop 38DS, 1 Infinite Loop, Cupertino, CA 95014

Closing the Gap, P.O. Box 68, Henderson, MN 56044

Compuserve, 5000 Arlington Centre Blvd., P.O. Box 20212, Columbus, OH 43220

Counsel for Exceptional Children, 1920 Association Dr., Reston, VA 22091

IBM Special Needs Systems, 1000 NW 51st St., Boca Raton, FL 33432

National Easter Seal Society, 230 West Monroe St., Suite 1800 Chicago, IL 60606

RESNA, 1101 Connecticut Ave., NW, Suite 700, Washington, DC 20036

Specialnet, 2021 K St., NW, Suite 215, Washington, DC 20006

TRACE Research and Development Center, 1500 Highland Ave., Room S-151, Waisman Center, Madison, WI 53705

BIBLIOGRAPHY

BERLISS, JAN. R., et al. Trace Resource Book: Assistive Technologies for Communication, Control & Computer Access. Madison, WI, 1991.

CHURCH, GREGORY, and GLENNEN, SHARON. The Handbook of Assistive Technology. San Diego, CA, 1992.

ENDERS, ALEXANDRA, and HALL, MARIAN. Assistive Technology Sourcebook. Washington, DC, 1990.

PFAFFENBERGER, BRYAN. Que's Computer User's Dictionary. Carmel, IN, 1991.

WALTER RUSS. The Secret Guide to Computers. Somerville, MA, 1991.

DINA LOEBL

CONGENITAL DISORDERS

See GENETIC DISORDERS

CONSUMERS

In the United States, definitions of disability and the services which respond to its existence have always been shaped by external political and socioeconomic forces. The Civil War, devastating in terms of casualties, produced the first pervasive government involvement in disability services. The efforts, by current standards, were crude and limited, but the budgets of many states were overwhelmed by large expenditures for prosthetic limbs. Wars have a cyclical place in the production of disability, and they produce medical advances in saving lives and, secondarily, in the rehabilitation of survivors.

From the mid-1800s onward, industrialization has had a more sustained effect on the production and management of disability. The Progressive Era harkened a new perspective on social responsibility toward growing numbers of people crippled by industrial accidents and occupational diseases. By the early 1900s, that number reached 14,000 workers annually, with a cumulative figure of 500,000 in the working-age population. In its wake came such organizations as the Federation of Associations for Cripples to make both the problem and proposed solutions known. Industrialization spawned the trade union movement, which pushed for workers' compensation legislation. The first such law was passed in 1908 for civil employees, and by 1920 almost every state had one.

World War I transformed the steady flow of industrial diseases and accidents to a flood of injuries and disabilities. By May 1919, when the American Expeditionary Forces returned, the number of casualties was 123,000. This era has been dubbed the "defect with a cash value" period. The criterion was ability to return to work. The loss of both eyes resulting in blindness was regarded at that time as prima facie evidence of inability to return, but the loss of one eye might not even necessitate a change in job. Measurement of functional loss was almost exclusively in terms of male remunerative work activity.

By 1940 the "rehabilitation rather than compensation" era was in full bloom, stimulated by recognition of needs for long-term care and for returning skilled and executive-level workers to their jobs rather than replacing them. In the mid-1930s the first major self/mutual help group was founded—Alcoholics Anonymous. It legitimized fellow sufferers as the primary sources of support if not cure. While medicine, following advances in science and industry, became more "high tech," awareness increased of the need to treat the whole person through comprehensive and not exclusively biomedical approaches.

The Depression had raised awareness of needs for social safety nets. President Roosevelt, himself a consumer of rehabilitation services due to adult-onset polio, rejected a national health plan but established the March of Dimes. This voluntary association paid for the total medical needs of people diagnosed with polio regardless of income. Beneficiaries did not have to sacrifice their privacy, or grovel, or do battle with a tightfisted bureaucracy when they were in weakened condition in order to get the help they needed. A generation of polio survivors who experienced this program that gave help without hassles grew up with the strength, expectations, and self-confidence required to provide leadership for a future consumer movement.

The only other disability group for which societal allowances have long been made is the blind. No group has had a more ambivalent history, from being considered the victims of most tragic of punishments (Oedipus) to the recipients of most blessed of inspirations (John Milton to Helen Keller). Blind persons were the first to have their own schools; the only disability group to have a specific federal income-tax deduction, a reserved job status (guaranteed vendor opportunities in buildings on federal property), and mail privileges (free matter for the blind); the first to have set-aside state "financial relief" funds and separate state agencies to serve them; and a long history of "designated codicils" in omnibus rehabilitation legislation.

Meanwhile, World War II had catalyzed further medical advances, and rehabilitation was recognized as a medical specialty. As psychosocially trained specialists joined the rehabilitation teams, the specialty became more multidisciplinary, and some attention was turned to acceptance of disablement, adjustment to losses and limitations, and coping with environmental demands as well as the attitudes and behavior of other people.

Through the 1950s, disability was seen as a tragedy to be contained as much as possible through rehabilitation services. Service consumers' attitudes toward themselves began to be acknowledged by the now diverse group of professionals providing treatment, but the importance lay mainly in the degree to which their feelings might influence motivation for prescribed treatment and improved functioning. The importance of their own decision-making expertise or the effects of other people's attitudes would not be widely recognized until the following decade. University training programs for physical and occupational therapists and rehabilitation counselors were being established, but many schools had explicit if not written policies against accepting students with disabilities. The psychological wisdom expressed at that time was that such students would "overidentify" with their patients or clients and would thus be rendered unhelpful. By the turn of the decade, a few programs were allowing students with disabilities into their programs but were watching them closely.

By 1960 the self-help movement that originated with Alcoholics Anonymous had gained sufficient number and diversity of spin-off programs (e.g., for overeating and gambling problems, or the need for support following discharge from psychiatric hospitalization) to be featured in the popular press. Widespread dissemination of information about the success of such groups planted seeds in the minds of people with disabilities who perceived that they also could benefit from mutual support. Those persons requiring substantial support to live outside of family or institutional settings were beginning to apply to universities for education that might prepare them for competitive employment. One of the earliest successful efforts began in 1962, when Edward Roberts, a person with postpolio quadriplegia and half-time tank respirator user, arranged to live in the university hospital as a way of attending the University of California.

In 1965 the riots in south central Los Angeles triggered reexamination of passive acceptance of second-class citizenship by ethnic and national minorities generally, and by women, people with disabilities, and elders. Two years later, Edward Roberts had drawn together a cluster of students with severe disabilities who were living in a designated area of the university hospital and getting the supports they needed for activities of daily living. By 1968 the federal government, via the Architectural Barriers Act, and individual states began enacting laws aimed toward reducing barriers to people with disabilities. For example, in California, a pioneering state in this regard, a 1968 statute promoted mainly by organized constituents with visual impairments focused on publicly funded structures.

In 1969 a similar law, promoted largely by advocates for people with mobility impairments, addressed barriers in privately owned public accommodations. Local lobbying committees had sprung into being as soon as the idea of civil rights was driven into the collective consciousness. Members were generally disability-service professionals and people with disabilities who were unemployed because of employer prejudice but who were eager to put their energies to use. The end of the decade saw the beginning of ombudsmen programs for consumers of disability services patterned after those that grew from Great Society projects for socially disadvantaged minorities.

Meanwhile, Edward Roberts and his fellow students were getting ready to graduate. The first generation of the Physically Disabled Students Program now needed support to move into the community, and the Berkeley Center for Independent Living was born. The two programs became prototypes for university- and community-based service agencies operated by and for people with disabilities. They are now seen collectively as the birthplace of the independent-living/disability-rights movement.

The 1970s saw the proliferation of self/mutual help groups and the beginning of multidisability coalitions clamoring for resources and rights. In 1973 an almost unnoticed provision of a rehabilitation act twice vetoed by President Nixon built on all that had gone before and catalyzed a social movement of national rather than local scope. Section 504 provided the federal enabling legislation sought by early activists with disabilities to encourage all states and municipalities to enact laws and ordinances ensuring people with disabilities access to public accommodations and programs. Fewer than fifty words became known as "the civil rights provision for people with disabilities":

> No otherwise qualified handicapped individual in the United States as defined in Section 7 shall, solely by reason of his handicaps, be excluded from participation in, be denied the benefits of, or be subjected to discrimination under any program or activity receiving federal financial assistance.

The foregoing came into being almost by accident. After two presidential vetoes, one sustained by the Senate, legislative staffers Jack Duncan (Senate) and Martin LaVor (House) went to work on a revision. Despite personal interests—Duncan has a disability and LaVor previously worked in rehabilitation—they virtually gutted the bill of anything that might elicit a third veto. Another staffer, Lisa Walker (Senate), reviewed the wreckage with dismay and said, "Surely no one would object to a statement that one shouldn't discriminate against them. . . ." The momentous passage was the trio's response to what seemed a reasonable expectation. There was no legislative history, not a word about it in the conference report, no debate on the floor. It was born in the absence of guidance like the appearance of a new quantum particle in a vacuum.

It took three years to turn these words into thousands of pages of regulations for dozens of federal agencies. Each agency resisted, and the task was completed only with sustained effort by the American Coalition of Citizens with Disabilities, the first cross-disability coalition. A Washington, DC-based demonstration led in part by disability activist Judith Heumann was quashed fairly quickly but not before it gained valuable media dissemination to feed the imaginations of local activists everywhere. A more successful San Francisco-based demonstration at the Federal Region X offices may have been supported by officials in part because by 1975 the California State Department of Rehabilitation was being directed by former service consumer Edward Roberts. Specialized commissions for the blind had long been headed by people who were blind or severely vision-impaired, but the general agencies had not had "disabled" representatives of the service population at the helm. Within a few years it became common for people with substantial disabilities to be preferentially recruited by elected officials to serve as appointed directors of public disability-related agencies. For example, directors of the federal Rehabilitation Services Administration have been drawn from the consumer population since President Nixon appointed Andrew Adams to the post. Max Clelland, who is a triple amputee, served as the head of the Veterans Administration under President Carter. In 1993 Judith Heumann, who had helped to lead a sit-in on Secretary Joseph Califano's residential lawn to force him to sign the 504 regulations for the Department of Health, Education and Welfare (now Health and Human Services), was appointed assistant secretary for the Office of Special Education and Rehabilitation Services by President Clinton. This is the highest governmental position dealing specifically with disabilities.

When, in 1977, Califano signed the regulations to the 1973 Rehabilitation Act, he also signed the regulations to the Education for All Children Act. Although the latter paralleled in spirit the struggle over rights captured in Section 504, it had a different history. Until the 1960s, elementary and secondary education for children was primarily a state and local activity. With the passage of the Elementary and Secondary Education Act (ESEA) in 1965, federal monies were to be allocated for educational materials based on the number of low-income children in each school district. Through amendments and reauthorizations over the next decade, funding for materials and training was extended to special-need children and special-education teachers.

These thrusts were parts of a sustained "parents' campaign" demanding an end to segregated education for children with disabilities and the beginning of "mainstreaming." In 1971–72, two landmark court decisions signaled the need for further, more encompassing legislative action. The first was *Pennsylvania Association for Retarded Children* (PARC) v. *Commonwealth of Pennsylvania*. In this case the plaintiffs, acting on behalf of fourteen students with mental retardation, brought a class-action suit against the commonwealth of Pennsylvania, arguing that the state had violated their due-process and equal-protection rights. The resulting consent agreement required Pennsylvania "to place each mentally retarded child in a free, public program of education and training appropriate to the child's capacity." The second case, *Mills v. Board of Education of the District of Columbia*, brought by the parents and guardians of seven children with mental retardation, charged that the defendant denied them publicly supported education. Together these legislative, judicial, and parental efforts resulted in the Education for All Handicapped Children Act, which required states, as a precondition for receiving federal funds, to ensure that they provide a free and appropriate education to all children with handicaps. Most important, this legislation enshrined the concept of "least restrictive environment" and the necessity of a written, agreed-upon individual education plan (IEP) negotiated by parents and educational administrators.

Crucial to the solidification of gains, for the translation of ideas into practice, was the passage of the Rehabilitation Comprehensive Services and Developmental Disabilities Act Amendments of 1978.

New coalitions were formed and specifics were added to the ideals of the 1973 provisions. Two elements pried the idea of disability farther from the medical model and medical dominion and helped to solidify a movement by creating and legitimating a cross-disability orientation and community. Functional limitations rather than medical categories were enshrined into law. Federal recognition was given to independent living as a legitimate nonvocational goal of rehabilitation services, and the first national institute devoted to research on disability was created (then the National Institute for Handicapped Research; now the National Institute for Disability and Rehabilitation Research). It was located in the Department of Education rather than with the National Institutes of Health in the Department of Health and Human Services.

Empowerment

The decade of the 1980s was one of people with disabilities digging in heels, consolidating constituencies, and delineating visions and missions. Many influences were involved. Not only was the general population aging, but also the old old, those over eighty-five, constituted the fastest-growing segment. Being old puts a population at risk for physical changes that are sociopolitically viewed as disabling. Also, the 1980s ushered in another significant epidemiological shift—large increases in the general rates of disability and the specific rates of disability-related chronic disease conditions as well as longer survival rates of people with existing disabilities. Moreover, three conditions were to emerge that would challenge traditional conceptions, measurements, service delivery, and research, each in its unique way: AIDS, Alzheimer's disease, and learning disabilities.

Accounts of people with disabilities began to appear in anthologies and in first-person narrations of disability experiences. Magazines for consumers of disability-related products and services began to appear. No universally accepted terms had yet been established, but a language shift away from familiar terms with pejorative connotations (e.g., "cripple") and the concept of politically correct language (e.g., person *with* a given disabling condition) emerged.

Substantial if not majority consumer representation on directorial and advisory boards began to be required for functions as diverse as independent living programs in local communities and national research advisories.

Such a body is the National Council on Disability, created by law for the primary purpose of overseeing the research activities within the Office of Special Education and Rehabilitation Services (OSERS) in the U.S. Department of Education. A disability research constituency began to emerge that formed the national Society of Disability Studies with intent to influence the relevance and utility of disability research funded or conducted by public agencies. Greater intertwining of the disability and research communities encouraged people with disabilities to shift from being only the objects of research and policy to being partners in policy-setting and research. "Participatory action research" and "consumer-oriented research and dissemination" were early attempts to designate the desired research topics and methods that are heavily influenced by representatives of the subjects of investigation or beneficiaries of the findings.

Meanwhile, building on the Vietnam War protest and other civil rights movements, disability activists took more systematically to the TV screens and the streets. The organization ADAPT became the most visible symbol when, in demanding access to mass transportation, member-demonstrators chained themselves to buses. At the end of the decade they turned their attention to the nursing home industry and a demand for a national system of personal assistant services. The students of Gallaudet University captured national attention for several days in their demand for a university president with a hearing impairment.

In 1988 the political constituency of people with disabilities was recognized for the first time and incorporated into a political campaign. The remarks of presidential candidate George Bush about bringing "the handicapped" into the mainstream are said to have shifted nearly half a million voters. The National Council on Disability originally drafted and spearheaded the Americans with Disabilities Act (ADA), which became law by George Bush's signature in 1990. In 1992 the ADA took force and, during that year's presidential campaign, the disability community, mostly through its now widespread media network, was the target of intensive campaigning.

Speculations on the Future

1. An irony exists in the fact that a federal law such as the ADA was envisioned by activists in the 1960s, when funds were flowing to programs countering social disadvantage and the United States considered itself an affluent society. By the mid-1970s, such funding had slowed so much that programs shrank because increases did not keep pace with inflation. The 1980s saw straightforward cuts. The longed-for federal statute became law in the 1990s, after U.S. economic status had eroded, competition for scarce jobs and resources had grown harsh, and the potential for backlash from newly displaced/impoverished people without disabilities had become great.

2. The independent-living and disability-rights movement may engender a return to a compensation rather than a rehabilitation era. This development has already begun in a subtle way within state-federal vocational rehabilitation programs as a result of changes in the Rehabilitation Act. In returning decision authority to consumers, much of the opportunity to get free professional expertise has been eliminated, too. Evaluative procedures that once helped consumers who wanted career-choice guidance are no longer authorized. As the process moves toward supplying whatever consumers request at intake without advice from vocational experts, and as professionally trained counselors reject working as functionaries and take jobs with more rewarding duties, the process may move to a "voucher" system more quickly than expected and to the dismay of some.

3. On the other hand, that disability is multidimensional and varies through time is better understood as a result of consumer involvement. The number of people with disabilities is fluid, not fixed. The number "43 million" is mentioned in legislation, but it is not a knowable reality. True disability is the result of interaction among individuals' physical-mental condition, personal resources, and the socio-political-economic environment. Conceptions of "disability culture" and "disability pride"

call for characterizing disability as a value-neutral experience.

4. Whether the events described in this entry are merely symbolic acts or whether they will usher in a new era of a prominent role for people with disabilities in the formulation of policies only time will tell. Prejudices and paradigms run so deep that even a revolution will not overturn them in a single generation. A process leading toward empowerment has, however, begun for people with disabilities.

(*See also:* ACCESSIBILITY; AMERICANS WITH DISABILITIES ACT; CIVIL RIGHTS; DISABILITY LAW AND SOCIAL POLICY; HISTORY OF REHABILITATION; INDEPENDENT LIVING)

RESOURCES

National Council on Disability, 1331 F St., NW, Suite 1050, Washington, DC 20004–1107
World Institute on Disability (WID), 510 16th St., Suite 100, Oakland, CA 94612

BIBLIOGRAPHY

ALBRECHT, GARY L. *The Disability Business—Rehabilitation in America.* Newbury Park, CA, 1992.
BERKOWITZ, EDWARD D. *Disabled Policy—America's Programs for the Handicapped.* Cambridge, Eng., 1987.
FOX, DANIEL M., and WILLIS, DAVID P., eds. "Disability Policy: Restoring Socio-Economic Independence." *The Milbank Quarterly* 2 (1989): Parts 1 + 2.
FREY, WILLIAM D. "Functional Assessment in the '80s—A Conceptual Enigma, a Technical Challenge." In *Functional Assessment in Rehabilitation,* eds. A. S. Halporn and M. J. Fuhrer. Baltimore, MD, 1984.
GRITZER, GLEN, and ARLUKE, ARNOLD. *The Making of Rehabilitation: A Political Economy of Medical Specialization.* Berkeley, CA, 1985.
PERCY, STEPHEN L. *Disability, Civil Rights, and Public Policy: The Politics of Implementation.* Tuscaloosa, AL, 1989.
POPE, ANDREW M., and TARLOV, ALVIN R., eds. *Disability in America—Toward a National Agenda for Prevention.* Washington, DC, 1991.
SCOTCH, RICHARD K. *From Goodwill to Civil Rights: Transforming Federal Disability Policy.* Philadelphia, PA, 1984.
———. "Disability as the Basis for a Social Movement: Advocacy and the Politics of Definition." In

Moving Disability Beyond Stigma: Journal of Social Issues, eds. Adrienne Asch and Michelle Fine. Vol 44 (1987):159–172.

SHAPIRO, JOSEPH P. *No Pity: People with Disabilities Forging a New Civil Rights Movement.* New York, 1993.

STONE, DEBORAH. *The Disabled State.* Philadelphia, PA, 1984.

TREANOR, RICHARD BRYANT. *We Overcame—The Story of Civil Rights for Disabled People.* Falls Church, VA, 1993.

WEST, JANE, ed. *The Americans with Disabilities Act—From Policy to Practice.* New York, 1991.

WOODWILL, GARY. *Independent Living and Participation in Research.* Toronto, Canada, 1992.

ZOLA, IRVING KENNETH. "Disability Statistics: What We Count and What It Tells Us—A Personal and Political Analysis." *Journal of Disability Policy Studies* 4 (1993):9–39

IRVING KENNETH ZOLA
CAROLYN L. VASH

CORONARY ARTERY DISEASE

Atherosclerosis of the coronary arteries (coronary artery disease) is the leading cause of death and disability in all industrialized nations. Coronary artery disease is a progressive, chronic disorder that may lead to myocardial ischemia, an imbalance between the myocardial requirement for nutritive blood flow and the capacity of the coronary circulation to provide flow (Squires & Williams, 1993). Impaired coronary blood flow may result from either obstructive atherosclerotic lesions and/or an impaired capacity of the coronary circulation to vasodilate. Sequelae of coronary artery disease include angina pectoris, myocardial infarction, sudden cardiac death, and congestive heart failure.

In the United States, 6.3 million persons have a history of coronary artery disease, with an annual treatment cost of approximately $56 billion (Bittner, 1994). Each year approximately 1.5 million persons suffer a myocardial infarction, 300,000 undergo coronary bypass surgery, and 250,000 have balloon coronary angioplasty (a surgical procedure where a balloon catheter is inserted into a partially occluded coronary artery with subsequent inflations and deflations to mechanically open the artery).

Coronary artery disease is not necessarily an in-

evitable consequence of a genetic predisposition and the aging process. Multiple environmental risk factors are suggested by the variation in incidence of coronary artery disease around the world. This is powerfully illustrated by the observation that migrants, on leaving an area of lower incidence of cardiovascular mortality, assume the higher incidence of their new country.

From 1981 to 1994 there was a 32 percent decline in the age-adjusted death rate from myocardial infarction in the United States. This welcome decline has resulted from factors such as improved medical and surgical treatment as well as reduced coronary risk factors in the population. For example, decreased smoking rates, lower average serum cholesterol concentrations attributed to lower dietary saturated fat and cholesterol intakes, and improved screening and treatment of hypertension have occurred since the 1960s. Despite this good news, coronary artery disease remains a formidable challenge. The purpose of this entry is to describe the pathogenesis, diagnosis, treatment, secondary prevention, and rehabilitation procedures used in coronary artery disease.

Pathogenesis of Atherosclerosis

Arteries undergo changes that are considered part of the normal aging process, such as thickening of the intima (the innermost layer of the arterial wall and the site for atherosclerotic lesions), loss of elastic connective tissue, an increase in calcium content, and an increase in diameter. In contrast, atherosclerosis is a pathologic phenomenon resulting in alteration of the arterial wall, which may lead to partial or total obstruction of blood flow in the major arteries, such as the coronaries (Squires & Williams, 1993). The disease is complex and not fully understood. Multiple risk factors have been identified and include cigarette smoking, a blood lipid profile with elevated low-density lipoprotein cholesterol and/or depressed high-density lipoprotein cholesterol concentrations, hypertension, sedentary lifestyle, family history, insulin resistance and diabetes mellitus, psychological disturbances, male gender, increasing age, and obesity.

The initial event in atherosclerosis is injury to the endothelial cells, which line the artery, from such factors as tobacco substances, blood lipids, elevated blood pressure, immune complexes, viruses, and vasoconstrictor substances. The metabolically active endothelium, when injured, becomes more permeable to substances from the blood, has an increased affinity for blood platelets, and becomes less able to vasodilate. Platelets adhere to the endothelium, forming small blood clots, and release growth factors and vasoactive substances. Growth factors promote proliferation (increased cell numbers and cell size) of tissue and cause the migration of smooth muscle cells and fibroblasts from the middle of the arterial wall to the intimal layer under the endothelium, where these cells accumulate cholesterol. Monocytes, from the blood, also adhere to the endothelium and take up cholesterol. Over time, cell proliferation continues, as does formation of fibrous connective tissue. Atherosclerotic lesions progress in size at variable rates and may become an impediment to adequate blood flow.

As a result of local stress on an atherosclerotic lesion, rupture of the plaque may occur, exposing the contents of the lesion to the blood, resulting in thrombus formation and further obstruction of the vessel. In addition to obstruction of blood flow by the bulk of the atherosclerotic lesion, vasospasm superimposed over the lesion may result in a further reduction in blood flow.

Diagnosis of Coronary Artery Disease

The physical examination is of only modest usefulness in the diagnosis of coronary artery disease (Giuliani et al., 1991). The presence of xanthelasma or tendinous xanthomas (cutaneous collection of cholesterol) is indicative of familial hypercholesterolemia with a high probability of premature coronary artery disease. Similarly, signs of congestive heart failure are often associated with coronary atherosclerosis. Identification of classic coronary risk factors is important for the prevention and treatment of the disease, but these factors are relatively insensitive markers of the presence of clinically important coronary artery disease.

The methods of diagnosis for this disease are, for the most part, directed toward identification of evidence of reduced coronary blood flow resulting in myocardial ischemia or myocyte necrosis (the death of myocardial muscle cells as a result of heart at-

tack). A careful history of symptoms of angina pectoris is often all that is required to make the diagnosis. Angina pectoris is generally described as a feeling of pressure, heaviness, fullness, squeezing, burning, or aching. Some patients experience difficulty in breathing, or dyspnea (anginal equivalent), probably due to increased left ventricular end-diastolic pressure, as the primary symptom. Locations of ischemic pain include the substernal region, jaw, neck, and left arm, although the sensation may occur in the epigastrium (the stomach area) and interscapular regions. Typical angina is usually provoked by exertion, emotions, cold or heat exposure, meals, or sexual intercourse, and is relieved by rest or nitroglycerin. If the symptoms are reliably reproduced and unchanging, stable angina is the diagnosis. Unstable angina is described as new onset of exertional symptoms, increasing frequency or intensity or duration of previously stable angina, or angina that occurs at rest. Unstable angina is believed to result from the development of partially occlusive, transient platelet thrombi or periodic coronary vasospasm mediated by local vasoconstrictors produced by the injured endothelium (Giuliani et al., 1991; Squires & Williams, 1993).

Ischemia results in progressive abnormalities of cardiac function that may be detected with specific tests. Ischemic stiffening of the left ventricle (diastolic dysfunction) and impaired systolic emptying may be determined with echocardiography or nuclear imaging techniques. Electrocardiographic evidence of abnormal repolarization (ST segment or T wave abnormalities) may be observed. Ischemia may also initiate ventricular arrhythmias.

Exercise may unmask the presence of myocardial ischemia by increasing myocardial oxygen requirement above the capacity of a diseased coronary circulation to deliver blood. Exercise testing is often used in the evaluation of patients with suspected coronary artery disease (Giuliani et al., 1991). Standard exercise testing is generally performed with a treadmill or cycle, with continuous multilead electrocardiographic monitoring and periodic blood pressure measurement. The exercise intensity is gradually increased, with an end point of fatigue or signs and/or symptoms of ischemia. The hallmark of ischemia is an exercise electrocardiogram with one or more millivolts of ST-segment displacement from the pre-exercise tracing. The development of typical angina pectoris during exercise is also a relatively sensitive marker for ischemia, although many patients will demonstrate electrocardiographic evidence of ischemia without the presence of angina (silent ischemia). A drop in systolic blood pressure during progressive exercise is suggestive of myocardial ischemia.

Imaging techniques that provide either myocardial perfusion information (thallium, technetium-99m sestamibi) or mechanical performance characteristics of the ventricles (echocardiography, technetium-99m pertechnetate) may be combined with exercise testing and substantially improve the predictive value of the test results. Myocardial perfusion testing distinguishes reversible flow defects (ischemia) from permanent defects (infarction). Tests of the mechanical performance of the heart during exercise provide left ventricular systolic and diastolic function information (ejection fraction) and regional wall motion analysis that also distinguishes infarction from ischemia. For patients who cannot exercise adequately, pharmacologic "stress" with vasodilators such as dipyridamole or adenosine that unmask an abnormal flow reserve due to coronary narrowing or a positive chronotropic agent (a drug which increases the heart rates) such as dobutamine may be combined with imaging techniques.

Since atherosclerosis is associated with calcium deposition in the vessel wall, techniques to detect coronary calcification may be helpful in the diagnosis of coronary artery disease. Ultrafast computed tomography of the heart allows visualization and quantification of coronary calcification and is under investigation as a diagnostic tool.

Direct visualization of the lumen of the coronary arteries with angiography is the "gold standard" for diagnosis of coronary artery disease. Discrete areas of stenosis are easily identifiable although, when compared to autopsy results, the coronary angiogram generally underestimates the severity of the lesions. Coronary angiography is generally reserved for patients with limiting symptoms or evidence of substantial amounts of myocardial ischemia and who are candidates for revascularization.

Acute myocardial infarction is the necrosis of myocytes resulting from prolonged myocardial ischemia caused by complete occlusion of a coronary artery (Squires & Williams, 1993). The immediate factor that causes the complete occlusion appears to be the rupture of an atherosclerotic lesion with subsequent thrombus formation. Lesion rupture with thrombus formation resulting in complete vessel occlusion often occurs in lesions that are only 20 to 40 percent occlusive before rupture and explains why many patients who experience acute myocardial infarction do not have a clinical history of myocardial ischemia or angina pectoris prior to their infarction. The diagnosis of acute myocardial infarction is based on symptoms of myocardial ischemia, electrocardiographic hallmarks (ST segment and T wave abnormalities, pathologic Q waves), and the presence of cardiac enzymes in the blood that provide direct evidence of myocyte necrosis. Some patients with acute myocardial infarction do not experience symptoms (silent myocardial infarction).

Myocardial infarction results in the loss of myocytes and the formation of a scar. For large infarctions, particularly with an anterior wall location, and for patients with multiple infarctions, the resulting interstitial fibrosis, myocardial slippage, and infarct area expansion over time may result in cardiomegaly and severely depressed left ventricular pump function. This scenario may lead to chronic heart failure, with an extremely poor prognosis.

Treatment and Secondary Prevention

The treatment of coronary artery disease may include the use of medications, revascularization procedures, risk factor modification, and transplantation (Giuliani et al., 1991; Pashkow & Dafoe, 1993). For patients with demonstrable myocardial ischemia, treatment with anti-ischemic medications is indicated. Long- or short-acting nitrates are vasodilators that decrease myocardial oxygen requirement (reduced preload and afterload) and potentially may increase myocardial oxygen supply. Calcium channel blocking drugs are also vasodilators and reduce coronary vasospasm. Beta adrenergic blockers reduce heart rate, blood pressure, and contractility (decrease myocardial oxygen requirement). They are also effective in reducing ventricular arrhythmias.

Angiotensin-converting enzyme inhibitors are powerful vasodilators and have been demonstrated to decrease infarct expansion. These agents, along with digoxin and diuretics, are effective in the treatment of chronic heart failure and have been shown to improve survival. Aspirin, and other platelet-active medications such as ticlodipine, are given to reduce platelet aggregation and the risk of thrombosis. Aspirin and beta blockers improve survival after acute myocardial infarction. In postmenopausal women who have coronary artery disease, estrogen replacement therapy should be considered. Oral administration of estrogen replacement improves the blood lipid profile, primarily by causing an increase in high-density lipoprotein cholesterol concentrations, and also increases coronary vasodilation. Antioxidants such as vitamins E, C, and beta carotene may be beneficial in reducing progression of atherosclerosis and are under investigation.

For patients with symptoms or demonstrable myocardial ischemia that is not adequately controlled with medications, revascularization with catheter-based techniques (percutaneous transluminal coronary angioplasty, atherectomy, laser angioplasty, rotablator, stent placement) or coronary bypass surgery using internal thoracic arteries or saphenous vein sections as conduits is extremely useful (Giuliani et al., 1991). A substantial restenosis risk (approximately 30% of patients) within the first six months with catheter-based treatments somewhat limits the usefulness of these procedures. Coronary bypass grafting improves survival for patients with triple vessel disease, particularly in the setting of depressed left ventricular function. The saphenous vein (a large vein used for coronary bypass graft surgery) grafts are prone to develop obstructive lesions over time. For patients with end-stage heart failure, cardiac transplantation is the treatment of choice. For patients with acute myocardial infarction, the prompt use of thrombolytic agents to obtain reperfusion of the occluded artery is extremely useful in reducing infarct size. For patients with postinfarction chest pain, coronary angiography and coronary angioplasty are often employed to open the culprit stenosis.

Aerobic exercise training (more than thirty minutes, more than three sessions per week, more than 50% of maximal exercise intensity) in patients with coronary artery disease usually results in a 20 percent to 30 percent improvement in exercise capacity (Squires, 1994). Habitual exercise may improve symptoms of exertional intolerance such as angina pectoris, effort-related dyspnea, and fatigue. For a given intensity of physical activity, exercise training usually results in a lower heart rate and a lower myocardial oxygen requirement. Thus patients may perform activities with less myocardial ischemia. Exercise apparently does not improve the coronary collateral circulation that can be visualized on coronary angiography, but a reduction in thallium-determined myocardial ischemia at maximal exercise intensity has been reported after a period of exercise training (Squires, 1994). Exercise on a habitual basis has also been shown to retard progression and increase regression of coronary atherosclerosis observed on serial angiography. Meta analyses of trials of exercise training after myocardial infarction show a 20 to 25 percent reduction in cardiac events (cardiac mortality, fatal reinfarction).

Modification of coronary risk factors is an extremely important part of the treatment for coronary artery disease (Bittner, 1994; Pashkow & Dafoe, 1993; Squires et al., 1990). Cigarette smoking after myocardial infarction is associated with progression of atherosclerosis. Saphenous vein graft disease is also increased in smokers compared with nonsmokers or past smokers. Cessation of smoking after myocardial infarction reduces total mortality by 20 percent to 50 percent. An adverse blood lipid profile is a powerful indicator of progression of disease. In human coronary angiographic trials of established coronary atherosclerosis involving very aggressive treatment of blood lipids with diet and/or medications, reduced progression of disease has been demonstrated. In a minority of patients, some degree of regression of lesions may occur with treatment. Aggressive treatment of elevated low-density lipoprotein cholesterol with drugs resulted in a 30 percent reduction in total mortality and a similar reduction in nonfatal coronary events over a five-year period (Scandinavian Simvastatin Survival Study Group, 1994). Epidemiologic data show that in patients with angina pectoris or myocardial infarction, adequate control of hypertension is associated with improved survival. Left ventricular hypertrophy resulting from hypertension is a strong predictor of cardiovascular death.

A sedentary existence is a prevalent risk factor. In addition to the benefits of exercise training for patients with coronary artery disease discussed previously, risk factor improvements from a physical activity program include reduced blood pressure, improved glucose tolerance, and lower body fat stores; improved blood lipid profile, more normal blood platelet function, and better psychologic profile (Squires et al., 1990).

Obesity is associated with other established risk factors, such as dyslipidemia (adverse blood lipid profile, such as elevated cholesterol and triglycerides, and a low concentration of high density lipoprotein cholesterol); insulin resistance and glucose intolerance; hypertension; left ventricular hypertrophy; blood platelet abnormalities; and a sedentary lifestyle.

Psychological disturbance is associated with a greater rate of rehospitalization after a coronary event. Patients with a high level of aggressiveness, hostility, and competitiveness are more likely to suffer a coronary event than their more tranquil counterparts. Social isolation is associated with a poor prognosis after myocardial infarction. For patients with coronary artery disease, the following risk factor goals are recommended:

- low-density lipoprotein cholesterol less than 100 mg/dL;
- high-density lipoprotein cholesterol more than 35 mg/dL;
- blood pressure less than 140/90;
- exercise of more than thirty minutes, more than three sessions per week;
- complete cessation of tobacco use;
- body weight less than 130 percent of ideal;
- fasting blood glucose less than 140 mg/dL;
- adequate stress management and coping skills.

Rehabilitation Issues

Cardiac rehabilitation has become an accepted component of patient care after myocardial infarction or coronary revascularization (Squires et al., 1990). The process of cardiac rehabilitation assists patients in returning to a productive and sastisfying lifestyle as soon as possible after recognition of the disease as well as secondary prevention of coronary atherosclerosis. Comprehensive programs involving a variety of health-care professionals are available in many hospitals and clinics. These highly organized programs generally follow guidelines provided by the American Association of Cardiovascular and Pulmonary Rehabilitation and provide supervised exercise training, risk factor modification, education, and counseling (American Association of Cardiovascular and Pulmonary Rehabilitation, 1995). Two important aspects of rehabilitation deserve further discussion: the psychological reaction to a cardiac event and adjustment to coronary artery disease, and impairment/return-to-work issues.

A cardiac event elicits intense emotional responses from patients (Pashkow & Dafoe, 1993; Squires, 1994; Squires et al., 1990). Estimates of psychological distress after myocardial infarction generally indicate anxiety in 20 percent to 40 percent of patients and depression in 30 percent to 50 percent. Patients with a history of previous psychiatric illness, a record of substance abuse, those who are socially isolated, and persons with repeated major losses in life appear to be more vulnerable to distress after a cardiac event. In addition, a disruption in family functioning that may result in role reversal between spouses, financial pressures, and disorganization may worsen the coping ability of the patient. Fortunately, most patients' psychological problems resolve spontaneously within three months of the event. Psychiatric intervention is indicated for patients with prolonged periods of anxiety, depression, or other obvious adjustment disorders. Cardiac rehabilitation programs, counseling, and support groups are effective in assisting patients and families in coping with a coronary event.

Physical impairment after myocardial infarction or coronary surgery may be related to the following factors: psychological status, left ventricular function and exercise capacity, the presence of myocardial ischemia or life-threatening arrhythmias, and the recovery period after the event (Pashkow & Dafoe, 1993). After myocardial infarction, patients are usually restricted from returning to their occupations for one to twelve weeks, depending upon the size of the infarct and the demands of the job. Return to work after coronary bypass surgery is generally recommended in six to twelve weeks from the surgery date. Some patients who are symptomatic with minimal exertion, or high-risk patients with profoundly reduced left ventricular performance with congestive heart failure may not be able to return to physically or psychologically demanding occupations or hobbies.

Although the vast majority of postinfarct patients do return to work, approximately 30 percent of all disability payments in the United States are attributed to coronary artery disease. Physical impairment may be quantified by exercise testing and comparison of exercise capacity with norms for age and gender as well as with the average energy demands of the patient's occupation. For patients with poor exercise capacities, a period of exercise conditioning potentially to improve exercise capacity should be carried out before a decision regarding disability is made. The following factors are predictive of a poor probability of return to work after a cardiac event:

- age of more than sixty years;
- severe left ventricular dysfunction;
- history of previous cardiac events;
- overprotective attitude of the primary physician and/or family;
- poor patient confidence in ability to perform the job;
- employer unwillingness to modify the job description/requirements;
- financial disincentives such as disability payments;
- poor patient job satisfaction.

A formal job evaluation, including the physical requirements, cardiovascular demands, psychological stressors, and environmental factors such as temperature, humidity, air quality, and shift changes may be necessary before some patients are allowed to return to work. Vocational counseling and potential job retraining are important components of comprehensive rehabilitation.

(*See also:* DISABILITY MANAGEMENT; PHARMACOLOGY; PHYSICIAN; PSYCHOSOCIAL ADJUSTMENT; STROKE; SURGERY; WELLNESS; WORK)

RESOURCE

American Heart Association, 7320 Greenville Ave., Dallas, TX 75231

BIBLIOGRAPHY

AMERICAN ASSOCIATION FOR CARDIOVASCULAR AND PULMONARY REHABILITATION. *Guidelines for Cardiac Rehabilitation Programs,* 2nd ed. Champaign, IL, 1995.

BITTNER, VERA. "Primary and Secondary Prevention of Ischemic Heart Disease." *Current Opinion in Cardiology* 9 (1994):417–427.

GIULIANI, EMILIO R.; FUSTER, VALENTINE; GERSH, BERNARD J.; McGOON, MICHAEL D.; and McGOON, DWIGHT C. *Cardiology: Fundamentals and Practice,* 2nd ed. St. Louis, 1991.

PASHKOW, FREDERICK J., and DAFOE, WILLIAM A., eds. *Clinical Cardiac Rehabilitation: A Cardiologist's Guide,* Baltimore, 1993.

SCANDINAVIAN SIMVASTATIN SURVIVAL STUDY GROUP. "Randomized Trial of Cholesterol Lowering in 4,444 Patients with Coronary Heart Disease: The Scandinavian Simvastatin Survival Study (4S)." *Lancet* 344 (1994):1383–1389.

SQUIRES, RAY W. "Mechanisms by Which Exercise Training May Improve the Clinical Status of Cardiac Patients." In *Heart Disease and Rehabilitation,* 3rd ed., eds. Michael L. Pollock and Donald H. Schmidt. Champaign, IL, 1994.

SQUIRES, RAY W., and WILLIAMS, WILLIAM L. "Coronary Atherosclerosis and Acute Myocardial Infarction." In *ACSM's Resource Manual for Guidelines for Exercise Testing and Prescription,* 2nd ed. Philadelphia, 1993.

SQUIRES, RAY W.; GAU, GERALD T.; MILLER, TODD D.; ALLISON, THOMAS G.; and LAVIE, CARL J. "Cardiovascular Rehabilitation: Status, 1990." *Mayo Clinic Proceedings* 65 (1990):731–755.

SUE, DARRYL Y. "Exercise Testing in the Evaluation of Impairment and Disability." *Clinics in Chest Medicine* 15 (1994):369–386.

RAY W. SQUIRES

CORRECTIONAL REHABILITATION

The men and women who live in correctional institutions present the same types of demands for rehabilitation services as people in our communities except for one important aspect: Their disabilities, physical and/or mental, overlay their tendency to disregard society's laws. They may have committed a crime because of poor judgment, or they may have lived most of their lives flagrantly disregarding the legal parameters of behavior. From the undersocialized individual who grew up in poverty with no one to teach prosocial values, to the white-collar criminal with a professional degree but who was addicted to drugs, all need rehabilitation during their incarceration. Which types of services to be offered and the "costs" of these services have become highly politicized. Should offenders have access to free college education when law-abiding citizens must borrow money for their children's education? Or should nonviolent offenders sit idly for the duration of their incarceration, with the desire to improve themselves so they can contribute to society when they are released, but not be afforded the opportunity to do so? While these issues are argued frequently by politicians and taxpayers, most correctional professionals agree that opportunities for rehabilitation are a crucial part of the correctional setting.

The pendulum on which the emphasis on "rehabilitation" swings has moved back and forth radically since the 1950s. In the "enlightened" 1960s, liberal penologists believed that we should "tear down the walls" and allow inmates to govern themselves (DiIulio, 1990). And they believed that offenders could be "cured" of their criminality in much the same way that physical ailments are cured. This philosophy has been countered by the "lock 'em up and throw away the key" approach (DiIulio, 1990).

Since the mid-1970s, an approach between these two extremes has been taken. That is, offenders should be housed in a safe, humane environment where they are held accountable for their behavior and offered opportunities to "rehabilitate" themselves. Other than mandatory work and some mandatory education classes, rehabilitation programs are voluntary for the most part. The spirit of the current correctional approach is that individuals are responsible for themselves. Hopefully they will choose to take advantage of programs that will help them get out of prison and stay out of prison. But if they fail to take advantage of these opportunities, they will bear the consequences.

Current Practices

The American Correctional Association publishes standards for operating correctional institutions. These standards are developed by working correctional professionals and decided by consensus. They reflect the most current views of sound correctional policy and practice. The current *Standards for Adult Correctional Institutions* (American Correctional Association, 1990) include specific criteria governing the classification process, in which the offender's level of security (low, medium, or high) is determined along with his or her needs for work programs, academic/vocational programs, and therapeutic programs. During the classification process the offender's need for rehabilitation is determined. Reading level, education level, and employment history are reviewed, and needed programs become part of the plan. Also, mental health needs are assessed through clinical interviews with psychologists and, in some cases, psychological testing is administered. Therapeutic programs such as individual and/or group therapy may become part of the inmate's plan. If any addictive behaviors (gambling, drugs, or alcoholism) are evident in the offender's history, then participation in these therapeutic programs is encouraged and expected.

Education/Vocational Rehabilitation. In many cases, adult offenders did not complete their high school education, and often, if they have a diploma, their reading levels are much lower than twelfth grade. Most adult offenders have followed a pattern of delinquency that escalated during their middle school years and included truancy from school and failing grades, even if they were intelligent enough to succeed. *Standards for Adult Correctional Institutions* (American Correctional Association, 1990) states that academic and vocational training programs must be licensed or approved by the state department of education. Additionally, all teachers (academic and vocational), supervisors, and administrators should be certified by the state and should receive additional training to meet the needs of inmates.

Mandatory Literacy Programs. The Crime Control Act of 1990 included language that required the federal prison system to mandate that offenders achieve literacy at the eighth-grade level (McCollum, 1992). Before that legislation, it was mandatory that offenders read at the sixth-grade level. Many studies have pointed to the positive relationship between education and vocational training and the offenders' postrelease success. Offenders who have education and job skills when they reenter the job market fare much better than those who do not have these skills.

In 1991 the Correctional and Sentencing Committee of the American Bar Association (ABA) voted to support the concept of mandatory literacy. They agreed that the standard of mandatory literacy in all state adult correctional institutions should be the high school diploma or the General Equivalency Diploma (GED). In February 1992 this recommendation was approved by the House of Delegates of the ABA, and it became official ABA policy.

Beyond mandatory literacy programs, offenders who participate in vocational training programs and college-level courses tend to adjust better to incarceration, are more likely to find and keep employment while in a halfway house, and earn more money after release (McCollum, 1992). Such rehabilitative opportunities have been shown to serve the individual and society as well.

Vocational Training. Adult correctional institutions offer vocational training opportunities for offenders who have never worked, and for offenders who cannot return to their previous trade or profession because they have been convicted of a felony. For example, offenders who were physicians or nurses who became addicted or who illegally sold controlled substances would be restricted from practicing medicine by their state licensing boards. These offenders must learn new skills for their reentry into the job market.

Sometimes offenders believe that the high-pressure job they held, such as stockbroker or attorney, led them to become overwhelmed and out of control and subsequently contributed to their alcoholism or drug dependence. They believe their best chance for success is to redirect their abilities into a vocational area they can handle more effectively. Many adult correctional institutions contract with local college faculty to provide vocational courses at the prison for inmates.

Prerelease Preparation. For a prisoner, other than the time of adjusting to prison when first incarcerated, the next most difficult time is during the months preceding release from prison and to a halfway house before full release to the community. Prerelease programs often include providing the offender with information about parole supervision, expectations of the halfway house, and counseling programs to address the individual needs of the offender. Many are anxious and find that reentering the family structure they left is not as smooth as they had thought.

While in a halfway house, the offender secures employment or continues working with vocational rehabilitation services to gain new skills. The purpose of the halfway house stay is to provide a transition period for the offender.

Rehabilitation Programs: Mental Health

Many resources are still directed toward providing rehabilitative services to offenders who are addicted to drugs or alcohol; guilty of sex offenses; or who have chronic physical or mental disabilities. Eventually the offenders with these problems will be released, and any gains that can be made toward their rehabilitation while they are incarcerated improve their chances for successful reintegration into their communities.

Drug and Alcohol Rehabilitation. In 1966 the Narcotic Addict Rehabilitation Act mandated that prisons provide treatment for addicts who were convicted of violations of federal law (Wallace et al., 1990). The drug treatment units were developed as therapeutic communities with an emphasis on group therapy and an aftercare program that included urinalysis and counseling while in the community. All evaluations of these programs concluded that offenders who had the benefit of this type of treatment in prison had better chances of postprison success (Wallace et al., 1990). In the mid-1980s such "rehabilitative" programs fell out of political favor, and therefore resources became scarce. But a few years later, a political and social "War on Drugs" began anew, and prisons again received resources for rehabilitative programs.

In 1985 the health care cost to diagnose, treat, and rehabilitate illegal-drug users was more than $2.2 billion (U.S. Department of Justice, 1992). In 1990, on an average day there were more than 200,000 men and women serving time for drug offenses in local, state, and federal correctional facilities. It is estimated that 30 percent to 60 percent of these inmates have a moderate to severe drug problem (U.S. Department of Justice, 1992).

The major therapeutic interventions available in drug treatment programs for offenders typically include individual counseling, group counseling, urine surveillance, and referral to a support group such as Alcoholics Anonymous (AA) or Narcotics Anonymous (NA). There are many therapeutic approaches that initially help offenders understand their substance abuse problem and need, such as drug education and family therapy. Additional programs help offenders control their addiction, such as behavior modification and relapse prevention training. Once the offenders have gained control, they participate in programs that enhance their ability to remain drug-free. These services include job training and placement, job-search skills, and training in life skills such as budgeting and parenting.

Most individuals who are convicted of a crime and have a significant drug and/or alcohol problem are required by the court to participate in a drug rehabilitation program. The setting in which the offender serves his or her sentence depends on the seriousness of the crime. If the crime is not deemed serious and the offender poses no risk to the community, the offender will likely participate in a community-based treatment program. If the offender is to be incarcerated but the sentence is for less than one year, the offender will serve the sentence in jail and participate in a program offered by that jail. If the sentence is for more than one year, the offender will serve the sentence in prison: a state institution for violation of state laws, and a federal correctional institution if a federal law was violated.

Community-based treatment programs operate through various government agencies and private organizations. More than two hundred exemplary programs are listed in the directory published by the National Criminal Justice Association (1991). Treatment Alternatives to Street Crime (TASC) programs were begun in 1972; in 1989, more than 125 TASC and similar programs were operational in twenty-five states. These community-based programs monitor the drug- or alcohol-dependent offender from the point of identification through the treatment process and follow-up care (U.S. Department of Justice, 1992).

Jails typically offer treatment programs of thirty days to six months' duration, depending on the average length of stay of the offenders. After treatment in jail, the offender receives follow-up care in the community.

Almost all state prison systems offer support groups such as AA and NA. Ex-offenders who are recovering addicts participate as volunteers to provide inmates with support and encouragement. Volunteers follow the released offender into the community to provide continuity of care (U.S. Department of Justice, 1992).

In 1988, the federal prison system developed a new comprehensive strategy to treat drug addiction. Since then, the federal prison system has opened residential treatment units in more than half of its sixty-six correctional institutions. The treatment program follows a "biopsychosocial" model, which is based on the premise that addiction results from a variety and combination of hereditary factors, psychological factors, and social factors (U.S. Department of Justice, 1991). With the philosophy of personal responsibility as the therapeutic basis for the program, offenders learn to identify and correct criminal thinking patterns; to identify reactive thoughts that lead to feelings of anger and depression; to communicate effectively; to identify situations that increase their vulnerability to using drugs or alcohol; and to create a healthy lifestyle. It takes six to twelve months to complete the program, which also has a strong aftercare component.

Sex Offender Rehabilitation. Probably no crime is more harrowing to the public than offenses committed by child molesters and sexual psychopaths. In many cases the report of the offense is accompanied by a history of the offender, which includes descriptions of previous accusations, arrests, and convictions for sex crimes. From 1988 to 1990 the population of sex offenders in U.S. prisons grew by 48 percent (Marques, 1994).

Until the early 1990s there was little optimism that sex offenders could be "rehabilitated." However, now there are indications that programs that use a relapse prevention approach and cognitive behavioral methods are having some success (Marques, 1994). This treatment philosophy is based on the theory that sexual deviancy is a deeply ingrained pattern of behavior that can be controlled but not "cured." Offenders are taught methods to help them gain control of their sexual deviancy and then taught to prevent relapsing or reoffending. They learn to appreciate the degree of psychological and physical pain they have inflicted on others and learn to recognize and avoid places and situations that could put them at risk of engaging in a sex crime again. They learn to use support systems in the community and learn where to turn for help if they begin to lose control.

In the federal prison system's sex offender treatment program, the offender is involved in individual therapy and group therapeutic approaches that include victim empathy groups, behavior therapy groups, anger management, and cognitive distortions groups. The offender lives in a therapeutic community atmosphere within the prison while participating in a twelve-month program. During this time the offender is also involved in work and education programs. Aftercare supervision is carefully coordinated with the supervising parole officer or law enforcement representative in the offender's community.

Rehabilitation for Offenders with Physical or Mental Disability. The Americans with Disabilities Act covers all Americans, law-abiding as well as offenders. Prison officials have additional demands to address when providing housing and programs for offenders with disabilities. Offenders who are physically disabled are frequently housed in correctional medical centers—correctional institutions that are secure from escape and that provide a range of medical care, from acute services such as surgical procedures to care for persons with chronic physical or mental illness. These medical centers offer a full range of rehabilitative activities such as physical therapy, occupational therapy, and vocational therapy.

Offenders who are mentally retarded are offered special education programs and vocational programs. The offenders with chronic mental illness who must remain on psychotropic medications have the opportunity to work in sheltered workshop-type settings within the institution. They participate in art therapy, life skills groups, and individual and group therapy. Of special concern is protection of these offenders from predatory inmates who would steal from or abuse them.

Inmates who are too mentally ill to be released to their communities upon completion of their prison sentence are referred to state psychiatric facilities for further care.

Rehabilitation: Special Populations

Two special populations that are growing faster than the general prison population are female offenders and the number of long-term inmates. Each of these groups presents new challenges for rehabilitative services.

Female Offenders. The population of female offenders "grew at a faster rate than the male population in seven of the ten years between 1981 and 1991" (Kline, 1992). More than 5,000 women were incarcerated in the federal prison system in 1991. These numbers represented a 254 percent increase in growth over the previous ten-year period. The growth rate for male inmates was 147 percent (Kline, 1992).

More than 80 percent of incarcerated female offenders are single parents (Bartolo, 1992). This contrasts starkly to male inmates, who generally have not been the head of a single-parent family before their incarceration. Rehabilitation programs for women need to be somewhat different from those offered to men, but neither population should be underserved. Because female offenders generally are more likely to react to their incarceration with depression and anxiety about their separation from their children than male offenders, and because female offenders seek mental health services more frequently than do male offenders, correctional institutions need to have sufficient staff to meet these demands (Bartolo, 1992). Parenting classes, vocational training programs that interest women, and therapeutic groups that deal with overcoming dependency issues and the trauma of physical and sexual abuse are all important aspects of rehabilitative programs for women.

Long-term Inmates. Inmates are considered to be "long term" if they will serve ten years or more of their sentence incarcerated. Because of modification of sentencing legislation, elimination of parole at the federal level, and establishment of mandatory minimum sentences for some offenses, the numbers of inmates who are going to serve ten years or more are growing (Gordon & Wallace, 1991). From 1989 to 1990 the number of inmates serving fifteen years or more grew from 2,308 (or 5.4% of the federal prison population) to 4,034 (or 8.0% of the federal prison population) (Gordon & Wallace, 1991).

Most inmates are concerned about keeping ties with their families over the long term of their sentence. If they are married, they worry that their spouse will divorce them. If they have elderly relatives, they worry that they will not survive until their release. Therapeutic programs directed at learning to control anxieties and worries and at maintaining mental and physical health are important.

Long-term inmates want to stay current with vocational skills and pursue education programs, not only for acquisition of these skills but also for the opportunity to keep busy and to help pass the time. Institution work programs afford the inmate the opportunity to work and to save money to reestablish a home upon release. Transition programs help the inmate adjust to increased freedom and familiarity with the community as he or she approaches the end of a long sentence.

Future of Correctional Rehabilitation

Rehabilitation programs for offenders have steadily improved in kind and quality since the 1950s. As our understanding of "criminality" increases, so does our ability to develop rehabilitative programs that address the causes and control of criminal behavior. From a humanitarian perspective, offering individuals an opportunity to correct their behavior and improve themselves is the right thing to do. And from a cost-benefit perspective, although it is expensive to offer rehabilitative programs, it is far cheaper than having every offender recidivate to prison. The time, money, and effort invested in developing and implementing correctional rehabilitative programs are society's demonstration of its optimism in itself.

(*See also:* ALCOHOL REHABILITATION; AMERICANS WITH DISABILITIES ACT; DRUG REHABILITATION; PSYCHIATRIC REHABILITATION; PSYCHOLOGY; VIOLENCE)

RESOURCES

American Correctional Association, 8025 Laurel Lakes Court, Laurel, MD 20707–5075

National Criminal Justice Association, 444 North Capitol St., NW, Suite 608, Washington, DC 20007

National Institute of Justice, 633 Indiana Ave., Washington, DC 20531

BIBLIOGRAPHY

AMERICAN CORRECTIONAL ASSOCIATION. *Standards for Adult Correctional Institutions,* 3rd ed. Laurel, MD, 1990.

BARTOLO, ANN D'AUTEUIL. "A Journey to Understanding and Change." *Federal Prison Journal* 3 (1992):15.

DIIULIO, JOHN J., JR. "Prisons That Work." *Federal Prison Journal* 1 (1990):7–9.

GORDON, JUDY, and WALLACE, SUSAN. "Long-Term Inmates: A Preliminary Look at Their Programming Needs and Adjustment Patterns." *Federal Prison Journal* 2 (1991):61–62.

KLINE, SUE. "A Profile of Female Offenders in the Federal Bureau of Prisons. *Federal Prison Journal* 3 (1992):33.

MARQUES, JANICE; DAY, DAVID; NELSON, CRAIG; and WEST, MARY ANN. "Effects of Cognitive Behavioral Treatment on Sex Offender Recidivism." *Criminal Justice and Behavior Journal* 21 (1994):29.

NATIONAL CRIMINAL JUSTICE ASSOCIATION. *Directory of State-Identified Intervention Treatment Programs for Drug-Dependent Offenders.* Washington, DC, 1991.

MCCOLLUM, SYLVIA. "Mandatory Literacy: Evaluating the Bureau of Prisons' Longstanding Commitment." *Federal Prison Journal* 3 (1992):33–36.

U.S. DEPARTMENT OF JUSTICE. *Drug Treatment Programs: Meeting the Challenge.* Washington, DC, 1991.

———. *Drugs, Crime, and the Justice System: A National Report.* Washington, DC, 1992.

WALLACE, SUSAN; PELISSIER, BERNADETTE; MCCARTHY, DANIEL; and MURRAY, DONALD. "Beyond Nothing Works: History and Current Initiatives in the Bureau of Prisons' Drug Treatment." *Federal Prison Journal* 1 (1990):23–26.

VICKI DELLINGER VERDEYEN

COUNSELING

See ADJUSTMENT SERVICES; CAREER COUNSELING; PSYCHOLOGY; REHABILITATION COUNSELING; SOCIAL WORK

CREDENTIALS

Credentialing in rehabilitation includes both the process of individual recognition and competence and the accreditation or approval of professional education programs that prepare individuals to work in rehabilitation settings. Credentials are available for professionals working in the broad field of rehabilitation (e.g., rehabilitation counselors, vocational evaluators, insurance rehabilitation specialists, physicians, physical therapists, occupational therapists) and for facilities (e.g., rehabilitation hospitals and community-based programs) serving individuals with disabilities. However, to limit the scope of the topic, rehabilitation counseling is used as an example in the discussion of credentialing that follows. The scope of this entry will include three main areas: the development and influences of credentialing/accreditation processes, the meaning of different types of credentials applicable to the rehabilitation counseling profession, and the implications of their importance in meeting the needs of individuals with disabilities. Refer to the specific professions of interest for details about the credentialing process for each respective discipline.

The rehabilitation counseling profession has been widely acknowledged as the leading specialty in the development of credentialing mechanisms through national certification and educational program accreditation—the cornerstones of the general counseling professionalization system (Brooks & Gerstein, 1990; Remley, 1992). The historical evolution of credentialing in rehabilitation counseling reviewed here is to provide a conceptual understanding of the interrelationships of these processes.

Since 1970, rehabilitation counseling has witnessed substantial credentialing progress; however, it has been predominantly isolated within its own particular arena. The profession of rehabilitation counseling has evolved from its early history as a legislatively based occupation that was practiced in a limited number of settings to its current status as a profession that is practiced in diverse settings employing various service delivery systems (Jenkins, Patterson, and Szymanski, 1992; Tarvydas & Leahy, 1993). This evolution has aided and been aided by the process of credentialing.

Even though the rehabilitation counseling profession was an early and innovative leader among counseling and related rehabilitation specialty groups in the establishment and refinement of national credentialing standards and processes, the rehabilitation counseling profession is challenged to maintain its vision and autonomy in the counseling professionalization movement. It has become difficult to respond effectively in the increasingly complex environment of agency and federal regulatory bureaucracy and the arena of professional counseling "turfdom."

Terminology

A professional credential is accorded to programs, agencies, or individuals who have earned the right to offer a particular type of service to consumers. Attainment of a credential results from successful mastery of criteria established by professional organizations, professional preparation programs, credentialing bodies, or a government agency. The purpose of a credential is to validate some combination of practice, education, and examination and is evidence to an employer or consumer that a practicing professional is competent to offer services (Carter el al. 1990). Credentials are often viewed as symbols that represent the maturity level of a profession. As professionalization brings sophistication to credentialing standards, responsibilities and commitments among the various professional groups become intertwined.

Within higher education, accreditation should be distinguished from certification and licensure. Whereas accreditation applies to the recognition of institutions or programs of study, certification, registration, and licensure apply only to individuals. Certification is the process by which states and professional bodies recognize the particular competence of individual practitioners. Registration is usually viewed as a precursor to certification and involves a "listing" or registry of individuals who meet particular standards or requirements and who desire to use a particular title in their professional practice. Licensure is the process by which states authorize individuals to practice an otherwise restricted profession and is commonly referred to as a "screening out" process, whereas certification is a "screening in" process (Jenkins, Patterson, and Szymanski, 1992). Since the mid-1980s, there has been a resurgence of both certification and licensure in the counseling field.

Accreditation

There is a long-recognized and arguably proper responsibility of institutions and program accrediting associations to assist in improving the quality of the enterprises of education programs in schools and colleges (Crosson, 1987). This responsibility has historically been achieved by program accreditation.

Programs of higher education and the higher ed-

223

ucation institutions as a whole are accredited by basically two types of accrediting bodies: those that provide specialized accreditation of professional schools and degree-awarding or diploma-granting programs, and those that accredit institutions as a whole.

Stephen M. Jung (1986) has written that one of the major mechanisms through which the U.S. postsecondary education community acts to verify and improve education quality is through nongovernmental accreditation. Richard G. Millard (1983) has provided a comprehensive overview of the development and value of an accreditation process and some of its strengths and benefits. Accreditation has long been recognized as a motivator and mechanism for institutional and programmatic self-study and change (Diamond, 1982; Healey, 1980; Warren, 1980).

But accreditation is more than a passive process for promoting self-improvement and gaining program recognition. In the past, accreditation has at times been conceived and practiced as the determination of whether an educational institution meets certain stipulated standards, primarily quantitative, such as the size and credentials of the faculty, the number of books in the library, and so forth (Crosson, 1987). This conception of accreditation came to be viewed as focusing too exclusively on the quantifiable resources and not paying sufficient attention to empirically based research needs in professional practice and trends within a profession. Unfortunately, outdated program goals and purposes continue to be the primary norms by which programs are evaluated.

Theoretically, accreditation is an organized, systematic process for recognizing professional preparation programs and the institutions with which they are affiliated for achieving and maintaining a level of integrity, performance, and quality worthy of recognition. In contrast to most other countries, it is primarily through nongovernmental, voluntary professional associations or service-oriented institutions that professional preparation standards are established and recognized in the United States (Carter et al., 1990).

Accreditation, as it applies to this entry, is a recognition process that relates to programs (e.g., graduate rehabilitation counselor education programs) and institutions (e.g., colleges and universities). The two fundamental purposes of the accreditation process are "to assure the quality of the institution or program, and to assist in the improvement of the institution or program" (Council on Postsecondary Accreditation, 1990, p. 108). The status of accreditation is conferred by a recognized accrediting body and signifies that the program or institution meets and continues to meet the published standards of the accrediting body.

It is important to distinguish program accreditation from other traditional forms of assessment, which are often aimed only at determining whether the outcome (the "finished product") meets certain standards. Assessment of this sort focuses on the project product evaluation and involves comparative rankings of a product, such as one might see in *Consumer Reports*. Such assessment of a product or outcome may also be employed as part of the evaluation of a program producing the outcome. In this case, the assessment of the product, whether comparative or not, plays only a part. In contemporary program accreditation, interest is not only in the success or failure of a program but also in the process of achieving that success or failure (Crosson, 1987).

What is it about the opportunity to obtain "credentials" that assumes (or assures) program quality and promotes confidence in college-bound students, their families, and government agencies? Even though accreditation standards are not widely understood by the general public, students and their parents look to program accreditation as an indicator of quality and stability, and programs respond to these concerns by listing their affiliations with various accrediting bodies in their promotional literature (Lawrence & Green, 1980).

One might also ask how strong the relationship is between accreditation and quality. Accreditation sometimes focuses on quantitative assessment of program performance against institutional objectives or against other program standards. In contrast, quality (e.g., wealth, beauty, and wisdom) exists on a continuum of subjectivity; we all think we know what quality is when we see it, but we frequently have difficulty describing it for others. The literature suggests that accreditation has departed from an earlier preoccupation with "minimum standards" focusing on quantity issues and moved toward (1) continued quality reevaluation and use of alternative assessment approaches; and (2) innovation, experimentation, and self-improvement in educational programs as the principal goals of evaluation (Lawrence & Green, 1980).

Changing political and social environments are now, as in the past, playing a central role in shaping both the form and emphasis of accreditation. In pursuing the goal of serving the public interest, ways must be identified that avoid compromising the essential characteristics of accreditation as a voluntary, self-regulating, nongovernmental evaluation procedure.

Various institutional factors have also stimulated increased use of accreditation beyond its initial purposes resulting in a significant growth in professional specialization, an increased need for legitimacy, and the determination of eligibility for federal funds (Bjork, 1985). There is an implied belief that institutional administrative attitudes can be changed by expanding—even manipulating—the purposes of accreditation; programs and departments have long recognized that accreditation or the implication of sanctions can serve as a useful level in accomplishing particular institutional or program ends.

The accrediting body for graduate rehabilitation counseling programs is the Council on Rehabilitation Education (CORE), which was incorporated in 1972. The purpose of CORE accreditation of rehabilitation counselor education (RCE) programs is "to promote the effective delivery of rehabilitation services to individuals with disabilities by promoting and fostering continuing review and improvement of master's degree level RCE programs" (Council on Rehabilitation Education, 1991, p. 2). The purpose of CORE was more than simply to grant recognition and ensure compliance with existing standards; it also was designed to foster continuing program improvement, to respond to consumer priorities, and to encourage reevaluation of education standards as demanded by emerging trends in the field (McAlees & Schumacher, 1975).

The CORE standards for RCE programs address several areas: (1) the articulation and fulfillment of the RCE program's mission; (2) program curricula; (3) the knowledge, skills, and job performance of graduates; (4) the composition, resources, and professional involvement of students; and (5) the program's internal support and resources, including architectural accessibility and faculty background, expertise, and composition.

Most accrediting bodies use a combination of self-study and site review as the major tools for completing the accreditation review process. However, CORE uses a combination of multigroup surveys, an extensive self-study document, and an off-site examination of evidence by several reviewers. The multigroup surveys are used to examine compliance with the standards following input from five referent groups: current program students, recent graduates of the program, employers of graduates, supervisors of student interns, and program faculty (Szymanski et al., 1992). Before 1995, site reviews were used when specifically requested by a program, when large discrepancies exist between the survey results and the self-study evidence, and for schools that are in the initial years of the accreditation process (Council on Rehabilitation Education, 1991). Beginning in 1995, site reviews are to be employed both for initial accreditation and re-accreditation, as required by the Commission on Recognition of Postsecondary Accreditation (Council on Rehabilitation, 1995).

The founders of CORE felt that accreditation would be of value to clients, agencies, and society. They asserted that accreditation would help agencies by furnishing them with a better basis from which to select their employees and would serve the taxpaying public by providing better-trained counselors to provide quality service (Linkowski & Szymanski, 1993). Another important aspect of the philosophy of CORE was the administrative and policy-making involvement of most of the pertinent groups (employers and supervisors), not just the professional organizations directly related to the interests of rehabilitation counselor education. Consumers, minority representatives, the public, and related organizations have been given representation on CORE and the Commission on Standards and Accreditation. This broad-based representation is not typical in that most accrediting bodies were and are composed primarily of academic personnel directly involved in professional training.

The CORE accreditation process has not survived and grown without its critics. When an accreditation body establishes standards or competencies related to specific areas of practice, it locks the profession into a prescribed academic curriculum, according to Kenneth R. Thomas (1987). This initiative is seen by many as a prerogative that has traditionally rested within universities. Thomas contends that establishment of "fixed" competency or course work requirements limits the ability of universities to respond to new directions in the field because faculty are too busy teaching "required" courses to offer innovative ones. When the concept of rehabilitation counselor accreditation was first developed, the hope was that it would establish reasonable standards for excellence as well as encourage innovation, positive program development, self-evaluation, and individuality; instead it has seemed to encourage uniformity and stagnation and to reward mediocrity (Thomas, 1987).

Accreditation is sometimes accused of not differentiating those programs that are "good" from those that are not. It promotes the notion that outstanding, excellent, good, and fair counselor training programs will all be given the same seal of approval. As a result, accreditation, like certification, primarily serves to encourage mediocrity. That is, it is much more important for lesser programs to be accredited than it is for prestigious ones, because accreditation allows lesser programs to become more prestigious (Thomas, 1987, 1993).

The CORE accreditation process has also been criticized as being divisive for the accreditation of counseling programs in general. During the early 1990s, the American Counseling Association (ACA) also held a series of meetings on professionalism, focusing on issues of accreditation, certification, and advocacy (Linkowski & Szymanski, 1993). Efforts have been made by various individuals and programs to reduce conflict regarding these issues through activities such as cooperation in joint site visits (Linkowski & Szymanski, 1993).

To add to the confusion and external pressures that were being experienced by CORE during this period, the Council on Postsecondary Accreditation (COPA), a national organization that reviewed and recognized accrediting groups, voted to dissolve as of December 31, 1993. Two new organizations have since emerged to carry out the functions formerly addressed by COPA: the Commission on Recognition of Postsecondary Accreditation (CORPA), and

the Assembly of Specialized Accrediting Bodies (ASAB).

Accreditation has at times been more concerned with process than with results and has tended to evaluate institutions and programs on the basis of resources (Council on Postsecondary Accreditation, 1990). Often accreditation has appeared to be more interested in professional status than in the quality of educational preparation for entry into the field. But accreditation has evolved, and, in this evolution, has moved from quantitative and prescriptive approaches to more qualitative standards and increased emphasis on peer judgment. It has moved from a primary emphasis on process and resources to increased attention to results and learning outcomes.

Institutions and programs using the accrediting process can move toward increased quality through constructive innovation while maintaining diversity and continuity. Accreditation has played an impressive role in raising the quality of postsecondary academic programs.

Certification

Since the mid-1970s, certification efforts in rehabilitation counseling have played a major leadership role in the professionalization process for the counseling and rehabilitation professions.

Although certification is a voluntary process, more counselors have come to recognize the need for such credentials in their work environment. While counselors seek certification for a variety of reasons, certainly the growing demands of their marketplace are a very important one. For a majority of counselors, however, accountability is the driving force behind their desire for certification. By achieving certification, a practitioner can assure the individuals and the community being served that acceptable standards for practice will be followed.

The Commission on Rehabilitation Counselor Certification (CRCC) is the oldest credentialing body in the counseling field (Commission on Rehabilitation Counselor Certification, 1993). Its program is an outgrowth of the professional concerns of two organizations: the National Rehabilitation Counseling Association (NRCA) and the American Rehabilitation Counseling Association (ARCA) which created the Joint Committee on Rehabilitation Counselor Certification. The Joint Committee was chartered as a not-for-profit organization in 1973 and then renamed the Commission on Rehabilitation Counselor Certification (CRCC).

CRCC is a nonprofit independent credentialing body and a member of the National Commission for Health Certifying Agencies (NCHCA), an independent regulatory body that oversees the certification processes of its member organizations. The CRC credential has achieved increasing national and international recognition during this time. CRCC certifies rehabilitation counselors throughout the United States and several foreign countries (Leahy & Holt, 1993).

The purpose of CRCC is to provide assurances that professionals engaged in the practice of rehabilitation counseling have met established standards at the time of entry into the profession and have maintained these standards throughout their careers. The standards for certification are established by a commission composed of a public member (representing consumers), a member-at-large, and individuals from eight professional organizations directly involved in promoting the profession of rehabilitation counseling.

The certification credential also serves other purposes. For example, it helps promote the counseling profession by increasing the visibility of certified practitioners to consumers, colleagues, and counselors in related fields. It also has had the effect of bringing clearer definition to the practice of rehabilitation counseling (Leahy & Holt, 1993). As a result, the rehabilitation counseling profession has been forced to reexamine itself continually in order to maintain appropriate service delivery goals. In an environment that changes almost daily, certification has often served as the only standard by which professional practices can be accurately measured in order to protect the consumer from unqualified practitioners.

Since the mid-1980s there has been a continual increase in the recognition of the CRC credential by workers' compensation regulatory bodies, an overall increase in new applications for certification, and a higher level of recertification for those already certified. In addition, CRCC has pioneered international certification efforts through establishment of the Canadian Certified Rehabilitation Counselor

(CCRC) credentialing system and established the Foundation for Rehabilitation Certification, Education, and Research.

While this historical review has mentioned important milestones and events, it must be emphasized that the leadership of individual professionals as well as individuals in voluntary and staff roles with CRCC are responsible for championing this movement (Leahy & Holt, 1993).

Licensure

Counselor licensure legislation has been intended to regulate the use of the terms by which a statute officially refers to professional counselors as well as to protect the practice of professional counseling as set forth in the definition and scope of practice of the profession. This combination of title and practice legislation is the most stringent form of credentialing and would prohibit anyone from practicing counseling unless fully qualified, regardless of formal professional title (Tarvydas & Leahy, 1993).

There are three types of licensure laws: title laws, practice laws, and title and practice laws. Title laws regulate the use of the title of a "profession," whereas practice laws define and protect a professional's "scope of practice." Title and practice laws regulate both. Licensure laws, regardless of type, uniformly address educational requirements by delineating specific course work or noting degrees that are acceptable; some licensure laws specify that individuals must have graduated from nationally accredited programs. In addition, experience requirements relate to the number of years counseling services have been provided and generally include a specified amount of supervised field experience following a specified training program (Tarvydas & Leahy, 1993).

Because some of these laws specifically address rehabilitation counselors, it is imperative that rehabilitation counselors become familiar with their own state licensure laws. Although most licensure laws are directed at counselors who provide private counseling services (e.g., mental health counseling and psychotherapy), other counselors may be included, intentionally or unintentionally, in the law. Rehabilitation counselors who work for the state–federal rehabilitation program are generally exempt from state licensure laws.

The early 1990s was a critical period for rehabilitation counseling in the resolution of licensure issues due to the developmental and political forces in the counseling professionalization movement. This movement has occurred amid growing societal concerns about the role of governmental regulatory efforts in promoting consumer well-being and access to minimal health care services (Tarvydas & Leahy, 1993). Ignoring or minimizing the opportunity provided in the professional counseling movement toward licensure is no longer possible without disastrous results for many rehabilitation counselors. In this sense, the licensure movement has both contributed to the course of professionalization in rehabilitation counseling and exposed the potential weaknesses of this group's fragmented professional identity.

Vilia M. Tarvydas and Michael J. Leahy (1993) indicate that the prevalence of "title only" bills and the frequent exemption of government employees have contributed to limited but shortsighted involvement of rehabilitation counselors in the licensure movement; rehabilitation counselors working in the state–federal system did not think the licensure movement would have an effect on their futures. Ironically, passage of the "qualified rehabilitation personnel" stipulations for employees under the 1992 amendments to the Rehabilitation Act may have a substantial effect on the upgrading of staff in these programs. In any case, it would seem that the potential decline of the state–federal service delivery system to one staffed by professionals with credentials less stringent than for other counseling service sectors will be questioned by the public and the consumers of services in this setting.

Two factors external to the profession make involvement of rehabilitation counselors within the licensure arena critical. One factor is the priority and attention given the professionalization drive within the ACA on behalf of its approximately 59,000 members. The other factor is the pressing need to provide an external, logical, and well-supported organizational structure for the profession of counseling to consumers, legislators, and third-party payers. Some form of organizational alliance is necessary to maintain credibility in the face of the increasingly critical analysis of mental health and medical services. If a cohesive, comprehensive struc-

ture or arrangement is not forthcoming, counseling is not likely to fare well among the highly competitive mental health and allied health professions in the projected alignments developing around models of managed care and a national health care program (Tarvydas & Leahy, 1993).

In the private sector, rehabilitation counselors have at times circumvented concern with counselor licensure laws by relying on the ability to redefine job titles of staff, and to preserve the ability to carry on "practice as usual." Moreover, the private practice of rehabilitation counselors has been fueled by third-party payments for vocational rehabilitation services by vendors who have established standards that have recognized "qualified providers" through adoption of established rehabilitation counseling credentials, such as the CRC. Although licensure laws have been a concern to those in private practice (those providing mental health rather than rehabilitation services), the movement toward practice legislation could remove the "perceived refuge" in the private rehabilitation sector (Tarvydas & Leahy, 1993).

Registration

The credential with perhaps the least importance, in the eyes of the public, is professional counselor registration. A number of state workers' compensation laws or regulations specify the education, training, and/or credentials an individual must possess to provide rehabilitation counseling services to workers with disabilities (Patterson, 1987). In these states, rehabilitation counselors register with the state workers' compensation agency by paying a fee and providing proof of their education and/or certification. Thus registration is merely a listing or registry of individuals meeting certain education and experience requirements for a particular title. Many states claim to have licensure bills but really provide only for a registration credential. Most of these states do not specifically include the Certified Rehabilitation Counselor (CRC) credential for the provision of rehabilitation counseling services; however, the actual services (i.e., scope of services) that may be provided may be legislated and will vary by state (Jenkins, Patterson, and Szymanski, 1992). In many of the states that have only the registration credential, continuing education units (CEUs) or proof that the credential has been maintained are required.

The Future of Credentialing

Many factors are in place for meaningful dialogue among rehabilitation professionals and those in other counseling constituencies to facilitate a more effective system of professional counseling credentialing. Credentialing activities in rehabilitation counseling, although internally significant for the profession, have resulted in progress in understanding or clarification of the underlying basis of the professional skill levels and competencies possessed by individuals working in both a rehabilitation or counseling setting. However, the development of credentialing has been complicated by the profession's continuing controversy regarding which term should receive primary attention—rehabilitation or counseling (Tarvydas & Leahy, 1993). The historical presence of two professional organizations illustrates the difficulty in attaining agreement regarding requirements for professional credentials. NRCA, a division of NRA, advocates the "rehabilitation core" perspective of the rehabilitation counseling profession. On the other hand, ARCA, a division of ACA, contends that rehabilitation counseling is a specialty area of practice within the profession of counseling.

Development of a consistent counseling licensure law based on national standards is a goal advocated by many (Hoggard, 1993). The rationale for a model law should include several important principles and characteristics: (1) counselors need to be recognized and protected as a group; (2) standards of ethics and practice would create visibility, credibility, and provide incentives to pursue professional excellence; (3) a national license says that each individual has met and passed the same requirements; and (4) a license based on recognized national standards could help provide opportunities for insurance reimbursement that may become crucial to the future of the rehabilitation counseling profession.

Kenneth R. Thomas (1987) has suggested that there appears to be a shift in the loyalties of rehabilitation counselors from the professional associations to CRCC and similar certification bodies. He suggested that because certification bodies deal only

in credentialing and do not foster the scientific or professional development of the field, such shifting of loyalties could have tragic long-term consequences for development of the profession and professional credentials. Credentialing bodies do not generally publish or support generation of scholarly journal articles, fund scientific research, conduct legislative activities, or distribute useful information on practice trends to current practitioners and prospective students and the public at large. In short, they provide few services and support activities that are necessary and expected in establishing a respected, recognized profession.

Legislatures and those involved in third-party payment for services are becoming increasingly disturbed with fragmented groups of professionals. Other counseling specializations are slowly coming to realize that such fragmentation may diminish opportunities for greater national acceptance of counseling services and for third-party reimbursement. It would seem unfortunate if rehabilitation counselors did not evaluate this issue of fragmentation among related professional groups to allow them to maintain their historic leadership in the counseling field.

If the futurists are even partially correct, American higher education will foster organizational restructuring, provide more emphasis on outcome-based evaluation of student learning, and stimulate more effective instructional delivery systems. Higher education will most likely see the development of a heavy reliance on telecommunications and computer systems, and an emphasis on and an expectation of a new level of competence in graduates. Response to these external factors will surely facilitate the continuing growth and value of professional credentials in the rehabilitation field.

(*See also:* ALLIED HEALTH PROFESSIONS; EVALUATION OF REHABILITATION PROGRAMS; FUTURE OF REHABILITATION; NURSING, REHABILITATION; OCCUPATIONAL THERAPY; PHYSICAL THERAPY; PHYSICIAN; PRIVATE SECTOR REHABILITATION; PSYCHOLOGY, REHABILITATION; REHABILITATION COUNSELING)

BIBLIOGRAPHY

BJORK, LARS G. *Environmental Change and Regulatory Reform in Postsecondary Institutional Accreditation.* Washington, DC, 1985.

BROOKS, DAVID K., and GERSTEIN, LAWRENCE H.

"Counselor Credentialing and Interprofessional Collaboration." *Journal of Counseling and Development* 68 (1990):477–484.

CARTER, MARCIA J.; UHLIR, G. A.; CISSEL, WILLIAM B.; and GREBNER, FLORENCE. *Professionalization: Whose Responsibility?* New Orleans, 1990.

COMMISSION ON REHABILITATION COUNSELOR CERTIFICATION. *The CRC Certification Process.* Rolling Meadows, IL, 1993.

COUNCIL ON POSTSECONDARY ACCREDITATION. *The COPA Handbook.* Washington, DC, 1990.

COUNCIL ON REHABILITATION EDUCATION. *Accreditation Manual for Rehabilitation Counselor Education Programs.* Champaign-Urbana, IL, 1991.

———. *Accreditation Manual for Rehabilitation Counselor Education.* Rolling Meadows, IL, 1995.

CROSSON, FREDERICK. "The Philosophy of Accreditation." *North Central Association Quarterly* 62 (1987):1–13.

DIAMOND, JOAN. "School Evaluation and Accreditation: A Bibliography of Research Studies." *North Central Association Quarterly* 56 (1982):427–437.

HEALEY, JAMES S. "Accreditation from the Other Side: A Study of the Accreditation Process and Its Effort on Three Schools." *Journal of Education for Librarianship* 21 (1980):146–158.

HOGGARD, KERRY. "Recognizing Professional Counselors: The Case for Credentials." *The Guidepost,* Aug. 1993, p. 5.

JENKINS, WILLIAM M.; PATTERSON, JEANNE B.; and SZYMANSKI, EDNA M. "Philosophical, Historical, and Legislative Aspects of the Rehabilitation Counseling Profession." In *Rehabilitation Counseling: Basics and Beyond,* eds. Randal M. Parker and Edna M. Szymanski. Austin, TX, 1992.

JUNG, STEVEN M. *The Role of Accreditation in Directly Improving Educational Quality.* Washington, DC, 1986.

LAWRENCE, JUDITH K., and GREEN, KENNETH C. *A Question of Quality: The Higher Education Ratings Game.* Washington, DC, 1980.

LEAHY, MICHAEL J., and HOLT, EDA. "Certification in Rehabilitation Counseling: History and Process." *Journal of Applied Rehabilitation Counseling* 24 (1993):5–9.

LEAHY, MICHAEL J., and SZYMANSKI, EDNA M. "Epilogue: Rehabilitation Counseling Credentialing." *Journal of Applied Rehabilitation Counseling* 24 (1993):79–80.

LINKOWSKI, DONALD C., and SZYMANSKI, EDNA M. "Accreditation in Rehabilitation Counseling: Historical and Current Context and Process." *Journal of Applied Rehabilitation Counseling* 24 (1993):10–15.

McALEES, DANIEL C., and SCHUMACHER, BROCKMAN. "Toward a New Professionalism: Certification and Accreditation." *Rehabilitation Counseling Bulletin* 18 (1975):160–165.

MILLARD, RICHARD M. "Accreditation." In *Meeting the New Demand for Standards: New Directions for Higher Education,* ed. Jonathan R. Warren. San Francisco, 1993.

PATTERSON, JEANNE B. "Certified Rehabilitation Counselors (CRC)." *Journal of Applied Rehabilitation Counseling* 18 (1987):45–47.

REMLEY, TED. "Rehabilitation Counseling's Leadership Role in Professionalism." *The Guidepost,* 1992, p. 3.

SZYMANSKI, EDNA M.; PATTERSON, JEANNE B.; LINKOWSKI, DONALD C.; BUTLER, AL J.; and SPINTO, JANE E. "Rehabilitation Counseling Accreditation: Comparison of Two Review Processes." *Rehabilitation Education* 6 (1992):283–287.

TARVYDAS, VILIA M., and LEAHY, MICHAEL J. "Licensure in Rehabilitation Counseling: A Critical Incident in Professionalization." *Journal of Applied Rehabilitation Counseling* 24 (1993):16–23.

THOMAS, KENNETH R. "Warning! Certification and Accreditation May Be Hazardous to Rehabilitation Counseling's Health." *Journal of Rehabilitation* 53 (1987):19–22.

———. "Professional Credentialing: A Doomsday Machine Without a Failsafe." *Journal of Applied Rehabilitation Counseling* 24 (1993):74–76.

WARREN, JONATHAN R. "Is Accrediting Worth Its Cost?" *American Association for Higher Education Bulletin* 32 (1980):11–15.

MARVIN D. KUEHN

CUMULATIVE TRAUMA DISORDERS (CTD)

See MUSCULOSKELETAL DISORDERS

D

DANCE/MOVEMENT THERAPY

Throughout recorded history, humanity has recognized the therapeutic and cathartic powers of dance. In discussing the utilization of dance in ancient Greece, the Dutch psychiatrist and dance advocate Joost Meerloo (1967) states, "The holy craze and abandonment of inhibitions had for them a reviving and healing action" (p. 45). The mystery dance of the Greeks was part of a drive for rejuvenation and a greater intensity of life. The dance history literature suggests that the dance event is one of the oldest forms of healing interventions and experiences known to humankind. Century upon century, in ancient and preindustrial cultures, ritualistic movement, trance excitation, and community exultation and release were forms generated and integrated into a culture's social organization. In Lois Ellfeldt's (1976) description of dance in preindustrial cultures, she writes, "Dance was not diversion or entertainment, but was a serious part of living. Power was gained from the rhythmic interaction of sound and movement, from the collective expression of emotion, and the cooperating members of the group had a strength greater than any one of the group" (pp. 38–39).

The American Dance Therapy Association (ADTA) has defined dance/movement therapy as "the psychotherapeutic use of movement as a process which furthers the emotional, cognitive and physical integration of the individual." Since its founding in 1966, this professional organization has helped the field to evolve by developing standards of practice, educational guidelines and competencies, and professional credentialing. Much of what has developed in the United States under the auspices of the ADTA and the various graduate-level dance/movement therapy programs is now being copied worldwide, as the model is regarded as highly effective and professional.

Dance/movement therapists work in a wide variety of therapeutic, educational, and clinical settings, assisting individuals in their emotional, psychological, mental, and physical growth and development. One of the primary goals of dance therapy is the changing of the movement behavior of clients or patients in treatment. Also, because of their skill in analyzing movement behavior, dance/movement therapists are able to assist in interpreting a client's

231

current state of health or dysfunction. Three basic assumptions are central to dance/movement therapy intervention: (1) that the movement expression of an individual is reflective of intrapsychic dynamics; (2) that a change in movement expression will result in a personality or behavioral change; and (3) that the greater the range of movement potential expressed, the better one is able to cope with the changes and stresses of one's environment.

Many clients or patients in treatment have extremely limited and fixed movement patterns, which often reflect an equally frozen emotional state. Wilhelm Reich (1972) theorized that defenses were rooted in the body as chronic muscular tension, stating that "every increase of muscular tonus in the direction of rigidity indicates that a vegetative excitation, anxiety or sexuality has become bound up" (p. 375), and that tension in specific body parts relates to the resolution of conflicts by the repression of basic affects (e.g., holding in the chest is considered indicative of repressed feelings of needing and longing).

Dance/movement therapy first gained recognition in psychiatric facilities in the 1950s and 1960s in Washington, DC, and in southern California based on its effectiveness in reaching patients who were viewed as isolated, withdrawn, and exhibiting fragmented thought and feeling. Trudi Schoop and Jeri Salkin began an innovative program at Camarillo State Hospital in Camarillo, California, working closely with psychiatrists and calling their method "body-ego technique." Marian Chace, a key pioneer in the field on the East Coast of the United States and a founding member of the ADTA, would initially form a relationship with a patient by physically externalizing his or her affect or mood as she perceived it and in so doing began to create an energy bond, or rapport, through a rhythmical interchange. From the establishment of an energy/movement relationship, the dance of self-expression, development, and mastery would begin. Her pioneering work at St. Elizabeth's Hospital in Washington, DC, became world-renowned.

Essentially, dance/movement therapy is involved with the psychodynamic/psychotherapeutic growth and change of individuals in treatment. However, though it utilizes the body's potential for physical expression, it is not a body manipulation therapy per se. Dance/movement therapy has evolved its own comprehensive body of knowledge and has a complex relationship to several areas of theoretical practice, certain elements of which add to its theoretical frame and help to define and refine its clinical application, interpretation skills, and educational imperatives.

The first area consists of various elements inherent in the nonverbal communication field, such as movement analysis, the relationship between speech and gesture, crosscultural communication and expression, and the mother-child bond/attunement/mirroring relationships. The second area consists of the so-called body therapies, particularly their concern with postural alignment and manifestation of personality and stress reduction. Since one aspect of dance/movement therapy treatment focuses on the expressive use of the body and the relationship between various levels of tension and functional movement, understanding what kinesiological, anatomical, and emotional factors contribute to an individual's functional movement behavior adds yet another dimension to the spectrum of expression interaction. Even though dance/movement therapists do not use physical therapy or massage therapy techniques, it is essential for them to understand the role of hands-on body work in assisting individuals to release blocked energy and reduce stress levels. The third area of influence is that of the creative process, that is, the utilization of dance as an art form that incorporates imaginative, nonlinear levels of cognition and expression. The fourth key area consists of developmental movement, particularly how it reflects and affects the totality of body-mind development. The fifth area encompasses concepts gleaned from psychodynamic and psychotherapeutic theory; particularly important are object relations and self-psychology and the dynamics of transference and countertransference.

Using the body and the voice as its fundamental means of communication and expression, dance/movement therapy is concerned with processes that lead to unblocking resistances manifested in a frozen musculature, a rigid response pattern, or frozen postural patterns. Any or all of these may limit an individual's range of feeling expression, perceptual reception, reality testing, interpersonal relating, self-esteem and self-concept development, and body image awareness and continuity.

Significant changes have been shown to occur as a result of therapeutic dance/movement treatment, particularly in the areas of body-image development, self-concept development, and the ensuing elements affected by these constructs. For example, clinical dance/movement therapy with exceptional and mentally, physically, or emotionally challenged children has resulted in increased attention spans, diminishment of impulse control issues, and greatly enhanced gross and fine motor development (Leventhal, 1980). Other research shows that as energy is expressed, released, and formed during dance/movement, general energy levels are increased; fragmentation is reduced; and, as body defenses diminish, feelings, thoughts, and actions become more integrated. Dance therapy treatment with the elderly has been shown to result in enhanced cardiovascular and respiratory function; increased development of strength, endurance, coordination, control, and balance; and development of receptive and expressive language (Leventhal & Schwartz, 1989).

Dance/movement therapists practice throughout the United States and in Canada, South America, Mexico, Asia, Africa, Israel, Australia, and Europe. The field appears to be growing worldwide in popularity, and new training programs were developed in the 1980s and 1990s in England, Greece, Australia, Mexico, France, Sweden, Israel, and Italy. It is a rewarding profession for the creative artist wishing to go beyond a performing career into the helping professions as well as for trained psychologists or counselors desirous of adding another dimension to their psychotherapeutic practice.

To become a professional dance/movement therapist a master's degree is required, either in dance/movement therapy or in a related field with additional graduate study in psychology and human development, movement analysis, research skills, and dance therapy theory and practice, along with a clinical internship. Two discrete credentials are awarded to qualified graduates and new professionals by the ADTA. The first is that of DTR, dance therapist registered. Individuals with this designation have successfully completed their graduate training and are qualified and prepared to work within a pro-

fessional treatment setting under supervision. The second credential is the ADTR: Academy of Registered Dance Therapists. Individuals within this designation have met additional requirements of the ADTA and are fully qualified to teach, provide supervision within the field, and engage in private dance/movement psychotherapy.

(*See also:* ART THERAPY; MUSIC THERAPY; RECREATION; WELLNESS)

RESOURCE

The American Dance Therapy Association, 2000 Century Plaza, Suite 108, Columbia, MD 21044-3263

BIBLIOGRAPHY

ELLFELDT, LOIS. *Dance from Magic to Art.* Dubuque, IA, 1976.

LEVENTHAL, MARCIA B., ed. *Movement and Growth: Dance Therapy for the Special Child.* New York, 1980.

———. "The Ancient Healing Art of Dance." In *Kinesis,* Australian Association for Dance Education, Fall 1987, Melbourne, Australia.

———. "Stages of Therapeutic Unfolding in Dance Movement." In *Research in Arts Medicine,* Chicago, IL, 1993.

LEVENTHAL, MARCIA B., and SCHWARTZ, JUDITH. "The Dance of Life: Dance and Movement Therapy for the Older Adult." *Topics in Geriatric Rehabilitation* 4 (1989):67–74.

LEVY, FRAN J. *Dance Movement Therapy: A Healing Art.* Reston, VA, 1988.

MEERLOO, JOOST. "Dance Craze and Sacred Dance." In *Creativity and Externalization: Essays on the Creative Instinct.* Assen, Netherlands, 1967.

REICH, WILHELM. *Character Analysis.* 1949. Reprint. New York, 1972.

STANTON-JONES, KRISTINA. *Dance Movement Therapy in Psychiatry.* New York, 1992.

MARCIA B. LEVENTHAL

DEAF-BLINDNESS

Deaf-blindness is a low-prevalence disability that creates serious barriers to the inclusion and full participation of the individual in community, social, and work life. Critically, the individual with deaf-blindness will have limited opportunity to communicate with a variety of people, access information, develop meaningful social relationships, orient to, and move about the environment. Planning services for this unique group of people requires sensitivity by the service delivery system to the individual issues specific to deaf-blindness, and the creation of alternatives to services that have been traditionally provided for individuals with other disabilities.

Defining the Population

The most noted person in history who was deaf-blind was Helen Keller, born in Tuscumbia, Alabama, in 1880. Ms. Keller shared with the world her experiences as a person with deaf-blindness, and it is her image that most people around the world associate with this disability. The population of individuals with deaf-blindness is, however, a very heterogeneous group with a wide range of visual, auditory, and cognitive abilities. These persons may have been born with this disability or may have acquired it—there are a variety of causes.

Worldwide, there are few definitive demographic data of the numbers, ages, and etiologies of individuals who are deaf-blind. In the United States the 1992 census report estimated 7,839 children and other youth who are under age twenty-two years who meet the federal definition of deaf-blindness (Bagley, 1992). It is estimated that there are 30,000 to 45,000 individuals in the United States who are deaf-blind (Watson, 1993), although there are no statistical data on the total population of adults who are deaf-blind.

Causes

The documented incidence of deaf-blindness in any given region of the world will differ depending on such variables as availability of medical services, genetic disorders that may be prevalent in a given region, prenatal care, viral epidemics, and immunization programs, as well as the presence of a system of identification and service delivery for individuals who are deaf-blind.

During the late 1950s and 1960s there was a worldwide epidemic of rubella, also known as German measles. From this epidemic large numbers of children were born with deaf-blindness because their mothers had contracted this virus during the first trimester of pregnancy. The birth of these children

called attention to the needs of individuals with deaf-blindness and was the most significant event in the development of services for this disability group.

Immunization for the rubella virus has been mandated for all school-age children in the United States since the 1970s. Therefore, this etiology is represented primarily in the age group of individuals born during the 1963–1965 national epidemic and is only rarely reported in the under-twenty-one-years population in the United States. It remains, however, significant in the population of deaf-blindness in other parts of the world.

Individuals who were born with congenital rubella syndrome presented characteristics such as glaucoma, cataracts, sensorineural hearing loss, varying degrees of mental retardation, and other physical and neurological impairments. As this group has reached adulthood, additional medical concerns have arisen in many individuals such as diabetes, thyroid conditions, and increased seizure activity (Parker, 1992).

In addition to the population of individuals who were born with congenital rubella syndrome, there are several trends that contribute to the incidence of deaf-blindness in the United States, in many other developed countries, and in some developing regions of the world. Looking at this cross section of individuals with deaf-blindness can help in understanding the various challenges in the delivery of education and rehabilitation services.

First, there has been a growing population of elderly individuals in society. In the United States, the population of individuals who are over fifty-five years is increasing, with the population of individuals who are over age eighty-five increasing more rapidly than any other segment of this population. With the loss of vision and hearing being among the top ten chronic conditions experienced by older adults (Bagley, 1992), it is anticipated this age group will represent a steadily increasing number of people.

Advances in medical technology have also resulted in improved diagnostic procedures and in a decrease in mortality of infants born with multiple disabilities. There are increasing numbers of children born very prematurely, or with rare genetic syndromes that contribute to their deaf-blindness, posing a unique set of medical challenges and other complications associated with low birth weight and multiple physical anomalies. In past decades in the United States and in countries having unsophisticated medical care, the survival of these children beyond infancy was unlikely. Additionally, they would not have received a diagnosis of deaf-blindness because of the lack of available clinical technology (Riggio, 1992). Improved diagnostic procedures such as visual evoked potentials (VEP) and auditory brainstem response (ABR) allow objective measures of vision and hearing acuities in children who would in the past have been considered to be untestable.

Individuals with Usher's syndrome comprise a large portion of the deaf-blind population in the United States. This is a genetic condition wherein children are born deaf or hard of hearing, and show evidence of retinitis pigmentosa (RP), usually during their teen years. RP is a progressive eye disease that is characterized first by reduction of visual fields, often referred to as "tunnel vision," and loss of night vision, which can eventually lead to extreme visual field loss and total blindness.

Implications of Deaf-Blindness

The senses of vision and hearing are commonly referred to as distance senses. These senses connect the individual with the world beyond his or her immediate body space. It has been estimated that up to 75 percent of information received by the brain is visual (Smith & Cote, 1982). This significant statistic combined with an understanding that language is learned primarily through the auditory modality offers a beginning understanding of the impact this disability creates on the individual's ability to communicate with other people, access information, develop meaningful social relationships, and orient to move about the environment.

Difficulties in communication pose the most significant effect on the development of social relationships and acquisition of information. Helen Keller once said that "blindness separates people from things, and deafness separates people from other people." This statement captures the impact of this dual disability on the social, emotional, and intellectual development of the individual.

In many yet more complex ways, the issues of deaf-blindness are likened to those faced by individuals who are deaf. Many people in the deaf community view themselves as members of a subculture not unlike other minority populations who speak a different or foreign language (Dolnick, 1993). People with deaf-blindness are a smaller and more diverse subculture within society. Not unlike ethnic minority groups, facility of communication is what often creates the desire to live and socialize with individuals who utilize like "languages." The ability to connect directly with another person without external interpretation allows an individual to develop meaningful social relationships.

Individuals who are deaf-blind may express and receive information in a variety of ways that typically are not used by people without this disability. The mode of communication used will vary depending on the amount of functional residual vision and hearing, the presence of intellectual limitations, and other physical disabilities. These modes may include sign language, augmentative communication devices, finger spelling, gestures, and other nontraditional forms of communication. Of great significance is the reliance of the individual, regardless of his or her communication skill level, on another person to access information about the environment and to receive personal feedback from others.

Educational and vocational training requires individual instruction by a person who is skilled in interpreting more than spoken words, as is typically the role of interpreters for people who are deaf or hard of hearing. Rather, the individual with deaf-blindness must have "interpreted" for them the entire context in which communication occurs.

Individuals with deaf-blindness require very specialized instruction to learn how to communicate and acquire functional living and vocational skills, areas that are not commonly included in the curriculum in schools or vocational training programs.

Instruction must be provided in a very consistent manner that allows maximum use of residual vision and hearing, utilizing appropriately adapted materials and technology. Such training must be provided on an individual basis.

The psychosocial implications of deaf-blindness are varied, depending on the age of onset of the disability, the etiology, and the presence or absence of other cognitive disability. The lack of immediate access to information and the availability of skilled individuals to interpret the context and content of communication will significantly influence how the person who is deaf-blind perceives himself or herself and others.

Family and societal attitudes about the person who is deaf-blind also significantly affect how a person who is deaf-blind develops both cognitively and socially. There is often a tendency by the individual who is sighted and hearing to withdraw from the person with deaf-blindness because of a fear of not knowing how to interact properly and the appropriate strategies for communication. This can create in the person who is deaf-blind a feeling of isolation and disconnection. The results of this isolation can range from the development of self-stimulatory behaviors to feelings of loneliness and depression (Sauerburger, 1993).

Development of Programs

Prior to the 1960s there existed in the developed world only isolated educational programs that served individuals with deaf-blindness, primarily in North America and Europe. Staff within these programs had available to them little formal training about this disability but nonetheless made a valiant effort to develop techniques for providing educational services.

During the late 1960s in the United States two significant pieces of legislation were passed that have served as the cornerstones in the development of services to people who are deaf-blind in that country and that have been looked on by many other countries as a model from which to develop their own services.

The birth of approximately 5,000 children during the rubella epidemic in the United States created an immediate need to develop specialized services to people who are deaf-blind. In 1968 the passage of the Elementary and Secondary Education Act created ten regional centers for services to children and youth with deaf-blindness. These centers served as a source of personnel training, technical assistance, and sponsorship for the development of educational programs for children who were deaf-blind. These

centers have evolved into the current fifty-state and multistate centers for services to children and youth with deaf-blindness.

In 1967 Congress passed the Helen Keller National Center Act to develop and enhance rehabilitation services for individuals who are deaf-blind. This piece of legislation resulted in the development of a rehabilitation center in Sands Point, New York, as well as ten regional offices staffed by rehabilitation consultants; a national training team; and provision of seed money for new program development.

These two efforts for children and adults with deaf-blindness have evolved into the current multifaceted service delivery system, which attempts to address the lifelong needs of individuals with deaf-blindness. The services provided through the nationwide system of single and multistate centers for services to infants, children, and youth with deaf-blindness, combined with those of the Helen Keller National Center, have assisted states in developing services that address the needs of children making the transition from education to adult services.

In the design and delivery of adult services to individuals who are deaf-blind it is important to acknowledge the range of abilities within this disability group. The disability of deaf-blindness cannot be considered the sum total of the disabilities of deafness and blindness. There are ranges of abilities— from individuals with profound levels of mental retardation and complex health care needs to those who can complete university courses of study with the proper support.

Periods of transition in the life of the person with deaf-blindness are especially critical, particularly for the largest segment of the emerging population who also have mental retardation. Although issues of transition are encountered throughout life, the transition from education into adult services is especially significant in the life of an individual who is deaf-blind. Typically, an individual will leave either home or a residential school where he or she has lived for many years surrounded by people who have learned to understand that person's modes of communication and behavior, and to interact in a manner which provides the person who is deaf-blind with the added information necessary to understand the context of daily life, giving them a feeling of safety and security.

During this period in life, when both living and work environments will change, the person without vision and hearing requires well-planned transitional services to alleviate anxiety, frustration, and lack of personal control in addressing the many facets of adult life (Riggio, McGinnity, and Gannon, 1985).

Designing services that will meet the needs of each adult person with deaf-blindness will require formal means of collaboration among service providers so the full range of services can be accessed. Typically, individuals with single disabilities receive services from an agency designated to provide services to meet their needs. A state department for persons with mental retardation will serve this segment of the disabled population; state services for the blind will serve those who have blindness as their primary disability, etc. The population of individuals with deaf-blindness, however, because of their range and severity of disability, will require creativity and collaboration to ensure that their needs are met by accessing all necessary services that will allow maximum participation in all aspects of daily life.

Due to the low prevalence of this disability, it is uncommon to find a single agency within a given area that can meet all of the service needs of a person with deaf-blindness. Services are most successfully provided when there is a designated lead agency with staff skilled in understanding the needs of a person with deaf-blindness and that can serve as the single entry point into the adult services system, without risk of no one agency realizing that responsibility. Generally, services for people who are blind, who are deaf, and who are mentally retarded are most commonly required to share responsibility for this program development. These agencies share responsibility in addressing the interpreter, mobility, vocational training, home management, and other services the individual will require. As the emerging population of children who are deaf-blind reaches adulthood, there will be increased collaboration with public health service providers for those individuals with chronic health care needs.

Because of the barriers imposed by limited access to information, it is necessary for the individual to have available ongoing support to function in day-to-day life. Services such as supported employment, orientation and mobility, home management, and independent living skills will enable the individual who is deaf-blind to minimize the necessity of assistive services; however, access to these services must be continued throughout life. Services provided by rehabilitation agencies typically encourage case closure and often do not provide these needed services.

Due to the lack of experience of many rehabilitation agencies in addressing the needs of individuals who are deaf-blind, potential for employment or success in community living is often underestimated. Specialists who are knowledgeable about this disability are needed to determine eligibility and are essential to assist the person who is deaf-blind in partnership with the responsible adult services agencies in the development of appropriate service plans.

The subgroup of individuals with Usher's syndrome can serve as an illustration of the complexity in design and delivery of appropriate services. Individuals with Usher's syndrome are usually brought up as people who are deaf or hard of hearing and regard themselves as members of this community. They have been educated in methods designed for individuals having deafness and hearing impairment. The onset of a vision loss creates the need for services for individuals with visual impairments, such as orientation and mobility services that assist the individual in developing skills necessary for independent travel. This condition additionally creates a great potential for a difficult psychological adjustment to loss of vision, an understandably very feared disability by individuals who are deaf, the need to shift from visual forms of communication to the use of tactual systems, and a need for genetic counseling, employment counseling, and training services that are responsive to the needs of individuals who are deaf-blind.

Other subgroups within the population present different yet equally complex challenges to the adult services system. To meet the needs of individuals who are deaf-blind adequately, the rehabilitation system must recognize and accommodate the needs of the individual to have available to him or her supports that cannot be time-limited.

Speculation for the Future

Current trends in education and rehabilitation have focused efforts on development of community-based services. The passage in 1990 of the Americans with Disabilities Act (ADA) and the subsequent Rehabilitation Act Amendment of 1992 speak to the right of all people with disabilities to full participation in all facets of work and community life. As students who are deaf-blind move from education into adult services, these systems must address this unique disability in new and creative ways.

In a U.S. federal policy statement issued in November 1992, states will now be mandated to report numbers of individuals with deaf-blindness. The ability to gather information about the adult population of individuals with deaf-blindness will significantly influence the process of planning services at state, regional, and national levels.

In addressing the future of services to individuals who are deaf-blind, we must look toward the development of support services that will allow these people to participate fully in community life. In preparing communities to meet the needs of individuals with deaf-blindness, an analysis of the availability of trained personnel to support the participation of individuals with deaf-blindness in that community is necessary.

As the development of community-based living and work options increase for individuals with deaf-blindness, the role of consumer groups such as the American Association for the Deaf-Blind, parent organizations such as the National Family Association for the Deaf-Blind, and professional organizations such as the International Association for the Education of the Deaf-blind will become more critical.

Consumer organizations will provide opportunities for social relationships among people who are deaf-blind and will influence policy at all levels within the service delivery system. Organizations such as the National Coalition on Deaf-Blindness will significantly affect the connection of all of the above groups for development and enhancement of the service delivery system. Such organizations remain watchful of the services offered to individuals who are deaf-blind and advocate appropriate legislative initiatives that will improve the quality of life for members of this disability group.

(*See also:* BLINDNESS AND VISION DISORDERS; COMMUNICATIONS DISORDERS; DEAFNESS AND HEARING IMPAIRMENT; KELLER, HELEN; MULTIPLE DISABILITIES; PSYCHOSOCIAL ADJUSTMENT)

RESOURCE

National Coalition on Deaf-Blindness, 175 North Beacon St., Watertown, MA 02172

BIBLIOGRAPHY

BAGLEY, MARTHA. "Population Trends and Life Span Issues for Individuals with Deaf-Blindness: Reaction Paper." *Proceedings of the National Conference on Deaf-Blindness: Deaf-Blind Services in the 90s.* Watertown, MA, 1992.

BARRETT, STEPHEN S. "Comprehensive Community-Based Services for Adults Who Are Deaf-Blind: Issues, Trends, and Services." *Journal of Visual Impairment and Blindness,* November 1992.

DOLNICK, EDWARD. "Deafness as Culture." *The Atlantic,* September 1993.

KONAR, VALERIE and RICE, B. DOUGLAS. *Strategies for Serving Deaf-Blind Clients: Eleventh Institute on Rehabilitation Issues.* Arkansas, 1984.

PARKER, STEVEN. *Congenital Rubella Syndrome: Health Care Challenges.* Watertown, MA, 1992.

REIMAN, JOHN and JOHNSON, PATTIE, eds. *Proceedings of the National Symposium on Children and Youth Who Are Deaf-Blind.* Monmouth, OR, 1993.

RIGGIO, MARIANNE. "A Changing Population of Children and Youth with Deaf-Blindness: A Changing Role of the Deaf-Blind Specialist/Teacher: Reaction Paper." *Proceedings of the National Conference on Deaf-Blindness: Deaf-Blind Services in the 90s.* Watertown, MA, 1992.

RIGGIO, MARIANNE; McGINNITY, BETSY; and GANNON, CHERYL. *Report on the Needs of the Deaf–Blind in Massachusetts.* Watertown, MA, 1985.

SAUERBURGER, DONNA. *Independence Without Sight or Sound.* New York, 1993.

SMITH, AUDREY and COTE, KAREN. *Look at Me: A Resource Manual for the Development of Residual Vision in Multiply Impaired Children.* Philadelphia, 1982.

STAHLECKER, JAMES; GLASS, LAURA; and MACHALOW, STEVEN, eds. *State-of-the-Art: Research Priorities in Deaf-Blindness.* San Francisco, 1984.

WATSON, DOUGLAS, and TAFF–WATSON, MYRA, eds. "A Model Service Delivery." Little Rock, AR, 1993.

MARIANNE RIGGIO

DEAFNESS AND HEARING IMPAIRMENT

Hearing loss may range from mild (difficulty with hearing soft sounds or inability to hear them) to profound (difficulty with hearing loud sounds or inability to hear them). Generally speaking, this group can be divided into persons who are either hard of hearing or deaf.

The term "hard of hearing" refers to a hearing loss from 25 decibels (db) (mild loss) to 90 db (severe loss). An individual with this degree of loss frequently communicates using a combination of strategies that rely on residual auditory ability enhanced by a hearing aid or assistive listening device and often supplemented through lipreading or other visual means.

The term "deaf" refers to a hearing loss greater than 90 db (profound hearing loss). Persons are considered "deaf" if their hearing loss is such that they are unable to hear or understand speech and must rely on vision for communication. Deaf persons in the United States, especially those who are born deaf or lose their hearing at an early age, generally prefer to communicate using American Sign Language (ASL), sign language interpreters, reading, writing, or other visual means. Deaf persons who lose their hearing later in life, sometimes referred to as "late deafened," may have different communication preferences and rely on residual hearing, lipreading, captioning, or perhaps signed English.

Number of Persons Who Are Hard of Hearing or Deaf

In 1987 the National Center for Health Statistics (NCHS) estimated that almost 21 million persons, or 8.8 percent of the U.S. population, had hearing problems (Table 1). Their data show that dramatic differences exist in the prevalence rates by age groups (Figure 1): Persons in their prime working years, eighteen to forty-four, and persons forty-five to sixty-four years of age were more than three and eight times, respectively, more likely to be hearing-impaired than persons under age eighteen. At the other extreme, persons sixty-five years or older were twice as likely to be hearing-impaired as persons between ages forty-five and sixty-four. The prevalence of hearing impairment is greater for males than for females and greater for whites than for blacks for all age groups (Table 2). These data were based on NCHS estimates of the number of persons with any type of hearing problem. The survey methodology did not permit for estimates by severity of the hearing loss to determine the number of Americans who are deaf or hard of hearing. A related study by Mitchell LaPlante (1988), however, does provide estimates based on severity of hearing impairment. He reports that there are an estimated 21,028,000 hearing-impaired persons, with an estimated 1,741,000 deaf persons and 19,287,000 persons with less severe hearing impairments among the noninstitutionalized population (Table 3).

Table 1. Estimates of the reported prevalence of hearing impairments in the population by age group, United States, 1987

Age Group	Number	Rate per Thousand
Total	20,994,000	88.0
Under 18 years	1,012,000	16.0
18–44 years	5,529,000	54.1
45–64 years	6,098,000	135.6
65 years or older	8,355,000	296.8
65–74 years	4,582,000	264.7
75 years or older	3,773,000	348.0

SOURCE: National Center for Health Statistics (1988).

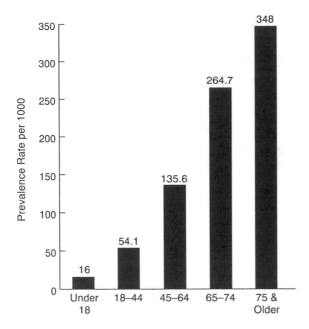

Figure 1. Estimates of the reported prevalence of hearing impairments in the population by age group, United States, 1987

SOURCE: National Center for Health Statistics (1988)

Communication Methods

People who are hard of hearing or deaf communicate with each other and with hearing people in a variety of ways, including speaking, speechreading, reading and writing, natural gestures, ASL, and Manually Coded English (MCE). The communication method or methods used depend on the individual's

training, when the hearing loss occurred, the degree and type of hearing loss, and the specific circumstances in which communication takes place.

Many people who become hard of hearing or deaf later in life maintain the ability to produce very clear spoken language but use special methods to understand the speech of others. Many people whose hearing loss occurs early in life may identify with Deaf Culture and prefer to use ASL primarily. Each person who is hard of hearing or deaf usually uses the specific combination of communication strategies that work best in a given situation. Generally, people who are hard of hearing and have mild to severe hearing losses rely on amplification for receptive communication. Persons who are deaf with severe to profound hearing losses more often rely heavily or entirely on visual methods of communication.

A wide variety of accommodations have been developed to assure accessible communication for persons who are hard of hearing or deaf. Many of these communication accommodations are inexpensive and easy to implement; some are more expensive and complex. A listing of the more frequent approaches would include the following:

1. Assistive listening devices/systems. In addition to the individual use of a hearing aid, several systems are widely used: the audio loop system, the wireless FM system, and the wireless infrared system.

2. Interpreters. Sign language and/or oral interpreters are regularly used to provide communication accessibility in conversations, meetings, and related

Table 2. Estimates of the reported prevalence of hearing impairments per 1,000 in the population, by age group and sex, by age group and race, United States, 1987

	Sex		Race	
Age Group	Male	Female	White	Black
Total	**103.1**	**73.9**	**96.3**	**38.7**
Under 45 years	47.5	31.6	43.4	18.7
45–64 years	184.3	91.1	144.1	72.0
65 years or over	346.1	261.9	308.2	162.0
65–75 years	331.8	211.3	274.7	141.2
75 years or over	373.7	333.2	361.2	197.7

SOURCE: National Center for Health Statistics (1988)

Table 3. Estimated distribution of the hearing-impaired population by severity of hearing impairment and by age group, United States, 1983–1985

Age Group	Deaf	Hard of Hearing
Total	1,741,000	19,287,000
Under 45 years	318,000	5,988,000
45–69 years	667,000	8,272,000
70–84 years	551,000	4,302,000
85 years or older	205,000	725,000

SOURCE: Mitchell LaPlante (1988)

situations. Depending on individual or group preferences, sign language interpreters most often use ASL or MCE. Oral interpreters most often are asked to mouth silently or paraphrase the spoken message. If requested, both approaches can include voice-interpreting the speech or signs of a person who is hard of hearing or deaf. Fees for interpreters generally range from fifteen to sixty dollars per hour, with a two-hour minimum.

3. Real-time caption services. Real-time captioning is used to display the text of a communication on a video monitor or projection screen immediately. Frequently used at large public meetings, real-time captioning is also used in some one-to-one situations. This type of translation service usually requires a skilled stenographer, video equipment, computer, and screen. Depending on group preferences and finances, many large public meetings with a mixed audience will include several large screens, one projecting the speaker with captions underneath and another projecting the interpreter or interpreters.

4. Captioning of television and movies. Captioning of television and movie productions is becoming commonplace, enabling viewers who use closed-captioning equipment to receive a word-for-word printed translation of the transmitted dialogue. Although not all productions are captioned, the percentage that are captioned is increasing at a phenomenal rate. In addition, federal law requires that all newly manufactured television sets with screens larger than thirteen inches must include a built-in decoder chip.

5. Telecommunication display devices (TDD).

The TDD (also called a teletypewriter, TTY, or teletext) is widely used for telecommunication purposes. Both the caller and the receiver can type and read their conversations as transmitted (Baudot mode) through the telephone. Recent innovations include the use of special software that permits the use of personal computers (ASCII mode) and/or a new generation of videotext machines that automatically adjust to either Baudot or ASCII modes for transmittal.

6. Telecommunication relay services. Telecommunication relay services, available in all fifty states, enable a person using a TDD to communicate with another person using a voice telephone. Using TDDs, voice operators at the telephone relay service act as a communication bridge between hearing people and persons who are hard of hearing or deaf by relaying TDD text to voice for the hearing party and relaying voice communication back to the party who is hard of hearing or deaf through typed TDD text (Figure 2).

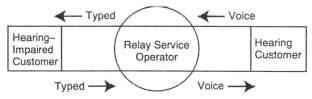

Figure 2. Telecommunications relay service

Rehabilitation System

Since its inception in 1920, the federal/state program of rehabilitation has driven the United States'

241

efforts to assist youth and adults who are hard of hearing and deaf to obtain the assistance needed to prepare them for the world of work and independent living.

Rehabilitation Outcome Data. National databases indicate that the fifty state rehabilitation agencies collectively serve more than 40,000 persons who are deaf or hard of hearing each year. Approximately two-thirds of these individuals receive some form of rehabilitation-sponsored training. There were substantial increases (17% and 30%, respectively) in the number of persons who are deaf and hard of hearing successfully rehabilitated between 1970 and 1985 (Table 4).

Model State Plan. Regulations governing the federal/state system require each state to design and implement a plan detailing how it will provide services to its residents who are disabled. Guidelines for serving this client population are presented in a special publication, *Model State Plan for the Rehabilitation of Individuals Who Are Deaf and Hard of Hearing* (Watson, 1990b). These guidelines provide a structure, a set of acceptable options, and numerous conceptions with which to build and direct a particular state's program of rehabilitation for these individuals. In addition to improvements in service delivery, these guidelines have also stimulated state rehabilitation agencies to make special efforts to recruit and employ program managers and counseling personnel trained and skilled in service to persons who are deaf or hard of hearing. As a result, most states now employ several specialists on staff to plan and provide quality services for this client population. Equally important, most states include people who are deaf or hard of hearing on their consumer advisory councils. In fact, many states now have a separate consumer advisory council that focuses only on issues related to the rehabilitation of deaf and hard of hearing persons. These consumer representatives have become important agents of change in the shaping and implementation of rehabilitation service systems in the various states.

Trained Rehabilitation Personnel. It is estimated that there are about 600 rehabilitation counselors skilled in serving people who are deaf and hard of hearing in the fifty states (Watson, 1990a). Many if not most of these trained counselors received their pre- or in-service training from one of the RSA-funded university training centers for rehabilitation counselors of the deaf (RCD), which are dispersed across the ten geographical regions of the United States. It is estimated that approximately 15 percent of these specialized counselors are themselves deaf or hard of hearing. To assure that these personnel are skilled in communication with their clients, many states have implemented a formal program to assess the sign communication skills of their personnel. In those instances where individuals need to improve their communication skills, many state agencies now sponsor their enrollment in appropriate training programs (sign communication proficiency training) for upgrading.

Delivery of Rehabilitation Services. The federal/state rehabilitation program has a long and distinguished record of special efforts to meet the rehabilitation needs of people who are deaf; efforts on behalf of people who are hard of hearing have too often focused on remediation of the hearing loss to the exclusion of addressing their many other rehabilitation needs. However, advocacy efforts by var-

Table 4. Number of deaf and hard-of-hearing clients successfully rehabilitated in 1970 and 1985

Group	1970[a]	1985[b]	Increase
Total	**14,334**	**17,908**	**24%**
Deaf clients	5,915	6,924	17%
Hard-of-hearing clients	8,419	10,984	30%

[a.] Jerome D. Schein and Marcus T. Delk (1974), p. 90
[b.] Rehabilitation Services Administration (1987), p. 81

ious consumer and professional groups have led to significant changes as the rehabilitation system has begun to recognize and deal with the broader needs of these individuals. An outline of selected program activities follows:

- Casefinding and transition from school to work. Each year an estimated 8,000 students who are deaf exit our secondary schools, seeking to make a satisfactory transition from school to work or postsecondary training. Cooperative efforts between secondary schools and rehabilitation in the transition of these students is a crucial part of the rehabilitation system. A study example found that within one year following graduation from high school, 85 percent of a national sample of young adults were receiving services from their state rehabilitation agency (El-Khiami, Savage, and Tribble, 1991). Two findings stand out: First, with rehabilitation assistance virtually the entire sample was enrolled in postsecondary training programs except for the 15 percent who requested assistance in obtaining employment; second, few of the students "got lost" in the transition process, indicating that the secondary education and rehabilitation partnership was successful in identifying and serving the needs of this cohort of students. Major gaps exist, however, since programs with fewer than ten students are less frequently contacted by rehabilitation personnel, and deaf youth with multiple and severe disabilities are sometimes poorly served by transition programs (Allen, Rawlings, and Schildroth, 1989).

- Rehabilitation sponsorship of postsecondary training. Students who are deaf and hard of hearing attend more than 150 colleges offering special programs in the United States. Between 60 and 75 percent receive some form of support from rehabilitation. In a U.S. Government Accounting Office audit of postsecondary programs for students who are deaf, it was found that although the proportions vary by program, 68 percent of the students were receiving rehabilitation assistance. Other studies have also found that rehabilitation is a major sponsor of deaf and hard-of-hearing postsecondary students (Allen, Rawlings, and Schildroth, 1989; Ragosta, 1990). Graduates from the nation's six federally funded programs were much more likely to have completed requirements for bachelor's or master's degrees, whereas graduates from other programs had earned vocational or associate's degrees (Table 5) (Schroedel & Watson, 1991; Watson, 1990a). The data highlight the central role that rehabilitation has assumed in the United States in cosponsoring and monitoring the progress of persons who are deaf and hard of hearing in postsecondary education and career preparation programs. Rehabilitation has become almost synonymous with career prepara-

Table 5. Percent distribution of respondents' highest completed degree by type of program funding

| | | Type of Program Funding | | |
Highest Completed Degree		Total	Federal	Nonfederal
	N	193	115	78
	Total	100.0	100.0	100.0
Vocational degree		34.7	31.3	39.7
Associate's degree		22.8	19.1	28.2
Bachelor's degree		26.4	38.3	9.0
Master's degree		7.8	8.7	6.4
No degree yet completed		8.3	2.6	16.7

SOURCE: John D. Schroedel and Douglas Watson (1991)

243

tion and training of youth and adults who are deaf and hard of hearing.

- Services for persons with severe and multiple disabilities. It is estimated that approximately one-third of the population have disabilities in addition to their hearing impairment. Special remedial services for these individuals often include independent living training, remedial education, sheltered or supported employment with the aid of job coaching, community-based rehabilitation, and social and recreational services (Watson, 1990). Unfortunately, the demand far exceeds current capacity to meet the diverse needs presented by this population subgroup. There is a continuing effort to obtain federal funding to support comprehensive programs in all ten federal regions of the United States.

- Public and private rehabilitation partnerships. It is estimated that several hundred programs nationwide provide daily rehabilitation services to persons who are deaf or hard of hearing. Ranging from locally funded deaf service centers to speech and hearing centers that also provide career counseling, placement, and related services, these programs are vital partners in our nation's rehabilitation system. An increasing proportion of such community service centers are operated and/or staffed by personnel who are themselves deaf or hard of hearing.

- Employment and earnings. The last national census of the deaf population conducted in the United States found that deafness is not "necessarily" or "in or of itself" a bar to employment; persons who are deaf held jobs in every industry and in most occupational categories, though not in the same proportions as workers in general (Schein & Delk, 1974). On average, workers who are deaf earned about 25 percent less than the national average. One study found that more than one-third of a national sample of deaf postsecondary 1984 graduates obtained professional and technical or management and sales jobs upon graduation (see Table 5). The average 1985 earnings of the group were approximately $14,000. The level of personal annual income appeared to be essentially determined by the level of completed degree: voca-

tional, $11,535; associate, $11,846; bachelor's, $16,007; master's, $20,472. These differences in earnings underscore the value that employers attribute to the various levels of education and training that graduates bring to the workplace.

These and other data suggest that persons who are deaf and hard of hearing in the United States do in fact have increased access to excellent employment opportunities. A careful reading of research literature on the socioeconomic attainments of the population from the mid-1970s to the mid-1990s suggests that, to a large degree, the question is not whether equal opportunities exist, but whether individuals take advantage of them to obtain the education and training needed for the demands of the contemporary labor market. In looking to the future, William B. Johnston and Arnold H. Packer (1987) report that more than half of the new jobs to be created in our economy by the year 2000 will require postsecondary training. While employment discrimination continues to exist, those persons who are deaf and hard of hearing who enter the labor force with the right education and training will have a greater likelihood of integration into the workforce on an equal footing with hearing peers. Those who lack strong educational and training preparation may not be able to compete for the best jobs.

Education for Deaf and Hard-of-Hearing Children

Dating from the 1817 founding of the American School for the Deaf in Hartford, Connecticut, by Thomas H. Gallaudet, the focus of U.S. educational efforts on behalf of children who are deaf and hard of hearing has emphasized placement in special schools. Even as late as the 1970s, up to 60 percent of these children were educated in such "center schools," where teaching personnel trained in education for the deaf provided specialized instruction. However, since the passage of P.L. 94-142 in the mid-1970s, a dramatic shift has led to more than 60 percent of children who were deaf being placed in public school programs. These placements are predicated on the assumption that communication access can be assured for these children by the use of education interpreters, notetaking, resource room teachers, assistive listening devices or systems, and related support services provided within the regular classroom. However, research data indicate that although physically housed in a regular public school with support services, a vast majority of these students are not placed in regular academic classes. Also, these dramatic changes have stimulated a growing groundswell of discontent from consumers and educators who believe that "mainstreaming" of hearing-impaired children is too often not in the best interest of the individual child. To assess and deal with these and other issues better, the U.S. Congress authorized a two-year study of the educational system. Selected findings of that study (COED, 1988) show that schools need to:

1. implement already available preventive and early identification procedures more widely;

2. issue appropriate guidelines for monitoring educational programs for persons who are deaf;

3. emphasize educational content rather than mere placement—to what is taught rather than where it is taught;

4. engage the active participation of parents and persons who are deaf—including those from minority and ethnic groups—in the decision-making process;

5. recognize that many of the needs of persons who are deaf are different from those of persons with other disabilities;

6. recognize that children who are deaf and hard of hearing represent a spectrum of diverse handicaps requiring that educational programs be tailored for the individual—whose needs change with time;

7. determine educational placements based on individual needs; for example, the concept of least restricted environment (LRE) is usually interpreted to be whatever comes closest to integration within the regular classroom, whereas for many children, regular classroom placement is not appropriate to meet their particular needs, while the appropriate LRE might be a special class or center school;

8. acknowledge that as many as 60 percent of teenagers are not qualified for college, yet no federal programs make provision for the comprehensive postsecondary training and education of this majority group;

9. encourage diverse, innovative, and high-quality research;

10. provide a wide range of educational opportunities for college students in various regions of the country;

11. put more emphasis on the training of adequate personnel for the specific and demanding task of participating in the education of children who are deaf and hard of hearing at various educational levels;

12. use, and encourage the use of, the diverse tools being provided by advancing technology, including computers and electronic equipment, and support use of TV closed captioning.

Providing the foundation for a reexamination of our educational practices and policies, the COED report and other findings have stimulated a vigorous movement within Congress to revise and otherwise mandate more effective national policies to guide the education of deaf and hard of hearing children in the United States. The most constructive aspect of these efforts is that the nation's attention and resources have been brought to focus on identifying and implementing more effective educational practices and programs for these children.

New Plans for People Who Are Deaf or Hard of Hearing in the United States

The 1990 passage of the Americans with Disabilities Act (ADA) has set forth far-reaching, fundamental changes in the nation's agenda for people who are deaf or hard of hearing. Empowered by ADA, consumers, and consumer organizations and their representatives are taking the initiative in advocating their rightful role in defining that agenda. Our review of these new plans will be limited to a listing of selected developments directly related to the areas of communication methods, the rehabilitation system, and education.

New Plans for Communication Methods:

• In addition to twelve Rehabilitation Services Administration (RSA)-funded regional programs to train rehabilitation interpreters, the Office of Special Education Programs (OSEP) has funded twelve grants to train educational interpreters. In combination, these two grant programs provide support for the pre- and in-service training of several thousand new and working interpreters each year in the nation's efforts to train the skilled personnel needed.

- National organizations for interpreter training (Conference of Interpreter Trainers—CIT) and professional interpreters (Registry of Interpreters for the Deaf—RID) are working together to develop and set minimum national standards for the education, training, and certification of professional interpreters.

- New developments are emerging for the use of personal computers for real-time captioning of individual and small group communication, videotext terminals that can readily interface with TDDs (Baudot) or other computers (ASCII), telecommunication relay services in all fifty states, and the further development of the picture telephone. These are but a few of the more promising examples of new developments to further enhance communication accessibility.

New Plans in the Rehabilitation System:

- The federal/state rehabilitation program has funded a national study on the rehabilitation service needs of hard of hearing and late-deafened individuals and has awarded grants to fund a five-year research project on hearing rehabilitation and a one-year grant to train rehabilitation personnel to work with clients who are hard of hearing or late-deafened.

- The Rehabilitation Research and Training Center for Persons Who Are Deaf or Hard of Hearing at the University of Arkansas published a 1993 edition of *Model State Plan for Deaf-Blind Persons*. Another group, at Northern Illinois University, is planning to develop a model state plan for low-functioning persons who are deaf. These new plans will be made available to guide the efforts of state rehabilitation agencies to improve their efforts on behalf of people who are

deaf-blind and/or deaf people who are severely and multiply disabled.

- Ten five-year funding grants were awarded in 1991 to establish and operate a national network of Regional Disability and Business Accommodation Centers (RDBACs). These programs were funded to provide technical assistance, advocacy, consultation, training, and related support to consumers with disabilities, rehabilitation personnel, and business and industry in the recruitment and employment of persons with disabilities. Otherwise referred to as ADA Technical Assistance Programs, their primary mandate is to assist consumers with disabilities, business and industry, and the rehabilitation system to work productively together to implement the intent of ADA fully. The challenge the field faces with this new initiative is to assure that these regional ADA centers also address the special needs of people who are deaf, hard of hearing, and/or late-deafened.

- The University of Arkansas—together with other consumer and professional organizations and representatives of business and industry—hosted a March 1993 national conference designed to foster more productive employment accommodations that address the special needs of deaf and hard-of-hearing persons, including those who are also members of racial and ethnic minority groups. These national conferences are being funded in part through the federal/state rehabilitation program. These cooperative efforts are but a few of the many activities under way to plan and implement more effective employment programs and services for the hearing-impaired population of the United States.

New Plans in Education:

- Congress has made major changes in policies and legislative mandates to improve educational services for hearing-impaired students and for other students with disabilities. Among other plans, Congress continues to seek ways to address many of the procedural problems identified in the 1988 COED report. Issues related to communication accessibility, appropriate educational placements (LRE); funding formulas, and numerous other policies are under review or being revised to reflect the views of consumers and parental concerns with existing laws.

- To achieve excellence in the education of deaf students, the Deaf Education Initiative collaboration has been established between State Directors of Special Education and the Conference of Executives of American Schools for the Deaf (CEASD). This initiative is directed to the development and implementation of national models and standards for educational programs for deaf students, personnel qualifications, educational interpreter training, partnerships/collaborations, resources, knowledge and understanding of deafness, and advocacy and networking. This new partnership is actively working to improve the quality of educational programming for deaf and hard-of-hearing children in the United States.

- In addition to the ongoing efforts to improve educational services for children who are deaf, there is a highly heightened awareness and plans to consider more appropriately the special needs of hard of hearing and/or late-deafened students served in the public school systems. Equally important, this includes older students enrolled in postsecondary training or education programs as well as younger children.

(See also: COMMUNICATIONS DISORDERS; DEAF-BLINDNESS; GALLAUDET UNIVERSITY; MULTIPLE DISABILITIES; SPECIAL EDUCATION; STATE–FEDERAL REHABILITATION PROGRAM)

BIBLIOGRAPHY

ALLEN, THOMAS T.; RAWLINGS, BRENDA W.; and SCHILDROTH, ARTHUR E. Deaf Students and the School-to-Work Transition. Baltimore, 1989.

BULLIS, MICHAEL B.; JOHNSON, BRIAN; JOHNSON, PATRICIA; and KITRELL, G. School-to-Community Transition Experiences of Hearing-Impaired Adolescents and Young Adults in the Northwest. Monmouth, OR, 1990.

COMMISSION ON EDUCATION OF THE DEAF (COED). Toward Equality: Education of the Deaf. Washington, DC, 1988.

EL-KHIAMI, AFAFE; SAVAGE, KENNETH; and TRIBBLE, LINDA. A National Study of Transition from School to Work for Deaf Youth. Little Rock, AR, 1991.

JOHNSTON, WILLIAM B., and PACKER, ARNOLD H. Workforce 2000: Work and Workers for the Twenty-first Century. Indianapolis, IN, 1987.

LaPLANTE, MITCHELL. National Health Interview Survey for 1983–1985. Washington, DC, 1988.

NATIONAL CENTER FOR HEALTH STATISTICS. Data from the National Health Survey. Hyattsville, MD, 1988.

RAGOSTA, MARJORIE. Progress in Education and Rehabilitation of Deaf and Hard-of-Hearing Individuals. Princeton, NJ, 1990.

REHABILITATION SERVICES ADMINISTRATION. Annual Report to the President and to the Congress: Fiscal Year 1987. Washington, DC, 1987.

SCHEIN, JEROME D., and DELK, MARCUS T. The Deaf Population of the United States. Silver Spring, MD, 1974.

SCHROEDEL, JOHN G., and WATSON, DOUGLAS. Enhancing Opportunities in Postsecondary Education for Deaf Students. Little Rock, AR, 1991.

U.S. GOVERNMENT ACCOUNTING OFFICE. Deaf Education: Costs and Student Characteristics at Federally Assisted Schools. Washington, DC, 1986.

WATSON, DOUGLAS. Deafness Rehabilitation: A Major Force in Services to Deaf People. In Marjorie Ragosta, Progress in Education and Rehabilitation of Deaf and Hard-of-Hearing Individuals. Princeton, NJ, 1990a.

———, ed. Model State Plan for the Rehabilitation of Individuals Who Are Deaf and Hard of Hearing. Little Rock, AR, 1990b.

WATSON, DOUGLAS, SCHROEDEL, JOHN G., and EL-KHIAMI, AFAFE. "A National Study of Postsecondary Education of Deaf Students." In Two Decades of Excellence: A Foundation for the Future, eds. Douglas Watson, Greg Long, Myra Taff-Watson, and Michael Harvey. Little Rock, AR, 1988.

DOUGLAS WATSON
MYRA TAFF-WATSON

DEINSTITUTIONALIZATION

Deinstitutionalization refers to the policy and philosophy in the fields of mental health and developmental disabilities of removing people from large public institutions, returning them to their communities, and providing them with services needed to live successfully in the society at large.

Prior to the late 1960s, there was widespread acceptance of the belief that people with psychiatric diagnoses, mental retardation, and related conditions belonged in institutions. From the middle of the nineteenth century until this time, the populations of state institutions grew at a steady pace. By 1955, state mental hospitals had reached their peak population of 558,922; in 1967, the population of state institutions for people with mental retardation peaked at 194,650.

The period from the 1960s to the 1990s marked a new era in society's treatment of people with disabilities. The era started with pleas for modest reform, but before long, parents formed organizations to advocate on behalf of their children with disabilities. The first national organization for people with mental retardation, the National Association for Retarded Children (now the ARC), was formed in 1950. Initially, parents came together to provide each other with mutual support, to share information, to sponsor fund-raising events, and even to operate special schools and programs. Parent groups gradually started to demand quality services.

Beginning in the 1970s, former mental patients and adults with mental retardation formed their own organizations to advocate on their own behalf. One of the most notable of these is People First, which, as the name implies, has demanded that people with mental retardation be afforded the same rights and privileges enjoyed by other members of society.

Exposés. The 1960s and 1970s witnessed a seemingly endless series of exposés of mental hospitals and state schools that captured widespread public attention.

Burton Blatt, a respected educator and researcher, closely followed the reactions of professionals and politicians to Robert Kennedy's scathing indictment of conditions in New York State's institutions following unannounced tours in 1965. Blatt knew the truth of what Kennedy had reported, and that Christmas, with a photographer named Fred Kaplan, Blatt secretly photographed the worst wards at five institutions in the Northeast. Their book *Christmas in Purgatory* and an article in *Look* magazine shocked America and fueled the growing disenchantment with institutions.

Reporter Geraldo Rivera's 1970 exposé of Willowbrook State School on Staten Island documented the same conditions found by Blatt and Kaplan. The artful documentary by Frederick Wiseman *Titticut Follies*, filmed at Bridgewater State Hospital in Mas-

sachusetts, focused public attention on dehumanizing conditions at mental hospitals.

Social Science Perspectives. In 1961, sociologist Erving Goffman described the devastating effects on the identity and self-esteem of inmates of mental hospitals and other institutions. Building on this work, professionals developed the principle of normalization as an alternative philosophy to social exclusion and segregation of people with disabilities. Two Swedish leaders, Karl Grunewald and Bengt Nirje, defined normalization as follows: "Making available to all mentally retarded people patterns of life and conditions of living which are as close as possible to the regular circumstances and ways of life of their society." Gunnar Dybwad and Wolf Wolfensberger popularized the concept in the United States.

Litigation. Just as other minority groups turned to the courts to achieve justice during the civil rights era, so people with disabilities and their families began to file suits in state and especially federal courts to challenge substandard conditions and to win the right to live in the community. In *O'Connor v. Donaldson,* handed down in 1975, the U.S. Supreme Court ruled that a "nondangerous" mental patient had a constitutional right to liberty and could not be warehoused in a state mental hospital. Federal judges in suits in Alabama (*Wyatt v. Stickney*), New York (*NYSARC v. Rockefeller*), Pennsylvania (*Halderman v. Pennhurst State School and Hospital*), and dozens of other states ordered state governments to reform their institutions and to provide services in the community. In case after case, judges required states to hire additional institutional staff, to halt such practices as seclusion, and to move at least some residents into smaller and more normalized community settings.

Legislation. Spurred by federal court cases, the U.S. Congress, from the early 1970s to the 1990s, passed a series of laws designed to reform institutions, fund community services, and protect people with disabilities from discrimination. Foremost among these are the federal intermediate care facilities for the mentally retarded program and the "Medicaid waiver," Section 504 of the Rehabilitation Act of 1973, the Developmentally Disabled Assistance and Bill of Rights Act, and the Americans with Disabilities Act.

Throughout much of the 1970s and 1980s, deinstitutionalization was extremely controversial. Many professionals were skeptical whether people with severe disabilities could live in the community; some parents worried that their children would be dumped into the streets without services; prospective neighbors and local politicians in some communities expressed stereotyped fears of people with psychiatric diagnoses or mental retardation. Despite the opposition, deinstitutionalization proceeded at a steady rate during the era. By 1986 the population of state and county mental hospitals had declined to 107,056, and by 1991, state institutions for people with developmental disabilities had declined to 80,269 people.

By the 1990s, the controversy surrounding deinstitutionalization had subsided. In developmental disabilities, an emerging consensus supports the right of all people to live in the community, and a number of states have either closed all of their institutions or announced plans to do so. While the field of mental health lacks consensus on deinstitutionalization, there is general support for the preferability of community settings over institutions.

Deinstitutionalization has passed its own set of challenges. First, many people, though physically placed in the community, are socially isolated. Attention today is focused on helping people to participate fully in the life of the community. Second, many so-called community facilities are large and share institutional characteristics. In some states, deinstitutionalization has meant "transinstitutionalization," or movement from one type of institution to another. Many states and service providers are exploring innovative ways of supporting children as well as adults to remain at home with their families.

(*See also:* CIVIL RIGHTS; DEVELOPMENTAL DISABILITIES; INDEPENDENT LIVING)

BIBLIOGRAPHY

BLATT, BURTON, and KAPLAN, FRED. *Christmas in Purgatory: A Photographic Essay on Mental Retardation.* Syracuse, NY, 1974.

BOGDAN, ROBERT, and TAYLOR, STEVEN J. *The Social Meaning of Mental Retardation: Two Life Stories.* New York, 1994.

GOFFMAN, ERVING E. *Asylums: Essays on the Social Situation of Mental Patients and Other Inmates.* New York, 1961.

ROTHMAN, DAVID J., and ROTHMAN, SHEILA M. *The Willowbrook Wars: A Decade-Long Struggle for Social Justice.* New York, 1984.

TAYLOR, STEVEN J.; BIKLEN, DOUGLAS; and KNOLL, JAMES, eds. *Community Integration for People with Severe Disabilities.* New York, 1987.

WOLFENSBERGER, WOLF W. *Normalization: The Principle of Normalization in Human Services.* Toronto, 1972.

STEVEN J. TAYLOR

DEMENTIA

See ORGANIC MENTAL SYNDROMES

DEPRESSION

See LOSS AND GRIEF; MOOD DISORDERS

DEVELOPMENTAL DISABILITIES

The term "developmental disability" came into use with the passage of the Developmental Disabilities Service and Construction Act of 1970. The initial definition of developmental disabilities included mental retardation, cerebral palsy, epilepsy, and other neurological conditions occurring prior to age eighteen years. In 1975 autism was added to the definition of developmental disabilities. Unlike many of the other terms referring to disabilities, developmental disabilities is not a classification or diagnostic term but rather a term functionally describing groups of persons who have had a disability from early years (Gollay, 1979; Kiernan, Smith, and Ostrowsky, 1986).

The origins of developmental disabilities are substantially different from other classifications of disabilities where there are uniform characteristics and established assessment procedures for determining the presence of persons with the condition. For developmental disabilities the focus is on functional capacities and similarities in need among persons who have had disabilities from birth or shortly after birth. The adoption of the term in legislation was a significant step toward the establishment of a functional capacity perspective rather than a deficit view of a disabling condition (Summers, 1981). Subsequent to the passage of the legislation there has been a growing emphasis on the use of functional criteria in defining disability (Schalock & Kiernan, 1990). The definition and classification systems used in mental retardation continue to influence heavily the definition, classification, and functional support needs of persons with disabilities (Grossman, 1983; Luckasson et al., 1992).

Developmental disability and mental retardation are not synonymous. Not all persons with the diagnosis of mental retardation should be considered as having a developmental delay, as in the case of persons with mild intellectual impairment who are working, living in the community, and participating in typical community activities. Conversely, not all persons having a developmental delay should be considered as having a cognitive limitation. Certain persons with cerebral palsy who have significant impairment in communication, self-care, work, and community living will not have any cognitive limitation but would be considered developmentally disabled (Kiernan & Bruininks, 1986).

This entry reviews the major categories of disability included under the term "developmental disabilities"; considers the incidence of developmental disabilities; discusses some of the current practices in providing services to persons with developmental disabilities; and provides an overview of some of the professional, governmental, and consumer organizations involved in providing supports and services.

Definition

Developmental disability has its origins in a person's early years. Thus such disabilities that are attributable to the aging process, trauma in adult years, substance dependence, and mental illness with onset in later years are not included in the scope of this entry. The current definition of developmental disability reflects a shift in thinking to emphasize supports rather than services, functionality rather than classification, independence rather than dependence, and inclusion rather than specialized or segregated programs (Bradley, 1992; Luckasson et al.,

1992). This shift was reflected in early 1990s federal legislation, including the Individuals with Disabilities Education Act, the Rehabilitation Act Amendments of 1992, the Americans with Disabilities Act, and the Developmental Disabilities Assistance and Bill of Rights Act.

The Developmental Disabilities Assistance and Bill of Rights Act defines developmental disability as a severe, chronic disability of a person that:

- is attributable to a mental or physical impairment, or a combination of mental and physical impairments;
- is manifest before twenty-two years of age;
- is likely to continue indefinitely;
- results in substantial functional limitations in three or more of the following areas of major life activities, including self-care, receptive and expressive language, learning, mobility, self-direction, capacity for independent living, and economic self-sufficiency;
- reflects the person's need for a combination and sequence of special, interdisciplinary, or generic care, treatment, or other services that are of lifelong or extended duration and individually planned and coordinated.

Three general components of the definition are important: cause or etiology; characteristics; and duration of needed services. In reference to cause, conditions that are attributable to prenatal, perinatal, or postnatal factors, including traumatic brain injuries that occur during childhood or adolescence years, are included. In regard to characteristics, persons with developmental disabilities reflect "substantial functional limitations" in three or more of the seven life activities contained in the above legislative definition. Although there is at present little agreement as to what constitutes a functional limitation, in general one meets this criterion if the person needs moderate to constant assistance to do the activity. The third component relates to the type of services required and the duration of service needs. This will be discussed in greater detail later; for the time being, it is important to remember that such persons frequently need multiple services provided by a number of different professionals and human service programs over an extended period of time, even a lifetime.

Disability Groupings

Table 1 organizes the categories of persons with disabilities into four impairment groups: cognitive/developmental, sensory/neurological, physical, and emotional/behavioral. Within each of these four impairment groups, there are a number of diagnostic conditions that have a likelihood of resulting in a developmental disability.

1. Cognitive/developmental impairment. Persons with mental retardation represent the largest group of individuals within this category. "Mental retardation refers to substantial limitations in present functioning. It is characterized by significantly subaverage intellectual functioning, existing concurrently with related limitations in two or more of the following applicable adaptive skills areas: communication, self-care, home living, social skills, community use, self-direction, health and safety,

functional academics, leisure, and work. Mental retardation manifests before age eighteen" (Luckasson et al., 1992).

Significantly subaverage intellectual capabilities as measured by the IQ assessment will generally result in a score of approximately 70 to 75 or below. This upper boundary of IQ is flexible to reflect the statistical variance inherent in all intelligence tests and the need for clinical judgment by a qualified psychological examiner. If a valid IQ score is not possible, significantly subaverage intellectual capabilities means a level of performance that is less than that observed in the vast majority (approximately 97%) of persons of comparable background. To be valid, the assessment of intellectual capabilities must be free from performance impediments caused by motor, sensory, emotional, language, or cultural factors (Luckasson et al., 1992).

The second consideration is the existence of limitations in adaptive skills. Limitations must occur in two or more applicable adaptive skills areas noted above (Ford et al., 1989). The general dimensions of adaptive skills correspond reasonably well to the

Table 1. Impairment groups and diagnostic conditions likely to result in a developmental disability

Cognitive/Developmental Impairment (CI)	Physical Impairment (PI)
Metabolic and immune deficiency disorders	Hemiplegia
Mental retardation	Cerebral palsy
Hydrocephalus	Muscular dystrophy
Down syndrome	Arthrogryposis
Other chromosomal anomaly	Congenital deformity of limb
Fetal alcohol syndrome	Multiple sclerosis
Multiple congenital anomalies	

Sensory/Neurological Impairment (SNI)	Emotional/Behavioral Impairment (ERI)
Disease of central nervous system (CNS)	Autism
Epilepsy	Behaviorally-emotionally impaired
Bilateral blindness	Dual diagnosis (mentally retarded/mentally ill)
Bilateral deafness	
Anencephalus	
Spina bifida (with or without hydrocephalus)	
Encephalocele	
Deformity of brain (microcephalus or congenital hydrocephalus)	

two basic concepts that have emerged from research on adaptive behavior: personal independence and social responsibility (Bruininks & McGrew, 1987; Bruininks, Thurlow, and Gilman, 1987; McGrew & Bruininks, 1989). Two significant reasons can be cited for the importance of limitations in adaptive skills as an accompaniment to the cognitive limitations. First, consideration of adaptive skills provides confirmation of the existence of functional limitations when the validity of the IQ score is in question. Second and more important, emphasizing the impact on adaptive skills reflects the linkage of these functional limitations to the need for services.

The diagnosis of mental retardation requires knowledge of the individual's capabilities and an understanding of the structure and expectations of the individual's personal and social environment. Thus the key elements in the definition of mental retardation are capabilities, environments, and functioning (Luckasson et al., 1992).

As was noted earlier, not all persons with a diagnosis of mental retardation would be considered as having a developmental delay. In some instances when there is a cognitive impairment but the life activity areas are not significantly impaired, the individual may be considered mentally retarded but not developmentally delayed. This is the exception rather than the rule, with most persons having a diagnosis of mental retardation also being considered as having a developmental delay and needing the interdisciplinary supports over a protracted if not lifelong period (Kiernan & Bruininks, 1986). For the definition of developmental disabilities, the parallels to the definition of mental retardation with the emphasis on functionality and early age onset are obvious.

2. Sensory/neurological impairment. Table 1 indicates that persons with sensory/neurological impairments are very heterogeneous, with disabilities ranging from sensory impairment (such as blindness or deafness) to brain deformities (such as microcephaly or hydrocephaly). For expository purposes, we will discuss epilepsy.

The Epilepsy Foundation of America provides the following general definition of epilepsy: a disorder of the central nervous system marked by sudden and periodic lapses of consciousness and distinctive disturbances in the electrical discharges within the brain. Many of these electrical disturbances result in a "seizure," but the qualitative and quantitative nature of the seizure depends on the nature of stimulation to the brain, the region (lobe) of the brain where disturbances start, and the severity and spread of the discharge. In a general sense, seizures are characterized by convulsions of the body's muscles, partial or total loss of consciousness, mental confusion, or disturbance of bodily functions.

Since most seizures-prone persons are not significantly cognitively impaired, it is important to realize that the vast majority of persons with epilepsy have no significant impairment in life activity areas and thus would not be considered to be developmentally disabled. However, if deficits do occur, they are often in the areas of learning, self-direction, independent living, and economic self-sufficiency (Schalock & Kiernan, 1990).

3. Physical impairment. Physical impairments relate to one's inability to execute proper muscular or bodily movement. In its extreme form, the impairment results in complete paralysis; more frequently, it results in partial paralysis. For purposes of explanation we will look more closely at cerebral palsy (CP).

CP is a general term referring to the results of damage to motor control centers in the brain. The condition affects muscle tone or the degree of tension in the muscles, which thereby interferes with voluntary movement and the expression of fine and gross motor development. The three major types of CP include (Kirk & Gallagher, 1989):

- Spastic cerebral palsy. Muscle tone is abnormally high (hypertonia) and increases during activity. Both muscles and joints are tight or stiff, and movements are limited in affected areas of the body.
- Athetoid cerebral palsy. Muscle tone is constantly changing, usually from near normal to high. Movements are uncoordinated, uncontrolled, and jerky.
- Ataxic cerebral palsy. An individual with this form of cerebral palsy has severe problems with balance and coordination but is usually ambulatory.

Persons can have one or a combination of these three types. Damage to the brain resulting in CP can occur before birth, during birth, or after birth due to an accident or injury.

Many additional problems can be associated with cerebral palsy, including cognitive deficits, seizures, and joint and bone deformities such as spinal curvature and contractures. Approximately 40 percent of persons with CP have normal intelligence, with the probability of normal intelligence decreasing as secondary problems increase (Kirk & Gallagher, 1989). Thus it is difficult to generalize regarding probable life activity deficits. A study of adults, however (Schalock & Keith, 1988), suggests that the most likely deficited areas include self-care, learning, mobility, independent living, and economic self-sufficiency.

4. Emotional/behavioral impairment. Our emotional state reflects what is happening to us; our feelings are tied to either external events or thoughts, and they are usually the result of a reasonable assessment of the importance these events have for our lives. But for some persons, emotion and its expression become divorced from reality or separated from logical action-reaction patterns. The net result is exaggerated mood swings, feelings separated from actions, and what many people frequently refer to as "inappropriate emotions." Among children the impairment is sometimes referred to as autism. Autism is characterized by poor interpersonal response patterns, impaired language, under- or overresponsiveness to sensory stimulation, emotional swings, and repetitive self-stimulatory or ritualistic behavior.

In the adult population, one is most likely to encounter the term "dual diagnosed," and it is this group that will be used as an example. A dual diagnosis involves a person with mental retardation who also exhibits a diagnosable form of mental illness. Such persons may constitute one of the most underserved populations (Reiss, Levitan, and McNally, 1982; Senatore, Matson, and Kazdin, 1985). A list of the most frequently reported mental illnesses in persons with mental retardation includes psychoses, anxiety disorders, personality disorders, transitional-situational conditions, and syndrome-associated behaviors such as stereotyped behaviors and confusional-aggressive episodes (Schalock & Kiernan, 1990). Ruth S. Luckasson and others (1992) report a 20 to 35 percent frequency rate of serious

mental illness in noninstitutionalized persons with mental retardation. Generally speaking, persons with a dual diagnosis are probably most limited in the life activity areas involving learning, self-direction, independent living, and economic self-sufficiency.

Prevalence of Developmental Disabilities

The prevalence of many disability conditions has presented a significant challenge to epidemiologists and researchers. Because of the partial inclusion of several diagnostic groups, onset occurring during the first twenty-one years of life, and the use of functional criteria to establish the classification, it is very difficult to establish the extent of developmental disabilities.

Some work has been done examining the prevalence of the categorical groupings making up the term "developmental disabilities" and then adjusting for those with multiple disabilities who would appear twice, as in the case of the person with mental retardation and cerebral palsy. Additionally, with a greater focus in early years on school performance, where there is a higher reliance on cognitive skills and the growing ability to assist persons with severe disabilities in accessing employment, community living, and recreation, there may be differences in the estimates for school-age and adult populations. William E. Kiernan and Robert H. Bruininks (1986), who reviewed a number of the studies of incidence and prevalence of the categorical groupings, and Robert L. Schalock and Kenneth D. Keith (1988), in Nebraska, estimated the presence of developmental disabilities in the school-age population as approximately 1.6 percent, and in the adult population as 1.49 percent. The discrepancy in the age groupings reflects the two factors noted above. These estimates have often served as the basis for state developmental disabilities councils' planning documents. With changes in technology and the effects of prevention and early intervention, these estimates may decline over time. However, traumatic injuries and a greater ability to recognize the developmental and psychiatric needs of persons with dual diagnosis may serve to raise the estimates. The estimates noted above are the most accepted estimates of developmental disabilities nationally.

Current Practices in Providing Services

Clustering persons with developmental disabilities into specialized settings, as in the case of institutions, sheltered workshops, and special schools, was felt to be the optimal way to provide supports in the early 1970s. With extensive documentation of the inadequacies of large institutions, there has been a shift in the focus of residential supports to group homes, apartments, and more recently home ownership for adults with developmental disabilities. For the child, the growing recognition of the role of the family and the natural home environment has been reinforced with efforts in early intervention, home care, and family support. It has now been well documented that persons with developmental disabilities are more appropriately served and supported in the community (Kline 1992).

The development of inclusive education has likewise raised serious questions as to the validity of the special schools, substantially separate educational experiences, and even the resource rooms for students with developmental disabilities. Research shows that children with severe disabilities when placed and supported in the regular school environment learn better, their presence does not impede the instructional environment for other students, and that upon graduation there are more positive outcomes for such students (Sailor et al., 1989). The growing awareness of the need to have a functional curriculum at the secondary level and to provide real work opportunities for students with disabilities has also been supported through extensive research in the transition from school to adult life process (Hasazi, Gordon, and Roe, 1985; Wehman et al., 1988). Those students who have a work experience in school are three times as likely to be employed one year after graduation as those who have not had such an experience (Hasazi & Clark, 1988).

Employment for persons with developmental disabilities has evolved from the belief that such persons could not work to one where there was a need for a specialized work setting, as in the case of a sheltered workshop, to the recognition, through supported employment, that with adequate supports persons with severe disabilities can work in real work settings (Kiernan & Stark, 1986; Rusch, 1990).

Demonstration projects and research have shown that persons with developmental disabilities can be employed in jobs (Kregel, Revell, and West, 1990; McGaughey et al., 1991). The train and place model of rehabilitation is being replaced with the place, train, and support design for persons with developmental disabilities (Schalock & Kiernan, 1990). More recently there has been a growing recognition of the role that coworkers, supervisors, and other naturally occurring supports can play in assisting persons with disabilities in becoming more integrated into the social fabric of the workplace (Hagner, 1992; Kline, 1992; Nisbet, 1992).

The changes in the service system reflect the move from dependence to independence, segregation to integration, facilities to supports, and specialization to generic resources in the community (Kiernan et al., 1993). The influence of the self-advocacy movement, with its emphasis on empowerment, choice, and control, is reshaping and will continue to reshape how services will be developed and offered in the twenty-first century for persons with developmental disabilities.

Professional, Governmental, and Consumer Organizations

By the very nature of the definition of developmental disabilities, a wide variety of professionals and paraprofessionals will be involved in providing supports and services. The interdisciplinary focus of the definition recognizes the need for medical, rehabilitation, educational, psychological, and social support professionals. At various points in the life planning and program development process, different professionals will play a more or less prominent role. During the early years social workers, psychologists, and health care professionals will often support families and persons with developmental disabilities through early intervention programs, family counseling, and health care supports. During the school years educators and related services personnel (physical therapists, occupational therapists, and speech therapists) will interact with the child and family in planning the educational program and in developing community experiences. In the adolescent and adult years rehabilitation counselors will often assist in career development and job placement as well as provide counseling support to the individual as the transition from school and family life to adult life progresses.

As is the case in most conditions that are chronic, episodic, and/or ongoing, supports will be necessary if the person is to be independent and included in normal community life. The relationship of the person with a developmental disability to the professional, particularly in the adult years, is one of a partnership where decision-making is the responsibility of the individual. In some instances, by the nature of the disability, the range of choices both available and able to be comprehended will be limited. The professional plays an important role in identifying and presenting options, and in assisting the individual to make choices and to implement those choices.

A number of resources exist for persons with developmental disabilities. At the federal level, within the Department of Health and Human Services, the Administration on Developmental Disabilities has the primary responsibility in assisting state developmental disabilities planning councils (DDPC) in developing state plans, protection and advocacy (P&A) agencies in assuring that the rights of persons with developmental disabilities are protected, and university-affiliated programs (UAP) in assuming leadership roles in developing services for persons with developmental disabilities through training professionals and paraprofessionals. Financial and health care supports are provided through the Social Security Administration. Social Security supplemental security income (SSI) and disability insurance (SSDI), along with Medicaid, offer a mechanism for financial support and health insurance. For the child with a developmental disability, parental income is calculated in eligibility determination for Social Security benefits, while for the individual over eighteen years of age, family income is not included in this process.

Within each state, in addition to the DDPC, P&A, and UAP (in almost all states), a number of state agencies support persons with developmental disabilities. Early intervention programs, often run in collaboration with state public health or state education agencies, offer services to children with a developmental disability from birth to three years of age. Local schools are required to provide education in the least restrictive environment for all children. Adults with developmental disabilities may receive services from the state mental retardation/developmental disabilities agency and the state vocational rehabilitation agency as well as from a myriad of recreation and housing resources at both the state and local levels.

A number of consumer advocacy groups have been actively involved in the passage of developmental disabilities legislation, including the Association for Retarded Citizens (now the Arc), the United Cerebral Palsy Association, the Epilepsy Foundation of America, the Autism Society of America, and the National Head Injury Foundation, to name just a few. Many of these national organizations have state and local chapters. More recently, self-advocacy groups such as People First have emerged to take a visible role in the formulation of developmental disabilities policy at both the state and national levels. A growing number of organizations, associations, and citizens are taking an active role in expanding services for persons with developmental disabilities.

In summary, the conception of developmental disabilities is undergoing tremendous changes (Summers, 1981; Schalock & Kiernan, 1990). Some of the changes are due to the current paradigm shift that emphasizes equity, inclusion, and support services within the community. Part of the changes also reflect a better understanding of the potential of persons with disabilities, especially when habilitation practices are based on functional skill training, use of prosthetics, and environmental accommodation and modification. And part of the changes are also due to a change in social and policy orientation that provides opportunities and support for persons with disabilities so that they, like the general population, can increase their independence, productivity, and community integration.

(*See also:* AUTISM; CHILDHOOD DISABILITIES; MENTAL RETARDATION; SPECIAL EDUCATION; SUPPORTED EMPLOYMENT)

BIBLIOGRAPHY

BRADLEY, VAL. *The Paradigm Shift.* Cambridge, MA, 1992.

BRUININKS, ROBERT H., and McGREW, KEVIN. *Explor-*

ing the Structure of Adaptive Behavior. Minneapolis, MN, 1987.

BRUININKS, ROBERT H.; THURLOW, MAUREEN; and GILMAN, CLARENCE J. "Adaptive Behavior and Mental Retardation." Journal of Special Education 21 (1987):69–88.

FORD, ARNOLD; SCHNORR, RICK; MEYER, LUANA; DAVERN, LAWRENCE; and DEMPSEY, PAUL. The Syracuse Community-Referenced Curriculum Guide. Baltimore, 1989.

GOLLAY, ELEANOR. The Modified Definition of Developmental Disabilities: An Initial Exploration. Columbia, MD, 1979.

GROSSMAN, HERB J. Classification in Mental Retardation. Washington, DC, 1983.

HAGNER, DAVID. "The Social Interactions and Job Supports of Supported Employees." In Natural Supports in School, at Work, and in the Community for People with Severe Disabilities, ed. J. Nisbet. Baltimore, 1992.

HASAZI, SUSAN B., and CLARK, GREG C. "Vocational Preparation for High School Students Labeled Mentally Retarded: Employment as a Graduation Goal." Mental Retardation 26 (1988):343–349.

HASAZI, SUSAN B.; GORDON, LARRY R.; and ROE, CHARLES A. "Factors Associated with the Employment Status of Handicapped Youth Exiting High School from 1979 to 1983." Exceptional Children 51 (1985): 455–469.

KIERNAN, WILLIAM E., and BRUININKS, ROBERT H. "Demographic Characteristics." In Pathways to Employment for Adults with Developmental Disabilities, eds. William E. Kiernan and Jack A. Stark. Baltimore, 1986.

KIERNAN, WILLIAM E.; SCHALOCK, ROBERT L.; BUTTERWORTH, JOHN; and SAILOR, WAYNE. Enhancing the Use of Natural Supports for People with Severe Disabilities. Boston, 1993.

KIERNAN, WILLIAM E.; SMITH, BETTY C.; and OSTROWSKY, MAURICE B. "Developmental Disabilities: Definitional Issues." In Pathways to Employment for Adults with Developmental Disabilities, eds. William E. Kiernan and Jack A. Stark. Baltimore, 1986.

KIERNAN, WILLIAM E., and STARK, JACK A. Pathways to Employment for Adults with Developmental Disabilities. Baltimore, 1986.

KIRK, SAM A., and GALLAGHER, JACK J. Educating Exceptional Children. Boston, 1989.

KLINE, JOSEPH. "Get Me the Hell Out of Here: Supporting People with Disabilities to Live in Their Own Homes." In Natural Supports in School, at Work, and in the Community for People with Severe Disabilities, ed. Jan Nisbet. Baltimore, 1992.

KREGEL, JIM; REVELL, WILLIAM G.; and WEST, MICHAEL. The National Supported Employment Initiative: Expanding Employment Opportunities for Persons with Severe Disabilities. Richmond, VA, 1990.

LUCKASSON, RUTH S.; COULTER, DAVID L.; POLLOWAY, ED A.; REISS, STEVE; SCHALOCK, ROBERT L.; SNELL, MARTI E.; SPITALNIK, DEBRA M.; and STARK, JACK A. Mental Retardation: Definition, Classification, and Systems of Support. Washington, DC, 1992.

McGAUGHEY, MARTHA J.; KIERNAN, WILLIAM E.; LYNCH, SHEILA A.; SCHALOCK, ROBERT L.; and MORGANSTERN, DARLENE R. National Survey of Day and Employment Programs for Persons with Developmental Disabilities: Results from State MR/DD Agencies. Boston, 1991.

McGREW, KEVIN, and BRUININKS, ROBERT H. "The Factor Structure of Adaptive Behavior." School Psychology Review 18 (1989):64–81.

NISBET, JAN, ed. Natural Supports in School, at Work, and in the Community for People with Severe Disabilities. Baltimore, 1992.

REISS, STEVE; LEVITAN, GREG W.; and McNALLY, ROBERT J. "Emotionally Disturbed Mentally Retarded People: An Underserved Population." American Psychologist 37 (1982):361–367.

RUSCH, FRANK R. Supported Employment: Models, Methods, and Issues. Sycamore, IL, 1990.

SAILOR, WAYNE; ANDERSON, JIM; HALVERSON, ARNOLD; DOERING, KATHY; FILLER, JIM; and GOETZ, LOUIS. The Comprehensive Local School: Regular Education for All Students with Disabilities. Baltimore, 1989.

SCHALOCK, ROBERT L., and KEITH, KEN D. Assessing the Impact on the Current System of Services and Clientele of Changing from a Categorical to a Functional Developmental Disabilities Definition. Lincoln, NE, 1988.

SCHALOCK, ROBERT L., and KIERNAN, WILLIAM E. Habilitation Planning for Adults with Developmental Disabilities. New York, 1990.

SENATORE, VICTORIA; MATSON, JOHN L.; and KAZDIN, ALAN E. "An Inventory to Assess Psychopathology of Mentally Retarded Adults." American Journal of Mental Deficiency (1985):459–466.

SUMMERS, JOSEPH. "The Definition of Developmental Disabilities: A Concept in Transition." Mental Retardation 19 (1981):259–265.

WEHMAN, PAUL; MOON, M. SHERYL; EVERSON, JOSEPH

M.; WOOD, WILLIAM; and BARCUS, JACK M. *Transition from School to Work: New Challenges for Youth with Severe Disabilities.* Baltimore, 1988.

WILLIAM E. KIERNAN
ROBERT L. SCHALOCK

DIABETES

See ENDOCRINE DISORDERS

DIALYSIS

See KIDNEY DISORDERS

DIGESTIVE DISORDERS

See GASTROINTESTINAL DISORDERS

DISABILITY

This entry discusses disability from a broad perspective, including medical, legal, and the general public's conceptualizations of the term. For a discussion of specific disabilities, disorders, or impairments, see ALZHEIMER'S DISEASE; ANXIETY DISORDERS; APHASIA; ARTHRITIS; AUTISM; BACK DISORDERS; BLINDNESS AND VISION DISORDERS; BLOOD DISORDERS; BURNS; CANCER; CHILDHOOD DISABILITIES; CHILDHOOD PSYCHIATRIC DISORDERS; CHRONIC FATIGUE SYNDROME; COMMUNICATION DISABILITIES; CORONARY ARTERY DISEASE; DEAF-BLINDNESS; DEAFNESS AND HEARING IMPAIRMENT; DEVELOPMENTAL DISABILITY; EATING DISORDERS; ENDOCRINE DISORDERS; GASTROINTESTINAL DISORDERS; GENETIC DISORDERS; GROWTH DISORDERS; HEAD INJURY; HUMAN IMMUNODEFICIENCY VIRUS DISEASE AND ACQUIRED IMMUNODEFICIENCY SYNDROME; KIDNEY DISORDERS; LEARNING DISABILITIES; MENTAL RETARDATION; MOOD DISORDERS; MULTIPLE DISABILITIES; MUSCULOSKELETAL DISORDERS; NEUROLOGICAL DISORDERS; NEUROMUSCULAR DISORDERS; ORGANIC MENTAL SYNDROMES; PAIN; PERSONALITY DISORDERS; RESPIRATORY DISEASE; SCHIZOPHRENIA; SICKLE CELL ANEMIA AND THALASSEMIA; SPINAL CORD INJURY; STROKE.

Disability is a condition that impairs or imposes restrictions on a person's ability to function at normal or expected levels of mental or physical activity. The term "handicap" is not synonymous with disability but refers to the presence of physical and social barriers constructed by individuals, institutions, and societies that prevent people with disabilities from participating equally or fully in their environments.

Disabilities may be apparent or hidden. Hidden disabilities (e.g., certain diseases such as diabetes, or learning impairments such as dyslexia) are conditions recognized by diagnosticians but that are not usually obvious to laypeople. There are three distinct origins of disability: congenital, developmental, and acquired. Congenital disabilities originate from hereditary genetic factors (e.g., cystic fibrosis); developmental disabilities occur prior to age twenty-two and are diagnosed from specific symptoms which can become more severe over time (e.g., epilepsy, cerebral palsy); acquired disabilities occur through accident, disease, or injury and prevent full physical and/or mental functioning (e.g., paraplegia and quadriplegia, severe brain damage).

The definition of disability and the discussion of its impact on the individual and society are examined from three perspectives: medical and/or rehabilitation, legal, and social. The medical and/or rehabilitation perspective of disability, whose objective is to heal, restore, and improve capabilities, focuses on functional limitations resulting from physical (e.g., mobility), sensory (e.g., vision, auditory), organic (e.g., diabetes, epilepsy, cerebral palsy), intellectual (e.g., learning), or psychiatric (e.g., schizophrenia, types of depression) impairment. A common objective of legal redress for people with disabilities is to seek financial support and social security. This is discussed and defined within the context of rights (or entitlements) and justice (or equality in a broad social context). Disability from the social perspective has two consequences: as a state or condition of "differentness" that engenders and sustains marginalization and/or exclusion in personal interactions, and as a condition in which public values and public policies determine the physical and behavioral requirements for participating in community life.

Medical and/or Rehabilitation Perspective

From the medical perspective, the principles of beneficence and nonmaleficence are the philosophical and ethical guidelines for diagnosis and treatment. Beneficence instructs to "do good," while nonmaleficence instructs to "avoid doing harm" to others

(Jonsen, Siegler, and Winslade, 1986). Using these guidelines, medical and rehabilitation professionals heal, restore, and provide optimum opportunity for functioning "normally" when diagnosing and treating people with disabilities. By definition, then, the goal of medical personnel is to reverse, eliminate, or control disability through treatment, habilitation, and rehabilitation. Pertinent *a priori* philosophical tenets in the field of rehabilitation have focused on facilitating a self-empowerment approach to rehabilitation service delivery that sets out four basic assumptions:

- Each individual is of great worth and dignity.
- Each individual should have equal opportunity to maximize his or her potential with societal help.
- Individuals strive to grow and change in positive directions.
- Individuals should be free to make their own decisions about the management of their lives (Dowd & Emener, 1978).

People with disabilities may or may not choose to maximize habilitative and/or rehabilitative potential. Choices depend on several factors: type and severity of the disabling condition, individual ego strengths, prognosis, ability to have autonomy in decision-making, familial and associate support systems, health care support systems, advocacy support, demographics (age, community treatment facilities, distance to major centers), financial status, and social status. William G. Emener, A. Patrick, and D. K. Hollingsworth (1984) define rehabilitation as "a process of helping handicapped individuals move from positions of dependency in their community toward positions of independency in a community of their choice" (p. 6). This premise promotes personal choice in quality of life for individuals and the support and service delivery systems that strive to facilitate independent living and autonomy. For people with severe disabilities, however (i.e., those considered unable to make personal choices intellectually or mentally, or those who are physically incapable of functioning without personal care attendants and assistive devices), the idea of independence and autonomy generates moral and ethical debates in quality-of-life issues. New medical techniques make it possible to practice active euthanasia by transplanting organs from "brain dead" infants to those born with organ defects, to create life in a test tube, or to end fetal life based on a prenatal diagnosis of severe mental retardation. Further, current debate focuses on whether medically assisted suicide should be allowed, and who makes the decision to end life because quality of life is absent. It is a mandate, however, for rehabilitation professionals, in partnership with medical diagnosticians, to be aware of and optimize every opportunity for the self-empowerment ideal so the "ability" rather than the "disability" of an individual becomes the focus for promoting sustainable quality of life.

Legal Perspective

From a legal perspective, disability is defined "in principle" by legislation that ensures the rights of individuals who have a disability (e.g., entitlement, compensation for injury, accessibility), and justice, which decrees full community participation of each citizen regardless of race, sex, ethnicity, religion, or physical or mental ability. In the United States, the Americans with Disabilities Act (ADA) (1990) provides for the integration into the workplace of, and public accessibility for, millions of Americans with disabilities. In Canada, inclusion for people with disabilities is a social and legal requirement under the Charter of Rights and Freedoms, as well as provincial, territorial, and federal human rights legislation. Globally, the Universal Declaration of Human Rights of the United Nations Charter, Article 55 (1) specifies that "the United Nations shall promote: universal respect for an observance of human rights and fundamental freedoms for all" (Brownlie, 1992). International protection of human rights is based on the 1948 U.N. foundation document, the *Universal Declaration of Human Rights* (Brownlie, 1992), which mandates specific rights and freedoms for all people under "Life," "Liberty," "Security of the Person," "Arrest and Detention," "Exile," and "Residence." In reality, these "in principle" defined and categorized rights have not specifically included people with disabilities, as they have not traditionally had a strong voice in advocating on their own behalf (Baker, 1993).

Many laws establish and perpetuate a social order

that reinforces a paternalistic or protectionist attitude toward disability. These laws concentrate on a person's inabilities rather than abilities. From this perspective, people with disabilities are defined as "unable," and therefore not entitled to, or capable of, making decisions for the management of their own lives (Rioux, 1993). For this reason in many societies people with disabilities are denied the fundamental freedoms outlined in the Universal Declaration of Human Rights. They are denied the right to live, are institutionalized against their will, violated and abused, detained because of mental and physical disorders, denied immigration and travel, and denied access to buildings and facilities for conducting business or obtaining an education.

Advocacy, activist, and litigation groups involved with disability issues focus on inclusion, integration, accommodation, and the removal of barriers that obstruct legal redress for people with disabilities. Legal definitions of equality for all do not necessarily translate into equity or fairness for people with disabilities. The process for enforcing legislation, removing barriers, and providing legal venues for ensuring full community participation is slow as the move from inequality (i.e., no provisions for legal redress), to equality (i.e., the right to legal redress), to equity (i.e., accommodation for accessibility, inclusion, and participation in society) becomes the goal of advocacy for people with disabilities. The impact of this movement on social policy and fiscal planning requires that supplements and corrections to the system of justice continue so that accessibility, self-sufficiency, and adequate financial resources for people with disabilities can be achieved. The translation of public will into social policy is an important objective of advocacy, activism, and litigation.

Social Perspective

From a social perspective, the culture and structure of societal institutions are influential in manifesting prejudice, stereotyping, discrimination, and stigma by reinforcing negative images of disability. Mass media imagery, naming language (Blaska, 1993; Zola, 1993), physical and literacy barriers to participation, discriminatory laws, and exclusion from basic organizations have perpetuated disability as "differentness" in physical, mental, and behavioral capacities (Bogdan & Biklen, 1977). The experiences of people with disabilities and their self-perceptions are influenced positively and/or negatively through interaction with others, by public attitudes, and by social policies.

Negative aspects of disability stem from social myths and assumptions. Research conducted by Michelle Fine and Adrienne Asch (1988) outlined the following set of basic assumptions about disability made by others and by people with disabilities:

- Disability is a biological condition that is synonymous with the person and therefore the cause of others' behaviors and attitudes.
- Problems encountered by the person with a disability are a result of the disability.
- People with disabilities are "victims."
- The disability of the person is central to his or her self-definition, social comparison, and reference group.
- Disability is synonymous with needing help and social support.

From these assumptions, people with disabilities can be considered as involuntary deviants. S. Becker (1963) defines deviance as "not a quality of the act the person commits, but rather a consequence of the application by others of rules and sanctions. The deviant is one to whom the label has been successfully applied." (p. 9) Hence some people with disabilities are devalued and devalue themselves because they do not present conventional images of human physique or behavior.

For some people with disabilities, coping and management strategies have been instrumental in alleviating the difficulties and resulting stigma associated with their condition or conditions. In part this is a result of a significant shift in the definition of disability as discussed by Harlan Hahn (1988), who notes that in the past disability was seen from the medical focus on functional impairments, or from the economic focus on vocational limitations. Hahn sees a new sociopolitical focus emerging that transcends the clinical and economic model limitations by "recognizing that the fundamental restrictions of a disability may be located in the surroundings that people encounter rather than within the [person with a disability]." (p 37)

It is difficult to forecast the ability of any person to adjust to a disability. Again, adjustment depends on factors such as the type and severity of the disability, the origin of the condition, support systems, self-perception stemming from social interaction with others, and the individual's ability to make autonomous decisions for the management of his or her life. However, as Harlan Hahn (1993) idealizes, "all persons may need to realize that the occurrence of disability is not necessarily a tragic fate. In many respects, it is also an opportunity to play a significant role in a major process of social change. [People with disabilities] have a unique chance to become involved in an historic struggle to extend and expand the definition of human rights. And there are perhaps few other activities that can provide greater meaning and purpose in life." (p. 224)

(*See also:* ABILITY; ADVOCACY; CIVIL RIGHTS; DISABILITY LAW AND SOCIAL POLICY; PHILOSOPHY OF REHABILITATION; PSYCHOSOCIAL ADJUSTMENT)

BIBLIOGRAPHY

Americans with Disabilities Act (ADA), P. L. 202–336, 1990.

BAKER, DAVID. "Human Rights for Persons with Disabilities." In *Perspectives on Disability*, 2nd ed., ed. Mark Nagler. Palo Alto, CA, 1993.

BECKER, S. *Outsiders: Studies in the Sociology of Deviance.* New York, 1963.

BLASKA, JOAN. "The Power of Language: Speak and Write Using Person First." In *Perspectives on Disability*, 2nd ed., ed. Mark Nagler, Palo Alto, CA, 1993.

BLAXTER, MILDRED. *The Meaning of Disability.* London, 1976.

BOGDAN, ROBERT, and BIKLEN, DOUGLAS. "Handicapism." *Social Policy* (March/April 1977):14–19.

BROWNLIE, IAN. *Basic Documents on Human Rights.* 3rd ed. New York, 1992.

DOWD, E. T., and EMENER, WILLIAM, G. "Lifeboat Counseling: The Issues of Survival Decisions." *Journal of Rehabilitation* 9 (1978):34–36.

EMENER, WILLIAM. "Empowerment in Rehabilitation: An Empowerment Philosophy for Rehabilitation in the 20th Century." *Journal of Rehabilitation* 57:2 (1991):29–34.

EMENER, WILLIAM G.; PATRICK, ADELE; and HOLLINGS-WORTH, DAVID K., eds. *Critical Issues in Rehabilitation Counseling.* Springfield, IL, 1984.

FINE, MICHELLE, and ASCH, ADRIENNE. "Disability Beyond Stigma: Social Interaction, Discrimination, and Activism." *Journal of Social Issues* 44:1 (1988):3–21.

HAHN, HARLAN. "Can Disability Be Beautiful?" *Social Policy* (1988):26–32.

————. "The Politics of Physical Differences: Disability and Discrimination." *Journal of Social Issues* 44:1 (1988):39–47. Ann Arbor, MI.

JONSEN, ALBERT R.; SIEGLER, MARK; and WINSLADE, WILLIAM J. *Clinical Ethics: A Practical Approach to Ethical Decisions,* 2nd ed. New York, 1982.

MARINELLI, ROBERT P., and DELL ORTO, ARTHUR E., eds. *The Psychological and Social Impact of Disability,* 3rd ed. New York, 1991.

NAGLER, MARK, ed. *Perspectives on Disability,* 2nd ed. Palo Alto, CA, 1993.

RIOUX, MARCIA. "Rights, Justice, Power: An Agenda for Change." *Perspectives on Disability.* 2nd ed., ed. Mark Nagler. Palo Alto, CA, 1993.

SCHWARTZ, HOWARD D. "Further Thoughts on a Sociology of Acceptance for Disabled People." In *Perspectives on Disability*, ed. Mark Nagler. Palo Alto, CA, 1990.

WORLD HEALTH ORGANIZATION. "International Classification of Impairments, Disabilities, and Handicaps: A Manual of Classification Relating to the Consequences of Disease." Geneva, 1980.

ZOLA, IRVING K. "Self, Identity and the Naming Question: Reflections on the Language of Disability." In *Perspectives on Disability*, 2nd ed., ed. Mark Nagler. Palo Alto, CA, 1993.

MARK NAGLER
WENDY WILSON

DISABILITY LAW AND SOCIAL POLICY

In its various forms, public policy both follows and leads public opinion about important social issues. The attitudes and actions of policymakers, whether they be elected representatives, public administrators, or judges, are forged in the context of economic, political, and social circumstances. At times, seemingly abrupt paradigmatic shifts occur, but even these are rooted in contextual themes. In hindsight, and sometimes contemporaneously, policy eras can be identified and analyzed, and these illuminate the interwoven nature of public attitudes, public behavior, and public policy.

And so it is with disability policy. Since its establishment, the federal government has viewed disability first as the unfortunate outcome of patriotic service, then as an unintended consequence of the industrial revolution, then as a cause for charitable treatment, and finally as an indication of membership in a minority group. (Table 1 lists statutes and judicial decisions relevant to each of these eras.) Each of these thematic policy eras reflects the larger reality of the time, and disability policy is particularly interesting because of this connection. There is perhaps no better example than disability policy to illustrate the changing nature of U.S. society over the course of its history. This entry provides a historical account of disability policy, drawing on this larger context.

Disability's Emergence in Federal Policy: National Defense and the Industrial Revolution

Prior to the turn of the twentieth century, almost all federal policy treated disability as a military matter. The government, beginning in 1776, demonstrated its commitment to honoring wounded Revolutionary War veterans by establishing a system of monetary compensation. Following every subsequent military engagement, attention was again turned to the needs of soldiers injured in service to their country. By 1890 more than 400,000 men were receiving disability pensions that were service-connected, and some were also provided with medical care. After World War I the country was ready to apply new training and counseling approaches to the personal and employment problems of veterans, and in 1918 the Soldier Rehabilitation Act established a program of vocational rehabilitation for military veterans to help them adjust to their return to civilian life (Obermann, 1965).

During this same period, there had been a building consensus that something must also be done to help victims of the "Industrial War" (Macdonald, 1944). Industrialization had produced significant changes in the basic structures of Western societies between the Civil War and World War I. Following centuries of relatively slow change in agrarian cultures, the industrial revolution spurred the rapid development of manufacturing facilities in cities and the mass movement of farm residents to the growing metropolises. The need for unskilled and semiskilled labor resulted in liberal immigration policies (Hays, 1957). Occupational injuries became an important social issue, contributing to the emergence of labor unions and prompting state governments to establish perhaps the earliest civilian disability programs—the states' workers' compensation systems. These programs were intended to spare employees and employers the need to litigate a worker's claim that an injury had resulted from employment—a process that in the past had often proven unfair to workers. Under the new scheme, an insurance program to which all employers contributed would compensate workers for their health care costs and provide them with compensation for their injuries (Berkowitz, 1987). A total of ten states had passed workers' compensation legislation by 1911, and ten years later, forty-five states and territories had programs (Obermann, 1965).

The triparte industrial employment policy formulated by federal policymakers called for safety programs to be implemented by private employers and workers' compensation to be provided by the states. A third component was a civilian rehabilitation program. Shortly after the passage of the 1918 Soldier Rehabilitation Act, legislators turned their attention to a bill to provide such services to civilians. In 1920 they passed the Civilian Rehabilitation Act, which provided grants to the states to implement this new federal priority. This new program faced challenges ranging from uncertainty regarding the nature of the rehabilitation process itself to a lack of adequately trained professionals (Obermann, 1965) but represented the first national commitment to the issues faced by ordinary citizens with disabilities. In later years there was significant pressure to expand both the clientele for the state/federal VR program and its offerings, but this expansion pressure had more in common with the philosophy of the welfare state than with an industrial employment policy.

The Welfare State and Disability

The American welfare state is a unique national response to industrialization, political upheaval, and

Table 1. Major statutes and court decisions related to disability

Statute/Court Decision	Major Provisions/Findings
National Defense/Industrial Revolution	
National Vocational Rehabilitation Act of 1920	Established state/federal system of rehabilitation services
Welfare State	
Social Security Act of 1935	Established federal/state system of health services for "crippled" children; permanently authorized civilian rehabilitation program
Wagner-O'Day Act of 1938	Authorized federal purchases from workshops for people who are blind
Randolph-Sheppard Act of 1938	Authorized program to employ people who are blind as vendors on federal property
Vocational Rehabilitation Act of 1954	Authorized innovation and expansion grants, and grants to colleges and universities for professional training
Wagner-Peyser Act Amendments of 1954	Required federal/state employment security offices to designate staff members to assist people with severe disabilities
Social Security Amendments of 1956	Established Social Security Disability Insurance Trust Fund and provided for payments to eligible workers who became disabled
National Defense Education Act of 1958	Authorized federal assistance for preparation of teachers of children with disabilities
Mental Retardation Facilities and Community Mental Health Centers Construction Act of 1963	Provided grants for construction of mental retardation research centers and facilities; provided for training of educational personnel involved with youth with disabilities; authorized grants to states for construction of community mental health centers
Mental Retardation Facilities and Community Mental Health Centers Construction Act Amendments of 1965	Established grant program to cover initial staffing costs for community mental health centers
Social Security Act Amendments of 1965	Established Medicaid program for elderly people and for blind persons and other persons with disabilities
Elementary and Secondary Education Act of 1965	Authorized federal aid to states and localities for educating deprived children, including children with disabilities
Elementary and Secondary Education Act Amendments of 1966	Created National Advisory Committee on Handicapped Children; created Bureau of Education for the Handicapped in U.S. Office of Education
Fair Labor Standards Amendments of 1966	Established standards for employment of workers with disabilities, allowing for subminimum wages
Elementary and Secondary Education Amendments of 1967	Authorized regional resource centers; authorized centers and services for deaf-blind children
Handicapped Children's Early Education Assistance Act of 1968	Established grant program for preschool and early education of children with disabilities
Vocational Education Act Amendments of 1968	Required participating states to earmark 10 percent of basic vocational education allotment for youth with disabilities

Table 1. Major statutes and court decisions related to disability (*continued*)

Statute/Court Decision	Major Provisions/Findings
Developmental Disabilities Services and Facilities Construction Amendments of 1970	Expanded services to individuals with epilepsy and cerebral palsy; authorized new state formula grant program; defined "developmental disability" in categorical terms; established state-level planning council
Javits-Wagner-O'Day Act of 1971	Extended purchase authority to workshops for people with severe disabilities in addition to blindness; retained through 1976 preference for workshops for people who are blind
Social Security Amendments of 1972	Extended Medicare coverage to individuals with disabilities; established Supplemental Security Income program for elderly people and for blind persons and other persons with disabilities
Small Business Investment Act Amendments of 1972	Established the "Handicapped Assistance Loan Program" to provide loans to nonprofit sheltered workshops and individuals with disabilities
Rehabilitation Act of 1973	Established service priority for people with severe disabilities; required Individualized Written Rehabilitation Plan; established Rehabilitation Services Administration in Department of Health, Education, and Welfare
Education Amendments of 1974	Required states to establish plans and timetables for providing full educational opportunities for all children with disabilities as condition of receiving federal funds
Headstart, Economic Opportunity, and Community Partnership Act of 1974	Required that at least 10 percent of children enrolled in Headstart be children with disabilities
Housing and Community Development Act of 1974	Established Section 8 housing program for low-income families, including individuals with disabilities and/or their families
Developmentally Disabled Assistance and Bill of Rights Act of 1975	Added requirement that state plan include deinstitutionalization plan; required states to develop and annually review rehabilitation plans for all clients
Education for All Handicapped Children Act of 1975	Established grant-in-aid program requiring free appropriate public education in least restrictive environment for all children with disabilities; authorized funding for preschool and early intervention programs
Rehabilitation, Comprehensive Services, and Developmental Disabilities Amendments of 1978	Established National Institute of Handicapped Research; established National Council on the Handicapped; authorized grant program for independent living services; replaced categorical definition of developmental disability with functional definition; established minimum funding level for protection and advocacy services
Department of Education Organization Act of 1979	Established Office of Special Education and Rehabilitative Services in new cabinet-level Department of Education
Job Training Partnership Act of 1982	Authorized training and placement services for "economically disadvantaged" individuals, including persons with disabilities

263

Table 1. Major statutes and court decisions related to disability (*continued*)

Statute/Court Decision	*Major Provisions/Findings*
Education of the Handicapped Act Amendments of 1983	Authorized grants for training of parents of children with disabilities
Developmental Disabilities Act of 1984	Shifted emphasis to employment in priority services; required Individual Habilitation Plan for consumers; increased minimum funding for protection and advocacy services
Rehabilitation Amendments of 1984	Established Client Assistance Programs as formula grant program; made National Council on the Handicapped an independent agency
Education of the Deaf Act of 1986	Updated statute establishing Gallaudet College and changed name to Gallaudet University; authorized Gallaudet University to operate demonstration elementary and secondary schools for deaf children; established Commission on Education of the Deaf
Rehabilitation Act Amendments of 1986	"Severe disability" definition expanded to include functional (as well as categorical) criteria; defined "employability" for first time; added formula grant program for supported employment; renamed research branch the National Institute on Disability and Rehabilitation Research
Developmental Disabilities and Bill of Rights Act Amendments of 1987	Raised minimum allotment levels for basic state grant program and protection and advocacy systems; increased minimum allotment for university-affiliated programs, basic state grant program, and protection and advocacy systems
Rehabilitation Act Amendments of 1992	Changed eligibility requirements and procedures for determining eligibility; strengthened requirements for interagency cooperation; strengthened consumer involvement requirements
Civil Rights	
Architectural Barriers Act of 1968	Required most buildings and facilities built, constructed, or altered with federal funds after 1969 to be accessible
Urban Mass Transportation Act Amendment of 1970	Authorized grants to states and localities for accessible mass transportation
Pennsylvania Association for Retarded Children v. Commonwealth of Pennsylvania (1972); *Mills v. Board of Education of the District of Columbia* (1972)	Applied equal protection and due process theories to establish that children with disabilities cannot be denied public education without due process
Rehabilitation Act of 1973	Prohibited disability discrimination in federally assisted programs and activities and federal agencies; required affirmative action programs for people with disabilities by federal agencies and some federal contractors; established the Architectural and Transportation Barriers Compliance Board
Developmentally Disabled Assistance and Bill of Rights Act of 1975	Described congressional findings regarding rights of persons with developmental disabilities; established funding for protection and advocacy systems

Table 1. Major statutes and court decisions related to disability (*continued*)

Statute/Court Decision	Major Provisions/Findings
Education for All Handicapped Children of 1975	Required states to establish policy assuring free appropriate public education for children with disabilities as condition for receiving Part B funds; established procedural safeguards, procedures for mainstreaming children with disabilities to the maximum extent possible, and procedures for nondiscriminatory testing and evaluation practices
Civil Rights Commission Act of 1978	Expanded jurisdiction of Civil Rights Commission to disability discrimination
Civil Rights of Institutionalized Persons Act of 1980	Empowered Department of Justice to bring suit against states for allegedly violating rights of institutionalized persons with disabilities
Child Abuse Prevention Treatment Act Amendments of 1984	Required states' child protection agencies to develop procedures for responding to reports that newborns with disabling conditions were being denied treatment; established conditions for requiring such treatment
Air Carrier Access Act of 1986	Prohibited disability discrimination in provision of air transportation
Protection and Advocacy for Mentally Ill Individuals Act of 1986	Authorized formula grant program for statewide advocacy services for persons with mental illness, provided directly by, or under contract with, the protection and advocacy system for persons with developmental disabilities
Television Decoder Circuitry Act of 1990	Required new television sets to have capability for close-captioned television transmission
Americans with Disabilities Act of 1990	Prohibited disability discrimination in employment, public services and public accommodations operated by private entities; requires that telecommunication services be made accessible

NOTE: Many of the statutes listed in this table have undergone numerous changes since first passage. Readers should consult other sources, such as U.S. Department of Education (1992) for information about the current status of these and other statutes. For more information about judicial decisions, consult Bonnie P. Tucker and Bruce A. Goldstein (1992).

economic deprivation. In the latter part of the nineteenth century there was a move afoot to strengthen the role of the federal government to preserve the nation's political stability and to protect citizens from economic and social risk. This followed a long period during which local communities and states were presumed to bear most of the responsibility of caring for those who, because of illness or other misfortune, were unable to provide for themselves (Tratt, 1989). Historical forces, including decades of industrial development in the Western countries, political revolution abroad and political turmoil at home, and the American Great Depression combined to support increased centralization of authority and, at the same time, broadened responsibilities for the federal government. Throughout the first half of the twentieth century, the national government expanded its reach into the daily lives of the citizenry.

For citizens with disabilities, this trend became

apparent as a series of initiatives providing services and benefits. These were intended, on the one hand, to repay a societal debt to those who had served in the work force (or in the military), and on the other hand, to provide a modicum of care for those who had little or no tie to the work force but were seen as deserving of compassion. The programs followed no master plan. A new service or benefit might be designed with almost no regard for what had come before. Almost randomly, policymakers funded institutional programs for people labeled mentally retarded or mentally ill; education and training services for people who were deaf, blind, or deaf and blind; and a federal-state system of services for "crippled" children.

These programs reflected the values of the time and thus favored some social roles over others, men over women, and some disabilities over others. Injured workers, who had contributed to the nation's economic well-being, could receive vocational rehabilitation services or disability insurance payments, while unemployed adults who became disabled could not. Men's benefits from Social Security Disability Insurance were (and still are) generally higher than women's, reflecting women's lower average income and shorter work histories. Similarly, there is a long-standing pattern of favored treatment for blind persons as opposed to individuals with other kinds of disabilities. The initiatives during the half century after the establishment of the civilian rehabilitation program greatly increased the federal presence in the lives of people with disabilities. The significant developments of this time included:

- The establishment of income maintenance programs. By 1972, two major income maintenance programs had been established. The first, Social Security Disability Insurance (SSDI), is a social insurance program to which employers and employees contribute to provide cash benefits to working individuals who develop a disability that prevents their continued participation in the work force, their spouses, or their dependents. The Supplemental Security Income (SSI) program is not tied to work force participation and is means-tested—that is, individuals are eligible for benefits only if they

have few other resources. These two programs are a significant part of the federal government's disability expenditures. In fiscal year 1990, approximately $24.8 billion was paid to 3 million individuals through SSDI, and about $12.9 billion was paid to 3.4 million individuals with disabilities through the SSI program (USGAO, 1992).

- A collection of habilitation, rehabilitation, and treatment programs. In keeping with the core liberal philosophy of this century, the government established a number of programs designed to provide basic services to people with disabilities. Some of these were directed at groups of individuals with specific disabilities. For example, the Randolph-Sheppard Act authorized the granting of vendorships in federal buildings to persons who are blind (U.S. Department of Education, 1992); and the Mental Retardation Facilities and Community Mental Health Centers Construction Act provided for the building of mental retardation centers (Scheerenberger, 1987). Other programs provided services to people with varying kinds of disabilities. The Wagner-Peyser Act Amendments of 1954, for example, required that employment security offices designate at least one staff member to assist individuals with any type of severe disability (U.S. Department of Education, 1992). In still other instances, people with disabilities were included as a target group for more general social legislation. In one example, the Housing and Community Development Amendments of 1974 specifically mentioned families with a disabled member as eligible for Section 8 low-income housing. Whatever their structure, these initiatives were ample proof that policymakers had recognized the potential for a significant federal role in assisting people with disabilities (U.S. Department of Education, 1992).

- The establishment of a strong federal commitment to educating children with disabilities. In 1965 the federal government acted on its long-time concern regarding the welfare of children with disabilities and other disadvantages and established the first federal grant program to assist states in their educational efforts (U.S. De-

266

partment of Education, 1992). In the next ten years, policymakers took a number of steps to strengthen the states' educational offerings to such children. The result of these efforts was a vastly expanded federal role in mandating and funding educational services to children who have disabilities. This commitment eventually led to the passage of the Education for All Handicapped Children Act of 1975.

These programs were established during a long period of economic prosperity, which provided an expanding tax base for government growth. They were examples of the dominant liberal philosophy of the time, a philosophy that stressed the role of a strong national government in providing social and economic security for the nation's citizens through social insurance, entitlements, and service delivery. At the same time, these policy initiatives illuminated the widespread public view toward people with disabilities as "deserving" of assistance, even though that assistance might be viewed by some recipients as demeaning, paternalistic, or misdirected. Most policymakers believed that people with disabilities suffered hardship through no fault of their own and that a wealthy nation such as ours should commit public resources to their sustenance, treatment, and rehabilitation. Policymakers were willing to devote federal resources to a collection of specialized services, to be controlled largely by professionals, for the betterment of individuals with disabilities. Such thinking was in keeping with public opinion of the time, although there was evidence that a rights perspective was beginning to take hold in some quarters.

The public investment in services for people with disabilities spurred the development of new professions, and rehabilitation counseling is illustrative of this process. As early as 1930 the government addressed the role of rehabilitation counselors (Obermann, 1965) and has adopted a singular role in their training and employment. Direct funding of academic programs has been authorized since 1954, and in the first twelve years of the program, more than three thousand counselors had been trained through federally funded programs (Walker, 1985). The Rehabilitation Services Administration continues to grant monies for student stipends and related costs.

Other professions, such as physical therapy and psychiatry, have experienced similar growth patterns, though with much less direct federal support (Gritzer & Arluke, 1985).

The influence of various interest groups has grown during this period. Professional groups, such as the National Rehabilitation Association, were among the first groups to work with legislators on disability issues, and they remain an important influence. Others soon formed as parents and other advocates discovered the benefits of political action. The parents' movement established the Association for Retarded Citizens (now called The Arc), a group that gained considerable power due to its competent representation of its constituents' interest in expanded services (Blatt, 1987). People with disabilities formed a number of associations, including the first significant national cross-disability group, the American Coalition of Citizens with Disabilities (Bowe, 1978). A panoply of organizations now exists, ranging from the Academy of Physical Medicine and Rehabilitation to the Epilepsy Foundation of America. These groups, however diverse in membership and purpose, form the backbone of the disability community and strive to serve the interests of people with disabilities.

The federal disability infrastructure grew substantially during the early part of the twentieth century, though in a haphazard way. The current structure reflects the facts that disability programs are among both the oldest domestic assistance programs and the least coordinated. By 1986 there were forty-four distinct funding sources for programs and activities, ranging from small, well-defined programs such as workers' compensation for longshore and harbor workers to complex mammoths such as Medicaid and SSDI (National Council on the Handicapped, 1986). Fourteen agencies—six independent executive agencies and five cabinet offices—were involved in conducting these activities. The Department of Education had the largest number of programs, but the most expensive are in the Health Care Financing Administration (HCFA; Medicaid and Medicare) and the Social Security Administration (SSA, Social Security Disability Insurance, and Supplemental Security Income). Oversight authority, too, has been widespread: six Senate committees and eight committees in the House of Representatives as well as the Joint Committee on the Library (of Congress) have had such authority. The irony here is that the agencies responsible for most of the federal monies devoted to disability—HCFA and SSA—did not view disability as an important part of their efforts; and the most prominent disability committees in the Senate and the House have had no jurisdiction over the most expensive disability programs (West, 1993). Nonetheless, the enormity of the federal disability infrastructure may be viewed as evidence of the importance of disability to the state and to those who experience it.

Civil Rights and People with Disabilities: The Paradigm Shifts

Gradually, people with disabilities began to view themselves, and to be viewed by others, as a minority group whose difficulties were caused more by societal prejudice and discrimination than by disability. This important paradigm shift is marked by three key events of the 1970s: court decisions based on the equal protection and due process principles; the passage of the 1973 Rehabilitation Act; and the growth of the disability rights movement. Each of these indicated a growing consciousness by people with disabilities, their advocates, and the larger society that the long pattern of paternalistic and dehumanizing practices typified by institutionalization and segregation should end.

The first events were court decisions that relied on the constitutional principles of equal protection and due process (Tucker & Goldstein, 1992; Turnbull, 1990). Following the logic of *Brown v. Board of Education*, these two cases—*Pennsylvania Association for Retarded Children (PARC) v. Commonwealth of Pennsylvania* and *Mills v. D.C. Board of Education*—established the right of children with disabilities to a free appropriate public education. These court decisions, together with congressional dissatisfaction with the states' progress in improving educational opportunities for such children, prompted passage of the Education for All Handicapped Children Act in 1975, which extended the role of the federal government in mandating and funding schooling for children with disabilities. Thus began the long process of integrating children with disabilities into the nation's schools, a process that continues today and

that has spawned another iteration of the education debate—whether special education should be replaced by a "full inclusion" strategy in which children with disabilities are educated, with necessary supports, alongside nondisabled children in their neighborhood schools (McDonnell et al., 1991).

During the same period, the Rehabilitation Act of 1973 became the first federal statute containing a title clearly patterned after civil rights legislation for racial minorities (Scotch, 1984). In Section 504 of the act, federal grantees were prohibited from discriminating against persons with disabilities in employment and in any other activity. Originated by congressional staffers, the section itself caused little controversy at the time of its passage. The implementation phase, though, was uproarious due to the government's lack of experience with such legislation, tactical delays by the administration, and the demands of the nascent disability rights movement. Later, the 1973 Rehabilitation Act and its regulations served as a partial blueprint for both the Education for All Handicapped Children Act and the Americans with Disabilities Act.

The disability rights movement was the third major contributor to the conceptual shift toward a minority group model. To speak of the "movement" as though it were a single entity is somewhat misleading. In reality, the disability rights movement was and is made up of literally dozens of organizations and hundreds, perhaps thousands, of individuals who are committed to establishing the legal rights of people with disabilities (Scotch, 1989). All of these advocacy efforts were grounded in the view that people with disabilities were struggling against almost overwhelming odds to overcome the effects of oppressive social biases, and knew that political action could bring changes in public policy. These forces come together in a loose and shifting coalition around various issues.

The passage of the Americans with Disabilities Act (ADA) of 1990 is the culmination of a quarter-century trend toward the establishment of legal protections for people with disabilities. The ADA prohibits discrimination and requires reasonable accommodation in employment, public accommodations, government services, some communication services, and public and private transportation systems. This far-reaching statute will eventually affect employers with fifteen or more employees, every state and local government entity in the United States, private providers of public accommodations, and major telecommunications networks (West, 1991). The ADA mandate, if enforced vigorously, should improve the quality of life for many individuals who have disabilities. It is unclear, however, whether the ADA is sufficient to remove completely attitudinal, educational, communication, and other barriers faced by people with disabilities. Some argue that it will help only those with the least severe disabilities and the best education and training, and that individuals who are "doubly disabled" by both impairments and poor education and job training require additional policy approaches (Burkhauser, 1992). The failure of the ADA to prohibit insurance practices that keep even employed disabled people uninsured or poorly insured is another concern (Turnbull, Bateman, & Turnbull, 1993).

The disability rights movement has forced a profound change in the way policymakers think about "disability." It is no longer an abstract concept that serves to demarcate the work-based economy from the needs-based economy (Stone, 1984), or a medical issue best addressed by the health care system. The word "disability" now reflects a new social construction of a minority group whose needs are best met, advocates argue, by a combination of legal protections against discrimination and specialized services (Jones, 1991; for a contrary view on specialized services, see Schriner, Rumrill, & Parlin, 1994).

The issue of disability in our society is thus a complex and difficult one. The long history of disability policy in the United States has institutionalized policy boundaries that distinguish those with disabilities from those without, leaving us stumbling over the meaning of equality for people whose disabilities have traditionally excluded them from society in what Martha Minow has called "the dilemma of difference" (Minow, 1990). At this point, our policy decisions leave us with disconcerting contradictions. We allow positive discrimination—through services and benefits designed especially for people with disabilities—while we prohibit negative discrimination. In a very real sense, we are using disability to get beyond disability. How will we resolve this dilemma? The dimensions of this problem involve both rights-based political orthodoxy and the need for society to understand the interconnectedness of individuals (with all their differences), families, and the larger community. The challenge is to promote the expansion of opportunities and access through broad-based accommodative and redesign strategies without further dividing those who have disabilities from those who do not. The sooner our society can recognize and accommodate individual differences without requiring the force of public policy to do so, the more successful we will have been.

(See also: ADVOCACY; AMERICANS WITH DISABILITIES ACT; CIVIL RIGHTS; HISTORY OF REHABILITATION; STATE-FEDERAL REHABILITATION PROGRAM)

BIBLIOGRAPHY

BERKOWITZ, EDWARD D. Disabled Policy: America's Programs for the Handicapped. Cambridge, Eng., 1987.

BLATT, BURTON. The Conquest of Mental Retardation. Austin, TX, 1987.

BOWE, FRANK. Handicapping America: Barriers to Disabled People. New York, 1978.

BURKHAUSER, RICHARD V. "Beyond Stereotypes: Public Policy and the Doubly Disabled." The American Enterprise. (Sept./Oct. 1992), pp. 60–68.

GRITZER, GLENN, and ARLUKE, ARNOLD. The Making of Rehabilitation: A Political Economy of Medical Specialization, 1890–1980. Berkeley, CA, 1985.

HAYS, SAMUEL P. The Response to Industrialism, 1885–1914. Chicago, 1957.

JONES, NANCY LEE. "Essential Requirements of the Act: A Short History and Overview." In The Americans with Disabilities Act: From Policy to Practice, ed. Jane West. New York, 1991.

MACDONALD, MARY E. Federal Grants for Vocational Rehabilitation. Chicago, 1944.

McDONNELL, ANDREA; McDONNELL, JOHN; HARDMAN, MICHAEL; and McCUNE, GALE. "Educating Students with Severe Disabilities in their Neighborhood School: The Utah Elementary Education Model." Remedial and Special Education 12 (1991): 34–45.

MINOW, MARTHA. Making All the Difference: Inclusion, Exclusion, and American Law. Ithaca, NY, 1990.

NATIONAL COUNCIL ON THE HANDICAPPED. Toward Independence. Washington, DC, 1986.

OBERMANN, C. ESCO. A History of Vocational Rehabilitation in America. Minneapolis, 1965.

SCHEERENBERGER, R. C. *A History of Mental Retardation.* Baltimore, 1987.

SCHRINER, KAY FLETCHER; RUMRILL, PHILLIP; and PARLIN, RUTH. "Rethinking Disability Policy: Equity in the ADA Era and the Political Meaning of Specialized Services for People with Disabilities." *Journal of Health and Human Services* (1994).

SCOTCH, RICHARD K. *From Good Will to Civil Rights.* Philadelphia, PA, 1984.

————. "Politics and Policy of Disability Rights." *The Milbank Quarterly* 67 (1989):380–400.

TRATT, WALTER I. *From Poor Law to Welfare State: A History of Social Welfare in America,* 4th ed. New York, 1989.

TUCKER, BONNIE P., and GOLDSTEIN, BRUCE A. *Legal Rights of Persons with Disabilities.* Horsham, PA, 1992.

TURNBULL, H. RUTHERFORD III. *Free Appropriate Public Education: The Law and Children with Disabilities,* 3rd ed. Denver, 1990.

TURNBULL, H. RUTHERFORD III; BATEMAN, DAVID F.; and TURNBULL, ANN P. "Family Empowerment." In *The ADA Mandate for Social Change,* ed. Paul Wehman. Baltimore, 1993.

U.S. DEPARTMENT OF EDUCATION. *Summary of Existing Legislation Affecting People with Disabilities.* Washington, DC, 1992.

U.S. GENERAL ACCOUNTING OFFICE (USGAO). *Social Security: Racial Differences in Disability Decisions Warrant Further Investigation.* Washington, DC, 1992.

WALKER, MARTHA LENZ. *Beyond Bureaucracy: Mary Elizabeth Switzer and Rehabilitation.* Lanham, MD, 1985.

WEST, JANE, ed. *The Americans with Disabilities Act: From Policy to Practice.* New York, 1991.

KAY FLETCHER SCHRINER
ANDREW I. BATAVIA

DISABILITY MANAGEMENT

Disability management is operationally defined as an active process of minimizing the impact of an impairment (resulting from injury, illness, or disease) on the individual's capacity to participate competitively in the work environment (Shrey & Lacerte, 1995). The concept is used in the context of the rehabilitation of workers with disabilities and industrial rehabilitation. When defining "disability management" it is important to distinguish among the related concepts "impairment," "disability," and "handicap," which the World Health Organization has defined as follows:

Impairment: Any loss or abnormality of psychological, physiological, or anatomical structure or function.

Disability: Any restriction or lack (resulting from an impairment) of ability to perform an activity in the manner or within the range considered normal for a human being.

Handicap: A disadvantage for a given individual resulting from an impairment or a disability that limits or prevents the fulfillment of a role that is normal (depending on age, sex, and social and cultural factors) for that individual.

Based on these definitions, one needs to understand that not all impairments result in a disability; nor do all disabilities necessarily result in a handicap. To prevent impairments and subsequent disabilities from becoming handicaps, it is necessary to manage all the forces and factors that physically or functionally compromise an individual's fulfillment of a specific role. That role, in the context of disability management, is competitive employment.

Basic Principles of Disability Management

The basic principles of disability management are:

1. It is a proactive (preventive) process—the early prevention or resolution of a disability requires the timely utilization of employer-based and community-based services and interventions.

2. It requires employer involvement, support, and accountability—the employer is a key participant in the disability management process, participating actively as a decision-maker, planner, and coordinator of interventions and services.

3. It requires early intervention and early return-to-work strategies (e.g., functional job analysis, physical capacity evaluation, physical reconditioning, job coaching, ergonomic job modifications, workstation modifications, safe work practices monitoring, etc.) designed to control employer costs while protecting the employability of the workers with disabilities.

Successfully managing the consequences of illness, injury, and chronic disease in the work force requires an accurate understanding of the types of injuries and illness that occur, the employer's timely response to the injury or illness, clear administrative policies and procedures, and the effective utilization of health care and rehabilitation services.

Controlling the cost of disability in business and industry and its ultimate impact on employee productivity is not a simple task. Complex and conflicting relationships exist among employer goals, resources, and expectations; the needs and self-interests of workers, health care providers, labor unions and attorneys; and the services available in the community. The ability of the employer to participate actively and effectively in this relationship will contribute to the control of costs as well as the protection of the worker's sustained employment.

Controversial Issues: Deinstitutionalization of the Injured Worker

The dramatic growth in facility-based work-hardening programs has led to the virtual institutionalization of the injured worker in America. The facility-based approach to rehabilitating injured workers is characterized by inherent problems of ecological validity for both the clinical staff and the injured worker. Treatment staff rarely have a true appreciation for the worker's actual job duties, labor relations issues, and the conditions in the work environment. Likewise, there is often concern among treatment staff regarding the validity of third-party job analysis data and distorted descriptions of job duties as reported by injured workers. Although clinicians may occasionally visit the worksite, they are rarely afforded sufficient time to assess the work environment, work culture, labor relations, and technological processes. These factors play a vital role in the development and implementation of effective work return plans.

Deinstitutionalization is a concept that many will relate to the dramatic changes in American mental health and mental retardation services that began in the 1970s. The warehousing of thousands of "deviant" individuals in segregated facilities had resulted in tremendous costs to society as well as losses in

human potential. Legislated rights to independent living and education led to the "mainstreaming" of these people into public school systems and communities. The Americans with Disabilities Act further protected the right to work of millions of persons with physical and mental disabilities.

The injured American worker continues to be institutionalized, despite lessons learned and research showing high correlations between lengthy work disruptions and low work return probability (Boschen, 1989; California Workers' Compensation Institute, 1985). Workers subjected to the institutional or facility approach to rehabilitation are inclined to take on institutional or maladaptive characteristics. Sterile clinical environments that simulate work activity are in sharp contrast with real work conditions in industry. Workers in facilities interact with other injured workers and with medical and allied health professionals rather than with coworkers, labor representatives, and supervisors. Facility-based work hardening merely simulates jobs; employer-based real work facilitates work adjustment. Employees in work-hardening programs receive wage replacement benefits; injured workers in industry-based work transition programs receive pay and fringe benefits. The employer is physically distanced from facility-based work-hardening services. At the worksite, the employer is directly involved in rehabilitation interventions. On-the-job rehabilitation interventions emphasize job retention, positive work adjustment, and accommodation as the primary methods of protecting the employability of workers with disabilities while concurrently reducing the financial liabilities of the employer.

Disability Management: Cost-Effectiveness and Cost Savings

The economics of accidents continues to place a financial drain on employers, insurance carriers, and persons with disabilities. This cost is often passed along to the consumer in the form of higher prices for goods and services and increased insurance premiums. In 1981 the Health Insurance Association of America estimated that accidents resulted in costs exceeding $83 billion for wage loss, medical expenses, fire losses, motor vehicle damage, indirect

271

work losses, and the cost of insurance administration (Matkin, 1986). In 1988, work accidents and injuries cost U.S. employers, workers, and society an estimated $47.1 billion. This represented a 35 percent increase from the $34.8 billion incurred in 1986 (Frieden, 1989). Monroe Berkowitz (1990) reported that the United States had experienced a 400 percent increase in workers' compensation and health care costs over the preceding fifteen years. As expenses for health care and insurance coverage continue to escalate, it becomes crucial that methods be developed for controlling these costs.

Major insurance carriers such as Employers Insurance of Wausau, Travelers, Hartford, and Metropolitan have found disability management to be an effective method of cost reduction. Gopal Pati (1985) reported that "the best predictor of successful rehabilitation potential is the amount of time that has elapsed from time of injury to referral." J. Gardner (1987) noted, "Vocational intervention at an early stage of the rehabilitation process is more likely to secure a timely return to work at a salary rate that is comparable to the pre-injury wage level." According to Steven Scheer (1990), the cost-effectiveness of early intervention with the physically or cognitively injured worker should not be underestimated. He concluded that vocational counselor involvement in the early stages of rehabilitation is prudent from medical, humanistic, and financial perspectives.

During the mid-1980s, the General Electric Company (GE) developed, implemented, and evaluated the Convalescent Assistance to Recovering Employees (CARE) Program. According to Dennis Stempien (1989), the mission of this program was to provide quality health care to injured or ill workers in a timely and coordinated fashion. Early intervention services coordinated by occupational health nurses yielded highly significant results. At one GE plant, the cost per employee consistently decreased each year, over a three-year period, in the areas of short-term disability (33% decrease), salary continuance and hourly sick pay (23% decrease), and workers' compensation (35% decrease).

According to a report in *National Underwriter* (1989), education about the rehabilitation process and early involvement of rehabilitation professionals are the key to solving system-related problems. This report, based on the 1989 Workers' Compensation Congress, called for legislators, injured workers, insurers, attorneys, employers, physicians, and others to be educated about "redirecting their primary attention to equitably resolving rehabilitation issues in a realistic fashion that eliminates the adversarial (litigious) approach." The report stressed the importance of "early, prompt, and realistic determinations of employee rehabilitation potential." A 1988 Florida study was cited, which concluded that evaluation for rehabilitation potential within six months of injury could save the employers and insurers nearly $6 million per year while possibly increasing the earnings of people with disabilities by $9 million per year.

Disability Management Programs at the Worksite

As a result of rapidly escalating workers' compensation costs and mandated disability program benefits, trends reflect that employers have begun to take a more active role in disability management. As a result, many employers have initiated disability management programs at the worksite (Schwartz et al., 1989). The following concepts are central to an effective disability management program in business and industry:

1. Early intervention strategies and early return-to-work programs result in decreased lost time, increased employer productivity, and decreased workers' compensation and disability costs. In nearly all research and writings, "early intervention" is considered to be the primary factor upon which the foundation of medical, psychosocial, and vocational rehabilitation is established (Lucas, 1987; Pati, 1985; Scheer, 1990; Wright, 1980). However, the successful management of disability also requires "early return-to-work" opportunities, accommodations, and supports (Habeck et al., 1991; Shrey & Olsheski, 1992).

2. Disability management requires an interdisciplinary disability management team. Members of this team often include employer representatives (e.g., safety managers, occupational health nurses,

risk managers, human resources personnel, and operations managers), labor union representatives, the worker's treating physician, a rehabilitation case manager, an on-site physical/occupational therapist, and the worker with a disability (Lacerte & Desjardins, 1993).

3. Employer-based disability management programs require joint labor-management support. Many unionized employers have successfully developed and implemented on-site disability management programs under the guidance and support of joint labor-management committees (Shrey & Bruyere, 1991).

4. Disability management interventions must be directed at both the individual and the work environment. The traditional approach to rehabilitation often ignores the fact that occupational disability may originate as much from environmental barriers as from the worker's personal traits. Workers dissatisfied with their jobs, supervisor-worker conflicts, and poorly designed workstations are among the many environmental barriers to disability management. In short, to maximize rehabilitation outcomes among injured workers, an equally balanced focus on the individual and the work environment is needed.

5. Case management services are necessary to facilitate the development and implementation of disability management strategies and return-to-work plans for workers with disabilities. The case manager serves as a central disability management team member by functioning as a liaison between employers, labor representatives, injured workers, community health care providers, and others.

6. "Occupational bonding" is the fundamental principle underlying an effective return to work program for employees with work restrictions (Shrey & Bruyere, 1991). Employer-based disability management interventions recognize and utilize the therapeutic value of the physical, psychological, social, and environmental dimensions of the workplace. Workers, despite their impairments, must continue to see themselves as valued employees who remain attached to the workplace. The concept of occupational bonding describes the relationship between the worker and employer. Disability management interventions introduced within the ecological con-

text of the workplace strengthen the bond between the worker with functional restrictions and the employer (Shrey, 1992).

7. Disability management is perhaps best characterized by employer-based transitional work programs. Transitional work is generally developed by integrating any combination of job tasks and functions that may be performed safely and with remuneration by an employee whose physical capacity to perform functional job demands has been compromised. Such programs are designed to encourage and support an injured employee's safe and timely return to work. They provide the worker with accommodations and an opportunity to "transition" back to work gradually through conditioning, safe work practices education, and work readjustment. Essential components of on-site programs include:

- objective worker evaluations;
- an analysis of job tasks and physical functions;
- designated jobs or work transition units;
- on-site clinical supervision;
- a gradual work return plan that increases the worker's capacity to return to full duty.

Job accommodations, as required under the Americans with Disabilities Act, often expand the range of transitional work options for an injured worker. Redesigned tools, ergonomically correct workstations, adaptive devices, and work schedule modifications are all effective disability management methods that enable the worker to perform essential job tasks (Gross, 1988). These same interventions can be utilized in a preventive manner to identify and redesign jobs that are likely to cause future injuries.

The importance of employer-based disability management programs for workers with injuries and disabilities cannot be underestimated. Disability is a complex phenomenon that cannot be holistically addressed by medical interventions alone. The multidisciplinary nature of disability requires timely medical, psychosocial, economic, and vocational interventions, with case management coordination. Delays in providing medical interventions to persons with impairments result in loss of function and reduced potential for physical restoration. Likewise, the failure to address the individual's multidimensional needs, through early interventions and coordinated disability management programs at the worksite, significantly jeopardizes rehabilitation success.

Time is the enemy of rehabilitation. Lost time translates into increased medical and rehabilitation costs. Early rehabilitation interventions have consistently contained the personal and economic costs of injury and disability. Timely disability management services benefit the government by turning "tax users" into "taxpayers." Such services benefit the insurance industry by reducing the liabilities otherwise associated with secondary disabilities, which often emerge when primary disabilities are not fully addressed. Disability management benefits employers and labor organizations by protecting the employability of experienced workers. More importantly, early rehabilitation interventions and employer-based disability management programs help preserve the integrity and economic security of the individuals whose lives, and families' lives, have become compromised by the consequences of injury and disability.

(*See also:* ASSESSMENT; ERGONOMICS; WORK)

BIBLIOGRAPHY

BERKOWITZ, MONROE. "Should Rehabilitation be Mandatory in Workers' Compensation Programs?" *Journal of Disability Policy Studies* 1 (1990):63–80.

BOSCHEN, KAREN. "Early Intervention in Vocational Rehabilitation." *Rehabilitation Counseling Bulletin* 32 (1989):34–45.

California Workers' Compensation Institute. "VR: 1985 Costs and Results." *CWCI Research Notes* (1985).

FRIEDEN, JOHN. "Cost Containment Strategies for Workers Compensation." *Business and Health* 7 (1989):48–54.

GARDNER, J. "Vocational Rehabilitation: Lessons for Employers." *Business and Health* 5 (1987):20–24.

GROSS, C. "Ergonomic Workplace Assessments Are the First Step in Injury Treatment." *Occupational Safety and Health* (May 16–19, 1988):84.

HABECK, ROCHELLE. "Managing Disability in Industry." *NARPPS Journal and News* 6 (1991):141–146.

HABECK, ROCHELLE; LEAHY, MICHAEL; HUNT, ALLEN; CHAN, FONG; and WELCH, EDWARD. "Employer Factors Related to Workers' Compensation Claims

and Disability Management." *Rehabilitation Counseling Bulletin* 34 (1991):210–226.

LACERTE, MICHEL, and DESJARDINS, LORRAINE. "Evaluation of Work Disability from a Worker-Work Environment Perspective." In *Principles and Practices of Disability Management in Industry,* ed. Donald E. Shrey and Michel Lacerte. Orlando, FL, 1993.

LUCAS, S. "Putting a Lid on Disability Costs." *Management Solutions* (April, 1987):16–19.

MATKIN, RALPH. "Employers, Insurers, and Vocational Rehabilitation: The Need for Cooperation." *Forum* 13 (1986):10–11.

PATI, GOPAL. "Economics of Rehabilitation in the Workplace." *Journal of Rehabilitation* (Oct.–Dec. 1985):22–30.

SCHEER, STEVEN. *Multidisciplinary Perspectives in Vocational Assessment of Impaired Workers.* Rockville, MD, 1990.

SCHWARTZ, GAIL; WATSON, SARAH; GALVIN, DONALD; and LIPPOFF, E. *The Disability Management Sourcebook.* Washington, DC, 1989.

SHREY, DONALD E. "Employer-Based Work Return Transition Programs and the Deinstitutionalization of America's Injured Workers." *Work Injury Management* 1 (1992):4–6.

SHREY, DONALD, and BRESLIN, ROBERT. "The Americans with Disabilities Act, Employer-Based Disability Management Strategies, and Work Return Transition Programs." In *The Americans with Disabilities Act: Access and Accommodations,* ed. Brian McMahon and Nancy Hablutzel. Orlando, FL, 1992.

SHREY, DONALD E., and BRUYERE, SUSANNE. "Disability Management in Industry: A Joint Labor-Management Process." *Rehabilitation Counseling Bulletin* 34 (1991):227–242.

SHREY, DONALD E., and LACERTE, MICHEL, eds. *Principles and Practices of Disability Management in Industry.* Orlando, FL, 1993.

SHREY, DONALD E., and MCMAHON, BRIAN. "The Americans with Disabilities Act, Disability Management, and the Injured Worker." *Journal of Workers Compensation* 1 (1992):9–29.

SHREY, DONALD E., and OLSHESKI, JERRY. "Disability Management and Industry-Based Work Return Transition Programs." In *Physical Medicine and Rehabilitation: State of the Art Review,* eds. Chrisanne Gordon and Paul E. Kaplan. Philadelphia, 1992.

STEMPIEN, DENNIS. *CARE Program: Executive Summary.* Fairfield, CT, 1989.

WRIGHT, GEORGE. *Total Rehabilitation.* New York, 1980.

DONALD E. SHREY

DISCRIMINATION

See AFFIRMATIVE ACTION; ATTITUDES; CIVIL RIGHTS; DISABILITY LAW AND SOCIAL POLICY; MINORITIES

DISEASE

For a general discussion of disabilities, disorders, and impairments, see DISABILITY.

DOWN SYNDROME

See GENETIC DISORDERS

DRUG REHABILITATION

The societal costs of substance use and abuse are staggering. Consider the following:

- In 1990, alcoholism and drug abuse cost the United States an estimated $169 billion (Doweiko, 1993).
- Of persons who are chemically dependent, thirty-four of every thirty-six will die due to their chemical dependence (George, 1990).
- Estimates of substance abuse among persons with disabilities range from 53 percent to 68 percent (Helwig & Holicky, 1994).
- In 1991, 22.5 percent of all deaths in the United States were linked to smoking (Inaba & Cohen, 1993).

Prevalence of Drug Use

During the 1970s and 1980s the growing epidemic of dependence on drugs became apparent to the American public. The use of illicit drugs plateaued in the early 1990s, according to a 1992 national household survey (National Institute on Drug Abuse, 1992). Even though the overall use of drugs leveled off, the number of persons using cocaine at least once per week increased from 662,000 in 1990 to 855,000 in 1991. In 1991, 19.5 million people had used marijuana at least once during the past year, while 5.3 million were using it once per week, and 3.1 million

persons were smoking it daily. The nonmedical use of tranquilizers increased from 1.3 percent in 1990 to 1.7 percent in 1991. For the first time in the history of this survey, questions relating to anabolic steroid use were included. An estimated 1 million persons were reported to have used steroids, 90 percent of whom were males.

Substance Abuse Versus Substance Dependence: A Distinction

A significant portion of Americans use drugs often enough to be classified as dependent. The *Diagnostic and Statistical Manual* (DSM-IV) distinguishes between drug abuse and drug dependence. The former is a maladaptive pattern of substance use manifested by recurrent and adverse consequences resulting from repeated use of substances. Dependence is a cluster of cognitive, behavioral, and physiological symptoms indicating an individual's continuing use of the substance despite those substance-related problems. In drug rehabilitation, the focus is generally on drug dependence, while prevention efforts are more focused on drug abuse.

Etiology, Diagnosis, and Prevention

The etiology of drug abuse can be classified into three categories: biological/genetic, psychological, and sociological. The biological/genetic view of drug abuse/dependence focuses on physiological processes that predispose an individual to develop a dependence on chemicals. Considerable work has been done in Scandinavian countries in tracing genetic factors in the development of drug dependence through the study of adopted individuals. Such studies have shown a rather strong relation between a family history of chemical dependence and development of such dependence in an individual. Psychological theories have generally focused on the individual's unique personality characteristics and their relationship to drug abuse/dependence. Jim R. Orford (1985), for example, points to a number of studies that indicate that early tendencies toward nonconforming behavior and membership in "fringe" groups are predictive of later difficulties with drugs. Sociological studies of the origins of substance abuse examine the role of memberships in certain groups on the incidence of abuse. Considerable evidence indicates that membership in certain minority groups increases one's risk for substance abuse (L'Abate, Farrar, and Serritella, 1992). Peer pressure among teenagers has been identified as playing a role in experimentation with drugs. Most authorities concede, however, that all of these factors contribute in varying degrees to the incidence of drug abuse/dependence. The difference of viewpoints on etiologies is one of the relative weight assigned to biological/genetic, psychological, or social factors.

The diagnosis of chemical dependence involves an examination of both the extent and the severity of use/abuse of substances. For an understanding of diagnosis, one must first be aware of the patterns of drug use (George, 1990). According to Ricky George, such patterns range from use to misuse to abuse and, finally, to dependence. Use is the taking of a chemical with or without accompanying problems; misuse is characterized by some adverse effects; abuse is chronic, ongoing misuse; and dependence is signaled by an intense urge or craving for altering one's moods. Professionals often differ, based on their own value systems, on what constitutes use, misuse, abuse, or dependence. According to George (1990), adverse consequences of drug abuse can be physical effects, behavioral problems, emotional problems, or social symptoms. Physical effects include liver, heart, and other internal physiological disorders. Behavioral changes involve a preoccupation with use and the behavior involved in attempts to control and/or deny the severity or extent of use. Emotional problems range from guilt or remorse over use of drugs, to psychiatric problems involving depression, to hyperexcitation, to hallucinations. Social symptoms involve disruptive relationships with family members or friends, school or work difficulties resulting from use, and legal problems.

According to Jason White (1991), questions regarding drug use should focus on the individual's current use as well as his or her history of use. These questions should concern the quantity used, the frequency of use, situations prompting use, and so on. The DSM-IV lists specific behaviors related to substance abuse as well as to dependence, but these lists should be used by people professionally trained in their use and application.

Prevention of drug abuse takes place at three levels: primary, secondary, and tertiary (L'Abate, Farrar, and Serritella, 1992). Primary prevention involves efforts focusing on people before they develop problems and on people who are at risk for developing drug abuse problems. "Just Say No" and other similar campaigns are examples of primary prevention programs. The Center for Substance Abuse Prevention is the federal organization charged with establishing and maintaining prevention programs in the United States. Examples of secondary prevention programs are employee assistance programs in industry. Such programs attempt to identify employees who are in the initial stages of problems with drug abuse and provide appropriate services to halt the progression of their problem. Tertiary programs are treatment programs per se that attempt to assist the individual's recovery from drug dependence.

Treatment Considerations

Treatment for chemical dependency is a multifaceted phenomenon. One of the major considerations in treatment, particularly in vocational rehabilitation settings, is whether the chemical dependence is the primary diagnosis or whether chemical dependence is a problem coexisting with and/or secondary to another physical or mental disability (Corthell & Brown, 1991).

Chemical Dependence as a Primary Condition. Luciano L'Abate, Jack E. Farrar, and Daniel Serritella (1992) state that treatment options for chemical dependence are determined primarily by the length and severity of the problem. For problems of longstanding duration that also involve dependence of a very severe nature, a full range of services in an inpatient facility may be required. Such services would typically involve medical detoxification, individual and group therapy, outside attendance in twelve-step groups, and relapse prevention. Less extreme dependencies of shorter duration may be treated on an outpatient basis. Most treatment programs have abstinence as a goal, and programs may require periodic urine testing to ensure compliance. Individual therapy, according to Lynn Ranew and Daniel Serritella (1992), involves three levels: education, skill-building, and insight-oriented counseling. Education consists of presenting material on the destructive nature of addiction and the goals of treatment. Skill-building assists the addict in acquiring skills for interpersonal functioning. Insight-oriented counseling involves working with addicts to enhance insight into the underlying problems that led to their initial addictive behavior. Group therapy assists addicts in observing the behaviors of other addicts, which may mirror their own behavior. Such groups can become very confrontational at times.

Addiction is a family disease (George, 1990; Ranew & Serritella, 1992). As a family disease, any treatment that does not address the needs of the addict's family is virtually ineffective. Like the addict, families must be educated, provided with new skills, and offered insight into family interaction patterns that may enhance or defuse the destructive behavior of the addict. Many family members believe "fixing" the addict will solve their family's difficulties. Such family members do not realize that certain behaviors within their unit may have promoted the addict's "using behavior."

Chemical Dependence as a Secondary Disability. There are two distinct instances in which chemical dependence is secondary to another, preexisting disability. The first is in the case of psychiatric conditions. Many individuals use drugs to self-medicate underlying affective or other psychiatric disorders (George, 1990; L'Abate, Farrar, & Serritella, 1992). If such an individual were withdrawn from drugs, psychiatric symptoms would most likely appear and/or intensify. Withdrawal from any drug in the case of a person with an underlying psychiatric condition should be attempted only under the guidance of a physician experienced in the treatment of such cases.

The second instance involves an individual with a physical disability who also has a drug abuse problem. As outlined by David Corthell and James Brown (1991) and Jo Anne Ford and Dennis Moore (1992), individuals with disabilities may be at a higher risk for developing drug abuse problems due to easy access to prescription drugs, attempts to deal with the stresses of disablement, enabling attitudes of associates, and atypical social experiences. In one study conducted by Ford and Moore (1992), 50 percent of applicants for vocational rehabilitation in one state had some type of substance abuse problem. Individuals with physical disabilities and substance abuse problems present a multitude of problems for drug treatment as well as for physical and vocational rehabilitation personnel. Few drug treatment facilities are equipped to provide effective services to such individuals. Yet drug abuse can prevent such persons from receiving an appropriate education, from living independently, from securing employment, and from engaging in other activities that would enable them to become functional members of society.

Organizations Related to Substance Abuse. Some of the most active and effective organizations in the area of substance abuse are self-help groups such as Alcoholics Anonymous, Narcotics Anonymous, and Cocaine Anonymous. All such organizations have central service offices willing to provide literature regarding their functions and services. A useful source for addresses of these offices is Yoder's *The Recovery Resource Book* (1990). States have departments of mental health that generally have separate branches for funding drug abuse programs within those states. Such programs receive a large portion of their funding from two federal agencies, the Center for Substance Abuse Prevention (CSAP) and the National Institute for Drug Abuse (NIDA). Within CSAP is the National Clearinghouse for Alcohol and Drug Abuse Information (NCADAI). This clearinghouse is the central source of statistics and other information on substance abuse.

A variety of professionals work in this area, with varying roles and responsibilities. Physicians are active in medical detoxification and psychiatric endeavors. Addictionology is a psychiatric subspecialty for physicians specifically interested in this field. Nursing, social work, family therapy, psychology, vocational rehabilitation counseling, and other health-related professions have specializations in the treatment of addictions.

Due to changes in funding formulas of private insurance companies, facilities are being encouraged to try alternatives to the twenty-eight-day inpatient treatment programs. By the year 2000 we will see the emergence of a very broad spectrum of treatment facilities and modalities available to drug abusers that will be more directed toward meeting the treatment needs of the individual and his or her family.

(*See also:* ALCOHOL REHABILITATION; FAMILY; PSYCHIATRIC REHABILITATION)

RESOURCES

Narcotics Anonymous (NA), P. O. Box 9999, Van Nuys, CA 91409

Resource Center on Substance Abuse Prevention and Disability, 1819 L St., NW, Suite 300, Washington, DC 20036

Wright State University, Projects on Drugs and Disability, School of Medicine, 3640 Colonel Glenn Highway, Dayton, OH 45435

BIBLIOGRAPHY

AMERICAN PSYCHIATRIC ASSOCIATION. "Diagnostic and Statistical Manual of Mental Disorders," 4th ed. Washington, DC, 1994.

CORTHELL, DAVID, and BROWN, JAMES, eds. *Substance Abuse as a Coexisting Disability.* Menomonie, WI, 1991.

DOWEIKO, HAROLD E. "Concepts of Chemical Dependency," 2nd ed. Pacific Grove, CA, 1993.

FORD, J. A., and MOORE, DENNIS. *Substance Abuse Resource and Disability Issues: Training Manual.* Dayton, OH, 1992.

GEORGE, RICKY. *Counseling the Chemically Dependent: Theory and Practice.* Englewood Cliffs, NJ, 1990.

HELWIG, ANDREW A., and HOLICKY, RICHARD. "Substance Abuse in Persons with Disabilities: Treatment Considerations." *Journal of Counseling and Development* 72 (1994): 227–233.

INABA, DARRYL, and COHEN, WILLIAM E. *Uppers, Downers, All Arounders.* San Francisco, 1993.

L'ABATE, LUCIANO; FARRAR, JACK; and SERRITELLA, DANIEL, eds. *Handbook of Differential Treatment for Addictions.* Boston, 1992.

LEWIS, JUDITH, A.; DANA, ROBERT Q.; and BLEVINS, GREGORY A. *Substance Abuse Counseling: An Individualized Approach.* Pacific Grove, CA, 1988. National Institute on Drug Abuse. *National Household Survey on Drug Abuse: Population Estimates, 1991.* Washington, DC, 1992.

ORFORD, JIM. *Excessive Appetites: A Psychological View of Addictions.* New York, 1985.

RANEW, LYNN F., and SERRITELLA, DANIEL. "Substance Abuse and Addiction." In *Handbook of Differential Treatment for Addictions,* eds. Luciano L'Abate, Jack Farrar, and Daniel Serritella. Boston, 1992.

WHITE, JAMES M. *Drug Dependence.* Englewood Cliffs, NJ, 1991.

YODER, BARBARA. *The Recovery Resource Book.* New York, 1990.

BOBBY G. GREER

DRUGS

See PHARMACOLOGY

DYSLEXIA

See LEARNING DISABILITIES

E

EATING DISORDERS

Eating disorders have become a major public health issue in the United States with consequences affecting the lives of many people, mostly young persons.

Anorexia nervosa. The best-known eating disorder, anorexia nervosa, is characterized by a refusal to maintain body weight over a minimal normal weight, a fear of weight gain or becoming fat even though underweight, a disturbance of body image, and amenorrhea. People with restrictor anorexia lose weight by pure dieting. People with bulimic anorexia also lose weight but have periodic binge eating and purging.

People with anorexia commonly have depressive symptoms when they are underweight and malnourished and, in many cases, when weight is recovered. They also have a high prevalence of obsessive-compulsive symptoms or disorders.

Bulimia nervosa. Bulimia nervosa is at least three times more prevalent than anorexia nervosa and is characterized by uncontrollable binge eating, and self-induced purging. People with bulimia purge themselves through vomiting, laxatives, or diuretics. Periods of binge eating are often interspersed with fasting and dieting, and weight fluctuations are commonly seen. The typical duration of illness prior to treatment is reported to be at least five years.

Patients with bulimia and people with bulimic anorexia frequently have problems with depression, anxiety, alcohol abuse or dependency, and impulse disorders. Mortality rates in anorexia are 5 to 20 percent, and bulimia nervosa also is associated with potentially life-threatening consequences.

Epidemiology

The prevalence of anorexia nervosa in the United States has been calculated to be 113.1 per 100,000, or 0.2 percent for females and 0.017 percent for males. The lifetime prevalence of bulimia nervosa in women is found to be as high as 19.6 percent, while in men the disease is much more rare. Though surveys in college populations place the prevalence of eating disorders at 4 to 13 percent using strict criteria, the prevalence is more likely to be closer to 1 percent in young adult and adolescent females.

Etiology

In the past, theories of the etiology of anorexia included family dysfunction and environmental pressures to maintain low weight (Strober & Humphrey, 1987). However, new data in animals and humans suggest that a disturbance of brain serotonin, which modulates appetite, could contribute to many aspects of the anorexia nervosa symptom complex. This finding is further supported by preliminary data showing that medications affecting the serotonin system have some efficacy in anorexia nervosa.

A number of points of evidence suggest a link between bulimia nervosa and substance abuse. Studies in humans suggest that the pathophysiology of bulimia nervosa involves alterations of certain central nervous system neurotransmitter systems, such as opioid and monoamine systems, which have been implicated in addictive, affective, and anxiety disorders.

Assessment and Treatment

The assessment of eating disorders involves a comprehensive evaluation that includes a complete history of weight, eating behavior, psychological functioning including perceptions of weight and shape, depression, and anxiety, a complete medical history and examination, and family and developmental history.

The treatment of anorexia can generally be divided into two stages. The first is refeeding and weight restoration. People with anorexia, particularly those with restricting anorexia, do not begin to gain weight consistently until they begin to eat approximately 50 kcalories per kilogram per day. It may take up to 100 kcal/kg/per day to maintain consistent weight gain and 50 kcal/kg/per day after weight recovery to maintain a normal weight. The second is maintenance of weight after weight gain, in an outpatient setting. Most patients with anorexia nervosa will gain weight with a well-designed nutritional program; however, there is no pharmacological agent that seems to affect the obsessional pursuit of thinness and fear of being fat. Pharmacological treatment is directed at accessory symptoms such as anxiety or depression. Only about 50 to 70 percent of people with anorexia are able to maintain a relatively normal weight after restoration of weight. It is common to see these severely ill patients gain weight in an inpatient treatment unit but rapidly lose weight after discharge.

The initial treatment of choice for bulimia nervosa involves a structured program that uses cognitive-behavioral, educational, and nutritional interventions in either a group or individual setting. For patients resistant to this approach, the use of antidepressant medications can help to decrease the frequency of binge eating and purging and, when outpatient treatment is unable to decrease severe bulimic behavior that is associated with severe medical instability or disabling depression, anxiety, or impulsive behavior, then a period of inpatient treatment should be implemented.

Social and Economic Impact of Eating Disorders

Little research has been done regarding the social, economic, and career complications of eating disorders. Studies of medical students with current or previous eating disorders report greater work, social/leisure, and overall social maladjustment than for those who did not have eating disorders. Social maladjustment was found to persist in both treated and untreated samples (Herzog, Pepose, Norman, and Rigotti, 1985).

Normative social functioning has been found in medical students with a history of anorexia nervosa (Herzog et al., 1985). This finding is in contrast to the findings of Donald M. Schwartz and Michael G. Thompson (1981), who, in their review of the literature from 1965 to 1977, found that only 55 percent of 478 patients for whom marital data were available were married or involved in a relationship. Data from other studies in this review suggested that even those who marry show poor personal and sexual adjustment.

People with anorexia were also found to be at the highest risk for unemployment (Bland et al., 1988). Other authors have found that 90 percent of their sample were successfully employed and also noted that the chronic and life-threatening nature of the illness does not interfere with the ability of a person with anorexia to work, even up to death from their illness (Schwartz & Thompson, 1981). These findings, however, do not address the quality of work of a person with anorexia, nor the issues of under-employment and career potential and their economic implications.

The issues of independence and community living in individuals with eating disorders are closely related to the level of impairment associated with their eating-disordered behavior. Individuals who are severely underweight or who engage in high rates of bingeing and purging generally require the structure of an inpatient or partial hospital setting. As a reduction in symptoms is achieved, transition to less structured settings offering greater independence can be achieved. The individual's ability to assume responsibility, problem-solve, and manage stress are key factors in their ability to live independently.

Often the transition from the highly structured treatment environment to the relatively unstructured home environment is a major factor contributing to high rates of relapse. The need for semistructured living arrangements in the community to provide an appropriate and flexible level of structure while encouraging independence is apparent. Currently, there is a scarcity of programs and resources to address this need, which adds substantially to the high economic and personal cost associated with eating disorders.

Current Controversies. Due to rapidly changing health care, a major challenge involves changing the treatment of eating disorders so that recovery can be a realistic expectation of patients. The growing body of evidence suggests that treatment for eating disorders is improving for both anorexia and bulimia nervosa. Unfortunately, our current method of inpatient treatment may take a number of months for subjects to achieve a normal weight with weight gain. The challenge will be to continue to provide effective treatment in less costly outpatient or partial hospitalization settings.

(*See also:* MOOD DISORDERS; PSYCHIATRIC REHABILITATION; PSYCHIATRY)

RESOURCES

American Anorexia/Bulimia Association, Inc. (AA/BA), 418 East 76th St., New York, NY 10021

National Anorexic Aid Society, Inc. (NAAS), P.O. Box 29461, Columbus, OH 43229

National Association of Anorexia Nervosa and Associated Disorders (ANAD), P.O. Box 7, Highland Park, IL 60035

Western Psychiatric Institute and Clinic, Center for Overcoming Problem Eating, 3811 O'Hara St., Pittsburgh, PA 15213–2593

BIBLIOGRAPHY

AMERICAN PSYCHIATRIC ASSOCIATION. *Diagnostic and Statistical Manual of Mental Disorders* (DSM-IV). Washington, DC, 1994.

BLAND, ROGER C.; STEBELSKY, GEORGE; ORN, HELEN; and NEWMAN, STEPHEN C. "Psychiatric Disorders and Unemployment in Edmonton." *Acta Psychiatrica Scandinavia Supplement* 388 (1988):72–80.

HERZOG, DAVID B., and COPELAND, PAUL M. "Eating Disorders." *New England Journal of Medicine* 313 (1985):295–303.

HERZOG, DAVID B.; PEPOSE, MAURA; NORMAN, DENNIS K.; and RIGOTTI, NANCY A. "Eating Disorders and Social Maladjustment in Female Medical Students." *Journal of Nervous Mental Disorders* 173 (1985):734–737.

JOHNSON, CRAIG; STUCKEY, MARILYN K.; LEWIS, L. D.; and SCHWARTZ, D. M. "Bulimia: A Descriptive Study Survey on 316 Cases." *International Journal of Eating Disorders* 2 (1982):3–16.

NORMAN, DENNIS K., and HERZOG, DAVID B. "A Three-Year Outcome Study of Normal-Weight Bulimia: Assessment of Psychosocial Functioning and Eating Attitudes." *Psychiatry Research* 19 (1986): 199–205.

SCHWARTZ, DONALD M., and THOMPSON, MICHAEL G. "Do Anorectics Get Well? Current Research and Future Needs." *American Journal of Psychiatry* 138 (1981): 319–323.

STROBER, MICHAEL, and HUMPHREY, LAURA L. "Familial Contributions to the Technology and Course of Anorexia Nervosa and Bulimia." *Journal Consulting Clinical Psychology* 55 (1987):654–659.

THEODORE E. WELTZIN
ELIZABETH BLOCHER McCABE
WALTER H. KAYE

ECONOMICS

Rehabilitation services are a large and growing component of the health and human services system of the United States. Since rehabilitation services are provided in many different settings, precise figures on the economic importance of these services cannot be obtained. Fragmentary information, however, confirms the multibillion-dollar scope of rehabilitation efforts. For example, payments by the Medicare program alone to rehabilitation units and/or facilities in fiscal 1990 totaled $1.68 billion (Bradley, 1994). Approximately the same amount of money in 1990 was paid by the federal government to states for the Vocational Rehabilitation (VR) program (Rehabilitation Services Administration, 1991). The state matching funds brought expenditures on the VR program to approximately $2 billion in total in that year. A 1991 survey of rehabilitation providers by the American Hospital Association (AHA) documents the rapid growth in rehabilitation services; from 1988 to 1990, inpatient admissions grew by more than 20 percent and inpatient days grew by about 15 percent, while outpatient visits increased by more than 40 percent in hospitals responding to the survey (American Hospital Association, 1993).

The large expenditures on rehabilitation services invite inquiry into their effectiveness and into the relationship of costs to benefits or effectiveness for these services. While strong evidence of cost-effectiveness has been reported from time to time in the popular literature, careful and comprehensive economic evaluations of rehabilitation services are not commonly found in the research literature. This entry focuses on the available findings in the research literature, the potential problems and limitations of completed research, and possible areas of new emphasis in future economic evaluations of rehabilitation programs.

The research literature on evaluation of rehabilitation programs ranges from highly focused studies of changes in program design (e.g., five-day vs. seven-day physical therapy), to assessments of the effectiveness of specific types of programs (e.g., pain management centers), to studies of rehabilitation services for specific groups of patients (e.g., stroke, traumatic brain injury), to evaluations of broad program initiatives such as the federal–state Vocational Rehabilitation (VR) system. A comprehensive annotated bibliography is provided in National Association of Rehabilitation Facilities (1994).

Studies vary widely in the amount of economic information they convey. Many studies are primarily concerned with measuring treatment effectiveness, where effectiveness is measured by functional scales such as the Disability Rating Scale (DRS) or the Functional Independence Measure (FIM). Other outcome measures have included frequency of community vs. institutional placement after treatment, return-to-work rates, and mortality rates. The problem of valuing these outcomes, either in monetary terms or in terms of a nonmonetary utility or value scale, is rarely considered.

Detailed information on costs is much less plentiful. Some studies look at resource-use measures, such as length of inpatient stay, as a proxy for costs. When cost information is included, it is usually restricted to the costs experienced by the specific program under study.

These limitations on the measurement of cost and the valuation of outcomes have diminished the significance of evaluation studies for health care policy decision makers. Other limiting factors in studies include study design problems and the lack of information on the *distribution* of benefits and costs among different constituencies (e.g., patients, taxpayers, insurance plans, employers).

Measurement of Costs

Measured costs of a rehabilitation intervention or service should include both direct service costs and costs of related services whose volumes are likely to be affected in a nonnegligible way by the intervention. For example, for an inpatient program, related costs would include costs of other in-hospital services and costs of services provided after discharge by other health care providers and institutions (e.g., nursing homes) as well as community agencies and programs (e.g., meals-on-wheels).

The cost measure should account for all resources used in delivering services, including both direct patient care and overhead support functions. Relevant costs are those that are incremental to the provision of services; that is, if no services had been provided, these costs would not have been incurred. In the case of overhead costs in particular, it may be difficult to measure these incremental costs; as a practical matter economists may be forced to rely on somewhat arbitrary allocation schemes for estimating these overhead costs. It is often convenient to use available data on charges or payments as proxies for costs, but possible errors in this method should be recognized in cases where charges are marked up substantially over costs, or payments (e.g., Medicaid rates) are substantially below costs.

Interventions that promote earlier hospital discharge and return to the community also often impose costs on patients' families that are difficult to measure. These costs may include goods and services that families pay for (such as home modifications and home health care), as well as in-kind services rendered free by the family. Precise measurement of in-kind service costs is difficult, but at a minimum the evaluator should measure the magnitude of these services in time units (e.g., hours per day), even if they cannot be combined with monetary cost measures for other services. Some researchers have also tried to develop comprehensive nonmonetary measures of these costs using "family burden" scales.

It is important to document the distribution of costs among different payers, particularly because payers are important health care decision makers. For example, if a state Blue Cross plan has to decide whether to pay for services at pain centers, the evaluator should be able to indicate the costs and savings to the Blue Cross plan of covering these services. Similarly, information about cost impacts on Medicare, Medicaid, and other state and local program budgets will be useful to political decision makers in drafting laws and regulations pertaining to coverage of rehabilitation services.

Outcome Measures

From a public policy standpoint, probably the most important outcome for rehabilitation programs is return to competitive employment by the client. While this view must surely derive from a political consensus about the social value of work, it is reinforced by the dismal labor market picture for persons with disabilities. According to the 1991 National Health Interview Survey data for the noninstitutionalized U.S. population, only 46.5 percent of the 23.6 million adults age eighteen to sixty-five with any activity-limiting chronic condition or impairment are in the labor force, compared with 79.5 percent for comparable persons without such health limitations. The corresponding figures for employ-

ment rates are 42.8 percent versus 75.7 percent. The disparity is, of course, far greater for adults with severe disabilities.

Studies of rehabilitation cohorts have often described return-to-work outcomes but have rarely attempted to measure the effects of specific treatment programs (versus no treatment or "standard" treatment) on the probability of this outcome. Thomas Mayer et al. (1987) examined return to work for treated versus untreated persons with on-the-job low-back injuries. Michael Picard et al. (1989) compared time to return to work for employed men with acute myocardial infarctions randomized between "usual care" and an occupational work evaluation program.

Results of these studies typically show positive effects of rehabilitation interventions on probability of employment or return to work. Usually this effect is measured over a fairly short follow-up period, such as one year or less.

The employment impacts of the VR program have been the subject of many studies. A very recent and comprehensive study was conducted by the General Accounting Office (1993). In that study, recipients of VR services were compared with persons accepted for VR who dropped out before receiving services using a merged database of Social Security earnings records and VR records. Among recipients of VR services, the study found modest but statistically significant employment gains for those classified by VR as "rehabilitated" at closure. These gains were highest at closure and declined steadily thereafter but remained statistically significant five years after rehabilitation. They were found for all major condition groupings (physical disabilities, emotional disabilities, mental retardation). VR recipients classified as "not rehabilitated" at closure, however, had employment records similar to the comparison group of VR dropouts. Since these "not rehabilitated" recipients are a substantial portion of all VR clients (about 30 percent when dropouts are excluded), and since they received services costing about two-thirds as much as those received by "rehabilitated" clients, an important question for future research is understanding why these services were not translated into subsequent employment gains.

Another important outcome measure related to

employment is the level of earnings. Here again evidence from studies comparing different treatment interventions or treatment versus control groups is very limited. The GAO VR evaluation study looked at earnings levels after rehabilitation, with the analysis limited to clients who reported at least some earnings. As in the case of employment, significant differences were observed between rehabilitated clients and dropouts, both at closure and five years later, while nonrehabilitated clients did not report higher earnings than dropouts. Among those with earnings, the differences in average earnings between rehabilitated clients and other groups did not decline substantially over time.

Evaluation researchers have recognized a number of other important dimensions of outcome in addition to employment and earnings. Improvements in functioning have been measured in units ranging from highly specific physiologic measures, such as grip strength (Jankowski & Sullivan, 1990), to measures of cognitive skills (Mackay et al., 1992), to broader functional assessment measures, such as independence in activities (Granger, Hamilton, and Fiedler, 1992), to overall health status or quality of life measures (Deyo et al., 1990). Since these units are nonmonetary, comparison to costs would be facilitated by converting them into monetary magnitudes (Cardus, Fuhrer, and Thrall, 1980). The task of doing this in a conceptually sensible way is challenging and rarely attempted. (As explained below, this difficulty also applies to earnings impacts of rehabilitation.) By contrast, outcome measures that reflect cost savings (such as reduced hospital stay) can be directly compared to program costs and have been computed in a number of studies (e.g., Mackay et al., 1992). Another type of monetary impact that has rarely been measured is rehabilitation impacts on disability benefit payments or other types of transfer payments. This oversight may be due to the erroneous presumption that transfer payments are not relevant to economic evaluations because they do not correspond to use of "real" resources.

Distributional issues are important in monetary benefit measurement, just as they are in cost measurement. State policymakers may care as much about increased state income taxes paid by rehabilitation clients as they do about the overall earnings gains of those clients. The distribution of transfer payment impact among different levels of government (particularly state vs. federal) is also important. Unfortunately, even among the economic evaluation studies that do estimate monetary benefits (such as service cost savings, increased earnings, and transfer payment savings), computations of fiscal impact on insurance programs or on local, state, and federal budgets have not been carried out.

The Need for Randomization in Evaluation Designs

Randomization of patients or clients into control and experimental groups is desirable in evaluation studies. It is also extremely rare (Ernst, 1990). Studies of new rehabilitation services are typically uncontrolled trials reporting on the experiences of the treated patients; in some cases comparisons are drawn to nonequivalent control groups or to past experience of similar patient groups before the service was available. These weak research designs leave unanswered serious questions about the internal validity of economic evaluation studies.

In the several large-scale evaluations of VR that have been undertaken, a number of ingenious strategies to control for nonrandom selection into the program have been employed. Statistical regression models have examined data on individuals and controlled for prior earnings in testing for effects of rehabilitation on postprogram earnings (Worrall, 1988). An innovation in a GAO study was to use as a control group individuals who were accepted for VR services but who dropped out of the program before receiving any services.

It is often feasible to use a randomized design to evaluate a new or existing service (see, e.g., Applegate et al., 1990), but randomization may be more difficult to achieve in the VR program. With a legal mandate to provide services, randomly denying services to eligible persons may not be politically feasible. With substantial excess demand for VR services, however, various access barriers effectively ration services (Salkever, 1994). Monroe Berkowitz (1988b) has observed that random rationing may indeed be feasible under such excess demand conditions. If random denial of services is not feasible, evaluators must content themselves with randomized comparisons of alternative service options such as the VR program with a private sector voucher option (Berkowitz, 1988b).

Cost-Benefit and Cost-Effectiveness Studies: Conceptual and Methodological Issues

Cost-benefit and cost-effectiveness studies bring together information on costs and outcomes of rehabilitation programs or services to assist policymakers in selecting among program options. In cost-benefit analysis, all costs and benefits are expressed in monetary terms, and a "net benefit" figure (dollars of benefit minus dollars of cost) is computed. It is common to assert that a positive net benefit figure indicates that an intervention is worth undertaking.

Incorporation of program cost figures into a cost-benefit analysis is obvious and direct. If the monetary cost of the program can be measured as $Y, this translates directly into a $Y loss of well-being for individuals in society (e.g., taxpayers); the "opportunity costs" of using resources to implement the program are $Y worth of other goods and services forgone.

Benefit measurement for rehabilitation programs is not straightforward, however. Monetary benefits have typically included dollars of service cost savings (due, for example, to reduced length of inpatient stay) and dollars of earnings (after rehabilitation) of the clients, but conceptually these two are not equivalent. While $X of service cost savings translate into $X of increased well-being for individuals (specifically, taxpayers or insurance-premium payers), $X of increased earnings cannot be directly translated into $X worth of increased well-being. A discussion of this point is provided in William Milberg (1988); the issue was first identified in the literature by Fritz Machlup (1965). Thus these two types of monetary benefits are "apples and oranges" and should not be added together; for the same reason, increased earnings and program costs are also "apples and oranges" and not simply positive "apples" versus negative "apples." Simply adding up increased earnings with other benefits and then subtracting costs to get a net benefit figure is conceptually incorrect.

The forgoing implies a need for caution in interpreting cost-benefit studies and a recognition that they are less definitive than they may appear. A full-scale "social" cost-benefit analysis that appropriately measures all costs and benefits on a "willingness to pay" basis is demanding and difficult to accomplish and has yet to be applied in the field of rehabilitation (Milberg, 1988). Nevertheless, analyses of costs and benefits can serve useful but more limited purposes in informing the policy debate. Information on increased earnings is useful at least as a measure of program effectiveness, even if it cannot be directly plugged into a net benefit figure. Information on tax payments by clients after rehabilitation and reduced receipt of transfer payments can help in describing the net fiscal impact of a program. In some unusual cases, the additional taxes paid and transfer payments saved might even exceed the cost of the program so that the program can be viewed as "paying for itself" and actually reducing the burden on taxpayers.

The difficulty in placing dollar values on important rehabilitation outcomes (e.g., employment status, increased levels of functioning in activities of daily living, participation in community activities) may lead program evaluators to opt for the more limited task of cost-effectiveness analysis, in which program costs are measured in monetary terms but effectiveness is measured in nonmonetary units (such as percent of people employed). While this may be justified on practical grounds, the more limited power of cost-effectiveness analysis should also be recognized. This type of analysis cannot indicate whether implementing a program is better than doing nothing. When comparing two alternative programs, if one is more effective and more costly than the other, cost-effectiveness analysis cannot determine which of the two programs to choose. (Some authors have used a cost-effectiveness ratio for this purpose, but this method is without logical basis; if one program's costs are 50% higher while its effectiveness is 40% higher, policymakers may find the extra costs of this program "worth" the extra benefits even though its cost-effectiveness ratio is lower.) Cost-effectiveness analysis also often relies on strong assumptions about interpersonal comparisons—for example, that one year of a specified level of improved functioning is of equal value across all program clients. Most published cost-effectiveness studies do not point out these limitations to the reader, and many ignore them, thereby arriving at policy recommendations that do not flow directly from their analyses.

The cost-benefit literature on the VR program amply demonstrates a number of these methodological difficulties. Relying on before-after earnings comparisons as their principal measure of benefit, studies conducted by state VR agencies invariably find that benefits exceed costs (Collignon, 1988). These studies vary widely in the inclusiveness of their cost measures. Studies that go beyond direct VR program costs to measure costs of services provided by other public or private agencies typically report smaller differences between benefits and costs. "Control group" issues discussed above also often undermine the internal validity of these studies.

Future Issues in Economics and Rehabilitation

Revisions in federal legislation have directed rehabilitation professionals and policymakers to a broad range of possible outcomes from rehabilitation services and away from a narrow focus on competitive employment or return to work as the primary program objective. Valued alternatives to competitive employment (e.g., supported work, volunteer work) have been defined and promoted with public funding. Inclusion and participation of individuals with disabilities in the mainstream of community life have become policy goals in their own right.

It is reasonable to expect that these policy trends will soon be reflected in the economic evaluation literature. This possibility means that greater attention will need to be paid to a broader range of outcome measures related to functioning in the community. For purposes of cost-effectiveness studies, measurement of these outcomes in nonmonetary utility terms will be a major challenge for cost-effectiveness researchers.

A more manageable task is to expand the scope and detail of measured costs and monetary outcomes (such as transfer payment impacts). With expansion of health insurance coverage under whatever version of health care reform is enacted, the fiscal and budgetary impacts of rehabilitation programs on insurers and government budgets will attract increased attention. Economic evaluators will hopefully devote greater efforts to these matters in their research.

(*See also:* DISABILITY MANAGEMENT; EVALUATION OF REHABILITATION PROGRAMS; FAMILY; PRIVATE SECTOR REHABILITATION; RESEARCH; STATE–FEDERAL REHABILITATION PROGRAM)

RESOURCES

American Rehabilitation Association (formerly National Association of Rehabilitation Facilities), 1910 Association Drive, Suite 200, Reston, VA 22091

Office of Health Policy and Research, American Academy of Physical Medicine and Rehabilitation, 122 S. Michigan Ave., Suite 1300, Chicago, IL 60603–6107

Rehabilitation Section, American Hospital Association, One North Franklin, Chicago, IL 60606–3401

BIBLIOGRAPHY

AMERICAN HOSPITAL ASSOCIATION. *Survey of Medical Rehabilitation Hospitals and Programs—1991.* Chicago, 1993.

APPLEGATE, WILLIAM; MILLER, STEPHEN; GRANEY, MARSHALL; ELAM, JANET; BEARER, TERINELL; and AKINS, DERENE. "A Randomized, Controlled Trial of a Geriatric Assessment Unit in a Community Rehabilitation Hospital." *New England Journal of Medicine* 31 (1990):1572–1578.

BERKOWITZ, MONROE, ed. *Measuring the Efficiency of Public Programs: Costs and Benefits in Vocational Rehabilitation.* Philadelphia, 1988a.

———. "Conclusion." In *Measuring the Efficiency of Public Programs: Costs and Benefits in Vocational Rehabilitation,* ed. Monroe Berkowitz. Philadelphia, 1988b.

BRADLEY, THOMAS. Prospective Payment Assessment Commission. Personal communication, March 1994.

CARDUS, DAVID; FUHRER, MARCUS; and THRALL, ROBERT M. *A Benefit-Cost Approach to the Prioritization of Rehabilitation Research.* Houston, 1980.

COLLIGNON, FREDERICK C. "Benefit-Cost Analyses Conducted by State Agencies." In *Measuring the Efficiency of Public Programs: Costs and Benefits in Vocational Rehabilitation,* ed. Monroe Berkowitz. Philadelphia, 1988.

DEYO, RICHARD A.; WALSH, NICHOLAS E.; MARTIN, DONALD C.; SCHOENFELD, LAWRENCE S.; and

RAMAMURTHY, SOMAYAJI. "A Controlled Trial of Transcutaneous Electrical Nerve Stimulation (TENS) and Exercise for Chronic Low Back Pain." *The New England Journal of Medicine* 322 (1990):1527–1634.

ERNST, EDZARD. "A Review of Stroke Rehabilitation and Physiotherapy." *Stroke* 21 (1990):1081–1090.

GENERAL ACCOUNTING OFFICE. *Vocational Rehabilitation—Evidence for Federal Program's Effectiveness Is Mixed.* Washington, DC: General Accounting Office, 1993.

GRANGER, CARL V.; HAMILTON, BYRON B.; and FIEDLER, ROGER C. "Discharge Outcome After Stroke Rehabilitation." *Stroke* 23 (1992):978–982.

JANKOWSKI, LEWIS W., and SULLIVAN, S. JOHN. "Aerobic and Neuromuscular Training: Effect on the Capacity, Efficiency, and Fatigability of Patients with Traumatic Brain Injuries." *Archives of Physical Medicine and Rehabilitation* 71 (1990):500–504.

MACHLUP, FRITZ. "Comments." *Measuring Benefits of Government Investments.* Washington, DC, 1965.

MACKAY, LINDA E.; BERNSTEIN, BRUCE A.; CHAPMAN, PHYLLIS E.; MORGAN, ANTHONY; and MILAZZO, LORAINE S. "Early Intervention in Severe Head Injury: Long-Term Benefits of a Formalized Program." *Archives of Physical Medicine and Rehabilitation* 73 (1992):635–641.

MAYER, THOMAS G.; GATCHEL, ROBERT J.; MAYER, HOLLY; KISHINO, NANCY D.; KEELEY, DENISE J.; and MOONEY, VERT. "A Prospective Two-Year Study of Functional Restoration in Industrial Low Back Injury." *Journal of the American Medical Association* 258 (1987):1763–1767.

MILBERG, WILLIAM. "Welfare Measurement for Cost-Benefit Analysis." In *Measuring the Efficiency of Public Programs: Costs and Benefits in Vocational Rehabilitation,* ed. Monroe Berkowitz. Philadelphia, 1988.

NATIONAL ASSOCIATION OF REHABILITATION FACILITIES. *Medical Rehabilitation Cost-Effectiveness and Cost Benefits: A Resource Guide,* rev. ed., Washington, DC, 1994.

PICARD, MICHAEL H.; DENNIS, CHARLES; SCHWARTZ, RICHARD; AHN, DAVID; KRAEMER, HELENA; BERGER III, WALTER E.; BLUMBERG, ROBERT; HELLER, ROBERT; LEW, HENRY; and DEBUSK, ROBERT F. "Cost-Benefit Analysis of Early Return to Work After Uncomplicated Acute Myocardial Infarction." *American Journal of Cardiology* 63 (1989):1308–1314.

REHABILITATION SERVICES ADMINISTRATION, U.S. DEPARTMENT OF EDUCATION. *Annual Report to the President and to the Congress Fiscal Year 1990 on Federal Activities Related to the Rehabilitation Act of 1973 as Amended.* Washington, DC, 1991.

SALKEVER, DAVID. "Access to Vocational Rehabilitation Services for Persons with Severe Disabilities: Analysis of the 1990 Developmental Disabilities National Consumer Survey." *Journal of Disability Policy Studies* 5 (1994):45–64.

WORRALL, JOHN D. "Benefit and Cost Models." In *Measuring the Efficiency of Public Programs: Costs and Benefits in Vocational Rehabilitation,* ed. Monroe Berkowitz. Philadelphia, 1988.

DAVID S. SALKEVER

EMPLOYEE ASSISTANCE PROGRAMS

There are at least 10,000 employee assistance programs (EAPs) in existence in the United States (DeCarlo & Gruenfeld, 1989). These programs have been shown to reduce medical costs, absenteeism, and tardiness; increase productivity and efficiency; and result in lower on-the-job accident rates, less turnover, and lower training costs (DeCarlo & Grunfeld, 1989). They have demonstrated a rehabilitation success rate of 70 to 80 percent and appear to enhance labor-management relations as well (Challenger, 1988).

The major ingredients of an effective EAP, according to Dickman (1988), are as follows:

- management and labor endorsements;
- establishment and dissemination of a comprehensive policy statement;
- confidentiality between worker and service provider;
- supervisory and labor steward training;
- consideration of financial aspects and insurance coverage;
- professional personnel;
- broad service components;
- accessibility of the program to the workplace;
- employee awareness of the scope and nature of services;
- program evaluation and revision to ensure service efficacy and cost-effectiveness.

Effective EAPs also practice early identification and remediation, provide proactive education and prevention programs, use quality treatment modalities that are also economical, and agree on the provision of a full array of follow-up and evaluative data (Challenger, 1988).

Items to be considered when establishing an EAP include range of services to be provided, staffing patterns, referral and counseling modalities, accessibility of services, utilization rate, feedback, promotional and educational materials and media, and indemnification of the program (Challenger, 1988; Rosenzweig & Kramer, 1992). Services provided through EAPs can vary, but some major issues dealt with are substance abuse (both worker and family), dysfunctional families, codependency, stress, and sexual problems (Dickman et al., 1988).

There are essentially four major models of EAP service delivery (Phillips & Older, 1988). The first is the internal program, which is characterized by coordination of all client activity from within the work environment. Some of these programs render all counseling, treatment, and/or social services within the organization, while others might refer out for services. The second type of service delivery is the service center program; this type occurs when the employer contracts with an independent EAP service provider, which provides diagnosis and referral to treatment sources within the community. There may or may not be an individual identified with the program at the workplace. The third type occurs when the EAP is located in a treatment or social service agency. These services can be offered at no cost or at a reduced cost negotiated in a service agreement between the employer/EAP and the agency. Finally, a limited number of EAPs are union-based. Services are rendered at the union office or hiring hall.

The majority of EAPs have a case manager to do case finding, intake, eligibility determination, assessment, counseling, development and implementation of treatment plans, provision and supervision of services or appropriate referral, monitoring of service effectiveness, closure determination, and post-services follow-up (Emener & Dickman, 1988). The case manager can be a professional rehabilitationist or a member of some allied profession such as social work or human resources with special training in EAP issues. Other professionals who might be involved include those in occupational medicine, personnel management, organized labor, and a diverse array of treatment agencies and specialties as might

be appropriate for the individual's unique needs (Roman, 1988). EAP personnel may be called on to work as part of a team or teams established to solve organizational problems as well. In that setting they may work closely with other departments, such as human resources, health and safety, employee relations, employee health benefits, occupational medicine, risk management, vocational rehabilitation, work and family therapy, wellness and stress reduction, training, production, finance, management information systems, engineering/ergonomics, and legal (Akabas, Gates, and Galvin, 1992; Yandrick, 1993).

While much of the information available describes the rehabilitation services provided by EAPs, their most important activities are in the areas of prevention and wellness. These efforts are typically directed at physical and mental health. They may include such components as weight reduction, stress management, antismoking campaigns, and a myriad of other "healthy" endeavors. The goals of prevention include reduction in the incidence of disability; demonstration to the workforce that the employer is concerned about employee well-being, resulting in increased morale and satisfaction; promotion of strategies for better means of performing jobs; and cost containment (Akabas, Gates, and Galvin, 1992). Prevention, when coupled with early intervention, is the real key to the overall cost-effectiveness of EAPs.

EAPs have been associated with disability management to include both resolution and prevention of dysfunction (Erfurt, Foote, and Heirich, 1992). The growth of disability management programs in the late 1980s and early 1990s resulted from an attempt to meet several goals simultaneously. Chief among those goals are the reduction in disability-associated costs, maintenance of a highly skilled work force, and conversion to a more diverse work population mandated by such civil rights legislation as the Civil Rights Act of 1964 and the Americans with Disabilities Act of 1990. As organizations try to meet these challenges, the establishment of disability management programs that include EAP principles, practices, and professionals will increase. Other issues being addressed regarding EAPs are an expansion of team efforts aimed at disability management (Yandrick, 1993), legal recognition of the professionalism of EAP personnel (EAPA Exchange,

1992), provision of services through managed care health programs (Zientel, 1993), and establishment of efficacious program evaluation methodology (Dickman & Emener, 1988; Emener & Yegedis, 1988; Jerrell & Rightmyer, 1988).

Most successful EAPs will continue to develop the following components: clear organizational commitment to a healthy workforce as expressed through explicit goals and objectives; a well-conceived strategic plan; uniformity and consistency in implementing the program; flexibility to allow for differences among employees; knowledgeable, experienced, and enthusiastic service providers; baseline data to inform program planning and enable evaluation; and formal program evaluation to assess how well the program is meeting its objectives and how best to modify it for the future (Akabas, Gates, & Galvin, 1992; Kelly, 1986).

(*See also:* DISABILITY MANAGEMENT; LABOR UNIONS; MANAGEMENT; PRIVATE SECTOR REHABILITATION)

RESOURCES

Alcohol and Drug Problems Association, 444 North Capital St., Department E, Washington, DC 20005

ALMACA (Association of Labor-Management Administrators and Consultants on Alcoholism), 1800 North Kent St., Suite 901, Arlington, VA 22209. Publishes the *Almacan.*

EAP Digest, Performance Resource Press, 1863 Technology Drive, Suite 200, Troy, MI 48083

Employee Assistance, 225 North New Rd, P.O. Box 2573, Waco, TX 76702–2573

Employee Assistance Professional Association, (EAPA), 4601 North Fairfax Drive, Suite 1001, Arlington, VA 22203. Publishes *EAPA Exchange* and the *Journal of Employee Assistance Research*

Employee Assistance Society of North America, 2145 Crooks Rd, Suite 103, Troy, MI 48084

National Association of Social Work, Occupational Social Work Task Force, 7981 Eastern Ave., Silver Spring, MD 20901

National Council on Alcoholism, 12 West 21st St., New York, NY 10010

National Institute on Alcohol Abuse and Alcoholism, 5600 Fishers Lane, Rockville, MD 20857

BIBLIOGRAPHY

AKABAS, SHEILA H.; GATES, LAUREN B.; and GALVIN, DONALD E. *Disability Management: A Complete System to Reduce Costs, Increase Productivity, Meet Employee Needs, and Ensure Legal Compliance.* New York, 1992.

CHALLENGER, B. ROBERT. "The Need for Employer Assistance Programs." In *Employee Assistance Programs: A Basic Text,* eds. Fred Dickman, B. Robert Challenger, William G. Emener, and William S. Hutchison. Springfield, IL, 1988.

DeCARLO, DONALD T., and GRUENFELD, DEBORAH H. *Stress in the American Workplace: Alternatives for the Working Wounded.* Fort Washington, PA, 1989.

DICKMAN, FRED. "Ingredients of an Effective Employee Assistance Program." In *Employee Assistance Programs: A Basic Text,* eds. Fred Dickman, B. Robert Challenger, William G. Emener, and William S. Hutchison. Springfield, IL, 1988.

DICKMAN, FRED; CHALLENGER, B. ROBERT; EMENER, WILLIAM G.; and HUTCHISON, WILLIAM S., eds. *Employee Assistance Programs: A Basic Text.* Springfield, IL, 1988.

DICKMAN, FRED, and EMENER, WILLIAM G. "Employee Assistance Programs: Basic Concepts, Attributes and an Evaluation." In *Employee Assistance Programs: A Basic Text,* eds. Fred Dickman, B. Robert Challenger, William G. Emener, and William S. Hutchison. Springfield, IL, 1988.

DICKMAN, FRED; EMENER, WILLIAM G.; and HUTCHISON, WILLIAM S., eds. *Counseling the Troubled Person in Industry: A Guide to the Organization, Implementation, and Evaluation of Employee Assistance Programs.* Springfield, IL, 1988.

EMENER, WILLIAM G., and DICKMAN, FRED. "Case Management, Caseload Management, and Case Recording and Documentation in Professional Employee Assistance Program Service Delivery." In *Employee Assistance Programs: A Basic Text,* eds. Fred Dickman, B. Robert Challenger, William G. Emener, and William S. Hutchison. Springfield, IL, 1988.

EMENER, WILLIAM G., and YEGEDIS, BONNIE L. "Program Planning and Evaluation of Employee Assistance Programs: Foundations and Concepts." In *Employee Assistance Programs: A Basic Text,* eds. Fred Dickman, B. Robert Challenger, William G. Emener, and William S. Hutchison. Springfield, IL, 1988.

ERFURT, JOHN C.; FOOTE, ANDREA; and HEIRICH, MAX A. "Integrating Employee Assistance and Wellness: Current and Future Core Technologies of a Megabrush Program." *Journal of Employee Assistance Research* (1992).

HAVRANEK, JOSEPH E. *Employee Assistance Programs: Benefits, Problems, and Prospects.* Rockville, MD, 1987.

———. "EPA Seeks Recommendations for 1993 L&P Agenda." *EAPA Exchange* (November–December 1992).

JERRELL, JEANETTE M., and RIGHTMYER, JONATHAN F. "Evaluating Employee Assistance Programs: A Review of Methods, Outcomes, and Future Directions." In *Employee Assistance Programs: A Basic Text,* eds. Fred Dickman, B. Robert Challenger, William G. Emener, and William S. Hutchison. Springfield, IL, 1988.

KELLY, KAREN E. "Building a Successful Health Promotion Program." *Business and Health* (March 1986).

MASI, D. A. *Designing Employee Assistance Programs.* New York, 1984.

PHILLIPS, DONALD A., and OLDER, HARRY J. "Models of Service Delivery." In *Employee Assistance Programs: A Basic Text,* eds. Fred Dickman, B. Robert Challenger, William G. Emener, and William S. Hutchison. Springfield, IL, 1988.

ROMAN, PAUL H. "From Employee Alcoholism to Employee Assistance." In *Employee Assistance Programs: A Basic Text,* eds. Fred Dickman, B. Robert Challenger, William G. Emener, and William S. Hutchison. Springfield, IL, 1988.

ROSENZWEIG, STEPHEN, and KRAMER, ERIC P. "Human Resources: Get with the Program." *Small Business Reports* 17(1992).

SWANBECK, J., and TREADWELL, J., eds. *Employee Assistance Programs: Helping the Troubled Employee.* Chicago, 1988.

YANDRICK, RUDY M. "In the Loop." *EAPA Exchange* (February 1993):10–13.

ZIENTEL, BOB. "Working Through Managed Care Roadblocks." *EAPA Exchange* (February 1993): 28–29.

JOSEPH E. HAVRANEK

EMPLOYMENT

See AFFIRMATIVE ACTION; CAREER COUNSELING; JOB PLACEMENT; PRESIDENT'S COMMITTEE ON EMPLOYMENT OF PEOPLE WITH DISABILITIES; WORK

EMPOWERMENT

See ADVOCACY; CIVIL RIGHTS; CONSUMERS

ENDOCRINE DISORDERS

The endocrine system consists of a hierarchical organization of glands that release hormones directly into the bloodstream, to be carried to target tissues, where they modulate biochemical processes that automatically compensate for environmental changes. The endocrine organs represent an initial line of defense against external or internal stress and also interface with the central and peripheral nervous systems. Control and coordination of growth, development, and reproductive function involves the appropriate activation and timing of diverse endocrine glands. Sustained disturbance of the minute-to-minute control of temperature regulation, metabolic rate, blood sugar, and electrolyte and mineral balance produces the clinical manifestations of endocrine disorders. Although many hormonal deficiencies or excess states are amenable to therapy and do not result in chronic disability, it is certainly recognized that diabetes mellitus burdens society with staggering costs in terms of morbidity, mortality, and direct and indirect medical expenses. Diabetes mellitus accounts for a disproportionate share of disability and rehabilitation requirements among the endocrine disorders.

This entry will highlight the common endocrine causes of disability, with an emphasis on diabetes mellitus. Current and future research issues will be mentioned.

Diabetes Mellitus

Diabetes mellitus, recognized more than 2,000 years ago, affected an estimated 7.2 million people in the United States in 1992, with a similar number estimated to be undiagnosed. Diabetes disproportionately affects minority populations, and its incidence increases with age. Several studies have shown the age-adjusted prevalence of diabetes mellitus among African Americans, Hispanics, and Native Americans to be 2 to 2.8 times that of the European-American U.S. population. These racial and ethnic minority groups are also at greater risk for diabetic complications.

Diabetes mellitus comprises chronic disorders characterized by elevated blood sugar and disturbance of fat and protein metabolism. Insulin, produced and released from the beta cells of the pancreas, maintains the blood sugar in a relatively narrow range following food intake. When insulin is absent or ineffective, high blood sugar levels appear. Classification of diabetes mellitus includes insulin-dependent diabetes mellitus (IDDM or Type I), noninsulin-dependent diabetes mellitus (NIDDM or Type II), diabetes recognized during pregnancy (gestational diabetes mellitus, GDM), and diabetes associated with other endocrine or genetic syndromes.

Individuals with IDDM are severely insulin-deficient and have classic signs and symptoms such as ketones in the urine; excessive thirst, urination, and appetite; and weight loss. They depend on insulin injections to prevent death from ketoacidosis and usually are diagnosed under age thirty. They account for 10 percent of all cases of diabetes in the United States.

People with NIDDM typically have milder symptoms; absence of ketones in the urine; and low, normal, or high insulin levels. They have insulin resistance and are not dependent on insulin injections for survival. They can be treated with oral hypoglycemic medication but may require insulin for adequate blood sugar control. NIDDM usually occurs in individuals over age forty and accounts for 90 percent of all cases of diabetes in the United States.

GDM affects 2 to 4 percent of pregnant women and usually is diagnosed during the second or third trimester.

Diabetes mellitus is diagnosed in adults and children who have a random plasma glucose level of 200 mg/dl or greater plus classic signs and symptoms. High-risk individuals (i.e., those with a family history of diabetes, obesity, or previous glucose elevation) should be screened. Two fasting plasma glucose levels of 140 mg/dl or greater are diagnostic of diabetes. Fasting plasma glucose levels of 115 mg/dl to 139 mg/dl are equivocal and require clarification by an oral glucose tolerance test (OGTT). All pregnant women are screened for GDM between twenty-four and twenty-eight weeks of pregnancy, and any abnormal result prompts a referral for an OGTT. There are different criteria for diagnosing diabetes mellitus, on the basis of an OGTT, in children, and nonpregnant and pregnant women.

Diabetic Complications

Diabetic complications can be thought of as acute or chronic. Poor metabolic control increases the risk of the acute complications of hypoglycemia, ketoacidosis, severe hyperglycemia and dehydration of the elderly (hyperglycemic, nonketotic state), complicated pregnancies, large-birth-weight babies, and congenital malformations.

Hypoglycemia usually occurs when the blood sugar falls below 50 mg/dl as a result of excessive insulin or oral medication action relative to the body's needs. The Diabetes Control and Complications Trial (DCCT) showed that one-third to one-half of intensive insulin-treated IDDM patients had at least one severe hypoglycemic episode over a three-year period, and the risk of hypoglycemic coma or seizure increased from 8 to 21 percent. Indeed, governmental concern over hypoglycemia has barred insulin-using individuals from interstate truck driving and commercial aviation. All individuals with diabetes should wear a medical alert tag or a bracelet specifying diagnosis and medication so that hypoglycemia can be readily identified and treated.

The chronic complications of diabetes mellitus involve diseases of the small and large blood vessels and nerves. Small-blood-vessel disease of the retina, proliferative diabetic retinopathy and macular edema, is the leading cause of acquired blindness in adults twenty-five to seventy-four years of age. After a period of thirty years, 20 to 60 percent of persons with diabetes have proliferative retinopathy, depending upon the age at onset of diabetes. Diabetic kidney disease or nephropathy results from years of metabolic insult, and diabetes is the leading cause of end-stage kidney disease. After fifteen years' duration, diabetic nephropathy occurs in 19 to 34 percent of people with diabetes. Kidney failure accounts for 10 to 40 percent of deaths in this group.

Diabetic neuropathy most commonly causes symmetric loss or distortion of sensation and/or weakness of the extremities (polyneuropathy). This may result in repeated painless trauma to the feet followed by infection, and ultimately amputation. The classical example of diabetic neuropathic joint disease, the Charcot joint, is thought to result from repetitive insensate microtrauma. Neuropathy may also involve the autonomic nerves and cause dysfunction of heart rate and blood pressure, gastric and intestinal motility, bladder emptying, and sexual response. Occasionally, larger, distinct nerves may be involved as a mononeuropathy. Involvement of cranial nerves with temporary paralysis of eye movement and double vision is a common example of a mononeuropathy. Some form of neuropathy is present in at least half the people with diabetes for twenty-five years. Autonomic neuropathy is observed in 20 to 40 percent of persons with diabetes, and impotence affects 35 to 75 percent of men with diabetes.

Large blood vessel disease manifestations are coronary artery disease, lower extremity arterial disease, and stroke. Individuals with diabetes are two to four times more likely to have coronary artery disease, with the excess risk being highest in those forty-five years old or younger. Fifty-five percent of all diabetic deaths and 25 to 50 percent of deaths in long-standing insulin-dependent diabetes mellitus are caused by cardiovascular disease.

Peripheral artery disease and lower extremity amputation are four and fifteen times, respectively, as common in persons with diabetes as in those without diabetes. The prognosis is poor after amputation, with a five-year survival rate of only 40 percent.

Stroke occurs two to six times more frequently in people with diabetes than in people without diabetes. The prevalence of stroke peaks in elderly persons with diabetes, 13 percent of whom reported having had this disability, according to a 1993 American Diabetes Association report.

Treatment

People with IDDM and GDM are treated with insulin, administered by subcutaneous injection or continuous infusion pump, and diet. Treatment for NIDDM emphasizes diet; weight control; exercise; and, when appropriate, oral hypoglycemic medication and/or insulin. One-quarter of people diagnosed with diabetes are not using any of the above treatments. In general, African Americans are more likely to be treated with insulin than oral medica-

tion, and Mexican-American persons with diabetes are more likely to be undertreated compared to African Americans or European Americans. Only half of all insulin users and 5 percent of noninsulin users perform self-monitoring of blood sugar. This is of concern because, in 1993, the DCCT conclusively demonstrated the benefit of strict blood sugar control in preventing or reducing retina, kidney, and nerve complications in IDDM. Results from a United Kingdom study investigating stricter blood sugar control by insulin or oral medication, when they are released, should reveal whether similar benefits can be expected in NIDDM.

Regular eye examinations and early detection of diabetic retinopathy are essential to prevent blindness. Aggressive laser therapy and retinal surgery can restore and preserve vision.

In 1994, the *New England Journal of Medicine* reported that a neutralizing antibody to a vascular growth factor present in the eye inhibited the stimulated growth of retinal blood vessel cells in culture. Further clinical trials are needed to assess whether blocking new blood vessel formation will prevent or slow the progression of diabetic retinopathy.

Aggressive treatment of hypertension and early diabetic nephropathy have been shown to delay the onset of diabetic kidney failure.

Addressing the issue of atherosclerotic risk factors would undoubtedly reduce the associated cardiovascular morbidity and mortality in NIDDM.

Newer treatment options include transplantation of whole-pancreas or isolated insulin-producing islet cells. As of 1994, these procedures were available only at a few specialized centers for appropriately selected individuals with IDDM. Restricted availability of donor tissue, use of immunosuppressive medications, and immune rejection are additional limiting factors.

Prevention of Diabetes

It is estimated that preventing obesity in the United States could reduce the incidence of NIDDM and GDM by 50 and 33 percent, respectively. Individuals at high risk for IDDM are participating in investigations aimed at suppressing the immune response to the pancreatic beta cell.

Facts and Figures about Diabetes Mellitus

Hospitalization. In 1992 there were approximately 372,000 hospitalizations due to diabetes per se, accounting for 2.3 million hospital days. Two-thirds of patients with diabetes were less than sixty-five years of age. There were more than 731,000 hospitalizations or six million hospital days for chronic complications in 1992. The rate of hospitalization for chronic diseases was 155 per 1,000 patients with diabetes versus 54 per 1,000 patients without diabetes, a threefold increase. Sixty percent of hospitalizations were due to cardiovascular complications, 7 percent for amputation, and 18.4 percent for neurological complications. On average, the length of stay was 2.8 days longer for patients with diabetes compared to patients without diabetes.

Nursing Home Stays. In 1992 there were 17.8 million nursing home days for 107,000 patients with diabetes. The rate of institutionalization increased twenty-fivefold for patients older than sixty-five years compared to those less than forty-five years of age. Individuals under forty-five years had an eightfold higher risk of institutionalization compared to people of the same age without diabetes.

Outpatient Care. Approximately 15.7 million outpatient physician visits, 5.7 million outpatient hospital visits, 647,000 emergency room visits, 500,000 home care visits, 1 million dietician or nutritionist visits, and 50 million purchases of prescriptions and supplies were due to diabetes in 1992.

Lost Productivity. One million work-loss days were due to diabetes in 1992, with three-quarters associated with individuals forty-five to sixty-four years of age with diabetes. One and one-half million days of restricted activity and 543,700 bed-loss days were reported by employed individuals with diabetes, compared to 7.6 million and 2.7 million days, respectively, in unemployed persons with diabetes.

Disability. A total of 47,800 workers were permanently disabled due to diabetes in 1992, 82.2 percent being people aged forty-five to sixty-four years.

Mortality. Diabetes is the seventh leading cause of death and the fourth leading cause of death by disease in the United States. In 1992, diabetes was the underlying cause of death of approximately 48,000 individuals and the contributory cause of death in an estimated 434,000 people. In individuals with IDDM, the acute complications of ketoacidosis, hypoglycemia, and infections account for 50 percent to 70 percent of deaths in those under twenty years of age. With increasing age, death from renal and cardiovascular disease predominates. In individuals with NIDDM, the leading cause of death is cardiovascular disease, accounting for 65 percent of deaths, with fewer than 5 percent attributed to renal disease.

Cost. The direct cost of medical care and the indirect cost of death or lost productivity due to diabetes totaled $91.8 billion in 1992. Direct medical costs increased from 2.2 percent of total personal health care expenditures in 1987 to 5.8 percent in 1992, an increase of 164 percent.

Rehabilitation Concerns

Sensory loss, abnormal sensation, or painful extremities from diabetic polyneuropathy, dermatome pain from diabetic nerve root involvement, entrapment neuropathy, quadriceps wasting due to diabetic amyotrophy, and postural hypotension due to autonomic neuropathy frequently involve the rehabilitation specialist. Recognition and treatment of mechanical foot deformity and abnormal gait can forestall the development of a neuropathic ulcer. Instruction in proper foot care and prevention of foot injury can reduce the incidence of amputation in individuals already predisposed to vascular disease and infection. Early management of the Charcot joint foot is directed at weight redistribution by orthotic shoes, walking cast, or short leg brace. Gait training can also prevent falls and hip fractures in individuals with impaired balance due to proprioceptive defects or transmetatarsal amputations.

Therapies and Treatment. Physical therapy is an important modality for restoring thigh muscle bulk and strength in diabetic amyotrophy. Most individuals improve within six to twelve months. Postural exercises, support stockings, and salt-retaining medication may be useful in postural hypotension. Treatment for carpal tunnel syndrome involves wrist supports, avoidance of extremes of wrist flexion and extension, and anti-inflammatory medication. More severe cases will require surgical decompression of the median nerve. Peroneal nerve entrapment produces sudden, painless foot drop. Trauma may also play a role because of the superficial location of the nerve near the fibular head. A fitted foot support permits independent ambulation. Slow recovery usually occurs, but residual weakness is common.

Treatment of nerve root pain involves similar modalities as in the person without diabetes, including transcutaneous electrical nerve simulation. Decreased thermal perception in the person with diabetes calls for heightened awareness to prevent burns from any treatment employing heat. Topical application of 0.075 percent capsaicin cream may be effective for localized pain. In general, nerve pain gradually resolves within months to a year.

Disability Act. The 1990 Americans with Disabilities Act denotes diabetes as a defined disability. This law makes it illegal to discriminate against any person with diabetes and supports employment of such an individual, consistent with the policy of the American Diabetes Association (ADA). The ADA monitors public health policy concerning diabetes, sets standards of care for people with diabetes, and provides a broad array of services to patients and health care professionals.

Thyroid Disorders

The main etiologies of excess thyroid hormone production (hyperthyroidism) are: Graves' disease, overactive multinodular goiter, and overactive solitary nodule. Deficiency of thyroid hormone (hypothyroidism) most commonly is caused by Hashimoto's thyroiditis and radioactive iodine-induced destruction after treatment for Graves' disease. The female-to-male ratio of most thyroid disease is about four to one. Hormonal assays permit precise diagnosis of thyroid dysfunction.

Proximal muscle exertional weakness can occur with hyperthyroidism or hypothyroidism. Excess thyroid hormone causes muscle wasting and calcium loss from the skeleton. Hypothyroidism is associated with muscle and joint aches and carpal tunnel syndrome. Autoimmune thyroid disease (Graves' disease, Hashimoto's thyroiditis) may be associated with eyeball protrusion and swelling of the orbit and eye muscle. Corneal irritation, double vision, de-

creased visual acuity, and visual field deficits may result. Therapy consists of topical medication, diuretics, oral corticosteroids, surgical orbital decompression, prisms, and eye muscle and eyelid surgery.

Hyperthyroidism is treated with antithyroid medication, radioactive iodine therapy, or surgical removal of thyroid tissue. Persistent hypothyroidism is treated with systemic thyroid hormone replacement. Restoration of a normal thyroid state reverses many of the manifestations of disordered metabolism. Aggressive treatment in an intensive care unit is required for the life-threatening extremes of severe thyroid hormone excess (thyroid storm) or almost complete absence of thyroid hormone (myxedema coma).

Adrenal Disorders

Intrinsic disease of the adrenal glands or of the controlling hypothalamic-pituitary unit results in over- or underproduction of adrenal hormones. Primary adrenal cortical (outer layer) insufficiency (Addison's disease) causes reduction in corticosteroid, salt-retaining, and androgenic hormones. The most common etiology is autoimmune adrenalitis, but tuberculous, fungal, cytomegalovirus, and HIV infections, as well as antituberculous and antifungal medications, are increasingly implicated. The manifestations are diffuse weakness, fatigue, hypotension, increased skin pigmentation, joint and muscle aches, and psychiatric complaints ranging from mild cognitive impairment to overt psychosis. Treatment consists of hormone replacement, increased dietary salt, and anticipation of augmented corticosteroid requirements during stress. A medical warning medallion may be life-saving.

Adrenal insufficiency also results from disruption of hypothalamic-pituitary function or after withdrawal from long-term pharmacologic doses of cortisone or prednisone. The clinical presentation, physical examination, and hormone levels permit differentiation from Addison's disease.

Diseases of adrenal cortical hormone excess are Cushing's syndrome (cortisol excess), Conn's syndrome (mineralocorticoid or salt-retaining hormone excess), and androgen excess. Benign and malignant adrenal tumors, and pituitary and other tumors oversecreting adrenocorticotropin (ACTH), are the neoplasms causing cortisol excess. Excessive levels of cortisol cause central obesity with wasting of the extremities; easy bruising; proximal muscle weakness; osteoporosis; and psychological disturbances such as emotional lability, depression, and psychosis. Treatment options are pharmacologic blockade of adrenal hormone production, surgical resection of the culprit adrenal or pituitary tumor, bilateral adrenalectomy, pituitary irradiation, and removal of sources of ectopic ACTH.

The physical stigmata of cortisol and androgen excess often persist for months after correction of the hormonal abnormality.

Pheochromocytomas are tumors of the adrenal medulla (inner core) that can occur sporadically or as part of a genetic syndrome (multiple endocrine neoplasia, neurofibromatosis, Von Hippel-Lindau syndrome). Signs and symptoms result from catecholamine excess and include headache, sweating, palpitations, tremor, hypertension, and orthostatic hypotension. Paroxysmal release of catecholamines, at times provoked by emotional or physical stress, is common. Prolonged exposure to high levels of catecholamines can induce cardiac arrhythmias, cardiomyopathy, and peripheral myopathy. Preoperative pharmacologic treatment followed by surgical resection of the tumor or tumors is usually curative for benign disease. Malignant tumors are treated palliatively with surgical debulking, pharmacologic inhibition of catecholamine production, and combination chemotherapy.

Pituitary Disorders

Pituitary insufficiency results from disruption of anterior and/or posterior function due to compression, invasion, infarction, or hypothalamic dysfunction or destruction. Disease states of the anterior pituitary are recognized by hypofunction of one or more target endocrine glands (gonads, thyroid, adrenal) and impaired growth if growth hormone deficiency occurs in childhood or adolescence. Intrinsic pituitary tumors may produce excessive amounts of a specific trophic hormone, resulting in a characteristic clinical syndrome (e.g., excessive growth hormone causes acromegaly) while at the same time compromising synthesis and release of other pituitary hormones. Loss

of posterior pituitary function secondary to stalk section or hypothalamic disease results in central neurogenic diabetes insipidus (impaired urine concentration due to lack of the antidiuretic hormone ADH). Tumors of pituitary or extrinsic origin may compress adjacent neurologic and/or vascular structures with manifestations such as headache, visual field defects, decreased visual acuity, and paralysis of extraocular muscles.

Treatment includes use of pharmacologic agents that shrink tumors and lower hormone overproduction, tumor resection, and irradiation. Target organ hormone deficiencies are treated with replacement hormones. Deficiency of ADH is managed with intranasal desmopressin (DDAVP). Long-term monitoring is essential, and all affected individuals should wear a medical alert tag or bracelet.

Calcium Disorders

Disorders of calcium excess (hypercalcemia) may affect 0.5 to 3 percent of the population. For nonhospitalized people, a benign overactive parathyroid state (hyperparathyroidism) causes 70 to 80 percent of the hypercalcemia. Fifty percent of inpatient hypercalcemia results from other malignancies. Benign hypercalcemia, frequently long-standing, may have no symptoms, or may be heralded by kidney stones, peptic ulcer disease, pancreatitis, or osteopenic fractures. It is most frequently discovered incidentally on multipanel blood chemistry testing. Hypercalcemia secondary to malignancy usually presents with a rapidly increasing level that impairs alertness and arousal and that occasionally causes personality and psychiatric disturbances. Constitutional complaints such as malaise, decreased appetite, and muscle and joint aches are frequently encountered.

Treatment is modified according to severity of hypercalcemia, clinical presentation, underlying cause, and coexisting illness. Maintaining hydration and kidney function and suppressing bone resorption with oral or intravenous diphosphonate medication are temporary measures. Definitive treatment consists of parathyroid surgery for hyperparathyroidism and tumoricidal treatment for cancer. Prognosis for benign parathyroid disease is excellent, but generally poor for hypercalcemia associated with malignancy. Women who have osteopenia benefit from exercise, normal calcium intake, and estrogen replacement, if postmenopausal.

Low levels of serum calcium (hypocalcemia) are most commonly due to underactivity of the parathyroid glands, chronic kidney disease, magnesium deficiency, or pancreatitis. Symptoms are those of neuromuscular irritability: tingling, numbness, or cramping. More severe and chronic hypocalcemia can cause personality and psychiatric disorders and seizures without loss of consciousness. Treatment consists of intravenous or oral calcium replacement and vitamin D derivative supplementation.

Conclusion

Endocrine disorders, by virtue of their multisystem effects, can present challenging therapeutic and rehabilitation considerations. The clinical spectrum spans acute, life-threatening illness to chronic neuromuscular and circulatory disease. Early diagnosis and treatment, especially with regard to diabetes mellitus, should reduce acute and chronic morbidity. Multidisciplinary evaluation and management is essential to ensure an optimal outcome for the person with complications due to diabetes mellitus.

(*See also:* AMPUTATION; BLINDNESS AND VISION DISORDERS; CORONARY ARTERY DISEASE; GASTROINTESTINAL DISORDERS; GENETIC DISORDERS; GROWTH DISORDERS; KIDNEY DISORDERS; MINORITIES; PHARMACOLOGY; STROKE)

RESOURCES

American Diabetes Association, Inc., 1660 Duke St., Alexandria, VA 22314

Juvenile Diabetes Foundation International, 432 Park Ave. South, New York, NY 10016

National Diabetes Information Clearinghouse, 1 Information Way, Bethesda, MD 20892

National Eye Health Education Program, National Eye Institute, National Institutes of Health, Box 20/20, Bethesda, MD 20892

BIBLIOGRAPHY

AIELLO, LLOYD P.; AVERY, ROBERT L.; ARIGG, PAUL G.; KEYT, BRUCE A.; JAMPEL, HENRY D.; SABERA, T. SHAH; PASQUALE, LOUIS R.; THIEME, HAGEN; IWAMOTO, MAMI A.; PARK, JOHN E.; NGUYEN, HUNG V.; AIELLO, LLOYD M.; FERRARA, NAPOLEONE; and KING, GEORGE L. "Vascular Endothelial Growth Factor in Ocular Fluid of Patients with Diabetic Retinopathy and Other Retinal Disorders." *New England Journal of Medicine* 331 (1994):1480–1487.

AMERICAN DIABETES ASSOCIATION. "Clinical Practice Recommendations 1995." *Diabetes Care* 18 (1995): 4–96.

———. *Diabetes 1993 Vital Statistics.* Alexandria, VA, 1993.

———. *Direct and Indirect Costs of Diabetes in the United States in 1992.* Alexandria, VA, 1993.

BARDIN, C. WAYNE., ed. *Current Therapy in Endocrinology and Metabolism,* 5th ed. St. Louis, 1994.

DIABETES CONTROL AND COMPLICATIONS TRIAL RESEARCH GROUP. "The Effect of Intensive Treatment of Diabetes on the Development and Progression of Long-Term Complications in Insulin-Dependent Diabetes Mellitus." *New England Journal of Medicine* 329 (1993):977–986.

KAHN, C. RONALD, and WEIR, GORDON C., eds. *Joslin's Diabetes Mellitus,* 13th ed. Philadelphia, 1994.

LEWIS, EDMUND J.; HUNSICKER, LAWRENCE G.; BAIN, RAYMOND P.; and RHODE, RICHARD D. "The Effect of Angiotensin-Converting-Enzyme Inhibition on Diabetic Nephropathy." *New England Journal of Medicine* 329 (1993):1456–1462.

MCDERMOTT, MICHAEL T., ed. *Endocrine Secrets.* Philadelphia, 1995.

SPANHEIMER, ROBERT. "Skeletal and Rheumatologic Complications of Diabetes." In *Advances in Endocrinology and Metabolism,* vol. 4, ed. Ernest L. Mazzaferri. St. Louis, 1993.

U.S. DEPARTMENT OF HEALTH AND HUMAN SERVICES, PUBLIC HEALTH SERVICE. *Diabetes Surveillance, 1993.* Atlanta, 1993.

WILSON, JEAN D., and FOSTER, DANIEL W., eds. *Williams Textbook of Endocrinology,* 8th ed. Philadelphia, 1992.

ELLIOT STERNTHAL

END STAGE RENAL DISEASE

See KIDNEY DISORDERS

ENGINEERING, REHABILITATION

Rehabilitation engineering is the branch of engineering that is concerned with the application of science and technology to improve the quality of life of individuals with disabilities. Areas addressed within rehabilitation engineering include wheelchairs and seating systems, access to computers, sensory aids, prosthetics and orthotics, alternative and augmentative communication, and home and work site modification. Because many products of rehabilitation engineering require careful selection to match individual needs and often require custom fitting, rehabilitation engineers have necessarily become involved in service delivery and application as well as research, design, and development.

History

While it can be argued that "rehabilitation engineering" has been practiced for centuries, it is generally agreed that the beginning of rehabilitation engineering as an organized discipline in the United States can be traced to our nation's attempts to deal with the loss of limbs and vision in thousands of U.S. veterans following World War II. In 1945 the surgeon general of the Army asked the National Academy of Sciences (NAS) to initiate a research and development program with the goal of improving prostheses by applying technology from other fields. The NAS established the Committee on Prosthetic Devices, a group of prominent surgeons, prosthetists, and engineers, to direct what came to be known as the Artificial Limb Program. The committee's name was later changed to the Committee on Prosthetics Research and Development (CPRD).

Key support for this program was provided by Congress. In 1948 it passed P.L. 729, authorizing appropriation of $1 million annually to the Veterans Administration (VA) for a research and development (R&D) program in the field of prostheses, orthopedic appliances, and sensory aids. Additional funds were provided in 1954 with passage of the Vocational Rehabilitation Act, which authorized the Department of Health, Education, and Welfare (DHEW) to support research and training that would lead to improvements in rehabilitation practices. Some of the latter funds were used to support projects of the Artificial Limb Program. These programs began a truly remarkable period of collaboration between the VA and the DHEW, with the CPRD assisting both by developing research needs, reviewing proposals, evaluating devices developed

through their R&D projects and programs, and disseminating results of these activities through workshops and reports.

One of the early projects of the Artificial Limb Program was evaluation of the practicality of the suction socket for above-knee amputations. Suction sockets did indeed prove to be a useful addition to the prosthetist's armamentarium, but the project was perhaps even more influential in establishing the need for close cooperation between prosthetist and physician. Suction sockets require a close fit without impairment of circulation, and it was quickly discovered that a successful result was more likely when a prosthetist-physician team was involved. This type of close working relationship between technologists and clinicians later became one of the guiding principles of the emerging field of rehabilitation engineering.

Two international tragedies furthered the development of rehabilitation engineering during the 1960s. Early in that decade, it was discovered that thalidomide, a sedative being taken by pregnant women for nausea, was causing severe congenital limb deficiencies in many children. Governments in Canada and Western Europe, where the problem was most acute, established centers to develop prostheses for these children. These programs were successful in developing artificial limbs that were small enough and light enough to be used for essential functions such as eating. Additionally, they attracted engineers to work in clinics as members, if not leaders, of clinic teams. Through this involvement, engineers became aware of the many other problems faced by children and soon began focusing their talents on seating, mobility, communication, and other aspects of rehabilitation for children.

The second tragic event was the Vietnam War. Improvements in evacuation techniques and field medical care implemented during this war greatly increased the survival rate of wounded soldiers. As a result, there was a dramatic increase in the number of U.S. servicemen returning home with a spinal cord injury. This situation in turn caused a dramatic shift in emphasis within the medical care facilities of the Veterans Administration, which was suddenly faced with the responsibility of providing appropriate care for these people. Engineering research and development programs within the VA, therefore, began to focus increased attention on wheelchairs, orthoses, and environmental control systems in response to this need.

The Artificial Limb Program had successfully demonstrated the benefits to be gained from a government-sponsored program of research, development, evaluation, and training directed toward a common goal. It had become apparent to many that there were other disabling conditions that could also benefit from such an effort. Accordingly, the CPRD organized and conducted a workshop in 1970 at Annapolis, Maryland, to develop a plan to apply engineering "to improve the quality of life of the physically handicapped through a total approach to rehabilitation, combining medicine, engineering, and related science." Rehabilitation engineering, a term coined by personnel of the DHEW, was thus born.

The workshop report recommended the formation of rehabilitation engineering centers (RECs) to be supported by the DHEW and to be complementary to work supported by the VA and others. The report formulated guidelines for establishing the centers and objectives to be achieved. It recommended that centers be established in institutions that already had demonstrated ability in rehabilitation engineering, were associated with a university with recognized excellence in medicine and engineering, and provided continuing rehabilitation services to patients in a clinical environment. The need for collaboration among physicians and allied health personnel with engineers and their allied technical persons was deemed to be indispensable.

The first two RECs were funded by the DHEW in 1971, at Rancho Los Amigos Medical Center in Downey, California, and Moss Rehabilitation Hospital in Philadelphia. Three more were added the following year, at the Texas Institute for Rehabilitation and Research in Houston, the Rehabilitation Institute of Chicago, and the Children's Hospital Center in Boston. The REC program was written into law by the Rehabilitation Act of 1973, which identified rehabilitation engineering as a priority of the R&D programs of the Rehabilitation Services Administration of the DHEW.

The Veterans Administration likewise funded engineering centers at VA medical centers in Hines, Illinois; Palo Alto, California; and Decatur, Georgia. Just as with those funded by the DHEW, these centers were established to support teams of engineers and clinicians to address established technology needs of persons with physical disabilities.

The National Institute of Handicapped Research (NIHR; currently the National Institute on Disability and Rehabilitation Research) was established as an autonomous agency in the Rehabilitation Act of 1978 to support many of the research and training activities previously supported by the Rehabilitation Services Administration. The NIHR and the VA jointly sponsored the Interagency Conference on Rehabilitation Engineering in 1978 and 1979. These conferences were in part an outgrowth of the Conferences on Systems and Devices for the Disabled, which began in Boston in 1974.

At the 1979 Interagency Conference, which was held in Atlanta, 150 persons met to found the Rehabilitation Engineering Society of North America (RESNA). Its stated mission was "to improve the quality of life of persons with disabilities in all possible ways; from recognition of their needs, through design, development, evaluation, and production of devices and modification of housing and transportation environments, to enhancing the effectiveness of the delivery system to meet their needs." From the outset, RESNA was intended to be a professional society that was open to all persons, including individuals with disabilities, who were involved in development and delivery of rehabilitation equipment.

Three subsequent pieces of legislation have furthered the field of rehabilitation engineering. A 1986 amendment to the Rehabilitation Act of 1973 required that each state vocational rehabilitation agency provide evidence that rehabilitation engineering services were being provided to beneficiaries within their state. This amendment resulted in a hiring surge of "rehabilitation engineers" by state vocational rehabilitation agencies. The Technology-Related Assistance for Individuals with Disabilities Act, referred to as the Tech Act, was passed by Congress in 1988. It supports the concept that assistive technology can remove some of the barriers that prevent people with disabilities from participating in education, gainful employment, independent living, and a higher quality of life. The Tech Act is important to rehabilitation engineering because it can refine the delivery system within each state to facilitate acquisition of assistive technology by end users. The Individuals with Disabilities Education Act (IDEA) of 1990 guarantees the right of children with disabilities to be placed in the least restrictive educational environment and allows for whatever supplementary aids and services, including provision of assistive technology, that are necessary to achieve this.

Education

Most of the engineers who gravitated into "rehabilitation engineering" in the 1950s and 1960s were graduates of traditional engineering programs and had little or no formal training in anatomy, physiology, disability, or rehabilitation. During this period, engineering faculties at a number of universities initiated research activities in selected areas of what we now call rehabilitation engineering. This initiative was due in part to the availability of federal funds, primarily in prosthetics research as previously described, and also due to and coincident with the establishment of biomedical engineering programs on many campuses. Interest was further boosted by the additional funds made available through the REC program, and today a number of universities offer courses and research opportunities in this field. Generally, these programs are available through departments of biomedical, electrical, mechanical, computer, or industrial engineering.

The need to train engineers to become members of a clinical team and provide rehabilitation engineering services to clients with disabilities was formally recognized in 1976. In November of that year, a government-sponsored workshop was held in Knoxville on rehabilitation engineering education. One of the workshop recommendations was federal sponsorship of pilot programs at three or four universities to train graduate students to assume a primary responsibility for the delivery of engineering technology to persons with disabilities. One such program was subsequently established at the University of Virginia in 1981. This program received federal support until 1988 and graduated twenty-eight students. Additional funding was made available in subsequent years, and federal funds are provided to support programs partially at several universities. In each case, graduates receive a certificate in rehabilitation engineering while earning a master's degree, generally in biomedical engineering.

Philosophy

Rehabilitation engineering involves development and provision of equipment to be used by people with disabilities. In most cases the equipment is intended to replace or substitute for a function (walking, talking, seeing, hearing, manipulating, etc.) that has been lost or impaired. How the equipment performs is of paramount importance, but in many cases how it looks and the image it conveys are equally important. Thus, many wheelchair riders select a particular chair not only for how it performs but also for how it defines them to others. A person with an amputation may select a myoelectric hand even though a body-powered hook may be more functional. A woman with cerebral palsy may prefer a communication device with a feminine voice output.

Because selection of this type of equipment (known collectively as assistive technology) is so highly personal, rehabilitation engineering recognizes the importance of involving individuals with disabilities in all phases of the development-provision process. This process begins with defining needs and identifying design specifications that are important to the individual with the disability, continues through the development and evaluation stages, and culminates with including the consumer with disability as an important member of the clinical team selecting equipment to satisfy his or her individual needs.

To maximize performance and ensure that equipment does not cause harm to the user, it is also essential that the rehabilitation engineer work closely with physicians and members of the allied health team who understand the broader implications of the disabling condition. As demonstrated with suction sockets, a close working relationship between technical and clinical persons is often essential to developing or providing a successful product. Hence the rehabilitation engineer must be able to work effectively as part of a team whose members differ widely in training, professional approach, and individual characteristics. Having clinical members on the team, however, does not relieve the engineer of his or her responsibility to have extensive knowledge relating to rehabilitation and disability.

Organizations

The major professional society for rehabilitation engineering is RESNA, which draws most of its members from the United States and Canada. Membership is open to all persons who are interested in assistive and rehabilitation technology. RESNA headquarters are in Arlington, Virginia. Most members of RESNA are also members of other societies particular to their professional affiliation. These include the following:

- Institute of Electrical and Electronic Engineers (IEEE)
- Biomedical Engineering Society (BMES)
- American Society of Mechanical Engineers (ASME)
- American Institute for Medical and Biological Engineering (AIMBE)
- Canadian Medical and Biological Engineering Society (CMBES)
- American Occupational Therapy Association (AOTA)
- International Society of Alternative and Augmentative Communication (ISAAC)
- American Speech and Hearing Association (ASHA)
- American Physical Therapy Association (APTA)
- American Congress of Rehabilitation Medicine (ACRM)
- International Society of Prosthetics and Orthotics (ISPO)
- National Association for Medical Equipment Services (NAMES)

Each of the above organizations addresses topics related to rehabilitation engineering in their publications and at their conferences.

Other societies specific to rehabilitation engineering have been formed outside of North America. RESJA, the Rehabilitation Engineering Society of Japan, was formed in 1991, and, like RESNA, is open to engineers, educators, and clinicians. It holds an annual conference and publishes a proceedings with abstracts printed in English. An association has also been formed in Europe to organize ECART, the European Conference for the Advancement of Rehabilitation Technology. These conferences were established to provide a common forum for all persons involved in the development and delivery of rehabilitation technology. In Australia, delegates to a 1993 rehabilitation technology conference resolved to form the Australian Disability Technology Association to conduct conferences every two years.

Significant Issues

Perhaps the most significant issue in rehabilitation engineering today is the lack of an established credentialing system for certifying professionals and accrediting service delivery programs. Initial efforts to create such a system have focused on certifying persons who provide assistive technology services. Assistive technology providers have a variety of professional backgrounds, including engineering, occupational therapy, physical therapy, speech pathology, and special education. While most persons are certified or licensed within their professions, it is not practical for all professional associations to incorporate assistive technology into their credentialing processes. Since RESNA's membership represents a majority of the disciplines involved, RESNA has assumed the lead role in developing a credentialing program for providers of assistive technology.

Credentialing is particularly key for rehabilitation engineers. While many engineers are currently providing assistive technology services, the lack of formal certification has made third-party reimbursement difficult to obtain. Other rehabilitation professionals receive reimbursement for their services because they are credentialed or licensed within their professional disciplines. Plans for credentialing rehabilitation engineers are still being developed, but the minimum requirements to achieve certification will likely include: (1) a bachelor's degree in engineering or a demonstrated basic knowledge of engineering; (2) completion of specified course work related to disability and rehabilitation; and (3) clinical experience in a service delivery program under the supervision of a certified rehabilitation engineer.

A second issue is the lack of adequate training programs for students interested in rehabilitation and assistive technology. As stated previously, only a few academic programs for rehabilitation engineering in the United States attempt to prepare engineers for clinical practice. Likewise, the technology content in the curricula of schools of medicine and allied health is minimal in most cases. Finding room in already crowded curricula will be difficult, and specialized skills in assistive technology may have to be taught at the continuing education level.

There are major barriers to bringing rehabilitation products to the marketplace. In many cases equipment is highly specialized, markets are small, and costs are high. In some cases these problems are due to the need to conduct large-scale clinical evaluations to prove safety and efficacy to the Food and Drug Administration. Product liability also drives costs up for many products. But funds to purchase assistive technology are limited; individuals with disabilities traditionally have had low average earnings; and third-party payers (insurance companies and government programs) continue to look for ways to reduce reimbursable expenses.

Another issue is roadblocks to obtaining funding for assistive technology, especially from government-funded programs. Federal and state support for individuals with disabilities continues to grow but becomes more complex each year. Congress has established more than thirty programs that affect Americans with disabilities. More than a dozen federal agencies are charged with managing these programs and monitoring implementation at the state level. The resulting patchwork quilt of programs presents a complex and often impenetrable maze to consumers and professionals alike.

Finally, at the other end of the development-provision process, funds for R&D are inadequate to address satisfactorily the many needs of individuals with disabilities. It has been estimated that more than 43 million Americans have disabilities. A significant number of these individuals have impairments that limit their participation in the full range of life's activities, and many could benefit from products and services provided by rehabilitation engineering. A survey conducted in the early 1980s found that the U.S. government spent about $66 million a year on R&D related to technologies for

disabilities. At that time, the government also spent about $36 billion a year to support the income of people with disabilities. Thus its R&D expenditures in this area represent only 0.2 percent of its support payments. By comparison, the government's total health care R&D accounts for about 2 percent of its total health care expenditures. Because rehabilitation engineering has demonstrated its potential to reduce costs by helping to put people with disabilities back to work, thereby making them more independent, additional expenditures in R&D would more than pay for themselves in the long run.

The Future

In his book *Cybernetics,* originally published in 1948, Norbert Wiener observed that the loss of a limb segment implied not only the loss of a mechanical extension of the stump and contractile power of its muscles but also the loss of cutaneous and kinesthetic sensations originating in it. He noted that prosthetists at that time were attempting to replace the first two losses, but replacing the third was far beyond their scope. He envisioned prostheses in which touch, pressure, position, and motion would be reported back to the amputee through mechanical vibrators on the skin or even through multiple electrodes applied to the ends of the cut nerves. Today, limb prostheses are vastly improved and more closely mimic the action of the missing limb, but prosthetists are still replacing only the first two losses. Sensory feedback, if provided at all, is provided in a very limited, rudimentary way that does not come close to replacing the sensations that have been lost.

This, then, is one of the future challenges for rehabilitation engineering; namely, to develop prostheses and other technologies for people with disabilities that restore functional abilities to levels that are at least as good as those in individuals without impairments. We have come a long way since World War II, but we still have a long way to go, in all areas of rehabilitation engineering, to achieve this goal. This must be, and will be, the goal toward which rehabilitation engineering will continually strive.

While one group of rehabilitation engineers will continue to advance the state of the art, another group will be in the front lines, as members of the clinical team, working to ensure that all individuals with disabilities receive equipment that is most appropriate for their particular needs. These engineers will be certified assistive technology providers, and they will be recognized as valued members of the team by all members of the rehabilitation community, including third-party payers who will reimburse them for the rehabilitation engineering services they provide.

It is unfortunate but true that the need for rehabilitation engineering will continue to grow. As medicine and medical technology continue to improve, more people will survive traumatic injury, disease, and premature birth, and many will acquire functional impairments that impede their involvement in personal, community, educational, vocational, and recreational activities. People continue to live longer lives, thereby increasing the likelihood of acquiring one or more disabling conditions during their lifetime. This presents an immense challenge for the field of rehabilitation engineering. As opportunities grow, more engineers will be attracted to the field—engineers who are looking for exciting technical challenges and opportunities to help people live more satisfying and productive lives.

(*See also:* AMPUTATION; ASSISTIVE TECHNOLOGY; PROSTHETICS AND ORTHOTICS; WHEELCHAIRS)

RESOURCES

RESNA, an interdisciplinary association for the advancement of rehabilitation and assistive technologies, 1700 N. Moore St., Suite 1540, Arlington, VA 22209-1903. Conducts an annual conference, publishes a newsletter and a journal, and provides general information on rehabilitation and engineering.

National Institute on Disability and Rehabilitation Research (NIDRR), U.S. Department of Education, 400 Maryland Ave., SW, Washington, DC 20202-2572. Funds a network of rehabilitation engineering centers and supports university programs leading to a master's degree in engineering with an emphasis on rehabilitation engineering.

Rehabilitation Research and Development Service, Department of Veterans Affairs, 103 South Gay St., Baltimore, MD 21202-4051. Funds projects at Veterans Administration medical centers related to re-

habilitation engineering and conducts an evaluation program for pre-commercial devices.

BIBLIOGRAPHY

EDWARD, J. W. "Historical Development of Artificial Limbs." In *Orthopaedic Appliances Atlas*, vol. 2, Ann Arbor, MI, 1960.

McLAURIN, COLIN A. "Rehabilitation Engineering." *Rehab Management* (August–September 1991):71–77.

OFFICE OF TECHNOLOGY ASSESSMENT, CONGRESS OF THE UNITED STATES. *Technology and Handicapped People.* Washington, DC, 1982.

SMITH, RAYMOND V., and LESLIE, JOHN H., eds. *Rehabilitation Engineering.* Boca Raton, FL, 1990.

WIENER, NORBERT. *Cybernetics or Control and Communication in the Animal and the Machine*, 2nd ed. New York, 1961.

DONALD McNEAL

EPILEPSY

See NEUROLOGICAL DISORDERS

ERGONOMICS

Ergonomics is the name given to an interdisciplinary field involving industrial and production engineers, work physiologists, medical and occupational health and safety professionals, design engineers, industrial hygienists, and all those concerned with the performance of humans at work, how they cope with the working environment, how they interact with machines, and, in general, how they deal with their surroundings. The term "ergonomics" is coined from the Greek words *ergon*, meaning work, and *nomos*, meaning natural laws. In essence, ergonomics may be defined as a scientific discipline primarily concerned with the application of natural laws governing human work.

Ergonomics may be defined in other ways. For instance, William T. Singleton (1972) defines ergonomics as the technology of work design. Ergonomics may also be defined as the application of technology to assist the human element in manual work.

Ergonomics is known by several other names, such as human factors and human-machine systems. In the United States the term "human factors" is more widely used. When ergonomics is applied to occupational settings as opposed to nonoccupational settings, such as homes, it is generally referred to as industrial ergonomics.

Even though the terms "ergonomics" and "human factors" are generally considered synonymous, many individuals prefer to make a distinction. These individuals associate the human factors with the behavioral factors of human performance, and ergonomics with the quantitative and/or health and safety aspects of humans at work in occupational and nonoccupational settings. The trend is toward the elements covered under "ergonomics."

The overall objective of ergonomics is to fit the tasks to humans to enhance their effectiveness in the workplace. This means that ergonomics aims at:

- eliminating or minimizing injuries, strains and sprains;
- minimizing fatigue and overexertion;
- minimizing absenteeism and labor turnover;
- improving quality and quantity of output;
- minimizing lost time and costs associated with injuries and accidents;
- maximizing safety, efficiency, comfort, and productivity.

Ergonomics is based on biological (natural) sciences. The main components of ergonomics are anatomy, physiology, psychology, medicine, and engineering. Anatomy is concerned with the structure of the human body and involves the study of human body size (anthropometry) and how the body responds when subjected to various internal and external forces (biomechanics). Physiology is mainly concerned with how the body functions when performing work (work physiology) or when subjected to different climatological factors (environmental physiology). Psychology is concerned with the behavioral responses of humans to work and environment and includes information processing and decision-making (skill psychology) and training, effort perception, and individual worker factors (occupational psychology). Medicine is concerned with the diagnosis, including developing invasive and noninvasive tests, and treatment of injuries (acute and chronic). Engineering provides information about the machinery and assists in adapting this equipment for human use. Engineering knowledge also assists in designing and developing equipment and devices that fit humans.

An Ergonomist's Definition of Disability

Disability is any restriction or lack of ability resulting from an impairment, to perform an activity in the manner or within the range of able-bodied persons (Mital & Karwowski, 1988). Impairment is any loss or abnormality of psychology or physiological functions or anatomical or physiological structures (Kroll, 1985). The impairment may be the result of a disease, an accident, or a congenital disorder. An individual with a disability, therefore, is a disadvantaged individual whose role is limited, or who is prevented from functioning as would a person without a disability.

Scope of Ergonomics

As stated earlier, ergonomics has several distinct but related goals. Its overall goal is to maximize workers' capabilities while ensuring their safety, comfort, efficiency, and effectiveness. During World War II and the adolescent years of its growth, ergonomics was primarily concerned with ensuring that human operators were able to get the "best" out of their equipment. The drive to increase efficiency led designers to know more about human capabilities, their limitations and responses to things and the environment. The study of human performance became the central issue. "Designing for humans" and "human use" became the primary expressions ergonomists and human factors specialists started using in describing their activities.

As ergonomics evolved, it became clear that job satisfaction, quality of life, operator comfort, safety, injury control, stress, productivity, and efficiency were all related. The role of ergonomics in containing costs, particularly those directly resulting from and attributable to injuries, absenteeism, retraining new hires, increased medical costs and liability insurance and punitive damages, started getting wide recognition. Today, ensuring maximum long-term health and safety of workers by preventing and/or controlling occupational injuries and illnesses, and accommodating persons with disabilities, are important and prominent goals of ergonomics. The role of ergonomics in controlling cumulative trauma disorders (CTD) of the upper and lower extremities and the costs associated with these disorders is an appropriate example of this relatively new emphasis.

Ergonomics in Rehabilitation

Rehabilitation aims at reducing the impact of disabling conditions on individuals and enabling them to achieve social integration. Comprehensive rehabilitation includes medical, social, vocational, and ergonomic rehabilitation. (In earlier models, ergonomic rehabilitation has been shown to be part of vocational rehabilitation. The sophistication necessary to integrate fully a person with disabilities in the society mandates that ergonomic rehabilitation be considered separately.)

From an ergonomics standpoint, rehabilitation is a process of recognizing and assessing functional limitations of persons with disabilities, and circumventing these limitations through design. One of the most prevalent techniques to accomplish this is through available motion inventory. The limitations of persons with disabilities are recognized by comparing their functional capabilities with those of people without disabilities. Once the limitations are determined, corrective actions are taken to design the external environment (design of the tools, equipment, work, and workplace) that alleviates or minimizes the adverse consequences of the disability.

Role of Professional and Governmental Organizations

Following are some of the major professional and governmental organizations active in the area of ergonomics and rehabilitation:

- National Institute on Disability and Rehabilitation Research, U.S. Department of Education
- National Institutes of Health, U.S. Department of Health and Human Services
- National Institute for Occupational Safety and Health, U.S. Department of Health and Human Services

- Human Factors and Ergonomics Society
- International Foundation for Industrial Ergonomics and Safety Research
- International Journal of Industrial Ergonomics

All these organizations realize the need to integrate people with disabilities socially and in the workplace. While the governmental organizations are funding rehabilitation ergonomics research, the professional organizations are active in disseminating the new knowledge. Passage of the Americans with Disability Act (1990) has accelerated accommodation of persons with disabilities in the workplace and has provided industry with a motive to recruit and retain workers with disabilities. These efforts are expected to accelerate in the future. Furthermore, the problems of persons with disabilities are likely to be attended by an interdisciplinary team comprising health, engineering, and vocational professionals.

(*See also:* DISABILITY MANAGEMENT; ENGINEERING, REHABILITATION; WORK)

RESOURCES

National Institute on Disability and Rehabilitation Research, U.S. Department of Education, 400 Maryland Ave., SW, Washington, DC 20202–2572

National Institutes of Health, U.S. Department of Health and Human Services, 5333 Westbard Ave., Bethesda, MD 20892

National Institute for Occupational Safety and Health, U.S. Department of Health and Human Services, Robert A. Taft Laboratories, 4676 Columbia Parkway, Cincinnati, OH 45226

Human Factors and Ergonomics Society, P.O. Box 1369, Santa Monica, CA 90406

International Foundation for Industrial Ergonomics and Safety Research, Dr. S. Dutta, Secretary, Department of Industrial Engineering, University of Windsor, Windsor, Ont. N9B 3P4, Canada

International Journal of Industrial Ergonomics, Elsevier Science Publishers, P.O. Box 211, 1000 AE Amsterdam, The Netherlands

BIBLIOGRAPHY

KROLL, J. "Disability Prevention and Rehabilitation." In *Encyclopedia of Occupational Health and Safety*, 3rd ed., ed. Luigi Parmeggiani. Geneva, 1985.

MITAL, A., and KARWOWSKI, W. "Rehabilitation: An

Urgent Need?" In *Ergonomics in Rehabilitation*, ed. A. Mital and W. Karwowski. London, 1988.

SINGLETON, W. T. *Introduction to Ergonomics*. Geneva, 1972.

ANIL MITAL

ETHICS

Rehabilitation is a multidisciplinary field whose goal is to empower and maximize the restoration of persons with disabilities physically, mentally, socially, vocationally, and economically and to help them gain control over their lives by minimizing dependence (Rehabilitation Act Amendments, 1992; Wright, 1980). This service system involves professionals with a diversity of skills, codes of ethics, education, and values working in a myriad of organizations. Value conflicts arise as professionals determine how best to serve people under the constraints of differing personal philosophies, public policy, codes of ethics, limited resources, and patient or client interest.

The purpose of this entry is to describe ethics in rehabilitation from a broad perspective that includes ethical theory, principles, and issues; ethical dilemmas; codes of ethics; ethics committees; and decision-making.

Ethics and Ethical Theory

Ethics, derived from the Greek word *ethos*, referring to character or customs, generally describes how to evaluate life through a set of standards and how to regulate behavior (Flew, 1984). Ethical theory is a systematic body of principles and rules that assists in determining the validity of moral arguments and justifies what is morally appropriate when value conflicts arise among different courses of action. Many types of ethical theories exist, such as hedonism, empirical naturalism, stoicism, Christian ethics, existentialism, behaviorism, and phenomenology (Edwards, 1972; Jones et al., 1977). The two prominent theories relevant to rehabilitation ethics are deontology and utilitarianism (Arras & Hunt, 1983).

The Greek word *deon* means duty. Deontology evaluates actions in terms of duty, obligation, and rights. Duty is independent of the concept of good, and some actions are right or wrong regardless of their consequences. For example, promises, contracts, justice, and truthfulness determine what is right; deception is wrong. Some deontologists base judgments about right and wrong on the Ten Commandments, natural law, intuition, or social contracts. Immanuel Kant introduced deontology through the concept of the categorical imperative. It states that a maxim or a rule must be applicable universally and in all situations to be followed. Therefore, it is binding with no exceptions and provides guidance on how one must act morally. Second, what is morally acceptable is contingent on the maxim/rule that influences one's will. Actions have moral worth if conducted by a person with good will. A person has good will if he or she can base that will on a valid rule. For example, the Golden Rule is a maxim from which other rules, such as truth-telling and fidelity, may be derived (Beauchamp & Childress, 1989).

Utilitarianism evaluates the worthiness of an action's consequences or the consequences of observing rules (Beauchamp & Childress, 1989). Morally right actions/rules are determined by nonmoral values such as pleasure, knowledge, health, or friendship. Utility is the underlying principle of this theory. Utility means that actions are good if they maximize the greatest good for the greatest number of people and minimize harm. Therefore, the end justifies the means. Some utilitarians believe that the greatest good—right or wrong—is determined by the intrinsic value produced by an action. Others believe that utility should be based on happiness or pleasure. An action should be performed if the sum of the happiness of all affected persons would be maximized by the performance of that action.

Principles

Five ethical principles apply to ethics in rehabilitation: beneficence, autonomy, nonmaleficence, justice, and fidelity (Beauchamp & Childress, 1989). Beneficence refers to promoting the welfare and interests of others—doing good. Nonmaleficence means avoiding or preventing intentional harm to others. Autonomy refers to respecting people's choices and the right to self-determination without controlling constraints. Justice means treating others fairly and involves the equitable allocation of scarce resources among competing persons or groups.

Fidelity refers to keeping promises, commitments, and obligations—explicit or implied—to others and abiding by rules and regulations.

Ethical Dilemmas

Ethical dilemmas arise when professionals must decide on a course of action that will best meet the needs of persons with disease or disability while fulfilling their duties of preserving life, reducing suffering, benefiting the sick, abiding by codes of ethics and organizational guidelines, and adhering to public policy. Conflicts may occur among any combination of ethical principles as well as among groups with different value systems. An ethical dilemma is defined as a situation in which (1) a person is faced with a choice between two mutually exclusive courses of action; (2) either course of action is supported by ethical principles; and (3) either course of action may have significant consequences (Harding, 1985; Kitchener, 1984).

Public Sector Rehabilitation

Henry Wong, Stanford Rubin, and Richard Millard (1991) identified thirty-eight ethical dilemmas encountered by rehabilitation counselors and independent living service providers employed in state rehabilitation agencies and centers for independent living that involve conflicts among the five principles mentioned above. Only the three most frequently encountered dilemmas, those involving conflict between autonomy and beneficence, will be discussed here.

Rehabilitating a client on Social Security disability income (SSDI) into competitive work sometimes conflicts with maximizing the client's financial security. For example, some clients receive more money and medical benefits on SSDI than they would by returning to work at minimum wage. Second, supporting a client's selection of a particular vocational objective may conflict with directing that client toward a more realistic vocational objective. Some clients may not be realistic about the types of jobs that are appropriate in light of their skills and limitations. Third, providing support for a specific type of training requested by the client may conflict with supporting the type of training recommended in the client's evaluation report. The medical and vocational assessment may determine jobs that contraindicate a client's educational choice.

Private Sector Rehabilitation

Since the 1970s there has been a rapid rise in opportunities for rehabilitation counselors in the private sector. The public and private sectors serve different populations and have differing philosophies. The goal of private sector rehabilitation, an insurance benefit provided to workers with industrial injuries, is to restore a client to the former level of vocational functioning or as close an approximation of that level as possible. Counselors may provide expert opinion, without providing rehabilitation services, or serve as expert witnesses. Consequently, the ethics of private rehabilitation have been questioned, since the rehabilitationist does not strive to restore an individual to maximum potential (Cottone, 1982; Kaiser & Brown, 1988; Nadolsky, 1986).

In private rehabilitation, professional judgments may influence the amount and duration of compensation payments as well as the magnitude of award settlements. Provision of medical and vocational case management services is routinely scrutinized by insurance representatives, attorneys, physicians, clients, rehabilitation supervisors, and administrative law judges, each with a different set of guidelines and/or needs (Matkin & May, 1981; Pape & Klein, 1986). Conflicts of interest may arise for the counselor when the above "masters" differ in their requests regarding the quantity or quality of service necessary to resolve a client's file. For example, a claims investigation may be requested under the guise of a rehabilitation evaluation, counselors may be asked to "document the file" without providing quality services, and overbilling may be suggested to meet a quota or to stay in business. Counselors may be pressured to "take sides" or provide a biased interpretation of a case for the benefit of the insurance carrier (Cottone, 1982). These practices pose dilemmas for the rehabilitationist due to conflicts among ethical principles.

Professionals in the field of "insurance rehabilitation" operate from a myriad of educational and experiential backgrounds, including nursing, business, rehabilitation counseling, and claims adjusting. This professional interdisciplinary team can produce a disjointed array of qualifications, competencies, and training needs. The answer to the question "Who is the client?" may differ depending on an individual's training and experience. For example, in the business world the client is the referral or funding source, whereas in rehabilitation the client is the person with the disability. Ethical questions regarding the role of the profit motive, the absence of professional supervision, and limited demands for accountability often arise—that is, conflicts between beneficence and justice (Matkin & May, 1981). The issues may be complicated by the professional isolation that results from the independence of fieldwork and the lack of a unified code of ethics.

Confidentiality is another ethical issue in the private sector. The counselor's report on the client's medical, vocational, and motivational status is based on information provided by the client and the rehabilitation team (e.g., physicians, employer, and therapists). Information is typically shared, with or without a release of information from the client. An ethical dilemma (i.e., fidelity vs. justice) occurs when incriminating information provided by the client, employer, and/or medical personnel is used by the insurance carrier to decrease benefits. Even though the client may be served by exposure of his or her concealment of increased independence and a productive lifestyle, the issue of whether the rehabilitation counselor should play a role in exposing that concealment remains unresolved (Kaiser & Brown, 1988).

Codes of Ethics

Formal codes of professional ethics are general prescriptive guidelines based on ethical principles that include sets of rules for behavior applicable to individuals or groups. These codes govern responsibilities, duties, and the quality of the relationship between the patient/client and the professional service provider. The advantages of codes of ethics are that they represent the general consensus on professional conduct by members of a particular professional group (Beauchamp & Childress, 1989). The disadvantages of such codes are that they cannot comprehensively cover all aspects of the professional relationship, may be contradictory in parts, and may

not clarify a clear direction when conflicts emerge. Only a few of the numerous codes in existence will be mentioned here. The reader is referred to Tom Beauchamp and James Childress (1983) for a full discussion of the Hippocratic oath, the American Medical Association Principles of Medical Ethics, and the American Nurses' Association Code for Nurses.

The Hippocratic oath, applicable to physicians, emphasizes above all to do no harm and to benefit the sick, not to give deadly drugs, to be just, and to avoid sexual exploitation.

The American Psychological Association's (APA) ethical principles of psychologists cover confidentiality, responsibilities and competencies, public statements, consumers' welfare, assessment techniques, research with human subjects, and the care and use of animals (American Psychological Association, 1992).

The Code of Professional Ethics for Rehabilitation Counselors emphasizes behaving in a legal, ethical, and moral manner; respecting the integrity and welfare of persons with disabilities; advocacy; confidentiality; acting with integrity in relationships; proper use of assessment measures; expanding research; and maintaining competency (Commission on Rehabilitation Counselor Certification, 1989).

Ethics Committees

Hospital ethics committees—also known as terminal care, prognosis, and/or optimum care committees—had their early development in the late 1970s in response to the case of Karen Quinlan. After being in a comatose state for more than ten years, Karen Quinlan had her respirator removed at the request of her father, who had petitioned the New Jersey Supreme Court to allow the removal (Mackay, 1988). The court had mandated that her parents and physician consult with the hospital ethics committee.

The role of ethics committees includes reviewing treatment decisions on terminally ill patients, reviewing medical decisions having ethical consequences, providing counseling to patients and their families, establishing treatment guidelines, and providing education to hospital staff and the general public about ethical problems (President's Commission, 1983). Committee members may include physicians, hospital administrators, attorneys, social workers, clergy, advocates, and hospital volunteers. Committee members—except physicians proven to have been negligent or to have shown a willful disregard for the patient's interests—have civil and criminal immunity from liability for their recommendations. Ethical dilemmas arise for these committees whenever professional values conflict with the patient's interests.

Robert Veatch (1977) found ethics committees primarily in hospitals with teaching programs and with more than 200 beds (i.e., in fewer than 1 percent of hospitals in the United States). The major benefits of ethics committees include decision-making, providing legal protection for hospital/medical staff, developing policy on life support, and serving as a forum for the discussion of professional disagreements.

Ethical Decision-Making

Rocco R. Cottone (1982) expressed concern about the ethical conduct of rehabilitation professionals. The need for ethics education for rehabilitation counselors has been indicated (Emener & Rasch, 1984; Rubin et al., 1991). Several medical ethics training programs exist from which rehabilitation ethics education draws guidance (Purtilo, 1983). These programs focus on ethical principles, issues, and ethical theory; critical–analytical problem-solving; codes of ethics and their limitations; and sensitizing students to ethical dilemmas and their own value systems (Bicknell, 1985; Welbourn, 1985).

Stanford Rubin et al. (1991) developed an ethics training program for rehabilitation counselors. It covers defining ethical principles and the concept of an ethical dilemma, the use and application of the Code of Professional Ethics for Rehabilitation Counselors in case management, and the application of a decision-making model.

The decision-making model is applied to ethical dilemmas encountered in rehabilitation based on Henry Wong (1990). Components of this model involve reviewing the case to determine the two courses of action, listing the reasons supporting and not supporting each course of action, identifying which ethical principles support each action and which are compromised, and writing a justification for the decision based on the above components.

Research indicates that graduates who have received ethics training have enhanced ethical decision-making ability compared to those who have not received such training (Baldick, 1980; Rest, 1984).

(*See also:* PHILOSOPHY OF REHABILITATION)

BIBLIOGRAPHY

AMERICAN PSYCHOLOGICAL ASSOCIATION. "Ethical Principles of Psychologists and Code of Conduct." *American Psychologist* (December 1992):1–15.

ARRAS, JOHN, and HUNT, ROBERT. *Ethical Issues in Modern Medicine*, 2nd ed. Palo Alto, CA, 1983.

BALDICK, THOMAS. "Ethical Discrimination Ability of Intern Psychologists: A Function of Training in Ethics." *Professional Psychology* 11(1980):276–282.

BEAUCHAMP, TOM, and CHILDRESS, JAMES. *Principles of Biomedical Ethics*, 2nd ed. New York, 1983.

———. *Principles of Biomedical Ethics*, 3rd ed. New York, 1989.

BICKNELL, DAVID J. "Current Arrangements for Teaching Medical Ethics to Undergraduate Medical Students." *Journal of Medical Ethics* 11 (1985):25–26.

COMMISSION ON REHABILITATION COUNSELOR CERTIFICATION. "Code of Professional Ethics for Rehabilitation Counselors—1989." Rolling Meadows, IL, 1989.

CORMIER, WILLIAM and CORMIER, LOUISE. *Interviewing Strategies for Helpers*, 2nd ed. Pacific Grove, CA, 1985.

COTTONE, ROCCO R. "Ethical Issues in Private-for-Profit Rehabilitation." *Journal of Applied Rehabilitation Counseling* 13 (1982):14–17.

EDWARDS, PAUL, ed. *Encyclopedia of Philosophy.* New York, 1972.

EMENER, WILLIAM, and RASCH, JOHN. "Actual and Preferred Instructional Areas in Rehabilitation Education Programs." *Rehabilitation Counseling Bulletin* 27 (1984):269–280.

FLEW, ANTHONY. A *Dictionary of Philosophy*, 2nd ed. New York, 1984.

HARDING, CHRISTOPHER G. *Moral Dilemmas.* Chicago, 1985.

JONES, WILLIAM; SONTAG, FREDERICK; BECKNER, MORTON; and FOGELIN, ROBERT. *Approaches to Ethics.* New York, 1977.

KAISER, JEANNE M., and BROWN, JOSEPH. "Ethical Dilemmas in Private Rehabilitation." *Journal of Rehabilitation* 54 (1988):27–30.

KITCHENER, KAREN S. "Intuition, Critical Evaluation, and Ethical Principles: The Foundation for Ethical Decisions in Counseling Psychology." *The Counseling Psychologist* 12 (1984):43–55.

MACKAY, ROBERT D. "Terminating Life-Sustaining Treatment—Recent U.S. Developments." *Journal of Medical Ethics* 14 (1988):135–139.

MATKIN, RALPH E., and MAY, V. ROBERT. "Potential Conflicts of Interest in Private Rehabilitation: Identification and Resolution." *Journal of Applied Rehabilitation Counseling* 12 (1981):15–18.

NADOLSKY, JULIAN M. "Ethical Issues in the Transition from Public to Private Rehabilitation." *Journal of Rehabilitation* 52 (1986):6–8.

PAPE, DEBORAH A., and KLEIN, MICHAEL A. "Ethical Issues in Rehabilitation Counseling: A Survey of Rehabilitation Practitioners." *Journal of Applied Rehabilitation Counseling* 17 (1986):8–13.

PRESIDENT'S COMMISSION FOR THE STUDY OF ETHICAL PROBLEMS IN MEDICINE AND BIOMEDICAL AND BEHAVIORAL RESEARCH. "Splicing Life." Washington, DC, 1982.

———. "Foregoing Life-Sustaining Treatment." Washington, DC, 1983.

PURTILO, RUTH B. "Ethics in Allied Health Education: State of the Art." *Journal of Allied Health* 12 (1983):210–221.

REHABILITATION ACT AMENDMENTS OF 1992, Pub. L. No. 102–569, 106 Stat. 4344. Washington, DC, 1992.

REST, JAMES R. "Research on Moral Development: Implications for Training Counseling Psychologists." *Counseling Psychologist* 12 (1984):19–29.

RUBIN, STANFORD; MILLARD, RICHARD; WILSON, CAROLYN; and WONG, HENRY. "An Introduction to the Ethical Case Management Practices Training Program." *Rehabilitation Education* 5 (1991):113–120.

VEATCH, ROBERT. "Hospital Ethics Committees: Is There a Role?" *Hastings Center Report* 7 (1977):22–25.

WELBOURN, RICHARD B. "A Model for Teaching Medical Ethics." *Journal of Medical Ethics* 11 (1985):29–31.

WONG, HENRY. "Ethical Dilemmas Encountered by Rehabilitation Counselors and Independent Living Service Providers." Ph.D. diss., Southern Illinois University at Carbondale, 1990.

WONG, HENRY, and MILLARD, RICHARD. "Ethical Dilemmas Encountered by Independent Living Service Providers." *Journal of Rehabilitation* 58 (1992):10–15.

WONG, HENRY; RUBIN, STANFORD; and MILLARD, RICHARD. "Ethical Dilemmas Encountered by Rehabilitation Counselors." *Rehabilitation Education* 5 (1991):19–26.

WRIGHT, GEORGE N. *Total Rehabilitation.* Boston, 1980.

HENRY D. WONG
ANN T. NEULICHT

ETHNIC ISSUES

See MINORITIES

EVALUATION OF REHABILITATION PROGRAMS

Evaluation efforts are becoming increasingly important in assessing what rehabilitation programs are doing for clients and if the services provided are doing what is intended. The Rehabilitation Act of 1973 (and all subsequent amendments) requires the evaluation of the delivery of rehabilitation services. In addition to the pressures of legislation, rehabilitation managers at all levels understand the need for evaluative feedback in making more informed decisions. The rehabilitation field has evolved into a very complicated human services program. No longer can problems be solved by informal decisions or a manager's past experience as a practitioner (Spaniol, 1985). Program managers are faced with a growing fiscal restraint among funding resources, skepticism about service interventions, and a demand for greater justification of program accomplishments.

While evaluation is considered important, it contains an element of anxiety. Program administrators are generally not enthusiastic about evaluation because many perceive it as an externally imposed requirement for which there is neither adequate preparation nor sufficient funding. Common fears of staff are that they may be fired, the program may be terminated, or that the evaluation information may be distorted or inappropriately used for political purposes (Boschen, 1984).

"Evaluation" is a term that can have different meanings to different persons and different programs.

In general, the word "evaluation" usually means judgment, or the determination of the relative value of some object, person, or idea. In regard to rehabilitation programs, evaluation includes a variety of different activities. In a general sense, the evaluation of programs can be defined as the systematic activities of collecting, analyzing, and interpreting program data to provide rehabilitation managers and other decision-makers with information in regard to the effectiveness and efficiency of programs, systems, and methods of service delivery. LeRoy Spaniol (1985) emphasized the continuous nature of program evaluation by defining it as a systematic, continuous process of providing information about the value of a program for purposes of decision-making.

As a decision-making tool, evaluation should be considered an essential part of the management process. Without knowing the current status of a program, it is difficult to establish meaningful goals, objectives, and strategies for the future. Effective program administration includes collecting, analyzing, and interpreting data by which to assess service needs, patterns of use, program outcomes, and the cost/benefit ratio of services offered (Posavec & Carey, 1985).

Purpose of Evaluation

Two general purposes commonly associated with the evaluation of rehabilitation services are program improvement and accountability. These purposes need to be designed into individual systems to reflect the organization's philosophy of rehabilitation/habilitation, client mix, accountability demands, the community or environment in which the organization exists, and the needs of the people being served (Commission on Accreditation of Rehabilitation Facilities [CARF], 1991). These purposes of program improvement and accountability generate yet another series of questions. What about efficiency, effectiveness, and the standards used? Consequently, these questions complicate matters and contribute to the general lack of consensus, understanding, and utilization of program evaluation. Some organizational structure is necessary from which to approach program evaluation (Garske, Trach, and Leung, 1992).

One assumption regarding rehabilitation program evaluation is that it is both formative and summative in nature (Scriven, 1967). Formative or "feedback" evaluation is used to assess program operations to provide data for decision-makers concerned with making the program more effective. This type of ongoing evaluation permits program changes as needed. On the other hand, summative evaluations assess the program outcomes. For example, assessments are made to determine if treatment goals have been accomplished or if a program is worth continuing. In other words, current and ongoing collection and use of data on rehabilitation serve both the function of program improvement and the assessment of program merit. Almost all evaluation models can be both formative and summative.

Evaluation Models

Some people have suggested evaluation models specific to rehabilitation services. A model offered by Le Roy Spaniol (1985) includes three basic concepts: purpose, context, and methodology. Purpose refers to the reason why an evaluation is undertaken. Examples of purpose may include program justification, planning and policy analysis, and organizational development. Context refers to the goal of an evaluation. The emphasis is on what the evaluation is attempting to achieve. For example, in a goal-oriented evaluation, context includes the mission statement, goals, and objectives of the program. The last concept, methodology, refers to the system of variables, criteria, tools, measures, design, data collection, and analysis system for judging the results and providing feedback used in evaluation. Spaniol further specified that there are four types of evaluation utilized in rehabilitation. These include:

1. Input types of evaluation
   A. Needs analysis
      The determination of client demographic and service needs characteristics.
   B. Social audits
      The determination of the availability, accessibility, and utilization of programs and services.
2. Process types of evaluation
   A. Case review
      The evaluation of individual case files, pri-

marily with reference to adherence to administrative and service delivery standards.

B. Case flow analysis

The analysis of the physical movement of clients through the rehabilitation process.

C. Continuous monitoring

The process by which information on program performance is collected and analyzed relative to a standard.

D. Task force or committees

E. Questions and answers

F. Intuition

3. Outcome types of evaluation

A. Goal review

The assessment of the relevancy and adequacy of the goals/objectives to the original needs.

B. Goal-oriented evaluation

The assessment of the extent to which goals/objectives have been met.

C. Generalized outcome evaluation (goal-free evaluation)

The assessment of the actual effects of a program in relationship to the original needs.

4. Systems type of evaluation

A. Cost-benefit analysis (higher-level efficiency)

A means of relating the cost of a program/project to the cost of an alternative program/project in terms of the total benefit to the client and the community.

B. Cost-effectiveness analysis (lower-level efficiency)

A means of relating the cost of a particular activity or project to effective performance or goal attainment.

C. Program analysis of service systems (PASS)

An evaluation system that objectively quantifies the quality of a wide range of human service projects, activities, and programs.

D. Operations research

An application of science and mathematics to coordination and problem-solving.

E. Contingency analysis

A simulation of a program before its implementation to assess its probable outcomes and implications for decision-making.

F. Systems analysis

The analysis of alternative approaches to defined goals.

Another evaluation model related to rehabilitation was offered by Kathryn A. Boschen (1984), who suggested that evaluation of a vocational rehabilitation program may reflect a desire for any or all of the following specific kinds of assessments:

• an evaluation of the need for the vocational rehabilitation program within the community (often used to justify the existence of a current service or the plans to institute a new service);
• a process evaluation of the program, examining program activities and the clientele served (for program monitoring);
• an evaluation of program outcome, documenting whether program goals and objectives are being met (to aid in the decisions about program change);
• an evaluation of program efficiency, investigating both the cost and the effectiveness of the service (for budgetary justification).

In view of the models presented above, there appears to be no one way of assessing program success or merit. In human service programs, evaluators should be careful not to get slowed in controversies about the evaluation processes. Because of the multiplicity of causes and effects of any activity, it is suggested, however, that no simple criterion can ever adequately reflect the operation of a program (Spaniol, 1975). Programs should attempt to be as comprehensive as possible in their evaluation efforts.

The models referred to above suggest a variety of assessment approaches that may be included in the evaluation of rehabilitation services. The following section will focus on some of the most common evaluation measures used.

Needs Assessment. Program planning and implementation cannot take place in a vacuum. A basic management error can occur when services are planned and delivered without assessing the needs of the target groups to be served. An evaluation of potential clients and service needs is important, along with the assessment of available resources. Generally, a needs assessment consists of procedures used together with information for planning to take place (Simon, 1989).

A variety of needs assessment approaches may be used. The most popular method for gathering information on needs is the survey method. Surveys may include mail and telephone questionnaires, structured personal interviews, and electronically activated technology (e.g., dial-up voting on public issues). The most popular types of surveys include key informant surveys, prevalence and incidence surveys, and community surveys. Key informant surveys attempt to acquire needs information from persons who are expected or known to be knowledgeable about the needs issue. Surveys designed to estimate only the number of individuals who became in need of services during a particular time period are called incidence surveys. Surveys to estimate the number of individuals in need of service are called prevalence studies. The community survey is a large-scale effort involving a general questionnaire for the population in a particular area (Region V Study Group, 1991).

Other needs assessment techniques in use, especially by state agencies, include analysis of existing data sources (e.g., social indicator analyses, epidemiological studies, rates under treatment studies, and case studies); group approaches (e.g., structural groups, community forums, and hearings); and techniques for identifying capacities to meet needs (e.g., resource inventories and provider surveys). Each needs assessment approach can be used to obtain understanding of need and the demands those needs might place on the agency and other service providers. Quite often more than one needs assessment method will be used.

Process Evaluation. The monitoring of program performance is an essential task of a rehabilitation agency. However, among some strategies used for evaluation, distinctions must be made between the ongoing, continuous monitoring of some index of agency performance and occasional possible ad hoc studies of current important issues. Characteristics that clearly lend themselves to monitoring include those client and service characteristics best handled in a good information system (e.g., numbers of admissions, numbers of services provided, and numbers of clients served). In general, monitoring works best if it is applied to indices considered important and relevant to their needs. In the public rehabilitation system, an example of process evaluation consists of the reporting of client case flow. George N. Wright (1980) defined case flow as the movement of

clients through successive stages of the rehabilitation process, from application for services to closure. Rehabilitation counselors regularly report case progress, which then is measured through a series of checkpoints. A state's public vocational rehabilitation process is categorized in stages. These stages are identified by a series of numbered statuses, which are represented by a two-digit code that is loaded into a computer for information storage and analysis.

Each state submits a plan for vocational rehabilitation every three years. Expressing the state's commitment to the requirements of the Rehabilitation Act, the plan serves as a major reference point for the Rehabilitation Services Administration (RSA) in monitoring the performance of the state related to client goals, program operation, and delivery of services. The major areas of monitoring are state plan compliance, eligibility, and internal fiscal controls. RSA uses two basic systems in this monitoring process: the State Plan Assurance Review (SPARS) and the Case Review System (CRS). Data regarding the total number of persons served, number of persons listed as rehabilitated, characteristics, and the time and resources used by the states are collated in the Rehabilitation Services Administration annual report to Congress and the president.

Outcome Evaluation. A goal-attainment model of evaluation is commonly used in rehabilitation to measure client progress. It is also well suited to assess program performance. Daniel W. Cook and Paul G. Cooper (1979) indicated that the logic behind this approach is readily apparent: The program is evaluated in terms of its effectiveness in meeting predetermined objectives. For all practical purposes, goal-attainment evaluation uses the ex post facto research design. This model focuses on the measurement of outcomes rather than inputs. Therefore, the emphasis is placed on clarification of program goals and objectives, and the evaluation of their accomplishment.

One way of classifying evaluation is by purpose. Evaluations may be conducted to make decisions about matters such as program changes, resources allocation, measuring accountability, and capacity-building. The goal attainment model seems especially well suited for capacity-building in that it facilitates the development of a database, improves the agency's ability to collect and assemble outcome data, and provides rapid feedback in regard to problems requiring technical assistance.

A goal-oriented management approach often used for planning and evaluating program goals and objectives is referred to as management by objective (MBO). The MBO approach is a results-oriented planning tool that originated in business but that has been adapted to human service settings. MBO as a management approach is best implemented throughout all levels of an organization, providing feedback to staff on their progress toward negotiated goals. MBO statements typically include time frames for completing each desired outcome (goal) and consist of the following information:

- mission—general philosophy and direction, which serves as a reference point for all organizational activities;
- goals—broad statements of accomplishment that contribute to the mission;
- objectives—specific operational procedures for attaining each identified goal;
- plan—activities and tasks undertaken to carry out each objective;
- performance review—informal checkpoints and formal evaluation procedures to assess progress toward carrying out objectives.

Cost-Benefit Analysis. Like other human service programs, rehabilitation programs are faced with the question of whether society is better off with the program than without it. In other words, do the total benefits outweigh the total costs? This type of question has become more significant because funding is becoming scarce and subject to more political scrutiny.

One attempt to demonstrate the fiscal worth of rehabilitation programs is cost-benefit analysis. Essentially, cost-benefit analysis has been used as a technique for evaluating policy options related to the allocation of resources between or among alternative programs. The intent is to consider all costs and benefits to obtain the best decision. Generally, costs as well as benefits are given a dollar value over time, and benefit over cost ratios are calculated. A ratio higher than 1 indicates the worth of the investment decision. As the ratio increases beyond 1, the value or worth of the program benefit increases.

While using dollar figures for rehabilitation benefits or costs is logical and economically useful, the cost-benefit analysis is not a perfect evaluation method. Placing a dollar figure on rehabilitation costs is in many cases much easier than placing a dollar figure on the benefits arising from a project. Problems arise when attempting to define what costs are and what benefits are in terms that are comparable. Costs are defined in economic terms, while benefits can be defined in economic, psychological, or social terms. Benefits are much more intangible and difficult to reduce to economic terms. Typical direct costs include medical costs, training, maintenance costs, or any case services that help individuals in a rehabilitation program. Indirect costs include staff salaries and building rent. Typical benefits to the individual with disabilities arise from increases in earnings, increased productivity, increased satisfaction with life, or less dependency on government aid.

Client Satisfaction Evaluation

In the past, the concept of normalization has been the philosophical and ideological cornerstone of human service programs. Normalization provided the impetus for the movement of hundreds of thousands of people from large, segregated facilities into community-based programs. In the late 1980s and early 1990s consumer empowerment became the driving force behind the development, implementation, and evaluation of human service programs. Program success is now being evaluated not only quantitatively but also qualitatively, through use of client satisfaction evaluation. Client satisfaction can be measured in a variety of ways. For example, individual satisfaction questionnaires and consumer monitoring systems are being used more often. The primary purpose is to ensure that services are responsive to the people who need them. At the agency level, responsiveness to the people receiving services can provide the opportunity to make program improvements. At the state or federal level, the results of consumer responses can help shape policy issues.

Client satisfaction is usually assessed by asking clients questions related to specific elements of the rehabilitation program. Instead of relying on closed-ended questions, such as those requiring a "yes" or a "no" response, the evaluator usually requests that clients indicate their degree of satisfaction with each area of service. Client satisfaction evaluation represents an inexpensive measure of the consumer perspective that could be used to validate or improve programs, predict consumer outcomes, improve public relations, and even facilitate program survival.

Evaluation Standards and Accreditation

The Rehabilitation Act of 1973 mandated development of program evaluation standards for the vocational rehabilitation (VR) program nationwide. The legislation called for development of a set of standards by which the impact of rehabilitation services could be assessed. The act emphasized the need for accountability of vocational rehabilitation programs. Nine "evaluation standards" were established as criteria for the evaluation of program effectiveness, to increase program accountability, and to encourage state VR agencies to begin a more comprehensive evaluation of their programs (*Federal Register*, 1974). The following nine program evaluation standards were developed:

- "to serve the target population equitably";
- "to place clients in relevant gainful employment";
- "to avoid undue delays in process";
- "to use resources efficiently";
- "to ensure manageable caseloads for counselors";
- "to ensure retention of the benefits achieved through rehabilitation";
- "to provide needed postemployment benefits";
- "to identify why clients are not successfully rehabilitated";
- "to ensure client participation with the written rehabilitation plan."

Since the development of these standards, attempts have been made to refine and improve them. By 1994, no changes had been made, nor had any other formalized comprehensive program evaluation system been developed. However, states are required to provide the Rehabilitation Services Administration (RSA) with statistical data on a regular basis. This reporting is followed by feedback and advice based on interstate comparisons. An emphasis on the "twenty-six" case closure criterion continues to play a significant role in these evaluations (Simon, 1989). The status "twenty-six" closure has been defined as a client placed in competitive employment for sixty days. Data related to this criterion can easily be gathered and analyzed. Unfortunately, a single criterion cannot be expected to provide answers readily to questions related to quality of client gains. Richard T. Walls and M. S. Tseng (1987) emphasized this growing concern for the need to develop outcome criteria that will more adequately represent client accomplishment. This increased concern continues to emerge as vocational rehabilitation begins to work more frequently with people with severe disabilities.

The Commission on Accreditation of Rehabilitation Facilities (CARF) is another organization with a major interest in program evaluation. CARF has published a set of guidelines for installing program evaluation in organizations serving people with disabilities, including standards for such systems. CARF surveys and accredits rehabilitation programs. It was formed in 1966 as a national, private, nonprofit organization to carry out the function of a quality control intermediary. CARF established and continues to refine a list of standards that are used by programs for self-evaluation and accreditation purposes.

According to CARF (1992), the organization's program evaluation system or systems should enable it to identify the results of services and the effects of the programs on the persons served. It is emphasized that program evaluation should measure outcomes following the delivery of services. For persons who are in programs for six months or longer, program evaluation should be used to measure progress in relation to overall program goals. CARF continually stresses that program evaluation information should be integrated into the organization's decision-making at all levels.

The CARF standards are meant to establish the expectations in regard to development, implementation, and utilization of a program evaluation system. However, the standards are not intended to provide a detailed guidance of a "how to do it" (CARF, 1991). Each program is expected to seek its own expertise.

Future Considerations

Given the resource requirements and time and energy commitments necessary, it must be asked whether an evaluation of rehabilitation services or programs will produce enough useful information to make it worth the investment of funds and staff time. The answer to this question will depend on whether the agency or program administrator and staff have learned to value and use evaluation information in their decision-making. It is clear that if evaluation is to become a useful management tool in rehabilitation, it must be seen in a more positive way. The demand for accountability and evaluation of rehabilitation services will continue to grow. Yet, program administrators are not generally enthusiastic about evaluation, since they may perceive it as an externally imposed requirement for which there is neither adequate preparation nor sufficient funding. Some administrators also think it is useless because it is insensitive to their programs' complexities, goals, work demand, and client characteristics (Schaloch & Harper, 1983). Staff are equally fearful about evaluation. Many fear that evaluation results will only be used against them rather than to help them perform their jobs.

For rehabilitation programs to continue to survive and improve in the twenty-first century, evaluation must become a higher priority and less of a burden. Evaluation must be seen as an ongoing process that relates directly to agency planning and implementation. Steven E. Simon (1989) suggested that evaluation that is designed to be an ongoing part of agency management and that is incorporated in organization development efforts should be effective in assuring the utilization of evaluation practices. This concept should allow the agency/program management cycle to operate according to its intent by encouraging continuous review and readjustment of programs. When program evaluation is clearly made part of the total agency management process, including integration into the performance evaluation system, utilization becomes a priority. Such an approach requires the involvement of all staff, especially top management. This approach should eliminate some threat and place all staff members in the best position for effective decision-making and control.

Training of current and future rehabilitation professionals in the areas of evaluation would appear to be a wise investment. Both preprofessional and in-service educational offerings should provide training opportunities in administration or management practices (e.g., planning and evaluation). Far too often, clinicians are moved into administrative positions with little or no training. They were trained to be clinicians, not administrators, program planners, or evaluators.

Another consideration relates to technology. In this age of abundant information, data collection and data reporting can be major burdens. As suggested by Charles V. Arokiasamy and others (1992), establishment of program evaluation systems has generally been labor- and time-intensive. They pointed out that computers can greatly ease these efforts. Establishing a program evaluation system includes data collection, data management, and data reporting. Computers and software are increasingly becoming more powerful and easier to use. Regardless of the agency size, great benefits can be realized by using computer systems for program evaluation.

Finally, this discussion in regard to evaluation must conclude with a focus on planning. The management cycle consists of program planning, implementation, and evaluation. While the need for quality evaluations is emphasized, it cannot be done without establishment of concrete objectives. It seems that rehabilitation programs, like many other human service programs, rarely have well-specified goals and objectives. While goals and objectives may exist, individuals may have only an intuitive feeling for why programs exist, what they are trying to accomplish, and how well they are doing (Spaniol, 1975). It is critical to develop clear and concrete goals and objectives. It is also critical that these directions should be developed via participatory management. One should encourage participation, openness, and active and constant communication throughout the ongoing planning, implementation, and evaluation process. Rehabilitation managers, staff, and consumers all have important roles to play in developing more effective and efficient rehabilitation services.

(See also: MANAGEMENT; RESEARCH, REHABILITATION; STATE–FEDERAL REHABILITATION PROGRAM)

BIBLIOGRAPHY

AROKIASAMY, CHARLES V.; BENSHOFF, JOHN J.; MCLEAN, LINDA S.; and MOSS, GREGORY L. "Computer Application in Program Evaluation: Basic Guidelines." *Journal of Rehabilitation Administration* 16 (1992):5–12.

BOSCHEN, KATHRYN A. "Issues in Evaluating Vocational Rehabilitation Programs." *Rehabilitation Psychology* 29 (1984):37–48.

COMMISSION ON ACCREDITATION OF REHABILITATION FACILITIES (CARF). *Program Evaluation: A First Step.* Tucson, AZ, 1991.

———. *Standards Manual for Organizations Serving People with Disabilities.* 1992 ed. Tucson, AZ, 1992.

COOK, DANIEL W., and COOPER, PAUL G. *Rehabilitation Counseling Research.* Baltimore, 1979.

Federal Register 39 (1974). Special issue on standards.

GARSKE, GREGORY G.; TRACH, JOHN S.; and LEUNG, PAUL. "Evaluation and the State/Federal Vocational Rehabilitation Program." *Journal of Vocational Rehabilitation* 2 (1992):9–16.

POSAVEC, EMIL J., and CAREY, RAYMOND G. *Program Evaluation: Methods and Case Studies,* 2nd ed. Englewood Cliffs, NJ, 1985.

REGION V STUDY GROUP. *Rehabilitation Needs Assessment for Vocational Rehabilitation Agencies,* Vol. 1, A *Guide to Needs in Rehabilitation Agency Planning.* Chicago, 1991.

SCHALOCK, ROBERT L., and HARPER, ROGER S. "Untying Some Gordian Knots in Program Evaluation." *Journal of Rehabilitation Administration* (1983): 12–19.

SCRIVEN, M. "The Methodology of Evaluation." In *Perspectives Curriculum Evaluation,* ed. Robert E. Stake. Chicago, IL, 1967.

SIMON, STEVEN E. *A Guidebook to Rehabilitation and Human Services Management: Fine-Tuning for Excellence.* Springfield, IL, 1989.

SPANIOL, LE ROY. *Program Evaluation Models for Rehabilitation: A Review of the Literature.* Madison, WI, 1975.

———. "A Program Evaluation Model for Rehabilitation Agencies and Facilities." In *Readings in Rehabilitation Administration,* ed. Ted F. Riggar and J. R. Lorenz. Albany, NY, 1985.

WALLS, RICHARD T., and TSENG, M. S. "Measurement of Client Outcomes in Rehabilitation." In *Handbook of Measurement and Evaluation in Rehabilitation,* 2nd ed, ed. Brian Bolton. Fayetteville, AR, 1987.

WRIGHT, GEORGE N. *Total Rehabilitation.* Boston, MA, 1980.

GREGORY G. GARSKE

EXERCISE

See CORONARY ARTERY DISEASE; RECREATION; WELLNESS

EXPERT WITNESS

See FORENSIC REHABILITATION

F

FACILITIES

The advent of rehabilitation services during the twentieth century required a corresponding creation and growth of facilities staffed and designed to deliver these services. Rehabilitation facilities have steadily grown and adapted to the continuing development of new rehabilitation technology and to public demands for greater individual personal freedom. State and federal regulations and laws also have influenced the operation and design of rehabilitation facilities. The range of facilities represents a varied industry and encompasses medical, vocational, and community services, all of which strive to restore persons with disabilities to their highest possible level of physical, psychological, social, vocational, recreational, and economic functioning. Additionally, some rehabilitation services are provided in facilities without walls—specifically those services that enhance an individual's personal freedom through home and community-based programs.

The diverse field of rehabilitation can be subdivided into three major subgroups, with the recognition that there is an interplay and mutuality of goals.

Those subgroups are medical, vocational, and residential/community.

Medical Rehabilitation

Medical rehabilitation represents an essential component of the health care continuum. These services are directed at minimizing physical, intellectual, and social consequences of disease, illness, injury, aging, and congenital conditions. The most common health conditions associated with medical rehabilitation include stroke, spinal cord injury, brain injury, orthopedic disorders, arthritis, amputation, back/neck pain, respiratory dysfunction, cardiac/pulmonary dysfunction, neurologic conditions, and cancer.

The primary goals of medical rehabilitation services are to maximize functional ability, restore or enhance vocational capabilities, improve quality of life, and prevent or reduce the need for costly long-term care or institutionalization.

The settings, or facilities, in which rehabilitation services are delivered have changed significantly since the emergence of medical rehabilitation in postwar America. The reconstructive care offered

317

wounded veterans of World War II focused on physical and occupational therapy in not-for-profit hospitals and a small number of freestanding rehabilitation hospitals.

Most commonly the first phase of medical rehabilitative care is provided to patients who arrive at acute care hospitals, general medical/surgical wards, trauma centers, and intensive care units for treatment of serious illness or injury. In a comprehensive acute rehabilitation inpatient setting, rehabilitative care is comprised of a number of medical specialties and allied health disciplines under the direction of a physician trained or qualified in physical medicine and rehabilitation. With this type of rehabilitative care, the focus is on recovery. In most cases, the facilities providing initial, intense rehabilitation services are freestanding rehabilitation hospitals or rehabilitation units in acute care hospitals. During the 1980s, the United States witnessed a rapid growth in the number of rehabilitation hospitals and rehabilitation units. According to the Health Care Financing Administration (HCFA), between 1985 and 1989 the number of rehabilitation hospitals increased approximately 84 percent; units increased by about 66 percent. By 1993 there were 169 freestanding rehabilitation hospitals with 19,286 beds in the United States.

Patients who enter rehabilitation hospitals or units come from short-term acute care hospitals, general medical/surgical wards, trauma centers, and/or intensive care units. These rehabilitation facilities are for patients who are still medically fragile, have severe functional impairments, and need the support of a medical facility. However, these patients have the potential for improving functional abilities at regular intervals. Freestanding rehabilitation hospitals and rehab units are accredited by the Commission on Accreditation of Rehabilitation Facilities (CARF), by the Joint Commission on Accreditation of Healthcare Organizations, and/or by the American Osteopathic Association. The standards and regulations that are required before accreditation occurs are: to provide close medical supervision; to have physicians available on a twenty-four-hour basis; and to have twenty-four-hour availability of registered nurses with specialized training and experience in rehab. The therapies required to be available and given

include physical, occupational, speech, and other daily therapies.

The outcome from these hospitals and units is improvement for the patient measured against her or his condition at admission. As improvements continue and realistic goals are reached, decisions about the patient's future are made, whether that be a move home with outpatient rehabilitation, or into a facility such as a skilled nursing facility.

Freestanding hospitals and units are at the beginning of the rehabilitation continuum. The next step across this continuum is for people with more severe disabilities who need longer but less intense care in facilities known as skilled nursing facilities (SNF). Patients entering skilled nursing facilities come from freestanding rehab hospitals and rehab units. In these facilities patients may stay longer but care may be less intense. An SNF has the staff and equipment to provide skilled nursing care and skilled rehabilitation services; within the rehab services they provide physical therapy, occupational therapy, and speech pathology therapy. SNFs may provide a comprehensive level of medical rehabilitation. Skilled nursing facilities are certified through Medicare. To obtain certification the facility must establish and meet minimum health and safety standards. Section 1819 of the law governing Medicare defines and identifies the requirements for SNFs. By 1993, 54 percent of all nursing homes in the United States were certified as skilled nursing facilities. While at an SNF evaluations are made to determine where the patient goes from there. The stay may be extended at the SNF; one can be sent back to a rehabilitation hospital or unit; or the patient may be sent home, to continue rehabilitation at an outpatient rehabilitation center.

Another option for patients and doctors is a long-term-care hospital. In 1993 there were 102 long-term-care hospitals, with 16,876 beds, in the United States. These are widely diverse institutions; one-third of all long-term-care hospitals are termed chronic disease hospitals (for patients seriously or terminally ill); the other two thirds of the hospitals include rehabilitation, psychiatric, pulmonary disease, and other specialty units within the hospitals. Many factors are involved in making a hospital a long-term-care hospital, the main factor being the length of stay of a patient. Medicare also has special standards for long-term hospitals, and they are excluded from the Medicare PPS (prospective payment system) if the hospital qualifies as a Medicare long-term-care hospital.

As in skilled nursing facilities, many patients may stay at a long-term-care hospital, are released to have outpatient rehabilitation at home, or are sent to an SNF. Once a patient is sent home, there are comprehensive outpatient rehabilitation facilities (CORFs), where they can continue the rehabilitation process. By definition a CORF is a facility primarily engaged in providing (by or under the supervision of physicians) diagnostic, therapeutic, and restorative services for the rehabilitation of persons with injury, disability, or sickness. CORFs provide services to people who periodically require a physiatrist or qualified rehab physician's attention. These services are comprehensive and are designed to help those who have not yet realized the goals of their rehab program. Patients at a CORF come from their homes or other residential settings. A person may need only one service a CORF provides; others may require all of the facility's services.

Standards and certification for a comprehensive outpatient rehabilitation facility are described in Section 1861(cc) of the law governing Medicare, although some states require separate and additional licensing for CORFs. The services a facility may provide, as stated by Medicare, include physicians' services, physical therapy, occupational therapy, speech pathology, and respiratory therapy. The facility may also provide prosthetic and orthotic devices, including testing, fitting, or training in the use of these devices; social and psychological services; nursing care provided by or under the supervision of a registered professional nurse; drugs and biologicals that cannot be self-administered; supplies and durable medical equipment; and any other items necessary for the rehabilitation of a patient. Outpatient departments of acute general or rehabilitation hospitals and outpatient rehabilitation centers also are sites for the provision of rehabilitation services. Often, rehabilitation at these facilities is a single service, such as physical therapy or occupational therapy, rather than a comprehensive treatment. The appropriate facility for any given patient is dependent on clinical, vocational, and residential factors, including the severity of the disabling con-

dition, the level of care required, the intensity of care needed, the support systems available to the patient, and insurance considerations.

Vocational Rehabilitation

Vocational rehabilitation facilities were developed in the United States to maintain a productive workforce. Training for employment and providing appropriate job placement were components of the vocational programs offered to employees injured on the job and veterans with disabilities. Additionally, vocational facilities often served as employers. Transitional employment leading to permanent job placement, and long-term employment for people with severe disabilities were made available through "workshop" settings. Much like medical rehabilitation, the field of vocational rehabilitation has expanded its range of services and broadened its clientele base to meet corresponding social trends.

Within the field of vocational rehabilitation there exists a difference of opinion on terminology in regard to facilities. Community Rehabilitation Programs (CRPs) offer a variety of employment and pre-employment services to individuals with a wide range of disabilities, including sheltered work, supported employment, work activities, and individual supported placements. Sheltered work provides paid employment and educational and therapeutic programs for workers with disabilities. In most cases, employment is transitional, leading to job placement. "Sheltered" implies that people with disabilities are protected from some of the aspects of commercial enterprise, while at the same time having the opportunity to build job skills and experience the atmosphere of the work environment. A work activity center (or rehab center) offers employment for workers with severe physical or mental impairments. Productivity is less important than the therapeutic activities offered in a work activity setting; transition to outside employment is not considered a viable alternative for many. Work activity centers are different from sheltered workshops. Sheltered workshops offer people with significant disabilities the training and experience that enable many to develop productive work skills, while work activity is primarily designed with therapeutic goals in mind. The workplace itself becomes a facility in the most recent of vocational rehabilitation trends. Supported employment is a form of vocational rehabilitation that takes place on-site, with a job coach provided by a rehab facility. Individuals with disabilities are integrated into the community workforce, work in competitive situations at wages that meet federal fair labor standards, and are supported with ongoing vocational and related services from their job coach.

Vocational rehabilitation programs offer diverse and comprehensive services to individuals with disabilities: career exploration, skill and potential assessment, advice and counseling on job selection, independent living skills development, training in prevocational skills, training for particular jobs, assistance in finding a job, and support once hired. These programs also provide employers with a range of services: identifying qualified applicants; conducting job analyses; suggesting ways in which a job may be restructured; assistance with employees injured on the job who are returning to work; identifying reasonable accommodations that enable particular individuals with disabilities to perform job functions; providing transitional and long-term support to individuals hired who have severe disabilities; and training other employees to work effectively with employees with disabilities.

Funding for community-based rehabilitation programs comes from several state and federal sources. Some funding is obtained through the Rehabilitation Act, the Developmental Disabilities Act, and the Job Training Partnership Act. Other funding comes from state and federal procurement programs that contract with community vocational rehabilitation programs to provide a service or to develop a product. To be eligible for these preferential contract opportunities, community programs must have a workforce whose composition is 75 percent individuals with disabilities. Finally, these community programs receive funding for federal projects to reach and serve special populations: minority individuals with disabilities, and individuals who are HIV positive or who have AIDS. Individuals may access assistance from community vocational rehabilitation programs directly, but usually they are referred by a state vocational rehabilitation agency office, another organization or agency, or a school. Nonetheless, once accepted for assistance, regardless of the refer-

ral source, public funds usually finance the services offered to an individual.

Just as community vocational rehabilitation programs offer a range of services, they also have the capacity to provide or to assist in securing a wide array of jobs in service industries and technical fields, white-collar and blue-collar. The size of a community and its local labor market will, of course, influence the number and nature of job-related experiences, training, and employment assistance a community vocational rehabilitation program is able to provide individuals with disabilities. With continuing interest in consolidating federal training and employment programs, community vocational rehabilitation programs will have expanded opportunities to offer their skills and expertise in assisting unemployed persons who do not have a disability to prepare for and obtain employment.

Residential/Community Rehabilitation

A national move began in the 1970s toward deinstitutionalization and led to a correlated advent and rise in the numbers of smaller residential settings for those with disabilities. Group homes are one example of this move; residences can be transitional as well as long-term. Other examples include supported living where persons with disabilities live individually or with roommates of their choice and have drop-in assistance to help with activities of daily living or instrumental activities of daily living, and assisted living where individuals with disabilities live in a communal environment that provides assistance to the residents. Community supports are any services or devices of a nonacute medical nature that enable an individual with physical, cognitive, mental, or sensory disabilities to live and function as independently as possible at home, at work, and/or in the community. Community-based services have become the predominant service delivery model for persons with disabilities since the early 1970s, with residential components as the cornerstone of the service delivery system. Supported employment and vocational supports that are brokered by rehabilitation providers are widely used. In both instances, providers have had to adjust from providing direct services in a separate, carefully controlled setting, to providing an array of services throughout the community.

In adapting to a community service model, rehabilitation providers have restructured their services; created new partnerships with business, family, consumers, and other funding agencies; restructured supervisory and administrative responsibilities; and retrained staff or hired new staff with skills and attitudes that encourage independence, freedom, and competence. Rehabilitation providers have also reallocated, relocated, or changed space use from large, separate facilities in which individuals lived or were trained for work, to smaller sites in integrated community settings. In so doing, rehabilitation providers have sometimes transitioned from being landlords and managing entire training operations or housing services, to providing services at sites owned or operated by others, a type of facility without walls.

The Americans with Disabilities Act of 1990 and its subsequent amendments have enlarged the potential for community supports as the United States moves toward greater equality for all citizens. This trend will continue to affect the way in which rehabilitation facilities are constituted. As barriers are removed for people with disabilities, rehabilitation facilities will increasingly move toward models integrated more fully into the community.

(See also: ALLIED HEALTH PROFESSIONS; CREDENTIALS; DEINSTITUTIONALIZATION; HOSPITAL, REHABILITATION; NURSING, REHABILITATION; REHABILITATION CENTER)

BIBLIOGRAPHY

AMERICAN REHABILITATION ASSOCIATION. Medical Rehabilitation Cost-Effectiveness, Cost Benefits and Outcome Studies: A Resource Guide. Reston, VA, 1994.
———. The American Rehab Guide to Assistive Technology. Reston, VA, 1994.
———. The Cost-Effectiveness and Cost Benefits of Rehabilitation. Reston, VA, 1994.
———. Trends in Medical Rehabilitation. Reston, VA, 1994.
———. Vocational Program Administrator's Handbook. Reston, VA, 1994.
———. General Facilities Survey. Reston, VA, 1993.
———. Survey of Industrial Rehabilitation Programs. Reston, VA, 1993.
———. CORFs: Who They Are and What They Do. Reston, VA, 1992.
———. National Scope Supported Employment Demonstration Project: Final Report. Reston, VA, 1991.
———. ADA Manual: Americans with Disabilities Act. Reston, VA, 1990.
———. Supported Employment Resource Guide. Reston, VA, 1990.
———. The Payers of Medical Rehabilitation: Eligibility, Coverage and Payment Policies. Reston, VA, 1989.
———. Medical Rehabilitation: What It Is and Where It Is—A Discussion. Reston, VA, 1988.
———. Statement of Principles Regarding Provision of Services to Patients in Medical Rehabilitation Hospitals and Units. Reston, VA, 1986.
———. Code of Ethics: Vocational Rehabilitation Facilities. Reston, VA, 1981.
KIERNAN, WILLIAM, and STARK, JACK, eds. Pathways to Employment for Adults with Developmental Disabilities. Baltimore, 1986.

CAROLYN ZOLLAR
PAT MORISSEY
KAREN O'DONNELL

FAMILY

The family has emerged as an important resource in the disability management and rehabilitation process. Traditional rehabilitation practice has focused almost exclusively on the individuals with disabilities themselves, while their families were infrequent partners. However, an expanded definition of disability emphasizes the resources of the familial environment and focuses on how the family can be of assistance throughout the disability experience and rehabilitation process. This entry will present an overview of the impact of illness and disability on the family, a discussion of the responses of the health care and rehabilitation systems to the family, and an explanation of the ways in which the rehabilitation system can facilitate rehabilitation goals.

Impact of Disability on the Family

To understand the impact of disability on the family, consideration must be given to the many determinants that can shape the family's response to major life losses. These include the family's prior experience with crises as well as the nature of the illness or disability and whether its onset was sudden or gradual, expected or unexpected. Other determinants of disability impact are cultural values, religion, coping options, and social supports available to the family. Also to be considered are the previous educational experiences of family members, and any prior interaction with health care and rehabilitation professionals (Power, 1991).

To these factors John Rolland (1987) has added three key variables that can also influence the family's response to an illness or disability. These variables, which form part of the family illness belief system, are (1) the family's beliefs about the cause of an illness or disability; (2) the family's multigenerational, evolutionary process with illness, loss, and crisis; and (3) the family's sense of mastery and control over the course of an illness. All of these elements not only can contribute to the impact of disability on the family but also can suggest whether the family can become a valuable resource or support system during the family member's treatment and rehabilitation process.

A number of theories attempt to explain the impact of trauma on family members in terms of specific but different stages (Power, 1991; Power, Dell Orto, & Gibbons, 1988; Reagles, 1982). Each stage has certain characteristics, which are determined by family priorities, composition, dynamics, and goals (Reagles, 1982). Sequential themes that are evident in most stage theories, however, are shock, denial, anxiety, fear, search for meaning, and eventually the reorientation of family life to the illness or disability event. In a family there may be varied reactions from individual family members. This variation limits the generalizability of stage theories to understanding how other families are dealing with even a similar trauma. Also, an illness or disability whose course of treatment, rehabilitation, and eventual recovery is predictable may generate a different reaction from family members than an illness or disability that has an uncertain process and outcome.

Another way to conceptualize the family's reactions to a trauma is to identify different emotions and coping mechanisms expressed by family members that may occur not in stages but at any time during the family member's treatment and rehabilitation. These emotions and coping styles may subside and then recur unexpectedly. Many emotions and behaviors of family members, such as anger, loss

of hope, and excessive alcohol or substance abuse, often can be seen as manifestations of individual coping styles. Coping strategies are efforts to manage stressful demands, and within a family, they may shift as the medical or rehabilitation status of the person changes. Family members may rely more heavily at certain times on one form of coping, for example, defensive strategies, and at other times on other forms, such as problem-solving strategies. Examples of problem-solving strategies are information-seeking, taking direct action, turning to others for help, a redefinition of the situation, and tension reduction techniques. In understanding family reactions as different emotions, behaviors, and coping styles, the family itself is viewed as a kaleidoscope producing at different times varied strategy patterns to deal with a trauma. The pattern itself can change as the disability situation changes.

A third way to understand a family's response to disability is in the context of definite time frames occurring from onset of the trauma throughout the course of treatment and rehabilitation. Each time frame can provoke definite emotions and adaptive tasks from family members. These time frames can be called "trigger" points, periods in which family members may be especially vulnerable to excessive stress and yet times when a series of tasks may have to be negotiated by them (Caroff & Mailick, 1985; Power, 1991). These trigger points are diagnosis, hospital treatment, discharge, and outpatient status (see Table 1, p. 323).

Understanding the family's reaction to a disability experience requires that rehabilitation personnel recognize that family behaviors are dynamic processes that may emerge, continue, and then wane over a course of time. From their extensive research with families, Sandra Gonzalez, Peter Steinglass, and David Reiss (1989) report that families are often reluctant to change their ways of handling disability, having developed a routine way of responding to the trauma during early or acute phases. Often family members are well aware of feelings of resentment, disappointment, anger, guilt, and helplessness regarding an illness or disability, and they can experience these feelings as unacceptable in light of the person's medical condition. These researchers also believe that families coping with a

Table 1. Times of family vulnerability to stress and necessary adaptive tasks

Trigger Points	Emotions	Adaptive Tasks
Diagnosis/beginning of treatment or rehabilitation	Shock; anger; intense anxiety; grief; guilt	Seek support; share feelings; neutralize environmental conditions; maintain family emotional equilibrium and family functions
Course of hospital treatment or rehabilitation	Grief; denial; anxiety; search for meaning	Seek understanding; communicate with health professionals; identify and develop coping mechanisms; recognize and organize personal and community resources; attempt to regulate one's feelings and actions
Discharge from the hospital and return to available family	Sadness; hope; anxiety over the future	Process information; recognize potential problems; respond to own family needs; avoid caregiver burnout; provide physical, emotional, and social support; accept responsibility; engage in planning and problem-solving
Outpatient status and continuation of treatment/rehabilitation	Anxiety; relief; lingering grief; expectations for the future	Reemphasize treatment-related information; involve returning family member in family life and responsibilities; help returning family member come to terms with perceived losses; facilitate positive reappraisal

SOURCE: Caroff and Mailick (1985), Power (1991)

chronic medical condition are often unable to find time for another disability-related activity, such as meeting with a family counselor or attending group meetings dealing with family adjustment issues. Effective intervention methods, consequently, are based on understanding all these behaviors, emotions, and accruing family needs.

To understand family reactions to illness and disability better, it is important that any perspective also conveys the reality that families are confronted with constraints against using coping resources or experiencing positive emotions leading to effective disability and family management. These constraints may be personal, such as internalized cultural values and beliefs that proscribe certain types of action or feeling, and personal agendas (e.g., fear of failure or unfinished business), or environmental (e.g., lack of available resources or negative, stereotypic attitudes from health professionals).

All of this information on family responses provides further knowledge about which responses facilitate the family's ability to cope and which do not. When family members attempt to normalize family life, change their own individual role expectations without making radical, external changes in their own environment (such as work and social activities), and renegotiate the role expectations that may be imposed by the implications of living with a disability (Hall, 1972), then the family itself can develop effective ways to deal with the illness or disability situation. The presence of these factors can also provide the impetus for both the utilization of community-based support systems and the pursuit of individual activities that bring personal satisfaction and relief to a demanding situation. On the other hand, if individual family members harbor their own grief, guilt, and anger and project these emotions in a negative manner onto each other and rehabilitation workers, or deny the family implications of the trauma, such as role reallocations and necessary changes in many family routines, then the family may never adjust to the disability experience. Refusal to accept some responsibility for caregiving duties or to acknowledge one's role in working toward family adjustment may also precipitate dysfunctional coping responses (Dell Orto & Power, 1994).

Responses of Health Care Providers to the Family

Fortunately, consensus has grown on the importance of family involvement in the rehabilitation process (Kelley & Lambert, 1992), but this perception has not been translated into steady, increased intervention efforts by rehabilitation and health care professionals. Attention to family concerns by health professionals has been generally uncoordinated and episodic. There are several reasons for this lack of familial consideration, such as the traditional, exclusive focus on the person with a disability, without consideration of the familial context in which a person lives; the lack of focus on the family in the training of rehabilitation and health care professionals; and the limited enforcement of rehabilitation policy that includes the provision of family services.

Until the middle 1980s, the definition of disability exclusively embraced the mental and physical limitations of the individual experiencing the disability. Disability was viewed primarily as a physiological deficit. Treatment efforts relied solely on person-centered approaches, and there was little attention to the interaction between individuals with disabilities and their immediate, available environments. How the family could be of valuable assistance during both treatment and rehabilitation was not given priority consideration. The implication was that the person with a disability was solely responsible for remedial efforts.

Similarly, the traditional training of rehabilitation and health care workers has followed curriculum guidelines mandated by respective accrediting organizations. Unfortunately, this curriculum has rarely included a family course that would enable students to provide meaningful support to families during the treatment and rehabilitation process. In fact, continuing education efforts sponsored by many professional organizations seldom include a family course.

Regarding policy development, the Rehabilitation Act of 1973, as amended, continued the authority for provision of services to family members as necessary to the adjustment or rehabilitation of persons with disabilities. However, these mandates have not become standard practice in every area of health care, treatment, and rehabilitation. Working with clients' families may not always be encouraged, and when it does occur, it is often a result of individual initiative and creative case-management techniques.

Often these factors have resulted in a lack of continued awareness of how a person's family can be a vital contributor to the accomplishment of rehabilitation goals. A characterization of many health care, rehabilitation, and human service responses to family needs and opportunities for involvement in the rehabilitation process can be expressed by the phrase "benign inattention but periodic intervention." Many professionals have not been aware of how the family is a vital component to rehabilitation efforts, and when efforts are attempted, they are usually periodic and regarded as incidental to the client's welfare.

The Rehabilitation System's Facilitative Response

Several trends have provoked renewed interest in and recognition of the essential role played by families during an individual's rehabilitation. These include the increased emergence of the independent living and client advocacy movements (Kelley & Lambert, 1992). During the 1980s, grass-roots groups of people with disabilities organized along single and cross-disability lines, forming statewide and national membership coalitions. These people worked along with parents of children with disabilities and with non-disabled advocates to urge for laws guaranteeing the right of access to education and employment. Health crises such as the growing incidence of people with HIV/AIDS and the large number of people with physical disabilities or living with Alzheimer's disease or psychiatric illness have contributed to the recognition of the importance of family involvement. The issue of client empowerment, which is finding its way into rehabilitation policy, will also stimulate additional attention to the family (Kelley & Lambert, 1992).

The prevalence of these crises and growing rehabilitation consumer advocacy and empowerment have challenged the health care and rehabilitation system to find cost-effective ways to deliver effective and comprehensive services. Cost-effectiveness calls for better coordination among all health care and rehabilitation professionals, creative case-management practices, and the utilization of all available resources for the individual's rehabilitation. To accomplish these goals requires a redefinition of the rehabilitation provider's role, a rethinking of the standard training curriculum for rehabilitation professionals, earlier intervention in the rehabilitation process by rehabilitation workers, and the implementation of a family-focused rehabilitation policy.

A redefinition of the rehabilitation worker's role implies that health care and rehabilitation workers develop a proactive approach to disability management rather than responding a long time after the onset of disability. Through a proactive approach, rehabilitation personnel can make contact with individuals and their families during in-hospital treatment. The establishment of an early client-family relationship can facilitate an ongoing working relationship that is essential during long-term treatment and rehabilitation.

Also, if the health care and rehabilitation system is to become more responsive to the family, then policymakers need to be aware of the family's changing and emerging needs. In the past, when consumer needs have been well articulated and promoted through strong advocacy efforts, change has become a reality, or at least a strong possibility. Consumer needs are often best expressed and promoted by consumer groups as well as national and state organizations and resources. Many of these organizations focus on a specific disability, such as head injury, mental retardation, mental illness, or multiple sclerosis (Dell Orto & Power, 1994).

The federal government has placed an emphasis on family support by establishing in the early 1980s a research and training center on families and disability. In 1992 this center, called the Beach Center on Family and Disability, was located at the University of Kansas. The center is engaged in such projects as family empowerment, family connection networks, family support coalitions, and the dissemination of rehabilitation literature related to family coping with disability and employment of people with disabilities. Researchers at the Beach Center

have also surveyed state disability laws and developed a model Disability and Family Support Act. Many states have adopted family support statutes that include the essential characteristics of the model, namely, a statement of family-oriented principles and goals, authorization of the program and assignment to a specific department, explanation of the type of services offered, a mandate for family participation at all levels of program policy making, and permanent budget authorization. As states adopt family support laws, they build on the model statute by ensuring that sufficient funding is available for family support programs (Turnbull, 1992).

How sufficient funding within states for family support programs can be ensured is one of many controversial issues regarding the family and rehabilitation. Laws that have been enacted in many states seek to expand the money available for these programs by supplementing, not supplanting, other state family benefits. But states face fiscal shortfalls and tremendous demands for no new taxes. Consequently, the funding of family support programs becomes a very thorny issue (Turnbull, 1992). Combined with this pervading concern are the related, conflicting issues of priority of available funding for family research, the building of awareness of the vital importance of family participation during the rehabilitation process, and the timing of rehabilitation intervention. Underlying these controversial issues is the question of who has professional responsibility for the family during both the medical treatment and the rehabilitation process. When families voice their concerns for the family member, whether during hospitalization or after discharge, professionals in the service delivery system (e.g., social workers, rehabilitation nurses, and rehabilitation counselors) could be designated to care for that family. For appropriate intervention the responses of the professionals should include communicating necessary information, conveying appropriate support, and assisting with adjustment concerns. But traditionally, as the rehabilitation process progresses, a confusing picture emerges, composed of different health care professionals who often have no established guidelines for family intervention. The provision of family services can generate conflict both between and within agencies if the focus is not kept on the needs of the person and the family.

A Future Perspective

Judging from the activities of advocacy movements, continuing efforts to pass and implement family-focused legislation, emerging rehabilitation practice, and increasing research efforts on the importance of family support, the future of family involvement in individual rehabilitation is bright. With the increasing emphasis on consumer and family empowerment and the emerging understanding of disability as an environmental problem as well as an individual one, the renewed attention to family support concerns is likely to intensify. Empowerment conveys responsibility, and people living with disabilities and their families will feel more comfortable to express their needs and to demand the necessary resources to reach their rehabilitation goals. Though "the complex problems associated with adjustment and outcomes in the rehabilitation process are inherently multidimensional in nature" (Kelley & Lambert, 1992, p. 115), family involvement does not contribute to the problem but actually offers one of many solutions. The family's role is not only an opportunity; it is a necessity. The further development of family support policies and their implementation by enlightened professionals will facilitate the appropriate rehabilitation of all people.

(*See also:* CAREGIVING; CONSUMERS; DISABILITY MANAGEMENT; LOSS AND GRIEF; PSYCHOSOCIAL ADJUSTMENT; RESPITE CARE)

RESOURCES

Beach Center on Families and Disability, c/o Institute for Life Span Studies, 3111 Haworth Hall, Lawrence, KS 66045

National Parent Network on Disabilities, 1600 Prince St., #115, Alexandria, VA 22314

BIBLIOGRAPHY

CAROFF, PHYLLIS, and MAILICK, MILDRED D. "The Patient Has a Family: Reaffirming Social Work's Domain." *Health and Social Work* 10 (1985):17–34.

DELL ORTO, ARTHUR E., and POWER, PAUL W. *Head Injury and the Family: A Life and Living Perspective.* Winter Park, FL, 1994.

GONZALEZ, SANDRA; STEINGLASS, PETER; and REISS, DAVID. "Family-Centered Interventions for People with Chronic Physical Disabilities" (unpublished monograph). Washington, DC, 1989.

HALL, DOUGLAS T. "A Model of Coping with Role Conflict: The Role Behavior of College Educated Women." *Administrative Science Quarterly* 17 (1972):471–489.

KELLEY, SUSAN D., and LAMBERT, SELDEN S. "Family Support in Rehabilitation: A Review of Research, 1980–1990." *Rehabilitation Counseling Bulletin* 36 (1992):98–119.

POWER, PAUL. "An Assessment Approach to Family Intervention." In *Family Interventions Throughout Chronic Illness and Disability,* eds. P. Power, A. Dell Orto, and M. Gibbons. New York, 1988.

———. "Family Coping with Chronic Illness and Rehabilitation." In *Handbook on General Hospital Psychiatry,* eds. Fiona K. Judd, Graham D. Burrows, and Don R. Lipsitt. Amsterdam, 1991.

POWER, PAUL; DELL ORTO, ARTHUR; and GIBBONS, MARTHA. *Family Interventions Throughout Chronic Illness and Disability.* New York, 1988.

REAGLES, SUSAN. "The Impact of Disability: A Family Crisis." *Journal of Applied Rehabilitation Counseling* 13 (1982):25–29.

ROLLAND, JOHN. "Family Illness Paradigms: Evolution and Significance." *Family Systems Medicine* 5 (1987):482–501.

TURNBULL, HENRY. *Families and Disability Newsletter.* Lawrence, KS, 1992.

PAUL W. POWER

FORENSIC REHABILITATION

Forensic rehabilitation refers to the application of rehabilitation principles in legal settings, usually to assess disability-related damages in personal injury litigation. This entry will discuss the relationship between rehabilitation and the courts, particularly the role of the rehabilitation consultant as expert witness and methods used by such consultants to assess various types of damages.

Rehabilitation experts are relatively new to the courtroom. Historically, rehabilitation counselors were trained specifically to work in public agencies and were often shielded from acting as expert witnesses in personal injury litigation. Nurses, the first rehabilitation professionals to work in the private sector, came into contact with the legal system on a large scale only in the late 1960s, when International Rehabilitation Associates, now Intracorp, was formed by an insurance company to help process and manage insurance claims. By the 1990s, private sector rehabilitation had extended into almost all areas of disability care, including that covered by workers' compensation, long-term disability insurance, Social Security disability insurance, standard health insurance, railroad (Federal Employees' Liability Act) and longshore workers' insurance, and under the Jones Act, as well as by damages awarded in personal injury litigation. Although there is considerable similarity across jurisdictions, there are a number of differences about which the rehabilitation expert should know before stepping into court.

For example, the word "disability" is defined differently in various systems. In public rehabilitation, disability usually refers to a medical condition that establishes a person's eligibility for rehabilitation services that may restore his or her ability to perform work. When the Social Security Administration determines that a person is disabled, however, the person is deemed unable to perform "substantial gainful activity" and may qualify for government support for living. In workers' compensation systems, some states have provision for permanent or temporary disability as well as partial or total. As this example shows, terminology can differ significantly, and it is important for the rehabilitation expert to understand the words used in a particular courtroom. A text such as the *Rehabilitation Consultant's Handbook* (Weed & Field, 1994) will provide the professional with a general understanding of these terms.

The rehabilitation professional need not be certified or possess a certain level of education to serve as an expert witness. According to *Kim Manufacturing v. Superior Metal Treating* (1976), an "expert witness is one who by reason of education or specialized experience possesses superior knowledge respecting a subject about which persons having no particular training are incapable of forming an accurate opinion or deducing correct conclusions." Therefore, an attorney may offer as an expert someone who would qualify as an expert in the workers' compensation systems of some states or as a vocational expert (VE) in the Social Security system.

Roles of the Rehabilitation Expert

There are generally two issues the attorney must address in the type of litigation that involves a rehabilitation expert: liability and damages. When a party is found liable, that party is determined to be at fault. The next task is to prove damages, or the costs associated with the incident. The rehabilitation expert will generally participate in the damages portion of litigation by assisting in two areas: (1) establishing the cost of future care, and (2) assessing the significance of the incident with regard to the person's ability to perform work (earnings capacity).

The rehabilitation professional may act as a consultant, which implies that he or she will work "behind the scenes" to assist the attorney with developing a case or reviewing the work of others. Although psychologists, rehabilitation counselors, neuropsychologists, physicians, therapists and others offer these services, this role is unique for rehabilitation nurses. In fact, many larger law firms employ nurses to conduct medical research, locate experts, develop deposition and trial questions, summarize medical records and depositions, and provide other litigation support services. The Legal Nurses Association is an excellent source of information for this alternative. A more common role for rehabilitation professionals is to act as the expert witness and develop opinions that will be offered as testimony. These opinions are usually in the realm of the two areas noted above.

One tool used to ascertain the costs of future care, particularly for serious medical conditions and catastrophic injuries, is the "Life Care Plan," developed by Paul Deutsch and John Raffa and first published in *Damages in Tort Action* (1981). The plan is organized in categories that outline expected treatment, start-and-stop dates, costs, and other information that will provide the jury with an understanding of the treatment plan (see Figure 1). The format is designed to facilitate the development of a comprehensive rehabilitation plan that includes the information necessary to project all treatment-related expenses and reach a "bottom-line" figure, usually with the help of an economist. For a more complete discussion of the use of such plans in rehabilitation, see the *Guide to Rehabilitation* (Deutsch & Sawyer, 1993).

Figure 1. "Life Care Plan" checklist

✔ **Projected evaluations:** Nonphysician evaluations, such as of the need for physical therapy, speech therapy, recreational therapy, occupational therapy, and music therapy. Dietary evaluation, audiology and vision examinations, and swallow studies, etc.

✔ **Projected therapeutic modalities:** Therapies needed based on the evaluations above. Consider a case manager to help control costs and reduce complications.

✔ **Diagnostic testing/educational assessment:** Testing, such as vocational evaluation as well as neuropsychological and psychoeducational levels.

✔ **Wheelchair needs:** Types and configurations of wheelchairs the client requires, e.g., power, shower, manual, ventilator, reclining, quad pegs, or recreational.

✔ **Wheelchair accessories and maintenance:** Bags, cushions, trays, etc.

✔ **Aids for independent functioning:** Include environmental controls, adaptive aids, and portable ramps.

✔ **Orthotics/prosthetics:** Include maintenance and replacement costs.

✔ **Home furnishings and accessories:** Such as a specialty bed to prevent skin problems.

✔ **Drug/supply needs:** Prescription/nonprescription drugs and supplies, including size and quantity.

✔ **Home care/facility care:** Include specialty programs and level of care required.

✔ **Future medical care—routine:** Includes medical specialties such as physical medicine, orthopedics, urology, internal medicine, vision, and dental as well as X ray, MRI, and lab.

✔ **Transportation:** Consider hand controls or a specialty van.

✔ **Health and strength maintenance:** Include specialty recreation such as adapted games, equipment, or annual dues for specialty magazines. Recreation wheelchairs should go on wheelchair page.

✔ **Architectural renovations:** Consider ramps, hallways, kitchen, fire protection, alternative heating/cooling, floor coverings, bath, attendant room, equipment storage, etc.

✔ **Potential complications:** Although not financially a part of the plan, list complications from poor rehabilitation.

✔ **Future medical care/surgical intervention or aggressive treatment:** Plans for additional surgeries such as cosmetic surgery, implants, radiation, etc.

✔ **Orthopedic equipment needs:** Identify Hoyer lift, walkers, standing or tilt tables, and body support equipment.

✔ **Vocational/educational plan:** Include costs of vocational counseling, job coaching, tuition, fees, books, supplies, and technology.

SOURCE: © 1994 by Roger O. Weed

Figure 2 outlines the components of one type of analysis used by rehabilitation professionals to assess earnings capacity.

Generally accepted methods for determining loss of earnings capacity include the following.

1. The most common method assumes the client has a work history. The professional scrutinizes vocational and medical records, perhaps supplementing them with testing, and provides a professional opinion regarding pre- and post-incident earnings capacity. Obviously this is not useful for a client with a limited or no work history.

2. The "Labor Market Access" method, developed by Timothy Field and Janet Field (1992), utilizes federal data regarding worker traits and the *Dictionary of Occupational Titles* (U.S. Department of Labor, 1991). A computer program matches various combinations of 70 worker traits to 12,741 job titles. This process identifies the number of potential pre- and post-incident jobs, their

Figure 2. The **RAPEL** method: A commonsense approach to earnings capacity analysis

Rehabilitation plan. Determine the rehabilitation plan based on the client's vocational and functional limitations, vocational strengths, emotional functioning, and cognitive capabilities. This may include testing, counseling, training fees, rehabilitation technology, job analysis, job coaching, placement, and other needs for increasing employment potential. Also consider reasonable accommodation. A life care plan may be needed for catastrophic injuries.

Access to the labor market. Determine the client's access to the labor market. Methods include the LMA92 computer program, transferability of skills (or worker trait) analysis, disability statistics, and experience. This may also represent the client's loss of choice and is particularly relevant if earnings potential is based on very few positions.

Placeability. This represents the likelihood that the client could be successfully placed in a job. This is where the "rubber meets the road." Consider the employment statistics for people with disabilities, employment data for the specific medical condition (if available), economic situation of the community (may include a labor market survey), and availability (not just existence) of jobs in chosen occupations. Note that the client's attitude, personality, and other factors will influence the ultimate outcome.

Earnings capacity. Based on the above, what is the pre-incident capacity to earn compared to the post-incident capacity to earn? Methods include analysis of the specific job titles or class of jobs that a person could have engaged in pre- vs. post-incident, the ability to be educated (sometimes useful for people with acquired brain injury), family history of pediatric injuries, and LMA92 computer analysis based on the individual's worker traits.

Special consideration applies to children, women with limited or no work history, people who choose to work below their capacity (e.g., highly educated people who are farmers), and the military-trained.

Labor force participation. This represents the client's work life expectancy. Determine the amount of time that is lost, if any, from the labor force as a result of the disability. Issues include longer time to find employment, part-time vs. full-time employment, medical treatment or follow-up, earlier retirement, etc. Display data using specific dates or percentages; for example, an average of four hours a day may represent a 50 percent loss.

SOURCE: © 1993 by Roger O. Weed

average and maximum earnings, and other information that can be used as a basis for the expert opinion.

3. To determine the earnings capacity of children and others who may not have ample work histories, an extensive review of the client's background may be useful. This review may include an analysis of the client's school records and the occupational and/or educational background of the parents and extended family, as well as educational or neuropsychological testing. In acquired brain injury pediatric cases, pre- vs. post-incident ability to be educated may be analyzed.

4. Another method, known as L-P-E, identifies the client's probability of life (L), labor force participation (P), and employment (E). For more in-

formation on this method, see *Economic/Hedonic Damages: The Practice Book for Plaintiff and Defense Attorneys* by Michael Brookshire and Stan Smith (1990).

Other references on assessing earnings capacity include *The Rehabilitation Consultant's Handbook* (Weed & Field, 1994) and "The Necessary Economic and Vocational Interface in Personal Injury Cases" (Dillman, 1987).

Another domain that some rehabilitation experts address is that of compensation for the loss of pleasures or choices in life, known as hedonic damages. Methods include describing to the jury the pain experienced by the client, his or her loss of access to the labor market, psychological effects, loss of consortium, and other factors. A chart developed by Brookshire and Smith (1990) may be used to provide the jury with guidelines for assessing hedonic damages.

Regardless of the type of damages, the expert must be able to quantify them in a way that provides the economist, if one is used, or the jury with the information necessary to project costs over time to determine the total amount to award the client if the party against whom the suit is lodged is found at fault. The basic information required includes start dates, stop dates, frequency and duration of treatment, and expense. For example, a client who requires psychological counseling for twelve months, one time per week, one hour per session, at a cost of $100 per hour will receive an award of $5200 to compensate for the expenses associated with this treatment.

The ethical rehabilitation professional who practices in forensic settings provides a valuable contribution by establishing a reasonable treatment plan, helping to settle personal injury litigation, or providing the jury with information on which to base an award. The domain is growing as more attorneys become aware of the value of the forensic rehabilitation expert to their cases.

(*See also:* ETHICS; LIFE CARE PLANNING)

BIBLIOGRAPHY

BROOKSHIRE, MICHAEL, and SMITH, STAN. *Economic/Hedonic Damages: The Practice Book for Plaintiff and Defense Attorneys.* Cincinnati, 1990.

DEUTSCH, PAUL, and RAFFA, FREDERICK. *Damages in Tort Action,* vols. 8 and 9. New York, 1981.

DEUTSCH, PAUL, and SAWYER, HORACE. *Guide to Rehabilitation.* New York, 1993.

DILLMAN, EVERETT. "The Necessary Economic and Vocational Interface in Personal Injury Cases." *Journal of Private Sector Rehabilitation* 2 (1987): 121–142.

FIELD, TIMOTHY, and FIELD, JANET. "Labor Market Access Plus 1992" (computer program). Athens, GA, 1992.

FIELD, TIMOTHY, and WEED, ROGER O. *Transferability of Work Skills.* Athens, GA, 1988.

Kim Manufacturing, Inc. v. Superior Metal Treating, Inc. 537 SW Reporter, 2d. 424 (1976).

U.S. DEPARTMENT OF LABOR. *Dictionary of Occupational Titles.* 4th ed., rev. Washington, DC, 1991.

WEED, ROGER O. "Earnings v. Earnings Capacity: The Labor Market Access Method." *Journal of Private Sector Rehabilitation* 3 (1988):57–64.

WEED, ROGER O., and FIELD, TIMOTHY. *The Rehabilitation Consultant's Handbook,* rev. Athens, GA, 1994.

WEED, ROGER O., and SLUIS, ANNE. *Life Care Planning for the Amputee: A Step by Step Guide.* Orlando, FL, 1990.

ROGER O. WEED

FUNCTIONAL ASSESSMENT

See ASSESSMENT; VOCATIONAL EVALUATION

FUNCTIONAL ELECTRICAL STIMULATION (FES)

Functional electrical stimulation (FES) is a medical and rehabilitation treatment that applies low levels of electricity to nerve, muscle, or other tissues to restore function and enhance health that has been lost due to disease or injury. More than two dozen different uses for the technique have been developed. When appropriately directed, electrical stimulation can activate nerves, initiate and sustain controlled muscle contractions, suppress abnormal or undesired nervous system activity, provide substitute sensory information, enhance tissue repair, and improve blood circulation.

Clinical trials of FES techniques were first reported in the eighteenth century, after investigators discovered that electricity could make frog muscles contract. By the 1950s, advancements in technology made the first cardiac pacemakers possible, introducing widespread clinical acceptance of FES. By the 1960s, research was initiated to study the use of electricity to restore functional movement to paralyzed limbs, resulting in the coining of the term "FES" later in that decade.

Functional electrical stimulation is used in an impressively broad spectrum of applications. To differentiate among FES treatments, one must know the purpose of the electrical stimulation, the intended patient population, the course of treatment, and the type of stimulator and electrode technology used.

All FES systems consist of a stimulator that generates electrical impulses, and one or more electrodes that transmit the electrical impulses to the body. Most stimulators are computer-controlled and portable. Some stimulators are implanted entirely within the body, such as a pacemaker. Electrodes are attached to an affected part of the body, depending on the specific application and technique. They may be placed on the skin, inserted through the skin, or implanted in the body.

For some persons with upper motor neuron paralysis due to spinal cord injury, stroke, head injury, cerebral palsy, or multiple sclerosis, FES can be used to activate the paralyzed muscles of the extremities, the respiratory system, and the bladder and bowel systems, increasing independence and enhancing quality of life. Sometimes such FES systems are called *neural prostheses* because they become a permanent substitute for the damaged neuromuscular system.

Some neural prostheses are more fully developed than others. For example, phrenic nerve pacers that replace ventilators and bladder stimulators that replace catheters have been commercially available since the early 1980s. However, neural prostheses for the upper and lower extremities have only recently achieved clinical acceptance. In 1993, the Food and Drug Administration (FDA) granted approval with conditions for an FES standing and walking system for persons with paraplegia that was developed at the University of Illinois at Chicago. Also in 1993, researchers from Case Western Reserve University commenced multicenter studies of an implanted FES hand grasp and release system for quadriplegics.

Electrical stimulation has many other uses for people with upper motor neuron paralysis. FES exercise equipment, such as a bicycle ergometer, is used to move paralyzed limbs against a programmed resistance. Such FES-induced movement may provide enhanced cardiovascular health, improved circulation, and increased bone strength. Electrical stimulation techniques are sometimes applied to enhance the healing of pressure sores that often occur when mobility is restricted. FES can also be used to counteract the negative effects of the spasticity that may occur as a result of upper motor neuron paralysis.

Additionally, an FES technique to induce ejaculation in males with neurological impairment, known as electroejaculation, is used at spinal cord injury clinics in conjunction with artificial insemination of the female partner to achieve pregnancy. Finally, investigators are studying how electrical stimulation can be applied to nerve grafts to enhance nerve regeneration for persons with spinal cord injury and other types of paralysis.

FES can also be used for people with sensory impairments to provide substitute sensory information. Electrotactile stimulation evokes a sensation of touch when tiny electrical impulses are applied to the skin. The technique can be used to code different types of environmental information for persons with impaired vision, hearing, or touch.

A cochlear implant is a widely available neural prosthesis that is used to stimulate the auditory nerve in people with sensorineural deafness. The implant restores a rudimentary sensation of hearing that improves lipreading ability. For persons with severe visual impairments, limited experiments have shown that electrical stimulation applied to the visual cortex can elicit visual sensations that may someday assist with mobility orientation.

Persons with partial refractory epilepsy may also benefit from FES. When applied to the vagal nerve, electrical stimulation reduces the occurrence of seizures. In the early 1990s the manufacturer of a vagal nerve stimulator submitted an application to the FDA; approval is expected before the end of the decade. In another application, adolescents with a spinal deformity such as scoliosis may benefit from electrical activation of the muscles surrounding the spine to reduce or eliminate the deformity.

In the early 1980s investigators developed an FES technique known as cardiomyoplasty for people suffering from ischemic heart disease and other types of severe heart failure. The latissimus dorsi muscle from the back is surgically removed and wrapped around the heart. Contractions of this muscle are rhythmically induced via electrical stimulation, causing a pumping action. A similar technique, dynamic myoplasty, is under investigation to help people with urinary or fecal incontinence. The surgically transferred muscle is wrapped around the sphincter and is electrically contracted to keep the sphincter closed.

FES is a multidisciplinary treatment modality, often involving surgeons, neurologists, physiatrists, nurses, occupational therapists, physical therapists, orthotists, and biomedical or rehabilitation engineers. On almost every continent there are major research centers fine-tuning existing techniques and launching new investigations to determine how FES can increase health and independence for persons with disability so they can better pursue their vocational, educational, and recreational goals.

In the United States, some of the major FES research centers are at Case Western Reserve University in Cleveland, Illinois Institute of Technology in Chicago, Louisiana State University in New Orleans, the University of Miami, and Wright State University in Dayton. Elsewhere, among the leading research centers are Ålborg University in Denmark; the University of Alberta in Edmonton; the University of Ljubljana in Slovenia; Tohoku University in Sendai, Japan; the University of Twente in Enschede, the Netherlands; and the University of Vienna in Austria.

By the year 2001 we will likely see several different FES products on the market that provide functional restoration of movement in the upper or lower extremities. Advances in orthotics to be used in combination with FES systems, sensors for force and position information, surgical muscle transfer techniques, and direct communication with the nervous system as a command control source will lead to greatly enhanced and more functional FES systems. Advances in semiconductor technology will complement implanted electrode and stimulator development, resulting in multiple-purpose and highly selective FES systems for motor and sensory restoration. As with any new medical technology, to be successful, the FES systems of the future must be accompanied by clear clinical outcomes measurements and favorable cost-effectiveness studies.

(*See also:* ASSISTIVE TECHNOLOGY; ENGINEERING, REHABILITATION; PHYSICAL THERAPY; PROSTHETICS AND ORTHOTICS; SPINAL CORD INJURY)

RESOURCES

Center for Neural Prostheses Research, Aalborg University, Department MIBA, Fredrik Bajersvej 7D, Aalborg 9220, Denmark

Institute for Rehabilitation Research and Medicine, Wright State University, 3171 Research Blvd., Dayton, OH 45420

Louisiana State University Medical Center, Depart-

ment of Orthopaedics, 2025 Gravier St., Suite 400, New Orleans, LA 70112

Miami Project, University of Miami, 1600 NW 10th Ave., Miami, FL 33136

Pritzker Institute of Medical Engineering, Illinois Institute of Technology, 10 W. 32nd St., E1-125 IIT Center, Chicago, IL 60616

Rehabilitation Engineering Center, MetroHealth Medical Center, Case Western Reserve University, 2500 MetroHealth Drive, Cleveland, OH 44109-1998

Tohoku University School of Medicine, Department of FES and Restorative Medicine, 2-1 Seiryo-maci, Sendai 980, Japan

University of Alberta, Physiology Department, 513 Heritage Medical Research Centre, Edmonton, Alberta T6G 2S2, Canada

University of Ljubljana, Faculty of Electrical and Computer Engineering, Trzaska 25, 61000 Ljubljana, Slovenia

University of Twente, Department of Electrical Engineering, P.O. Box 217, Enschede 7500 AE, The Netherlands

University of Vienna, Department of Biomedical Engineering and Physics, AKH Ebene 4/L, Waehringergeurtel 18-20, A-1090 Vienna, Austria

BIBLIOGRAPHY

AGNEW, WILLIAM F., and McCREERY, DOUGLAS B., eds. *Neural Prostheses: Fundamental Studies*. Englewood Cliffs, NJ, 1990.

BAKER, LUCINDA L., ET AL. *Neuromuscular Electrical Stimulation: A Practical Guide*. Downey, CA. 1993.

DURFEE, WILLIAM K., ed. "Special Issue on Practical Functional Electrical Stimulation." *Assistive Technology* 4 (1992):1–48.

MADDOX, SAM. "FES." In *Spinal Network: The Total Wheelchair Book*, 2nd ed. Boulder, CO, 1993.

STEIN, RICHARD B.; PECKHAM, P. HUNTER; and POPOVIC, DJAN B., eds. *Neural Prostheses: Replacing Motor Function After Disease or Disability*. New York, 1992.

YARKONY, G. M.; ROTH, E. D.; CYBULSKI, G. R.; and JAEGER, R. J. "Neuromuscular Stimulation in Spinal Cord Injury: I: Restoration of Functional Movement of the Extremities." *Archives of Physical Medicine and Rehabilitation* 73 (1992):78–86.

———. "Neuromuscular Stimulation in Spinal Cord Injury: II: Prevention of Secondary Complications." *Archives of Physical Medicine and Rehabilitation* 73 (1992):195–200.

JEANNE O'MALLEY TEETER

FUTURE OF REHABILITATION

Traditionally, rehabilitation has been a reactive rather than a proactive profession. Rehabilitation laws, significant program developments, rehabilitation education, and similar activities have been based on past experience, often with little thought given to future needs. For example, the earliest rehabilitation efforts, in the 1920s, were aimed at rehabilitating World War I veterans and unemployed industrial workers who had experienced physical disabilities. Later, as public and professional awareness of other disability types grew and attitudes changed, additional disability groups were added to the rehabilitation caseload. Support for persons with mental illness and mental retardation expanded in the 1930s and 1940s, as did rehabilitation services for individuals with sensory problems (blindness and deafness). The classification of disabilities has expanded to include substance abuse (alcoholism and drug addiction), Acquired Immune Deficiency Syndrome (AIDS), posttraumatic stress disorder, eating disorders, and a range of disorders with varied causes and implications. Unfortunately, the rehabilitation system and rehabilitation professionals are ill-prepared to serve these new disability groups, in part because of the lack of concern for future implications.

It has been suggested (Arokiasamy et al., 1988) that there are three major reasons for study of the future: "To prepare for inevitable futures, to avoid undesirable futures, and to plan desirable futures" (p. 318). Despite the importance of understanding the future, relatively few studies in rehabilitation have attempted to be predictive.

There is agreement in rehabilitation that several issues will profoundly affect its future. Those issues include changes in the nature of work in the United States; growing diversity in the workforce; changes in the nature of disability; advances in rehabilitation and medical technology; and alterations in the nature of strategies of service delivery.

Changes in the Nature of Work

The United States has moved from an industrially based manufacturing economy to a business-centered service economy, with the majority of jobs in the service sector. Changes in the nature of jobs will continue to grow as the economy shifts. Increasingly, service sector jobs will require technological training, familiarity, and skills to operate computerized equipment. Many jobs will be communication- and information-based, requiring increased levels of education for entry-level jobs. These jobs will appear simple but will make high knowledge and flexibility demands as workers are forced to keep up with the booming electronic age. The phrase "computer skills required" will be found in advertisements for jobs of all types. Jobs requiring college degrees will increase from 22 to 30 percent by the year 2000 (Coates, Jarratt, and Mahaffie, 1990; Riggar, Eckert, and Crimando, 1993). The educational requirements for better jobs will grow steadily, implying that persons with disabilities will need continued access to educational opportunities.

While many jobs will continue to be available in large corporations, the greatest job growth will be in small, developing companies with fewer than 100 employees. The Americans with Disabilities Act (ADA) now holds small firms (those with at least 15 employees) to the same standards of nondiscrimination on the basis of disability as larger firms. Because little is known about the culture and attitudes of small employers toward persons with disabilities, it is difficult to predict how these employers will respond to the mandates of the ADA. Some employers may be very responsive, while others may not be. However, it is well known that attitudes toward people with disabilities improve with familiarity. As more workers with disabilities enter the workforce, greater and more positive acceptance should occur.

Larger companies such as DuPont, IBM, and Eastman Kodak have demonstrated a substantial commitment to hiring and retaining workers with disabilities. Company records suggest that employees with disabilities have similar production, absenteeism, and turnover rates when compared to able-bodied employees. It is anticipated that large companies will continue to employ large numbers of persons with disabilities.

Growing Diversity in the Workforce

The work force will grow increasingly diverse, but one of the most profound changes will be its aging. By the year 2000, 11 percent of the work force will be fifty-five or over, and 51 percent will be thirty-five to forty-five years of age. The baby-boom generation (those born after 1945 to 1964) is the largest age cohort and has had the fewest number of offspring per person in history. The first of the baby-boom generation will retire shortly after the turn of the century, and few replacement workers will be available.

Older workers are more likely to become disabled as a result of the aging process. Many disabilities will be minor (e.g., hearing loss or visual loss), but other disabilities will be major, necessitating involvement with private or public rehabilitation systems. Older individuals with disabilities will use greater numbers of assistive devices, thereby boosting technology development.

Return to work as a rehabilitated worker is closely linked to timeliness of rehabilitation service and the amount of time spent receiving rehabilitation services. Older workers will naturally have slower recovery and recuperation times, which then may jeopardize successful rehabilitation and return to work. Companies will provide wellness programs ranging from blood pressure screening and smoking cessation programs to full-scale fitness programs to combat health- and disability-related problems in the aging workforce.

The age of the workforce will directly affect training for and provision of rehabilitation services. Many rehabilitation practitioners, administrators, and educators joined the rehabilitation field in the "Golden Era of Rehabilitation" in the 1960s and 1970s and will leave the field in large numbers through retirement and career shifts in the near future. Many of those departing will be senior staffers with a wealth of years of experience.

Changes in the Nature of Disability

It is estimated that at least 43 million people in the United States have disabilities; however, only 33 percent of people with disabilities are employed. Minorities are thought to fare less well: Only 16.4 percent of African Americans with disabilities are employed, for example. By the year 2050, one-half of the population will be African American, Hispanic, Native American, or Asian American. Except for Asian Americans, minorities tend to be less

well educated and consequently qualify for the lowest-paid, highest-risk jobs. They are more apt to suffer disabling injuries on these jobs and less likely to have health care coverage. If disabled, they will more likely become clients of the state-federal vocational rehabilitation system than of private sector rehabilitation. Moreover, the poverty in which many minorities live results in higher levels of stress and more incidence of stress-related disabilities. The trend toward a multicultural society will mean that rehabilitation counselors' responsibilities will become increasingly diverse, requiring cultural sensitivity and second-language skills.

Emphasis on serving people with severe disabilities will continue to drive service delivery, and the nature of these severe disabilities will become increasingly complex. For example, a growing number of people who survive traumatic brain injury are being served in a variety of community facilities. Formerly, placement would have been limited to residential institutions. People with traumatic brain injury (TBI) require a wide array of services and have diverse, individualized needs. Rehabilitation practitioners serving this population will be confronted with pediatric clients, clients dependent on advanced technologies, and clients who require highly specialized professional services.

Significantly higher rates of alcohol and drug-related problems exist among people with disabilities (Greer, Roberts, and Jenkins, 1993). The dual diagnosis of substance abuse and other disabilities slow the rehabilitation process, hinder community reentry, and may increase the risk of additional disabling injury.

The issues concerning multiple disabilities and dual diagnoses will not be solved easily, and as life-saving technology and the world of work become more complex and as the definition of disability continues to expand (e.g., AIDS), so, too, will these issues. Rehabilitation services will become more labor-intensive, involving extended and costly acute and multidisciplinary services in specialized settings. As implementation of the ADA impacts on environmental barriers, people with severe disabilities will be able to function in the community with the support of attendant and independent living services.

AIDS will present continued challenges for rehabilitation. A diagnosis of AIDS implies physical illness and the eventuality of death, and also carries with it considerable long-term psychological and vocational implications. Rehabilitation practitioners will be obliged to work with consumers diagnosed with AIDS. Simultaneously, there will be complicated ethical dilemmas concerning confidentiality and disclosure.

Advances in Rehabilitation and Medical Technology

Technological advances have been called the great equalizer for people with disabilities. Print reading computer scanners, speech synthesizers, and computerized Braille printers have expanded communications options for people with visual impairments. With the implementation of the ADA, a national relay system of Telephone Devices for the Deaf has been established, also expanding communication and access for people with deafness or other hearing impairment. Developments in microchip technology, refinement and size reduction of electric motors, and advances in biotechnology (e.g., moving prosthetic limbs) have fostered advances in mobility, communications, and daily living activities for people with disabilities.

Advances in computer technology will have implications for people with disabilities and for rehabilitation counselors. Immediate access to information and resources can be provided by computer networks via databases, on-line discussion groups, and text files. A computerized human resource directory can be extremely useful when installed on staff computers, and these directories can help rehabilitation practitioners become oriented to the services provided in the area.

As more rehabilitation practitioners become involved with computer networking, a number of possible outgrowths can develop. On-line discussion groups will become national and international in nature, providing rehabilitation administrators and practitioners with access to and exchange with national and international leaders. Access to such leaders and databases can provide answers to questions from disability law to medication interactions through on-line help and expertise. This immediate access to help and expertise could positively influence the effectiveness and efficiency of rehabilitation service delivery.

Technology is the application of science to industrial or commercial objectives. Rehabilitation technology ranges from elaborate computer systems and assistive devices to simple activities such as placing blocks under a desk to make it accessible for a person with a disability. As the tenets of the ADA continue to mandate that employers provide reasonable accommodations to people with disabilities, the onus will be on the rehabilitation profession to advocate for both employees and employers. Rehabilitation practitioners will be charged with finding reasonable, affordable, and practical rehabilitation technology to accommodate people with disabilities in the work force, keeping in mind that each consumer has a unique mix of functional abilities and limitations. Increasingly, vocational rehabilitation professionals will find themselves authorizing plans and facilitating technology-based accommodations. As this participation becomes more involved, vocational rehabilitation professionals will be responsible for the success of such accommodations. Greater demand for and utilization of high-tech assistive devices should reduce costs.

Ironically, the computerized workplace may increase the incidence of certain kinds of disability. Increased utilization of keyboards, video display units, and scanning equipment will result in an escalation of visual, neuromuscular, and cerebral difficulties. Rehabilitation practitioners of the future will see more cases of hand and wrist injuries stemming from repetitive motion (e.g., carpal tunnel syndrome), visual disturbances, and head and neck pain. These problems may be reduced if staff training programs are developed, furniture and equipment are redesigned, and jobs are modified to protect the worker.

Alterations in the Nature and Strategies of Service Delivery

The 1992 amendments to the Rehabilitation Act have notable implications for rehabilitation service delivery.

The purpose of these amendments is to empower individuals with disabilities to: (1) maximize their employment, economic self-sufficiency, independence, and inclusion and integration into society; (2) ensure that the federal government plays a leadership role in promoting the meaningful and gainful employment and independent living of individuals with disabilities; and (3) assist states and service providers in these efforts. The Rehabilitation Act amendments have streamlined the intake process and made eligibility requirements less stringent, suggesting a future of easier access and participation in a less bureaucratized state-federal rehabilitation system. The amendments place emphasis on the outcome of the rehabilitation intervention and reduction of time to closure as well as the quality of that closure. With passage of the ADA and reauthorization of the Rehabilitation Act through the amendments of 1992, the federal government has reaffirmed its commitment to the disability rights movement, focusing on the empowerment and collective rights of people with disabilities. This movement away from the traditional policy of assisting people with disabilities to one of advocating for their rights will eventually leave the transitional phase, and rehabilitation and accommodation will become unquestioned rights.

The Rehabilitation Act amendments have influenced the independent living movement, and will continue to guide the provision of independent living services in the future. Title VII of the 1992 amendments promotes the philosophy of independent living, a philosophy that affirms consumer control, peer support, self-help, self-determination, equal access, and advocacy. The amendments provide funds to states for (1) expansion and improvement of independent living (IL) services; (2) support of statewide IL center networks; and (3) improvement of relationships among state IL programs, IL centers, and state IL councils. The amendments also establish the statewide independent living councils, and standards and assurances for centers of independent living. This recommitment to the independent living movement reinforces the trend toward the integration and full inclusion of people with disabilities into American society.

Labor and management have taken a more active role in managing disability, and as health-care costs rise and third-party coverage declines or is limited, disability management will play a more prominent role in rehabilitation. Disability management aims at promoting return to work in the quickest, most cost-effective manner. Multidisciplinary, goal-directed teams plan, coordinate, and implement services with the worker with a disability. As labor and management take on this active role, they will realize the cost-effectiveness of the prevention of disability, and prompt treatment and rehabilitation of injured and disabled workers.

Rehabilitation programs may be provided increasingly through state funding if there are reductions of federal money and support. However, if state programs downsize to meet budget restrictions, a shift of consumers to the private sector may occur. Private sector rehabilitation will continue to thrive if it provides efficient, top-quality rehabilitation services.

The 1975 Education for All Handicapped Children Act gave considerable impetus to the consumer movement and rehabilitation and should continue to have significant influence in the rehabilitation of children and youth. Mainstreaming students with disabilities into the normal classroom is no longer an isolated concept but one that has become widely accepted. However, in many cases a disparity arises when students with disabilities who have had the same educational opportunities as their non-disabled peers do not experience the same equality in placement in post-high school opportunities (i.e., entry-level jobs and/or college). Many emerging issues exist in the preparation of students for work or college beyond high school, including: "self-determination, the school's responsibility for initial placements, continued educational engagement of at-risk students and service coordination necessary for the meaningful implementation of the transition requirements of the Individuals with Disabilities Education Act (IDEA). Responding to these issues will require leadership on federal, state, and local levels" (Ward & Halloran, 1993, p. 4).

Supported employment has been a key strategy in the transition from school to work for many youngsters with disabilities. Supported employment centers on integrated, paid employment with ongoing available support, especially for individuals with the most severe disabilities (Rogan & Murphy, 1991). A basic guiding principle has been unconditional inclusion as opposed to the traditional vocational rehabilitation concept of potential employability as a criterion for eligibility for services. As Pat Rogan and Stephen Murphy (1991) write, "The important issue should not be whether one has potential, but in what community job and with what supports can one best apply the potential one possesses." Considering the growing consumer rights and advocacy movement for people with severe disabilities, and the government's support of those rights, the concept of "unconditional inclusion" will eventually replace the traditional concept of "employability."

The workers' compensation system in this country will likely undergo significant change. John Finch (1993) notes that workers' compensation and industrial rehabilitation tend to be seen as driving employer and health-care costs up rather than down. As long as the workers' compensation system is managed separately in each state and is perceived as an excessive expenditure by state legislators, there will be continual danger of benefit reduction. Many states will enact new workers' compensation laws to control increasing costs. Lowered benefits will result in more workers returning to work at a faster pace as secondary gains are reduced. In some states workers in smaller companies and selected occupations may not be eligible for workers' compensation coverage. Rehabilitation practitioners may play a significant role in unifying the disjointed national workers' compensation system by conveying the rehabilitation principle that industrial rehabilitation is focused on return to function and work as opposed to simple reduction of medical problems.

Conclusion

Constant change in rehabilitation can be predicted with certainty. History suggests that rehabilitation practitioners will continue to face budget cutbacks, resulting in staffing shortages, growing caseloads, and changes in the structure and function of the rehabilitation system. How will rehabilitation prepare for the advent of these changes in a proactive way?

Two strategies in particular may apply. The first involves networking with other rehabilitation professionals, facilities, agencies, consumers, and professional disciplines to provide access to vital information and resources pertinent to the delivery of efficient and effective rehabilitation services.

The second means of meeting the upcoming needs in rehabilitation will be continuous education and learning. Without qualified staff members the rehabilitation system cannot hope to meet the changing needs of consumers and the changing demands of society. Human resources development, including education and training, can improve individual, group, and organizational effectiveness in rehabilitation and can better prepare rehabilitation professionals to cope with constant, inevitable change.

(*See also*: ASSISTIVE TECHNOLOGY; CONSUMERS; INDEPENDENT LIVING; TECHNOLOGY AND DISABILITY)

RESOURCES

Council of State Administrators for Vocational Rehabilitation (CSAVR), 1055 Thomas Jefferson St., NW, Suite 301, Washington, DC 20007

Equal Employment Opportunity Commission, Review and Appeals Division, 1801 L St., NW, Washington, DC 20507

Job Accommodation Network (Jan), 918 Chestnut Ridge Rd, Suite 1, P.O. Box 6080, Morgantown, WV 26506–6080

National Clearinghouse of Rehabilitation Training Materials, 816 West 6th St., Oklahoma State University, Stillwater, OK 74078

National Council on Disability, 1331 F St., NW, Suite 1050, Washington, DC 20004–1107

National Rehabilitation Association, 633 South Washington St., Alexandria, VA 22314

President's Committee on Employment of People with Disabilities (PCEPD), 1331 F St., NW, Washington, DC 20004–1107

Rehabilitation Services Administration, Division of Research and Development, U.S. Department of Education, 330 C St., SW, Room 3324, Washington, DC 20202

Resource Center on Substance Abuse, Prevention for People with Disabilities, 1331 F St., NW, Suite 800, Washington, DC 20004

U.S. Department of Education, Office of Civil Rights, 330 C St., SW, Room 5431, Washington, DC 20202

World Institute on Disability (WID), 510 16th St., Suite 100, Oakland, CA 94612

BIBLIOGRAPHY

AROKIASAMY, CHARLES V.; LEJA, JAMES A.; AUSTIN, GARY; and RUBIN, STANFORD E. "The Study of the Future: A Contemporary Challenge for the Rehabilitation Counseling Profession." In *Contemporary Challenges to the Rehabilitation Counseling Profession,* eds. Stanford E. Rubin and Nancy M. Rubin. Baltimore, 1988.

COATES, JOSEPH F.; JARRATT, JENNIFER; and MAHAFFIE, JOHN B. *Future Work: Seven Critical Forces Reshaping Work and the Work Force in North America.* San Francisco, 1990.

FINCH, JOHN. "Workers' Compensation Administrator's Column: A Call to Action." *Journal of Rehabilitation Administration* 17 (1993):178–179.

GREER, BOBBY G.; ROBERTS, ROB; and JENKINS, WILLIAM M. "Substance Abuse Among Clients with Other Disabilities." *Rehabilitation Education* 4 (1993):33–40.

RIGGAR, THEODORE F.; CRIMANDO, WILLIAM; and PUSCH, BURTON D. "Learning Never Ends: Human Resource Development." *Journal of Rehabilitation Administration* 17 (1993):38–48.

RIGGAR, THEODORE F.; ECKERT, JOHN M.; and CRIMANDO, WILLIAM. "Cultural Diversity in Rehabilitation: Management Strategies for Implementing Organizational Pluralism." *Journal of Rehabilitation Administration* 17 (1993):53–61.

ROGAN, PAT, and MURPHY, STEPHEN. "Supported Employment and Vocational Rehabilitation: Merger or Misadventure?" *Journal of Rehabilitation* 57 (1991): 39–45.

WARD, MICHAEL J., and HALLORAN, WILLIAM D. "Transition Issues for the 1900s." *OSERS News in Print* (Fall 1993):4–5.

JOHN J. BENSHOFF
KAREN E. BARRETT

G

GALLAUDET UNIVERSITY

Established in 1864, Gallaudet University, in Washington, DC, remains today the only four-year liberal arts university in the world for deaf and hard-of-hearing students.

Gallaudet University serves as a national and international educational institution of higher education and a community of information on deafness and research. The university offers more than eighty undergraduate and graduate degree programs and numerous summer and continuing education programs.

History

In 1864 Congress authorized the board of directors of the Columbia Institution for the Instruction of the Deaf and Dumb ". . . to grant and confirm such degrees in the liberal arts and sciences as are usually conferred in colleges." On April 8, 1864, President Abraham Lincoln signed the charter, giving birth to what is known today as Gallaudet University.

Long a small liberal arts college unknown to the world at large, Gallaudet College began to expand in the mid-1950s and, with the support and encouragement of the U.S. Congress, underwent a multimillion-dollar construction program. At the same time, academic programs were expanded and the faculty strengthened. This expansion permitted the college to serve a larger number of students, and international students were admitted. The college was accredited in 1957, and in 1986 Gallaudet gained university status.

In 1988, the "Deaf President Now" student protest, which had the support of the faculty, staff, and alumni and which shut down the university for one week, captured world attention. This protest brought to the fore for the first time the status of deaf people and issues related to deafness. The results of that protest were the selection of the university's first deaf president since its founding and the appointment of a majority of deaf and hard-of-hearing members to the Board of Trustees.

Current Status

Gallaudet University remains a federally supported, private, multipurpose educational institution and resource center serving deaf and hard-of-hearing

339

people around the world through a full range of academic, research, and public service programs.

Gallaudet University is located on two campuses and has an on-campus enrollment of about 2,200 students. The original and main ninety-nine-acre campus, known as Kendall Green, is in northeastern Washington, DC. The second, smaller, nine-acre campus, in the northwestern section of the city, is home to the School of Preparatory Studies and other programs, including the English Language Institute, which offers full-time instruction in English as a second language, American Sign Language, and cultural studies to international deaf students. The university offers associate, baccalaureate, master's, and doctoral degrees through the following schools: College of Arts and Sciences, School of Communication, School of Education and Human Services, School of Management, and School of Preparatory Studies. Graduate studies programs admit hearing as well as deaf and hard-of-hearing students.

The College for Continuing Education (CCE) offers adult and family education and training programs. It provides seminars, materials, and information to regional constituencies through the university's eight regional centers in cooperation with local colleges and universities. It shares the university's accumulated knowledge, research, and resources with people in all walks of life and typically reaches about 55,000 persons. The CCE will be an integral part of the university's new $17 million Conference Center for Training and Development on the main campus.

The university also has a precollege program that includes two tuition-free, federally funded national model schools for deaf children: the Kendall Demonstration Elementary School and the Model Secondary School for the Deaf. Through these schools and its regional network, the precollege outreach unit develops and disseminates educational curricula and materials to schools and programs for deaf children across the nation.

Gallaudet University is a member of the Consortium of Universities of the Washington Metropolitan Area, allowing Gallaudet students to take courses at any of the more than a dozen other member colleges or universities. Gallaudet University is also a member of the Washington Research Library Consortium.

The university is accredited by the Middle States Association of Colleges and Schools, and many of the university's graduate-level programs are accredited as well by their respective nationally recognized professional associations.

Other important components of the University are the following:

The Gallaudet Research Institute is a leader in deafness-related research, and its demographic reports are recognized as the authoritative source for data on the deaf school population in the United States.

The International Center on Deafness (ICD) is committed to the dual objective of developing closer bonds among nations and upgrading educational, cultural, social, and vocational opportunities for deaf and hard-of-hearing people. Through exchange programs, training programs, seminars, conferences, and cooperative research, the ICD seeks to promote mutual sharing of programs and information.

The National Center for Law and Deafness serves as a national clearinghouse on legal issues and deafness. It provides technical assistance, workshops, classes, and a local legal services clinic.

The National Information Center on Deafness provides information on all aspects of deafness and hearing impairments to a national and international clientele.

Gallaudet is actively involved in developing and applying technology to aid the nation's estimated 21 million to 24 million citizens who are deaf or hard of hearing.

The university's library contains the largest collection of deafness-related resources in the world, and in its archives are materials dating back to 1546.

Contributions of Faculty

Gallaudet University has a collegiate faculty of 270 members, of whom 37 percent are deaf or hard of hearing. Fifty-six percent of the faculty hold earned doctorates. In addition to their teaching responsibilities they are involved in a broad range of research, scholarship, and creative activities that encompass a full range of societal issues to more direct deafness-related issues. Examples of this include the compilation of deaf historical data, deaf cultural research and studies, bilingual studies,

American Sign Language research, study of the attributes of successful deaf managers and entrepreneurs, compilation of bibliography of hearing children of deaf adults/parents, and development of deaf studies curriculum guides. Linguistics issues in deaf education, bilingualism and language acquisition, language contact in deaf communities, American Sign Language interpreting and deaf culture, multicultural issues in deafness, and maintaining deafness-focused records of genealogical value are other examples.

Communication among faculty, staff, and students at Gallaudet is through use of both sign language and written and spoken English. As a result, students are able to participate fully in all aspects of campus life and thereby acquire the comprehensive education and experience that is the goal of a liberal arts education.

Contributions of Graduates

The Gallaudet University Alumni Association (GUAA), founded in 1889, is governed by a nationally elected board of directors and has sixty-six chapters in the United States, Canada, and Japan. Approximately half of Gallaudet's alumni are members. The GUAA is an active partner of the university and funds fellowships to encourage deaf people to continue their studies at the doctoral level. The association also supports cultural activities of benefit to deaf people and recognizes exemplary service and achievement through annual national and international awards. The alumni office serves the university's more than 11,000 alumni scattered around the world and is located in a restored nineteenth-century Queen Anne style wooden building that was Gallaudet's first gymnasium, known as "Ole Jim."

Four of five Gallaudet graduates enter managerial or professional occupations. Gallaudet alumni generally earn more in their lifetimes than do other deaf people and are recognized as national and international leaders of the deaf community and assume leadership roles in education, science, law, the arts, and business. They hold high state and federal positions, administer school and state educational programs, serve on advisory boards, and edit leading publications in the field.

The Future

As the university looks to the future, it is faced with powerful new forces that are generating changes in society against a backdrop of an increasingly diverse nation and an increasingly interconnected world. The university must redefine what the best education for deaf and hard-of-hearing students is and chart bold new directions to guide its future.

Toward that end, Gallaudet must give its students the opportunity to experience those intellectual and practical challenges that lead to productive work, community service, and personal satisfaction. Learning at Gallaudet will continue to occur not only in the classroom but also through many other academic and extracurricular activities. And Gallaudet will value and nurture its wealth of cultural, linguistic, and ethnic diversity, all of which enriches the university's community.

(*See also:* DEAFNESS AND HEARING IMPAIRMENTS)

BIBLIOGRAPHY

ATWOOD, ALBERT W. *Gallaudet College, Its First One Hundred Years.* Gallaudet College, Washington, DC, 1964.

BORTNER, JUDY. "New Life for 'Ole Jim'." *Gallaudet Today* 9 (1979).

GALLAUDET UNIVERSITY. "Gallaudet University, A Tradition of Excellence." Washington, DC, December 1993.

GANNON, JACK R., *Deaf Heritage, A Narrative History of Deaf America.* National Association of the Deaf, Silver Spring, MD, 1981.

Research, Scholarship and Creative Activity at Gallaudet 1991–92. Compiled by Susan J. King. Gallaudet University, Washington, DC, 1993.

I. KING JORDAN

GASTROINTESTINAL DISORDERS

The dimensions of digestive diseases are staggering. One in ten Americans suffers from a digestive problem. Twenty million persons have a chronic digestive disease. Digestive disorders are the number one cause of hospitalizations and surgeries in the United States. Each day an estimated 200,000 Americans miss work due to digestive problems. The direct and indirect cost of digestive diseases in the United

States annually is fifty billion dollars (1994). Digestive diseases account for 14 percent of all disability claims, 11 percent of all disability days, and 13.6 percent of all hospitalizations for working persons. Among employed males, digestive diseases were the leading causes of disability (18%) in 1988. They were the second leading cause of disability in females.

The six principal gastrointestinal (GI) diagnoses causing disability are gastritis/duodenitis, gallbladder disease, gastric and duodenal ulcers, appendicitis, digestive cancer, and hepatitis. Together, these caused 78 percent of all GI disability (1988). Peptic ulcer and gastritis were more frequent in men, and diarrhea and enteritis more frequent in women. Digestive diseases, because of their relatively high frequency throughout the working years, combined with moderately long periods of disability, are of major importance, although they lack the dramatic impact of accidental injury in youth and heart conditions at older ages.

Peptic Ulcer

These benign ulcers of the stomach and duodenum derive their name "peptic" from their association with acid—pepsin juice active in their formation. In the past they had been thought to be caused by excessive acid production or excess use of aspirin or arthritis medications. Recent research has associated peptic ulcers with a bacterial parasite (H. pylori) present in the mucus on the surface of the lower third of the stomach.

Diagnosis of peptic ulcer is made by barium meal upper gastrointestinal X ray or by endoscopy (fiberoptic exam under conscious anesthesia of the surface of the stomach and duodenum). Therapy from 1930 to 1970 was by surgical gastric resection and/or vagal nerve resection to suppress gastric acid production. Therapy since the 1970s has been by suppression of stomach acid by antihistamines, H_2 receptor blocker pills. Research since 1989 has found that treatment with antibiotics clears the stomach bacterial parasite (H. pylori), heals the ulcers, and prevents future ulcer formation in 85 percent of patients.

Prevention of peptic ulcer is by early detection of H. pylori infection and early treatment with antibi-otics. For ulcers caused by excess aspirin or arthritis medication, prevention is by lesser doses of pain medication.

The effects of pain medications and antibiotics bring the issue of stress as causative agent into question. Most experts agree that cigarettes, excess caffeine, excessive aspirin and arthritis medication, and irregular eating habits are predominant factors in ulcer formation in those susceptible.

In the past, disability from peptic ulcer disease had been mostly from the side effects of stomach operative resection and/or vagal nerve resection performed for chronic, painful ulcers and for bleeding ulcers. Such operations were successful in stopping the pain and bleeding, but created a whole new set of disability symptoms—nausea, a chronically full feeling, loss of appetite, weight loss (often severe), and small stomachs that overfilled and then "dumped" the contents by vomiting or diarrhea. Three-fourths of people with "dumping syndrome" showed reduction in work capacity.

A whole generation of persons operated on from 1930 to 1970 for ulcers have high rates of continuing disability. Disability rates for ulcer operations are higher in countries with extensive social service disability systems, such as Germany and Russia. Ulcer recurrence rates do not depend on the duration of work disability, but rather on smoking status and type of medical or surgical therapy. Other factors relating to the duration of postoperative disability are the patient's age, additional diseases, postoperative complications, socioeconomic level, and patient motivation. Interestingly, younger physicians and family physicians give more time off for the same illness than do specialists.

Current Therapy. Eighty percent of persons with selective vagal surgical ablation to suppress gastric acid will return to work in four to six weeks. As a consequence of H_2 blocker therapy and antibiotic therapy of H. pylori, there will be a predictable drastic reduction of the rates of gastroduodenal ulcer recurrence, chronic duodenal scarring, and chronic pain with subsequent decrease in the need for drastic surgery in peptic ulcer patients. The quality of life is expected to return to normal for most peptic ulcer patients, and the need for more disability days and permanent disability to be reduced drastically. The limiting factors in such a good future prognosis will be the availability of adequate medical care and patient compliance with medical therapy.

Areas of Future Research. The long-term prevention and cure of ulcers by antibiotics is being studied and is promising. Vaccines given either orally or by injection for protection against *H. pylori* gastric infections are being investigated and would be future tools for public health treatment of large populations. At present there are no satisfactory ways to reverse the symptoms of "dumping" after surgical resection of the stomach.

Gallstones

Twenty-five million Americans—more than 10 percent of the population—have gallstones. Every year, one million more people are diagnosed with gallstones. Six thousand people will die from gallstone complications this year. Gallstone disease costs Americans $1.5 billion annually. Each year 500,000 persons have their gallstones removed. It is the fifth most common operation in the United States.

Gallstones are lumps of solid material that form in the gallbladder, precipitated from chemicals in the bile. Stones form because bile is oversaturated with cholesterol, or because the gallbladder does not empty properly, or because the bile becomes infected. Gallstones are more common with obesity; diabetes; for those on a high fat diet; and with American Indians.

Symptoms. A great many people have gallstones but do not have symptoms—so-called silent gallstones. However, during an acute attack of gallstones, there is severe, steady pain in the upper abdomen for minutes to hours, with nausea and vomiting and often fever and yellow jaundice.

Diagnosis. Diagnosis is made by clinical exam with laboratory assistance of ultrasound of the gallbladder. Occasionally an X-ray picture of the gallbladder and bile ducts is necessary. This is done by needle injection into the liver or by a flexible tube passed through the mouth and stomach to inject dye into the opening of the bile duct. This procedure is termed endoscopic retrograde cholangiopancreatography (ERCP).

Therapy. Surgical removal of the gallbladder (cholecystectomy) is by far the most common type of treatment for persons who develop gallstone complications. Recent advances in laparoscopic surgery allow gallbladder removal quickly, safely and with only one to three days in the hospital. The low incidence of complications and a quick return to work after such a laparoscopic surgery are encouraging.

Ultrasonic fracture of gallstones (lithotripsy) is practiced at some centers, but the procedure still leaves the gallbladder intact so that gallstones can reform after the procedure. Laparoscopic gallbladder surgery has leapfrogged over medical therapy, chemical dissolution of gallstones by catheter placement in the gallbladder, and lithotripsy to be the treatment of choice for inflammation of the gallbladder (cholecystitis).

Complications and Disability. Without surgery, chronic gallbladder disease leads to recurrent episodes of pain; fever; jaundice; and, in a small percent of cases, gallbladder cancer.

A person can live quite well without a gallbladder. However, the chronic discharge of bile into the upper digestive tract increases twofold the risk of gastritis (inflammation of the stomach lining) and esophageal reflux (heartburn). These postoperative symptoms often cause dyspepsia and a five- to ten-pound weight loss, but rarely any disability.

Complications of surgery, whether open or of the laparoscopic type, are fortunately uncommon but can be devastating and deadly—infection, jaundice, and liver failure. Remedial surgery is often the therapy of choice in these situations, with dietary and nutritional support adjunctive.

Inflammatory Bowel Disease (IBD)

This is a collection of chronic inflammatory diseases that involve the digestive tract, and include ulcerative proctitis, chronic ulcerative colitis, and Crohn's disease of the large and small bowel. It is not known what causes these diseases. Their treatment is based on observation, but the outcome of such treatment cannot be predicted.

Crohn's disease may affect any part of the bowel, from the mouth to the anus, and it involves the full thickness of the bowel wall. Ulcerative colitis affects the inner surface (mucosa) of the colon. Ulcerative colitis can be cured by surgical excision of the colon, whereas Crohn's disease cannot be surgically cured. Ulcerative colitis rates have been stable for decades, whereas Crohn's disease new-case rates have been rising dramatically in the Western world since the early 1940s.

Both types of IBD occur predominantly in Western or developed countries. People of Jewish ancestry have an unusually high frequency of both diseases, while persons of African or Asian ancestry have low incidences. There appears to be a genetic factor as well as an environmental factor that causes the disease, and very often a trigger factor for specific relapses. Both diseases affect both sexes equally and all age groups. IBD affects one in five hundred persons in the United States.

Both diseases cause inflammation of the bowel surface, with resulting diarrhea with mucus and blood, variable weight loss, weakness and dehydration, and, in Crohn's disease, abdominal pain. When IBD occurs in children, it can cause growth retardation. Parallel models of inflammatory diseases of the digestive tract occur in many animals, and the approach in diagnosis and therapy is similar to that in humans.

Diagnosis. This is made by complete history and exam, and confirming evidence of barium X rays and/or endoscopic exam of the colon and intestine. There is no known prevention for IBD and no way to test for those susceptible to IBD.

Therapy. This is aimed at suppressing the severity of each flare-up of IBD and avoiding known triggers for it (e.g., ibuprofen). Control of IBD symptoms is achieved by regulation of diet and medication. The patient is advised to avoid anything he or she knows to be irritating. Meanwhile, good nutrition should be maintained with repletion of any weight loss or nutritional deficiencies (e.g., folic acid, magnesium, calcium). Predigested nutritional supplements are used liberally by mouth and day/ night feeding tubes. At various times in the course of IBD, bowel rest and total parenteral nutrition or oral supplemental alimentation may be used.

Medications. Basic medications include corticosteroids, antibiotics for acute and chronic inflammation, and anti-inflammatory agents (Azulfidine and 5-ASA), and immunosuppressive drugs. Hospital-ization for control of active IBD is often warranted and successful.

When medical and nutritional therapy is inadequate, surgery may be used to control the disease or remove other irreversibly damaged segments of bowel. Surgery for ulcerative colitis is needed in only 20 percent of patients and usually involves resection of the damaged colon. Surgery for Crohn's disease usually is only for complications such as bowel obstruction, or gastrointestinal bleeding, or to resect a permanently damaged segment of bowel. When surgery is necessary, the results are good and the quality of life is improved.

Sometimes a colostomy or ileostomy (opening into the abdomen to drain feces from the colon or small intestines with an external bag device) may be necessary. The freedom from pain, frequent trips to the bathroom, and embarrassing incontinence make this type of surgery worthwhile.

Psychological and social aspects of disability are especially important factors in IBD. There are major differences here for disability as seen by the IBD patient, by caregivers, and by agencies charged with managing the disability caused by IBD. A patient may sense a disabling dysfunction pertaining to basic human cleanliness, such as anal incontinence, leakage of odor from ostomy, sexual dysfunction or loss of sexual attractiveness, or fear of incontinence.

Weakness or loss of energy, slowness of action, and loss of mental motivation may be sensed by the IBD patient, but only weight loss and anemia can be measured by a certifying agency.

In a disease involving relapse, such as IBD, loss of health security is the reason patients are often afraid to risk a new job, with possible loss of health benefits. Promotions may be declined if it means the patient will be moved from the vicinity of a familiar bathroom, or if he or she must present in front of people when an incontinence episode might occur. IBD patients often sense loss of well-being and personhood. These factors are not immediately evident to the caregiver or disability screener, unless they are probed. Health security in a full sense is essential for full work performance.

Disability and Rehabilitation. IBD comprises chronic diseases that have relapses of various durations and severity for the life of the patient. IBD patients have normal length of life; the few deaths from IBD and associated bowel cancer are offset by the somewhat lower incidence of cardiovascular disease because of mild malnutrition and associated low serum cholesterol.

Each year in Germany, 3 percent of all employees with IBD are granted disability pensions (1987). An American survey of 1200 IBD patients showed that a total of 8 percent received disability payments (1987). This is a lifetime average: three-quarters with Social Security, and one-quarter via private pensions.

German social security statistics show that 7 percent of IBD patients undergo job rehabilitation each year; 87 percent were still employed before rehabilitation and 72 percent improved after rehabilitation; 84 percent went back to the same job after rehabilitation. The success rate for rehabilitation was slightly lower with IBD than with other major diseases in the social security system. IBD patients had a greater need for medical and vocational measures, and yet fewer than 5 percent of German IBD patients became permanently disabled and fewer than 10 percent of IBD patients were unemployed (1975).

The benefits are evident for vigorous medical and vocational rehabilitation begun early in the IBD disability, and reinforced as the disease relapses.

Ostomics

These may be created after bowel or bladder surgery or cancer surgery. In the 1950s, U.K. studies showed that one of the more common causes of death for persons who had had ostomies was suicide. Since then, improved surgical ostomy techniques; new and easier-to-use appliances; and, more recently, continent ileostomy and ileoanal anastomosis have made the life of IBD patients close to normal.

Preoperative planning for the ostomy includes patient education and patient participation in choosing the ostomy site, appliances, etc. Enterostomal therapists are specially trained medical staff members who themselves have had an ostomy. They are the primary teachers and organizers of postoperative education and support for the new ostomy patient. Ostomy support groups meet regularly and have hospital visitation programs in most major hospitals and communities. They are invaluable for the patient's full recovery of health and self-worth.

Functional Gastrointestinal (GI) Disorders

These are defined as variable combinations of chronic and recurrent gastrointestinal symptoms not explained by structural or biochemical abnormalities. They include symptoms attributed to the pharynx, esophagus, stomach, gallbladder, small and large intestines, and anorectum. A recent study reported 30 percent of Americans as having at least one of the twenty functional GI syndromes in the prior three months. Females reported greater frequency of swallowing disorders, irritable bowel, functional constipation, and abdominal pain. Males reported greater frequency in aerophagia and functional bloating. The study reports that all symptoms, except for incontinence, decline with age. Low income is associated with greater symptom reporting. Work/school absenteeism and physician visits are more frequent in those having a functional GI disorder. The greatest rates of absenteeism are associated with fecal incontinence and more painful functional GI disorders.

Evaluations of patients with functional diet disorders reveal organic diseases such as acute cholecystitis, peptic ulcer, colon cancer, and lactase deficiency. Prior studies have noted the incidence of functional GI symptoms, identical for patients who did see a doctor and for patients who did not make office visits. Those who came in for office visits for evaluation often had associated anxiety and depression.

The financial impact for the diagnosis and care of functional GI symptoms is staggering. Medication use is into the hundreds of millions of dollars for self-care of these disorders. There is still controversy among physicians as to how extensive the workup should be to rule out organic diseases in patients with functional GI disorders. For now, there is more controversy than consensus for therapy of such patients. Therapies are wide-ranging, and range from tranquilizers, antimotility drugs, acupuncture, and individual psychotherapy, to judicious neglect.

Resource, Future Developments, and Issues in Gastroenterology

Dramatic breakthroughs have occurred in the area of digestive and liver diseases since the early 1970s. The results have been as follows:

1. Dramatic control of peptic ulcer disease and reflux esophagitis by acid-suppressing drugs, resulting in a rapid decline in the number of hospitalizations and duration of hospitalizations for peptic ulcer, as well as a rapid decline in the number of cases of gastric resection for intractable ulcer disease. This has resulted in many fewer persons becoming disabled as a result of stomach resection.

2. New understanding of peptic ulcer disease caused by the parasite *H. pylori*. The 14-day antibiotic therapy for peptic ulcer results in cures in 85 percent of cases.

3. The 87 percent decrease in the number of deaths from Crohn's disease because of modern medical therapy with antibiotics and immunosuppressant drugs as well as modern surgery. Parenteral nutrition and the "artificial gut" have prevented deaths from a short bowel. Patients are able to go back to gainful employment with a full family life.

4. Organ transplant surgery is a fact of life for chronic and terminal liver diseases for which there was no medical or surgical hope. There is excellent one-year and five-year survival data for liver transplants. This has changed the therapy of liver diseases from hopeless to hopeful.

5. Parenteral nutrition programs for both short-term therapy and chronic maintenance have improved patient survival and quality of life. They are an integral part of preoperative and postoperative care.

We can look forward to the medical and surgical developments in organ transplants for end-stage diseases of the pancreas as well as total gut transplants for patients with congenital or acquired digestive disorders. New vaccines will be developed for treatment of hepatitis C. There will be widespread application of hepatitis B vaccines, with eradication of hepatitis B and associated liver cancer. There will be developments in the area of *H. pylori* treatment, with probable oral vaccinations for eradication of *H. pylori* infections.

We all look forward to the day when the dreaded enigma of inflammatory bowel disease will be understood, giving us therapies for complete cure and prevention of IBD. Until such time we will rely on successful programs of long-term medical and surgical treatments. We need common sense rehabilitation programs based on medical/clinical and psychosocial criteria aimed at restoring patients to gainful work and complete family life.

(*See also:* ENDOCRINE DISORDERS; PHARMACOLOGY; PSYCHOSOCIAL ADJUSTMENT; SURGERY; WELLNESS)

RESOURCES

Center for Ulcer Research and Education Foundation (CURE), 1166 San Vincente Blvd., Suite 304, Los Angeles, CA 90049

Crohn's and Colitis Foundation of America, 386 Park Ave. South, New York, NY, 10016–7374

Functional Brain—Gut Research (for functional GI disorders), University of North Carolina, School of Medicine, 420 Burnett-Womack Building, Chapel Hill, NC 27599–7080

The American Liver Foundation, 1425 Pompton Ave., Cedar Grove, NJ 07009

The National Digestive Diseases Education Information Clearing House, 2 Information Way, Bethesda, MD 20892

The Simon Foundation for Continence, P.O. Box 835, Wilmette, IL 60091

United Ostomy Association, 2001 West Beverly Blvd., Los Angeles, CA 90057

BIBLIOGRAPHY

AMERICAN MEDICAL ASSOCIATION. *Guides to the Evaluation of Permanent Impairment*, 4th ed. Chicago, 1993.

CUNNICK, W. R.; EIDE, K.; SMITH, J.; "Digestive Disease as a National Problem, IV; Disability Claim Study of Digestive Diseases." *Gastroenterology* 54 (1968):246–252.

ORCES, H.; FELDMAN, J.; GARDNER, B.; and ALPHONSO, A. "Analysis of Patient Disability After Curative Resection for Colonic and Rectal Cancer." *American Journal of Surgery* 131 (1976):98–102.

SHERLOCK, SHEILA, ed. *Diseases of Liver and Biliary System*, 8th ed. Oxford, England, 1988.

SLEISENGER, MARVIN H., and FORDTRAN, JOHN S. *Gastrointestinal Disease*, 4th ed. Philadelphia, 1989.

SONNBERG, A. "Disability and Need for Rehabilitation Among Patients with Inflammatory Bowel Disease." *Digestion* 51 (1992):168–178.

STOWE, STEPHEN, and REDMOND, STEPHEN. "An Epidemiologic Study of Inflammatory Bowel Disease in

Rochester, New York—Hospital incidence." *Gastroenterology* 98 (1990):104–110.

STOWE, STEPHEN; STORMONT, JAMES; SHAH, ASHOH; CHESSIN, LAWRENCE; SEGAL, HARRY; and CHEY, WILLIAMS. "Communitywide Analysis of IBD in Rochester, New York—January, 1975–December, 1989." *Canadian Journal of Gastroenterology* 7 (1993):149–154.

WILLETT, W. C.; STAMFER, M.; MANSON, J. A.; and VAN ITALLIE, T. "New Weight Guidelines for Americans Justified or Injudicious." *American Journal of Clinical Nutrition* 53 (1991):1102–1103.

STEPHEN P. STOWE

GENETIC DISORDERS

Genetic conditions are common causes for disability, especially severe disability. Genetic conditions that cause a variety of physical and intellectual disabilities may be due to chromosome problems, gene disorders, and conditions that arise from an individual's genetic makeup that lead to susceptibilities or tendencies to have certain kinds of problems.

Biologic Overview

The total genetic composition of an individual is established when sperm and egg nuclei fuse after fertilization. The genetic makeup of a person ordinarily consists of forty-six chromosomes comprised of twenty-three chromosome pairs, one of each pair derived from each parent. The genetic information is packaged within the chromosomes, which are made up of DNA and protein, but the sequence of DNA determines the individual's genetic endowment. Specific DNA segments that control cell and body structures and biologic functions are called genes. An individual's total genetic endowment consists of many genes, perhaps more than 100,000. The DNA in turn consists of chemical compounds called bases that specify the genetic code; the genetic information is translated into various cell capabilities.

Every nucleated body cell contains a copy of the entire genetic material, and although an average size adult consists of about 70,000 billion cells, each cell functions in a specialized way and uses only a fraction of the total genetic complement within its nucleus.

The genetic material is the blueprint for cell function; for embryonic, fetal, and childhood growth and development; and for a lifetime of biological functioning. Genes operate at specific times in embryonic development; some groups of cells influence other cells by synthesizing chemical signals that affect adjacent or remote groups of cells. Genes must function in the correct time and place within the developing organism. Critical functions in development occur during limited periods of opportunity. Once a development period is past, the embryo cannot repeat the step it has missed. Such key intervals make the embryo vulnerable to environmental insults that can affect it adversely at a critical developmental stage.

Environmental agents can mimic genetic effects by adversely affecting embryonic development. For example, the basic architecture of the central nervous system is organized between eighteen and twenty-eight days of embryonic development, when the neural tube forms. Errors made in the formation of the neural tube will lead to permanent problems of the back, spine, or brain and, although possibly amenable to surgical amelioration, never to biological correction. The formation of the neural tube is under the control of several groups of genes, but in addition some individuals require high levels of a B vitamin, folic acid, to form a neural tube properly. The environment can also adversely affect the neural tube, and at least one anticonvulsant, valproic acid, can disrupt neural tube development. Thus neural tube defects, which include spina bifida, meningomyelocele (a protrusion of meninges and spinal cord through a defect in the spinal column), and related malformations, can occur because of gene abnormalities, or because of an inadequate amount of folic acid, or because of an environmental insult. Differentiating the actual tube defect in any specific case is a major challenge.

The culmination of the complicated and essential processes of embryonic and fetal development, all of which are controlled by gene activity, is the birth of an individual capable of biological function for seven to ten decades. If the genetic makeup of a conceptus contains qualitative or quantitative errors of significance, the individual may not successfully complete embryonic or fetal development at all. More than 50 percent of conceptions have major growth or developmental problems and die in the first week or weeks of embryonic existence. Some conditions, even those that are associated with high in-utero mortality, may still be compatible with life and can result in problems evident at birth; however, many genetic conditions may not manifest themselves until later infancy, or childhood, or even adult life.

Chromosome Disorders

Chromosome disorders result from additional chromosomal material or from missing or rearranged chromosomal material in an individual's body cells. If the chromosomal change is only in some cells rather than every cell, the individual is described as a mosaic.

A chromosome is a very compact package of DNA that is wrapped in and around protein so that any abnormality of chromosome number or structure, visible at the light microscope level, involves a significant amount of DNA and, therefore, a large number of genes. The impact of chromosome abnormalities upon the individual is generally significant.

The best known and most common type of chromosome abnormality is trisomy 21, or Down syndrome. In this condition the affected individual has three number 21 chromosomes in all or most body cells, rather than the correct number of two number 21 chromosomes. The chromosome composition, or karyotype, in Down syndrome is 47,XX (for a female) or XY (for a male) +21. Two number 21 chromosomes are derived from one parent and one number 21 is derived from the other parent, instead of the normal situation of one number 21 chromosome being derived from each parent. Trisomy 21 provides an excellent example of variability between individuals with the same condition. About 80 percent of conceptions with trisomy 21 spontaneously die in utero. The surviving Down syndrome children have certain features in common but will vary as much from each other in performance as do children in the "normal range." Cognitive function can be in the low normal range of intelligence down to the profound and severe level; most individuals are in an intermediate range.

Other than the extra chromosomal material, there is virtually no finding that every Down syndrome person will have. About one-half will have a heart abnormality, 5 percent to 6 percent may have a bowel obstruction, most Down syndrome children will be shorter than their siblings, but individual differences are considerable. Although three number 21 chromosomes are the cause of Down syndrome, the remainder of the genetic material will also affect the expression of the condition. Two or 3 percent of children with Down syndrome are mosaics for trisomy 21, with some cells with trisomy and some normal cells. When the only children to have chromosome analysis for Down syndrome were those with obvious, or at least suspicious, clinical findings of the condition, the finding of mosaicism for Down syndrome did not correlate very well with expression of the condition with regard to intellectual handicap or physical problems.

It is far more difficult to predict outcome when mosaicism is discovered by chance during prenatal diagnosis, when the clinical findings are not apparent. Infants with fewer than 40 percent of cells with trisomy 21 have had prominent findings of Down syndrome, while others, with more than 75 percent of cells with trisomy 21, have no obvious clinical findings or mental handicap. The same is true for other chromosomal mosaics. It is likely that mental development varies with the percent of brain cells affected with the chromosome abnormality.

Although trisomy 21 may occur in children whose parents are of any age, the frequency of the condition increases with parental age, especially maternal age. This finding is true for most chromosome abnormalities and is the reason for considering prenatal diagnosis for women who are thirty-five years of age or older. The risk for Down syndrome is about one in 1,667 at a maternal age of twenty, and about one in seven at age fifty.

Unfortunately, there is no cure for Down syndrome, although surgical and medical intervention as necessary, and educational support, can make a significant difference for the child and family. Prenatal diagnosis can detect trisomy 21 in utero, the extent of physical problems can be evaluated by ultrasound examination, and the family can be prepared emotionally for the condition, but prevention is limited to pregnancy termination.

The consequences of other numerical chromosome abnormalities, excepting sex chromosome abnormalities, are generally more severe than trisomy

21. Chromosomal gains or losses on a scale less than an entire chromosome generally have consequences proportional to the amount of chromosomal material involved. Rearrangements of chromosomes where there appears to be no missing or additional chromosome material may lead to problems because of altered relationships between genes within the affected area.

Parents who have a child or fetus with a chromosome abnormality have about a 1 percent recurrence risk for chromosome abnormalities in each future pregnancy.

Sex Chromosome Disorders

One pair of chromosomes in the human set consists of the sex chromosomes. In females these are ordinarily two medium-size chromosomes called X chromosomes. In males the sex chromosomes consist of one X chromosome, derived from the maternal parent, and a much smaller chromosome called the Y chromosome, which is derived from the paternal parent. The X chromosome contains considerable essential genetic information, and at least one X chromosome is necessary for the survival of a cell or of an individual; the Y chromosome contains genetic information that results in male development, but a Y chromosome is not necessary for survival of a cell or a person. The presence of only one X chromosome in males has significant consequences; whatever information is contained in the single X chromosome of a male will be expressed. Females have two X chromosomes and, therefore, two opportunities to have "correct" genetic information for each gene on the X.

Numerical abnormalities of sex chromosomes may result in mild disabilities, such as learning disorders. Some sex chromosome problems may result in sterility, but individuals with numerical abnormalities of sex chromosomes are generally able to function within the mainstream of the population. However, individual scores on performance tests of persons with abnormalities of sex chromosomes are often lower than other siblings in the same family. Persons with sex chromosome abnormalities generally have no problems with gender identification.

The sex chromosome abnormality called Turner's syndrome represents a broad spectrum of consequences for the individual. Turner's syndrome occurs when all or many of an individual's cells contain only one normal X chromosome and there is no other normal sex chromosome (karyotype 45,X). This condition is found in about one in each 3,000 newborn female infants; however, it is much more common during fetal development because more than 90 percent of fetuses with this condition spontaneously die in utero. In spite of a high in-utero death rate, infants who do come to term are generally healthy. This chromosome disorder, unlike all the other sex chromosome abnormalities, does not vary in frequency with parental age, nor does it have an elevated recurrence risk for future pregnancies. It may result from a problem of chromosome division in the cells of the early embryo. Girls with Turner's syndrome are invariably quite short throughout life, and most do not go through puberty without treatment with supplementary female hormones. Height can often be increased to close to five feet by pharmacological treatment, with growth hormone supplemented by an anabolic steroid. Girls with Turner's syndrome may have life-threatening heart problems that should be evaluated in the neonatal period. For the most part, girls with Turner's syndrome do well and blend in with the general population. Although most girls with this condition do not generate eggs, several women with Turner's syndrome have had successful pregnancies using donor eggs.

In the past, certain patterns of behavior were attributed to individuals with various types of sex chromosome abnormalities. Some of the more common sex chromosome abnormalities include the numerical problems designated as 47,XXX ("triplo-X"), 47,XXY (Kleinfelter Syndrome), and 47,XYY (no specific name). It is certainly possible that an individual with a sex chromosome abnormality may differ in behavior from siblings, but it is not possible to make infallible generalizations about the behavior of an individual on the basis of sex chromosome composition alone. Learning disabilities may be more likely, but individuals with these numerical abnormalities of sex chromosomes generally function in the normal range of cognitive development.

All chromosomes abnormalities can be detected by prenatal diagnosis, but prevention is limited to pregnancy termination. A supportive environment, appropriate educational strategies, and indicated medical and surgical intervention will optimize the outcome for the individual with a chromosome abnormality, but the basic chromosome makeup of a person cannot be corrected.

Gene Disorders

The sequence of bases in the segment of DNA that comprises one gene specifies a code that is transcribed and translated into a functional compound. Human genes tend to be large; they average about 16,000 bases long (16 kilobases, Kb), although only part of the gene, the exons, actually code for a final product. Introns are sequences of bases that intervene between the exons. Introns are part of the gene but generally don't become translated into a product. The gene is linear and codes for linear products, but the linear gene product may assume a folded structure before being able to function. Sometimes two or more separate gene products must interact to form a functional structure. In this instance two different genes are necessary to make one functional product. Even a change in one base can significantly alter a gene product. A one-base change is called a point mutation, but many other alterations in a gene are possible. These can include duplications and deletions of segments of DNA, inversions of sequences, and translocated and inserted sequences; any of these changes is called a mutation. Some changes will result in an altered gene product; others may lead to no gene product at all. Sometimes an altered gene product will function as well as the "original" or offer some advantage, but most altered gene products function less well than the normal gene product, and some are not able to function at all. Small changes in a gene, especially in a noncritical area, may not lead to any changes of significance and may be biologically tolerated. Such changes in noncritical areas of the gene will lead to small but insignificant changes in the gene product. However, many small changes lead to genetic diversity in the population and among individuals. The accumulated subtle differences lead to diversity in physical appearance and result in each individual being biologically unique; this is evidenced by the lack of interchangeability of body parts or organs, even between related persons, unless the immune system is artificially suppressed.

The only individuals with the same genetic makeup are identical twins. Identical twins result from the splitting of an early embryo that derives from a single fertilized egg nucleus. Other individuals, even siblings, are essentially unique. Every individual results from a random mix of paternal and maternal genes, so it is not surprising that most genetically determined conditions occur without a prior positive history in a family. Inherited conditions can result from new mutations or from new combinations of genes received from "normal" parents.

Gene disorders are quite diverse in severity and in the effects caused, but they generally occur in three basic patterns of inheritance that are called Mendelian inheritance.

- Conditions that require that only one altered gene be expressed in the individual are called dominant conditions. Many dominant conditions occur as new mutations and, therefore, occur without prior history.
- Conditions that require both genes of a pair to be altered for the condition to manifest itself are called recessive conditions. Recessive conditions are apt to affect siblings, but parents generally have no manifestation of the condition, although each parent is a carrier for the gene. Recessive conditions also often happen without prior family history for the condition.
- Conditions that are determined by genes on the X chromosome are called sex-linked. Most sex-linked conditions are recessive in expression. Males will show these conditions because they have only one X chromosome. A number of essential genes are located on the X chromosome; as a result, males are much more likely to have disabilities determined by sex-linked genes. Sex-linked conditions can be dominant or recessive in expression. Dominant and recessive conditions that are not sex-linked are called autosomal conditions.

Recessive Conditions

Hundreds of conditions follow the pattern of autosomal recessive inheritance. There are no practicable tests for the carrier state for most of these conditions. As a result, often the first evidence for a couple to be at risk is the discovery of an affected child. Four examples will be used to illustrate the variation of autosomal recessive conditions: PKU, cystic fibrosis, sickle cell disease, and lysosomal storage diseases.

PKU or phenylketonuria affects about one in 20,000 infants. These children lack an enzyme that metabolizes an amino acid, phenylalanine. Phenylalanine is an essential dietary ingredient because it is a building block of human and animal protein and cannot be synthesized de novo. However, high levels of phenylalanine and its by-products are neurotoxic and cause irreversible mental retardation and seizures. If a child is identified with PKU in the first months of life, and put on a diet very restrictive in phenylalanine for life, he or she can otherwise be totally normal. A lifelong diet virtually free from meat and dairy products is heroic but possible.

The availability of diagnosis and treatment for PKU motivated the first population-based newborn screening for a genetic disease. This successful program has been a model for screening and intervention in genetics. Most states test every newborn infant for PKU and institute treatment as soon as possible for those affected. Treatment and follow-up for adolescents and adults can be a problem, however, because health insurance may not cover the special dietary products or blood phenylalanine monitoring. Simple carrier testing of the general population for PKU is not yet available, but prenatal diagnosis is possible. As with all autosomal recessive conditions, once parents are identified as carriers, each pregnancy has a 25 percent chance for resulting in an affected child.

Cystic fibrosis affects about one child in 2,000. The gene for cystic fibrosis is 250 Kb long and consists of twenty-four exons. Mutations anywhere in the gene can cause the disease. The most common site of mutation is known and can be screened by molecular techniques. Mutations at other sites in the gene require laborious analysis and may be missed. Cystic fibrosis adversely affects all the secretory glands of the body and can lead to digestive problems and difficulties in keeping air passages in the lungs free from mucous plugs. Cystic fibrosis does not cause mental retardation but can lead to lifelong disability and dependence on constant medical in-

tervention in many cases. The standard, current treatment consists of antibiotics and pulmonary treatment to prevent pneumonia, and oral intake of enzymes with food to aid in digestion. The condition often leads to premature death from complications, generally of the lungs. Experimental treatments of the lung with synthetic gene product are in progress. Population screening for the mutation that causes cystic fibrosis is possible and can identify about 80 percent of the mutations that lead to the condition. The other 20 percent of carriers have a mutation elsewhere in the gene, and these may be missed during screening. Prenatal diagnosis for the condition is possible if the mutation is identified.

PKU and cystic fibrosis occur in all groups of people but are more common in persons of European ancestry than in people of African ancestry. In contrast, sickle cell disease occurs in people of southern and eastern Mediterranean ancestry, but is much more common in people of African ancestry. In the United States about 1 in 600 African Americans has sickle cell disease. The gene for beta hemoglobin is small (1.6 Kb) and is completely sequenced. Sickle cell disease is always due to the same point mutation and can be identified by molecular gene testing as well as by gene product analysis. Nonetheless, the clinical expression of the condition is very variable and can range from anemia to more serious problems, including circulatory complications that may be life-threatening. Sickle cell disease is treatable, but a cure is possible only at great risk. Bone marrow transplant can potentially cure sickle cell disease by replacing the marrow of an affected individual with normal marrow. However, the mortality from this method is more than 30 percent, and patients and professionals seem unenthusiastic about such a risky approach. Newborn screening for sickle cell disease has been instituted in many states because early detection of the condition and subsequent daily treatment with antibiotics prevent infant and childhood death from infections associated with the disease.

Sickle cell disease represents one of the inherent properties of inherited conditions, namely that some diseases disproportionately affect an identifiable subset of the population. Such group-clustered diseases are challenging from a social, ethical, and political perspective and require significant sensitivity when one is considering programs or interventions.

PKU, cystic fibrosis, and sickle cell disease are serious conditions, but early identification and early treatment can lessen the burden of the disease on the individual, the family, and society. The lysosomal storage diseases are a group of serious illnesses that result from enzyme deficiencies within cells. Cells are unable to break down various intracellular chemicals that accumulate within cell structures called lysosomes; this accumulation eventually leads to cell death. Lysosomal storage diseases often result in progressive loss of physical and intellectual capabilities and ultimately result in death. These conditions are theoretically amenable to enzyme replacement therapy or gene therapy, but they are almost invariably fatal. Prenatal diagnosis is possible but generally only after one affected child is already born.

Although many of these conditions are eventually lethal, affected individuals can live for years with slow progression, including plateaus and exacerbations, of the disease over decades. Conditions of this type challenge the commitment and sincerity of educational programs aimed at helping people with disabilities. Teachers become discouraged when they realize that the disease is progressive. Abandonment by the professional, educational, and medical communities is a real problem with individuals that are so affected.

Dominant Conditions

Dominant conditions arise from new mutations or are inherited from an affected parent. Dominant conditions can vary in severity even when the mutation in the gene is the same from parent to child. An affected parent has a 50 percent risk for each child to receive the abnormal gene. Two autosomal dominant conditions will be used for illustration: neurofibromatosis (NF) and Huntington's disease (HD).

NF affects about one in 3,000 persons. The condition is associated with multiple tumors, including skin and nerve sheath tumors, some of which may become malignant. Occasionally but not typically the condition leads to mental retardation. Some individuals with NF have only large tan freckles (café

au lait spots), while others, even in the same family, may have multiple disfiguring skin nodules, skeletal deformities, and life-threatening tumors. The gene has been identified on a molecular level; however, treatment is still symptomatic.

Huntington's disease is an example of a late-onset condition. It affects about one in each 40,000 persons, but onset is typically after a person's reproductive years. The molecular nature of the gene is known, but no treatment exists. Affected individuals slowly lose function in the central nervous system; they have impaired speech, impaired coordination, movement problems, and altered mental thought processes. Many individuals who develop HD live productive lives before symptoms limit function; nonetheless, HD is viewed with greater fear and apprehension than most other inherited conditions. This attitude seems to be a problem for professionals as well as for persons and families living with the effects of HD.

Sex-Linked Conditions

The majority of sex-linked disorders are recessive and primarily affect males. If a woman is a carrier, 50 percent of her sons will receive the affected sex-linked gene and develop the condition, and 50 percent of her daughters will be carriers, like their mother. Two sex-linked conditions will be used for illustration: X-linked mental retardation (or "Fragile X" syndrome, "FraX") and hemophilia.

FraX syndrome affects about one in 1,500 in males. The condition derives its name from the finding, with light microscopy, of an apparent chromosome break, near the end of the long arm of the X chromosome, in many males affected with the condition. The fragile site or break is not always present in all affected persons and is sometimes seen in female relatives. Although some females show the mental retardation, many do not. Symptoms include mental retardation, especially disproportionate delays in expressive language, and sometimes "autistic" behavior. There are no absolute identifying physical findings, but some males have prominent jaws and ears and develop large testicles (macroorchidism) after puberty. The gene is altered by a series of tandem base repeats in the DNA near the end of the long arm of an X chromosome. The longer the sequence of repeated bases, the more severe the expression of the condition and the more likely the fragile site on the X chromosome will be visible with light microscopy. An explanation for differences in the length of the base segment repeats in the same family is not clear, but the more repeats the greater the likelihood of a person being affected, including females. There is no cure for FraX syndrome. Treatment is educational and supportive.

Classical hemophilia is due to an absence of clotting factor VIII. Factor VIII is controlled by a large gene that consists of twenty-six exons and is about 186 KB long. Mutations can occur anywhere in the gene, and each affected family seems to have a unique or "private" mutation that is peculiar to the one family. This makes testing for the gene difficult and time-consuming until the specific mutation is discovered. Males affected with factor VIII deficiency have severe problems with bleeding and can have loss of joint function because of spontaneous bleeding. Treatment has been available for many years, although a cure is not available. Until 1985, treatment was with factor VIII extracted from human blood, but since 1986, treatment has been with "synthetic," genetic-engineered factor VIII. Before 1986, factor VIII was extracted from pooled donor blood, it required 1,000 to 2,000 donors for one treatment vial. A bleeding episode might require six or a dozen or more treatments to achieve control of bleeding, thus exposing the recipients to thousands of donors. As a result, many males who received pooled factor VIII before 1986 also received the human immunodeficiency virus (HIV) and now have AIDS. This has been a sobering complication in genetic replacement therapy.

Novel and Non-Mendelian Inheritance

Several non-Mendelian mechanisms for inheritance have been discovered. Mitochondria are DNA-containing, self-replicating, cell organelles that are essential for the respiratory function of every cell. All of a person's mitochondria are derived from the egg cytoplasm; therefore they are all maternal in origin. At least one condition of blindness (Leber optic atrophy) is due to a mutation in the maternal mitochrondrial DNA. This is called mitochrondrial inheritance. Conditions inherited in this manner can affect every child of an affected mother.

Some genes are affected by the sex of the parent who has donated the gene to the child. This mechanism is called imprinting. An example of imprinting is afforded by two dissimilar conditions resulting from what seems to be a deletion of bases in the gene, depending on whether the gene comes from the mother or the father. In Prader-Willi syndrome, a paternally derived deletion in a small area of a number 15 chromosome leads to obesity and mental retardation but reasonable language and social skills. When the same deletion is derived from the maternal 15, the condition is called Angleman syndrome. The latter condition is associated with severe mental retardation, an unusual type of shaky gait (ataxia), and virtually no expressive language. Probably most genes do not undergo imprinting, but it is a complication that makes analysis of gene structure and function difficult.

Still another novel mechanism for inheritance is called unparental disomy. This condition happens when one parent is the source of both chromosomes in a group and the other parent, for reasons not understood, has not contributed a chromosome in that group. This condition can be a mechanism for a child developing a recessive condition when only one parent is a carrier—that is, the parent who has contributed both chromosomes in the group.

Effects of Multiple Genes and Genetic Susceptibility

Single gene disorders are amenable to study by family history and molecular analysis of affected persons and their relatives. Conditions that are associated with multiple genes or even the entire genetic makeup are much more difficult to analyze. Because genes enter into new and unique combinations in each individual, predictions about general outcomes, rather than the operation of a single gene, are virtually impossible. Since the mid-1970s, maternal serum folic acid level has been suspected in playing a role in the development of neural tube defects such as spina bifida in some families. Formation and closure of the neural tube are dependent on a number of genes; increased intake of folic acid can prevent at least 70 percent of these defects. Although the mechanism of action is not known, the empiric data have motivated enactment of public health measures to increase the folic acid intake of women who are likely to become pregnant.

Susceptibility to cancer, heart disease, hypertension, diabetes, and other common diseases probably stems from clusters of genes, but analysis and exact prediction of outcomes for such wide spectra of genes await future analysis.

Screening for Genetic Disease

The success of some types of widespread population screening for inherited diseases has made this a popular approach with broad health appeal. A successful screening program should be based on a reliable test, easily applied on a wide scale, that has few false positives and few or no false negatives. Needless to say, there should be an available and acceptable intervention that appreciably changes the outcome of the illness. As is often the case, though, diagnostic capabilities outstrip treatment possibilities. Many genetic tests will be available as a result of the federally sponsored Human Genome Project, which is an international effort to identify all base sequences in each human chromosome and, therefore, in every gene. However, carrier screening and presymptomatic testing for genetic disease or predisposition to disease must be viewed with caution. In the past, individuals discovered to be asymptomatic carriers for recessive conditions have been subjects of prejudice and discrimination, and have found the process embarrassing at best or even emotionally handicapping. There has been very mixed acceptance of presymptomatic testing for serious diseases, such as Huntington's disease and hereditary cancer in individuals who are at risk for having the genes for these conditions.

During a period of transition in methods for paying for health care, any circumstance that could identify a person or a family to be at increased risk for special health care needs, habilitation, or rehabilitation service may be a real disincentive for the family to seek testing.

There is also a strong emotional component for any disease or condition that seems to be "preprogrammed" in nature and that may not be controllable by lifestyle or behavior. Parents can experience immobilizing guilt if a child is found to have an inherited disease. Working with such families requires sensitivity and skill in alleviating guilt and in educating the parents so their efforts with the affected family members can be productive and positive.

Support for the Severely Affected Individual

In a society that no longer tolerates depriving seriously affected persons of oxygen, water, food, warmth, and basic comfort, individuals with serious problems will survive, sometimes indefinitely. Infants with severe disabilities, such as those with lysosomal storage diseases or some severe chromosome disorders, may survive to school age and beyond. Families have appropriately become strong advocates for their children, but often when resources seem scarce, services for people with disabilities shrink. A quarter of a century of emphasis on the utilization of the least restrictive environment for children with disabilities has led us, in some instances, to a cynical use of mainstream education with heterogeneous grouping of students without regard to the needs of persons with physical or mental disabilities. Federal and private funds for categorical diseases put one worthy group against another, but when attempts are made to combine diverse conditions under the rubric of "genetics," the emotional impact of individual conditions is lost and funding is diminished. Professionals, educators, counselors, and clinicians all have difficulty facing progressive diseases for which palliation, or making the person comfortable, is the only available strategy. This situation warrants efforts to recognize and support families and affected individuals who must cope with the condition, sometimes for many years. A commitment to the humanity and worth of every person must be maintained by caregivers and educators.

Organizations Relevant to Genetics

The multimillion-dollar Human Genome Project ("HUGO"), funded through the National Institutes of Health, is an exciting basic science adventure, but it does not provide service or intervention with genetic disorders. The derived benefits from this project are in the future. Three percent of the HUGO budget is set aside for studies involving ethical issues evoked by new genetic technology, but the diagnostic capabilities of the project will precede any treatment possibilities by many years. Federal and state funding for genetic services has come through maternal and child health block grants and short-term funds for special projects of regional and national significance from the Bureau of Maternal and Child Health. For many years the National Foundation-March of Dimes has funded activities in genetics, but their supported activities are now mostly research and educational. Parent support groups have become active; each has a specific disease focus, but coalitions of such groups have been organized. The Alliance of Genetic Support Groups is notable in this regard.

Genetic services are not yet integrated into mainstream medicine; knowledge of genetics is not yet viewed as a relevant component of medical practice, nor of education, nursing, social work, or other disciplines that will deal with individuals who have genetic conditions. Nevertheless, the HUGO Project will produce information about human disease and predisposition to disease that will challenge science, medicine, and education for the next century.

(See also: DEVELOPMENTAL DISABILITIES; GROWTH DISORDERS; MENTAL RETARDATION; RESPIRATORY DISEASE; SICKLE CELL ANEMIA AND THALASSEMIA)

RESOURCES

Alliance of Genetic Support Groups, 35 Wisconsin Circle, Suite 440, Chevy Chase, MD 20815

American College of Medical Genetics, 9650 Rockville Pike, Bethesda, MD 20814–3998

March of Dimes Birth Defects Foundation, 1275 Mamaroneck Ave., White Plains, NY 10605

BIBLIOGRAPHY

ALLIANCE OF GENETIC SUPPORT GROUPS. Directory of National Genetic Voluntary Organizations and Related Resources (see RESOURCES), 1992.

BEHRMAN, R. E., and KLIEGMAN, R. M. Nelson Essentials of Pediatrics, 2d ed. Philadelphia, 1994.

LEWIN, B. Genes V. Oxford, England, 1994.

MILUNSKY, A. Heredity and Your Family's Health. Baltimore, 1992.

WAGNER, R. P.; MAGUIRE, M. P.; and STALLINGS, R. L. Chromosomes. New York, 1993.

R. STEPHEN AMATO

GROWTH DISORDERS

In children, a fundamental yet sensitive assessment of health is the process of growth, including head circumference, weight, and linear stature. The latter is first measured in terms of "length" in the infant and then by "height" in the older child and adolescent. Linear growth arguably reflects health status better than the other two growth measurements; head growth is highly prioritized, and weight can fluctuate dramatically with acute illness.

Disorders of growth may first bring the child to the attention of pediatric health care providers and others. The short-statured or growth-retarded child is brought in more often than is the child with excessive growth, but both types of growth disturbances may signal underlying disease, and each has unique physical, emotional, and psychosocial complications.

The definition of the abnormally growing child is variable and depends on geographic, community, and societal norms, but most pediatric endocrinologists consider the child to have abnormal growth if the height or weight falls outside 2.0 standard deviations from the mean for age and gender, thus less than the third percentile or greater than the ninety-seventh percentile. Therefore, standardized growth charts for the population served are required.

Short children may be proportionally or disproportionally small. Often the terms "midget" or "dwarf," respectively, are used broadly, albeit imprecisely and inappropriately, to describe these growth patterns. Similarly, the child with excessive growth is often labeled a "giant."

Types and Etiologies of Growth Disorders

A complete discussion of all etiologies of short stature is beyond the scope of this entry; reviews are available (Grunt & Schwartz, 1992). However, in broadest terms, the growth-retarded child may be categorized into one of three groups: (1) intrinsic short stature; (2) constitutional delay in growth and development (CDGD); and (3) systemic disease-related.

The child with intrinsic short stature usually is

growing to his or her fullest potential; greater height is limited due to familial/genetic or perinatal factors such as intrauterine growth retardation caused by a variety of conditions. In these children skeletal maturation (bone age) is usually commensurate with chronologic age. A subgroup is often referred to as having "significant idiopathic short stature." Children with CDGD are often "late bloomers" and typically achieve an eventual final adult height within the range of normal, with a corresponding late-adolescent growth spurt; in extreme cases growth may continue beyond age twenty. In CDGD bone age is usually within 75 percent of chronologic age. Children with significant nutritional or emotional illness; major skeletal, cardiopulmonary, gastrointestinal, or renal disease; or underlying endocrine disorders comprise the group with systemic disease–related growth retardation. Primary bone and cartilage disorders can cause disproportional growth of the limbs as seen in achondroplasia and similar conditions, grouped together as chondrodystrophies. Endocrine disorders include, but are not limited to, growth hormone (GH) deficiency or inactivity, hypothyroidism, rickets, and glucocorticoid excess, and in girls, Turner's syndrome (gonadal dysgenesis) as well as other more uncommon disorders.

The child with tall stature usually follows a familial pattern. Somewhat more serious genetic conditions associated with tall stature include Klinefelter syndrome (in boys) as well as Marfan syndrome and homocystinuria, which share many physical characteristics. Metabolic conditions that lead to tall stature in childhood include simple obesity, hyperthyroidism, precocious puberty, and rare cases of GH excess.

Evaluation of the Child with a Growth Disorder

Many children with significant growth disorders are vulnerable to diverse developmental, social, and educational problems, substantiating the importance of a multidisciplinary treatment approach that includes a comprehensive psychological and medical assessment. This includes a thorough history, beginning with the perinatal history, including birth weight and length. Abnormal neonatal edema in a female may lead to a diagnosis of Turner's syndrome. The longitudinal growth pattern is essential: during childhood, the growth needed to maintain height relative to peers is approximately two to three inches per year. Although an increase or decrease in growth on the growth chart is common in the first year or so of life, normal growth curves are usually maintained after age two. A history of central nervous system injury or insult may indicate disorders of the hypothalamic-pituitary axis. A complete and careful physical examination will assess for proportional growth, limb lengths, neurologic and intellectual development, and pubertal development as described by James Tanner (1975), as well as for characteristic physical signs suggesting a specific illness, condition, or eponymic syndrome.

Diagnostic laboratory evaluation begins with radiographic assessment of bone age. In the growth-retarded child, other screening parameters include general blood tests to assess anemia, inflammation, kidney and liver function, and measurement of thyroid hormone and thyroid stimulating hormone. In significantly short girls, a complete karyotype (chromosomal characteristics of a cell) is warranted to exclude gonadal dysgenesis (defective development of the reproductive glands that produce gametes and include the ovaries and testes) and its variants. After other conditions are excluded, formal evaluation of the child's pituitary secretory dynamics may be warranted. Plain lateral skull X rays will screen for intracerebral calcifications, as might be seen in craniopharyngiomas, the most common form of tumor involving the pituitary gland. Although pituitary anatomy is evaluated definitely with magnetic resonance or computed tomography, these tests are best used after a functional pituitary hormone irregularity is documented.

The diagnostic evaluation of the tall child usually can be guided by the history and physical examination; laboratory studies can confirm a diagnosis of hyperthyroidism or precocious puberty. Assessment of skeletal maturation remains an integral tool. Evaluation for GH excess can be difficult but involves measurement of insulin-like growth factor-I (IGF-I) and GH levels after an oral glucose tolerance test, which remained the standard in the early 1990s.

Disability and Rehabilitation Issues

Society's perception of stature is pervasive; "heightism" describes society's bias toward taller stature. One study of business graduates found a 12.4 percent higher salary in "taller" vs. "shorter" graduates of the same business school (Feldman, 1975). Even our daily lexicon is guilty as we may "belittle" or denote "shortcomings" in others.

Short or tall stature is not a disease in itself but may reflect underlying pathology. Short-statured children have normal overall intelligence compared to normal-statured peers (Siegel, Clopper, and Stabler, 1991). Interestingly, some studies have suggested diminished academic performance in short children, but this may represent observer bias (Siegel, Clopper, and Stabler, 1991). Older studies have suggested specific behavior and "dependency" problems in select groups of growth-retarded children (Roizen, Ekwo, and Gosselink, 1990). Delayed motor skills have been noted in some children with achondroplasia.

Low self-esteem leading to decreased social interactions that result in further social isolation and poor self-image have been described in short children. Short children may become class or neighborhood "pets" or "mascots," may be the target of verbal or physical abuse by peers, or may become "Napoleonic" themselves; becoming a "class clown" is another compensation mechanism. Social isolation may be more apparent in those with skeletal dysplasias, but positive parental attitudes play a vital role in limiting this in these or other short children (Ablon, 1990; Boulton et al., 1991). Before adolescence, most growth-retarded children rate their popularity and physical appearance as satisfactory; social maladaptations become more apparent during adolescence (Siegel, Clopper, and Stabler, 1991).

Parental concerns are often not those immediately addressed by the health care team; tangible "reality" issues encompass physical and emotional limitations such as mobility (learning to ride a bicycle or drive an automobile), dating and marriage, and the ability to find adequate housing (Ablon, 1990). These concerns may be valid, as shown in follow-up studies of adults with growth disorders treated with GH as children: unemployment, marriage rates, and heterosexual relationships were less than national averages, although level of education was similar (Dean et al., 1985; Stabler, 1991). Similar outcomes were reported in follow-up of children with CDGD. Patients with achondroplasia had similar educational experiences as their same-sexed siblings, but while affected males had slightly lower (but statistically insignificant) "occupational scores" compared with their brothers, affected women had significantly lower scores than their nonaffected sisters (Roizen, Ekwo, and Gosselink, 1990). Interestingly, perceived differences may only be highlighted when short or tall patients are treated with GH, androgens, or estrogens, as the "abnormality" is reinforced by virtue of its treatment (Boulton et al., 1991).

Treatment of Growth Disorders

The advent of recombinant DNA technology has resulted in potentially unlimited supplies of human GH. Sufficient quantities are now available not only for the long-term, uninterrupted treatment of GH-deficient children but also for children with Turner syndrome, renal failure, and other non-GH-deficient growth disorders. As of the early 1990s, many of these uses of GH remained in the research setting. Low-dose oxandrolone and estrogen for growth promotion in CDGD and idiopathic short stature have been used for many years.

Children with metabolic bone disorders such as achondroplasia should be considered in a special category for therapy. Leg lengthening is a controversial approach to the treatment of short stature in achondroplasia; an increase of as much as 30 percent of lower limb length may be achieved. The results seem to be quite favorable in Europe (Aldegheri et al., 1988; Vilarrubias, Ginebreda, and Jimeno, 1990); however, there continues to be a question of psychological benefit (Cattaneo et al., 1988; Csapo, 1991). The treatment of children with tall stature is also controversial. Physicians rarely become involved with this problem. If the diagnosis of Marfan syndrome or a pituitary irregularity has been excluded, treatment usually involves large doses of gender-appropriate sex hormone therapy. Rare cases of limb shortening have been described (Grunt & Schwartz, 1992).

Advocacy Groups

In the United States there are several support groups for people with growth disorders, including the Human Growth Foundation, the Turner Syndrome Society, the Little People of America, Klinefelter Syndrome and Associates, the Magic Foundation, the National Marfan Foundation, the Association for Children with Russell-Silver Syndrome, and others.

Future Issues

Increased availability of biosynthetic GH therapy has been associated with increased demand. Many children who do not have classical hypopituitarism may respond to GH therapy. There are those who arguably suggest that children who are "handicapped" (arbitrarily defined as including those whose height is below the first percentile) and GH-responsive are entitled to treatment (Allen & Fost, 1990).

Issues of ethics and expenses for therapies of growth disorders are likely to be raised more often in the future. The annual cost of GH therapy approached $20,000 in 1993; society may feel that there are more appropriate medical uses for such large sums of money. Clinical use of growth-hormone-releasing hormone IGF-I and other growth factors needs to be investigated. Many individuals with growth disorders will benefit most from psychological support. Others may benefit from medical treatment. The responsibility of the health care profession is to determine the most appropriate treatment program for each individual.

(*See also:* CHILDHOOD DISABILITIES; ENDOCRINE DISORDERS; GENETIC DISORDERS; PSYCHOSOCIAL ADJUSTMENT)

RESOURCES

Association of Children with Russell-Silver Syndrome, 22 Hoyt St., Madison, NJ 07940–1604

Human Growth Foundation, 7777 Leesburg Pike, Falls Church, VA 22043

Klinefelter Syndrome and Associates, P.O. Box 119, Roseville, CA 95661–0119

Little People of America, Inc., P.O. Box 9897, Washington, DC 20016

National Marfan Foundation, 382 Main St., Port Washington, NY 11050

Noonan Syndrome Society, 1278 Pine Ave., San Jose, CA 95125

The MAGIC Foundation, 1327 North Harlem Ave., Oak Park, IL 60302

Turner Syndrome Society, 1550 Wayzata Blvd., 768-214, Wayzata, MN 55391

BIBLIOGRAPHY

ABLON, JOAN. "Ambiguity and Difference: Families with Dwarf Children." *Social Science & Medicine* 30 (1990):879–887.

ALDEGHERI, ROBERTO; TRIVELLA, GIANPAOLO; RENZ-BRIVIO, LODOVICO; TESSARI, GIULIO; AGOSTINI, SAULO; and LAVINI, FRANCO. "Lengthening of the Lower Limbs in Achondroplastic Patients: A Comparative Study of Four Techniques." *Journal of Bone & Joint Surgery—British Volume* 70 (1988):69–73.

ALLEN, DAVID B. and FOST, NORMAN C. "Growth Hormone Therapy for Short Stature: Panacea or Pandora's Box?" *Journal of Pediatrics* 117 (1990):16–21.

BOULTON, T. J.; DUNN S. M.; QUIGLEY, C. A.; TAYLOR, J. J.; and THOMPSON, L. "Perception of Self and Short Stature: Effects of Two Years of Growth Hormone Treatment." *Acta Paediatrica Scandinavica-Supplement* 377 (1991):20–27; discussion 28.

CATTANEO, R.; VILLA, A.; CATAGNI, M.; and TENTORI, L. "Limb Lengthening in Achrondroplasia by Ilizarov's Method." *International Orthopaedics* 12 (1988):173–179.

CSAPO, MARG. "Psychosocial Adjustment of Children with Short Stature (Achondroplasia): Social Competence, Behavior Problems, Self-Esteem, Family Functioning, Body Image, and Reaction to Frustrations." *Behavioral Disorders* 16 (1991):219–224.

DEAN, HEATHER J.; MCTAGGART, TERRI L.; FISH, DAVID G.; and FRIESEN, HENRY G. "The Educational, Vocational, and Marital Status of Growth Hormone-Deficient Adults Treated with Growth Hormone During Childhood." *American Journal of Diseases of Children* 139 (1985):1105–1110.

FELDMAN, SAUL D. "The Presentation of Shortness in Every-day Life—Height and Heightism in American Society: Toward a Sociology of Stature." *Life Styles: Diversity in American Society*, eds. Saul D. Feldman and Gerald W. Theilbar. Boston, 1975.

GRUNT, JEROME A. and SCHWARTZ, I. DAVID. "Growth, Short Stature, and the Use of Growth Hormone: Considerations for the Practicing Pediatrician." *Current Problems in Pediatrics* 22 (1992): 390–412.

ROIZEN, NANCY; EKWO, EDEM; and GOSSELINK, CAROL. "Comparison of Education and Occupation of Adults with Achondroplasia with Same-Sex Sibs." *American Journal of Medical Genetics* 35 (1990):257–260.

SIEGEL, P. T.; CLOPPER, R.; and STABLER, B. "Psychological Impact of Significantly Short Stature." *Acta Paediatrica Scandinavica—Supplement* 377 (1991):14–18.

STABLER, BRIAN. "Growth Hormone Insufficiency During Childhood Has Implications for Later Life." *Acta Paediatrica Scandinavica—Supplement* 377 (1991):9–13.

TANNER, JAMES M. "Growth and Endocrinology of the Adolescent." *Endocrine and Genetics Diseases of Childhood and Adolescence*, ed. Lytt I. Gardner. Philadelphia, 1975.

VILARRUBIAS, J. M.; GINEBREDA, I.; and JIMENO, E. "Lengthening of the Lower Limbs and Correction of Lumbar Hyperlordosis in Achondroplasia." *Clinical Orthopaedics* (1990):143–149.

CAMPBELL P. HOWARD
I. DAVID SCHWARTZ

359

H

HEAD INJURY

In the United States, the leading cause of death and disability among people under twenty-four years of age is head injury, also commonly known as traumatic brain injury or acquired brain injury. A traumatic head injury occurs every fifteen seconds, with a death every five minutes (*Interagency Head Injury Task Force Report*, February 1989). Although definitions vary according to source, a head injury is usually considered a traumatic injury to the brain, either open or closed. An open head injury is usually the product of penetrating or acceleration-deceleration injury of the head, with traumatic damage to the brain and a visible, open wound. An acceleration–deceleration injury to the brain occurs when a seated human being is rapidly accelerated in the horizontal plane with the body restrained. A deceleration injury is caused by the transition from uniform linear motion to a maximum deceleration or jolt to the brain. A closed head injury is usually a by-product of acceleration or deceleration of the brain, accompanied by a blow to the head, such as

may be experienced when the head strikes a windshield of a car in a crash.

Head injury is so frequent that it causes a major treatment need. Estimates made in the early 1990s suggest that as many as two million persons experience head injury in the United States each year; as many as 30 percent of these are severe enough to warrant extended medical treatment and rehabilitation. Head injury causes 50,000 deaths in the United States each year (*Interagency Head Injury Task Force Report*, February 1989). Estimates of the incidence of cerebrovascular accidents and related acquired brain injuries place their occurrence at five times the rate of traumatic brain injury. The National Head Injury Foundation has labeled head injury "the silent epidemic."

It was not until the 1980s that head injury became recognized as a particular injury or set of injuries requiring specialized intervention. This sudden rise of a new disability group has been dramatic, and for many observers was unforeseen. Before 1980, according to incidence statistics published by the National Head Injury Foundation, as many as 90 percent of all persons experiencing serious head injuries—most often incurred in automobile crashes—died at the scene of the crash. By 1990 the number had reversed; as many as 90 percent of all persons experiencing serious head injuries lived to reach the hospital. The overwhelming number of persons surviving head injuries in the 1980s is directly attributable to the use of and improvement in emergency evacuation procedures, the availability of life support equipment in most communities, and a concomitant advance in medical technology to treat persons with moderate or severe head injuries.

Two reasons predominately explain why head injuries have reached such epidemic proportions in our society. First, technology has outpaced our evolution and education about prevention. Although remarkable treatment advances began to be made in the 1980s, sufficient means to protect the brain from the kinds of high speeds and hard surfaces that are now commonplace in our world have not been developed, and we haven't as a nation adequately addressed this fact. Head injury is overwhelmingly a problem of young adults, who are risk takers in our mobile society. Second, we live in a world that is becoming increasingly violent.

Causes of Head Injury

The statistics on head injuries frequently mirror accidental-injury statistics. In the United States, most deaths from automobile crashes are caused by traumatic brain injury. Fifty-one percent of traumatic brain injuries are motor vehicle–related; 21 percent are the result of falls; 12 percent are the result of assaults and violence; and 10 percent are related to sports activities (New Jersey Safe Kids Campaign, 1992; WHO, 1991). Males of all ages are more likely to sustain head injuries than females, and young adults are the most at risk.

Primary and Secondary Injuries. The mechanism of brain injury can be considered to be a process. The initial injury occurs, which then sets in motion a sequence of pathological processes that create secondary damage (brain ischemia). Impact is followed by bleeding, which puts pressure on some parts of the brain and restricts blood flow to others. The brain swells, which forces it against the hard and sometimes sharp inside of the skull and the leather-like dura mater (a membrane that envelopes the brain and spinal cord). This causes contusions or lacerations. Metabolic changes then destroy cell membranes, which causes further edema and reduced blood flow. Loss of consciousness often occurs, but there can be significant brain damage without loss of consciousness.

Head injuries can be either closed injuries (diffuse axonal injuries) or open, focal injuries large enough to be seen by the naked eye. Diffuse, closed brain injuries may not be readily visible and can be the result of trauma, such as when an infant is shaken. At times the mechanism of injury is not immediately apparent. Head injuries may result from comparatively minor incidents, or the onset of symptomatic difficulties may not occur until several hours after injury. Generalized dysfunction often accompanies focalized brain damage because no part of the brain is completely independent of the other parts.

Effects of Head Injury

Head injury often produces catastrophic effects on the individual experiencing the injury and his or her family. Effects of head injuries are often unrecognized or misdiagnosed. Especially in the case of closed head injuries (injury to the brain without a fracture or surface wound to the skull), substantial behavioral, cognitive, or other difficulties may arise in the days, weeks, or months following the injury. The person injured may be unaware of the reason for the subsequent difficulties in keeping up in school, getting along at work, or maintaining family relationships. These difficulties are often thought to require methods other than those best used to treat head injury (e.g., behavioral difficulties that are neurogenic in origin may require different treatment than behavioral difficulties that are psychogenic in origin). Treatments that may not satisfactorily resolve difficulties arising from head injury include counseling, psychiatric intervention, disciplinary or "reality" treatments, and others. If the presenting problem is head injury, treatment should be structured according to the neurologic need as well as the psychiatric need.

Physiological/Physical. Physiological effects of head injury vary, of course, according to the injury itself, but several are common. Closed head injuries frequently result in edema resulting from trauma to the brain as the swollen or contused brain tissue impinges upon sharp bony protrusions within the skull. Prominent physiological effects include edema, frequent seizure disorders, paralysis of certain extremities, reduced respiratory capacity, and reduced strength. Since the brain controls functioning according to certain localities, specific localized damage often results in concomitant physiological difficulties.

Prominent physical consequences include gait disturbances, learning and vision impairments, various forms of paralysis of extremities, and others. Head injury, however, is characteristically associated less with physical impairment than with physiological, cognitive, and behavioral impairments.

Cognitive. Cognitive impairment is among the more noticeable effects of head injury, especially when the injury is localized in frontal, temporal, or upper sites of the brain. Prominent characteristics include slowed information processing, speech difficulties (mostly expressive—except for the slowness, receptive language remains intact), loss of short-term memory capabilities, and loss of what is known as executive function, which includes sequencing ability, planning ability, understanding of "self" in relation to the environment, and understanding of subtlety, especially in social relationships.

Early data describing deficits resulting from head injury focused on cognitive and behavioral impairments, primarily because these deficits are so readily observed. Recovery data, therefore, focused on cognitive impairments and recovery from them, using data obtained from repeated measures of academic achievement or commonly used measures of intelligence. Results from early studies showed a recovery curve in which maximal recovery from head injury was obtained at eighteen to twenty-four months post-injury. Frequently citing results from studies in this genre, major insurance carriers have limited funding for most rehabilitation to twenty-four months or so after injury.

Behavioral. Behavioral effects of survivors of head injury vary greatly across the continuum of recovery. In the coma phase the person is passive but may occasionally strike out unexpectedly. In re-

covery from coma, the acute phase, the person may become agitated both verbally and physically and will often strike out unpredictably. It is not uncommon for persons with highly restrained patterns of behavior before their injuries to speak loudly, using obscene language. This behavior, when it happens, is transitory and will pass as the person improves after injury. At this stage, environmental manipulations are more likely to produce needed behavioral change than direct efforts to modify behavior. If behavior modification techniques are used, they should be oriented more to simple operant conditioning or stimulus control techniques than to higher-order conditioning. In this regard, involvement of both the family and the person with the head injury is crucial for the design of the most effective treatment intervention.

As functioning levels improve after injury, behavioral difficulties are more often associated with impulse control (e.g., disinhibition) and impairments in judgment. Survivors of head injury may misinterpret actions of others, misapply emotional states (e.g., experience anger at a happy occasion, etc.), and become confused in social situations that require subtlety in understanding. The rehabilitation discipline that most closely speaks to this last dimension has become known as "pragmatics," the discipline of understanding nonverbal communication, such as behavioral cues from others. At higher levels, behavioral difficulties are best met by a combination of behavior modification and counseling to retrain the combination of insight, self-awareness, and behavior patterns that can lead to appropriate adjustment.

Psychological. The most significant psychological deficits after injury are in self-esteem, executive function, and judgment. Survivors of head injury are profoundly affected by their injuries, but they are often not aware of their deficits. One result of this pattern is a complex set of psychological difficulties in a survivor who resists treatment, believing that he or she does not need intervention. It is common to attribute this refusal of limitations to "denial," as the term is commonly used psychologically, when in fact the refusal is neurogenic in origin, not psychogenic. Therefore the refusal to accept limitations and accept treatment is part of the recovery process.

One characteristic, particularly of frontal injuries, is lack of self-awareness. Treatment designs with a primary focus on helping the person with a head injury gain self-esteem are often accompanied by improved outcomes in other therapeutic areas.

Rehabilitation

As many as half of all head injuries have few or no long-term medical or treatment needs. Of the half that remain, about one fourth need sophisticated retraining to regain the functioning necessary to live and work independently. Persons who have experienced head injury are often treated in rehabilitation programs, which should be community-based and should include the person with head injury and his or her family in all aspects of rehabilitation. The goal of head injury rehabilitation is to return the individual with a head injury to community living and competitive employment or school.

Assessment. Assessment of potential rehabilitative need should begin early in the course of treatment. Two diagnostic instruments are used most widely: (1) the Glasgow Coma Scale, which measures responsiveness in the early hours after injury, and (2) the Rancho de Los Amigos Scale, known widely as the "Rancho" Scale. The Rancho Scale estimates functioning from level 1 through level 8. Level 1 is "unresponsive to pain." Levels 1 and 2 are customarily thought of as "coma." Levels 3 and 4 describe head injury survivors who are awake, somewhat confused, and who have erratic angry outbursts. These persons are usually served in hospital-based rehabilitation programs, often referred to as "acute" rehabilitation. In acute rehabilitation, the focus is on skill retraining and development, such as a physical therapist encouraging standing balance or a neuropsychologist focusing on control of behavioral issues. Levels 5 through 7 generally describe the head injury survivor who is able to function but who exhibits difficulty with memory, judgment, and the tasks of daily living. These persons are served in rehabilitation environments that offer a mixture of the structured acute setting and yet provide an increasingly greater degree of independence. Such environments are usually referred to as "transitional" or postacute settings. Levels 6 through 8 describe persons who are best served in outpatient settings, often living at home or in group settings, able to drive their own cars, and who respond well to methodologies that promote their ultimate full return to independent living and competitive employment.

The Rehabilitation Team. Persons with severe or moderate head injury frequently experience difficulty living independently and getting and holding a job. Rehabilitation addresses these areas through several treatment disciplines, including the following:

Physical therapy
Occupational therapy
Neuropsychological services
Behavioral psychological services
Counseling and peer counseling
Vocational services
Speech-language pathology services
Social and family services
Neuropsychiatric services
Medical services
Therapeutic recreation

Because the efforts of the rehabilitation team must be coordinated to be effective, the team is usually organized around a clinical or team director (who may be called a case manager). The survivor's day is organized around a series of treatment or training appointments with team members, who then gather together periodically to discuss the person's progress in rehabilitation.

Teams use a process that is usually called "interdisciplinary," which means that the team meets together to set goals for each person's rehabilitation and periodically to discuss progress toward these goals. Starting in the 1990s, teams organized around new concepts that are variations on the interdisciplinary theme. Examples include the "transdisciplinary" team, in which therapeutic specialists combine to cotreat on certain goals, and the "curriculum" approach to rehabilitation, in which the goals of rehabilitation are arranged according to certain sets of prearranged milestones to make the team more efficient but still tailor rehabilitation to the individual.

Community-based rehabilitation is more effective and useful than hospital-based rehabilitation in returning the person with head injury to independent living and employment. Community-based programs frequently are described as "nonmedical" or "developmental" in nature. The primary differences between medical and nonmedical models are not the treatment personnel or the organization of the program but the nature of rehabilitation goals (greater functionality), different supervision of the team, and greater use of paraprofessional treatment personnel. Self-directed rehabilitation is now emerging, with the person with head injury contributing his or her own input in planning and organizing his or her own rehabilitation.

Life After Injury

The overwhelming twin goals of all survivors and their families are (1) to be able to live normally (not always "independently," although many will be independent) again, and (2) to be able to work—to be gainfully employed.

Community Living. Beginning with studies such as the one produced by the Missouri Governor's Task Force on Head Injury in 1986, it has been apparent, however, that most survivors of head injury do not obtain independent living situations after their injuries, with or without rehabilitation (although rehabilitation clearly improves the chances at a positive ultimate solution). Most eventually live with their families. A few live in nursing homes or group living settings. Increasingly, housing for survivors of head injuries is developing around the concept of "supported living" in apartments, group homes, and similar arrangements. Supported living arrangements provide some degree of protection and structure while still allowing for privacy and social interaction. Several communities offer supported apartments specially adapted for the survivor of head injury. Some survivors of head injury who would previously never have been able to live independently are now able to do so because of advances in the art and science of rehabilitation. Personal care services and family support systems are emerging as important components of community living.

Employment. In the United States, adults will change jobs several times during their working years. The "typical" person with head injury is likely to be considerably more variable still, experiencing greater levels of difficulty in obtaining and holding employment. For this reason, vocational rehabilitation services are vitally important.

Vocational services are increasingly being structured around supported systems, some of which stem from home and some from work. "Supported employment" is a system whereby a "job coach" develops the competitive or sheltered worksite, trains the injured individual in the specific job, then accompanies the individual to the worksite and "coaches" him or her regarding specific behaviors that promote long-term work and employability.

There is increasing interest in employee-supported networks in which vocational specialists train other employees at the worksite to become "mentors" of the person with head injury. This technique is proving to be acceptable financially as well as being more normalized, and it is becoming increasingly popular among survivors of head injury. Self-esteem, self-direction, and dignity are significant goals of vocational services.

Prevention

Once destroyed, brain cells cannot be rejuvenated. Prevention is the only way to avoid brain injury. Since injuries, like diseases, occur in highly predictable patterns, they are controllable and in many cases can be prevented.

Head injury prevention efforts have taken three forms: engineering and technological strategies, legislation and enforcement strategies, and public awareness and educational strategies. Engineering and technological advances include air bags in automobiles, improved bike helmets, and shredded tire surfacing under playground equipment. Legislation and enforcement strategies include child safety seat and safety belt laws, motorcycle and bike helmet laws, and stiffer drunk-driving enforcement. Public awareness and education efforts such as helmet drives, bike safety rodeos, and "take a seat" campaigns are being conducted at the state and community level across the country. In addition, injury prevention through education has become the focus of several national organizations.

The National Head Injury Foundation's Be Head-Smart[SM] Campaign, launched in 1992, seeks to alter behavior through education, thereby reducing the incidence of traumatic brain injury. The Safe

Kids Campaign chose two major high-risk activities for head injury as the focal points for its 1993 injury prevention efforts: automobile occupant safety and bike safety. Finally, the World Health Organization chose the prevention of violence and negligence as the focus for World Health Day in 1993.

Head Injury Movement. The emergence of the head injury phenomenon has been accompanied by the development of a movement regarding head injury services and prevention, spearheaded by the National Head Injury Foundation (NHIF). Founded in 1980 in Boston, the NHIF has become the major voice of the consumer movement in head injury service provision in the United States as well as a leader in coordinating prevention efforts, and in the early 1990s it began organizing international efforts in the field as well. By special resolution, the U.S. Congress designated the 1980s as "The Decade of the Brain," recognizing the need for a significant movement toward public assistance, public housing, and increased treatment services in all aspects of national, state, and community life for people with head injury.

Research

Much research needs to be undertaken to understand the damaged brain and the healing process. The last great frontier may be the complete understanding of the brain and its functions. Scientific advances in neuroregeneration, cell implantation, pharmacological intervention, and adaptive technology must be promoted through increased support for research at the basic to the applied level if improved outcomes are to be achieved.

Advances seem possible in several areas of research, such as plasticity (reforming of neural pathways), neuronal budding, regeneration, and electrical stimulus of muscle tissue. Much of the research in neural changes is conducted with laboratory animals; a significant amount of the muscular stimulus and related work is being accomplished with human subjects. Perhaps major advances will occur in the field of head injury as well, and one day it will no longer be incurable.

(*See also:* BEHAVIOR THERAPY; FAMILY; PSYCHOLOGY; PSYCHOSOCIAL ADJUSTMENT)

RESOURCE

National Head Injury Foundation, Inc. (NHIF), 1776 Massachusetts Ave., NW, Suite 100, Washington, DC 20036

GEORGE A. ZITNAY

HEALTH

See WELLNESS

HEARING

See AUDIOLOGY; COMMUNICATION DISORDERS; DEAFNESS AND HEARING IMPAIRMENT

HEART DISEASE

See CORONARY ARTERY DISEASE

HEMOPHILIA

See BLOOD DISORDERS; GENETIC DISORDERS; HUMAN IMMUNODEFICIENCY VIRUS AND ACQUIRED IMMUNE DEFICIENCY SYNDROME

HISTORY OF REHABILITATION

Persons who are perceived to be significantly different from others in some important aspect have been negatively valued in most cultures in ancient and modern times. Historical changes in society's response to differences and disabilities attest to economic, cultural, scientific, and religious influences.

Wolf Wolfensberger (1972) described the major historic roles of persons perceived as deviant. He classified society's efforts to deal with deviancy into four categories: destruction of deviant individuals, segregation, reversal of the condition, and prevention of deviancy.

In Greece and Rome, among Eskimos, and in Nazi Germany, infanticide, abandoment, and extermination were practiced. During the Middle Ages and in early America, persons with disabilities were viewed as offensive or frightening and were removed from the mainstream of society. Religious beliefs held that deviancy was a punishment of the persons or of their parents. Belief in witchcraft was common in Puritan America; persons with mental illness and certain physical disabilities were thought to be possessed by Satan. Humanitarism grew with the advent of the Industrial Revolution as the incidence of occupational injuries increased, along with public awareness of them. World War I created national sympathy for disabled veterans, leading to the establishment of federal rehabilitation policy for military and civilian personnel. Eventually attempts began to be made to reverse disabling conditions through medical and educational means. Today, prevention of disability is viewed primarily as a problem of societal attitudes.

A roll call of early heroes and heroines in the shift of societal attitudes from segregation to reversal of deviances includes Thomas Hopkins Gallaudet (1787–1851), who brought manual communication to Americans with hearing and speech impairments; Louis Braille (1809–1852), who developed a touch system for reading; Samuel Gridley Howe (1801–1876), who opened the Perkins Institute for the Blind and created one of the first workshops for the visually impaired; Harvey Wilbur (1786–1852), who opened an experimental school for retarded children in New York; Dorothea Dix (1870–1951), who championed the building of mental hospitals so that mentally ill persons could be removed from jails; Edgar James Helms (1863–1942), who founded Goodwill Industries; Bell Greve (1894–1957), who established the Sunbeam Circle for bedfast children in a Cleveland, Ohio, hospital; Jeremiah Milbank (1887–1972), who established the Red Cross Institution for Crippled Soldiers and Sailors and became a great benefactor of rehabilitation facilities; and Dr. Fred Albee (1876–1945), who provided an array of services at his Reconstruction Hospital to return veterans who were seriously disabled to useful civilian life (Dean, 1972).

Government's Responsibility to Its People

Political and social influences near the end of the nineteenth century led to the federal government's assuming responsibility for dealing with societal problems. Progressives believed that the federal government should guarantee economic opportunity and assist casualties of the economic system. In 1913 the first federal income tax was collected to pay for past, present, or future wars. The first workers' compensation law was passed in 1910 as a result of the large numbers of persons disabled by industrial accidents.

The shift in the national attitude toward one shared responsibility by all for the misfortunes of some was also evident in the compulsory education, vocational education, and special education movements, which proclaimed education as a right of every citizen. The Smith-Hughes Act of 1917 made federal funds available to states to create vocational education programs. Testing, counseling, and training were coming into their own, sparked by the belief that residual capacities could be developed into vocational effectiveness. The National Defense Act of 1916 created the authority to assist soldiers in reentering civilian life by offering instruction in agriculture or "mechanical arts" (Obermann, 1967). The United States entered World War I in April 1917, and the stage was set for the first federal rehabilitation legislation.

The Soldier Rehabilitation Act passed in June 1918 authorized the Federal Board of Vocational Education to offer vocational rehabilitation to veterans who were disabled. A vocational rehabilitation act for civilians was not enacted until two years later, however, when pressure from states that had passed vocational rehabilitation and workers' compensation laws contributed to the passage of the Smith-Fess Act, which affirmed the federal role in promoting the welfare of disadvantaged people. State boards of vocational education were to be the implementing agencies of the new law, and each state had to be wooed into matching federal funds. The early vocational rehabilitation program suffered under an administration that understood the problems of school-age youth more easily than those of persons with disabilities.

In the earliest days of a federal-state rehabilitation effort, several leaders advanced and expanded the concept that rehabilitation was a "complex and specialized personal service" (Obermann, 1967). These leaders emphasized the importance of sound counseling and physical restoration before training was undertaken. Among these leaders were John A. Kratz, who was chief of the Vocational Rehabilitation Division of the Federal Board of Vocational Education for many years (1920–1947); Tracy Copp (1878–1955), one of the original "rehabilitation agents"; Oscar Sullivan (1881–1955), who directed the program in Minnesota and proposed a national system of disability insurance fifteen years before the Social Security Act was passed; William F. Faulkes (1877–1961), who directed the Wisconsin Vocational Rehabilitation program and was the first president of the National Rehabilitation Association; and Dr. John Stanley Coulter (1888–1976), who instituted the first program in physical medicine, at Northwestern University Medical School (Dean, 1972).

Until the Depression, help to disadvantaged persons was still considered by the majority of U.S. citizens as charity. The lesson that hard times could fall upon worthy and deserving people also had not been learned. With the Depression a change in public attitudes ushered in the New Deal and the welfare state, with a new understanding that every citizen had a right to economic opportunity and self-esteem. The United States had held to a frontier tradition in which no person in a free state could claim assistance from or be required to aid others. But in 1933, unemployed millions turned to the federal government for help. Three powerful economic currents converged within the next decade: industrialization, modern medical science, and the rise of the welfare state (Hughes, 1986). In 1935 the Social Security Act addressed the problems of unemployment, old age, poverty, and blindness. It abandoned federal programs for health and disability, but it did make vocational rehabilitation a permanent program.

World War II not only increased demands for products, it also created opportunities for persons with disabilities to enter the workforce. Rehabilitation came to be recognized as a means of enhancing the economy. A new federal agency had been formed in 1939, and the Office of Vocational Rehabilitation found the new Federal Security Agency more compatible with its own philosophy (Walker, 1985). Economic, political, social, and administrative entities were in place for the growth of rehabilitation.

In 1943 the Vocational Rehabilitation Amendments, called the Barden-LaFollette Act, authorized major extensions of the rehabilitation program. For the first time, mentally retarded and mentally ill persons could be served. The law authorized the first federal subsidy for medical care. Until 1943, applicants had been refused services because of physical impairments requiring surgery or medical treatment. Federal funds could now be used to provide such medical services if prompt restoration to work was expected.

The rapid development of the vocational rehabilitation program during World War II was characterized by its outreach into other agencies and organizations. By 1947 the Office of Vocational Rehabilitation had formal cooperative agreements with nineteen organizations concerned with disability (Obermann, 1967). Rather than monitoring and regulating, the Office of Vocational Rehabilitation took the role of initiating, stimulating, and coordinating efforts of the entire community.

The Rise of Medical Science and Rehabilitation

One product of World War II was the formalization of physical medicine and rehabilitation as a medical specialty. Several visionary physicians, including Dr. Howard Kessler (1896–1978), an orthopedist who had been a strong advocate of rehabilitation programs since 1931, were drawn into the rehabilitation of veterans. Dr. Kessler and Dr. George Deaver had met at the Institute for the Crippled and Disabled in New York in 1934. Dr. Kessler implemented the concept of a comprehensive medical-social-psychological-vocational approach to disability before physical restoration was authorized in federal legislation (Dean, 1972).

Another pioneer in physical restoration was Dr. Frank Krusen (1898–1973), who was the first president of the American Academy of Physical Medicine and who established a department of physical medicine at the Mayo Clinic. Dr. Krusen and Dr.

Kessler joined their efforts with those of Dr. Howard Rusk (1901–1989), a colonel in the Air Force who demonstrated the effectiveness of physical medicine with injured pilots. After the war, Rusk and his colleagues had difficulty selling their medical colleagues on the rehabilitation concept; however, each persisted in separate locations to promote an approach that took the whole person into account, not just an injured part.

Physical and occupational therapy as well as prosthetics and orthotics continued to draw attention and funding after World War II. The United Mine Workers established a welfare and retirement fund that provided funding for several hundred disabled miners needing comprehensive restorative care. Throughout Appalachia hospitals were established where Dr. Warren Draper (1883–1970), Dr. Rusk, Dr. Kessler, and Dr. Donald Covalt demonstrated the effectiveness of physical medicine approaches. In 1944 the American Medical Association created a specialty board on physical medicine. The physiatrists were to become the strongest advocates for federal support of rehabilitation services.

Breakthrough Years

The postwar expansion of the federal role in medicine and hospitals had done little in terms of federal funding for rehabilitation, however. In 1950 a new public assistance law was added to the Social Security Act. In 1953 Dwight D. Eisenhower, the first Republican president since 1933, found himself in search of a way to reduce dependency. His attention was drawn to the vocational rehabilitation program and its dynamic director, Mary Switzer (1900–1970).

The Vocational Rehabilitation Amendments of 1954 were signed into law by President Eisenhower in August of that year. The law recast the role of the federal government in the field of rehabilitation by establishing a working partnership between public and private organizations, initiating a federally assisted research program, and training professionals to staff public and private rehabilitation programs (Dean, 1972). The amendments also expanded the types of services (e.g., work evaluation and work adjustment) and authorized the construction of rehabilitation facilities.

Mary Switzer surrounded herself with talented staff in these years of expansion: Dr. James Garrett was recruited to direct the research program; Henry Redkey was the rehabilitation facility specialist; and Emily Lamborn, Donald Dabelstein, Joe Hunt, and Russell Dean were her closest colleagues (Walker, 1985). Mary Switzer's principal allies outside the agency were Howard Rusk and Henry Viscardi, who was born without legs and whose experiences led him to found a center where persons with disabilities were helped to work in industry (Walker, 1985). Federal funds for rehabilitation increased fivefold in the next ten years as a result of Mary Switzer's entrepreneurship. The steady expansion of rehabilitation programs to new client populations marked a shift in government priorities to the providing of human services without an insistence on decreasing dependence (Rusalem, 1976).

The 1965 Vocational Rehabilitation Amendments ensured the continuation of growth, extending services to those with social disabilities and providing for extended evaluation to determine the rehabilitation potential of clients who were severely disabled. By 1966 the vocational rehabilitation bonanza was at its height. Within one year state rehabilitation agencies had twice as much money for services as in 1965 (Walker, 1985). Mary Switzer testified that public attitudes had evolved from compassion without action, to willingness to act for economic reasons, to willingness to act for social reasons. She interpreted these golden years as evidence of an advanced civilization ordering its system so that all persons with disabilities would be restored as fully as possible, without regard for economic benefit.

From Disability to Disability Rights

A war, an election, an administrative reorganization, and Mary Switzer's retirement in 1970 brought an end to the record growth of public rehabilitation programs. The promises of the Great Society had been broken, and restrictive management policies tended to disregard the rights of persons with disabilities. The welfare state never received the massive doses of vocational rehabilitation that Mary Switzer intended (Hughes, 1986).

Independent living had been discussed in 1960,

yet under federal law, vocational rehabilitation could not serve persons with little prospect of being employed. Throughout the 1960s, people with disabilities who left hospitals found themselves isolated in communities. A group of wheelchair users and blind students at the University of California at Berkeley were inspired by students' rights activists and formed an organization to hire attendants and readers (Owen, 1992). Independent living for those with disabilities would soon become known as a movement.

Early leaders in the independent living movement were Ed Roberts, who also directed California's vocational rehabilitation program for several years, and Judy Heumann, who battled on the East Coast for access to the community.

The Rehabilitation Act of 1973 placed emphasis on expanding services to clients with more severe disabilities, but a proposed independent living program was deleted. Important civil rights provisions were enacted in sections 501, 502, 503, and 504 of Title V of the act, all focused on expanding the employment opportunities of persons with disabilities. The focus of rehabilitation was changing from the individual with a disability to the environment and the elimination of discriminatory practices. Disability rights advocates grew in number and in expertise. Lex Frieden became the director of the National Council on Disability, an independent federal agency created in 1978 to recommend policy initiatives to the president and Congress. Researchers, including Carolyn Vash, Gerben DeJong, Irving Zola, Frank Bowe, and Margaret Nosek, collected data that described the restrictiveness of environments in which persons with severe disabilities lived.

In 1990 the Americans with Disabilities Act (ADA) was passed by an overwhelming majority of both the House and the Senate. The act proclaims participation in the mainstream of daily life as an American right. Earlier federal laws that led to the ADA, in addition to the Rehabilitation Act of 1973, were the Architectural Barriers Act of 1978, the Education for All Handicapped Children Act of 1975 (now called the Individuals with Disabilities Education Act), the Development Disabilities Assistance and Bill of Rights Act of 1975, the Civil Rights of Institutionalized Persons Act of 1980, the

Voting Accessibility for the Elderly and Handicapped Act of 1984, the Air Carriers Access Act of 1986, and the Fair Housing Amendments of 1988 (West, 1991). The ADA articulates goals for the nation that foster independence and integration, affording persons with disabilities antidiscrimination protection comparable to that provided women and members of minority groups.

As the legislative basis for disability rights developed, the research and training aspects of the federal rehabilitation movement continued to mature. Early educators, including Tamara Dembo and Beatrice Wright, provided a conceptual framework for rehabilitation counselor education. Soon accreditation standards and certification standards were developed by educators and practitioners to assure quality in federally funded rehabilitation counselor education programs. Marceline Jacques, George Wright, and Brockman Schumacher led university efforts to construct curricula for rehabilitation counseling.

Research and training centers also contributed to what was known about rehabilitation of people in specific disability categories or with particularly difficult problems. Rehabilitation of disabled persons in minority groups within the United States became the focus of a research and training center at Howard University, where Sylvia Walker directed studies related to the employment and access to rehabilitation services of such persons.

William Anthony, at Boston University, led national research and training efforts to rehabilitate persons with psychiatric disabilities. Deinstitutionalization had been followed by attempts at community-based treatment, but the lack of clearly defined goals for psychiatric rehabilitation prompted Anthony to develop principles and programs of living, learning, and working skills. The psycho-social rehabilitation model emphasized resocialization, skill-building, and community support.

As the importance of disability in the workplace became increasingly evident, disability management became a new emphasis within rehabilitation. The approaches developed within the public rehabilitation program began to address employer sensitivity to the costs of injury and disability. Rehabilitation practitioners began to practice industrial rehabilitation models centered in the employment setting. Increasingly, the relationship between employer and employee has come to be seen as the best predictor of maintenance of employment after work injury or onset of disability. Information from international expert and information exchange programs support the global need for cost-effective programs to reduce the loss of work potential as a result of disability (Habeck, Shrey, and Growick, 1991).

The Rehabilitation Movement in the Twenty-first Century

Following the passage of the ADA, limited funding, personnel, and public awareness led to delays in the reauthorization of the Rehabilitation Act. Clients of the vocational rehabilitation system identified control and the extent of services to be the major issues. After two years of discussion, a series of public hearings, and a summit conference conducted by disability rights activists, the Rehabilitation Act was signed by President Bush in October 1992. The purpose of the act was to provide a coordinated, effective, efficient, and accountable program of vocational rehabilitation. A philosophy of independent living is apparent within the act, and empowerment of clients is a central concept.

The future of vocational rehabilitation rests on the capacity of clients, providers, administrators, and the public to deliberate and to make hard choices. Technological advances in medicine, assistive devices, and supported employment make it possible for most people with disabilities to work as long as there is a job available. What criteria should be used to allocate rehabilitation resources? Who should receive the benefits of personal assistance services, rehabilitation technology, and job coaches if funding is diminished?

Perhaps progress toward a more inclusive environment for all will make it possible to find ways to maximize the potential of all citizens. Perhaps the "tools, strategies, technology, and aids now considered part of accommodating people with disabilities may come to be viewed as conveniences for anyone who wishes to use them" (Owen, 1992). If so, Wolfensberger's conception of deviancy will become a celebration of diversity, and the mission of reha-

bilitation will be realized beyond even the dreams of Mary Switzer.

(*See also:* AMERICANS WITH DISABILITIES ACT; CIVIL RIGHTS; CONSUMERS; DISABILITY LAW AND SOCIAL POLICY; INDEPENDENT LIVING; RUSK, HOWARD; STATE–FEDERAL REHABILITATION PROGRAM; SWITZER, MARY)

BIBLIOGRAPHY

ANTHONY, WILLIAM. *The Principles of Psychiatric Rehabilitation.* Baltimore, 1980.

DEAN, RUSSELL. *New Life for Millions.* New York, 1972.

HABECK, ROCHELLE; SHREY, DONALD; and GROWICK, BRUCE. "Special Issue on Disability Management and Industrial Rehabilitation." *Rehabilitation Counseling Bulletin* 34 (March 1991):178–181.

HUGHES, JONATHAN. *The Vital Few.* New York, 1986.

OBERMANN, C. ESCO. *A History of Vocational Rehabilitation in America.* Minneapolis, 1967.

OWEN, MARY JANE. "Consumer Perspective on the Preparation of Rehabilitation Professionals: Perplexing Paradox or Refreshing Paradigms?" In *Journal of Vocational Rehabilitation* 2 (1992):4–11, eds. Paul Wehman, Susan Hasazi, and Martha L. Walker. Stoneham, MA.

RUBIN, STANFORD E., and ROESSLER, RICHARD. *Foundations of the Vocational Rehabilitation Process.* Austin, TX, 1987.

RUSALEM, H., and MALIKIN, D. *Contemporary Vocational Rehabilitation.* New York, 1976.

WALKER, MARTHA L. *Beyond Bureaucracy: Mary Elizabeth Switzer and Rehabilitation.* Lanham, MD, 1985.

WEST, JANE. *The Americans with Disabilities Act.* New York, 1991.

WOLFENSBERGER, WOLF. *Normalization.* Toronto, 1972.

MARTHA LENTZ WALKER

HIV

See BLOOD DISORDERS; HUMAN IMMUNODEFICIENCY VIRUS AND ACQUIRED IMMUNE DEFICIENCY SYNDROME

HOME CARE

See CAREGIVING; FAMILY; INDEPENDENT LIVING; PERSONAL ASSISTANCE SERVICES

HOMELESSNESS

The threat of homelessness looms over the lives of many Americans, and perhaps none feel so vulnerable as persons with mental or physical disabilities. While research on homelessness has expanded enormously since the early 1980s, most studies have focused on characteristics of homeless persons, particularly their severe mental problems, and how these characteristics may have contributed to their situation. This entry will describe how and why the plight of homeless persons reached crisis proportions by the 1980s, what is known about the extent of homelessness among persons with disabilities in the United States, disability as both cause and consequence of homelessness, and efforts to alleviate the problems of homeless persons with disabilities.

Homelessness Persons with Disabilities

It is perhaps well known by now that the homeless population in the United States is diverse and, contrary to earlier stereotypes of older white skid row male alcoholics, contains a large proportion of women and children as well as young adult men who are African American or Hispanic. The more recent stereotype of homeless persons as consisting largely of severely mentally ill persons has fallen under the weight of repeated findings from epidemiological studies that only about one-third of single homeless adults have a severe mental illness such as schizophrenia or manic-depressive disorder. This proportion rises to one-half if heavy use of drugs and alcohol is included (McCarty et al., 1991; Tessler & Dennis, 1989).

The extent of homelessness in the United States is pervasive, affecting an estimated 700,000 persons on any given night (Congressional Budget Office, 1990) and including persons in rural and suburban areas as well as the nation's cities (Foscarinis, 1991). In a national survey of 1,507 American households, 14 percent of respondents reported that they had been homeless at some time in their lives (Link et al., 1992).

All attempts at estimating the number of homeless are plagued by the lack of a standard agreed-upon definition of homelessness. While homelessness is typically defined as sleeping in public spaces or shelters, the number of homeless individuals increases dramatically if persons who are living doubled up with family members or friends are included, with estimates as high as a ratio of twenty to one arising from a survey of public housing units in New York City (Hopper, 1989).

From the perspective of persons with mental or physical disabilities and with few resources, the threat of homelessness can be particularly acute. While there are no known estimates of the prevalence of homelessness among the 48 million Americans with mental or physical disabilities, studies suggest that persons with severe psychiatric disorders are more likely than their counterparts who are not mentally ill to experience homelessness and housing instability. Ezra Susser and colleagues (1991) examined 337 persons admitted to a New York State psychiatric hospital and found three-month, three-year, and lifetime prevalence rates of homelessness of 19 percent, 25 percent, and 28 percent, respectively. The 28 percent lifetime rate is exactly double that reported in the national household survey by Bruce Link and his colleagues cited above. Other studies of people with severe mental illness have come to similar conclusions.

Unfortunately, there are no known studies of rates of homelessness among persons with physical disabilities. Unlike persons with severe mental illness, who are identifiable by a set of diagnostic criteria typically applied during hospitalization, persons with physical disabilities are treated in a variety of settings and are more difficult to identify for sampling purposes since they are a more diagnostically diverse population embracing disabilities arising from birth defects, injuries, and chronic conditions such as arthritis or obstructive pulmonary disease.

A caveat must be added to this discussion: for persons with adequate income and support—whether disabled or not—homelessness is not likely to be a threat. Of the approximately 2 million persons diagnosed with schizophrenia in this country, fewer than 8 percent are estimated to be homeless at any given time, and nearly one-half live with their families (Cohen & Thompson, 1992). Thus the primary risk factors for becoming homeless are poverty and lack of affordable housing (Shinn, 1992).

The Role of Deinstitutionalization in the Homeless Crisis

In discussing the origins of homelessness, it is useful to distinguish between two interrelated levels of causation—social structural causes and individual or person-centered causes. The former refers to macro-level social change and shifts in government policies that foster homelessness; the latter refers to characteristics of individuals or events in their lives that may precipitate the loss of housing. Clearly, the two levels are linked—a decline in the availability of affordable housing can force an individual in crisis to seek public shelter or live on the streets. In this context, individual problems may increase the risk of homelessness when housing is scarce and costly.

There is virtual consensus among researchers and policymakers that the roots of this crisis can be traced to a reduction in the supply of low-income housing units that coincided with an increase in the need for such housing as the proportion of Americans living in poverty increased (Institute of Medicine, 1988; McChesney, 1990). This tragic clash of low supply-high demand reached crisis proportions in the early 1980s. An Institute of Medicine report also cites a tightening of eligibility criteria for public assistance programs and a decline in the purchasing power of these benefits during the 1980s; this further exacerbated the plight of poor people (Institute of Medicine, 1988).

Nevertheless, there is a widespread perception, fueled in part by the visibility of the mentally ill homeless person on urban streets, that homelessness is largely the result of deinstitutionalization.

Deinstitutionalization refers to a policy shift in the delivery of mental health services beginning in the late 1950s that led to a sharp decrease in the number of patients in public mental hospitals, from a high of 559,000 in 1955 to a low of 130,000 by 1980. This shift was precipitated by growing confidence that psychotropic drugs and community treatment could satisfactorily replace the dehumanizing conditions common to so many of the state hospitals in the late 1950s. Unfortunately, a lack of community treatment programs, rehabilitative housing, and other supportive services for persons with mental illness made deinstitutionalization a problem rather than a solution for many.

There is little empirical evidence that deinstitutionalization is a significant cause of homelessness in the United States (Cohen & Thompson, 1992; Kiesler, 1991). First, the depopulation of public mental hospitals took place long before the crisis began to peak in the early 1980s. Second, as stated earlier, the majority of homeless persons are *not* diagnosed with mental illness. Put another way, even if deinstitutionalization had not been implemented, larger social forces would have produced a homeless crisis in this country (Cohen & Thompson, 1992).

Nevertheless, the policy of deinstitutionalization has created severe problems for persons with mental illness discharged from hospitals, who are burdened by their disability, by a lack of income and social supports, and by stigma. The ongoing effects of deinstitutionalization can be seen in shorter hospital stays following psychiatric admissions and the growing number of young persons with chronic mental illness who have never been hospitalized (Pepper, Kirschner, & Ryglewicz, 1981). The dramatic decline in single-room-occupancy hotels combined with increasing restrictions in eligibility for social welfare benefits has forced many persons with mental illness to seek refuge in public shelters or to live on the streets.

Homelessness and Disability: Cause or Consequence?

There are no longitudinal studies documenting the role of various societal and individual factors in increasing the risk of homelessness; cross-sectional studies tend to overrepresent the long-term homeless and underrepresent persons who are short-term or episodically homeless. In considering the role of physical disability as a primary cause of homelessness, surveys of homeless persons have shown that they seldom mention poor health as a reason for their homelessness—only about 4 to 7 percent of homeless respondents cite this as a primary factor (Jahiel, 1992), and for only 3 percent is it the most important factor (Institute of Medicine, 1988). Marilyn Winkleby and Randall White (1992) found that only 5 percent of homeless persons surveyed in California reported having a physical impairment that preceded their homelessness. Two-thirds of these homeless persons with a disability cited injuries as the cause of their disability. Compared to the remaining members of the sample, they tended to be older and to have worked full-time before their physical problem began. Persons in the sample with no physical or mental impairments preceding their homelessness tended to be from an ethnic minority group, to be married, and to have lower educational attainment, thus reinforcing the view that poverty plays a prominent role in causing homelessness, particularly among African Americans and Hispanics (Winkleby & White, 1992).

The impact of physical disability is considerably greater when it is considered as a contributory rather than as a prime cause of homelessness. James D. Wright (1989) asserted that poor physical health contributed to homelessness for about 21 percent of all homeless persons, and Elmer L. Struening (1988) found that 15 percent of homeless adults in New York City reported having a disabling condition before they became homeless.

The extent to which mental disability contributes to homelessness is difficult to ascertain. While estimates of the prevalence of mental problems among homeless persons can vary depending on diagnostic criteria and the sample and site of the study, there is widespread agreement that these problems are far greater among homeless people than in the general U.S. population, though this gap narrows when homeless people are compared with their poor but domiciled counterparts. As discussed earlier, mental disability may increase the risk of becoming homeless, since housing with adequate support services for persons with mental disorders is quite scarce. Young adults with dual diagnoses—chronic mental illness and substance abuse—are particularly difficult to treat and to place in supportive housing after treatment. Many have exhausted family and other sources of social support and have little recourse left other than public shelters or encampments.

While many studies have documented the existence of mental and physical problems in homeless populations around the country, few have identified the extent to which these problems actually resulted from, or have been seriously exacerbated by, homelessness. Given the stress of extreme poverty and of a life exposed to the elements, the risk to physical and mental health can be easily imagined.

For a significant minority of homeless persons who are mentally ill—estimated to be as high as 40 percent (Sosin, Colson, and Grossman, 1988)—the first psychiatric hospitalization came after they became homeless rather than vice versa. When we consider less severe mental disorders such as personality disorders or subclinical depression, the proportions grow much higher (Padgett & Struening, 1991). It is perhaps easier to see how the traumatic experience of homelessness may lead in time to antisocial behavior (which may be adaptive to life on the streets or in shelters), to depressive symptoms, and to substance abuse. One study that attempted to identify both the antecedents and the effects of homelessness found that the highest rates of alcohol abuse, illegal drug use, and psychiatric hospitalization were found among persons who have been homeless five years or longer (Winkleby & White, 1992).

Several studies of physical problems of homeless people have been published (Breakey et al., 1989; Brickner et al., 1985; Gelberg & Linn, 1989; Institute of Medicine, 1988; Jahiel, 1992; Ropers & Boyer, 1987; Struening & Padgett, 1990; Wright & Weber, 1987), and the prevalence of disability in this population is extensive. In a survey of 1,260 homeless adults in the New York City shelter system in 1987, one-fifth reported that they had a disease, injury, or handicap that restricted their daily life (Struening, 1988).

Much of the data on physical health problems have come from the national network of programs known as the Health Care for the Homeless (HCH) projects sponsored jointly by the Robert Wood Johnson Foundation and the Pew Memorial Trust beginning in 1983 (Brickner et al., 1985). Physical health problems most frequently found among homeless people include injury-related orthopedic problems, hypertension, diabetes, asthma, and arthritis—all conditions that are exacerbated by a homeless existence. Illnesses such as flu, bronchitis, and skin and dental problems are also prevalent, and the incidence of tuberculosis and AIDS among people who are homeless is increasing (Institute of Medicine, 1988).

Perhaps the most striking evidence of the impact of homelessness on health can be found in traumatic injury rates. The Institute of Medicine (1988) reported that 23.4 percent of homeless clients of the

HCH programs had some type of traumatic injury requiring treatment, and the medical records of a San Francisco hospital emergency room revealed that 30 percent of homeless persons treated there presented with traumatic injuries (Kelly, 1985). Among a sample of homeless adults in New York City, traumatic injuries accounted for 39 percent of all emergency room visits and overwhelmed all other presenting problems, including physical illnesses (Padgett & Struening, 1991). Rates of injuries were high in a sample of 269 homeless adults in the Los Angeles area, with 30 percent reporting a broken bone during the previous two months (Ropers & Boyer, 1987).

Mental and Physical Comorbidities Among the Homeless

Evidence from existing studies indicates that 50 to 75 percent of homeless persons report having serious alcohol, drug, or mental (ADM) problems and/or physical problems. Multiple coexisting conditions, or comorbidities, are common in this population (Drake, Osher, and Wallach, 1991; Struening & Padgett, 1990; Winkleby & White, 1992). Examples of this phenomenon include "dually diagnosed" persons who have a mental disorder and also abuse drugs or alcohol; alcohol abusers who suffer from physical complications of alcoholism such as liver and digestive problems; and persons with physical disabilities who abuse drugs or alcohol. Unfortunately, researchers have not been able to identify how, if at all, these coexisting problems contribute to homelessness for persons afflicted with them.

The impact of coexisting physical and mental problems among homeless persons poses a significant threat to their well-being. In addition to comorbidity of drug or alcohol abuse found among homeless persons with mental illness, those suffering from ADM problems are also at greater risk of poor physical health (Struening & Padgett, 1990; Wright & Weber, 1987) and more likely to experience traumatic injuries and victimization by others (Padgett & Struening, 1992). Clearly, an accurate picture of the health consequences of homelessness requires examining the extent of comorbidities in this population.

Benefits, Services, and Programs

Like their domiciled counterparts who are poor, homeless persons who are disabled are eligible under federal statutes to receive benefits from Social Security Disability Insurance (SSDI) or from Supplemental Security Income (SSI), federal programs administered by the Social Security Administration. In both programs, disability is defined as the inability to engage in any substantial gainful activity by reason of medically determinable mental or physical impairments that can result in death or that have a duration of twelve months or longer. While SSI is considered particularly valuable to homeless people, application procedures and benefit levels vary considerably among states, and eligibility determination is a lengthy and discouraging process, although there have been attempts in some states to streamline the process for homeless persons. SSDI, which also provides persons who have disabilities with case benefits, is limited to persons with work histories who have paid Social Security taxes, a barrier to poor persons who have worked at low-wage, part-time, or transient jobs where such taxes were not deducted.

Access to medical care is a critical problem for homeless persons with disabilities. While persons applying for Medicaid benefits are no longer required to have a permanent address, eligibility is still difficult to establish. Persons receiving SSI or Aid to Families with Dependent Children (AFDC) are routinely eligible for Medicaid, but studies have shown that a surprisingly low proportion of homeless persons are enrolled in Medicaid. Only 12.3 percent of adult shelter residents in New York City were enrolled in Medicaid in 1987 (Struening, 1988).

Even persons with Medicaid coverage face barriers such as the shortage of primary care physicians and of clinics who accept Medicaid and treat people who are homeless. For the approximately one-third of homeless men who are veterans, a wider array of health services is available through VA hospitals and clinics. However, only about 3 percent of homeless men in New York City reported using these services in 1987 (Struening, 1988). A lack of proximity to areas where homeless persons live renders many VA medical centers inaccessible or inconvenient for homeless persons.

Estimates of the proportion of homeless persons receiving government benefits vary enormously because of state- and city-level differences in eligibility criteria and depending on the site of the study. For example, James D. Wright (1989) reported that 18 percent of disabled homeless clients of the Johnson-Pew HCH programs were receiving SSDI benefits and 48 percent were receiving SSI benefits. However, 40 percent of clients with physical disabilities received neither SSI nor SSDI, and 25 percent did not receive any form of social benefit or entitlement. Among general shelter residents in New York City, the proportion of persons enrolled in these programs was found to be much lower: only 3.1 percent were enrolled in SSI and 2.3 percent enrolled in SSDI in 1987 (Struening, 1988).

Regardless of the site, the number of homeless persons enrolled in entitlement programs is invariably lower than the number who are eligible, thus raising the question of barriers to access. The most comprehensive national effort to increase access to services for the homeless began with the passage of the Stewart B. McKinney Homeless Assistance Act in 1987. The McKinney Act authorized $364 million in funding in 1988 for aggressive outreach programs to provide health and mental health services for more than 230,000 homeless persons in forty-two states (National Directory of Homeless Health Care Projects, 1989). Although the McKinney program is widely viewed as a positive step, health services for homeless persons remain severely underfinanced, and budgetary constraints make it unlikely that homeless persons with disabilities will experience substantive improvements in health care in the near future. As is the case for the poor in general, virtually the only avenue for medical help for many remains the hospital emergency room (Padgett & Struening, 1991).

For homeless persons disabled by mental illness, a number of recommendations have been made by public and private organizations and by advocates for homeless people (Foscarinis, 1991; Hopper, 1990), but the obstacles are many. State and local governments must grapple with the cost of reinstitutionalizing homeless people who are mentally ill who need help but who cannot get access to community-based treatment. Meanwhile, political pressures continue to mount from community groups opposing halfway houses in residential neighborhoods, thereby slowing the much-needed expansion of supportive housing for homeless people who are mentally ill. Despite the efforts of two task forces on homeless mentally ill persons commissioned by the American Psychiatric Association in 1984 and 1989, little headway has been made in improving treatment continuity and access to outpatient services for those in need.

As described by John K. Wing and Brenda Morris (1981), the homeless person with chronic mental illness may experience three types of disability: (1) primary disability, arising from the symptoms of the illness; (2) secondary disability, arising from the individual's coping and adaptive resources; and (3) tertiary disability, arising from externally imposed "disablement" or societal stigma. These three types of disability, which may also be applicable to the homeless person with physical disabilities, must be addressed simultaneously if services are to be effective and humane.

Conclusion

Research has demonstrated that mental or physical disability is rarely the sole cause of homelessness and is more likely to be one of many factors contributing to homelessness among the very poor. At the same time, homelessness can lead to disability due to the greater risk of injuries and of physical illness experienced by homeless people. Furthermore, homeless persons may become disabled by depression or substance abuse exacerbated by stress. Given the extreme circumstances of their lives, homeless persons may be more appropriately viewed as adaptive survivors than as helpless victims partially or wholly to blame for their plight.

While outreach programs tailored to the physical and mental health needs of homeless persons with disabilities exist in many cities and states, their effectiveness is compromised by a lack of public funding and by a severe shortage of affordable housing and rehabilitative services. National health care reform programs under discussion in the 1990s may enhance access to medical care, but more intensive outreach, casework, and acute-care and rehabilitative services will still be needed by many people with disabilities who are homeless.

376

(See also: DEINSTITUTIONALIZATION; PSYCHIATRIC REHABILITATION)

BIBLIOGRAPHY

BREAKEY, WILLIAM R.; FISCHER, PAMELA J.; KRAMER, MORTON; NESTADT, GERALD; ROMANOSKI, A. J.; ROSS, A.; ROYALL, R. M.; and STINE, O. C. "Health and Mental Health Problems of Homeless Men and Women in Baltimore." *Journal of the American Medical Association* 262 (1989):1352–1357.

BRICKNER, PHILIP W.; SCHARER, LINDA K.; CONANAN, BARBARA; ELVY, ALEXANDER; and SAVARESE, MARIANNE, eds. *Health Care of Homeless People.* New York, 1985.

COHEN, CARL I., and THOMPSON, KENNETH S. "Homeless Mentally Ill or Mentally Ill Homeless?" *American Journal of Psychiatry* 149 (1992):816–823.

CONGRESSIONAL BUDGET OFFICE. "Preliminary Cost Estimate for the Homeless Outreach Act of 1990." Unpublished manuscript, 1990.

DENNIS, DEBORAH L.; BUCKNER, JOHN C.; LIPTON, FRANK R.; and LEVINE, IRENE S. "A Decade of Research and Services for Homeless Mentally Ill Persons." *American Psychologist* 46 (1991):1129–1138.

DRAKE, ROBERT E.; OSHER, FRED C.; and WALLACH, MICHAEL A. "Homelessness and Dual Diagnosis." *American Psychologist* 46 (1991):1149–1158.

FOSCARINIS, MARIA. "The Politics of Homelessness: A Call to Action." *American Psychologist* 46 (1991): 1232–1238.

GELBERG, LILLIAN, and LINN, LAWRENCE S. "Assessing the Physical Health of Homeless Adults." *Journal of the American Medical Association* 262 (1989):1973–1979.

HOPPER, KIM. "The Ordeal of Shelter." *Notre Dame Journal of Law Ethics and Public Policy* 4 (1989):301–323.

———. "The New Urban Niche of Homelessness: New York City in the Late 1980s." *Bulletin of the New York Academy of Medicine* 66 (1990):435–450.

INSTITUTE OF MEDICINE. *Homelessness, Health and Human Needs.* Washington, DC, 1988.

JAHIEL, RENE. "Health and Health Care of Homeless People." In *Homelessness: A National Perspective,* eds. Marjorie J. Robertson and Milton Greenblatt. New York, 1992.

KELLY, JOHN T. "Trauma: With the Example of San Francisco's Shelter Programs." In *Health Care of Homeless People,* eds. Philip W. Brickner, Linda K. Scharer, Barbara Conanan, Alexander Elvy, and Marianne Savarese. New York, 1985.

KIESLER, CHARLES A. "Homelessness and Public Policy Priorities." *American Psychologist* 46 (1991): 1245–1252.

LAMB, HAROLD R. "Deinstitutionalization and the Homeless Mentally Ill." *Hospital and Community Psychiatry* 35 (1984):899–907.

LINK, BRUCE; MOORE, ROBERT; SCHWARTZ, SHARON; STRUENING, ELMER L.; and STUEVE, ANN. "Public Reactions to Homeless People: Compassion Fatigue?" Paper presented at the annual meeting of the American Public Health Association, 1992.

MCCARTY, DENNIS; ARGERIOU, MILTON; HUEBNER, ROBERT B.; and LUBRAN, BARBARA. "Alcoholism, Drug Abuse, and the Homeless." *American Psychologist* 46 (1991):1139–1148.

MCCHESNEY, KAY Y. "Family Homelessness: A Systemic Problem." *Journal of Social Issues* 46 (1990): 191–205.

NATIONAL DIRECTORY OF HOMELESS HEALTH CARE PROJECTS (Section 340, Public Health Service Act). Washington, DC, 1989.

PADGETT, DEBORAH K., and STRUENING, ELMER L. "The Influence of Alcohol, Drug, and Mental Problems on Use of Emergency Room Services by Homeless Adults in New York City." *Hospital and Community Psychiatry* 42 (1991):834–38.

———. "Victimization and Injuries Among the Homeless: Associations with Alcohol, Drug, and Mental Problems." *American Journal of Orthopsychiatry* 62 (1992):525–534.

PEPPER, BERT; KIRSCHNER, M.; and RYGLEWICZ, H. "The Young Adult Chronic Patient: Overview of a Population." *Hospital and Community Psychiatry* 32 (1981):463–469.

ROPERS, RICHARD H., and BOYER, RICHARD. "Perceived Health Status Among the New Urban Homeless." *Social Science and Medicine* 24 (1987):669–678.

SHINN, MARYBETH. "Homelessness: What Is a Psychologist to Do?" *American Journal of Community Psychology* 20 (1992):1–24.

SOSIN, MICHAEL R.; COLSON, P.; and GROSSMAN, S. *Homelessness in Chicago: Poverty and Pathology, Social Institutions, and Social Change.* Chicago, 1988.

STRUENING, ELMER L. *A Study of Residents of the New York City Shelter System in 1987.* New York, 1988.

STRUENING, ELMER L., and PADGETT, DEBORAH K. "Physical Health Status, Substance Use and Abuse, and Mental Disorders Among Homeless Adults." *Journal of Social Issues* 46 (1990):65–81.

SUSSER, EZRA, S.; SHANG, P. LIN; and CONOVER, SARAH A. "Risk Factors for Homelessness Among

Patients Admitted to a State Mental Hospital."
American Journal of Psychiatry 148 (1991):1659–
1664.

TESSLER, RICHARD, and DENNIS, DEBORAH. *A Synthesis of NIMH-Funded Research Concerning Persons Who Are Homeless and Mentally Ill.* Rockville, MD, 1989.

WING, JOHN K., and MORRIS, BRENDA. "Clinical Basis of Rehabilitation." In *Handbook of Psychiatric Rehabilitation Practice,* eds. John K. Wing and Brenda Morris. Oxford, Eng., 1981.

WINKLEBY, MARILYN A., and WHITE, RANDALL. "Homeless Adults Without Apparent Medical and Psychiatric Impairment: Onset of Morbidity Over Time." *Hospital and Community Psychiatry* 43 (1992):1017–1023.

WRIGHT, JAMES D. *Address Unknown: The Homeless in America.* New York, 1989.

WRIGHT, JAMES D., and WEBER, E. *Homelessness and Health.* New York, 1987.

DEBORAH K. PADGETT

HOSPICE

Most people do not want to die alone in a sterile, impersonal surrounding, hooked up by tubes to machines and cut off from their family and friends and everything that is familiar. Nor do they want to die in pain. They would prefer, if possible, to spend their last days at home, alert and free of pain, among people and things they love. Hospice is dedicated to making this possible.

Bringing death out into the open and making sickness and loss a time of sharing and remembrance have been difficult. And while the hospice experience may not be for everyone, those who choose it find the specialness of caring for a loved one and the richness of sharing memories of youth, trials, and joys a rewarding experience never to be forgotten.

Hospice Is a Special Kind of Caring

Hospice programs provide a special kind of care for dying people and their familes that:

1. treat the physical needs of the patient and his or her emotional and spiritual needs;
2. take place in the patient's home, or in a home-like setting;
3. concentrate on making patients free of pain and as comfortable as possible so they can make the most of the time that remains to them;
4. consider helping family members an essential part of its mission;
5. believe the quality of life to be as important as the length of life.

Receiving hospice care is always a choice for patients and families who have decided to alleviate aggressive curative or life-extending treatment for their terminal illness, and want to concentrate on quality of life, pain and symptom management, and psychosocial and spiritual support services for themselves and their families.

Hospice recognizes dying as part of the normal process of living and focuses on maintaining the quality of life. Hospice affirms life and neither hastens nor postpones death. Hospice exists in the hope and belief that through appropriate care and the promotion of a caring community sensitive to their needs, patients and their families may be free to attain a degree of mental and spiritual preparation for death that is satisfactory to them. Hospice offers palliative care to terminally ill people and their families without regard for age, gender, nationality, race, creed, sexual orientation, disability, diagnosis, availability of primary caregiver, or ability to pay.

The Hospice Interdisciplinary Care Team

A highly qualified, specially trained team of hospice professionals and volunteers work together to meet the physiological, psychological, social, spiritual, and economic needs of hospice patients and families facing terminal illness and bereavement. Core team members and their qualifications include:

1. the patient's attending physician;
2. hospice physicians with palliative care training;
3. registered nurses with demonstrated experience and practice in pain and symptom management and assessment;
4. social workers with a master's degree and clinical experience appropriate to the counseling and casework needs of the terminally ill;
5. spiritual counselors with appropriate education and experience in pastoral counseling;

6. trained volunteers supervised by a volunteer co-ordinator who has a demonstrated ability in organization, communication, and managing people.

Hospice uses specialized team members to meet specific needs of each patient as outlined in the patient's plan of care. These team members include allied therapists, art and music therapists, dieticians, pharmacists, and nursing assistants. This team works together to develop a plan of care and to provide services that will enhance the quality of life and provide support for the patient and family during the terminal illness and the bereavement period.

Hospice provides palliative care to terminally ill patients and supportive services to patients, their families, and significant others twenty-four hours a day, seven days a week, in both home and facility-based settings.

The National Hospice Organization (NHO) defines palliative care as treatment that enhances comfort and improves the quality of a patient's life. No specific therapy is excluded from consideration. The test of palliative treatment lies in agreement among the patient, the physician, the primary caregiver, and the hospice team that the expected outcome is relief from distressing symptoms, easing of pain, and enhancement of quality of life. The decision to intervene with an active palliative treatment is based on the treatment's ability to meet the stated goals rather than its effect on the underlying disease.

The Interdisciplinary Team Plan of Care

The hospice interdisciplinary team collaborates continuously with the patient's attending physician to develop and maintain a patient-directed, individualized plan of care. The plan of care is based on interdisciplinary team assessments that recognize the patient's and family's psychological, social, religious, and cultural variables and values. At a minimum, the plan includes patient and family problems and needs; realistic and achievable goals and objectives; the frequency and mix of services and the level of care to be provided; agreed-upon outcomes; prescribed and required medical equipment; and patient and family understanding of and agreement and involvement with the plan of care.

Hospice History

Hospice is a thoroughly modern concept of care that derives its name from the Latin word *hospes,* which means "to be both host and guest."

Dr. Cecily Saunders is generally credited with establishing the modern hospice movement in Great Britain in the 1960s. The basic concept—care in a special facility that addressed the social, emotional, and spiritual needs of the dying—was readily received and gratefully embraced by those it sought to serve.

It was not long before the hospice concept spread to the United States. It was largely a grassroots movement that developed outside the conventional health care delivery system. These early hospices survived on shoestring budgets and were almost entirely dependent on charitable contributions and volunteer staff to provide the intensive and personalized care central to the hospice concept.

Hospice developed in the United States as a concept of care rather than as a place for care; from the beginning the focus has been care in the patient's home. During the 1970s, hospice leaders began meeting regularly to formulate model standards for guiding development of hospice care. Creation of NHO in 1978 provided a national forum for advocacy for terminally ill persons, and discussion, education, and support of quality standards for hospices.

In 1983 Congress expanded Medicare coverage to include hospice care. Many private insurers, recognizing not only the compassion associated with hospice care but also its cost-effectiveness, began offering hospice benefits. Many states now provide hospice benefits under Medicaid.

Current Hospice Patients

Hospice care continues to grow as part of the mainstream health care and social service systems in the United States. Since the first hospice program provided care for patients in Stamford, Connecticut, in 1974, community-based replication of programs and services increased to a recognized 1,935 hospice programs providing care in 1992, up from 1,874 operational and/or planned programs in 1991, 1,604 programs in 1990, and 1,529 in 1989. The majority of hospice programs are Medicare-certified, with 72 percent indicating current or pending certification.

The majority of hospice programs are also small, not-for-profit, community-based organizations, with operational budgets of fewer than $500,000.

According to the 1992 NHO census, hospice programs and professionals provided care to more than 246,000 patients in 1992, up from 210,000 patients in 1990, 186,000 patients in 1989, 177,000 patients in 1987, and 158,000 in 1985, the first year of the NHO census.

Nearly consistent with past census estimates, the 1992 statistics indicate that 53 percent of hospice patients were male and 47 percent were female. Of the male patients, 68 percent were sixty-five years of age or older, 23 percent were forty-five to sixty-four, 8 percent were eighteen to forty-four, and 1 percent were between birth and age seventeen. Of the female patients, 72 percent were age sixty-five or older, with 21 percent being between forty-five and sixty-four, 6 percent eighteen to forty-four, and 1 percent between birth and age seventeen.

The majority of hospice patients (55%) indicated that they lived with their spouse, while 20 percent lived with children, 10 percent lived with a significant other person, 10 percent lived alone, and 5 percent lived with parents while receiving hospice care. (This response reflects only living arrangements, not the designation of a primary caregiver.)

According to the 1992 NHO census, the majority (78%) of patients receiving hospice care had a disease diagnosis of cancer, 10 percent had heart-related diagnoses, 4 percent were receiving care for AIDS, 1 percent had renal diagnosis, 1 percent had Alzheimer's disease, and 6 percent had other diagnoses.

Paying for Hospice Care

Initial funding for a hospice may come from grants, contributions from private foundations, local government funds, and individual contributions. The majority of hospice programs depend on philanthropic support to provide comprehensive quality hospice care. Ongoing financial support is often received through local fund-raisers, by memorial gifts, voluntary contributions, and fees for patient services.

Reimbursement for hospice services may come from Medicare, Medicaid, or private insurance.

As noted earlier, the Medicare hospice benefit was established in 1983, making all Medicare recipients eligible to receive hospice care as a covered Medicare benefit. Under this benefit, hospice care coverage includes nursing services on an intermittent basis; physician services; drugs, including outpatient drugs for pain relief and symptom management (a patient may be asked to pay 5% of the cost of outpatient drugs or five dollars for each prescription, whichever is less); physical therapy; occupational therapy; speech-language pathology; home health aide and homemaker services; medical supplies and appliances; short-term inpatient care, including respite care (a patient may be asked to pay 5% of the Medicare rate for respite care); and medical social services and counseling.

Anyone covered by Part A of Medicare is eligible to receive hospice care related to terminal illness when all three of the following conditions are met: (1) the patient's physician and hospice medical director certify that a patient is terminally ill (a life expectancy of six months or less); (2) the patient chooses to receive care from a hospice instead of standard Medicare benefits; and (3) care is provided by a hospice program certified by Medicare.

Medicare pays covered costs for two ninety-day periods, one additional thirty-day period, and an unlimited extension if the patient is recertified as terminally ill. The patient may stop hospice care at any time and return to cure-oriented care. The Medicare hospice benefit does not pay for treatments or services unrelated to the terminal illness. Any attending physician charges would continue to be reimbursed in part through Medicare Part B coverage. However, the standard Medicare benefit program still helps pay covered costs necessary to treat an unrelated condition.

While each hospice has its own policies concerning payment for care, it is a principle of hospice to offer services based on need rather than the ability to pay.

Hospice Care Settings

The focus of hospice care is to enable an individual to remain in the familiar surrounding of his or her own home as long as is possible and appropriate. Hospice care plans reflect efforts staff and volunteers make to maximize patient independence, deliver services at the convenience of the patient, family, and caregiver, arrange respite services for caregivers, bridge gaps in the patient's caregiving network, and adapt the home environment to meet the patient's physical needs.

Because a person's home may not be his or her personal residence, a hospice program may, as an alternative, offer home care services in a variety of facility settings appropriate to the patient's care needs.

Cost-Effectiveness of Hospice Care

A number of studies have examined the cost of hospice care relative to conventional care. Together these studies provide strong evidence that hospice is a less costly approach to care for persons who are terminally ill when the service delivery and payment systems reinforce incentives to manage care and cost appropriately.

The two largest studies—the Medicare Hospice Benefit Program Evaluation and the National Hospice Study (NHS)—both found savings to Medicare associated with hospice care relative to conventional care. The most recent of these—the Medicare Hospice Benefit Program Evaluation—found that for the first three years of the hospice benefit, Medicare saved $1.26 for every $1.00 spent on hospice care.

Hospice—Quality of Life

There is reasonably strong evidence that hospice provides better quality of life for both patients and caregivers. The evidence might provide stronger support consistent with anecdotal evidence collected from states and other sources were it not for the extraordinary difficulty in scientifically evaluating quality of life.

The lack of evidence showing quality of life to be greater for hospice patients than for nonhospice patients is a function of the enormous difficulty researchers have in evaluating and assessing quality of life, particularly for terminally ill patients, because of the subjective nature of care and the mental and physical effort required to complete questionnaires. In addition, the small sample size of some studies makes it particularly difficult for researchers to find statistically significant differences between the two types of care.

Based on available data, significant differences were found in five of the fifteen measures used to evaluate quality of life for hospice and conventional care patients. For four of these five measures, hospice was found to be significantly superior. These included measures of pain, satisfaction with interpersonal care, satisfaction with involvement in care, and the measure called "quality of death." For the fifth measure in which a significant difference was noted—measure of the patient's social involvement with the support system—hospice was found to be significantly better than conventional care for all but the last week of life.

Significant differences in favor of hospice were also found in four measures used to evaluate the quality of life of the primary caregiver. Primary caregivers for hospice patients were found to be less anxious and more satisfied with their involvement in care than were their nonhospice counterparts.

Locating a Hospice Program

Hospice programs exist in most urban areas throughout the country. Through the NHO help line, anyone can call their 800 number to locate a hospice program providing services to the terminally ill and their families in their respective location. This help line service also provides general information on hospice care, along with referral to additional organizations and agencies offering specialized care for patients and families.

(*See also:* CAREGIVING; FAMILY; LOSS AND GRIEF; PSYCHOSOCIAL ADJUSTMENT; QUALITY OF LIFE; RESPITE CARE)

RESOURCES

Children's Hospice International, 700 Prince St., Alexandria, VA 22314

Hospice Education Institute, 190 Westbrook Rd, Essex, CT 06426–1511

National Hospice Organization, 1901 North Moore, Suite 901, Arlington, VA 22209

BIBLIOGRAPHY

AMADO, ANTHONY. "Comparative Utilization Study: Hospice vs. Certified Home Care Users." Detroit, MI, November 10, 1990.

BROOKS, CHARLES. "A Comparative Analysis of Medicare Home Care Cost Savings for the Terminally Ill." *Home Health Care Services Quarterly* 10 (1989):79–96.

BROOKS, CHARLES, and SMYTH-STARUCH, KATHLEEN.

"Hospice Home Care Cost Savings to Third-Party Insurers." *Medical Care* 22 (1984):691–703.

CARNEY, KIM. "An Economic Perspective on Hospices." In *Socioeconomic Issues of Health.* Chicago, 1981.

CARNEY, KIM, and BURNS, NANCY. "Economics of Hospice Care." *Oncology Nursing Forum* 18 (1991):761–768.

GAUMER, GARY, and STAVINS, JOANNA. "Medicare Use in the Last Ninety Days of Life." *Health Services Research* 26 (1992):725–742.

GREER, DAVID. "An Alternative in Terminal Care: Results of the National Hospice Study." *Journal of Chronic Diseases* 39 (1986):9–26.

KIDDER, DAVID. "The Effects of Hospice Coverage on Medicare Expenditures." *Health Services Research* 27 (1992):195–217.

LUBITZ, JAMES, and RILEY, GERALD. "Trends in Medicare Payments in the Last Year of Life." *The New England Journal of Medicine* 328 (1993):1092–1096.

MOR, VINCENT, and KIDDER, DAVID. "Cost Savings in Hospice: Final Results of the National Hospice Study." *Health Services Research* 20 (1985):407–421.

MOR, VINCENT; WEICHTEL, THOMAS; and KIDDER, DAVID. "Patient Predictors of Hospice Choice, Hospital Versus Home Care Programs." *Medical Care* 23 (1985):1115–1119.

MUURINEN, J. "The Economics of Informal Care, Labor Market Effects in the National Hospice Study." *Medical Care* 24 (1986):1007–1017.

SCHAPIRA, DAVID; STUDNICKI, JAMES; BRADHAM, DOUGLAS; and WOLFF, PETER. "Intensive Care, Survival, and Expense of Treating Critically Ill Cancer Patients." *Journal of the American Medical Association* 269 (1993):783–786.

STODDARD, SANDOL. *The Hospice Movement: A Better Way of Caring for the Dying.* New York, 1974.

WALLSTON, K., et al. "Comparing the Quality of Death for Hospice and Non-Hospice Cancer Patients." *Medical Care* 26 (1988):177–182.

GALEN MILLER

HOSPITAL, REHABILITATION

Rehabilitation hospitals provide comprehensive physical and cognitive rehabilitative services to persons with a variety of disabling conditions. Individuals frequently admitted include persons with traumatic brain injury, spinal cord injury, stroke, joint replacement, hip fracture, multiple injuries, or neurological conditions, including multiple sclerosis and amyotrophic lateral sclerosis (Lou Gehrig's disease). Such facilities are sometimes freestanding but at other times exist as distinct units within acute-care hospitals. Rehabilitation hospitals may be a singular organization or be part of a regional or nationwide corporation. Like other hospitals, many are not-for-profit, but an increasing percentage are for-profit.

Rehabilitation hospitals have developed since the early 1940s to serve the needs of various patient populations. Early leaders in the field included Howard A. Rusk, M.D., at New York University, who developed hospital programs of early ambulation and therapy for individuals with medical conditions such as stroke. During the same period, Frank H. Krusen, M.D., developed rehabilitation care at the Mayo Clinic. Because of their leadership and teaching, rehabilitation services have developed into an integral part of the inpatient treatment of individuals with chronic disease and disabilities. Since the early 1970s there has been rapid expansion in the number, variety, and specialization of rehabilitation hospitals. Especially significant is the development of specialized programs for individuals following traumatic brain injury and spinal cord injury.

Persons appropriately served in rehabilitation hospitals must have medical conditions that lead to functional limitations in areas such as mobility, communication, thinking, and activities of daily living. Since rehabilitation is a learning process, the individual must be capable of learning. Persons served in inpatient rehabilitation must also be medically stable and engage in at least three hours of therapy per day.

The size, scope, and specialization of services available within rehabilitation hospitals vary. Rehabilitation units within acute-care hospitals tend to have generic programs designed to meet the needs of individuals with moderately disabling conditions, particularly resulting from stroke or orthopedic conditions. Freestanding rehabilitation hospitals offer greater specialization and more diverse services for individuals with catastrophic disabling conditions such as traumatic brain injury or spinal cord injury. Unique services such as adapted drivers' training, rehabilitation engineering, aquatic therapy, and horticultural therapy are often available. Freestanding rehabilitation hospitals also often have state-of-the-art technology available.

As freestanding hospitals have increased their

affiliations with acute-care hospitals and hospital systems, the distinctions between rehabilitation units and hospitals are less significant. The size and scope of the rehabilitation program, rather than the setting in which it is provided, decide the degree of specialization offered.

The complement of services provided within a rehabilitation hospital varies with availability of resources and the needs of the individual served. A constant is the provision of care by a multidisciplinary team. Rehabilitation nurses care for the acute medical needs of the patient and focus on improving patient function. The nurses provide patient and family education regarding the individual's disability, remaining abilities, and adaptive measures. Physical therapy concentrates on the improvement of mobility and balance of the individual served. Occupational therapy focuses on increasing the patient's independence with activities such as dressing, bathing, and eating. Speech pathology helps with thinking and communication deficits.

Psychology helps the patient and family deal with emotional and cognitive issues. The social worker or case manager coordinates patient services and prepares the patient for discharge. Recreational therapy uses recreational activities to foster the individual's progress in rehabilitation and to redevelop his or her capabilities with leisure activities. The vocational specialist helps prepare the patient for return to work or school.

Medical care within rehabilitation hospitals is generally directed by an attending physician in physical medicine and rehabilitation (physiatrist). A neurologist, orthopedic surgeon, or other specialist occasionally directs medical services within rehabilitation programs.

Regular, periodic team conferences are held to ensure coordination of the rehabilitation effort. Such conferences allow for an exchange of information about individual patient needs and progress. Patient and family participation and integration in rehabilitation occur through conferences and rounds. Families are encouraged to participate actively in the rehabilitation program to ensure continuity of care upon discharge.

Economic forces and medical developments are leading to more rehabilitation services being provided in an outpatient or home setting. Full integration of individuals with disabilities into their communities is receiving increasing emphasis. Rehabilitation facilities often serve as the catalyst for establishing community alternatives for persons with disabilities.

The Joint Commission on Accreditation of Healthcare Organizations (JCAHO) accredits rehabilitation hospitals. JCAHO focuses on enhancing organizational performance, especially concerning quality patient outcomes. Rehabilitation programs can also voluntarily seek accreditation from the Commission on Accreditation of Rehabilitation Facilities (CARF). CARF emphasizes three areas: Persons served make significant functional progress, they participate as an active member of the rehabilitation team, and care is provided in a safe and secure environment.

Reimbursement constraints and industry trends are causing rehabilitation facilities to examine the populations served as inpatients. Facilities are being challenged to provide care in less costly settings while ensuring comparable outcomes. Patients who traditionally have been treated as inpatients are now being served in less intense programs or at home. Community residential programs are being established for patients who require a higher level of support and service than can be provided in their home.

Many factors will influence the future growth and development of rehabilitation hospitals. Limited staff resources, particularly with physical and occupational therapists and rehabilitation nurses, could impede the development of rehabilitation services. Health care reform, at both the state and national levels, will likely decide how readily the average citizen can access rehabilitation services. The ability of rehabilitation facilities to quantify clinical outcomes and the total cost benefit of rehabilitation services will influence the degree to which insurers will be willing to pay for rehabilitation care for their beneficiaries.

(*See also:* FACILITIES; HEAD INJURY; NURSING, REHABILITATION; OCCUPATIONAL THERAPY; PHYSICAL THERAPY; PHYSICIAN; PHYSICAL THERAPY; REHABILITATION CENTER; REHABILITATION PSYCHOLOGY; RUSK, HOWARD; SPINAL CORD INJURY; STROKE)

RESOURCES

American Academy of Physical Medicine and Rehabilitation, 122 South Michigan Ave., Suite 1300, Chicago, IL 60603–6107

American Congress of Rehabilitation Medicine, 5700 Old Orchard Rd, First Floor, Skokie, IL 60077–1057

American Hospital Association—Rehab. Section, 840 North Lake Shore Drive, Chicago, IL 60611–2431

Association of Academic Physiatrists, 7100 Lakewood Bldg., Suite 112, 5987 East 71st St., Indianapolis, IN 46220

Commission on Accreditation of Rehabilitation Facilities, 101 N. Wilmot Rd, Suite 500, Tucson, AZ 85711

Joint Commission on Accreditation of Healthcare Organizations, One Renaissance Blvd., Oakbrook Terrace, IL 60181

Bibliography

Commission on Accreditation of Rehabilitation Facilities. 1993 *Standards Manual for Organizations Serving People with Disabilities.* Tucson, AZ, 1993.

DeLisa, Joel A., and Gans, Bruce M., eds. *Rehabilitation Medicine Principles and Practice,* 2nd ed. Philadelphia, 1993.

Eckenhoff, Edward A.; Hamilton, Byran B.; and Watkins, Ruth Ann. "Medical Rehabilitation in the 1980s." *HLM Review* (Spring 1981):55–61.

Joint Commission on Accreditation of Healthcare Organizations. *Physical Rehabilitation Services: Accreditation Manual for Hospitals, 1993.* Oakbrook Terrace, IL, 1993.

Kjellstand, Leslie. *Rehabilitation: The Quest for Quality of Life.* Austin, TX, 1992.

Kottke, Frederic J., and Lehmann, Justus F., eds. *Krusen's Handbook of Physical Medicine and Rehabilitation,* 4th ed. Philadelphia, 1990.

Krusen, Frank H. "Historical Development in Physical Medicine and Rehabilitation During the Last Forty Years." *Archives of Physical Medicine and Rehabilitation* (January 1969):1–5.

Mullner, Ross; Nuzum, Frank J.; and Matthews, Dale. "Inpatient Medical Rehabilitation: Results of the 1981 Survey of Hospitals and Units." *Archives of Physical Medicine and Rehabilitation* 64 (1983):340–345.

Richard Paul Bonfiglio
Jan Loeffler Bergen

HOUSING

A large and growing population of people with disabilities cannot be accommodated by most of the housing built in the United States today. Unable to find appropriate housing, many people with disabilities and older people live in housing that limits their independence and self-sufficiency. As their abilities decline with age, they are often forced to give up even this inadequate housing for the services and more accessible environments found in special group living facilities or nursing homes.

Adequate housing is a basic but often difficult need to fulfill for people with disabilities. Although there are laws such as the Americans with Disabilities Act (ADA, 1990), which establishes minimum accessibility standards for public and commercial facilities, and the Fair Housing Act amendments (FHAA, 1988), which require improved accessibility in multifamily housing projects, the private housing industry has not responded with dwellings designed to meet the functional needs of people with disabilities and older people. However, a growing movement toward universal design in housing is addressing the problem. Universal design regards most special needs as part of overall consumer needs. It addresses the issues with design features that are universally usable, aesthetically pleasing, and therefore more broadly marketable.

Housing as a Basic Need

Without adequate housing, a person—regardless of ability—is deprived of independence, self-determination, and personal security. For people with disabilities, performing simple tasks of daily living such as bathing, dressing, and meal preparation may be an extremely time-consuming activity, even under the best of circumstances. These tasks become an insurmountable burden in a nonsupportive or inaccessible environment; force people to rely on expensive personal care attendant services; and prevent other essential life activities, such as pursuit of job opportunities. In too many cases people with disabilities must turn to special, more institutional housing programs and privately or publicly funded caregivers when a more accessible home may be all they need to achieve self-reliance. What may be an easily accommodated disability becomes a major personal barrier as well as a drain on local services and facilities.

People with disabilities need accessible environments and support services in varying degrees, depending on their type and level of disability. A common misconception is that having a disability means using a wheelchair, so adapting housing has typically meant building ramps and widening doors. The ADA, which prohibits discrimination against people with disabilities, recognizes these categories of impairment: mobility (people using wheelchairs, and others who walk with difficulty and may use crutches, canes, walkers, etc.), visual (partial or complete vision loss), hearing (partial or complete deafness), and cognitive (learning disabilities, mental illness, etc.). Also included are people who are temporarily impaired because of injury, people who have reduced stamina and agility, people whose illnesses are not immediately visible (heart disease, arthritis, etc.), and people who are perceived as being impaired (elderly people, small people, and those with disfigurement). When survivors of traumatic injury as well as the aging population in this country are included, the number of people covered or potentially covered by disability legislation is considerable.

Within the design and construction community there is a general lack of awareness as to the range of disabilities people experience, and correspondingly the range of accommodations that may be needed. Simply adding ramps to existing structures is not always appropriate nor always desirable. For persons with mobility impairments, accessible housing includes features such as wide doorways, level entrances, lowered light switches, raised receptacles, bathrooms with maneuvering room, lowered countertops, and accessible emergency exits. For visually impaired people it may mean audible signals, preventing hazardous protruding objects, large-type signs and dials, and protected edges at drop-offs. For hearing impaired people text telephones and visual signals for alarms and doorbells may be necessary. Most if not all of these elements are a benefit to other users, and if sensitively designed and integrated into housing they become marketable features that can make housing universally usable.

Why Housing Has Not Met the Needs of People with Disabilities

Conventionally built housing has not recognized people with disabilities as potential home buyers for many reasons. First, this market has been invisible and silent. Few people like being singled out as having a disability or being old, and they may be reluctant to call attention to their needs, especially for personal home adaptations, such as to a bathroom. Not finding appropriate housing and other limiting experiences have led some to feel powerless and disconnected. Some do not consider themselves as having a disability or feel embarrassed and that "special" or "handicapped" housing is stigmatizing. Because they are a disparate and diverse group, surveying people with disabilities is challenging, and few if any companies have the time, interest, or know-how to conduct effective market research among this group. As a result, businesses have had to rely on second-hand and sometimes clinical information provided by advocates and caregivers, and people with disabilities have not had a powerful effect on the building practices of the housing industry except indirectly, through legislation.

Furthermore, information about accessible design is not always readily available to the public. In pursuing housing, people with disabilities often must take it upon themselves to consult specialists, independent living centers, government publications, or the builders themselves, who may not know how to address a particular need anyway. This lack of sufficient information, combined with reticence by many people with disabilities, often reinforces a "make do" response from both homeowner and builder, thus perpetuating the myth that all housing should be built for young, able-bodied people.

It is difficult to assess the true number of people who, at one time or another, have a disability or the extent of the disability. In the United States that number exceeded 46 million in 1994. Since this number is based on limited measures, it includes only the most easily identified people. Some people, using a broad definition of disability, state that the actual number was vastly larger. Almost everyone has a family member or acquaintance who needs some form of assistance or adaptation, whether it be eyeglasses, hearing aids, help with steps, or more involved assistance. It is also known that the number of people with disabilities will only grow as our population ages and as advances in emergency rescue, medical procedures, and assistive technology further extend and improve lives. Market research that is directed to the general housing market, focusing on home size, price, and aesthetic and trendy features, has missed the more pragmatic and functional needs of this growing population. Little has been done industrywide to educate architects, designers, and builders about universal "adaptive" designs by way of university departments of design, trade publications, or word of mouth.

Typically, accessibility information available to designers and builders has focused on the most severely affected people whose needs seem "special." The emphasis too often is on special designs in special locations for special people. Most known examples are special-purpose housing projects contracted by individuals, disability service providers, or government agencies. Unfortunately, limitations in both funding and information for such projects create housing that is institutional or clinical in nature and not saleable on the open market.

Since the 1960s, minimum accessibility standards, upon which most state and local building accessibility codes are built, have inadvertently stereotyped accessible housing within the construction community. Accessible housing laws almost always require a small percentage of rental units (usually 5%) to be wheelchair-accessible but little or nothing else. Application of minimum accessibility standards has also been haphazard and inadequate, sometimes owing to a misunderstanding of the purpose and need involved. Some accessibility specifications have resulted in unpopular, ugly, and obtrusive features such as stainless steel grab bars and lengthy outdoor ramping. These unpopular units in some locations have been made less desirable by owners who adapted only small, one-bedroom units, precluding their use by families and those who need live-in companions. Minimum requirements for accessible units have resulted in a focus on compliance rather than an effort to provide accessible, affordable, and marketable housing that can accommodate all users.

Inadequate information, individual reticence, disability stereotyping: each of these factors contributes to the problem of ensuring sufficient housing for people with disabilities and for elderly people. It is fair to say that the market does not design and build accessible housing that responds to the needs of people with disabilities. Historically, developers have feared that the features necessary to make housing accessible will cost more, look aesthetically unpleasant, not be marketable to people without disabili-

ties, and present liability problems. With limited training, hands-on experience, and information generally consisting of special clinical examples, the risk of trial-and-error construction for builders may be too great to speculate on accessible housing.

How Legislation and Adaptable Housing Have Addressed These Problems

Americans seeking housing alternatives can benefit from more than three decades of accessibility and antidiscrimination legislation. Discriminatory practices against people with disabilities had prevented many from pursuing educational and employment opportunities. For those not already affluent, this often meant a lower-income existence. However, beginning with accessibility standards and legislation in the early 1960s, local, state, and now national codes and laws have gradually enfranchised this formerly disenfranchised group. The Architectural Barriers Act of 1968 requires accessibility in all federally assisted buildings; Section 504 of the Rehabilitation Act of 1973 and the Uniform Federal Accessibility Standards require accessibility for all federally assisted programs; the Education for Handicapped Children Act of 1975 requires equal access to educational settings for children with disabilities; the Fair Housing Act amendments of 1988 prohibit housing discrimination and require minimum or basic accessibility in large numbers of units in all covered multifamily-dwelling projects; and finally, the Americans with Disabilities Act (ADA) of 1990 prohibits discrimination on the basis of disability in almost all public or privately sponsored programs, services, or activities. This major civil rights law established the ADA Standards for Accessible Design (ADASAD) for accessibility in all new or existing buildings nationwide. These new standards either match or exceed the latest ANSI accessibility standards. With time, the ADASAD specifications are replacing existing local and state codes.

Along with these advances, the deinstitutionalization movement has moved many people with disabilities from large institutions into private settings, requiring that they be served with housing and support services in their local communities. Nationwide independent living programs are establishing centers where people with disabilities can find assistance or learn how to get the services they need to live independently in their communities. These trends are adding to the pressure for a broad variety of accessible and more usable housing in every price range and location. Additional alternatives include supportive living environments and community housing projects.

Another factor influencing housing is that more people with disabilities are graduating from schools and universities as trained professionals and skilled workers. They are moving up in the economic system to become taxpayers, thus creating a market for more appropriate housing.

The Future of Accessible Housing

Increasing numbers of people with disabilities, greater awareness of common needs in housing, new laws, improved attitudes, and advanced technologies have provoked important changes in our social system, and reciprocally, in our expectations for housing. These changes are defining a need for at least two types of accessible housing: a percentage of special housing designed specifically for people with particular types of disability; and large numbers of conventional but more universally usable housing units available on the open market in every price range, style, and location.

It has long been recognized that many of the features required for accessibility make life easier and more convenient for everyone. A person does not have to have a disability to benefit from "universal design." This approach argues that accessible features should and can be provided everywhere, eliminating the stigma associated with special features provided for people who are regarded as "handicapped," "disabled," or "elderly." In addition to the features described earlier in this entry, this would include careful design that meets and exceeds minimum accessibility standards; site placement that enables ground levels to meet interior floor levels (vehicles, rather than people, climb heights); removable vanity cabinets; and reinforced walls that could accept grab bars if needed. Adaptable housing ensures that some common access features are installed at construction time, others will be made adjustable, while others still could be added or removed when needed by particular occupants. Houses with these features do not look different, nor do they cost significantly more, as experience has proven.

The movements toward adaptable housing, equal program access, independent living, assistive technology, and fulfilling the rights of people with disabilities have brought people with disabilities into the mainstream of society. As outspoken advocates and consumers with political and economic power, this diverse population is finally being recognized as a potentially powerful market. When the housing industry accepts the reality that disability is a normal condition of life rather than a unique and tragic event, accessible housing will likewise enter the mainstream of design, building, and marketability.

(*See also:* ACCESSIBILITY; AMERICANS WITH DISABILITIES ACT; ARCHITECTURAL ACCESSIBILITY; DISABILITY LAW AND SOCIAL POLICY; HOMELESSNESS; INDEPENDENT LIVING; QUALITY OF LIFE)

RESOURCES

Adaptive Environments Center, 374 Congress St., Suite 301, Boston, MA 02210

Center for Universal Design (Center for Accessible Housing), School of Design, NC State University, P.O. Box 8613, Raleigh, NC 27695–8613

Excel Homes (modular universal home manufacturer), RR#2 P.O. Box 683, Liverpool, PA 17045

Fair Housing Information Clearing House, P.O. Box 6091, Rockville, MD 20850

Home Depot (universal homes program), 3030 North Rockey Point Drive, West, Suite 300, Tampa, FL 33607–5903

Home Store (modular universal homes), P.O. Box 300, Whately, MA 01093

U.S. Department of HUD–Fair Housing Office, 451 7th St., SW, Room 2535, Washington, DC 20410–2000

BIBLIOGRAPHY

ADAPTIVE ENVIRONMENTS CENTER. *A Consumer's Guide to Home Adaptation.* Boston, 1989.

BARRIER FREE ENVIRONMENTS. *Accessible Housing Design File.* New York, 1991.

BARRIER FREE ENVIRONMENTS FOR U.S. DEPARTMENT OF HOUSING AND URBAN DEVELOPMENT. *Adaptable Housing: Marketable Accessible Housing for Everyone.* Washington, DC, 1987.

———. *Universal Design: Housing for the Lifespan of All People.* Washington, DC, 1988.

LIEBROCK, CYNTHIA, with BEHAR, SUSAN. *Beautiful Barrier-Free: A Visual Guide to Accessibility.* New York, 1992.

MACE, RONALD L.; HARDIE, GRAEME J.; and PLACE, JAINE P. "Accessible Environments: Toward Universal Design." In *Design Intervention: Toward a More Human Architecture,* eds. Wolfgang E. Preiser et al., New York, 1990.

RACINO, JULIE ANN; WALKER, PAMELA; O'CONNOR, SUSAN; and TAYLOR, STEVEN, eds. *Housing Support and Community: Choices and Strategies for Adults with Disabilities.* Baltimore, 1993.

WYLDE, MARGARET; BARON-ROBBINS, ADRIAN; and CLARK, SAM. *Building for a Lifetime: The Design and Construction of Fully Accessible Homes.* Newton, CT, 1994.

RONALD L. MACE

HUMAN IMMUNODEFICIENCY VIRUS DISEASE AND ACQUIRED IMMUNE DEFICIENCY SYNDROME

The human immunodeficiency virus (HIV) causes a chronic, progressive immune deficiency disorder called HIV disease (HIVD); certain clinical patterns of advanced HIVD are called the acquired immune deficiency syndrome (AIDS). HIV is transmitted in blood and blood products, semen, and vaginal secretions; it therefore passes from person to person largely during anal, vaginal, or oral sexual intercourse, needle sharing (in using injected drugs), the transfusion or transplantation of infected blood or tissues, and accidents in health care. Transmission of HIV through nonintimate personal contact—air, water, shared facilities, respiratory secretions, or inanimate objects (except needles and related medical equipment)—does not occur. Shortly after infection, a period of unopposed replication allows HIV to infect a large proportion of immunologically competent cells; thereafter, in most infected people, the virus induces a gradual, progressive, but nonlinear decline in the number and function of those cells. The resulting deficiencies in tumor surveillance and control of infectious pathogens produce the most striking and consistent features of HIVD: opportunistic infections and neoplasms. HIV also infects neural tissue; lesions in the central nervous system, spinal cord, and peripheral nerves lead to characteristic clinical syndromes.

HIVD generally appears clinically in a series of relatively orderly, predictable phases or stages, which occur sequentially:

1. Acute (primary) HIVD. Usually self-limited, this protean illness (the symptoms of which are best described as "flulike" or "monolike") coincides with the rapid proliferation of HIV in a newly infected person; it precedes the development of specific antibodies to HIV, and therefore of a positive serologic test, by several weeks, and is difficult to recognize or diagnose. People with primary HIVD have very high concentrations of HIV in blood and body fluids, despite the absence of a positive antibody test.

2. Chronic asymptomatic HIVD. The longest period of a person's experience with HIV, this phase is defined by the simultaneous presence of clinical silence and progressive immunologic deficits. It may last more than a decade (though the range is broad; some people progress beyond asymptomatic disease in fewer than two years). People with chronic asymptomatic disease ordinarily feel and look well, the only evidence of their HIVD being a positive antibody test; the important "visible" clinical features are psychological, so people who do not know of their HIV infection have no symptoms. Disability at this time is psychological rather than physical. Immunologic changes are predictable but not inevitable; long-term "nonprogressors" (a very small percentage of all people with HIV) may retain normal immune function for twelve or more years. Although nonprogressors may have strikingly better cellular and antibody responses to HIV than most people, other variations in the course of HIVD, and therefore of the duration of the asymptomatic period, seem more related to strain variations in HIV itself than to either host factors or cofactors. The colloquial term "HIV positive," used to refer to people with chronic asymptomatic HIVD, is inadequate as a descriptor of the process, because it fails to describe the presence of an ongoing immunologic disorder. The point of "early intervention" therapy is to stabilize immune function by restricting the replication of HIV during this phase.

3. Chronic symptomatic HIVD. Once immunologic function is impaired further, physical symptoms develop. The manifestations of chronic symptomatic disease vary, but usually include (1)

constitutional symptoms—notably fever, night sweats, anorexia, and weight loss; (2) enlarged lymph nodes in multiple sites; and (3) a variety of recurrent disorders of skin (including, e.g., folliculitis, seborrheic dermatitis, and herpes zoster) and mucous membranes. Both the pattern and the individual illnesses may complicate a person's psychological adjustment to HIV, and both may also render people temporarily physically disabled. This phase generally lasts from three months to about three years.

4. Advanced HIVD/AIDS. AIDS is a clinical diagnosis, made by the presence of any of the tumors, infections, neuropsychiatric disorders, or wasting included in the surveillance definition established by the Centers for Disease Control and Prevention (CDC). For terminologic and conceptual consistency, the name "advanced HIVD" includes AIDS. The most important clinical patterns include (1) opportunistic infections—illnesses caused by organisms usually incapable of causing disease but given potency by the reduction of immunologic function—in the lung, brain, gastrointestinal tract, skin, or elsewhere; (2) cancers, which progress quickly in the absence of immunologic control (notably lymphomas, which are typically aggressive and resistant to usual treatments, and Kaposi's sarcoma, a skin tumor); (3) dementia and a number of disorders of central or peripheral nerves; and (4) wasting, with an extreme loss of lean body mass. In addition, the CDC now accept a reduction of helper lymphocytes (the primary "target cell" for HIV) to fewer than 200/mm³ as evidence of AIDS. Of the preceding, the most common sources of short-term disability are opportunistic infections, especially pneumonia and meningitis. But neurologic and malignant diseases, as well as the profound clinical effects of wasting, gradually occupy higher proportions of the time between opportunistic illnesses and thus are responsible for substantial components of disabilities.

The treatment of HIVD remains unsatisfactory, though improving. Attempts to control HIV have not been successful in living people; antiretroviral drugs, most of which are reverse transcriptase inhibitors, fail alone or in combinations to eliminate HIV, permanently paralyze its replication, or prevent its clinical effects, though they may delay the development of serious symptoms and improve the quality of life (if the toxicities of the drugs do not impede it). Theoretically, drug therapy directed against HIV might best begin before, rather than in reaction to, damage to the immune system; unfortunately, though, the most basic and important questions about timing the initiation of treatment remain to be answered, and the best sequence of primary and secondary agents is still controversial. The most promising approach is one in which combinations of antiretroviral drugs are employed in an individualized fashion, the specific therapy in any person determined by objective measurements of viral burden. Greater success has occurred with effective regimens to prevent many opportunistic infections (such as pneumonia caused by a parasite, *Pneumocystis carinii*, and disseminated infection with *Mycobacterium avium intracellulare*) and to treat many more. Taken together, antiviral and antimicrobial strategies have materially reduced hospital time, improved quality of life, delayed serious disease, and preserved performance status for most people with HIVD. At the same time, it is equally important to recognize that drug toxicities contribute meaningfully to the pattern of disability for many people with HIV.

There is much more to treating HIVD than medical therapies. A case management approach, in which people with HIV work in partnership with a variety of helping professionals (including counselors, therapists, nutritionists, social workers, and others), works best. Involving people with HIV in their own care helps them retain some control of what can otherwise seem a monolithic opponent in a battle where only the process, and not the outcome, is in doubt. Psychological assessment and management are important throughout, and strategies to provide social support are essential.

Patterns of Disability in HIVD

Patterns of disability are more useful concepts than phases of disease. Although there is a general consistency to the effects of any given "stage" of HIVD, there is also extraordinary variability. Different people with the same level of helper lymphocytes may have very different experiences; whereas most people with helper cell counts below 50/mm³ develop recurring significant illnesses, some retain both well-being and clinical stability. The types of disability noted below, then, do not necessarily correlate directly with the phases of disease described previously.

Psychological Disability. As is true of people with most other chronic illnesses, people with HIV complain bitterly of the disappearance of certainty in their lives and of the readjustments, changes, and discomforts created by its loss. These difficulties are particularly pertinent during the asymptomatic phase, when uncertainty is greatest. Anxiety, depression, and inability to sleep are common, and two-thirds of people with HIVD receive prescriptions for anxiolytic, antidepressant, or hypnotic drugs. Both these psychological symptoms and the toxicities of psychotropic agents can reduce attention span, restrict the speed and accuracy of thinking, and limit mental flexibility and creativity. The intensity of these effects is grossly unpredictable, and may change in the context of other life events; accordingly, the severity of the resulting disability likewise is variable and subject to the influence of occurrences in relationships, employment, and finance as well as disease.

Inhumane, prejudicial, and disrespectful attitudes toward people with HIV often contribute to alienation, depression, self-doubt, fear, and anxiety. Despite the improvements consequent to the passage of legislation such as the Americans with Disabilities Act (ADA) and the amelioration of hard sentiments among most Americans, people with HIV still feel unwelcome or despised in some homes, workplaces, and institutions. Some individuals with HIV have enormous psychological resiliency, regardless of their earlier life experience; some have more limiting psychological history and greater vulnerabilities. This internal psychological climate certainly warms and cools in the setting of the reactions and assistance provided by friends, family, peers, and agencies; those relational and social variables also shift with time. Accordingly, the specific combination of symptoms, reactions, and adjustments is hard to anticipate; it always reflects a changing reality. That a certain degree of psychological disability represents the conjoined effects of HIV, adjustments to having HIVD, psychological history, and social and relational support explains its richness and texture. Pro-

viding any of a number of medical, social, psychological, and support services may materially lessen the effects of any degree of psychological disability.

Occasional Systemic Illness. Constitutional symptoms during the chronic symptomatic phase (and thereafter) can limit or preclude many personal or occupational activities for days to months. Even if there is no identifiable underlying opportunistic infection, the fever and night sweats directly attributable to HIVD cause sleeplessness and exhaustion that prevent usual work, study, and social life. During this time, formal criteria may or may not justify a diagnosis of AIDS and therefore may or may not support applications for a variety of entitlement services.

Complicating illnesses can interfere with ability for various periods. Shingles (a reactivation of *varicella* [chicken pox] virus infection) causes pain and rash in the cutaneous distribution of a spinal nerve; although antiviral therapies improve the symptoms and limit their duration, many patients with shingles will be unable to perform their usual jobs for days to weeks. Recurrences of oral *herpes simplex* infection or aphthous stomatitis (canker sores) can make speech and swallowing painful or impossible.

When constitutional symptoms are not troubling and no complications are present, people with this pattern of disability may feel healthy and be able to work normally. But the presence of even intermittent physical complaints can exacerbate and complicate the psychological stress they feel and disturb the balance of their adjustment. Physical symptoms undermine the ability of a person with HIVD to manage anxiety, depression, loneliness, or sleeplessness; patients who did not require psychotropic medication before may need medications now. These drugs can produce side effects that add reversible components to the total pattern of disability.

Chronic Illness. As HIVD progresses, constitutional symptoms become more predictable. Lymph nodes are commonly enlarged, and visible or tender nodes cause both physical and psychological distress. Many patients will have started taking antiretroviral medications or prophylactic antibiotics to prevent opportunistic infections, and a significant minority will be enrolled in research trials that require time away from school or work. Depending on the pattern and tempo of illness, people may or may not be able to work in their usual occupations with some accommodations. The degree of disability, however, may vary on a daily basis; work attendance, study habits, and capacity to complete activities of ordinary living are decidedly unpredictable.

At this time many employers feel frustration: accommodations and understanding do not necessarily produce predictable work performance. The volatile combination of changing abilities, irregular attendance, varying accommodations, the concerns of coworkers, and the strong desire of many people with HIVD to continue working often causes tension in the workplace. At the same time, the personal and social environment for people with HIVD commonly becomes turbulent as well; friends and family grow concerned about imbalance in their loved one's life, and their expectations about medical care and rest may conflict with the patient's wish to remain active, working, and involved in activities.

Chronic Illness with Intermittent Acute Complications. Chronic illness, with its unpredictability, can be interrupted at intervals by acute complications (major infections, cycles of chemotherapy, or recurrences of neurologic conditions). Significant opportunistic infections, including pneumonia, meningitis, or retinitis can require hospitalization, prolonged outpatient therapy, or repeated clinic visits. There may be new medications (with new toxicities), referrals to different consultants, and a variety of diagnostic tests and procedures, which create substantial demands on time and resources and cause prolonged absences. When only a single major complication occurs (usually a first occurrence of *pneumocystis* pneumonia), an employee may return to work and a previous pattern of performance, or may do so with temporarily augmented accommodations. But a series of complications often heralds permanent disability or withdrawal from school.

Occasional Serious Illness. In this uncommon but important pattern, rare episodes of serious illness, sometimes requiring hospitalization or intensive therapy, punctuate long periods of good health. Usually an opportunistic infection resolves with treatment, and prophylactic therapy prevents recurrences. Increasingly flexible antiretroviral drug therapy, combined with more prophylactic antibiotics, has allowed more patients to maintain this pattern

of disability for long periods. Eventually a pattern of chronic illness replaces it—but while it lasts, employees are often able to maintain their usual work performance.

Progressive Chronic Illness. Eventually most patients develop significant wasting, permanent (though fluctuating) disability, and ongoing illness, interrupted by major crises demanding hospitalization or residential care. This progressive pattern brings escalating limitations in physical ability. Very few employees can continue work.

A significant minority of people with advanced HIVD develop dementia. Its frequency and severity have been reduced by antiretroviral therapies, which seem to reduce the impact of HIV on cognition and affect. Nonetheless, dementia remains a terrifying and disabling feature of advanced HIVD. It reduces performance status for individuals with any other disabling condition. The disabling results of combining dementia with sensory loss (especially blindness) are more than additive.

The progressive phase is exceedingly difficult, both for people with HIVD and for their partners, families, friends, coworkers, supervisors, and employees. As disability terminates employment, it also disconnects relationships; hospitalization, residential care, or hospice services may further remove people from predictable surroundings and usual caregivers. Negative attitudes about HIV, homophobia, and other prejudices can, of course, contribute to growing isolation. The fear of retribution or rejection can prevent people with HIVD from disclosing the reason for their absences and limitations and, therefore, from having access to accommodations and services they desperately need.

Disability and Rehabilitation Services

Management of people with HIVD responds to the chronicity, progressiveness, and predictable pattern of the illness; at each phase, specific assessments and interventions, including disability and rehabilitation services, are required. In general, the evaluation of their disabilities and the provision of appropriate accommodations and rehabilitation services are not different in content, process, or character from efforts made for individuals with other disabilities. Many of the disabilities associated with HIVD are not specific to HIVD; the limitations produced by recurrent pneumonias, lymphoma, or dementia closely resemble those occurring in other settings, and many of the needs are similar as well. The great bulk of accommodations or rehabilitation services needed by people with HIVD will not be conceptually or procedurally unique.

Nonetheless, there are special challenges in responding effectively to the disabilities and needs of people with HIVD. Both patients and providers of services must simultaneously manage their own fears and feelings, the reactions and questions of coworkers and colleagues, and the disability or rehabilitation needs identified. In both workplaces and service agencies, a clear, humane, respectful HIV policy is important. A strong positive statement allows an employer or service agency to express its commitment to meeting the needs of people with HIV. Statements that say only that discrimination will not occur are simply affirmations of intent to obey the law. Policies that affirm an employer's intent to welcome, accommodate, and enable people with HIVD contribute to a positive work environment, and similar policies in health care or rehabilitation facilities create safety for people with HIVD.

The fear of casual contagion (that HIV might be acquired by ordinary interpersonal contact) remains significant in many workplaces. Despite the reasonable assurance of public health officials and supervisors, some employees will directly or indirectly express concern about the presence of a person with HIVD. Having a carefully written policy helps produce consistency, and well-trained managers bring sensitivity and leadership. Having antidiscrimination laws that prohibit actions against an employee with HIVD does not prevent informal discrimination, and the most informal actions of all—among employees as peers—can be the most hurtful and restricting. These same fears may interfere with the willingness, effectiveness, or compassion of clinicians or support personnel who provide rehabilitation services.

In health care facilities, there are rational concerns about accidental transmission of HIV during the routine performance of job duties; guidelines issued by the CDC and the Occupational Safety and Health Administration (OSHA) should be followed whenever occupational transmission is a possibility.

Although most disability and rehabilitation services will not involve invasive procedures, all service providers having direct physical contact with patients should observe prescribed universal precautions then current.

A more general prejudice against people with HIVD, based on judgment about its acquisition, can also obstruct efforts to provide humane conditions and reasonable accommodations. The association of HIV with sexuality, needle sharing, and illicit drugs collaborates with the discomfort many Americans feel about sex (especially homosexuality), human differences, and drug use to produce moralistic attitudes, hurtful statements, and abusive treatment. Discomfort with people who are, or who are perceived to be, gay, lesbian, or bisexual underlies much mistreatment. When homophobia unites with the fear of casual contagion, there is potential for injustice, including verbal or physical violence. Similarly, people with HIVD face prejudice in their attempts to find medical, social, and disability services. Gay and bisexual men with HIVD may have had difficulty feeling safe with community services in the past, and building trust in service providers may take time. Racial prejudice is also an important barrier: African-American and Hispanic people are disproportionately affected by HIVD (not because of the biological correlates of ethnicity, but because of the social limitations determined by race in our society).

Working with people who have HIVD thus creates special training and support needs. Learning about HIV as a transmissible (but not contagious) virus and understanding the spectrum of clinical patterns and disability needs are the easier parts. Only marginally more difficult is discovering how to reduce occupational risks. The most demanding training is preparing to work with people whose differences sometimes stimulate powerful feelings and fears. Clarifying attitudes and values is essential to this preparation; self-assessment, discussing issues in small groups, or working through concerns with a trusted mentor may be successful. Working effectively with people with HIVD requires that we manage our own beliefs and attitudes about race, sexuality, and intimacy. We must confront the connections we make between behavior and illness, and the moral tone we attach to those associations. Regardless of the tenacity of our own beliefs, we must dispense with the arrogance of presuming to judge the nature or behavior of another; people with HIVD must not encounter opprobrium from service providers, nor should they be frightened by our fears or embarrassed by our gossip. The most carefully designed programs and services will fail if patients are offended or made to feel unsafe.

Providers of disability services confront other important challenges. People with HIVD are often young; they may not have the social supports, financial resources, insurance, or developmental maturity to manage disabilities effectively. Service providers have to make adjustments: Dealing with dementia in an eighty-year-old is different from managing the uncertain and variable course of that disability in a twenty-nine-year-old. Some people with HIVD have had virtually no access to medical or social services; some, especially injecting drug users, have criminal records and histories of negative interactions with society's systems. Many people with HIVD have nontraditional families: gay men with partners; unmarried women with children; people, young or old, who no longer feel connected to their families of origin. These families, regardless of their description and legal status, are often vital and loving companions; their support is essential, and acknowledging their presence and role is important.

Although the pattern of disability observed over time may be one of gradual and progressive decline, the day-to-day balance of capacity and challenge in the life of a person with HIVD changes frequently. Therefore it is often not possible to plan with accuracy the intensity of accommodation needed. The most useful and reasonable approach is to make "best guess" plans that include contingency strategies to allow for acute adjustments when some usual activity (walking, climbing steps, carrying materials, word processing) is impossible on any given day. Sometimes the pattern of intermittent acute illness requires more intensive accommodations temporarily; during convalescence from a complication, some people with HIVD receive home or outpatient therapies, including intravenous medications, that interfere with some, but not all, abilities and require some, but not all, of the patient's time. In the workplace, these treatments may demand a private place and time. If needles are used in treatments, there

must be safe disposal procedures and containers. The reality of hyperacute changes in functional capacities, work performance, and accommodation needs can influence the perceived effectiveness of disability services; it may also discourage practitioners who attempt to rehabilitate people with HIVD when today's regression in ability obscures the memory of yesterday's progress. Flexibility is thus required in evaluating people with HIVD and in adjusting to shifts and fluctuations in their patterns.

A final challenge concerns confidentiality of information. The threat of unwanted disclosure of the diagnosis (and of other personal characteristics that others might assume) is of the loss of relationships, family, housing, and livelihood. In most states, statutory protection of confidential information concerning HIVD is specific and strong; penalties for unauthorized disclosure are significant. For both legal and humane reasons, providers and agencies serving persons with HIVD must attend carefully to these requirements and restrictions. Confidentiality about the personal history of people with HIVD may be difficult to maintain, especially in a small office or agency. Curiosity, carelessness, misguided good intentions, and the need for power and control (usually disguised as "need to know") are enemies of privacy. The connection of HIVD to such deeply interesting human behaviors as sexual intercourse fuels speculation about employees' personal lives. But service providers and employers must always adhere strictly to the letter and spirit of statutes and ethical guidelines when handling confidential information.

(*See also:* ATTITUDES; CAREGIVING; DISABILITY MANAGEMENT; HOSPICE; LOSS AND GRIEF; PHARMACOLOGY; PSYCHOSOCIAL ADJUSTMENT; QUALITY OF LIFE)

RESOURCES

Business Responds to AIDS Resource Center, P.O. Box 6003, Rockville, MD 20849–6003

CDC National AIDS Hotline, American Social Health Association, P.O. Box 13827, Research Triangle Park, NC 27709

Impact AIDS, Inc., 369 18th St., San Francisco, CA 94110

National Leadership Coalition on AIDS, 1730 M St., NW, Suite 305, Washington, DC 20036

Office of HIV/AIDS Education, American Red Cross

National Headquarters, 1709 New York Ave., NW, Washington, DC 20006

BIBLIOGRAPHY

BATESON, MARY CATHERINE, and GOLDSBY, RICHARD. *Thinking AIDS: The Social Response to the Biological Threat.* Reading, MA, 1988.

COHEN, PHILIP T.; SANDE, MERLE A.; and VOLBERDING, PAUL A. *The AIDS Knowledge Base.* Waltham, MA, 1990.

CRIMP, DOUGLAS. *AIDS: Cultural Analysis, Cultural Activism.* Cambridge, MA, 1989.

DEVITA JR, VINCENT T.; HELLMAN, SAMUEL; and ROSENBERG, STEVEN A. *AIDS: Etiology, Diagnosis, Treatment, and Prevention,* 2nd ed. Philadelphia, 1988.

PRESTON, JOHN. *Personal Dispatches: Writers Confront AIDS.* New York, 1991.

SONTAG, SUSAN. *AIDS and Its Metaphors.* New York, 1989.

VOLBERDING, PAUL. "HIV Infection as a Disease: The Medical Indications for Early Diagnosis." *Journal of AIDS* 2 (1989):421–425.

WACHTEL, TOM; PIETTE, JOHN; MOR, VINCENT; STEIN, MICHAEL; FLEISHMAN, JOHN; and CARPENTER, CHARLES. "Quality of Life in Persons with HIV Infection: Measurement by the Medical Outcomes Study Instrument." *Annals of Internal Medicine* 116 (1992):129–137.

RICHARD P. KEELING

HUMAN RESOURCE DEVELOPMENT

Pivotal to the efficiency and effectiveness of rehabilitation service delivery is the quality of the personnel working within the systems (rehabilitation agencies, facilities, and companies) providing the services. The Rehabilitation Act of 1954 legislatively appropriated federal funds for research (to generate and develop new knowledge) and education and training of personnel (to impart and infuse new knowledge) within rehabilitation systems. Thus, from the early 1950s through the early 1980s, education and training (preservice, in-service, and continuing education) were the primary forums for the development of rehabilitation personnel.

In understanding the richness of human resource development in the field of rehabilitation, it is important to note the distinctive denotative and connotative features and characteristics of training, education, and development.

Training. Training (*a*) involves the act or process of directing or informing, usually by means of instruction, discipline, or drill; (*b*) targets employees who are passively involved in the training tasks and activities; (*c*) is typically designed to enable trainees to perform their current jobs at a higher level; and (*d*) aims to enhance consistency and reduce individualism among the trainees.

Education. Education (*a*) is designed to enhance overall knowledge and performance; (*b*) is focused on the individual needs of the employee (as opposed to training, where the focus is on the needs of the job and job requirements); (*c*) is designed to support future, expanded jobs and job requirements; and (*d*) tends to broaden individual differences among workers.

Development. Development (*a*) includes activities that are more future-directed; (*b*) is less specific and more difficult to measure; and (*c*) typically is focused on facilitating individual and organizational change.

Training might involve short programs designed to teach employees what they need to do to comply with new policies and procedures; education, a graduate course on ethics offered by a nearby college or university; and development, an in-service program on time management taught and facilitated by an expert/consultant.

Throughout the late 1980s and the early 1990s, all sectors of the field of rehabilitation experienced reductions in available resources, increased demands to serve new client populations, and increased pressures for greater accountability and cutbacks in management. This prompted numerous controversies as to the relative and comparative value of training, education, and development. Moreover, research documented the importance and necessity of having cooperative and synergistic relationships not only among training, education, and development but also among these three components and those of policy, administration, management and supervision, and day-to-day operations.

In the later 1980s, stronger and more cooperative relationships among the Rehabilitation Services Administration, the Council of State Administrators of

Vocational Rehabilitation, and the National Council on Rehabilitation Education led to numerous coordinated initiatives, which culminated in annual conferences designed to make concrete a "human resource development model" of training, education, and development activities. In addition, enhanced strategic involvement from professional organizations (such as the National Rehabilitation Association and its professional divisions), other systems groups (such as the National Association of Rehabilitation Facilities), and private sector rehabilitation entities (such as the National Association of Rehabilitation Professionals in the Private Sector) strengthened the human resource development movement in the field of rehabilitation.

It is expected that as the field of rehabilitation moves toward the year 2000, the spiraling rate of change will reveal (a) new client disability groups in need of rehabilitation services; (b) new workforce groups with increased educational, age, and cultural diversity among them; (c) new and enhanced credentialing criteria (e.g., for certification, licensure, and accreditation); and (d) new service delivery technologies. Thus, the need for a human resource development approach to training, education, and development as a central and integral entity of all rehabilitation agencies, facilities, and companies will continue. Also by the year 2000, human resource development initiatives will likely be more active in the areas of planning, development, and implementation.

(See also: CREDENTIALS; MANAGEMENT)

RESOURCES

Council of State Administrators of Vocational Rehabilitation, P.O. Box 3776, Washington, DC 20007

National Council on Rehabilitation Education, Department of Special Education, Utah State University, Logan, UT 84322–2870

Rehabilitation Services Administration, U.S. Department of Education, Office of Special Education and Rehabilitation Services, 400 Maryland Ave. SW, Washington, DC 20208

BIBLIOGRAPHY

EMENER, WILLIAM G.; LUCK, RICHARD S.; and SMITS, S. J., eds. *Rehabilitation Administration and Supervision.* Baltimore, 1981.

NAGLER, MARK. *Perspectives on Disability,* 2nd ed. Palo Alto, CA, 1993.

RIGGAR, TED F., and LORENZ, J. R., eds. *Readings in Rehabilitation Administration.* Albany, 1985.

WRIGHT, GEORGE N. *Total Rehabilitation.* Boston, 1980.

WILLIAM G. EMENER

HUMAN SERVICES

There is no single definition of human services that would satisfy all of the experts in the field. Yeheskel Hasenfeld's (1983) definition of human services as activities designed to protect or enhance the personal well-being of individuals is a broad one that encompasses a wide spectrum of services. A narrower definition, favored by some, would limit human services to activities designed to help people overcome the immediate effects of illness, disability, and economic dependency. Paul Schmolling and his colleagues (1993) proposed a definition that falls between the very broad and narrower ones; in their view, human services are organized activities that help people who are unable to meet their own needs play a useful role in society. These persons in need may be living with mental, emotional, or physical disabilities, or they may be victims of adverse social and economic circumstances. Considering that the criminal justice system and social welfare programs are included in the definition, it is obvious that human services cover a lot of ground, and taken together, constitute a major industry. In fact, about 12 percent of all employed people in the United States work in human services, either providing direct services or administering them (Hasenfeld, 1983).

It is important to note also what human services are *not*. The kinds of help given by family, friends, and peer groups are not included. The term "human services" implies that the benefits are provided by some sort of formal organization, be it an agency, bureau, school, clinic, hospital, or nursing home. These organizations may be sponsored—that is, organized and funded—by private citizens, religious and paternal groups, or by government. They may be profit-making, but most are operated on a nonprofit basis.

In the past, religious organizations and the family were the main providers of help to persons in need. A significant historical trend has been the increasing role of government, especially in industrialized nations, in providing human services. It cannot be said that governments were motivated entirely by deep concern for unfortunate citizens. Early welfare legislation was designed as a means of social control when periods of economic instability, famine, and epidemics threatened to destroy the existing social structure (Schmolling, Youkeles, and Burger, 1993). The Elizabethan Poor Law of 1601 reduced the emphasis on repressive and punitive measures that typified earlier legislation. Although some harsh measures were included, particularly in regard to vagrants, its historical importance rests on the fact that government accepted a positive obligation to help those who could not help themselves. The modern welfare state was initiated by Otto von Bismarck for similar reasons. During the 1880s the German leader adopted a program of social welfare legislation, including health insurance, accident insurance, and old-age and disability pensions. His intent was clearly to present an alternative to socialism, thereby preserving the property-holding, capitalist system.

In the United States, the federal government did not assume significant responsibility for human services until the 1930s—that is, not until large numbers of destitute unemployed were on the verge of revolt. During the administration of Franklin D. Roosevelt, Congress enacted the Social Security Act in 1935, which provided financial assistance to the elderly, dependent children, and persons with physical disabilities. Many additional programs were developed in subsequent decades. Among the most important were the Medicare and Medicaid programs (1965), which provided medical insurance to elderly and low-income persons, respectively. Another important milestone was enactment of the Supplemental Security Income (SSI) program (1972), which gives monthly cash benefits to people who are sixty-five or older, *or* are blind, *or* who have a disability *and* limited resources and incomes. During the 1970s and 1980s the general thrust of legislation and court decisions was to end discrimination against persons with disabilities in regard to educa-

tion, employment, services, and benefits. The intent was to begin admitting Americans with disabilities into the mainstream of life.

Early historical efforts were devoted mainly to helping dependent persons survive by providing them with food, clothing, and shelter. Institutional settings such as prisons and asylums made little distinction among various kinds of inmates and tended to provide minimal custodial care. Gradually the idea took hold that many of the beneficiaries might be treated or rehabilitated to improve their functioning. Ideally, the goal of modern rehabilitation efforts is to bring about the maximal degree of self-sufficiency possible for each person with a disability. In reality, serious obstacles prevent full accomplishment of this goal. One of these is the lack of sufficient funding. For example, some school systems have not yet made the physical renovations or provided the special equipment needed by children with disabilities. In fairness, it must be recognized that the expenses involved are considerable and would impose a strain on a tight school budget. There is also a danger of a loss of community support if the demands of social activists for persons with disabilities seem unreasonable or take funding away from other good causes.

Another unresolved problem preventing full rehabilitation of some individuals is that the social security and medical insurance regulations tend to discourage some people with disabilities from seeking full employment. If they earn above a certain amount, there is a risk of losing government support. It is ironic that the systems designed to help take away the incentive to become self-supporting. Many people with mental or developmental liabilities remain stuck within the system, sometimes because family members fear the loss of security provided by the benefits.

Since the 1960s there has been a softening of negative societal attitudes toward people with disabilities. There is abundant evidence, reviewed by Adrienne Asch (1984), that people with disabilities arouse strong negative emotions in able-bodied people, including anxieties about vulnerability and weakness. However, there is an increasing willingness on the part of the general public to accept people with disabilities into schools, colleges, and the workplace. The able-bodied person is learning to get beyond another's disability and relate on the basis of shared human feelings and desires. Hopefully, this process will accelerate as there is increasing contact between the two groups. The processes of mainstreaming and normalization are expected to continue for the foreseeable future, as is the tendency to view persons with disabilities as consumers of human services. As Robert Burgdorf (1980) noted, the history of society's treatment of people with disabilities can be summed up in two words: "segregation" and "inequality." There is every reason to expect that society has entered a new, more positive phase in its treatment of persons with disabilities.

(*See also:* ATTITUDES; CAREGIVING; CIVIL RIGHTS; CONSUMERS)

BIBLIOGRAPHY

ASCH, ADRIENNE. "The Experience of Disability: A Challenge for Psychology." *American Psychologist* 39 (1984):551–552.

BURGDORF, ROBERT L., JR. *The Legal Rights of Handicapped Persons.* Baltimore, 1980.

HASENFELD, YEHESKEL. *Human Service Organizations.* Englewood Cliffs, NJ, 1983.

SCHMOLLING, PAUL; YOUKELES, MERRILL; and BURGER, WILLIAM. *Human Services in Contemporary America,* 3rd ed. Pacific Grove, CA, 1993.

PAUL SCHMOLLING

HUNTINGTON'S DISEASE

See GENETIC DISORDERS; NEUROLOGICAL DISORDERS

I

INDEPENDENT LIVING

It is generally acknowledged that the first independent living program was started in Berkeley, California, in 1972 by Ed Roberts and other disability rights activists who were looking for alternatives to institutional living. Like programs that were started later in 1972 in Houston and Boston, the Berkeley independent living program provided support services in a residential setting for people who wanted more control over their lives than was typically available in long-term-care institutions. In 1972, with little in the way of community-based service options or accessible housing available to people with disabilities, independent living services almost had to be provided in residential settings.

Funding of Independent Living Centers

Securing support for activities designed to promote development of services programs operated by and for people with disabilities got under way in earnest during the 1970s. After several unsuccessful attempts, disability rights advocates were successful in getting federal funding for independent living ser-

vices through inclusion of Title VII in the 1978 amendments to the Rehabilitation Act of 1973. Although the Title VII authorization included provisions for funding both independent living services, under Part A of the act, and start-up money for independent living centers, under Part B of the act, funds were appropriated initially only for Part B. In 1979, Part B funding was provided for ten independent living centers in different parts of the country. However, as indicated by Ted Thayer and Douglas B. Rice (1990), many saw Part A as a means for ongoing support of independent living services, with Part B viewed as merely "start-up" or "seed" money.

Since 1978, appropriations for Title VII, Part B, have increased at a very modest rate from year to year. However, distribution of funding across states has not been uniform. The way the Title VII regulations were written gave state vocational rehabilitation agencies first right of refusal over administration of Part B funding. In a few states, the vocational rehabilitation agencies relinquished any control of Part B funding and allowed the funds to go directly to the independent living centers without passing through the state agency. In most states, the state vocational rehabilitation agency accepted

Part B funding and assumed responsibility for granting it to consumer-controlled independent living centers—giving the state agency considerable control over the way in which those centers operated. In a very few states, the state vocational rehabilitation agency used Part B funds to support delivery of independent living services by agency personnel and did not provide any funding to consumer-controlled independent living centers. As a result, there were a few states in which no consumer-controlled independent living centers were established prior to the 1992 Rehabilitation Act amendments.

No funds were appropriated for Part A of Title VII until 1986, when $11 million was appropriated for purchase of independent living services—roughly $200,000 per state. However, the way the implementing regulations for Part A funding were written still allowed state vocational rehabilitation agencies considerable latitude in the allocation of Part A funds. The regulations required that only 20 percent of Part A funds be committed to purchase of services from consumer-controlled, community-based agencies such as independent living centers. In a number of states, minimal amounts of the Part A funding found their way to independent living centers. The largest share of the funds was used by state vocational rehabilitation agencies to purchase durable medical equipment, home modification services, and other products and services often furnished through more traditional medical and vocational rehabilitation service providers. In other states, almost all of the Part A funding went to the direct purchase of services by the state vocational rehabilitation agencies from independent living centers through fee-for-service or contractual agreements.

Another factor contributing to the differences in funding for independent living centers from state to state has been the commitment of state funds. In a number of states, such as New York, California, Illinois, and Pennsylvania, advocacy efforts by disability groups have resulted in commitment of state general revenue funds to support centers, usually in conjunction with the state vocational rehabilitation agency. Although fiscal problems in some states, most notably California and New York, threatened this support in the late 1980s and early 1990s, the commitment of these funds during the early years of the movement was crucial to the development of a statewide network of independent living centers in these states. In many states, the commitment of state funding for independent living centers has been very modest, and relatively fewer centers have been established in these states. In quite a number of states, no state funding has been committed to support centers, and development of statewide networks of independent living centers has simply not occurred in these states.

With the initiation of federal support for centers, it has been explicit that centers are expected to engage in resource development rather than relying solely on federal support. In some respects, independent living centers represent an organizational hybrid in the disability-related service milieu. While receiving some support from federal and, in some cases, state agencies—not unlike state vocational rehabilitation boards or other public entities—centers are also expected to behave in an entrepreneurial fashion through revenue-generating activities that include establishing fee-for-service programs and other fund-raising activities. In this regard, centers are expected to behave like public agencies with regard to reporting requirements and other accountability procedures while also behaving like free-enterprise operations by operating efficient and effective programs that generate revenue to support services. While not intending to imply that public agencies are never—and private businesses are always—efficient, it is clear that some centers have struggled with problems related to satisfying public agency reporting requirements while also trying to build resource capacity through more entrepreneurial endeavors.

Notwithstanding the hybrid nature of independent living centers, the boards and staff of centers have become increasingly adept at fund-raising and resource development in the years since the establishment of the first centers. By the early 1990s, centers had become involved in a variety of revenue-generating activities. These efforts included selling services to those public and private agencies serving people with disabilities, marketing services related to compliance with the Americans with Disabilities Act, and selling durable medical equipment and other products through for-profit and not-for-profit subsidiary businesses. Other innovative funding approaches are discussed later in this entry.

Independent Living Services

Like the independent living movement itself, the mix of independent living services provided by centers continues to evolve. As mentioned earlier, the first independent living programs offered services in residential settings where people with disabilities could take advantage of shared services, such as personal assistance and meal preparation. At the time the first centers were started, there was little in the way of community-based services and few accessible housing options. For many people with disabilities, the only living options available involved family support or institutional living in nursing homes or state-operated facilities.

The development of residential options in non-institutional settings, such as group homes and apartment complexes, was a step forward for people with severe disabilities who had few options available to them. However, as the independent living philosophy evolved, it became increasingly clear that programs that fostered services in segregated living arrangements—in which people with disabilities were not integrated with other people with and without disabilities—were not promoting full inclusion. Residential facilities, no matter how well operated, that provided living options only for people with disabilities were vulnerable to becoming disability "ghettos" that contributed to social isolation and disengagement of people with disabilities from the larger community. Over the years since the independent living movement was founded, leaders in the movement became increasingly vocal in their opposition to residential options that segregated people with disabilities. Such opposition was targeted not only at institutional settings such as nursing homes, previously the only option available to many persons with disabilities, but also at publicly funded housing that was restricted to certain populations, such as "the elderly and disabled." This philosophical stand against segregated housing had the effect of moving independent living centers away from residential services and toward development of community-based service programs that could be delivered to anyone in the community with a disability, regardless of his or her living arrangements.

Today, independent living centers, operating as not-for-profit corporations, provide a wide range of services to cross-disability service populations. Determinations about the types of services to be offered by each center are made by governing boards composed of a majority of persons with disabilities who live in the area served by the center. Although there are service variations from center to center, all centers receiving federal funding through Title VII of the Rehabilitation Act must provide four core services: (1) information and referral; (2) peer counseling; (3) independent living skills training; and (4) individual and systems advocacy.

Information and referral services constitute a large portion of many centers' service activities, particularly in smaller centers with staff and budget limitations that restrict the volume of direct services that can be offered. Providing information about housing, transportation options, income support programs, and other service programs addresses a critical need for persons with disabilities who may have little knowledge or fragmented service systems. Likewise, by offering independent living skills training provided by center staff, volunteers, and consultants, centers can assist persons with disabilities in acquiring skills that enhance their abilities to live independently. Such skills might include managing a personal budget, using the public transportation system, or supervising a personal assistant who comes into the home intermittently. Like other programs offered by centers, the range of independent living skills training provided varies according to the preferences and expressed needs of persons with disabilities living in communities served.

The peer counseling concept has always been surrounded by some controversy. Since the notion of peer counseling was first introduced in the early years of the independent living movement, some individuals from more established counseling fields have been critical of this approach. This criticism is based on narrow interpretations of what "counseling" is and who may do it. These narrow interpretations have been codified in some states that have imposed legal restrictions on use of the term "counselor." In a few states, only persons with specific types of credentials can refer to themselves as counselors and offer counseling services. In response to these types of restrictions, independent living centers use terms such as "peer visitor" to describe staff with disabilities who provide assistance and support to other individuals with disabilities who are coping with physical and attitudinal barriers that diminish opportunities for optimal independence. The peer counselor approach is grounded in the notion expressed by Edward V. Roberts (1979) that "those who know best the needs of disabled people and how to meet those needs are the disabled themselves." Today, the value of peer counseling as an important tool in adjusting to disability has been documented (Barker, Altman, and Youngdahl, 1987; Shreve, 1991), and the requirement for peer counseling services as a core service of independent living centers is indicative of the level of acceptance of this approach by federal funding agencies.

Individual and systems advocacy, the fourth core service that must be offered by federally funded independent living centers, has also been somewhat controversial. Individual advocacy, or activities designed to assist an individual consumer in dealing with barriers to programs or services, generally has been accepted as an important service by most persons, including representatives of public or private funding and regulatory agencies vested with oversight responsibility for independent living centers.

Questions have been raised, however, about systems advocacy activities and the legitimacy of such activities as "services." These questions have been raised particularly with regard to aggressive advocacy efforts, such as street rallies, sit-ins, and the occupation of buildings by persons with disabilities who are trying to draw attention to policies and regulations that may detract from their efforts to attain optimal independence. Such high-profile advocacy efforts typically attract a good deal of media attention, which in turn leads to questions about public support for organizations that may be engaged in activities that may be perceived as civil disobedience. It has been the position of leaders in the independent living field that people with disabilities should draw upon the full array of weapons in the advocacy armamentarium—including civil disobedience as well as legislative activism—to fight against disability-based discrimination in programs and services. The inclusion of the broad definition of advocacy (i.e., including both individual and systems-targeted efforts) as a required core service of federally funded independent living centers provides tacit rec-

ognition of advocacy as a true "service" to persons living in areas served by independent living centers.

Beyond the four core services required of all federally funded independent living centers, the range of services offered by centers varies considerably. Some centers offer sign language interpreter services, while others offer reader services for persons with visual impairments; some centers operate large-scale personal assistance service programs, while others coordinate transportation services for persons living in underserved rural areas. One of the strengths of independent living centers has been their ability to respond to needs and service preferences of individuals in diverse communities. Rather than a "cookie cutter" approach to service development and delivery, in which each center mimics the others in its state or region, independent living centers tend to display considerable variation in service programs, staffing arrangements, and other characteristics. These variations allow for appropriate responses to consumers in communities with different levels of service available to the specific segments of the disability population served and create opportunities for innovation that may be lacking in more proscribed service models.

Research on Independent Living

Research on implementation of the independent living philosophy has been under way since the early years of the movement. Seminal research was done by Gerben DeJong in the late 1970s, comparing the "independent living paradigm" to the "medical rehabilitation paradigm." DeJong's comparisons of the two approaches to disability-related programs helped to crystallize fundamental distinctions in the manner in which services are organized and delivered. According to DeJong's analyses, while traditional rehabilitation approaches tend to define problems faced by people with disabilities as stemming from individual impairments that minimize functional capabilities, the independent living approach defines the problem in terms of hostile environments and attitudes that force persons with disabilities to be dependent on medical and vocational rehabilitation professionals, family members, and others whose interventions are required to overcome barriers. In the traditional rehabilitation model, the emphasis is on "fixing" the individual with an impairment, whereas in the independent living model the emphasis is on changing the environment to eliminate or reduce barriers to participation by persons with disabilities. Whereas traditional rehabilitation models assign the role of patient or client to the person being served, the independent living model suggests that individuals be viewed as consumers or users of services who should be the driving force in determining how services are delivered. And in terms of outcomes, traditional rehabilitation models are targeted at optimizing self-care or securing gainful employment, while the independent living model targets maximizing all options for full integration of persons with disabilities into all aspects of community life. DeJong's original research contrasting these service paradigms has provided a sound basis for ongoing efforts to explore the philosophical constructs of the independent living movement. Refinements on DeJong's original work have been made by Margaret Shreve and June Kailes (1994).

Since earlier research by DeJong, Susan Pflueger, and others, research on independent living services has been continuing at several locations. The first federally funded research and training center on independent living (RTC-IL) was established at the University of Kansas at Lawrence in 1980. James Budde, Mark Mathews, and others at the Kansas RTC did much of the early work on center organization, including working with the field to develop early standards against which the performance of federally funded centers could be assessed. In 1985, the Independent Living Research Utilization (ILRU) program in Houston, Texas, obtained funding from the National Institute on Disability and Rehabilitation Research (NIDRR) for a second RTC-IL. ILRU's early research, led by Margaret Nosek and Marcus Fuhrer, focused on refining the definition of independence so that the efforts of independent living centers and other service organizations working to foster independence could be understood better. In 1990, the World Institute on Disability (WID) in Oakland, California, received funding from NIDRR to establish an RTC-IL specific to public policy issues relating to persons with disability. WID's efforts, led by Simi Litvak, Judy Heumann, and Ed Roberts, have resulted in a number of key policy recommendations around programmatic issues in delivery of independent living services.

In early 1994, NIDRR convened a group of people knowledgeable about independent living and the operation of centers to secure advice on future research priorities for the field. Among the proposals emerging from this meeting were: (1) recommendations for further research on personal assistance services and their role in fostering independence; (2) access to health care and the influence of insurance restrictions on health care services and independence for persons with disabilities; and (3) ways to enhance management of independent living centers and to promote development of optimal service programs for people with disabilities who may be currently underserved by centers, including people with mental health and cognitive disabilities as well as people from racial and ethnic minority groups. As of late 1994, these recommendations were being considered by NIDRR leaders charged with developing research priorities for the immediate future.

Developments and Critical Issues Facing the Field

Although the independent living movement is relatively young—the first programs having been established in the early 1970s—considerable progress has been made in advocating for greater consumer control and direction in programs serving people with disabilities, including independent living centers and other service programs. This progress is reflected in the 1992 amendments to the Rehabilitation Act of 1973. With the 1992 amendments to the act, consumer control of centers was further strengthened through direct funding of independent living centers in most states. While this change places greater responsibility on centers to use federal funds responsibly, it also affords them the opportunity to plan and implement programs and services with far less involvement of state vocational rehabilitation agency staff who, in some cases, were more comfortable working in the traditional rehabilitation model rather than the independent living model approach to services. Other changes resulting from the 1992 amendments explicitly define "consumer control" as it relates to centers, a significant change over the vague definition of consumer control included in the act prior to 1992. This definition mandates that persons with disabilities be a majority of individuals constituting governing boards, management staff, and overall staff of independent living centers eligible for federal funding.

A very significant change resulting from the 1992 amendments to the Rehabilitation Act of 1973 relates to establishment of Statewide Independent Living Councils (SILCs) charged with preparing plans for development of independent living services in each state. As with board and staff of centers of independent living centers, each SILC must be comprised of a majority of persons with disabilities. To avoid conflict of interest, the voting majority of persons with disabilities serving on the SILC cannot include staff of independent living centers or employees of state agencies, including vocational rehabilitation agencies. The SILCs are vested with substantial authority, since the plans developed by each SILC govern development of independent living services in each state, including decisions regarding establishment of new centers. As of July 1, 1995, each SILC is required to prepare a three-year plan for independent living services in the state in which it operates. Joint approval for the statewide independent living plans is vested with both the chair of the SILC and the head of the "designated state unit(s)," meaning the head of the vocational rehabilitation agency and in many states the heads of both the general vocational rehabilitation agency and the head of the vocational rehabilitation agency serving adults who are blind. This represents a major advance in consumer control by giving the heads of consumer-controlled entities—the SILCs—equal authority with the heads of state agencies in planning service programs. Many in the independent living movement are urging even greater consumer control over the planning of independent living services by advocating for approval of statewide independent living plans solely by the chair of the SILC.

The establishment of consumer-controlled SILCs has brought with it new challenges for the field. These include the need for research on how to foster optimal functioning of the SILCs so that adequate training can be developed to allow individuals serving on SILCs to fulfill their responsibilities. When the 1992 amendments took effect in late 1993, many people appointed to SILCs by governors of various states, or their designated representatives, had little understanding of the roles they were expected to fill or the authority that has been vested in them to set the agenda for independent living service development for entire states. Training of persons serving in the crucial role of SILC member is of paramount importance, and training is being provided through the National Council on Independent Living (NCIL), ILRU, and others.

In addition to the challenges posed by changes in the Rehabilitation Act amendments of 1992, other critical issues are facing the independent living field. These include health care reform, establishment of adequate personal assistance services (PAS), addressing the needs of underserved populations, development of training opportunities for the field, and exploration of more effective governing structures to support development of independent living centers. Health care reform is a critical issue for persons with disabilities. Many individuals with disabilities are unable to secure adequate health insurance coverage because of preexisting conditions and find themselves faced with the prospect of declining attractive job offers so they can continue to be eligible for public health programs. Still other individuals with disabilities are denied employment because of the concerns of potential employers regarding escalating health insurance premiums associated with hiring someone with a "preexisting condition." For independent living centers, with their commitment to hiring people with disabilities, the health care reform issue has particular poignancy as they find themselves faced with escalating costs for premiums, and in some cases, making the choice between dropping insurance coverage for staff or substantially curtailing services in order to cover rising health insurance costs.

Similarly, the personal assistance service (PAS) issue is of paramount concern to the field. After years of fighting to "demedicalize" PAS so that reasonably priced service systems could be developed using persons without specialized health care credentials, the independent living field found itself arguing on behalf of inclusion of PAS in health care reform proposals as an approach to developing a national plan for PAS. Many leaders in the field believed it to be worth the risk of "remedicalizing" PAS to some degree if a national plan for providing much-needed PAS services could be included in the health care reform package. The availability of adequate support services is critical in ensuring optimal independence of persons with disabilities in home, work, and other settings. Because of this, efforts to secure or expand funding for PAS is likely to remain a "front burner" issue.

With regard to underserved populations (e.g., persons from ethnic or racial minority groups, persons with mental health or cognitive disabilities, older persons with disabilities), Gerben DeJong (1979) documented the origins of the movement with college-age European-American persons, most of whom had physical disabilities. This constituency has been slow to change since the early 1970s, but change is occurring. New federal initiatives have been designed to give priority to development of independent living services for underserved groups. More and more diversity is seen in the ranks of the movement. However, additional work needs to be done on ways in which the independent living philosophy, with its emphasis on consumer control and direction, can be used effectively with diverse groups of people with disabilities, including individuals who may have cognitive or mental impairments that influence judgment and decision making. True cross-disability representation has not yet been realized by the movement.

Research on effective ways for addressing training needs of the field is also a high priority. Standardized entry-level training has not been developed for the field, and on-the-job training continues to be the primary approach to prepare people for jobs in independent living centers (Smith et al., 1991; 1994). With rapid advances in learning technology, including breakthroughs in distance learning methods, training programs can be developed that are not limited by physical barriers that persist on many college campuses and in other learning settings, or by the high costs associated with replication of support systems (e.g., PAS, accessible housing and transportation) required for many persons with disabilities to access learning opportunities. Such research should be pursued aggressively.

Finally, research on governing structures that retain the important ingredient of consumer control but that truly foster effective and sustained development of independent living centers and services needs to be undertaken. Data gathered by ILRU, as well as anecdotal reports from the field, indicate that problems related to board and staff interactions continue to threaten ongoing operation of many centers. There are at least some indications that board structures that are somewhat different from the traditional nonprofit governing structure may work effectively in creating stable and effective governance of centers. Research on this issue is lacking, but it should be done so the field is aware of options for organizational governance that may help centers avoid some of the turmoil that has occurred in different locales when governing board problems have occurred, often resulting in interruption of consumer services.

There are still major barriers to full participation of persons with disabilities that must be overcome through the efforts of independent living centers and other groups and organizations. With the prohibition against operating residential facilities, independent living facilities are faced with trying to find other approaches to addressing inadequacies in accessible housing stock. Innovative projects in places such as Denver, Colorado, and Toledo, Ohio, are testing new approaches to addressing accessible housing shortages and providing other necessary services (Smith et al., 1994). Other centers have initiated entrepreneurial ventures involving sales of durable medical equipment and consumable medical supplies as well as marketing of ADA services and other disability-related services, such as home modifications (Smith et al., 1994). It remains to be seen how successful these ventures are in generating the resources necessary to assure continuation of high-quality consumer-directed services that result in optimal independence. However, the independent living movement can be expected to make significant contributions to improving the lives of people with disabilities well into the twenty-first century.

(See also: ADVOCACY; CONSUMERS; PERSONAL ASSISTANCE SERVICES; STATE-FEDERAL REHABILITATION PROGRAM)

RESOURCES

ILRU, 2323 S. Sheperd, Suite 1000, Houston, TX 77019

Independent Living Branch, Rehabilitation Services

Administration, U.S. Department of Education, 330 C St., SW, Room 3326, Washington, DC 20202

National Council on Independent Living, 2111 Wilson Blvd., Suite 405, Arlington, VA 22201

RTC-IL, University of Kansas, 1052 Dole, Lawrence, KS 66045

World Institute on Disability, 510 16th St., Suite 100, Oakland, CA 94612

BIBLIOGRAPHY

BARKER, LINDA TOMS; ALTMAN, MAYA; and YOUNG-DAHL, ANDREA. *Dimensions in Peer Counseling: Observations from the National Evaluation of Independent Living Centers.* Houston, 1987.

DEJONG, GERBEN. "Independent Living: From Social Movement to Analytic Paradigm." *Archives of Physical Medicine and Rehabilitation* 60 (1979):435–446.

ROBERTS, EDWARD V. "Foreword." In *Independent Living: Emerging Issues in Rehabilitation*, ed. Susan Pflueger. Washington, DC, 1977.

SHREVE, MARGARET. *Peer Counseling in Independent Living Centers: A Study of Service Delivery Variations.* Houston, 1991.

SHREVE, MARGARET, and KAILES, JUNE. "Independent Living and Traditional Paradigms" (adapted from original work by Gerben DeJong, 1979). In *Independent Living and the Rehab Act Training Manual for the NCIL/ILRU National Training and Technical Assistance Project.* Washington, DC, 1994.

SMITH, LAURA W.; SMITH, QUENTIN W.; RICHARDS, LAUREL; FRIEDEN, LEX; and KING, KYM. "Independent Living: Moving into the 21st Century." *American Rehabilitation* 20 (1994):14–22.

SMITH, QUENTIN W.; RICHARDS, LAUREL K.; NOSEK, MARGARET A.; and GERKEN, LAURIE. "Education and Training Needs of Independent Living Center Managers." *Rehabilitation Education* 5 (1991):101–111.

SMITH, QUENTIN W.; RICHARDS, LAUREL K.; REDD, LAURIE G.; and FRIEDEN, LEX. "Improving Management Effectiveness in Independent Living Centers Through Research and Training." *OSERS* VI (1994):30–36.

THAYER, TED, and RICE, DOUGLAS B. *Vocational Rehabilitation Services in Independent Living Centers: Report from the Study Group, 17th Annual Institute on Rehabilitation Issues.* Fayetteville, AR, 1990.

QUENTIN W. SMITH
LEX FRIEDEN
LAUREL RICHARDS

INDUSTRIAL REHABILITATION

See DISABILITY MANAGEMENT; EMPLOYEE ASSISTANCE PROGRAMS; PRIVATE SECTOR REHABILITATION

INFORMATION RESOURCES

Knowledge of disability issues and rehabilitation interventions empowers service providers and consumers to make effective decisions. In this information age, the amount and types of information available have expanded dramatically, as have the methods used to communicate it. Accessing the wealth of information available is sometimes frustrating. Huge printouts of data, unsorted articles, and dispersed information sources are being channeled into formats that people can readily use. An "information industry" has grown up around the task of translating cold data into understandable and usable information. Disability and rehabilitation information resources include (1) other people who know what you need to know; (2) print materials such as books, articles, and policy manuals of interest to you; (3) textfiles similar to books or articles that can be accessed from your computer; and (4) databases you can search or analyze.

In the local community, information resources include the library, the network of human service professionals, and news media. On a larger scale, regional or national centers and clearinghouses provide rehabilitation and disability information. These information centers help in the management of information by classifying documents and providing a usable interface. The centers differ in the types of information they handle and the methods of access. Table 1 presents a summary of some major rehabilitation and disability information resources, which are listed and discussed in detail below.

1. Rehabilitation research and training centers are designed to (*a*) conduct research that produces new knowledge to improve rehabilitation services, minimize effects of disabling conditions, and promote independence, and (*b*) institute training programs that enable wide application of research findings. Each center concentrates its research and

Table 1. Rehabilitation information sources, types of information available by source, and methods of access

Information Resources	Types of Information	Methods of Access
Rehabilitation research and training centers (e.g., ILRU)	Notebooks, books, articles, brochures, training materials, posters, video/audiotapes, software	Phone, fax, TDD, mail, computer bulletin board
Rehabilitation engineering centers (e.g., Trace)	Notebooks, books, articles, brochures, training materials, posters, video/audiotapes, software	Phone, fax, TDD, mail, computer bulletin board
Disability and Business Technical Assistance Centers (DBTACs)	Notebooks, books, articles, brochures, training materials, posters, video/audiotapes, software	Phone, fax, TDD, mail, computer bulletin board
National Rehabilitation Information Center (NARIC)	Documents and bibliographic information	Phone, fax, TDD mail, computer bulletin board
ABLEDATA	Product information, fact sheets, articles	Phone, fax, TDD, mail, computer bulletin board, CD ROM
Clearinghouse on Disability Information	Newsletter, lists of organizations and programs, guides to disability legislation	Phone, fax, TDD, mail, computer bulletin board
Job Accommodation Network (JAN)	Worksite accommodation information, video/audiotapes, brochures, ADA fact sheets, accessibility guides	Phone, fax, TDD, mail, computer bulletin board
Project Enable	Files of legislation- and disability-related information, software, graphics files, public/private messages, conference information	Computer bulletin board

training on a particular aspect of disability or rehabilitation. For example, the Research and Training Center on Independent Living (ILRU) is a national resource center for information, research, training, and technical assistance on such topics as community living, transition, assistive equipment, underserved populations, and service coordination among agencies. In addition to developing resource materials, this information center responds to individual inquiries related to independent living. There are about 40 rehabilitation research and training centers throughout the U.S.

2. Rehabilitation engineering research centers are operated in collaboration with institutions of higher education or nonprofit organizations. They conduct research, demonstration, and training activities in the area of rehabilitation technology and its impact on the lives of people with disabilities. They develop and disseminate models for applying technology and scientific knowledge to environmental barrier removal, service delivery, employment, and independent living needs. The Rehabilitation Act allows centers to be developed in the areas of early childhood services, education, employment, and independent living. For example, the Trace Center is a rehabilitation engineering research center that studies high-tech communication aids, computer control mechanisms, and accessibility of computers and other electronic equipment. Information can be obtained there on such topics as adaptive toys, screen readers, head pointers, keyboard adaptations, character recognition scanners, speech synthesizers, and other communication devices. There are about 20 rehabilitation engineering research centers throughout the U.S.

3. Disability and Business Technical Assistance Centers (DBTACs) provide information, training, and technical assistance to employers, people with

disabilities, and others with responsibilities under the Americans with Disabilities Act (ADA). The ten centers, such as the Mid-Atlantic ADA Information Center, are central information sources on ADA issues of employment, public accommodations, public services, and communications. The services provided by these regional centers vary, but all centers focus on the four core areas of individualized response to queries, referral to local specialists, ADA training, and technical assistance on compliance with the ADA.

4. The National Rehabilitation Information Center (NARIC) is a library established to enhance the use of rehabilitation and disability information. They collect and disseminate books, journal articles, and audiovisuals that result from federally funded rehabilitation research. They also update and maintain REHABDATA, a searchable database of their collection of documents. NARIC services include providing answers to simple questions over the phone, photocopying documents, and conducting REHABDATA and ABLEDATA (see next item) searches on a fee-for-service basis. In 1994 the NARIC collection included more than 43,000 documents on such topics as physical disability, independent living, employment, mental retardation, medical rehabilitation, assistive technology, psychiatric disabilities, special education, and public policy.

5. ABLEDATA is a national database of information on assistive technologies and rehabilitation equipment. Manufacturers are contacted yearly and requested to submit and update product information. Each record contains information on the product, cost, and company. More than 20,000 products and over 3,000 companies were represented in the database in 1994. Information is also available on "do it yourself" devices. The database can be searched by keyword (e.g., generic name, brand name, manufacturer) through a CD ROM.

6. The Clearinghouse on Disability Information is a service that focuses on federal disability legislation, funding for programs to serve individuals with disabilities, medical and scientific developments, incidence information, and national, state, and local programs and services for people with disabilities. They publish guides on legislation, listing of public and private organizations that serve people with disabilities, and a quarterly newsletter.

7. The Job Accommodation Network (JAN) is a consultant service that provides information on the Americans with Disabilities Act and workplace accommodations for people with disabilities. The consultants query the caller about the nature of the job, the essential functions to be accommodated, the functional capacities of the worker, and other relevant information. An individualized search for product information is conducted, and recommendations are given to the caller. JAN also provides information on public programs such as the Job Training Partnership Act, Supported Employment, Projects with Industry, and Targeted Jobs Tax Credit.

8. Project Enable is an electronic bulletin board that allows users to exchange messages, donate and receive computer files, form discussion groups, search text files, and locate rehabilitation information. Enable is a twenty-four-hour-a-day service that was developed to encourage information exchange among rehabilitation professionals and people with disabilities. Information files are sorted and categorized so that users can access them quickly. The text of the ADA and the Rehabilitation Act, for example, can be searched on-line or downloaded to the user's computer. Text files of newsletters, disability-related articles, legislation, and policy are available. Users can also access software files, training materials and information, lists of programs and services, and graphics files. Many of Enable's users are members of discussion groups. They post and read messages that address a particular topic. This kind of informal interaction fosters rapid exchange of new information.

These eight types of information centers are invaluable resources for people with disabilities, service providers, employers, and researchers. There is a large corpus of rehabilitation and disability information that can be accessed in a variety of ways. The interfaces between the person who needs to know and the information are continually improving. The staffs of these information centers are committed to widening the gateways to expanded information dissemination.

(*See also:* ASSISTIVE TECHNOLOGY; COMPUTERS; REHABILITATION RESEARCH)

RESOURCES

ABLEDATA and National Rehabilitation Information Center (NARIC), 8455 Colesville Road, Suite 935, Silver Spring, MD 20910-3319

Job Accommodation Network (JAN), 806 Allen Hall, West Virginia University, Morgantown, WV 26506

RICHARD T. WALLS
DENETTA L. DOWLER

INJURED WORKER

See DISABILITY MANAGEMENT; EMPLOYEE ASSISTANCE PROGRAMS, PRIVATE SECTOR REHABILITATION

INTERNATIONAL REHABILITATION

Worldwide, there are more than 500 million people with disabilities—people with physical, sensory, and/or mental conditions that limit the way they carry out their daily activities. The vast majority live in developing nations and without access to rehabilitation services of any kind.

Major international efforts have been in progress to improve the quality of life for people with disabilities and their families. These efforts have shifted in direction over time to emphasize societal change, the realization of equal opportunities, and the attainment of civil and human rights.

The Philosophical Framework

The United Nations International Year of Disabled Persons (IYDP) in 1981 and the Decade of Disabled Persons, 1983–1992, marked turning points in the international movement to meet the needs and aspirations of people with disabilities. These international advocacy efforts represented a change in public consciousness. Action shifted from an emphasis on meeting the special needs of people with disabilities through individually tailored programs of rehabilitation, toward a global philosophy of modifying society to include and accommodate the needs of all citizens, including people with disabilities. During this period, disability issues became focused on actions to achieve social change in human rights, accessibility, employment, education, leisure, recreation, sports, and cultural life. The voices of people with disabilities and their international organizations soared during the decade, emphasizing the crucial role of people with disabilities themselves in bringing about social change.

Historical Perspective and the Shift to Community-Based Services

The international rehabilitation movement had its roots in North American and European technical exchanges that began in the 1920s, following the conclusion of World War I. Young soldiers were returning to civilian life physically and/or psychologically traumatized. Developments in orthopedic and psychiatric medical specialties led to interdisciplinary techniques for minimizing the impact of their chronic conditions.

The international rehabilitation movement was stimulated by the creation in 1922 of Rehabilitation International (RI) and the concurrent development of other international organizations specializing in particular aspects of disability.

The need to expand rehabilitation efforts intensified following the end of World War II. The medical specialty of physical medicine and rehabilitation emerged, coupled with adapted vocational counseling approaches to return disabled clients to work.

A broadening of rehabilitation-related disciplines and specializations occurred during the 1950s, the 1960s, and the 1970s. Professional and paraprofessional roles evolved within the allied health fields of physical therapy, occupational therapy, special education, and prosthetics and orthotics. By 1969 Rehabilitation International was able to convene the first international review of how multidisciplinary rehabilitation services could be delivered within a variety of development and resources circumstances. This led to the subsequent evolution of concepts for community-based and low-cost service delivery in developing regions.

By the conclusion of the 1970s the efficacy and the sustainability of specialized institution-based rehabilitation and special education were being significantly challenged. New trends linking the provision of needed rehabilitation measures within primary health and community care systems were emerging, and concepts of deinstitutionalization and mainstreaming in education were gaining prominence.

The international movement to foster deinstitutionalization of care, particularly for children and adults with developmental disabilities and mental handicaps, facilitated normalization of daily living. Family- and community-based service delivery systems emerged.

Preoccupations have shifted at the international level from the provision of specialized institution-based services to support for family- and community-based initiatives. Specialized institutions are more and more utilized in a supporting capacity for people with multiple disabilities and the most specialized needs. Emphasis is retained on achieving the broadest possible participation within all aspects of societal life, and the delivery of rehabilitation services in the most effective manner to the broadest possible constituency of people with disabilities.

The Disability Rights and Independent Living Movements

At the same time, with the emergence in social service programs of consumer and client participation as a potent force for change, a consumer movement of people with disabilities emerged and began to coalesce at the international level. Disabled People International (DPI), which is best representative of this international trend, was born in 1981, the International Year of Disabled Persons (IYDP). It expanded in scope, activity, and membership throughout the Decade of Disabled Persons, giving voice to a growing movement for self-advocacy among people with disabilities.

DPI has become a powerful voice in the shift of consciousness from public policy based on expenditures through social programs for passive dependency, to activation of people with disabilities, enabled and empowered to participate in all aspects of societal life. An international independent living movement, based on these principles and the philosophy that people with disabilities themselves

should be the primary shapers of decisions that most directly affect their lives, has come into being.

International Disability Organizations

Scores of international organizations are active in the disability field, including among the most prominent: the World Blind Union, the World Federation of the Deaf, the International Federation of the Civilian Disabled, the World Veterans Federation, the International League of Societies of Persons with Mental Handicap, the World Confederation for Physical Therapy, the World Federation of Occupational Therapists, the International Cerebral Palsy Society, the International Rehabilitation Medicine Association, the International Federation for Physical Medicine and Rehabilitation, Rehabilitation International, and Disabled People International. The International Council on Disability (ICOD) provides an umbrella framework for coordination of international nongovernmental advocacy in the disability field and has worked with the U.N. disability program to promote this coordination since the ICOD's creation in 1953.

International nongovernmental organizations in the disability field have worked together to achieve recognition of the rights of people with disabilities through a series of international declarations, conventions, and the proclamation by the United Nations of the IYDP in 1981 and the Decade of Disabled Persons, 1983–1992.

Subsequently, the Asia and Pacific region of the United Nations, through the U.N. Economic Commission for that area, adopted a second Decade of Disabled Persons, for the period 1993–2002. The emphasis of this second decade will be on action and implementation of the concepts promoted during the global decade.

Legislative Developments

A series of international declarations on the rights of people with disabilities has been adopted parallel to the development of the international rehabilitation and disability rights movements. These declarations have changed in perspective as the broader awareness of disability as a socially defined set of interactive conditions has emerged.

Major international declarations in the disability field include:

- the International Declaration on the Rights of Disabled Persons, adopted in 1975 by the United Nations;
- the International Declaration on the Rights of Mentally Retarded Persons, adopted in 1971 by the United Nations;
- the International Convention on the Rights of the Child, which includes the "special needs of children with disabilities," adopted in 1990 by the United Nations;
- the International Convention on Vocational Rehabilitation of Persons with Disabilities, adopted by the International Labor Organization in 1983 to ensure participation in employment without discrimination for persons with disabilities.

Major legislation adopted at the national level includes, for example, the Americans with Disabilities Act (1990) in the United States.

U.N. World Program of Action

Most important, the United Nations adopted the World Program of Action for the Decade of Disabled Persons, which focused on disability prevention, rehabilitation, and equalization of opportunities.

Prevention encompasses primary health care, prenatal care, immunizations, safety regulations and prevention of accidents, and prevention of disability resulting from environmental pollution and armed conflict—that is, reduction of the causes of physical, sensory, and/or mental impairment.

Rehabilitation is a process enabling persons with disabilities to reach their optimal physical, sensory, intellectual, and social functioning levels. Rehabilitation includes measures to restore functions or to compensate for loss of functions or abilities. It includes a wide range of medical, social, educational, and vocational measures.

Equalization of opportunities refers to a process whereby the various systems of society and the environment, such as service, information, and documentation, are made available to all people, including and particularly people with disabilities. People with disabilities have the same right as other members of their societies to remain within their local communities and to receive the support they need within the ordinary systems of education, health, employment, and social service.

International Standard Rules on Equalization of Opportunities

The 1993 session of the U.N. General Assembly adopted international Standard Rules on the Equalization of Opportunities for Persons with Disabilities. These rules help governments to achieve comprehensive national disability programs and true equality of opportunity for people with disabilities and their families. The purpose of the rules is to ensure that girls, boys, women, and men with disabilities, as members of their societies, may exercise the same rights and have the same obligations as others. The rules are intended to remove any obstacles to achieving this purpose. Special attention is anticipated for groups in particularly difficult circumstances, including women, children, elderly persons, poor people, migrant workers, persons with multiple disabilities, ethnic minorities, and refugees with disabilities. The United Nations is monitoring the implementation process throughout the world.

The U.N. standard rules request U.N. member states to ensure:

- awareness in society about persons with disabilities, their rights and potential;
- provision of effective medical care and rehabilitation to persons with disabilities;
- supply of support services, including assistive devices to assist people with disabilities to achieve independence in daily living;
- accessibility to make the physical environment accessible and to provide access to information and communication;
- education of persons with disabilities as an integral part of the general education system;
- equal opportunities for productive employment and participation in the labor market;
- provision of Social Security and income maintenance as needed by persons with disabilities;
- full participation in family life, including the potential for marriage and parenthood;
- participation in cultural, recreational, and sports activities on an equal basis;

- participation in the religious life of their communities for people with disabilities;
- creation of a legal basis for measures to achieve the objectives of full participation and equality for persons with disabilities.

Future Directions

Implementation of the standard rules throughout the world will have a decisive impact on the future quality of life of persons with disabilities.

Adoption of the international symbol of access to denote public buildings and facilities free of architectural barriers to persons with disabilities required more than twenty years of effort. Now the use of ramps, elevators, accessible toilets, telephones, and drinking fountains is becoming widespread as awareness and attitudes change worldwide. Similarly, we must expect that the effort to achieve the purposes of the Standard Rules will extend well into the next century.

People with disabilities will continue to be among those groups in society at most risk. The challenge will be to harness the scientific, technological, and communications revolutions now in progress and transform the nature of work and information communication throughout the world to include and serve the needs of people with disabilities. They must become part of all activities aimed at furthering human development.

Improvements in world output in the future are predicated on improvements in people's capacities as competitiveness, productivity, skilled labor, and knowledge-based management and employment become the keys to economic growth. That is precisely what rehabilitation is about: the maximizing of independent functioning capacity, the improvement in capacity, skill, and knowledge. A prominent American sociologist with a disability, Professor Irving Kenneth Zola, put the issue clearly:

"Only when we acknowledge the near universality of disability and that all of its dimensions are a part of the social process, will it be possible to fully appreciate how general public policy can affect this issue. . . . [We must] promulgate a concept of special needs which is not based on breaking the rules for the few but on designing a flexible world for the many. What is done in the name of disability today, will have meaning for all of the world's tomorrows."

(*See also:* ADVOCACY; CIVIL RIGHTS; HISTORY OF REHABILITATION; PHILOSOPHY OF REHABILITATION)

BIBLIOGRAPHY

HAMMERMAN, SUSAN R. "Future Trends and Disability Policy from an International Perspective." *Futures Research Quarterly,* 1990 (6):39–43.

———. *Rehabilitation for the Disabled: Social and Economic Implications of Investments for this Purpose.* United Nations Department of Economic and Social Affairs, ST/ESA/65. New York, 1977.

HAMMERMAN, SUSAN R., and MAIKOWSKI, STEPHEN, eds. *The Economics of Disability: International Perspectives.* New York, 1981.

REHABILITATION INTERNATIONAL. *International Statements on Disability Policy.* New York, 1981.

UNITED NATIONS. *Standard Rules on the Equalization of Opportunities for Persons with Disabilities.* New York, 1994.

———. *World Programme of Action Concerning Disabled Persons.* New York, 1983.

ZOLA, IRVING K. "Toward the Necessary Universalizing of a Disability Policy." *The Milbank Quarterly* 67 (1989):401–427.

SUSAN R. HAMMERMAN

J

JOB ACCOMMODATION

See DISABILITY MANAGEMENT; PRESIDENT'S COMMITTEE ON EMPLOYMENT OF PEOPLE WITH DISABILITIES; REASONABLE ACCOMMODATION

JOB PLACEMENT

Placement in vocational rehabilitation refers to the employment of persons with disabilities in suitable jobs. In spite of how simple this sounds, there has been much confusion about what placement really is. It has been defined as the entire rehabilitation process, but it has also been defined as the primary outcome of that process (Vandergoot, 1987). Placement is viewed as one of the critical outcomes of vocational rehabilitation services and as part of the process leading to independence and enhanced quality of life for persons with disabilities. Employment is a significant need of all persons and not just of those with disabilities. Placement in a job represents the beginning, or the renewal, of a person's career.

Placement Models

There are many placement models and programs that are designed to provide job opportunities to persons with disabilities. In the selective placement model the counselor actively intervenes with employers to persuade them to hire persons with disabilities. The person with a disability, or consumer, is merely the recipient of services. The counselor is responsible for organizing all needed services and "selects" the job that best matches the skills and abilities of the consumer.

In direct contrast is client-centered placement. The counselor is a facilitator or teacher, helping the consumer to select and follow through with services and employment efforts to whatever extent possible. The consumer assumes most of the responsibility for finding employers and is encouraged to make all decisions about types of jobs to pursue and needed services.

The assisted placement model combines aspects of the previous models and adds a third person, often called a placement specialist. This professional provides information to the consumer and counselor so that their decisions reflect the types of jobs available

413

and so the consumer is prepared accordingly. The specialist will contact employers to gain interviews for the consumer and may also teach the consumer job-seeking skills so he or she can develop additional job leads.

Placement models also differ in how services are arranged and sequenced. Competitive placement uses a train-place-follow-up process. This reflects traditional vocational rehabilitation in which most services occur before employment, usually in special, segregated settings designed for persons with disabilities. Supported placement, however, uses a place-train-follow-up approach. This model offers most services in regular, integrated work settings after employment occurs. For example, a job coach frequently works side by side with a new worker until he or she has learned to do job tasks independently at a competitive rate. The outcomes in these two models are the same, but the location where services are provided is quite different.

Other placement models are based on the belief that certain consumers cannot work in competitive jobs due to the limitations resulting from their disabilities. Sheltered employment is provided in special settings that primarily employ persons with disabilities. These workers may be paid less than the minimum wage if their productivity is less than that expected of competitive workers in the community. These placements have been faulted for their segregated nature and low pay.

Homebound employment is a model established for persons who, due to their disabilities, need to work from their homes. Perhaps accessible transportation is not available, or the consumer may not have the stamina to travel. The person can be self-employed at almost any type of business or work for someone else. Computers and information exchange technology permit working at home in ways never before possible. Quality homebound employment may provide greater numbers of placements in the future as this technology develops and becomes cheaper.

All these approaches enable persons with disabilities to compete with others for jobs and, therefore, have an impact on the supply side of the labor market. Dennis D. Gilbride and Robert Stensrud (1992) suggested that other strategies are needed to have an effect on the demand side of labor markets that will create jobs for consumers. The model is designed to change work environments to fit persons with disabilities rather than changing them to fit existing jobs. Projects With Industry (PWI) are employer-rehabilitation partnership programs that employ persons with disabilities. Companies and rehabilitation agencies work together to identify jobs, provide training, and assist consumers in other ways to be successful workers.

The Americans with Disabilities Act (ADA) provides opportunities for promoting these demand-side models. Rehabilitation professionals can provide valuable services needed by employers, which can lead to the creation of job opportunities for consumers at the same time. The ADA requires that companies with more than fourteen employees accommodate the needs of qualified persons with disabilities. Accommodations can include modifying jobs by reducing hours, changing schedules, and revising job descriptions. However, other accommodations may require special expertise that rehabilitation professionals can provide. Rehabilitation engineers have devised many innovative tools, equipment, and work environments to overcome the functional limitations of persons with disabilities and enable them to perform work tasks on a competitive basis. Such specialized accommodations are known as assistive technology. Since federal legislation was passed in 1988, assistive technology has become more available and, in many cases, less expensive. Assistive technology can consist of highly sophisticated, specially designed electronic hardware such as voice-activated environmental controls, software that enables persons to access computers by bypassing keyboards, or simple physical adaptations such as blocks to raise the height of desks to accommodate a wheelchair.

The ADA focuses on much more than hiring persons with disabilities. All businesses must provide the same support to current workers with disabilities as they do to other workers. While some workers with disabilities may be very happy performing in an entry-level job for their whole careers, others will want to advance as fast as they can. Therefore, employers should provide the same career growth opportunities to all workers. Counselors should learn the laws and regulations that govern employment of people with disabilities, and use company and community resources on their behalf. With the support of the ADA and other recent legislation, more complete placement service models are now possible by combining initiatives that affect both the supply and the demand sides of labor markets.

The Employment Needs of People with Disabilities

For years, the most underemployed and unemployed group of U.S. citizens has been people with disabilities. Even during the decade of the 1980s, when virtually all disadvantaged groups improved their labor market participation rates, the gap in participation between persons with disabilities and others actually widened (Bennefield & McNeil, 1989). A Harris poll commissioned by the National Council on Disability (Louis Harris & Associates, 1986) provided evidence about how the lack of involvement in the economic and social mainstream has affected the persons with disabilities' quality of life. For those who were able to work, a majority held only part-time jobs and did not have access to health insurance. Their income lagged behind that of others and actually increased at a slower pace while it was increasing for most other disadvantaged groups. Although people with disabilities made up 8.6 percent of the population, they comprised 21.9 percent of persons at or below the poverty level. As they became older, they worked less and less (U.S. Census Bureau, 1986). Also, more than 500,000 Americans each year experienced a disability that kept them out of work an average of at least five months, and almost half of these never returned to work at all (Hester & DeCelles, 1985).

There are a variety of resources established to assist persons with disabilities. These may overlap and, at times, may even conflict with one another. Workers' compensation is provided if the disability is the result of a work-related illness or injury. Social Security Disability Insurance provides benefits for those whose disabilities prevent them from working for at least a year and who are qualified to receive them through their past work. Short- and long-term disability benefits are usually obtained as part of fringe benefit packages provided by employers to employees who acquire a disability from any activity, work-related or not.

These benefits are usually integrated so that a person does not receive more than he or she could earn from work. However, the income from these benefits is tax-free, and medical benefits are typically part of the package. Thus these benefits are valuable and, justifiably, can reduce a person's motivation to return to work. It has become difficult to find the right balance of needed support for those who have acquired a disability along with appropriate incentives to encourage them to return to work in some capacity. Many persons with disabilities have meager incomes, but it is possible for some to receive sufficient income due to disability such that work becomes unnecessary. In either case, the existence of disability significantly alters quality of life, at least in terms of how the majority in our society experiences it.

A variety of public and private service programs provide placement assistance to persons with disabilities. The federal and state governments collaborate in providing publicly supported vocational rehabilitation services to persons usually aged fourteen or older who qualify. The Rehabilitation Act Amendments of 1992 made it much easier for people with disabilities to become eligible. A comprehensive continuum of services is provided, ranging from evaluation, education, transportation, training, counseling, placement, and follow-up, among others, depending on need. These services are usually offered through nonprofit rehabilitation programs and paid for by the state. Counselors from state agencies usually serve as case managers, or coordinators of services, ensuring that consumers receive all needed and available services as close to their homes as possible.

Return-to-work programs for injured or ill workers have become a major growth area in rehabilitation, and placement has been a primary focus of these organizations, which are usually established as for-profit programs. Funding usually comes from insurance companies. It has been estimated that more than $100 billion are spent annually on costs related to workplace disabilities (Schwartz, 1984). Recognition of these high costs has prompted a great deal of interest in preventing disability and minimizing its impact when it does occur. Although some research is available, it is difficult to find information that can guide efforts to return persons back to productive work after they have been forced to take time off due to a disabling event.

Studies have been done, however, to identify important features of workplace disability management programs (Gottlieb et al., 1988; Gottlieb et al., 1987). Individuals responsible for providing medical care must coordinate their interventions with those who are responsible for providing vocational services. Ideally, a case manager coordinates all services, maintains communications, and assures that all appropriate resources are used. If a company is using a private or public rehabilitation program to enhance its own in-house efforts to manage disability, coordination of services becomes more difficult but can still be maintained.

The worker should be viewed as a key decision-maker in all steps of the rehabilitation process. Companies should fully explain to employees all their rights and responsibilities and keep them informed of new developments. Employees should be made aware of the disability program, in writing, at the time they are hired and again when a disability occurs. If a union is present, the bargaining agreement should detail how the company and the union will work together to ensure a conflict-free rehabilitation process. This is critical because involvement of an attorney and subsequent legal action appear to reduce greatly the chances of successful return to work (Vandergoot, 1991).

Vocational rehabilitation intervention should begin as soon as possible after a disability occurs and be coordinated with medical services. All parties need to agree on the goal of return to work at the outset of treatment. Management should communicate to employees that they are committed to the maintenance of their health, the prevention of illness or injury, and their speedy return to work. If injury or illness should occur, regular contacts between company personnel and the worker are desirable.

Especially in return-to-work situations, a careful balance of disability and other benefits must be maintained during the rehabilitation process to assure that all necessities are provided and the basic standard of living of the worker is maintained without creating a potential disincentive to going back to work.

Disability management programs are a continuum of services that begin for all employees as soon as they are hired and continue throughout their tenure. Prevention activities include safety instruction and precautions, health and wellness programs, medical screening, and timely medical care. Other vocational services and techniques should be available as well, including work hardening, light duty, flexible hours, job accommodations and restructuring, retraining, or even outplacement to a new company if another job assignment is not possible.

Labor Markets as a Conceptual Framework for Placement

Placement happens when a person is offered and accepts a job. An employer makes a decision to select an applicant, and an applicant decides to accept the job offer. These decisions seem simple but, if made well, they usually result from a long and difficult search process. In our economy, this searching is conducted in labor markets. To understand how placement occurs, therefore, and to plan services that take advantage of how labor markets work, it is necessary to understand labor markets.

Labor markets simply attempt to put the right persons in the right jobs. Just as supermarkets exist to help people select foods quickly and easily, labor markets exist to help employers and applicants find each other quickly and easily. Two decision-makers are involved—employers who select applicants, and applicants who select employers. Employers create the demand for workers, while applicants are the supply of workers available to fulfill the demand.

Markets exist to facilitate exchanges of needed resources. While money is exchanged for food in supermarkets, information helpful to make decisions is exchanged in labor markets. The quality of decisions improves along with the investment in information, which can be costly in time and money. Applicants and employers want to make the best decisions without a great deal of cost. Employers bear many costs when recruiting and hiring workers. They use many sources to create an applicant pool. Even though rehabilitation agencies, as one source of applicants, usually provide free services for placing a worker, they still must show that they provide cost-effective services. Cost reductions might result from sending prescreened and trained applicants more frequently than any other source. Providing

416

follow-along services and accommodations are other possible cost reduction tactics. In any situation, the agency must remember that employers, as "customers," have alternatives to "buying" from them. Helping employers wisely manage these costs, therefore, provides opportunities to rehabilitation professionals to assist persons with disabilities to obtain employment. Providing labor market-oriented placement services, therefore, requires that rehabilitation professionals view their "customers" as both employers and persons with disabilities and organize services accordingly.

Placement Services to Employers

What are the labor-market needs of employers? Employers want to obtain productive workers through an efficient and effective hiring process. This desire suggests incentives that rehabilitation programs can offer employers, including: (1) low-cost access to job candidates; (2) applicants who are prescreened; and (3) follow-up and support for long-term success (Vandergoot et al., 1993; Young et al., 1986).

Services should help the employer hire the right person and, after the person is hired, provide appropriate follow-up. Using the labor market model suggests that the place-train or place-train-maintain supported employment models of service delivery make the most "market" sense. Supported employment has defined the types of support that can be included in follow-up. These are coaching, coworker instruction, crisis intervention, job modification, site accommodations, identification and use of natural work site supports such as coworker mentors, and transportation assistance. There are no limits to the types of placement support that could be provided to help a consumer and employer achieve successful employment. Therefore, the groundbreaking service delivery approaches developed through supported employment should be extended to all placements. Employers do not distinguish between "competitive" and "supported" jobs, and neither should the rehabilitation community. All jobs should be equally valued and supported with any needed and reasonable service and accommodation.

When rehabilitation professionals understand they are in the business of "selling" employee recruiting services to employers, they will use job development strategies that avoid appeals to goodwill and refute the image that rehabilitation and employment of people with disabilities are a charity. Rehabilitation professionals, and the persons they represent, will, instead, be recognized as valuable resources by employers. This will make it easier to do job development because employers will always have a need for good workers.

A positive image of the capabilities of people with disabilities, and the valuable services provided by rehabilitation professionals, must be emphasized in all public relations and contacts made with employers. Marketing strategies must be used to identify the needs of employers and show how these needs can be met through the assistance of placement services. Rehabilitation professionals also must see the usefulness of using approaches similar to the sales techniques used in the business world. These approaches are valued by employers. Should not these techniques be used for promoting employment of people with disabilities as much as or even more than for selling soap? It has been difficult for rehabilitation professionals to harmonize "sales" techniques with their focus on counseling and providing support services to people with disabilities. However, placement is a critical outcome, which most people with disabilities are very interested in achieving. Employers will understand marketing and sales techniques when used to promote employment for people with disabilities. These approaches are part of their world, and rehabilitation professionals concerned about placement should take advantage of this situation.

Placement Services to Persons with Disabilities

Most people who come to vocational rehabilitation programs want to work (Roessler & Schriner, 1991). Some may appear "unmotivated" for a variety of reasons, including their desire to maintain their security obtained through disability benefits. Other persons will not be able to find jobs because they do not have the skills for the jobs in demand. However, there is a variety of behaviors besides work skills that employers also value. These include interpersonal skills, general appearance, compatibility with supervisors, compliance with instructions, punctuality, safety/accident prevention, dependability, attendance, work skills, work habits, work attitudes, and overall work performance (Vandergoot et al., 1993).

Employers also indicate that they value applicants who could demonstrate good job-seeking skills (Young et al., 1986). Employers seem to use ability in this area to indicate work potential. Rehabilitation professionals need to provide services to equip consumers with a variety of on-the-job skills as well as job-seeking ability.

One of the goals of vocational rehabilitation often thought to be necessary to achieve successful placement is work readiness. Theoretically, a person is work ready when he or she can do one job, but limiting a consumer to only one job in the labor market greatly reduces his or her chances of being successful. The more jobs a person can be "ready" for, the more likely he or she will become employed. The difficulty for rehabilitation professionals is to find the right balance of "readiness." This can be determined only in light of local labor market conditions. When jobs are readily available or when a person is skillful in a wide variety of jobs, placement is easier. However, it takes only one job for success. How much preparation, training, and education should be provided is difficult to decide. Providing unnecessary services that really do not contribute to a consumer's ability to compete in the labor market is costly to the consumer and to society. However, not equipping a consumer with needed competitive capability exposes him or her to a long, difficult, and potentially unsuccessful job search. This experience could result in diminishing a person's motivation to such an extent that he or she may drop out and never seek employment again.

To make wise decisions, consumers and professionals need accurate, up-to-date, and comprehensive labor market information. Obtaining and using this information in appropriate ways is the responsibility of the professional. Being a labor market expert should be one of the hallmarks that distinguishes a rehabilitation professional from other human service professionals.

One of the first steps in using information appropriately is to identify the skills and abilities the consumer has to offer the labor market. The consumer should be evaluated and assessed to determine his or her current functioning and knowledge. This pro-vides the rehabilitation professional with the ability to tailor service delivery to an individual's unique needs, defined in terms of what the local labor market requires.

If the consumer has worked previously, the evaluation process can begin with a transferability-of-skills analysis. This helps to identify skills learned on previous jobs that can be applied to other occupations. These skills must still be evaluated and confirmed since the onset or progression of disability may have changed these capacities. For persons who do not have a work history, more traditional evaluation approaches can be used to provide an opportunity to explore their potential in the labor market fully. Efforts should be made to identify a broad range of labor market possibilities, allowing the consumer to pursue as many jobs as possible.

The next step after evaluation is to develop a rehabilitation plan that specifies job goals or a cluster of related jobs. Instead of specifying goals in terms of jobs, it might be wiser to set goals that feature aspects of jobs that will meet consumers' specific needs, such as location, hours, and income. Other needs, such as interests, skills, and career ambitions, also should be considered. These needs become more focused as consumers become more aware of labor market opportunities through their job search. Therefore, goals should be revised regularly to take advantage of new information.

It is critical that employment objectives include income needs. Many individuals with disabilities run the risk of losing disability income and medical benefits if they become employed. It becomes important that the income they earn offsets the loss of these benefits as well as costs associated with transportation, clothing, and food. It is conceivable that consumers will become "unmotivated" to work when they realize that the jobs available to them will not improve their financial well-being.

This assessment process will reveal a consumer's potential "worth" in the labor market. An incentive to motivate a consumer is to show him or her how participation in rehabilitation activities could increase income. This can set the stage for determining what training, education, or other learning activity might help the consumer be more competitive in the labor market. Successful completion of training indicates to employers that the consumer can learn and is able to see something through to the end. It provides a positive springboard for placement. Another alternative is to consider on-the-job training (OJT) provided by employers. This can circumvent the sometimes long process of completing an educational or vocational training program and provide income for the consumer at the same time. Most employers expect to provide orientation, and even training, to new employees if they have met basic entry requirements. Specific skills unique to a particular employer often have to be learned on the job anyway. Experience with supported employment documents the willingness of employers to allow rehabilitation training resources to be used on the job. OJT has been shown to be a very powerful training technique.

Along with learning new work skills, the consumer also needs to learn how to use the labor market effectively through advanced job search techniques. Some consumers will be able to learn on their own using self-study guides, while others will require intensive tutoring or class work. A person seeking a job as a skilled craftsworker will use different strategies than one who is seeking general clerical work. Job search skills instruction must be tailored for labor markets, and instructional materials should reflect this point.

The job search can be difficult in terms of the time and effort needed. The consumer and professional should prepare a formal placement plan with a full set of objectives to be achieved, including income, location, and types of jobs desired. A list of companies to be contacted should indicate those that are to be called by the rehabilitation professional and those to be contacted by the consumer. This will vary depending on the capability of the consumer. The time frame in which contacts are to be made should be stated to ensure that accountability is built into the process. The plan should be in the form of a contract. The counselor and consumer need to meet regularly to share information and revise the plan as new information becomes available.

Looking for jobs is not easy. Most searchers experience many more rejections than job offers, which can seriously reduce the desire to continue. Job searchers need to recognize that (1) many contacts are needed to obtain one offer, (2) each rejec-

tion reveals new information for use in further searching; and (3) each contact brings the searcher one step closer to an actual offer. Consumers need to realize that this is how labor markets work and are not to take rejections personally.

After employment begins, the counselor has the opportunity to serve the consumer and employer together through follow-up services. Contacts should be set up in advance with both, particularly if the counselor had a prior relationship with the employer. Scheduled contacts usually can be made by telephone, which preserves everyone's time. This is fine for routine follow-up, but the counselor also must be available for emergencies or to handle unforeseen circumstances. The ability to respond quickly and efficiently separates the rehabilitation counselor from other employment resources available to employers and will lead to repeat placement opportunities.

A last service, and one that is rarely provided, is to assist the consumer to plan for career development. In many ways this can take the form of the placement plan but spread out over a longer period of time, probably not to exceed six months. The consumer should explore ways to advance with the current employer, but moving to other employers that can better address the consumer's needs should also be considered. The current employer can be included in the planning process. Upgrading good workers is of interest to most companies. The primary responsibility for carrying out and revising this plan will rest with the consumer.

(See also: CAREER COUNSELING; DISABILITY MANAGEMENT; REASONABLE ACCOMMODATION; SUPPORTED EMPLOYMENT; WORK)

BIBLIOGRAPHY

BENNEFIELD, R. L., and McNEIL, J. M. Labor Force Status and Other Characteristics of Persons with a Work Disability: 1981–1988. Washington, DC, 1989.

GILBRIDE, DENNIS D., and STENSRUD, ROBERT. "Demand-Side Job Development: A Model for the 1990s." Journal of Rehabilitation 58 (1992):34–39.

GOTTLIEB, AMY; VANDERGOOT, DAVID; and LUTSKY, LARRY. "Directions of Disability—From Neglect to Priority." Business and Health 5 (1988):26–29.

GOTTLIEB, AMY; VANDERGOOT, DAVID; and SMART,

LANA. *Managing Disability in the Work Place*. New York, 1987.

HESTER, EDWARD J., and DECELLES, PAUL G. *The Worker Who Becomes Physically Disabled: A Handbook of Incidence and Outcomes*. Topeka, KS, 1985.

LOUIS HARRIS & ASSOCIATES. *The ICD Survey of Disabled Americans*. New York, 1986.

ROESSLER, RICHARD T., and SCHRINER, KATE F. "The Implications of Selected Employment Concerns for Disability Policy and Rehabilitation Practice." *Rehabilitation Counseling Bulletin* 35 (1991).

SCHWARTZ, GAIL. "Disability Costs: The Impending Crisis." *Business and Health* 1 (1984):25–28.

U.S. CENSUS BUREAU. *Disability, Functional Limitations, and Health Insurance Coverage: 1984–85*. Washington, DC, 1986.

VANDERGOOT, DAVID. "Vocational Rehabilitation: Current Practices and Research Needs." *Journal of Job Placement* 3 (1987):21–28.

———. *Return to Work Practices in the Rehabilitation of Workers' Compensation Claimants*. New York, 1991.

VANDERGOOT, DAVID; STANISZEWSKI, STEPHANIE; and GANY, VICTOR. *Employer Perceptions of Supported Workers*. Albertson, NY, 1993.

YOUNG, JUDY; ROSATI, ROBERT; and VANDERGOOT, DAVID. "Initiating a Marketing Strategy by Assessing Employer Needs for Rehabilitation Services." *Journal of Rehabilitation* 52 (1986):37–41.

DAVID VANDERGOOT

JOINT DISORDERS

See MUSCULOSKELETAL DISORDERS; ARTHRITIS

K

KELLER, HELEN

Helen Adams Keller (1880–1968) was an author, lecturer, and humanitarian whose life and work not only greatly improved the lives of countless individuals with disabilities around the world, but also dramatically altered the public perception of what it means to live with disabilities. Ravaged by a sudden brain fever that has never been definitely diagnosed, she was left blind and deaf at nineteen months, after which she could communicate only through hysterical laughter or violent tantrums. With the help of her teacher, Anne Mansfield Sullivan, Helen Keller learned to communicate with the outside world by reading Braille and writing on her specially designed typewriter. Helen and her teacher's relationship was the subject of *The Miracle Worker*, a 1960 Pulitzer Prize-winning play and a 1962 film of the same name by William Gibson. In 1902–1903, with the help of John Macy (who married Anne Sullivan in 1905), Helen Keller wrote and published *The Story of My Life*. By 1904, Helen Keller had graduated with honors from Radcliffe College at Harvard University, after which she dedicated the remainder of her life to the betterment of persons with disabilities.

During World War I, Helen Keller began her global crusade on behalf of blind and visually impaired persons by affiliating herself with two organizations: the American section of the British, French, and Belgian Permanent Blind War Relief Fund (the Fund), and the American Foundation for the Blind (AFB). In 1916 she assisted in the establishment of the American branch of the Fund, which was created to rehabilitate veterans of World War I who had lost their vision in combat; and in 1921 she began work for the newly created American Foundation for the Blind, whose primary purpose was to educate and rehabilitate blind persons in the United States.

In 1925 the Fund, with Helen Keller heading its American section, changed its name to the American Braille Press for War and Civilian Blind (ABP), and by 1927 it had distributed more than 19 million pages of Braille print in five French, English, and Serbian periodicals and in Braille books. At the end of the 1920s, ABP's productions were being distributed free of charge to blind persons in thirty countries in Africa, Asia, Europe, and Latin America.

By 1935 Helen Keller was helping to administer an ABP operation that had founded or equipped two printing plants in Belgium, two in France, and one each in Brazil, Colombia, Poland, Portugal, and Yugoslavia. Two years later, ABP introduced the first talking books in Europe, and in 1940 it developed a new apparatus for teaching Braille so blinded soldiers could learn to read Braille easily.

In 1945 Helen Keller was elected ABP's counselor for international relations, and in 1946 the American Braille Press changed its name to the American Foundation for Overseas Blind (AFOB). In the same year, Helen Keller made her first trip under its auspices to Great Britain, France, Italy, and Greece. By the late 1940s she had visited Australia and the Far East as an emissary for AFOB. AFOB was providing services for blind and visually impaired persons in Asia, Africa, Europe, and South America in the form of special apparatuses, written materials, food, and clothing; and thousands of health workers were receiving training to improve conditions for the blind in their countries. Training of indigenous health workers, a method of self-help strongly advocated by Helen Keller and AFOB, is recognized as the most effective method of sustainable international development. In late 1949 AFOB sponsored the International Conference of Workers for the Blind at Oxford University, and education and rehabilitation leaders from fifteen countries joined Helen Keller to plan joint activities and to coordinate a global strategy.

In 1951 Helen Keller took a 25,000-mile tour of Africa for AFOB and, later that year, helped establish the World Conference for the Welfare of the Blind. The following year, the Association for the Chinese Blind merged with AFOB, and shortly afterward Helen Keller spent three months advocating the cause of blind people in the Middle East and North Africa. By 1955, while she was on a 40,000-mile, five-month speaking tour through Asia, AFOB began training programs for teachers of the blind in Chile, Finland, Greece, Iceland, Italy, Portugal, and Turkey; opened vocational training centers and schools for the blind in Egypt, Ethiopia, Iran, Iraq, Jordan, Kuwait, Lebanon, Nigeria, and Rhodesia (now called Zimbabwe); and home teaching and rehabilitation services were developed in Syria. The three months spent in the Middle East and North Africa in 1952 had opened the region for AFOB within three years.

Throughout the 1950s AFOB, under Helen Keller's leadership, opened permanent country offices in Uganda, Philippines, and Chile (to serve the South American region), and she continued her public advocacy on behalf of blind persons in Sweden, Norway, and Denmark. In 1956 AFOB sponsored the first rehabilitation center for blind and visually impaired individuals in Israel, and by 1958, integration of blind children with sighted children in public schools in Israel began. In 1959 AFOB initiated, as a tribute to the leadership and inspiration of Helen Keller, the World Crusade for the Blind, which was designed to expand public awareness of and support for AFOB's programs and to carry on her international work.

Throughout the 1960s AFOB continued to expand its programs, but in 1961 Helen Keller suffered a stroke and retired from public life. At the time of her retirement, AFOB was operating programs in seventy nations around the world. In 1962 it opened a regional office in Beirut to serve the Middle East and North Africa; this represented the culmination of an initiative begun ten years earlier by Helen Keller. That same year saw 500 teachers in India receiving training from AFOB to enroll 9,000 blind children in schools for sighted children. In 1963 schools for the blind were established in Iran, Ethiopia, and Saudi Arabia. In 1964 she traveled to Washington, DC, where President Lyndon Johnson awarded her the Medal of Freedom, the highest honor given in the United States to a civilian. She died on June 1, 1968.

Helen Keller's legacy continues to inform the education and rehabilitation community as well as those individuals and organizations who are striving for the prevention of blindness on a global scale. Efforts toward this goal continue, with ninety-five Helen Keller namesake organizations providing services to blind and visually impaired persons. The American Foundation for the Blind, with which Ms. Keller was affiliated from its first days, works exclusively in the United States, with six regional offices providing education and rehabilitation, talking books, special equipment, and medical referrals for blind and visually impaired persons. AFOB (the vehicle for Helen Keller's international efforts) changed its name in 1976 to Helen Keller International and administers blindness prevention, treatment, and education and rehabilitation programs for people afflicted with nutritional blindness (xerophthalmia), trachoma, and river blindness (onchocerciasis) as well as those in need of primary eye care, training, and cataract surgery.

(*See also*: BLINDNESS AND VISION DISORDERS; DEAF-BLINDNESS; DEAFNESS AND HEARING IMPAIRMENT; GALLAUDET UNIVERSITY; MULTIPLE DISABILITIES)

RESOURCES

American Foundation for the Blind, 15 West 16th St., New York, NY 10011

Helen Keller International, 90 Washington St. (15th Floor), New York, NY 10006

Perkins School for the Blind, 175 Beacon St., Watertown, MA 02172

BIBLIOGRAPHY

HARRITY, RICHARD, and MARTIN, RALPH G. *The Three Lives of Helen Keller*. New York, 1962.

KELLER, HELEN. *Optimism: An Essay*. New York, 1903.

———. *The World I Live In*. New York, 1908.

———. *The Song of the Stone Wall*. New York, 1910.

———. *Out of the Dark*. New York, 1913.

———. *Peace at Eventide*. London, 1932.

———. *Helen Keller in Scotland*. London, 1933.

———. *Helen Keller's Journal*. New York, 1938.

———. *Let Us Have Faith*. New York, 1941.

———. *Teacher: Anne Sullivan Macy*. New York, 1955.

———. *The Open Door*. New York, 1957.

———. *Helen Keller. Her Socialist Years*, ed. Philip S. Foner. New York, 1967.

———. *Midstream: My Later Life*. New York, 1968.

———. *My Religion*. New York, 1974.

———. *The Story of My Life*. New York, 1976.

LASH, JOSEPH P. *Helen and Teacher: The Story of Helen Keller and Anne Sullivan Macy*. New York, 1980.

CHRISTOPHER CAIAZZA

KIDNEY DISORDERS

Professionals treating individuals with kidney disease define rehabilitation broadly to include vocational, physical, and psychological restoration. Enlightened renal professionals view the goal of treatment for kidney disease as rehabilitation or achievement of the highest possible level of independence and quality of life.

Many kidney disorders affect rehabilitation. Chronic urinary tract infection, kidney stones, urinary incontinence, and congenital abnormalities of the urinary tract can affect emotional well-being, socialization, and absenteeism and performance in school or work. There are little data on how these diagnoses affect one's emotional state and quality of life. Research has shown that kidney failure or end stage renal disease (ESRD) can significantly affect the various components of rehabilitation.

Diagnosis and Etiology of End-Stage Renal Disease

Typically, physicians diagnose ESRD when an individual's kidney function is at or below 10 percent of normal. Primary causes of kidney failure include hypertension, diabetes, and chronic glomerulonephritis (Bright's disease), a non-bacterial inflammation of the kidneys' capillaries (glomeruli). Additional causes include recurrent bacterial kidney infection called pyelonephritis, congenital abnormalities, exposure to environmental hazards, misuse of over-the-counter and illegal substances, HIV, trauma to the kidneys or circulatory system, and hereditary conditions. Prevention of kidney disease is possible by taking over-the-counter medications correctly, avoiding high-risk behavior, reducing exposure to environmental hazards, and controlling hypertension. In cases that cannot be prevented, early intervention can maximize treatment benefits.

Treatment of End Stage Renal Diseases

The person with progressive renal disease must follow a prescribed diet and medication regimen. In addition, once kidney failure has occurred, the individual has three choices for treatment: hemodialysis, peritoneal dialysis, or transplantation. A nephrologist, nurses and other patient caregivers, a clinical social worker, a registered dietitian, and a transplant surgeon along with ancillary staff as needed form the ESRD treatment team.

Hemodialysis. Hemodialysis is a process of filtering the blood from the body through a dialyzer to remove toxins and excess fluid. The dialysis machine pumps the cleansed blood back to the body.

Dialysis treatments provide only about 15 percent of healthy kidneys' function. Chronic outpatient hemodialysis can be performed in a clinic or at home. The average time spent on dialysis in the United States is three hours per session three times weekly. Patients' work schedules and preferences may be considered in scheduling treatments in a clinic. In larger communities, usually at least one facility provides evening dialysis to accommodate employed patients. Home hemodialysis is an option for persons who have a partner to help with the treatment. This requires extensive training for the individual and partner, both of whom must be on-site during treatment. Home hemodialysis affords greater flexibility than center dialysis since it can be scheduled to complement work schedule and lifestyle. The person on dialysis must follow the prescribed treatment length and frequency to maximize health and rehabilitation potential.

Peritoneal Dialysis. Peritoneal dialysis removes the body's waste products and excess fluid from the blood through a process of fluid exchanges done inside the body's peritoneal cavity. There are two types of peritoneal dialysis. Continuous ambulatory peritoneal dialysis (CAPD) exchanges, performed four times daily, take approximately thirty minutes each. Continuous cycling peritoneal dialysis (CCPD) requires a machine to perform the exchanges during an eight- to ten-hour period nightly. Assistive devices are available to allow persons with functional and visual limitations to perform peritoneal dialysis, but some manual dexterity is required. The individual on peritoneal dialysis performs his or her dialysis independently at home. Compliance with the prescribed treatment regimen is essential to assure adequate dialysis and maximize rehabilitation potential.

Transplantation. Kidney transplantation requires major surgery to remove one kidney from a donor, either living or cadaveric, and place it into a recipient. Success rates are approximately 85 percent for living related donor transplants and 75 percent for cadaveric donor transplants. These have improved by use of improved medications that suppress the body's immune system. A transplant recipient must take antirejection medications as long as the donor kidney is functioning and maintain regular contact with his or her nephrologist and/or transplant team.

History of Rehabilitation in End Stage Renal Disease

ESRD is the only disease that entitles an individual to Medicare coverage despite age and receipt of Social Security disability benefits. Before the 1972 legislation that extended Medicare coverage to these persons, dialysis treatment was too expensive for most. There were few dialysis facilities, and all persons with ESRD were not offered treatment. Selection committees accepted a person partly on potential for rehabilitation, including vocational rehabilitation (DeNour et al., 1977–1978). During the congressional debate over whether to extend Medicare coverage to those with ESRD, testimony stated that many ESRD patients could return to work and productive lives if provided access to treatment. It was predicted that 60 percent could return to work with retraining, while most of the remaining would need none (Gutman & Amara, 1978). These predictions proved optimistic. In 1988, a total of 72 percent of the 77,000 working-age persons with ESRD were unemployed (USRDS, 1993; Vachon, 1992). Some variation between predicted and actual rehabilitation statistics can be accounted for by changes in population demographics. Before 1972, persons with ESRD were better educated, wealthier, younger, and had less severe comorbidity (Ferrans & Powers, 1985; Gutman & Amara, 1978).

Effects of Comorbidity and Aging on Rehabilitation. Research shows that multiple diagnoses decrease one's rehabilitation potential. More than 80 percent of employed patients have ESRD as their single diagnosis (Antonoff & Mallinger, 1990). Persons with diabetes, the fastest growing segment of the ESRD population, made up more than 34 percent of new patients initiating ESRD treatment in 1990 (USRDS, 1993). Diabetic ESRD patients are less likely to be employed (Rasgon et al., 1993). In 1990, approximately 29 percent of all those with ESRD were 65 years or older. Increasing age is positively correlated with unemployment among those with ESRD (Friedman & Rogers, 1988). In spite of increasing age and comorbidity of the population,

424

Nancy G. Kutner, Donna Brogan and Brooke Fielding (1991) estimate that at least one-third of those working-age unemployed persons with ESRD could be vocationally rehabilitated. Most of the remainder can live active, productive, and satisfying lives.

Effects of Education and Occupation on Rehabilitation. The most reliable indicator of employment potential for someone with ESRD is his or her level of education (Julius et al., 1989). Many studies report that occupation before the onset of illness is related to vocational rehabilitation. Blue-collar patients have greater difficulty maintaining employment, especially if the job is physically demanding (Gutman & Amara, 1978; Kutner & Cardenas, 1982). Unemployed persons with ESRD are likely to score lower on both the Karnofsky scales of functional status (Rasgon et al., 1993) and in professionals' assessments of functional ability (Friedman & Rogers, 1988).

Effects of Modality on Rehabilitation. Treatment modality appears to affect vocational rehabilitation potential and quality of life. Of the 167,440 persons receiving ESRD treatment in 1990, about 1 percent were treated by home hemodialysis. Ten percent were on peritoneal dialysis. Sixty percent were on center hemodialysis. Another 27 percent had functioning transplants. The modality of 3 percent was unknown (USRDS, 1993). Objective assessment suggests that those with transplants function at a higher level and have a higher quality of life than those on dialysis. A 1988 study showed that 74 percent of those with kidney transplants could work. Of those on center dialysis, 25 percent could work, and 59 percent of those on home dialysis could work. Those on CAPD could work in more physically demanding jobs than those on home hemodialysis (Rubin et al., 1990). Self-selection of and physician bias in recommended treatment may explain some variation in vocational potential.

Disincentives to ESRD Patient Rehabilitation

There are four broad categories of disincentives to ESRD patient rehabilitation: financial, attitudinal, educational, and lack of opportunity.

Financial Factors. The average annual cost for a person on dialysis is $30,000. Hospitalization and surgery for a kidney transplant can cost $60,000, and transplant medications cost a minimum of $800 monthly. Although 93 percent of all those with ESRD are eligible for Medicare, most of them are dependent on Medicare as their primary insurance. Medicare does not cover some expenses related to dialysis and transplantation, such as take home medications and transportation, and even those that are covered leave a 20 percent balance due. Many depend on Medicare as their only insurance because of preexisting condition exclusions and costly premiums for available high-risk insurance. They must choose between dialysis, with ongoing Medicare coverage, and a transplant, with potential loss of Medicare after three years. Any national health care reform will probably have an impact on those with ESRD.

Those diagnosed with ESRD are considered disabled by the Social Security Administration (SSA). If they meet other eligibility criteria, they are eligible for Social Security Disability Insurance (SSDI) or Supplemental Security Income (SSI). The main reason cited for reluctance to enter the workforce among those on dialysis is concern that they may lose disability payments (Antonoff & Mallinger, 1989). The ease of access to SSDI benefits for those with ESRD could influence them to choose disability rather than struggle to maintain employment.

Attitudinal Factors. Those with ESRD may become debilitated due to lack of physical activity. They may become comfortable in the "sick role" and dependent on others. Persons with ESRD who have high dependency needs are less likely to work (DeNour & Czackes, 1975). Many underestimate their rehabilitation potential.

The person with ESRD must deal with many feelings associated with illness and treatment. Depression is the most common reaction to loss of kidney function. It can result from facing one's mortality, changes in life expectations and goals, and dependence on a life-sustaining treatment and medical staff. Dietary and fluid restrictions, fluctuations in physical strength and endurance, altered body image, and changes in family and community roles also lead to depression. Depression can limit the ESRD patient's interest in activities and life, including the desire for interpersonal relationships and community and vocational involvement. It can also affect one's ability to perform household tasks and activities of daily living. Even survival on dialysis has been linked to cognitive depression. However, support groups are effective in reducing depression and improving survival (Peterson, 1991). Regulations mandate the role and presence of clinical social workers in dialysis and transplant facilities. One of their roles is to provide patient and family counseling to aid with adjustment to illness. However, caseloads and job demands are increasing, and these workers frequently spend less time attending to clinical responsibilities.

Educational Factors. Late referrals into the renal care system do not allow pretreatment intervention of those with ESRD, when rehabilitation potential is greatest. Blue-collar workers with ESRD historically have lower rehabilitation rates than workers in less physically demanding jobs (Ferrans & Powers, 1985). However, when provided predialysis intervention, they were twice as likely to return to work than those who did not receive pretreatment intervention (Rasgon et al., 1993).

The dialysis staff is often uneducated about ways to motivate persons to achieve greater rehabilitation and may place these individuals in dependence-independence double binds. Those with ESRD may be asked to comply with the dialysis regimen, be tolerant of limited flexibility in dialysis scheduling, and accept the dependent role as an uneducated, passive receiver of the dialysis treatment. While away from the center, they are encouraged to function independently and be productive. Staff may underestimate both the rehabilitation potential of those with ESRD and how functional rehabilitation, including exercise, contributes to the rehabilitation effort. Persons in ESRD treatment want enhanced interaction with their renal team, especially the physician. They also want to interact with their peers. They need this level of education and encouragement to attempt rehabilitation (Oberley, 1991).

The Rehabilitation Services Administration (RSA), the federal oversight agency for state vocational rehabilitation (VR) programs, was established to serve the rehabilitation needs of people with disabilities. Priority is given to those with "severe" disabilities, including ESRD. According to 1990 data compiled by the RSA, only 1 percent of those with ESRD sought VR assistance. Only half of those were accepted for services. Once accepted, 50 percent had successful closures. Those with ESRD state that VR counselors do not understand their illness and their special needs, providing some concrete services but few jobs (Brown & Ryersbach, 1980).

Frequently, employers believe myths about the high absenteeism, low productivity, high turnover rates, and high costs associated with hiring persons with disabilities. One study found that in the first six months after returning to work, those with ESRD had not missed one day because of illness (Friedman & Rogers, 1988). In general, 95 percent of employees with disabilities have less than average or average absenteeism, 91 percent have average or better productivity, and 88 percent have less than average turnover. Ninety percent of companies surveyed that hire workers with disabilities saw no increase in insurance costs, and 80 percent of all employment accommodations for workers with disabilities cost less than $500 (Frierson, 1990). There can be financial benefits associated with hiring and providing accommodations for employees with disabilities.

Lack of Opportunity. High unemployment affects those with ESRD. When assessing the employment potential of ESRD patients, the general labor market is probably more important than the person's diagnosis.

Some barriers limit access to employment. These can include transportation barriers, architectural barriers, and communication barriers. ESRD facilities may impose additional barriers to rehabilitation by prescribing inadequate dialysis, resulting in physical complications.

Organizational Participants in ESRD Rehabilitation

Several organizations are involved in ESRD rehabilitation. Renal professional organizations include the Renal Physicians Association; the National Renal Administrators' Association; the American Nephrology Nurses' Association; the National Kidney Foundation's professional councils, including the Council of Nephrology Nurses and Technicians, the Council of Nephrology Social Workers, the Council on Renal Nutrition, and the scientific councils consisting of medical specialists. Professionals belonging to these organizations are encouraged to participate in ESRD patient rehabilitation by federal mandate. In addition, most of the organizations are engaged in projects that influence rehabilitation.

Several agencies serve the rehabilitation needs of those with ESRD. Agencies having mandates to serve the rehabilitation needs of those with ESRD include the Social Security Administration (SSA), the RSA, and the eighteen ESRD networks of the Health Care Financing Administration (HCFA) that gather data, monitor treatment quality, encourage patient education and modality selection to enhance rehabilitation, and refer to vocational rehabilitation programs.

Voluntary health organizations are actively involved in ESRD patient rehabilitation. These include the National Kidney Foundation (NKF) and its fifty-two local affiliates serving specific geographic areas and providing patient, public, and professional education and advocacy. Besides other topics, the NKF has published educational materials related to rehabilitation, including brochures on exercise, employment, coping with illness, and sexuality. Several NKF affiliates have undertaken educational projects to enhance job readiness skills, dispel employer myths, and enhance professionals' awareness of programs and quality of life potential of those with ESRD. In addition to other patient services programs, the American Kidney Fund (AKF) has provided professional education programs on rehabilitation.

The most active ESRD consumer group is the American Association of Kidney Patients (AAKP). This organization has published relevant patient education materials related to coping with illness, employment rights, and adequacy of treatment.

What Changes Should Be Made

Advocacy for policy change is needed. Universal health insurance coverage is needed to eliminate disincentives in the Medicare and insurance system. Congress should consider increasing the substantial gainful activity (SGA) level for those with ESRD to the SGA level used for people who are visually impaired, or reducing SSDI benefits on a sliding scale

basis for those who return to work, similarly to how SSI has successfully treated persons with disabilities who work.

Greater emphasis on functional rehabilitation is required to maximize fitness and quality of life of each person with ESRD. This should include regular assessments of functional status and exercise training needs. When medically necessary, physicians should routinely refer those with ESRD for the full range of therapies provided through rehabilitation service agencies and hospitals.

Peer and professional support and education should be available when needed by those with ESRD. Staff should have qualifications and be employed in sufficient numbers to meet the demand. Patient role models should be sought. Peer group and individual counseling should be used to encourage ESRD patients to participate in valued home and community activities. There should be pretreatment education and counseling to encourage those who are active and working to maintain this level of activity and employment.

Further research is needed. The ESRD community should seek baseline data on the rehabilitation status of ESRD patients to allow adequate evaluation of intervention programs. Data collected should include functional status, employment status, and quality of life outcome measures. The renal community should seek both SSA data on numbers of ESRD patients receiving disability income and RSA data on numbers of ESRD patients referred for employment and their outcomes. The HCFA should report the results of the ESRD networks' progress toward meeting rehabilitation goals.

Finally, coordination of efforts is essential. The renal treatment team, public agencies such as the SSA, the RSA, and the HCFA, voluntary health organizations, and consumer groups must coordinate efforts to educate patients, professionals, and current and potential employers. An "expert committee" with representation from each organization and agency should study issues of rehabilitation. Both vocational rehabilitation counselors and ESRD professionals should understand ESRD patients' special needs and the opportunites available to them to help them achieve their goals.

Much has been done in the short history of the Medicare ESRD program to provide innovations in medical treatment. There has been less attention to those factors that contribute to the individual's quality of life, one component of which is rehabilitation. Maximal rehabilitation of all ESRD patients is a laudable, attainable goal, and efforts must be undertaken by all concerned parties if it is to be achieved.

Finally, coordination of efforts is essential. The renal treatment team, public agencies such as the SSA, the RSA, and the HCFA, voluntary health organizations, and consumer groups must coordinate efforts to educate patients, professionals, and current and potential employers. An "expert committee" with representation from each organization and agency should study issues of rehabilitation. Both vocational rehabilitation counselors and ESRD professionals should understand ESRD patients' special needs and the opportunities available to them to help them achieve their goals.

RESOURCES

American Association of Kidney Patients (AAKP), 111 S. Parker St., Suite 405, Tampa, FL 33606

American Kidney Fund (AKF), 6110 Executive Blvd., Suite 1010, Rockville, MD 20852

American Nephrology Nurses' Association (ANNA), Box 56, Pitman, NJ 08071

American Society of Nephrology (ASN), 1101 Connecticut Ave., NW, #700, Washington, DC 20036

National Kidney and Urologic Diseases Information Clearinghouse, Box NKUDIC, 9000 Rockville Pike, Bethesda, MD 20892

National Kidney Foundation, Inc. (NKF), 30 E. 33rd St., 11th Floor, New York, NY 10016

National Renal Administrators Association (NRAA), 1555 Connecticut Ave., NW, Ste 200, Washington, DC 20036

Rehabilitation Services Administration (RSA), Program Administration Division, 330 C St., M. E. Switzer Building, Washington, DC 20202

Social Security Administration (SSA), Office of Disability, Security West Building, 1500 Woodlawn Drive, Baltimore, MD 21241

BIBLIOGRAPHY

ANTONOFF, ARLENE, and MALLINGER, MARK. "Quality of Work Life of the Renal Patient." *Perspectives* 11 (1990):43–53.

BROWN, CATHY J., and RYERSBACH, VERA. "Vocational Rehabilitation for Dialysis and Transplant Patients." *Health & Social Work* 5 (1980):22–26.

DENOUR, ATARA K., and CZACKES, J. WALTER. "Personality Factors Influencing Vocational Rehabilitation." *Archives of General Psychiatry* 32 (1975):573–577.

DENOUR, ATARA K.; SHANAN, JOEL; and GARTY, ICHAK. "Coping Behavior and Intelligence in the Prediction of Vocational Rehabilitation of Dialysis Patients." *International Journal of Psychiatry in Medicine* 8 (1977–78):145–157.

EVANS, ROGER W. "The Quality of Life Assessment and the Treatment of End-Stage Renal Disease." *Transplantation Reviews* 4 (1990):28–51.

FERRANS, CAROL E., and POWERS, MARJORIE J. "The Employment Potential of Hemodialysis Patients." *Nursing Research* 34 (1985):273–277.

FRIEDMAN, NATHALLE, and ROGERS, THERESA F. "Dialysis and the World of Work." *Contemporary Dialysis & Nephrology* 19 (1988):16ff.

FRIERSON, JAMES G. "Make Way for the Disabilities Act." *Best's Review* 91 (1990):15ff.

GUTMAN, ROBERT A., and AMARA, A. H. "Outcome of Therapy for End-Stage Uremia." *Postgraduate Medicine* 64 (1978):183–194.

JULIUS, MARA; KNEISLEY, JILL D.; CARPENTIER-ALTING, PATRICIA; HAWTHORNE, VICTOR M.; WOLFE, ROBERT A.; and PORT, FRIEDRICH K. "A Comparison of Employment Rates of Patients Treated with Continuous Ambulatory Peritoneal Dialysis v. In-center Hemodialysis (Michigan End-Stage Renal Disease Study)." *Archives of Internal Medicine* 149 (1989):839–842.

KUTNER, NANCY G.; BROGAN, DONNA; and FIELDING, BROOKE. "Employment Status and Ability to Work Among Working-Age Chronic Dialysis Patients." *American Journal of Nephrology* 11 (1991):334–340.

KUTNER, NANCY G., and CARDENAS, DIANE D. "Assessment of Rehabilitation Outcomes Among Chronic Dialysis Patients." *American Journal of Nephrology* 2 (1982):128–132.

OBERLEY, EDITH T. "A Patient Review of the ESRD Program: Part II." *Nephrology News & Issues* 5 (1991):18–27.

PETERSON, R. A. "Psychosocial Determinants of Disorder: Social Support, Coping, and Social Skills Interactions." In *Handbook of Behavior Therapy and Psychological Science: An Integrative Approach*, ed. P. R. Martin. New York, 1991.

RASGON, SCOTT; SCHWANKOVSKY, LENORE; JAMES-ROGERS, ANNETTE; WIDROW, LESLIE; GLICK, JEFFREY; and BUTTS, EDMUND. "An Intervention for

Employment Maintenance Among Blue-Collar Workers with End-Stage Renal Disease." *American Journal of Kidney Diseases* 22 (1993):403–412.

Rubin, Jack; Case, Gay; and Bower, John. "Comparison of Rehabilitation in Patients Undergoing Home Dialysis." *Archives of Internal Medicine* 150 (1990):1429–1431.

United States Renal Data System (USRDS). *1993 Annual Data Report*. Bethesda, MD, 1993.

Vachon, R. Alexander. "Rehab: Should We Just Give Up?" *Nephrology News & Issues* 6 (1992): 25ff.

Beth Witten
Karren King

L

LABOR UNIONS

Labor unions have a tradition of representing the worker—fighting for their rights and for safe and healthy work environments, and advocating good jobs, good pay, and good benefits. Historically, that role included assisting workers (union members) who had become disabled and were seeking to return to work following the provision of rehabilitation services. Union assistance often included negotiating retraining of injured workers as well as job site accommodation.

Physical and mental rehabilitation services to union members typically are provided in three ways: through a third party (e.g., private rehabilitation facilities) under the provisions of a labor-management agreement; through state workers' compensation programs for work-related disabilities; and/or through state vocational rehabilitation agencies. The role of labor unions is one of resource identification, referral, and monitoring rather than provision of direct rehabilitation services, with the exception of job placement services through local labor unions.

When policy changes were adopted by the AFL-CIO central body in the late 1980s, the union role in employment expanded to include helping people with disabilities make their initial entry into the job market. The role and influence of organized labor is significant in that labor unions represent an estimated 17 million to 18 million workers in a variety of settings. The AFL-CIO policy is presented in *Working Together: The Key to Jobs for Workers with Disabilities* (AFL-CIO, 1988). Anticipation of the enactment of the Americans with Disabilities Act (ADA) of 1990, prohibiting discrimination in employment and other settings, was a major influence in the policy change. However, labor unions played a lead role in advocating protection of the rights of workers with disabilities even earlier, working through legislative channels and collective bargaining and other labor-management cooperative agreements. Federal and state legislative activities included working for reform in occupational health and safety laws, in state workers' compensation programs, and in wage and hours laws. To implement the AFL-CIO policy and in response to the passage of the ADA, a nationwide program that focuses on

431

employment was organized in 1992 through the 86 affiliated international unions and will involve state- and local-level training of union officers and staff in accommodating workers with disabilities.

Labor unions have demonstrated their commitment to expanding employment opportunities for workers with disabilities through special program initiatives and through a series of pilot demonstration projects, some operating as national networks and others operating in selected locations in states or communities. These programs and projects include the following:

- the International Association of Machinists Center for Administering Rehabilitation and Employment Services (IAM CARES), which operates job placement and training services programs in several locations;
- the Human Resources Development Institute (HRDI) Handicapped Placement Program, which operates a network of services in five locations: Baltimore, Houston, St. Louis, St. Paul, and Helena, Montana. The program assists workers and candidates with disabilities to enter the workforce and return to the work force; it also provides disability management, job search, and contract language advice as part of the AFL-CIO employment and training program;
- the American Federation of State, County, and Municipal Employees (AFSCME), which carries out a series of disability-related activities at the international level; conducts an annual program to recognize and award affiliates with exemplary programs serving workers with disabilities; and publishes and annually updates a comprehensive manual for AFSCME affiliates, *Fighting for the Rights of Disabled Workers*;
- an early intervention program, designed to provide services to workers with a recently acquired disability, is operated jointly by the AFL-CIO HRDI and the Columbia University Workplace Center and has the participation of many international unions, including the International Brotherhood of Electrical Workers and the Service Employees International Union.

Areas of Controversy

There are controversial issues pertaining to the union role. Labor union involvement in rehabilitation programs and services, particularly vocational rehabilitation, pertains mostly to the training or retraining and employment of workers with work-related disabilities. The reentry of workers disabled by non-work related accident or disease and the initial entry of worker candidates with disabilities represent separate considerations involving controversial issues. For example, in their collective bargaining agreement, unions likely have negotiated a return-to-work program for members with disabilities. Such action may include retraining, job transfer, and/or job restructuring or related worksite accommodation. To achieve successful return to work, waivers of seniority or promotion and transfer rights may be required, thus generating a possible infringement on the rights of other workers.

For worker candidates with disabilities the waivers and related accommodation are even more complex and controversial, especially in a period when job reduction and layoffs are more common than new hiring. In a 1989–1990 state and national study (Whitehead, 1990), local unions were found to be much more reluctant to grant waivers or make other concessions and accommodations to permit hiring of new workers. The impact of the Americans with Disabilities Act (ADA) should lessen this resistance and require both labor unions and employers to be more responsive. The ADA also should aid the return to work of workers with disabilities.

Union Role in the Future

Additional expansion of the labor union role in rehabilitation will require the formation of an effective partnership of union, management, and rehabilitation. One benefit of the enactment of the ADA and other federal initiatives (e.g., the Social Security Act Work Incentives and Rehabilitation Act Projects with Industry) in the late 1980s is that the working relationship among the three groups has improved significantly in many states and localities.

Finally, there are two special programs, generally operated jointly by union and management, that are particularly important because they aim to ensure that rehabilitation has a long range effect:

- apprenticeship programs offer people an opportunity to get jobs at higher skill levels and better pay, but people with disabilities often have been excluded from these training opportunities because of entry requirements and lack of knowledge of apprenticeship availability. Unions in many states have a joint responsibility with employers to establish and coordinate apprenticeship programs through state councils;
- employee Assistance Programs (EAP), originally designed to provide support for the worker with special personal problems (e.g., substance abuse and domestic conflict), are operated as independent entities by management (employers) in cooperation with labor unions in more than 7,000 locations (West Virginia Research and Training Center, 1986). The EAP model could address the critical need of some workers with severe disabilities for ongoing support that would ensure job retention.

Organized labor has a challenging opportunity to support the major rehabilitation initiative generated by the ADA. However, based on the results of national studies (Whitehead 1990), without special incentives, including funding, the support it offers may be minimal.

(*See also:* AFFIRMATIVE ACTION; AMERICANS WITH DISABILITIES ACT; DISABILITY LAW AND SOCIAL POLICY; DISABILITY MANAGEMENT; EMPLOYEE ASSISTANCE PROGRAMS; ERGONOMICS; FORENSIC REHABILITATION; JOB PLACEMENT; PHILOSOPHY OF REHABILITATION; VOCATIONAL ASSESSMENT; WORK)

RESOURCES

For more information on model programs described, contact:

International Association of Machinists Center for Administering Rehabilitation and Employment Services (IAM CARES), 1300 Connecticut Ave., NW, Washington, DC 20036

AFL-CIO Human Resources Development Institute (HRDI), 815 16th St., NW, Washington, DC 20006

American Federation of State, County, and Municipal Employees (AFSCME), 1625 L St., NW, Washington, DC 20036

Columbia University Workplace Center, 622 West 113th St., New York, NY 10025

BIBLIOGRAPHY

AFL-CIO. *Working Together: The Key to Jobs for Workers with Disabilities.* Washington, DC, 1988.

AFL-CIO HRDI. *Serving Persons with Disabilities.* Washington, DC, 1988.

AMERICAN FEDERATION OF STATE, COUNTY, AND MUNICIPAL EMPLOYEES. "Employee Assistance Programs: Making Them Work for Members." *AFSCME Steward* (Fall 1984):75.

———. *Fighting for the Rights of Disabled Workers: An AFSCME Guide.* Washington, DC, 1988.

DOHERTY, ROBERT. *Industrial and Labor Relations Terms: A Glossary.* Ithaca, NY, 1989.

ENTEEN, ROBERT; HERMAN, ROBERT; and TRAMM, MELVIN. *Affirmative Action for the Disabled: A How-to Manual for Labor Unions.* New York, 1979.

MAINSTREAM, INC. *A Working Agreement: Unions and Affirmative Action.* Washington, DC, 1988.

MENNINGER RESEARCH FOUNDATION. *Preventing Disability Dependence: Return-to-work Studies.* Topeka, KS, 1987.

SCHUSTER, MICHAEL. *Union-Management Cooperation: Structure, Process and Impact.* Syracuse, NY, 1984.

SIEGEL, IRVING, and WEINBERG, EDGAR. *Labor-Management Cooperation: The American Experience.* Kalamazoo, MI, 1982.

SONNENSTAHL, WILLIAM, and TRICE, HENRY. *Strategies for Employee Assistance Programs: The Crucial Balance.* Ithaca, NY, 1986.

WEST VIRGINIA RESEARCH AND TRAINING CENTER. *Final Report: Employee Assistance Programs for the Developmentally Disabled.* Morgantown, WV, 1986.

WHITEHEAD, CLAUDE. *Final Report and Recommendations: Training and Employment Services for Handicapped Individuals.* Washington, DC, 1981.

———. *Labor Unions and Disability: Suggestions for Expanding Employment for Persons with Disabilities.* Hudson, FL, 1990.

CLAUDE W. WHITEHEAD

LANGUAGE DISABILITIES

See COMMUNICATION DISABILITIES

LAW

See DISABILITY LAW AND SOCIAL POLICY

LEARNING DISABILITIES

Learning disabilities (LD) are characterized by specific and severe underachievement (i.e., a discrepancy between learning potential as measured by intelligence tests and academic performance) in language (aphasia), reading (dyslexia), writing (dysgraphia), mathematics (dyscalculia), spelling, and/or reasoning. Children with learning disabilities can have from borderline intelligence to above-average learning capacity. Many theorists maintain that a true learning disability represents delayed or irregular development resulting from dysfunction of the cerebral cortex, which is responsible for language, higher-order cognitive abilities, and information processing. In addition to specific learning problems, learning disabilities may involve attentional, social, emotional, memory, and perceptual-motor problems and hyperactivity. The Education for All Handicapped Children Act of 1975 (P.L. 94-142) characterized learning disabilities as a "disorder in one or more of the basic psychological processes involved in understanding or in using language . . ." and excluded learning problems due to ". . . visual, hearing, or motor handicaps, of mental retardation, or emotional disturbance, or of environmental, cultural, or economic disadvantage" (Federal Register, 1977, p. 65083). Considerable debate over this definition led to the formation of the National Joint Committee for Learning Disabilities (NJCLD), which included the major learning disabilities organizations (the Learning Disabilities Association of America, the Council for Learning Disabilities, the Council for Exceptional Children, the Orton Dyslexia Society, the American Speech-Language-Hearing Association, the National Association of School Psychologists, and the International Reading Association). In 1989, the NJCLD issued a consensus definition that reaffirmed that the cause of learning disabilities is intrinsic (neurological dysfunction) but added that learning disabilities could occur across the life span.

The P.L. 94-142 and NJCLD definitions are routinely used to justify placement and funding decisions in the United States. Nevertheless, the parent-led Learning Disabilities Association and others have criticized these definitions for "blaming the victim" and for overemphasizing verbal, academic-related problems.

Diagnosis

Learning disabilities are the fastest-growing group of disabilities in the United States. Prevalence estimates vary widely, reflecting differences in diagnostic criteria. The U.S. Department of Education (1989) reports that about 5 percent of students have learning disabilities. Seventy percent of students with learning disabilities are boys, and 80 percent have reading as the primary problem.

Differential diagnosis of learning disabilities (from other, non-neurologically related learning problems) is difficult. More than 50 percent of students in learning disabilities school programs may be misdiagnosed (Shepard & Smith, 1983). Critics argue that diagnosis is based on tests that are inadequate, invalid, unreliable, and culture-biased.

As firm evidence of neurological impairment is often unavailable, assessors may interpret "soft signs" (e.g., abnormal eye movements, poor gross and fine motor coordination, perceptual deficits) as symptoms of underlying central nervous system disorders related to the person's learning difficulties. Given the lack of independent evidence of dysfunction, many researchers caution turning symptoms into causes. Several postmortem and advanced brain scanning studies revealed atypical brain morphology and cerebral activity in some persons with learning disabilities.

Etiology

Learning disabilities are heterogeneous and probably have many root causes. Certain genetic disorders are related to learning disabilities and mild mental retardation (e.g., neurofibromatosis, Fragile X), and there is increasing evidence of hereditability of developmental dyslexia. Adverse prenatal conditions (e.g., maternal intake of nicotine, alcohol, and drugs; nutritional deficiencies) associated with low birthweight are related to lags in infant motor development and subsequent mild reading delays. Perinatal assaults such as intracranial hemorrhaging and oxygen deprivation may result in later learning problems. Postnatal factors related to learning disabilities include (1) ingestion of toxins (e.g., lead paint); (2) illnesses producing high fevers and biochemical imbalances; (3) head injury; and (4) chronic ear infections, malnutrition, deprivation, and stress.

Intervention

P.L. 94-142 (and similar legislation in other countries) mandates that every student with disabilities have an individual educational plan specifying clear instructional objectives and needed services. The "least restrictive setting" principle requires that students with learning disabilities be included in the regular classroom as much as possible; they may visit a resource teacher for part of the day or may receive one-to-one tutoring. Students with more serious learning and behavior problems may be placed in a segregated special education classroom with a specially trained teacher and a low student-to-teacher ratio. Many students with learning disabilities improve in settings that maximize individualized instruction.

In their daily practice remedial educators primarily apply an individualized "clinical teaching" model that involves four decision-making stages: (1) assessment; (2) planning; (3) teaching; and (4) evaluation. Information from the previous day's evaluation is used to design the next day's cycle.

Teachers use various strategies to remediate learning disabilities. "Indirect" approaches focus on the presumed underlying neurological, perceptual-motor, or cognitive deficits, while "direct" instruction addresses the target academic problem. A nationwide longitudinal evaluation, Project Follow-Through, found that behavioral direct instruction was superior to other popular strategies in averting academic delays in at-risk children (Newman, 1992).

Amendments to P.L. 94-142 (P.L. 99-457, 1986) emphasize prevention, early intervention, and family involvement. Preschool education for economically disadvantaged children results in meaningful long-term educational and social benefits (Berrueta-Clement et al., 1984).

Implications

Learning disabilities are associated with extensive life-span problems. Children and adolescents with learning disabilities who experience years of failure and rejection in school often have emotional and behavioral difficulties, inadequate social and problem-solving skills, and low self-confidence and intrinsic motivation. Many adults with learning disabilities mask and compensate for their disabilities, but reading and perceptual-motor difficulties are major career impediments. Social skill deficits hamper relationships. Transitional programs for adolescents with learning disabilities emphasize community living and social and vocational skills training, with the goals of competitive employment and maximum independence. Special college and vocational programs and funding are available for adults with learning disabilities.

Despite the increase in specialized service for adults with LD, many of them are not enrolled in state vocational rehabilitation programs. The potential negative impact of their attentional, memory, and social deficits on training and employment may not be readily apparent or considered serious enough to warrant rehabilitation services. Studies of vocational outcomes reveal that many adults with learning disabilities are unemployed, or underemployed in low-paying, part-time positions; they frequently change jobs that are often obtained through family or friends. Successful adults with learning disabilities are self-empowered and driven; establish clear goals; savor their work; cope well with their disabilities and adversities; persevere until desired results are achieved; and create, accept, and use (but do not become dependent on) available supports (Gerber, Ginsberg, and Reiff, 1992). These findings suggest that high school, transitional, and adult programs should be proactive rather than reactive and focus on training success-oriented skills, such as goal-setting, establishing support networks, and persistence.

Controversial Issues and Future Directions

Controversies and unresolved issues in learning disabilities abound and include (1) definition and inclusion criteria; (2) prevalence; (3) causes (internal vs. external); (4) the validity and biases of the tests used for diagnosis; (5) the impact of learning disabilities on females; and (6) class placements (special versus inclusive education). Researchers have yet to demonstrate the efficacy of many popular treatments such as diets, megavitamin therapy, perceptual-motor training, patterning, and special lenses.

Future efforts are needed in:

1. determining possible genetic and other causes of learning disabilities;
2. providing early identification of risk factors to prevent learning disabilities;
3. accurately diagnosing neurological impairment and differentiating learning disabilities from other learning problems;
4. developing and evaluating effective inclusive and special educational interventions, social skills training, and treatments for behavior problems;
5. training more effective teachers;
6. fulfilling the potential of computer-assisted instruction;
7. expanding programs for preschoolers, adolescents, adults, and families.

(*See also:* APHASIA; ASSESSMENT IN REHABILITATION; CHILDHOOD PSYCHIATRIC DISORDERS; DEVELOPMENTAL DISABILITIES; MENTAL RETARDATION; NEUROLOGICAL DISORDERS; SPECIAL EDUCATION)

RESOURCES

American Speech-Language-Hearing Association, 10801 Rockville Pike, Rockville, MD 20852

Council for Exceptional Children, 1920 Association Drive, Reston, VA 22091–1589

Council for Learning Disabilities, P.O. Box 40303, Overland Park, KS 66215

International Reading Association, 800 Barksdale Rd, P.O. Box 8139, Newark, DE 19714–8139

Learning Disabilities Association of America, 4156 Library Rd, Pittsburgh, PA 15234

National Association of School Psychologists, 8455 Colesville Rd, Suite 100, Silver Spring, MD 20910

Orton Dyslexia Society, Chester Building, Suite 382, 8600 LaSalle Rd, Baltimore, MD 21286–2044

BIBLIOGRAPHY

ADELMAN, HOWARD S., and TAYLOR, LINDA. *Learning Problems and Learning Disabilities: Moving Forward.* Pacific Grove, CA, 1993.

BERRUETA-CLEMENT, JOHN R.; SCHWEINHART, LAWRENCE J.; BARNETT, W. STEVE; EPSTEIN, ANN S.; and WEIKERT, DAVID P. *Changed Lives: The Effects of the Perry Preschool Program on Youths Through Age 19.* Ypsilanti, MI, 1984.

Education for All Handicapped Children Act of 1975. P.L. 94-142, 94th Cong. (1975).

Education for All Handicapped Children Act Amendments of 1986. P.L. 99-457, 99th Cong. (1986).

FEDERAL REGISTER. "Definition and Criteria for Defining Students as Learning Disabled." 42 (1977): 65083.

GERBER, PAUL J.; GINSBERG, RICK; and REIFF, HENRY B. "Identifying Alterable Patterns in Employment Success for Highly Successful Adults and Learning Disabilities." *Journal of Learning Disabilities* 25 (1992):475–487.

KAVALE, KENNETH A.; FORNESS, STEVEN R.; and BENDER, MICHAEL, eds. *Handbook of Learning Disabilities, Vol. II, Methods and Interventions.* Boston, 1988.

LERNER, JANET. *Learning Disabilities: Theory, Diagnosis, and Teaching Strategies,* 5th ed. Boston, 1989.

NEWMAN, BOBBY. *The Reluctant Alliance: Behaviorism and Humanism.* Buffalo, NY, 1992.

SHEPARD, LORRIE A.; and SMITH, MARY LEE. "An Evaluation of the Identification of Learning Disabled Students in Colorado." *Learning Disabilities Quarterly* 6 (1983):115–127.

U.S. DEPARTMENT OF EDUCATION. *To Assure the Free Appropriate Public Education of All Handicapped Children: Eleventh Report to Congress on the Implementation of the Education of the Handicapped Act.* Washington, DC, 1989.

MAURICE A. FELDMAN

LICENSURE

See CREDENTIALS

LIFE CARE PLANNING

Life Care Planning (LCP), its concepts and methodologies, has progressed dramatically. For many entering the field of case management in recent years, these concepts seem to be an inherent part of the field of rehabilitation and the various professional groups within that field. In addition to being employed by the practicing professional, LCP extensively requested by insurance carriers, attorneys, and other third parties interested in the catastrophic injury case. The many case management professionals moving into the field have too little understanding of the developmental processes and professional contributions that have been influential in bringing the life care planning methodology to its current state. To understand and appreciate life care planning and its future directions fully, it is important to have a historical understanding of its development and an appreciation for how life care planning differs from the techniques generally applied to case management before its inception.

A review of the literature reveals that the first published work on life care planning, as it applies to catastrophic case management, appeared in the late 1970s and early 1980s (*Damages in Tort Actions*, Deutsch & Raffa, 1982). Preliminary research and development came about for a variety of reasons:

1. A recognition that individuals and families with catastrophic disabilities (particularly in the pediatric area) needed a concise summary of a future plan that they could take away from an evaluation for guidelines and reference.

2. The importance to have a means by which practitioners could communicate to all parties involved in an injury case what precise needs are dictated by the onset of a disability. The advantage of the LCP is its ability to convey this information in a clear, concise, and precise fashion.

3. Catastrophic case management dictated the need for planning and prevention, rather than the more traditional approach of reacting to circumstances, which then dictated immediate needs.

4. Life care planning was designed to break disability down into its most basic components and allow for complex concerns to be assessed more carefully, with a view toward prevention of problems and complications rather than management by chaos.

5. The basic methodology provided for an evaluation that took into consideration the injury or disability; the needs, goals, interests, and preferences of the individual; the needs of the family; and the realities of the geographical region in which the individual and family resided. This planning process did not take into consideration budget requirements during the initial process. A plan could not be de-

veloped based on budget but had to be based on the above factors, with budget a consideration only at the point at which implementation of the plan was being accomplished.

Unquestionably, rehabilitation professionals were involved in the concept of case management prior to the mid-1970s, but no clearly defined methodology for disability analysis, consistent with the concepts of life care planning, was present prior to that time.

In its early stages, the foremost application of life care planning was through consultation. Consultation, primarily with insurance carriers and attorneys involved in litigation, became a major developing area of practice for the rehabilitation professional. As a result, litigation and the demands generated by its participants significantly influenced life care planning and greatly enhanced its credibility and acceptance. Increasingly, life care planning became an integral part of case management, with more and more individuals recognizing the importance of advanced planning rather than attempts to manage disability through a spur-of-the-moment process. As more and more individuals outside the rehabilitation field, but influential in disability management, began to recognize the broad complexities involved in disability management and long-term planning, there came about an increasing recognition of the broad gap between the role of treating physicians and the role of rehabilitation professionals involved in case management. The importance of understanding these different roles is critical to appreciating the valuable contribution made by the case manager. In part this distinction has been verified in six separate rulings by federal district appeals courts that have redefined independent medical exams and the ability of individual state courts to order these exams. In these rulings the redefinition of the independent medical exam included the ability of courts to order examinations by rehabilitation psychologists, rehabilitation nurses, and rehabilitation counselors. These appeals courts affirmed that an independent body of knowledge was being brought to the courtroom, by individuals with expertise in rehabilitation and case management, that was not generally available to juries through traditional medical testimony. As such professional recognition began to distinguish the value of the rehabilitation professional's role in case management, more and more individuals became involved in life care planning, and an increasing number of team approaches between physicians and health-related professionals developed.

The Case Management Movement and Life Care Planning

Life care planning and its related methodologies, concepts, and applications are at a critical point in development. This has been brought about in large part by the case management movement. An increasing number of individuals from a broad range of backgrounds have pushed to enter the field of case management, and the development of the certification process (CCM) has spurred growth dramatically. Use of life care plans and a focus on a common set of methodologies and terms will bring better understanding as well as greater consistency to the field.

Individual case managers have a critical need to know and understand the medical aspects of disability and the means by which we can set up programs to plan for and prevent the onset of problems or complications. They have a critical need to understand the methodological steps for case management planning while also understanding resource development and the best means by which to keep up with reference material and research literature that is critical to proper life care plan development.

A marriage between life care planning and case management seems natural if health professionals are to provide the best possible preventive services to the patients and families to whom their fields are dedicated. Keep in mind that the most critical aspect of life care planning is the development of a consistent methodology for analyzing the needs dictated by the onset of a disability. This is far more critical than the format of the charting system used to communicate conclusions and recommendations.

In addition to its primary role in case management, life care planning is also being applied to the following:

1. the setting of monetary reserves by personal injury or casualty carriers in catastrophic injury cases;
2. insurance case management where utilization by

adjusters and supervisors allows for better understanding and planning of future needs;
3. the development of structured annuities for settlement or trust management;
4. facility discharge planning.

The Life Care Planning Process

Life care plans are designed to address all of the needs dictated by the onset of a disability through life expectancy, taking into careful consideration the process of aging as it combines with disability to create changing needs. The plan is preventive in nature as opposed to reactive. Issues and programs geared toward prevention must be applied not only to patient care but also to appropriate maintenance of equipment and supplies. The plan must take into consideration not only the disability but also the individual's goals and desires, as well as family needs and the most appropriate manner to deal with geographic issues (such as the availability of programs, suppliers, or other services in the individual's home region). The case manager will find that the life care plan lessens the complexities of providing services throughout the case management process. The plan is a living or dynamic document that can be revised as phase changes are dictated by such events as progression through the postacute rehabilitation process, completion of educational programs, or issues of aging as it combines with disability.

The life care plan must always be specific to the individual and not generalized to a specific injury. The issue of consistency in life care planning applies to the methodology used in data collection and disability/patient analysis and not to making the same recommendations based on disability issues alone.

The first step in the process is the collection of all medical, psychological, and rehabilitation data pertinent to the individual's injury and treatment. If involved in litigation, then also available in the case will be depositions of health care professionals, which can greatly add to the availability of information. Consideration should be given to obtaining school records (primarily for patients twenty-five years of age or younger), as well as work history data. The review of available information is then supplemented by an on-site evaluation of the patient. Whenever possible, a family member should

438

be present to provide a more independent and objective perspective on the patient and the history of disability. This family member can also be critical in providing premorbid (preinjury) history.

The interview should provide for the collection of data in the following areas:

1. a medical and social history;
2. the history of accident;
3. initial treatment;
4. rehabilitation program since onset of injury;
5. prior medical history;
6. the individual's objective description of chief complaints;
7. the subjective description of physical limitations and restrictions;
8. any environmental influences or work settings that may exacerbate disability;
9. current medical treatment, including the names of physicians, their phone numbers, frequency of visits, and costs per visit;
10. any health-related professional treatment being provided, such as physical or occupational therapy;
11. the complete medication regimen;
12. activities of daily living;
13. social activities;
14. personal habits;
15. socioeconomic status;
16. state or federal agency involvement in rehabilitation;
17. past education and training;
18. past military experience;
19. past employment history;
20. behavioral observations made by the rehabilitation examiner;
21. a complete list of all supplies;
22. a complete list of all equipment;
23. a detailed review of all specific information related to the disability (e.g., review of all cognitive, behavioral, social, psychological, and motoric deficits secondary to a head injury or the level of lesion, pattern of paralysis and sensory loss, bowel programming, and bladder programming secondary to spinal cord injury).

Areas that must be covered in a life care planning process include the following (Figure 1, p. 440):

1. Projected evaluations. This covers all health-related professional evaluations that must occur on a periodic basis. This may include physical therapy, speech therapy, occupational therapy, recreational therapy, or a wide range of related intervention strategies.

2. Projected therapeutic modalities. Therapeutic modalities represent the actual provision of therapeutic services, as separate from the evaluation schedule. Again, these are focused on health-related professional services and are separate from medical services.

3. Diagnostic testing/educational assessment. This area deals primarily with future test assessment, which may be needed in support of the planning process. For the pediatric case this includes educational assessments, and for the adolescent adult patient this includes vocational testing before retraining or similar activities are considered.

4. Wheelchair needs. The focus here is on the type and configuration of wheelchair required, based on the disability, patient status, and the goals to be achieved.

5. Wheelchair accessories and maintenance. This area is a clear example of the preventive techniques employed in life care planning. Accessories may include, but are not limited to, wheelchair cushions for prevention of decubitus ulcers, lap tables, a wheelchair backpack, and other custom features to make the wheelchair more practical for the individual. Maintenance on the chair is done on a routine basis so that delays caused by more expensive breakdowns can be avoided.

6. Aids for independent function. Aids designed to allow more independent function by individuals who have significant motoric restriction are reviewed and recommended in this area. Only those aids that are realistically going to be used by an individual should be included.

7. Orthopedic equipment needs. This area covers a specific orthopedic or exercise equipment that may be required in a home care plan. Items such as walkers, standing tables, parallel bars, or related durable medical equipment should be included here.

8. Orthotics and/or prosthetics. This deals with orthotic or bracing needs, as well as prosthetic or limb replacement requirements. Detailed information on the type of orthotic device or prostheses is

Figure 1. Life Care Plan checklist

- ✔ Projected evaluations. Have you planned for different types of nonphysician evaluations (e.g., physical therapy, speech therapy, recreational therapy, occupational therapy, music therapy, dietary assessment, audiology, vision screening, swallow studies)?
- ✔ Projected therapeutic modalities. What therapies will be needed (based on the evaluations above)? Will a case manager help control costs and reduce complications? Is a behavior management or rehab psychologist, pastoral counselor, or family education consultant appropriate?
- ✔ Diagnostic testing educational assessment. What testing is necessary and at what ages? Vocational evaluation? Neuropsychological? Educational levels? Educational consultant to maximize the provisions of Individuals with Disabilities Education Act (IDEA)?
- ✔ Wheelchair needs. What types and configuration of wheelchairs will the client require: power? shower? manual? specialty? ventilator? reclining? quad pegs? recreational?
- ✔ Wheelchair accessories and maintenance. Has each chair been listed separately for maintenance and accessories (bags, cushions, trays, etc.)? Have you considered the client's activity level?
- ✔ Aids for independent functioning. What can this individual use to help himself or herself? environmental controls? adaptive aids? omni-reachers?
- ✔ Orthotics/prosthetics. Will the client need braces? Have you planned for replacement and maintenance?
- ✔ Home furnishings and accessories. Will the client need a specialty bed? portable ramps? Hoyer or other lift?
- ✔ Drug/supply needs. Have prescription and nonprescription drugs been listed, including size, quantity, and rate at which to be consumed? All supplies such as bladder and bowel program, skin care, etc.?
- ✔ Home care/facility care. Is it possible for the client to live at home? How about specialty programs such as yearly camps? What level of care will he or she require?
- ✔ Future medical care—routine. Is there a need for an annual evaluation? Which medical specialties? orthopedics? urology? internal medicine? vision? dental? lab?
- ✔ Transportation. Are hand controls sufficient, or is a specialty van needed? Can local transportation companies be used?
- ✔ Health and strength maintenance. What specialty recreation is needed? blow darts? adapted games? rowcycle? annual dues for specialty magazines? (Specialty wheelchairs should be covered in the area on wheelchairs.)
- ✔ Architectural renovations. Have you considered ramps, hallways, kitchen, fire protection, alternative heating/cooling, floor coverings, bath, attendant room, equipment storage, etc.?
- ✔ Potential complications. Have you included a list of potential complications likely to occur, such as skin breakdown, infections, psychological trauma, contractures?
- ✔ Future medical care/surgical intervention or aggressive treatment. Are there plans for aggressive treatment? Or additional surgeries such as plastic surgery?
- ✔ Orthopedic equipment needs. Are walkers, standing tables, tilt tables, body support equipment needed?
- ✔ Vocational/educational plan. What are the costs of vocational counseling, job coaching, tuition, fees, books, supplies, technology, etc.?

SOURCE: © 1989 by Paul M. Deutsch; Roger O. Weed; Julie A. Kitchen; and Anne Sluis provided, along with replacement schedules and maintenance information.

9. Home furnishings and accessories. Often the catastrophically injured individual residing at home will have special needs such as an electrical hospital bed, hydraulic patient lifts, suction equipment, feeding pumps, or a range of related requirements that are dictated by the disability. These are carefully assessed and outlined at this stage of the process.

10. Drug and supply needs. This represents a detailed list of the pharmaceuticals, nonprescription drugs, and supplies utilized by the individual. A great deal of detail is collected on all of these requirements, and the data are presented by unit size, per unit cost, monthly cost, and annual cost.

11. Home care/facility care. This needs to be one of the more carefully researched aspects of the life care plan if for no other reason than the high cost of services in this area. The decision as to home placement versus facility placement must be made carefully, and its impact on the patient's physical and psychological well-being, as well as the impact on family, has to be evaluated carefully. When home care is instituted, one must consider the home health practices guidelines established in the state of residence. Careful assessment, based on these guidelines, must be made concerning level of care (RN, LPN, CNA) and intensity (schedule) of care.

12. Future medical care—routine. Routine medical services provided as a standard of care in following certain catastrophic disabilities are outlined here by the case manager. In addition, routine follow-ups as specifically recommended by treating physicians, even if they are generally known as a standard of care, are to be included. This may involve routine annual reevaluations at a spinal cord injury clinic for the patient with spinal cord injury, or it can include routine physician evaluations, X rays, laboratory studies, or related medical support services.

13. Future medical care/surgical intervention or aggressive treatment. This area can only include specific recommendations by treating physicians for aggressive care or surgical intervention. This stage of the process cannot be completed by the life care planner/case manager based on routine assumptions of follow-up.

14. Potential complications. In dealing with this issue, it is important for the rehabilitation professional to understand that one cannot accurately determine the frequency, severity, or date of occurrence of a complication. As a result, an economist cannot include this issue in the assessment of the cost involved in the life care plan. Nevertheless, providing information on the most frequently encountered complications and their per incident cost will help rehabilitation professionals fulfill their role as educators. It is important for all parties to understand that a primary purpose of a life care plan is to set up programs designed to prevent the very kinds of complications outlined at this stage. Although no guarantee of prevention can be given, certainly the prognosis for reducing frequency and severity of complications when a proper life care plan is implemented is good. It is also important for all parties to understand that case managers cannot accurately cost out all future complications, and a separate fund must be considered to deal with these issues.

15. Transportation. The best means of providing barrier-free transportation will vary from disability to disability; this should be outlined carefully here. A special vehicle or vehicle modifications are needed; their specific purpose, cost, and availability can be presented here. In addition, all maintenance of adaptive equipment related to transporation should be outlined. All specifications for provision of various transportation should be outlined in this area.

16. Architectural renovations. This area deals specifically with the steps necessitated by the disability for achieving a barrier-free home environment. When completing this assessment, one should keep in mind not only the physical aspects that dictate the architectural changes but also the psychological influences. It is not enough that there is an available attendant to help the individual with a disability meet his or her needs. To the extent that architectural renovations can be provided that will allow the individual to participate more actively in self-care or to control his or her life and environment more actively, then a very positive psychological outcome can be achieved. Recommendations from the American National Standard Institute (ANSI, 1961) should be carefully considered. In addition, there is a wide range of literature on architectural renovations from which one can draw the necessary supportive data (Deutsch & Sawyer, 1985).

17. Vocational/educational plan. This is an effective and appropriate way of communicating specific vocational recommendations, particularly as related to training, job coaching, supported work programs, or transitional work programs. An alternative is to compile a separate appendix to the life care plan, often referred to as a vocational work sheet (Deutsch & Sawyer, 1985).

18. Recreational and leisure time activities. This area recognizes that the plan must deal with all aspects of the individual's life, including any adaptive equipment to allow him or her to participate in recreational and leisure time activities. This may involve special wheelchairs, adaptive games, adaptive sports equipment, special-need summer camps, and/or related recommendations that will allow for participation in these areas.

(*See also:* ADVOCACY; ASSESSMENT; DISABILITY MANAGEMENT; ECONOMICS; FAMILY; FORENSIC REHABILITATION; INDEPENDENT LIVING; PEDIATRIC REHABILITATION; PRIVATE SECTOR REHABILITATION; QUALITY OF LIFE)

BIBLIOGRAPHY

DEUTSCH, PAUL M. "Update and Research on Costs of Case Management." In *Damages in Tort Actions*, Vols. 8 and 9. New York, 1984.
———. "Ventilator Dependency." In *A Guide to Rehabilitation*. New York, 1987.
———. *A Guide to Rehabilitation Testimony: The Expert's Role as an Educator*. Orlando, FL, 1990.
———. "Life Care Planning: Its Growth and Development." *Viewpoints: An Update on Issues in Head Injury Rehabilitation*. San Marcos, TX, 1992a.
———. "Life Expectancy in Catastrophic Disability: Issues and Parameters for the Rehabilitation Professional." *NARPPS Journal & News*. Athens, GA, 1992b.
———. "Profile." *The Case Manager* (1992c). Little Rock, AR.
———, ed. *The Rehab Consultant*. Orlando, FL. 1989–1991.
DEUTSCH, PAUL M., and FRALISH, KATHLEEN. *Innovations in Head Injury Rehabilitation*. New York, 1988.
DEUTSCH, PAUL M., and KITCHEN, JULIE A. *Life Care Planning for the Ventilator-Dependent Patient: A Step-by-Step Guide*. Orlando, FL, 1989.

DEUTSCH, PAUL M.; KITCHEN, JULIE, A.; and CODY, STUART L. *Life Care Planning for the Brain-Damaged Infant: A Step-by-Step Guide*. Orlando, FL, 1989a.
DEUTSCH, PAUL M.; KITCHEN, JULIE A.; and MORGAN, NANCY. "Life Care Planning and Catastrophic Case Management." *Head Injury Reporter* 1 (1988). Lynn, MA.
DEUTSCH, PAUL M., and RAFFA, FREDERICK. *Damages in Tort Actions*, Vols. 8 and 9. New York, 1982.
DEUTSCH, PAUL M., and SAWYER, HORACE W. *A Guide to Rehabilitation*. New York, 1985.
DEUTSCH, PAUL M.; SAWYER, HORACE W.; JENKINS, WILLIAM M.; and KITCHEN, JULIE A. "Life Care Planning in Catastrophic Case Management." *Journal of Private Sector Rehabilitation* (1986). Athens, GA.
DEUTSCH, PAUL M.; WEED, ROGER O.; KITCHEN, JULIE A.; and SLUIS, ANNE. *Life Care Planning for the Head Injured: A Step-by-Step Guide*. Orlando, FL, 1989a.
———. *Life Care Planning for the Spinal Cord Injured: A Step-by-Step Guide*. Orlando, FL, 1989b.
GOODALL; DEDRICK; ZASLER; KREUTZER; and RIDDICK, SUSAN. "Survey of Case Manager Training Need" (accepted for publication in *Brain Injury*). 1992.
KITCHEN, JULIE; CODY, STUART; and MORGAN, NANCY. *Life Care Plans for the Ventilator Dependent Quad: A Step-by-Step Guide*. Orlando, FL, 1990.
Nicholson v. B. J. Blachly and International Rehabilitation Associates, Inc. NARPPS News (April/May 1988). Athens, GA.
PARKER, R., and HANSEN, C. *Rehabilitation Counseling*. Boston, 1981.
RIDDICK, SUSAN; and ROUGHAN, JAN. "The Ultimate Discharge Plan: The Case Management Approach to Life Care Planning." *Continuing Care Magazine* (October 1992). Waco, TX.
ROUGHAN, JAN. "Case Management: Definition, Process, and Perspective." *The Case Manager* (April, May, June 1990). Little Rock, AR.
WEED, ROGER. "Life Care Planning Questions and Answers." *Life Care Facts* 1 (1989):5–6.
———. "Marketing of Life Care Planning Services." *Life Care Facts* 2 (1990a):1–2.
———. "Marketing of Private Sector Rehabilitation Services." *PRSG Newsletter* (June 1990b):4–5.
———. "Presenting the Rehabilitation Consultant at Trial." *Trial Diplomacy Journal* 13 (1990c):212–226.
———. "The Role of the Rehabilitation Expert." In

PESI *Georgia Proof of Personal Injury Damages.* Eau Claire, WI, 1990d.

———. "Graduate Rehabilitation Counselor Training for the Private Sector." *Private Rehabilitation Suppliers of Georgia Newsletter* (1991a). Atlanta, GA.

———. "Support for Recreation and Leisure Time Activities in Life Care Plans." In *The Rehab Consultant.* Orlando, FL, 1991b.

———. "Economist's Role and Ethical Issues in Life Care Planning." *Orthotist & Prosthetist Business News* 1 (1992a):4.

———. "Figure 1—Life Care Plan Checklist." *The Case Manager* (1992b). Little Rock, AR.

———. "Orthotist and Prosthetist Roles in Life Care Plans." *Orthotist & Prosthetist Business News* 1 (1992c):4.

———. "Rehabilitation Consultants at Trial." *The Neurolaw Letter* 1 (1992d):1, 6.

———. "Working with the Life Care Planner." *Orthotist & Prosthetist Business News* 1 (1992e):5.

WEED, ROGER, and FIELD, TIMOTHY. *Rehabilitation Consultant's Handbook.* Athens, GA, 1990.

WEED, ROGER, and RIDDICK, SUSAN. "Life Care Plans as a Case Management Tool." *The Case Manager* (1992). Little Rock, AR.

WEED, ROGER, and SLUIS, ANN. *Life Care Plans for the Amputee: A Step-by-Step Guide.* Orlando, FL, 1990.

PAUL M. DEUTSCH

LIVER DISORDERS

See ALCOHOL REHABILITATION; GASTROINTESTINAL DISORDERS

LOSS AND GRIEF

Most of the literature on loss and grief is based on the reaction to the death of individuals in close relationship to the patient or client. There are many parallels between loss of a loved one and loss in disability. As with grief due to death, disability may be permanent, involving losses in roles, changes in relationships with others (such as from being a caregiver to a care recipient), changes in social expectations, and so on, all of which interact to cause grief. This entry describes three major classes of theoretical models of grief and summarizes suggestions for intervention based on these models.

Theoretical Models of Grief

Classic models of grief are based on theories rooted in the psychodynamic tradition, whereby the loss of an attachment object (i.e., a dear person, ability, possession) causes depression (Bowlby, 1980; Kübler-Ross, 1969). Such theories suggest that individuals must pass through stages or phases of grief before experiencing recovery. These stages involve shock and denial of the loss, protest against the loss (anger, searching behavior), and, eventually, acceptance of the loss.

Loss-depression Models. It is clear that loss-depression models that involve stages have some major limitations. First, they suggest that individuals must accept the loss and return to a prior emotional baseline, as would be the case with a major clinical depression. However, there is evidence that most people are permanently affected by the loss, making changes in their worldview and thus their personality to accommodate the loss. Although one may have some emotional resolution, the baseline would rarely be the same.

Second is the assumption that people must go through the stages in a fixed way to accept the loss. Most revisions of such models acknowledge some flexibility in the sequence of stages. Still, there are data that suggest that not only do people experience considerable fluidity in their mood during bereavement, but also there are enormous differences among individuals in the emotional impact of loss. Moreover, evidence from the studies of Camille B. Wortman and Roxanne Silver indicate that severe depression after loss is an indicator of difficulties in recovery over time and should not be considered typical. Many individuals may never feel depressed or angry in response to a loss.

Third, loss and depression models are based on the idea that finding meaning in the loss is an important predictor of resolution. However, many people do not find meaning, even after decades, and make good adjustments, while others who find meaning may be no better off emotionally. A fourth problem with loss-depression models is that they tend to gloss over individual differences in the experience of grief, and it is quite obvious that people vary within and across cultures in their experience. Helping professionals and even significant others may attempt to force or encourage emotional reactions such as depression that might not otherwise be experienced. This effort can engender guilt or other negative responses, feeling one has not suffered enough. Finally, the link between the survivor and the loss is crucial. For example, in bereavement due to death, the loss of the spouse is associated with different responses from those associated with the loss of a child, even an adult child. Causes of the loss, such as murder or suicide, are related to prolonged grief, when compared to long-term illness.

Stress-coping Models. Stress-coping models (Lazarus & Folkman, 1984; Pearlin, 1990) address the variability within bereavement. Unlike the primary focus on the individual's emotional state and reactions in the loss-depression models, the focus here is on assessment of coping style and resources, and enhancement of these to facilitate recovery and adjustment. These models are based on the idea that individual differences exist in coping styles and that people's coping resources predict recovery. Those with many resources, such as high income, high levels of education, belief in an orderly world, high levels of beliefs of mastery, and internal locus of control should have less difficulty recovering from loss. However, these models have not been shown empirically to work well in explaining effects of grief and recovery. Results by Camille B. Wortman and Roxanne Silver show that individuals with high levels of resources have more difficulty adjusting to grief, especially early on, than individuals with few resources.

Although stress-coping theories reflect the issues of grief more realistically than loss-depression models because of the focus of the former on individual variability, there are theoretical problems with both sets of models. First, both groups of models assume that a return to baseline emotional functioning signals recovery, but empirical research suggests that most people will not have a complicated bereavement but will nevertheless change. Second, loss-depression and stress-coping theories are based on a limited cultural base of understanding and tend to miss the mark in non-Western cultural groups. In some non-Western cultural groups, for instance, widows achieve a permanent change in social status, or families permanently enshrine the images and memories of their deceased members. Third, these theories are based on a medical model of intervention for health purposes and may take away from grief manifestations of the individual's self-expression and self-recovery. For instance, problems can arise when others expect that one should be depressed after a loss, should get over it after some specified time, or should rely on support groups and not deal with the loss independently. Fourth, there is growing evidence from empirical studies that these theories do not reflect the reality of dealing with loss.

Trauma-reintegration Models. Theories of grief that currently best fit the data are those in which the prediction of resolution of loss is viewed as based on the level of psychological trauma experienced due to the loss (Parkes, 1987; Epstein, 1992). Major losses are seen as more extreme adaptations of normal adjustments made to life changes and transitions throughout the life span in which individuals continue to reintegrate senses of self in relation to the world. Colin Parkes suggests that the loss causes extreme distress when it (1) is diametrically opposed to the individual's worldview (i.e., a view of the world as safe and predictable, as a place where one's actions reap specific benefits, and as controllable); (2) affects the individual permanently; (3) occurs suddenly. According to this model, which has been successfully applied to disabling conditions, if the individual's worldview is consonant with the loss, there is less difficulty integrating it emotionally. Those who are extremely distressed may never be able to integrate the loss into their worldview. Those who can revise their worldview to integrate the loss experience some distress as well, but once it is integrated, the distress is reduced.

The process of integrating the loss takes time—distress occurs because individuals need repeated experiences with attempting to integrate the loss in the worldview, and it is difficult to change the view for several reasons. One is that the worldview was effective before (i.e., nothing challenged it previously). Another is that people seek to incorporate their experiences into the view, regardless of the adequacy of the fit, because of long-standing habit.

Finally, others around them and the very culture itself may perpetuate the old worldview and fail to support or otherwise resist their attempts at change.

The trauma-reintegration models incorporate some of the best features of the loss-depression and stress-coping models and have empirical support from a variety of studies. As with the loss-depression models, the trauma-reintegration models acknowledge the role of depression, anger, and other emotional reactions, and these are viewed as symptoms of the struggle to integrate the loss. They are not necessary, though, for reintegration to occur. Similar to the stress-coping models, there is wide variability in response to loss, but individuals are not attempting to reachieve some baseline of functioning; rather, they strive forward on personal paths of growth. Paradoxically, there is a simultaneous inner circular process in which they may seem to regress or confront old losses again in a new way.

The major difficulty with these models is to identify what is "normal" from what may be pathological. Opponents would cite the need to identify outliers requiring more intensive support or treatment. Supporters of the trauma-reintegration models would probably argue that loss and reintegration are universal and inherent in the very fabric of life, and the question of normality is not very relevant. Without loss, change and adaptation would probably not occur.

Interventions for Loss and Grief

Interventions have been developed and successfully employed to assist individuals in their coping and adjustment to loss, despite problems with the models on which they have been based. Within the field of disability and rehabilitation, issues of grief and loss may apply to the patient or client, his or her family, and significant others.

Concurrent Emotional Disorders. The most common emotional disorder co-occurring with grief is depression. The majority of those experiencing grief often score within normal limits or at worst in the mild range on depression symptom inventories. Examination of symptom patterns reveals some overlap between grief and depression, namely, sadness, crying, insomnia, fatigue, and other physical symptoms, but grief rarely involves a pervasive negative

self-image, persistent hopelessness, and thoughts/plans of suicide, which can occur in depression.

When severe symptoms do arise in disability or when other symptoms persist or accumulate to moderate depression levels, individuals should be evaluated by a mental health professional for major depression, and treated as clinically depressed even if the onset was triggered by adjustment to a disabling condition. Without assessment and treatment, depression can complicate grief issues, lead to long-term emotional adjustment problems, and significantly impair functional and physical recovery. Treatment may consist of medication and/or short-term psychotherapy. Even when depression might have a neurological basis, as with multiple sclerosis and stroke patients, the treatment recommendations are the same.

Anxiety and posttraumatic stress are relatively infrequent but may be present in persons suffering the loss of a limb or disability from a traumatic injury (brain, spinal cord, and/or orthopedic) and who have some recollection of the traumatic event. Adaptation to typical posttraumatic symptoms involves a shift in worldview from being a victim to being a survivor. The recovery parallels closely that predicted by the trauma-reintegration models of grief described earlier, and as the general model suggests, many may recover, but remnants of grief may recur with anniversaries and other reminders of the loss, including the disability itself. In the case of traumatic brain injury, cognitive deficits may make the reintegration process more difficult. As with depression, severe anxiety beyond that of typical acute posttrauma symptoms should be evaluated by a mental health professional and, as indicated, treated as an anxiety disorder to facilitate both the grief process and physical rehabilitation. Anxiety treatment may include medication and/or short-term psychotherapy.

More severe psychiatric symptoms, such as psychotic features, are rare in disability outside of individuals with prior psychiatric problems or as medication side effects. When these symptoms are present, evaluation and appropriate treatment are essential.

Typical Grief Reactions. Even though the loss-depression models have their theoretical limitations, they have generated much clinical lore on typical

445

emotional reactions to grief and loss in disability. Negative reactions include shock, denial, anger, sadness, and fear; positive ones include acceptance, peace, and hope. Sharing information about typical emotional reactions with patients does considerable good. Many patients experience types or degrees of emotion they may not have encountered before, and the information may be reassuring.

Another ingredient in positive emotional adjustment, perhaps attributable to the classic grief models, is the importance placed on a positive, warm, and supportive environment. Patients who tend to regress emotionally or behaviorally need this safe environment to work toward emotional and cognitive reintegration. There are some individuals whose current loss with a disability may uncover unresolved issues with prior losses, a fruitful issue for more supportive, long-term psychotherapy.

Coping Styles. To cope with loss, as identified by the stress-coping models, some individuals rely on emotional expression (ritual expression, crying, talking about the loss), some on social support (family, friends, confidant or confidante, therapists, other patients, support groups), some on behavioral methods (diversion, recreational interests, helping others, physical activity), some on cognitive means (self-talk, positive thinking, information, planning, imagination), some on spiritual beliefs and actions (prayer, Scripture reading, clerical visits, rituals, spiritual company), and some on avoidance (alcohol, drugs, prolonged denial, rationalization, wishful thinking). Except for avoidance, which usually indicates poor coping, means should be made available to individuals with disabilities to rely on methods that work best for them. Methods used to deal with past losses may provide suggestions for current coping. Families and rehabilitation environments may need to be creative to enable individuals to engage in effective coping, and flexible to make new means available as they progress in independence. When coping methods begin to fail, or in the case in which the disability robs the person of a primary coping technique (e.g., ability to work or participate in sports), experimentation with new coping methods may be necessary.

The Larger Framework of Adjustment. Trauma-reintegration models have the most clinical and empirical support in providing the best "big picture" of adjustment and focus on the importance of individuals' abilities to adjust by their perceptions of the world and their relationship to it.

For example, one group that would be targeted by most professionals to suffer extreme distress in disability are those who were previously only marginally coping due to chronic stress, dysfunctional relationships, addictions, personality disorders, isolation, psychiatric problems, or economic difficulties. These individuals would not only lack sufficient resources to help them adjust to disability in a positive way, but also they often struggle to survive in rigid, overly controlled ways. For them, disability seriously disrupts a barely controllable world.

On the other hand, most models of loss and depression or of stress and coping would not predict that those who are also at risk for psychological distress may be at the other end of the spectrum— economically successful, staunchly independent, successful in a narrow band or arena of life. Despite many personal and social resources, and a strong sense of control of the world around them, disability may come as a major shock and disruption to these individuals.

How they deal with the grief and loss of a disability would vary, according to reintegration models, based on the interaction of their previous worldview and the nature of the disability, and the ease with which these two factors can be incorporated into a sense of self. For some, a disability may be temporary, and they eventually re-create the old world order. For others, some parts of the old world remain (economic success, renown, business opportunity), but they must make major adaptations to return to it (slower pace, delegation of authority). They lower personal aims and values to be more consistent with their physical and functional realities, and successfully adjust. For still others, a disability is the loss of a most treasured resource (an athletic body, a beautiful face, a talented voice, a sharp mind), and to adapt successfully, they must alter their worldview radically (e.g., learning to accept dependence on others over previously valued strong individualism).

Some people fail to adapt because they fail to revise their model of the world and reintegrate a sense of self consistent with it. As with others who have significant, and especially if enduring, problems in adaptation, these individuals are candidates for longer-term psychotherapy.

Prevention. The major contribution of trauma-reintegration models is to provide a framework for understanding the characteristics of individuals who are likely to adapt to loss successfully. This approach leads not only to treatment of individuals experiencing difficulties but also to developing models of prevention. The most critical characteristics of people who adapt well to disability seem to be: (1) a positive sense of self; (2) a balanced view of control between oneself and the external world; and (3) the flexibility to apply this view to life's changes and transitions. Numerous empirical articles in the literature demonstrate and discuss the buffering effects of positive self-esteem and self-efficacy in adaptation to illness and disability. Individuals with these characteristics adapt more easily, demonstrate more effective coping behavior, and physically recover more quickly or suffer less physical illness.

The ultimate way to enable people to cope with disability would be to foster development of the characteristics that would minimize adverse reactions should disability develop. It is, of course, a monumental and perhaps idealistic task to work through families, schools, communities, employers, and society at large to foster personal growth, self-esteem, and effective, flexible coping. Preventive education could focus on teaching basic trauma-reintegration principles as a general means of coping with the much more common losses that people experience—breakup of relationships, victimization by petty crime, or deaths of loved ones. Individuals then begin to develop the fundamental skills to cope with more significant losses such as a disability.

The Americans with Disabilities Act is another avenue of and motive for prevention. Educating people about others' disabilities may force some shift in worldview to see others as whole, functional persons despite a significant disability. Self-perception and the perception of others are intimately related.

Although most of the suggestions have focused on adults with disabilities and their adjustment, many of the same general issues apply to family members and to children, both as having disabilities themselves and as having parents or siblings with disabilities. We have included a few of the more important issues relevant to these special populations.

Families. The same theoretical models and basic principles applying to grief issues affecting individuals with disabilities also apply to spouses and other family members. Most of the clinical and research literature focuses on the family as caregivers, their emotional adjustment, and long-term functional adjustment. The caregiver role is paradoxical in a couple of ways. First, caregiving is not solely related to the degree of disability. Some caregivers are willing to provide or are capable of providing more care than others, based on feelings of affection, a sense of personal duty, or cultural expectations. Second, caregiving roles often conflict with other family roles—as spouse, lover, and wage earner. Necessary role changes and/or role conflicts can be major sources of family tension.

Emotionally, family members may experience reactions similar to those of persons with disabilities. Problems can arise when the roles of persons with disabilities in the relationship have changed. For instance, if the spouse with a disability was the former primary source of emotional support, the other spouse must seek some new or less gratifying sources of support, such as extended family, friends, or professionals. Problems can also arise when emotional reactions of families are not consonant with the expectations or capabilities of the member with a disability to adapt, such as when the individual with a disability experiences strong emotions and a spouse denies the disability. Finally, difficulties may occur after patients return home from the hospital and much of the professional support decreases or is eliminated, and the family's genuine experience of change really begins.

Family interventions follow the same guidelines provided above for persons with disabilities—complicating factors need assessment and treatment as indicated, typical recovery issues require time and general support. Special concerns in rehabilitation should be to keep family members involved (some more actively and others less so, depending on the nature of the family system), and resources for family support should be increased rather than decreased when patients return home.

Children. The general consensus of the literature on children's adaptation to loss with disability is that they (the degree varies with age) tend to mirror, or are at least be heavily influenced by, the reactions of those around them. That is, if family members panic, they are likely to be distressed; if peers are loving and supportive, they are more likely to develop positive self-esteem despite any disability. As family members they may be neglected as adult adjustment issues take more of center stage. In such instances, decreased school performance, psychiatric symptoms, physical complaints, and behavioral problems may arise.

Interventions with children with disabilities should focus on developing a supportive environment in medical treatment and rehabilitation, involving and fostering positive adjustment in the family, education at the child's level of understanding, and, if possible, education of significant peers. For children of other family members with disabilities, involvement in the rehabilitation process at their level of understanding is essential to prevent or minimize their adverse reactions.

Conclusions

We have discussed three major classes of models that describe the process of grief: loss-depression models, stress-coping models, and trauma-reintegration models. Although the first two sets of models have some clinical support and have generated useful interventions for patients and families, they lack empirical verification. Trauma-reintegration models highlight the degree of psychological trauma experienced by the person with a disability and help identify some of the intrapersonal factors that predict successful adaptation to loss as well as those that complicate grief.

We have also provided general guidelines for interventions with patients, families, and children. Numerous specific examples and illustrations of excellent intervention strategies exist in the literature on disability, and some of these are listed in the Bibliography.

Loss and grief affect all of us at different moments in our lives. If there is one thing they promote in all of us, it is a chance to look anew at ourselves, others, and our beliefs about the world around us. As painful as it may be, loss and grief can spur us on to change, growth, and personal development if seen in their proper context.

(*See also:* AGING; ANXIETY DISORDERS; CAREGIVING; FAMILY; MOOD DISORDERS; PSYCHOSOCIAL ADJUSTMENT)

BIBLIOGRAPHY

BOWLBY, JOHN. *Attachment and Loss.* Vol. 3, *Loss: Sadness and Depression.* New York, 1980.

COMMITTEE ON HANDICAPS. "Caring for People with Physical Impairment: The Journey Back." *Report of the Group for the Advancement of Psychiatry* 135 (1993).

EPSTEIN, SEYMOUR. "Coping Ability, Negative Self-Evaluation, and Overgeneralization: Experiment and Theory." *Journal of Personality and Social Psychology* 62 (1992):826–836.

GILEWSKI, MICHAEL J.; FARBEROW, NORMAN L.; GALLAGHER, DOLORES E.; and THOMPSON, LARRY W. "Interaction of Depression and Bereavement on Mental Health in the Elderly." *Psychology and Aging* 6 (1991):67–75.

KÜBLER-ROSS, ELISABETH. *On Death and Dying.* New York, 1969.

LAZARUS, RICHARD S., and FOLKMAN, SUSAN. *Stress, Appraisal, and Coping.* New York, 1984.

MARINELLI, ROBERT P., and DELL ORTO, ARTHUR E., eds. *The Psychological and Social Impact of Disability,* 3rd ed. New York, 1991.

PARKES, COLIN M. *Bereavement,* 2nd ed. Independence, MO, 1987.

PEARLIN, LEONARD. "The Study of Coping: An Overview of Problems and Directions." In *The Social Context of Coping,* ed. John Eckenrode. New York, 1990.

STROEBE, MARGARET S.; STROEBE, WOLFGANG; and HANSSON, ROBERT O., eds. *Handbook of Bereavement: Theory, Research, and Intervention.* New York, 1993.

VANDENBOS, GARY R., and BRYANT, BRENDA K., eds. *Cataclysms, Crises, and Catastrophes: Psychology in Action.* Washington, DC, 1987.

WORTMAN, CAMILLE B., and SILVER, ROXANNE G. "The Myths of Coping with Loss." *Journal of Consulting and Clinical Psychology* 57 (1989):349–357.

MICHAEL J. GILEWSKI
ELIZABETH M. ZELINSKI

LUNG DISEASE

See RESPIRATORY DISEASE

M

MAINSTREAMING

See DEINSTITUTIONALIZATION; NORMALIZATION AND SOCIAL ROLE VALORIZATION; TRANSITION FROM SCHOOL TO WORK

MANAGEMENT

Caring for human beings victimized by a trauma or born with physical or mental conditions is no small task. Managing rehabilitation facilities with an eye to restoring dignity and with a vision focusing on the total human being in order to minimize life's disruptiveness and to promote what Charles Dougherty (1991) calls "happiness," "freedom," and "fairness" is a challenge. It is a monumental task for those who provide services at a time when all of us are expected to do more with less. Rehabilitation costs money, but quality rehabilitation saves money.

The objective of this entry is to describe the role of management in not-for-profit (NFP) institutions such as rehabilitation agencies and facilities, independent living centers, and other entities engaged in the task of providing quality care to individuals in need with a focus on returning them to the fullest extent of productivity possible. This task is accomplished through planning, organizing, controlling, and directing with the goals of caring, nurturing, developing human capabilities, and returning people to the mainstream of life. Additionally, the role of visionary leadership will be described, because, as facilities continue to provide services in a rapidly changing society, with scarce resources that have to be managed carefully, managing institutions requires creative leadership on the part of both laypeople and professionals. In this connection, major management tools, techniques, and activities that may be considered by managers who are striving for excellence in service will be discussed.

Management and Rehabilitation: The Connection

The term "management" means many things to many people. In everyday life it is common to hear about "managing our life," "managing our time," "managing our money," "managing our own affairs," "managing our habits," and "managing our house-

449

hold." Some people think of management as applicable only to the running of a business that is trying to make a profit. The fact is, wherever there are human activities, there is management. It can be viewed as a means of getting things done using people. Here management will be defined as a process by which we create, maintain, and nurture an environment in which people work efficiently and effectively. Thus management is present in hospitals, schools and colleges, farms, government, parks and recreational areas, charitable organizations, law offices, religious organizations, and, of course, rehabilitation. Profit-making businesses are not the only ones that use management concepts.

Wherever there is a need (1) to achieve a goal using people; (2) to make well-coordinated efforts; (3) to maximize the value of money and other resources; (4) to provide quality goods and services; (5) to balance ethics and economics; (6) to design viable working relationships such as partnerships; (7) to respond to the needs and pressures of society; and (8) to create and provide programs to improve conditions of human life, management is needed.

Rehabilitation is a management process of planning, organizing, controlling, and directing activities and tasks in a well-coordinated manner so that individuals with disabilities can return to productive work and live as independently as their capabilities allow. The focus is on the total human being—his or her physical, social, and mental well-being. Furthermore, it has rightly been claimed repeatedly that "rehabilitation facilities are more than factories for treatment, they are social institutions through which the moral values of a nation are expressed" (Nichols, 1992).

Besides this system of caring for the total human being, health care organizations in general and rehabilitation facilities in particular require a unique kind of team approach in which many professionals from varied fields work together as a team to provide services. The team consists of physicians and nurses along with physical therapists, occupational therapists, psychologists, rehabilitation counselors, recreational therapists, rehabilitation engineers, vocational specialists, placement specialists, various federal and state rehabilitation agencies, and, of course, attorneys, insurance companies, and other third-party providers. It is not often recognized that the individual seeking the service is not always the one who pays the bill. Many entities are involved in the satisfactory conclusion of each case. The facility administrator, who provides the overall leadership that keeps a facility vital; the supervisors and employees, who are engaged in the performance of daily duties; and the consultants, who provide services on a required basis, have the monumental managerial task of creating an environment of quality service.

Society's increased pressure on rehabilitation to return people with disabilities to the mainstream with maximum restoration of abilities and skills requires tremendous service, accountability, responsibility, and performance. NFP organizations are torn between maintaining the economic viability of the facilities and meeting the ever-increasing needs of individuals with disabilities, who require financial resources and a dedicated, competent staff.

The Evolution of Management: From Asylums to Human Resource Centers

Rehabilitation facilities have emerged from a rich tradition of care that has been shaped by our culture, governmental forces, philanthropists, volunteers, professional groups, community attitudes, economics, and family structures. As people with disabilities have evolved from objects of pity, charity, dependence, and segregation into untapped human resources seeking dignity, independence, integration, and employment, so has the rehabilitation facility. It has evolved from an asylum into a human resource center where people can be developed and nurtured as assets. The rehabilitation facility was once a place where "undesirables" with physical and mental disabilities were confined for custodial care. Away from the mainstream of society, segregated, and at times forgotten, facilities did not provide much care, and their inhabitants were limited to a minimal physical human existence. The manager's role was perceived as being that of a caretaker whose duties consisted of feeding the residents, heating the building, providing security, and protecting and sheltering the residents. The first improvement on this agenda came with the help of the religious community, some caring physicians, and selected community-minded individuals, families, and friends. The emphasis of the facilities they established was primarily medical; they did not, by and large, focus on employment, al-

450

though some of them did provide employment for "blinds" or "deafs" within the facilities.

During the middle and late nineteenth century, a movement emerged that emphasized the notion that "the poor or sick" deserved more help. Workshops, schools, and other units were founded, including the School for the Deaf started by Thomas Gallaudet, the Perkins Institute for the Blind, the Massachusetts School for Idiots and Feeble-Minded Youth, Goodwill Industries, the Salvation Army, the Society of St. Vincent de Paul, and many others. The facilities that emerged in the twentieth century to provide services for people with disabilities find their roots in these earlier efforts.

In the United States there are more than six thousand NFP rehabilitation facilities. Many of these are accredited, and as nonprofits they are governed by volunteer boards of directors. With few exceptions, their leaders and staffs come from varied backgrounds with a strong orientation to human service. Financial management historically has not been a major concern. "Save the client at any cost" has been the motto. Sound business practices have often not been followed. Many facilities have been so consumer (client) oriented that research, evaluation, and financial issues have not received great attention. Typically, facility personnel receive low wages and benefits, and working conditions vary greatly. Often they receive much less than those working for state or county governments, let alone private for-profit rehabilitation facilities and private sector businesses. Upward mobility is limited, and employee turnover is high. Employee morale and staff burnout are major sources of concern. Limited financial resources, high turnover, and low morale are the kinds of internal challenges facility management must attend to and overcome in order to provide quality care and services.

Rehabilitation facility administrators face the following managerial challenges:

1. Increased competition for funding sources. While there may be money, access to funding sources is extremely complex. Facilities cannot depend on a single source of revenue anymore. They not only need to seek new financial resources but also must demonstrate the highest level of fiduciary responsibility in terms of cost containment and control of the resources they already have.

2. Attracting qualified professionals and reducing staff turnover by providing better working conditions, including staff training and development, are critical areas of concern. Facilities compete with for-profit rehabilitation facilities, private sector businesses, and the government to recruit individuals who are technically competent and have the highest level of human sensitivity. This requires leadership and financial resources that yesterday's "caretakers" simply cannot supply.

3. Serious conflicts exist between rehabilitation facilities and state agencies. Vying for funding for technology and needing to care for a population with more severe disabilities, who at times require state-of-the-art services, creates increasing tensions between these two entities. Resources must be shared, and state regulations that lead to some of these conflicts need reevaluation. New legislative initiatives are needed to establish fee structures that reflect the true cost of care to the facilities.

4. Rising expectations by clients and their advocates and the emergence of a consumer movement that demands the highest level of quality, professionalism, and efficiency in the delivery of care. An active consumer movement requires better planning and marketing by the facilities. Some facilities do this, but many do not. Such activities assist facilities in communicating to the community about the value of their services and mobilizing resources to meet the challenge head-on. The consumer movement, which demands accountability from the facilities, can be the same driving force not only in mobilizing resources but also in demanding more thoughtfulness and businesslike accountability from the state legislators who have created some of the difficulties. The legislators need to realize that their responsibilities do not end with the passing of laws. They must make provisions to pay for the cost of implementing legislation.

Role of Management in Rehabilitation: Creative Leadership

Facilities are human resource centers. They are very much like the small or medium-sized businesses in their communities. They need to utilize the principles of sound management practices to provide quality care. A badly managed business cannot provide this care. Therefore creative leadership with vision is required more than ever to meet the challenges of the remainder of the twentieth century and beyond. What should be the focus of creative leadership?

1. Strategic Planning

    There is an urgent need for facilities to engage in strategic planning, which is basically the creation of a realistic game plan, a road map to follow to produce results. The tasks constituting strategic planning are as follows:

    A. Define a mission.

    B. Translate the mission into specific short-run and long-run performance goals, and revise them as needed.

    C. Assess the current programs: improve or change them; look for opportunities and threats.

    D. Perform environmental scanning to study community moods and perceptions affecting the facility and the people it has served; monitor consumer demands and new government initiatives.

    E. Assess internal abilities and organizational structure to see if current resources can help achieve the mission.

    F. Develop priorities and plans, and ensure that the roles of the board of directors, top management, middle management, lower management, and staff are clearly defined and monitored.

    G. Implement the plan, and follow up through proper reviews to see if goals have been achieved. If not, corrective action must be taken.

    Such a planning process does not always guarantee success, but it minimizes risks and provides a facility with an opportunity to evaluate itself through meaningful participation by staff and consumers alike.

2. Facility Planning and Change

    It is clear that successful facilities do plan and carefully introduce change. Things can change quickly, but people change slowly. Before people change, they go through a period of psycho-

logical transition. Facilities go through similar transitions. A skillful leader minimizes risks, introduces change gradually, and gets people involved in crafting a program for change. Things that need to be considered include the following:

A. Focus

    • What are our objectives for change?

    • Are the objectives clear to all members?

    • Have we tried something like this before?

    • What have we learned?

    • How shall we evaluate our efforts?

    • Are the necessary resources available?

B. Structure

    • Does the change follow the organization's mission and values?

    • Have community factors been considered?

    • Have communication channels been established?

    • Does the change affect other parts of the organization?

C. Planning

    Does the change fit in with our short-term and long-term goals?

    • If not, what changes are necessary?

    • Is the change realistic (technically, schedule, people, cost)?

    • How much time will the change take?

    • Has the road map been adequately defined and communicated?

D. People

    • Are responsibilities clear?

    • How will the work atmosphere be affected by the change?

    • Have individual needs been addressed?

    • Has needed training been defined and planned for?

    • What is the reward system for accepting and supporting change?

E. Problems

    • What is the procedure for resolving problems and issues?

F. Output

    • Is this the best use of available effort/energy? (cost/benefit analysis)

    • Are there other alternatives?

As our society changes, it is clear that our rehabilitation facilities will also change. An analysis such as this provides valuable information and increases consumer confidence in the leadership of the facilities and the people they have served.

3. Performance Evaluations

Performance evaluations (PE) are extremely useful tools not only for evaluating performance but also for developing and motivating employees. A feeling of accomplishment is critical. Professionals and staff alike appreciate receiving feedback on the job, positive as well as negative. Proper PE not only raises individual morale but also improves the overall effectiveness of a facility (because its goals are accomplished through the efforts of people). It is crucial that personnel know they are contributing to the achievement of goals and helping the facility stay in business. A well-thought-out PE process disciplines facility management to define its objectives, set individual objectives, and evaluate results. Additionally, it requires the development of current job descriptions, specific job-related standards of performance, methods of keeping performance records, assessment of customer feedback, and meaningful discussion. The traditional goals of PE have been control and documentation, which often have been accomplished in a dictatorial fashion. This must change. The modern approach takes into consideration control and documentation. But it also emphasizes a collaborative approach to human development. The role of an evaluator is one of a mentor, coach, and invaluable partner in measuring progress. Rehabilitation change can be measured; such measurement is a valuable management tool in providing quality care.

4. Quality

The lifeblood of a rehabilitation facility is the quality of the people it has served. In our society many people with disabilities have been ill prepared for independent living and working. Family breakdown, limited transportation, inaccessible housing, improper and, at times, out-of-reach medical costs, and poverty have handicapped them. For many, rehabilitation facilities signify hope and a door to freedom. The serious responsibility that such expectations imply can be handled by making a commitment to quality and ensuring that quality efforts work and are properly implemented. Quality is not a program;

it is an attitude. It means giving clients what they want and deserve within the boundaries of ethics and limited resources. Quality is enhanced by good management, the ingredients of which include the following:

A. Visionary leadership that emphasizes consistency, reliability, and backup for the services provided.

B. Recognition of the fact that those who use services are customers. However, there are other customers as well—physicians, payers, families, vendors, and employees. If you do not treat your employees fairly, they in turn may not treat the customers fairly. It is an act of careful balancing.

C. A bias for action not only in solving problems but also in preventing them and in discharging responsibilities on the basis of teamwork and participation.

D. Commitment of the facility to provide a "safety net" of care. Management at all levels must be supportive, responsive, and committed to providing resources and making such provisions part of the strategic plan outlined above.

E. Ongoing improvement efforts are not considered additional responsibilities. Contrary to popular belief, they are part of the job and require doing what you are doing currently but doing it *differently*.

F. Empowering people with a team concept from the beginning and providing them with tools, time, training, information, and proper orientation. Combating bad work habits is part of good management.

Role of Professionals

The role of professionals is challengingly clear. If rehabilitation facilities are to be viewed as centers for human development, then visionary leadership is required from everyone. Such leadership will emphasize collaboration, strategic planning, a culture of teamwork, gradual introduction of change to balance economic needs and human needs, performance evaluations, staff development, organizational reviews, and total dedication to quality as part of the job. Such leadership will also be flexible.

Equipped with these management tools, the leaders will speak to the consumers with authority and credibility. The community will know that the facility has done its homework. As a result, the help will come; let's hope it will come to those who need it most. Rehabilitation facilities symbolize hope. Management symbolizes the vision needed to keep that hope alive.

(*See also:* EVALUATION OF REHABILITATION PROGRAMS; FACILITIES; HUMAN RESOURCE DEVELOPMENT; HUMAN SERVICES; INDEPENDENT LIVING)

BIBLIOGRAPHY

ALBANESE, ROBERT. *Management: Toward Accountability for Performance,* 2nd ed. Homewood, IL, 1975.

ANTHONY, WILLIAM P.; PERREWE, PAMELA L., and KACMAR. *Strategic Human Resource Management.* Fort Worth, TX, 1993.

DOUGHERTY, CHARLES J. "Values in Rehabilitation: Happiness, Freedom, and Fairness." *Journal of Rehabilitation* 53 (1991):7–12.

GARVIN, DAVID A. "Competing on the Eight Dimensions of Quality." *Harvard Business Review* 65 (1987):101–109.

JONES, C. T., and BRABHAM, R. "An Overview of the Rehabilitation Facilities Movement." In *Rehabilitation Facilities: Preparing for the 21st Century,* Switzer Monograph. Reston, VA, 1992.

MCFARLAND, DALTON. *Management: Principles and Practices.* New York, 1974.

MEWG, FREDERICK E. "Resource Development and Rehabilitation Capacities." In *Rehabilitation Facilities: Preparing for the 21st Century,* Switzer Monograph. Reston, VA, 1992.

NADOLSKY, JULIAN M. "The '1984' Crisis in Rehabilitation." *Journal of Rehabilitation* 30 (1984):4–5.

NICHOLS, NANCY A. "Profits with a Purpose: An Interview with Tom Chapman." *Harvard Business Review* 70 (1992):86–95.

PATI, GOPAL C., and ADKINS, JOHN I., JR. *Managing and Employing the Handicapped: The Untapped Potential.* Lake Forest, IL, 1981.

RAKICH, JONATHAN S.; LONEST, BEAUFORT B.; and DURR, KURT. *Managing Health Services Organizations.* Philadelphia, 1985.

SHAW, KENNETH, J. "The Value of Rehabilitation Facilities." In *Rehabilitation Facilities: Preparing for the 21st Century,* Switzer Monograph. Reston, VA, 1992.

SPIEGEL, ALLAN D.; PODAIR, SIMON; and FIORITO, EU-NICE. *Rehabilitating People with Disabilities into the Mainstream of Society.* Park Ridge, NJ, 1981.

TAYLOR, LEWIS J.; GOLTER, MARJORIE; GOLTER, GARY; and BACKER, THOMAS E. *Handbook of Private Rehabilitation.* New York, 1985.

THOMPSON, ARTHUR, JR., and STRICKLAND, A. J. III. *Strategic Management: Concepts and Cases,* 5th ed. Homewood, IL, 1990.

GOPAL C. PATI

MANIC DEPRESSION

See MOOD DISORDERS; PSYCHIATRY

MASSAGE THERAPY

Massage therapy is the systematic application of various manual soft tissue manipulations that may positively affect the health of a patient (Gerwitz, 1993; Hungerford, 1992; Zerinsky, 1987).

These manipulations have effects on the musculoskeletal, circulatory, respiratory, lymphatic, nervous, endocrine, digestive, urinary, integumentary, immune, and limbic systems. As a result, many pathologies can be treated with this type of therapy. Treatment plans can be created for traumas ranging from a fracture to recovery from cardiac surgery as well as a number of diseases from AIDS to Parkinson's disease. Five major Swedish massage manipulations form the basic foundation of massage therapy.

Effleurage: This is a superficial stroke that is performed on large areas of the body, increasing blood and lymph circulation. Effleurage can be used as a transitional movement and for tissue assessment.

Petrissage: More localized than effleurage, this also serves as a circulatory stroke. Two specific types of petrissage are compression and kneading.

Friction: This consists of parallel or transverse movement of tissues enpinged between the patient's bones and the therapist's hand. Friction is the stroke of choice in medical massage therapy and can be administered to bony attachments, joints, ligaments, and muscle bellies to break down adhesions, scar tissue, or cause local hyperemia.

Tapotement: This is a high-frequency application

of pressure and the only stroke in which the practitioner's hands break contact with the client. Tapotement is generally used for muscle contracture or postural drainage. The duration of application will directly affect targeted muscles: Fewer than ten seconds will stimulate, ten to sixty seconds will relax, and more than one minute will exhaust.

Vibration: Similar to tapotement, vibration utilizes high-frequency application of pressure. However, in this stroke physical contact is maintained between therapist and client. Vibration can be used as a neural stimulant, an aid in intestinal peristalsis, or in postural drainage. Duration of application is also subject to the same time parameters as tapotement, from ten to sixty seconds.

Biochemical processes, stress, anxiety, and poor sleeping habits can be positively affected by receiving regular massage treatment (Gerwitz, 1993).

Also in the repertoire of the massage therapist are evaluation, muscle testing, mobilizing, and stretching techniques. Use of heat and cold is also common. Massage therapy as a practice is not limited to the aforementioned methods. As in other medical professions, specialization is possible.

Research at the University of Miami School of Medicine Touch Research Institute indicates many benefits in treating various pathologies through the use of massage therapy. Premature newborns who received three fifteen-minute daily massages consisting of light effleurage and passive range of motion showed a 47 percent higher weight gain than the non-massaged control group (Gerwitz, 1993). Serotonin levels, natural killer cell number, and natural killer cell cytotoxicity were all shown to increase with regular massage sessions on seronegative gay men.

Massage therapy has also been shown to be beneficial in the treatment of depression and adjustment disorders in hospitalized children and adolescents.

Indications and Contraindications

Massage therapy plays a very important role in rehabilitation, though there are contraindications. When formulating a treatment plan, four basic categories should be examined to rule out anything that might jeopardize the patient's well-being. First, medication therapies can be adversely affected by the increase in circulation resulting from massage. The specific pathology should be thoroughly researched to eliminate the possibility of any proliferation. Additionally, one stroke might be contraindicated for a disease, whereas a dissimilar stroke may be indicated for that same illness. Last, massage can positively or negatively affect a pregnancy. Such factors as body position, type of stroke, location of stroke, and stage of pregnancy are all considerations. A careful medical history should be completed prior to any massage treatment. Massage can be prescribed by a physician.

There are many indications for massage therapy due to the wide scope of bodily systems that may be positively affected. The therapist may also combine techniques to achieve specific goals. These factors allow the therapist versatility in deciding what can be treated and how to treat it.

Before devising a plan, the therapist must review several considerations. What is the etiology of the particular disease? Can a cure be expected, or is the goal to enhance the patient's quality of life? Is the illness or trauma chronic or acute? Which strokes will benefit, and will they treat symptoms or the cause? Will this be adjunctive or primary therapy?

Frequency and length of sessions differ according to the pathology being treated and the goals of therapy. An average session lasts for one hour. However, frequency of treatments can range from weekly to daily sessions.

Taking indications and contraindications into account, let's briefly examine a possible treatment plan for Parkinson's disease. The etiology of Parkinson's is a deficiency of the neurotransmitter dopamine in the mid-brain, with no known cure. Symptoms include various muscular dysfunctions which lead to rigidity, atrophy, decreased nourishment of skeletal muscles, tremors, and poverty of movement. In addition, slowness of bowel habits, constipation, slow urinary action, and possible fluctuations in blood pressure may be present (Duvoisin, 1991). This basic information will inform the therapist that massage will not be the primary treatment because massage cannot administer to a dopamine deficiency. However, massage can address the resulting symptoms through effleurage, petrissage, and stretching techniques (Zerinsky, 1987). Massage can administer to slow bowels, constipation, and decreased urine output as well. One contraindication is the patient's state of muscular hypertension and sensitivity that will bar the use of friction and tapotement. If there is high blood pressure, this might rule out treatment of the abdomen for constipation.

Credentialing and Practicing

Credentialing of a massage therapist varies from state to state. In 1993 eighteen states, including Hawaii, Washington, Oregon, Utah, New Mexico, Texas, North Dakota, Nebraska, Iowa, Arkansas, Louisiana, Florida, Ohio, New York, Maine, New Hampshire, Rhode Island, and Connecticut, required a license to practice massage therapy. To obtain a license, a candidate must prove education in anatomy, physiology, pathology, basic and medical massage, first aid, and CPR. Fifty-six accredited schools exist in the United States, and many opt to teach additional course work such as kinesiology, psychology, and various Eastern techniques. Most states require classroom time of 500 to 1,000 hours. In addition, students participate in a practicum defined by the individual state offering licensure. Finally, candidates must pass a state board exam to receive their credentials. Further regulations are often required by many local towns and counties.

In states that do not offer licensure, there are statewide and local regulations for practice. Oftentimes statewide organizations and societies offer services to local therapists, health professionals, and communities.

The American Massage Therapy Association (AMTA) is the leading national body representing the field of massage therapy. In 1993 the AMTA had 15,000 active members. National certification is offered by the AMTA to monitor therapists' education in states that do not require licenses. Other association responsibilities include national and local education conferences, lobbying, research funding, educational accreditation, member services, and to act as a recourse directory for persons seeking massage therapy. The AMTA is divided into regional and state chapters. To maintain a "good standing" status, continuing education requirements must be met by each member.

Massage therapists practice in hospitals, doctors' offices, rehabilitation centers, health facilities, and their own offices.

(*See also:* PHYSICAL THERAPY; PAIN; QUALITY OF LIFE; WELLNESS)

RESOURCES

AMTA-American Massage Therapy Association, 820 Davis St., Suite 100, Evanston, IL 60201

ABMP-American Bodywork and Massage Professionals, P.O. Box 1869, Evergreen, CO 80438-1869

OMTA-Ontario Massage Therapist Association, 456 Danforth Ave., Toronto, ON, Canada, M4K 1P4

TRI-Touch Research Institute, University of Miami School of Medicine, P.O. Box 016820, Miami, FL 33101

BIBLIOGRAPHY

BALOTI, LAWRENCE, D. *Massage Techniques.* New York, 1986.

CREWS, MARY, and ROSEN, RICK. *A Guide to Massage Therapy in America.* Evanston, IL 1993.

DUVOISIN, ROGER C. *Parkinson's Disease.* New York, 1991.

FELTMAN, JOHN., ed. *Hands-on Healing: Massage Remedies for Hundreds of Health Problems.* Emmaus, PA, 1989.

GERWITZ, DAN, ed. *Touchpoints: Touch Research Abstracts,* Vol. 1. Miami, 1993.

HUNGERFORD, MYK. "A Patient's Notes: Massage Therapy After Open Heart Surgery." *Massage Therapy Journal* 31 (1992):71–72.

SPACK, JOHN F. "Legislative Time Capsule: 1993 Massage Laws." *Massage Therapy Journal* 32 (1993):79–81, 120–127.

ZERINSKY, SIDNEY S. *Introduction to Pathology for the Massage Therapist.* New York, 1987.

STEPHEN R. KOEPFER

MEDICAL REHABILITATION

See PHYSICIAN

MEDICATION

See PHARMACOLOGY

MENTAL ILLNESS

See ANXIETY DISORDERS; CHILDHOOD PSYCHIATRIC DISORDERS; HOMELESSNESS; MOOD DISORDERS; ORGANIC MENTAL SYNDROMES; PERSONALITY DISORDERS; PSYCHIATRY; SCHIZOPHRENIA

MENTAL RETARDATION

There are several commonly used definitions of mental retardation (MR). The American Association for Mental Retardation (AAMR) defines the term as involving "significantly subaverage intellectual functioning, existing concurrently with related limitations in two or more of the following applicable adaptive skill areas: communication, self-care, home living, social skills, community use, self-direction, health and safety, functional academics, leisure, and work. Mental retardation manifests itself before age 18" (AAMR, 1992). Similarly, the *Diagnostic and Statistical Manual* (DSM-IV-1994), published by the American Psychiatric Association, describes mental retardation as (*a*) significantly subaverage general intellectual functioning (for children and adults an IQ of 70 or below on an individually administered IQ test; for infants a clinical judgment of significantly subaverage intellectual functioning); (*b*) concurrent deficits or impairments in adaptive functioning (i.e., the person's effectiveness in meeting the age and cultural standards in areas such as communication, daily living skills, personal independence, and self-sufficiency); and (*c*) onset before age 18.

Incidence/Prevalence

The incidence (number of new cases) of mental retardation is estimated at approximately 125,000 births per year. The prevalence of mental retardation (total number of people with this disorder) is approximately 3 percent of the total population of the United States.

Diagnostic Instruments

Because mental retardation is defined by both a person's level of intellectual functioning and adaptive behavior, two types of assessments are employed. The Stanford-Binet and the Wechsler Scales are the most commonly used instruments for assessing intellectual functioning. These tests have been criticized for their lack of cultural neutrality and fairness, specifically because a disproportionate number of minority children are diagnosed as educable mentally retarded. The System of Multicultural Pluralistic Assessment was developed in an attempt to alleviate some of the problems associated with this test bias (Mercer & Lewis, 1978).

A variety of diagnostic instruments are available to assess adaptive behavior, including the AAMD (American Association of Mental Deficiency) Adaptive Behavior Scales, the Spitzer and Williams Structured Clinical Interview, and the Vineland Adaptive Behavior Scales. Typically, this type of assessment presents a profile of a person's behavioral strengths and weaknesses. For example, the Vineland Scales describe the individual's level of communication, daily living, socialization, and motor skills while also yielding an adaptive behavior composite score.

Classification

Persons with mental retardation are categorized by severity level, typically using an individual's score on a standard test of intelligence such as the Wechsler Scales. Using the Wechsler, a person would be considered mildly retarded with an IQ between 55 and approximately 69, moderately retarded with an IQ of 40 to 54, severely retarded with an IQ of 25 to 39, and profoundly retarded with an IQ of 0 to 24. Educators frequently use a somewhat different system, consisting of three categories: (1) educable mentally retarded (IQ 50 to approximately 70); (2) trainable mentally retarded (IQ 30 to 50); and (3) severely mentally retarded (IQ below 30).

Individuals falling into the mild level are considered capable of learning basic academic and vocational skills and living at least semi-independently. Persons in the moderate and severe categories usually are able to learn basic social, communication, and self-help skills but typically can't live independently. Persons in the profound category may be able to learn some basic self-help skills but require constant supervision and care.

Etiology and Outcomes

The specific causes for the cognitive and behavioral deficits of individuals diagnosed as having mental retardation are known in fewer than 50 percent of cases. Causes are either organic or psychosocial in nature or both. Among the organic causes are genetic and chromosomal anomalies, maternal infections (viral, bacterial, and protozoan), and maternal use of drugs. Psychosocial causes encompass environmental factors such as poverty, parental neglect, and abuse.

Down syndrome and Fragile X are the two most common chromosomal disorders that result in mental retardation, typically of a moderate to severe variety. Down syndrome, associated with abnormalities of the twenty-first chromosome, occurs in from 1 in 800 to 1 in 1,200 live births (Matson & Mulick, 1991). Women over thirty-five or under seventeen years of age are at increased risk for having a child with Down syndrome. In addition to exhibiting cognitive deficits, individuals with this disorder have a variety of recognizable physical characteristics, including slanting, almond-shaped eyes, a small head flattened in the back, small ears with earlobes often missing, a flattened nose, and underdeveloped nasal bones and jawbones (Baroff, 1986). Fragile X occurs usually in males, with an incidence of 1 in 346 live births. The degree of retardation is typically less severe than in Down syndrome. Physical characteristics of this syndrome include enlarged testes, ears, head, and jaw.

There is a multitude of genetic causes of mental retardation. The most common is phenylketonuria (PKU), which occurs in about 1 in 14,000 live births. The individual is unable to convert the amino acid phenylalanine into tyrosine, resulting in a toxic level of phenylalanine in the bloodstream. As a consequence, brain damage occurs. Typically, children with PKU have blond hair and blue eyes, a small head, and widely spaced teeth. Additionally, the urine tends to have an odd odor. Diet therapy, if begun at birth, can prevent or at least moderate the degree of retardation. If untreated, a PKU child will be severely retarded.

Neural tube defects (NTDs) are a group of polygenetic congenital anomalies that affect the closure of the neural tube. This disorder occurs in 1 in 1,000 live births. One variety, spina bifida, often results in hydroencephaly, which can be treated surgically.

A variety of factors affecting the prenatal intrauterine environment can be associated with decreased cognitive functioning: Malnutrition, disease (e.g., diabetes), drugs (e.g., alcohol, nicotine, cocaine), infections (e.g., rubella, HIV, syphilis, herpes), and other toxins affecting the mother may have deleterious effects on the growing fetus. Fetal alcohol syndrome (FAS) now occurs in about 1 to 2 of every 1,000 live births in the United States. Characteristics of FAS include retardation, distinct facial malformations, central nervous system disorders, and sensory and organ defects.

Perinatally, a number of factors, such as placental insufficiency, abnormal labor and delivery, and intraventricular hemorrhages, can produce MR, although relatively speaking these causes do not account for a large number of cases. Postnatally, insults such as head injuries and infections (e.g., meningitis and encephalitis) also occasionally cause mental retardation. Additionally, environmental deprivation, in the form of psychosocial disadvantage, abuse and neglect, and severe social or sensory deprivation, may lead to less than optimal cognitive functioning. Severe environmental stress during infancy probably also has adverse effects on early brain development. Mild mental retardation, which describes about 75 percent of the individuals with mental retardation, is thought by many to be entirely or at least partially environmentally produced, although others suggest that the low IQ is related to normal polygenetic transmission and inheritance.

Prevention and Treatment

Three types of prevention are commonly referred to in the literature: primary, secondary, and tertiary (Matson & Mulick, 1991). Primary strategies prevent the occurrence of mental retardation, secondary strategies prevent the full expression of the disorder, and tertiary strategies are directed at optimizing the potential of a person who has already manifested mental retardation.

Primary and secondary prevention efforts are commonly focused before conception, before birth, or shortly after birth. Prior to or after conception, the likelihood of some chromosomal and gene abnormalities can be determined through family information, physical exams, and chromosomal studies. Amniocentesis and other medical diagnostic procedures such as ultrasonography, amniography, and fetoscopy can be used to detect the presence in the fetus of a variety of abnormalities associated with mental retardation. Using information derived from these procedures, a variety of strategies can be implemented, including abortion, early dietary treatment, and surgery. Prenatal health care, including general dietary education, can also reduce the risk of some forms of mental retardation. The provision of health and parenting information is important after the child is born.

Early intervention and special education are forms of tertiary prevention aimed at the infant and young child. An individual educational program (IEP) is developed after a child is assessed as mentally retarded or being at risk for mental retardation. IEPs specify short- and long-term educational goals to be pursued and outline specific intervention strategies to be employed. Behavior modification programs have been found to be very successful in teaching a wide variety of adaptive behavior skills to individuals with severe or profound handicaps. For adults with a mild level of mental retardation, supported employment and occupational training are used to promote optimal functioning within the community.

Organizations

There are numerous professional, governmental, and parental organizations designed to assist individuals with mental retardation and their families.

Professional. The American Association on Mental Retardation (AAMR), formerly known as the American Association on Mental Deficiency (AAMD), is an interdisciplinary organization consisting of professionals from a variety of fields, including education, psychology, and medicine. This association's activities include developing definitions and classification systems to facilitate diagnosis, treatment, and intervention. The AAMR publishes manuals and other materials containing information on terminology and classification (AAMR, 1992). In addition, the AAMR actively promotes scholarly research on mental retardation.

The Association for Retarded Citizens (ARC) consists of parents and professionals who promote services, conduct research, enhance public understanding, and catalyze supportive legislation for individuals with mental retardation. The ARC works on local, state, and national levels. The Council for Exceptional Children (CEC) is comprised of educators concerned with educational issues affecting children with mental retardation. Specifically, this organization attempts to clarify educational definitions used to identify an individual's program eligibility, publishes journals, provides teaching materials, and lobbies for federal assistance programs.

Other professional organizations that work to promote intervention research, new legislation, and advocacy include the Accreditation Council on Services for People with Developmental Disabilities, the Mental Retardation Association of America, the National Down Syndrome Congress, the National Down Syndrome Society, and the National Association of Developmental Disabilities (for further information see Burek, 1993).

Governmental. The President's Committee on Mental Retardation, initiated by John F. Kennedy, advises the president of the United States in the area of mental retardation, distributes research information to the general public, and directs federal policies and initiatives. The National Institute of Child Health and Human Development, established in 1962, is the main federal agency responsible for promoting basic and applied research programs on mental retardation and other developmental disabilities.

Parental. Parental organizations, including Down Syndrome International, the Federation for Children with Special Needs, and Pilot Parents, educate parents about development disabilities, offer support, and provide information on how to access services and resources (for further information see Burek, 1993).

Issues and Challenges

A variety of issues and challenges confront professionals in the area of mental retardation, particularly issues related to identification, diagnosis, treatment, service provision, advocacy, and legislation.

Identification. Although there are more than 200 types of biologically based syndromes, approximately

75 percent of persons with mental retardation do not manifest a clearly identifiable cause. This group of people has more complex causes, stemming in part from psychosocial factors. To provide a framework for understanding this group, researchers have developed a "new morbidity" model of mental retardation. This model examines the dynamic relationship between environmental (drugs, alcohol, adolescent parenting) and biological (low birth weight, prematurity) factors associated with poverty and their causal link to developmental difficulties (Baumeister, Kupstas, and Klindworth, 1991). In addition, the federal government is sponsoring a large national research effort, called the Human Genome Project, to map the human chromosome. This project's goal is to determine the precise location and molecular structure of the genetic materials that make up the human chromosome (Lee, 1991). Research on the "new morbidity" model and in the area of molecular genetics has considerable potential for identifying previously unknown causes of mental retardation.

Diagnosis. Historically there has been a continuing debate concerning the emphasis placed on IQ scores in defining mental retardation. Increasingly, the importance of social competence is being stressed by organizations such as the American Association on Mental Retardation (AAMR, 1992). According to Stephen Greenspan and James M. Granfield (1992), social competence includes both intellectual (practical and social intelligence) and nonintellectual (temperament and character) components. Consistent with this perspective, deficits in both intellectual and instrumental competence are now considered critical to the diagnosis of mental retardation.

In addition, there is considerable professional concern about diagnostic overshadowing and misdiagnosis. Diagnostic overshadowing occurs when mental retardation is accompanied by an undetected and untreated mental illness. Even when a mental illness is identified, the presence of a developmental disability often overshadows the concern about an individual's mental illness and frequently prohibits appropriate treatment interventions (psychotropic drugs) due to detrimental side effects. Due to restricted training and a lack of knowledge regarding the other area of expertise, professionals in both

mental retardation and mental health have been very slow to acknowledge that individuals with mental retardation have psychiatric problems. Misdiagnosis is a problem, particularly when an individual manifests autistic behaviors or sensory-motor handicaps. Differentiation between mental retardation and other developmental disorders such as autism and deafness is critical if appropriate treatments are to be developed.

Finally, the act of labeling an individual as mentally retarded continues to be controversial. The assignment of the label "mentally retarded" is defended on the grounds that it facilitates the provision of treatment and services. However, opponents point out that the label of mental retardation can also stigmatize, limiting society's full acceptance of an individual.

Treatment. The use of aversive programming is a particularly controversial treatment issue. Since the advent of behavior modification, aversive procedures have been utilized to control a variety of maladaptive behaviors of persons with mental retardation, particularly self-injurious behaviors (e.g., head banging, biting), stereotypy, and social aggression. A wide variety of aversive techniques have been employed, including shock, taste and aromatic substances, response cost, time-out, overcorrection, and extinction. The use of aversive techniques has been defended on the grounds that maladaptive behaviors cannot always be controlled by less restrictive procedures and that without such control the development of adaptive behavior would be unlikely. Many professionals have criticized the use of punishment procedures as unethical and inhumane. A variety of alternatives to aversive programming have been recommended, including the use of positive reinforcement, instructional control, pharmacological intervention, and gentle teaching. (For further discussion see Harris & Handleman, 1990.)

Provision of Services. Service providers have been confronted with myriad questions, such as: Are all eligible individuals being identified in every state? Are some individuals in need of services overlooked due to variability in state criteria and cutoffs? States vary in the criteria, such as measured intelligence, adaptive behavior, and academic achievement, used to determine service eligibility. Although IQ is commonly employed as a criterion, cutoffs for qualification vary by state (Frakenberger & Harper, 1988). As a consequence, many individuals in need of services are probably not being identified.

A further question concerns whether individuals are being provided with the best possible services. Since the early 1960s, professionals have supported moving individuals from large institutions into smaller, community living arrangements, specifically because it was felt that such settings could offer more flexible, individualized care, training, and education. Programming has been guided by a normalization principle—making as available as possible the conditions of normal living to persons with mental retardation—and a developmental model that emphasizes the provision of programs appropriate to each person's developmental level. However, concerns abound about the quality of community education, vocational training, and medical and residential programs.

Advocacy. Citizen and legal advocacy has been critical to the development of services for individuals with mental retardation. As a consequence of a strong advocacy movement, many important pieces of legislation have been passed. For example, the Developmental Disabilities Assistance and Bill of Rights Act of 1975 established advocacy services for persons with developmental disabilities in every state. Effective community action facilitated the enactment of the Education for All Handicapped Children Act of 1975. This act ensured free and appropriate education for all children with handicaps and provided due process steps for obtaining services. Advocacy has been and continues to be essential in establishing and protecting the basic human rights of persons with mental handicaps.

Social and Legal Issues. Through litigation, a variety of rights, such as the right to treatment and the right to education, have been established. Despite major advocacy efforts, the rights of individuals with mental handicaps are not yet fully acknowledged by society and/or not always clearly established in law. For example, issues relating to marriage and sterilization continue to be sources of controversy. With regard to matrimony, thirty-eight states and the District of Columbia either prohibit or restrict marriage for individuals diagnosed with mental retardation. These statutes are based on the assumption that individuals with mental retardation cannot provide

informed legal consent to marry and would not make successful marriage partners, even though there is evidence that this often is not the case. Supporters of involuntary sterilization view it as a strategy for preventing mental retardation. Opponents contend that sterilization laws are discriminatory and violate the basic rights of persons who are retarded. In response to these concerns, states have recently developed guidelines concerning formal hearings and the justification of the need to sterilize an individual. Other social and legal issues faced by individuals with mental retardation relate to discrimination in employment and housing, and their rights when entering into contractual arrangements.

Future issues. Several critical issues are beginning to emerge in the field of mental retardation. Professionals are now recognizing that the human immunodeficiency virus (HIV) is likely to emerge as a major cause of mental retardation. Research indicates that 90 percent of children infected in utero with HIV experience neurodevelopmental difficulties (Cohen, 1992). Prevention and successful treatment of HIV infection will certainly influence the future incidence of mental retardation. In the areas of prevention and intervention, genetic research will also play a large role in determining not only how genes produce mental retardation but also how gene therapy might foster healthy outcomes. The Human Genome Project should be particularly helpful in this regard.

Several laws enacted in the late 1980s and early 1990s should affect the welfare of both children and adults with mental retardation. The expansion of early intervention programs presents a major challenge to service providers. The Education of the Handicapped Act Amendments of 1986 (P.L. 99-457) extends the provision of public education to include all eligible children from three to five years of age and also assists states in developing and implementing programs for eligible children from birth to three years. Despite federal and state efforts to extend services, governmental cutbacks and the increasing national deficit have deterred the full implementation of these programs.

Another federal law that should make some difference is the Americans with Disabilities Act (ADA) of 1990. This federal law is a groundbreaking piece of legislation that protects against discrimination any individual who is substantially limited in daily living by a physical or mental disability. The ADA addresses discrimination in the employment setting and provides support for increasing affirmative action activities, access to public facilities, and transportation, as well as for developing telecommunication networks. Also provided are advocates with the legal support to promote implementation of these activities. As in the past, the future welfare of persons with mental retardation will be enhanced to the extent that there can be an effective and balanced coalition of local community and governmental advocacy and action.

(See also: AMERICANS WITH DISABILITIES ACT; AUTISM; BEHAVIOR THERAPY; DEVELOPMENTAL DISABILITY; GENETIC DISORDERS; NORMALIZATION; SPECIAL EDUCATION)

BIBLIOGRAPHY

AMERICAN ASSOCIATION OF MENTAL RETARDATION. Mental Retardation: Definition, Classification, and Systems of Support, 9th ed. Washington, DC, 1992.

AMERICAN PSYCHIATRIC ASSOCIATION. Diagnostic and Statistical Manual of Mental Disorders, 4th ed. Washington, DC, 1994.

AMERICANS WITH DISABILITIES ACT OF 1990, P.L. 101-336, 42 U. S. C. 12101–12231 (enacted July 26, 1990).

BAROFF, GEORGE S. Mental Retardation: Nature, Cause, and Management, 2nd ed. Washington, DC, 1986.

BAUMEISTER, ALFRED A.; KUPSTAS, FRANK D.; and KLINDWORTH, LUANN M. The New Morbidity: A National Plan of Action. Newbury Place, CA, 1991.

BRADDOCK, DAVID. Federal Policy Toward Mental Retardation and Developmental Disabilities. Baltimore, 1987.

BUREK, DEBORAH M. Encyclopedia of Associations. Detroit, 1993.

COHEN, HERBERT J. "HIV Infection and Mental Retardation." In Mental Retardation in the Year 2000, ed. Louis Rowitz. New York, 1992.

FRAKENBERGER, WILLIAM, and HARPER, JERRY. "States' Definitions and Procedures for Identifying Children with Mental Retardation: Comparison of 1981–1982 and 1985–1986 Guidelines." Mental Retardation 26 (1988):133–136.

GREENSPAN, STEPHEN, and GRANFIELD, JAMES M. "Reconsidering the Construct of Mental Retardation: Implications of a Model of Social Competence." American Journal of Mental Retardation 96 (1992): 442–453.

HARRIS, SANDRA L., and HANDLEMAN, JAN S. Aversive and Nonaversive Interventions: Controlling Life-Threatening Behavior by the Developmentally Disabled. New York, 1990.

LEE, THOMAS F. The Human Genome Project: Cracking the Genetic Code of Life. New York, 1991.

MATSON, JOHNNY L., and MULICK, JAMES A. Handbook of Mental Retardation, 2nd ed. Elmsford, New York, 1991.

MERCER, JANE R., and LEWIS, J. SOMPA: Student Assessment Manual. New York, 1978.

THOMAS L. WHITMAN
CYNTHIA L. MILLER
DEIRDRE E. MYLOD

METABOLIC DISORDERS

See DEVELOPMENTAL DISABILITIES; ENDOCRINE DISORDERS; GENETIC DISORDERS; MENTAL RETARDATION

MINORITIES

While it is true that individuals with disabilities who are members of racial and minority groups experience the same disadvantages as other individuals with disabilities, these individuals face special and unique problems because of socioeconomic factors. In addition, prejudice and discrimination continue to exclude a great number of minority persons from full participation in all aspects of society.

Health problems and low socioeconomic status adversely affect large numbers of African Americans, Native Americans, and other persons from diverse cultural backgrounds. For example, since the 1970s there has been a marked increase in the number of Asians and persons of Hispanic descent coming to the United States. Large numbers of these persons are outside of the health care, educational, and rehabilitation systems. Many are refugees from rural settings who have come to live in urban settings that are at best unfamiliar and at worst hostile.

In such bleak surroundings, the impact on the family unit of an individual with a disability is formidable. The high cost of care, medication, and/or aids (such as wheelchairs) to assist the individual with a disability in gaining any degree of independence frequently cannot be afforded. This situation creates the necessity for a greater degree of public assistance to the family of the minority person with a disability and takes time away from the family that could normally be used for wage earning.

A minority person who becomes disabled frequently finds that his or her job is not accessible, especially if it is in an older establishment, where the barriers to access are the most numerous. If this individual is the head of the household, then the entire economic structure of the family is destroyed. A minority adult with a disability is frequently unable to become totally integrated into community life because his or her range of mobility in the community is restricted. Research conducted by Bobbie J. Atkins (1988), and Faye Z. Belgrave and Sylvia Walker (1991) reveals that minority persons frequently have more severe disabilities than European Americans, are more dependent on public transportation, and are less likely to be involved in the rehabilitation process.

Inadequate education, inaccessible health care, lack of employment opportunities, and poverty are among the factors contributing to the escalation of disability rates in minority populations compared to nonminority populations (Asbury et al., 1991; Walker, Orange, and Rackley, 1993). A disproportionate number of minority individuals with disabilities are unemployed or economically disadvantaged. An interpretation of 1990 census figures by Frank Bowe (1992) indicates that unemployment rates for Hispanics, African Americans, and other minority groups were consistently above the rate for the general population. Research by R. U. Burkhauser, R. H. Haveman, and B. L. Wolfe (1990) and a number of other investigators has revealed that the employment and income levels of minority people with disabilities are alarmingly low (Asbury et al., 1991; Morgan & O'Connell, 1987). Although the collective energy, time, and effort invested by disability advocates during the 1980s has brought about an awakening among the American public to the true needs of this at-risk population, the economic well-being of people with disabilities has worsened despite legislation and other efforts to prevent such circumstances. In addition, disability rates have escalated more rapidly among minority groups than within the general population. African Americans age sixteen to sixty-four constitute a larger segment of the disabled population than do any other ethnic group, and the number of Hispanics with disabilities is also increasing rapidly (Asbury et al., 1991). While the precise rate of disability among Asian Americans is unknown, there is a dire need to provide services for this unique population as well. The severity of disability among Native Americans is substantial. Since disability is perpetuated and aggravated by low socioeconomic status, a substantial number of individuals with disabilities tend to be poor and thus need a complex array of services. From the time of birth, the risk of acquiring a disability is greater for minority individuals than for the general population, and the multiple effects of minority group membership, poverty, and disability result in an increased likelihood of congenital disability (Walker, Orange, and Rackley, 1993).

Minority individuals with disabilities tend to be concentrated in specific geographic locations. A number of important findings have been made relative to the geographic distribution of disability among ethnic minority groups in the United States (Asbury et al., 1991; Walker et al., 1986). The midwestern region had the highest proportion of people with mental disorders (32.4%). The South and the Midwest were tied for first place with regard to the percentage of people with nervous disorders (23.6%). At least 50 percent of African-American subjects with disabilities resided in the southern region of the United States. Many Pacific Islanders and Asian Americans with disabilities are clustered in various geographic locations, including a number of cities in the northeastern, mid-Atlantic, and western regions of the United States. This distribution of disability suggests a greater need for rehabilitation and independent living services to specific minority populations in those areas.

Income is a major yardstick of the economic independence and potential for social mobility of any group. Historically, the family income levels of African Americans and other non-European-American persons have been influenced by the work experience patterns and education levels of family members (U.S. Department of Commerce, 1989) and by general discriminatory practices in the workplace. Income trends have shown that the poverty rate for minority families has consistently been higher than that of their European-American counterparts. A

1989 population survey revealed the vast contrasts in the income levels of European Americans, African Americans, Native Americans, and Americans of Hispanic descent (Asbury et al., 1991). While Asian Americans are perceived as having higher income levels than other minority groups, there is considerable variability in income based on country of origin within Asia. For example, the income levels of Vietnamese, Filipinos, and Cambodians are considerably lower than those of persons of Japanese or Chinese descent.

A number of studies have examined the status of minority persons with disabilities in the rehabilitation system (Atkins, 1980, 1986; Lawrence Johnson and Associates, 1984; Walker et al., 1986). Research conducted by Bobbie J. Atkins (1980) compared African Americans to European Americans using data from all of the states and territories participating in the public rehabilitation program. Findings revealed unequal treatment of African Americans in all major dimensions of the public vocational rehabilitation process. For example, a larger percentage of African-American applicants were not accepted for services. Of the applicants accepted for services, the African Americans whose cases were closed with the designation "successfully rehabilitated" were more likely than those of European Americans to be in the lower income levels. African-American rehabilitants were provided less training and education even though their needs were greater because of lower preservice educational levels. These findings were consistent with research conducted by Faye Z. Belgrave and Sylvia Walker (1991).

Similar trends were noted regarding the rehabilitation services available to other minority groups. M. H. Cooney (1988) found that the counseling needs of Hispanic clients were not being sufficiently met. The importance of developing culturally relevant delivery systems for Hispanics has not been adequately recognized by rehabilitation policymakers (Leal, 1990; Leal-Idrogo, 1993). Specific problems facing Hispanics in the rehabilitation system include the following:

1. They tend to be identified as ineligible for services more frequently than non-Hispanic clients.

2. They remain in the referral and application status and/or in the guidance and counseling status longer than non-Hispanics.

3. Their time in training is substantially less than that of non-Hispanics (Leal, 1990).

Given the increase in the Hispanic population anticipated in the 1990s, the gap between services provided and need is likely to grow even wider.

There is a scarcity of published literature relative to the utilization of vocational rehabilitation services by Hispanics. Mitchell P. LaPlante (1988) estimated that more than 2 million Hispanics had work-related disabilities in the late 1980s. Preliminary findings suggest that this targeted group has limited acceptance into and success in vocational rehabilitation (VR) systems. A. Leal-Idrogo (1993) explored this issue and found that 49,630 Hispanics applied for vocational rehabilitation services in 1989. Of those 49,630 applicants, 22,927 (46%) were not accepted for services, while 26,703 (54%) were accepted into the VR system. Despite the fact that 54 percent were accepted for services, only 17,543 were successfully rehabilitated. The remaining Hispanic applicants accepted for services (9,250) were not rehabilitated or their cases were cited as closed.

Similar problems have been identified relative to Native Americans with disabilities. Clayton O. Morgan and others (1986) reported that vocational rehabilitation programs are largely unsuccessful with Native Americans, particularly those with severe disabilities on rural reservations. Although Native Americans are eligible for services, vocational rehabilitation programs tend not to meet their needs. Unemployment among Native Americans with disabilities may be as high as 80 percent in communities where they must compete with able-bodied persons for jobs (Joe, 1991; Morgan et al., 1986).

Vocational rehabilitation systems have traditionally been unresponsive to the needs of Native Americans regardless of geographical location (Marshall, Johnson, & Lonetree, 1993). For example, J. M. Fischer (1991) discovered that at one northwestern state agency the total expenditure for Native Americans was $1,858 per person as compared to $3,938 per person for non–Native Americans. Although the sample size was small (n = 137), this study did provide critical information relative to the inequities between non–Native Americans and Native Americans in the VR service delivery system. At the University of Northern Arizona and the University of Arizona, important efforts have been made to identify the unique and diverse needs of persons with disabilities from the more than 300 sovereign nations of Native Americans located in various parts of the country.

Fong Chan and others (1988) estimated that as many as 73,834 Chinese Americans have disabilities and could potentially benefit from rehabilitation services; however, services are underutilized. Asian Americans often encounter difficulty communicating with rehabilitation counselors. Cultural differences and lack of acceptance of Western counseling techniques also reduce the participation of Asian Americans in the rehabilitation process (Woo, 1991). Research indicates that as many as 50 percent of the rehabilitation cases involving Asian Americans are terminated prematurely (Chan et al., 1988; Leung & Sakata, 1988; Marshall, Wilson, and Leung, 1983). The cases of Asians, like those of Hispanics and African Americans, are often closed with the status "failure to cooperate," "unable to locate," or "disability too severe" (Leung & Sakata, 1988; Marshall, Wilson, and Leung, 1983).

Minority persons with disabilities (including African Americans, Hispanic Americans, Native Americans, and Asian Americans) represent a substantial proportion of the disabled population. The 1992 amendments to the Rehabilitation Act contain a number of mandates that are relevant to the needs of persons with disabilities in multicultural communities, including a mandate for increased service to multicultural, ethnic, and racial populations with disabilities. Specifically, the 1992 amendments require rehabilitation agencies to reduce the discrepancies in service delivery to ethnic groups, respond to the changing demographic composition of the United States, and increase the number of rehabilitation personnel from multicultural communities. The independent living movement has also resulted in increased access to services for persons from minority communities.

The Role of Minority Persons in the Independent Living Movement and the Rehabilitation System

As professionals in the National Rehabilitation Association (NRA) and other professional associations, as advocates and service providers, and as educators and researchers, minority persons have made considerable contributions in the disability and rehabilitation field. The role of minority persons in professional organizations such as the National Rehabilitation Association may be traced to 1969, when a number of activists organized the Council of Non-White Rehabilitation Workers. These individuals were among those who placed pressure on the National Rehabilitation Association to recognize the fact that the needs of non-European-American individuals with disabilities are multidimensional and complex. During the 1969 NRA annual conference in New York City, this group submitted a list of demands to the NRA that included the following:

1. That its members be involved in the decision-making process within the NRA at the legislative, administrative, and consultative levels.
2. That its members be given a 50 percent voting membership in the NRA board of directors and subdivisions.
3. That federal/state rehabilitation funds be allocated to non-European-American communities and other rehabilitation agencies for the purpose of meeting the rehabilitation needs of minority communities.
4. That a major effort be made to recruit and train numerous rehabilitation personnel from minority groups.

The National Rehabilitation Association responded to these demands by implementing several resolutions, and a division dedicated to the consideration of minority issues was ultimately established within the association (the National Council of Multicultural Disability Concerns).

Within the rehabilitation and independent living movements, a number of advocates and service providers have made major contributions to holding these systems more accountable in responding to the needs of minority consumers with disabilities. Some such efforts have been made in connection with the Center for Independent Living in Berkeley, California, the first independent living center established in the United States. Others have been made through the Center for Disability and Socioeconomic Policy Studies (CDSPS) at Howard University, whose activities focus on issues relating to minority persons with disabilities, including African Americans, Hispanic Americans, Asian Americans, and Native Americans. A component of the CDSPS, the Howard University Research and Training Center for Access to Rehabilitation and Economic Opportunity, implements research and training activities that facilitate the attainment of maximum potential by economically disadvantaged and minority persons with disabilities. The program of the center is founded on the premise that, given the compounding effects of minority group status, economic hardship, and disability, an interdisciplinary collaborative approach is the best vehicle to respond effectively to the needs of the targeted population. The program encompasses three focal areas: (1) assessing (through research) the specific needs of minority persons with disabilities and the economically disadvantaged; (2) reducing barriers through the provision of supportive services; and (3) facilitating greater client independence and employment through training and self-advocacy. Research and training activities are conceived as a coordinated, interrelated, interdisciplinary set of projects.

Minority Persons with Disabilities in the Future

Paul Leung (1993) addressed the changing demography of the United States and how it will affect state and federal vocational rehabilitation. The ethnic, racial, and cultural composition of the United States has changed significantly since the 1970s. Vocational rehabilitation as well as other service delivery programs must respond to these demographic changes to be effective.

Given the rapid increases in the minority populations of the United States, it is projected that by the year 2000 approximately one-third (86 million) of the total population will be members of ethnic minority groups (U.S. Congress, 1990). Of this pop-

ulation, a disproportionate number of individuals will have disabilities (Walker, Orange, and Rackley, 1993).

Research conducted by the Hudson Institute (1987) revealed several startling trends about the American work force as the year 2000 approaches. In addition to technological developments and shifts in international competition and demography, a number of other factors will change the nation's economic and social landscape. The following trends were cited in the Hudson Institute report (1987):

1. The population and the work force will grow more slowly.
2. The average age of the work force and the population will rise, and the pool of young workers entering the labor market will shrink.
3. More women will enter the work force.
4. Immigrants will represent the largest share of the increase in the population and the work force since World War I (a projected 600,000 documented and undocumented immigrants).
5. By the year 2000, the number of new entrants into the work force who are members of minority groups will double.

In spite of the potential for increased employment, Hispanics and many other recently arrived immigrants are disproportionately represented at the lower end of the economic spectrum and among unemployed individuals with disabilities. The jobs of the future will demand much higher skill levels than the jobs of today; few will be available for those who cannot read, follow instructions, and use mathematics. These trends will lead to more joblessness among the least skilled and less joblessness among those with educational and economic advantages, challenging policymakers in a number of ways. They will need to find ways to stimulate growth and balance the world economy, increase productivity in the service industries, maintain the dynamism of an aging workforce, and reconcile the conflicting needs of women, work, and families.

The educational preparation of all present and future workers must be improved. Furthermore, given the pressing societal and economic demands—including the shrinking number of young people, the rapid pace of industrial change, and the ever-

466

increasing skill requirements of the emerging economy—economically disadvantaged and ethnic minority workers with disabilities must be fully integrated into the economy and their potential fully utilized as soon as possible. One of the most amazing changes of the 1990s with respect to the possibility of gainful employment by persons with disabilities is the emergence of high-technology equipment and software that is able to do what some disabilities prevent. Access to technology by minority persons with disabilities will expand their capabilities and render them more likely to be employed successfully.

Scientific advances and medical research have resulted in many thousands of individuals surviving who would not have survived in the past. Similarly, organ transplants and expert surgery provide the potential to extend life to a degree unimaginable in the past. Now consideration must be given not only to the length of life, but to its quality as well.

(*See also.* ATTITUDES; CIVIL RIGHTS; CONSUMERS; ECONOMICS; FAMILY; STATE-FEDERAL REHABILITATION PROGRAM; WORK)

BIBLIOGRAPHY

ASBURY, C. A.; WALKER, S.; MAHOLMES, V.; RACKLEY, R.; and WHITE, S. *Disability, Prevalence, and Demographic Association Among Race/Ethnic Minority Populations in the United States: Implications for the 21st Century.* Washington, DC, 1991.

ATKINS, BOBBIE J. "The Participation of Blacks as Compared to Whites in the Rehabilitation Program." *Dissertation Abstracts International* 40 (1980):3854.

———. "Innovative Approaches and Research in Addressing the Needs of Non-White Disabled Persons." In *Equal to the Challenge*, eds. S. Walker, F. Z. Belgrave, A. M. Banner, and R. W. Nicholls. Washington, DC, 1986.

———. "Rehabilitating Black Americans Who Are Disabled." In *Building Bridges to Independence*, eds. S. Walker, J. W. Fowler, R. W. Nicholls, and K. A. Turner. Washington, DC, 1988.

BELGRAVE, FAYE Z., and WALKER, SYLVIA. "Predictors of Employment Outcomes of Black Persons with Disabilities." *Rehabilitation Psychology* 36 (1991):111–119.

BOWE, FRANK. *Black Adults with Disabilities: A Portrait.* Washington, DC, 1992.

BURNHAUSER, R. V.; HAVEMAN, R. H.; and WOLFE, B. L. "The Changing Economic Condition of the Disabled: A Two Decade Review of Economic Well Being." Paper presented at the National Council on Disability Symposium on Writing National Policy on Work Disabilities, Washington, DC, 1990.

CHAN, FONG; LAM, CHOW S.; WONG, DANIEL; LEUNG, PAUL; and FANG, X. S. "Counseling Chinese Americans with Disabilities." *Journal of Applied Rehabilitation Counseling* 9 (1988):21–24.

COONEY, M. H. "Training Students to Work with Hispanic Clients." *Rehabilitation Education* 2 (1988): 35–38.

FISCHER, J. M. "A Comparison Between American Indian and non-Indian Consumers of Vocational Rehabilitation Services." *Journal of Applied Rehabilitation Counseling* 22 (1991):43–45.

HUDSON INSTITUTE, THE. *Workforce 2000: Work and Workers for the Twenty-first Century.* Indianapolis, IN, 1987.

JOE, J. R. "Vocational Rehabilitation and the American Indian: Where Is the Innovation?" In *Future Frontiers in the Employment of Minority Persons with Disabilities*, eds. S. Walker, F. Z. Belgrave, R. W. Nicholls, and K. A. Turner. Washington, DC, 1991.

LAPLANTE, MITCHELL P. *Data on Disability from the National Health Interview Survey, 1983–1985.* Washington, DC, 1988.

LAWRENCE JOHNSON and ASSOCIATES. *Evaluation of the Delivery Services to Select Disabled People by the Vocational Rehabilitation Service System: RSA-300 Data Analysis.* Report submitted to the Department of Education, Office of Special Education and Rehabilitative Services, Rehabilitation Services Administration, Washington, DC, 1984.

LEAL, ANITA. "Hispanics and Substance Abuse: Implications for Rehabilitation Counselors." *Journal of Applied Rehabilitation Counseling* 9 (1990):52–54.

———. "Vocational Rehabilitation of People of Hispanic Origin." *Journal of Vocational Rehabilitation* 3 (1993):27–37.

LEUNG, PAUL. "A Changing Demography and Its Challenge." *Journal of Vocational Rehabilitation* 3 (1993):3–11.

LEUNG, PAUL, and SAKATA, ROBERT. "Asian Americans and Rehabilitation: Some Important Variables." *Journal of Applied Rehabilitation Counseling* 14 (1988):74–78.

MARSHALL, C. A.; JOHNSON, S. R.; and LONETREE, G. L. "Acknowledging our Diversity: Vocational Rehabilitation and American Indians." *Journal of Vocational Rehabilitation* 3 (1993):12–19.

MARSHALL, C. A.; WILSON, J. C.; and LEUNG, P. "Value Conflict: A Cross-Cultural Assessment Paradigm." *Journal of Applied Rehabilitation Counseling* 14 (1983):74–78.

MORGAN, C. O.; GUY, E.; LEE, B.; and CELLINI, H. R. "Rehabilitation Services for American Indians: The Navajo Experience." *Journal of Rehabilitation* 52 (1986):25–31.

MORGAN, J., and O'CONNELL, J. C. "The Rehabilitation of Native Americans." *International Journal of Rehabilitation Research* 10 (1987):139–149.

THAYER, J. D. *Annual Report*. Prepared for Rehabilitation Services Administration. Washington, DC, 1989.

U.S. CONGRESS. *Public Law 101-476: Individuals with Disabilities Education Act*. Washington, DC, 1990.

U.S. DEPARTMENT OF COMMERCE. *Labor Force Status and Other Characteristics of Persons with a Work Disability: 1981–1988*. Washington, DC, 1989.

WALKER, MARTHA L. "Effective Approaches to the Education of Black Americans with Disabilities." In *Building Bridges to Independence: Employment Successes, Problems, and Needs of African Americans with Disabilities*, eds. S. Walker, J. W. Fowler, R. W. Nicholls, and K. A. Turner. Washington, DC, 1988.

WALKER, S.; AKPATI, E.; ROBERTS, V.; PALMER, R.; and NEWSOME, M. "Frequency and Distribution of Disabilities Among Blacks: Preliminary Findings." In *Equal to the Challenge*, eds. S. Walker, F. Z. Belgrave, A. M. Banner, and R. W. Nicholls. Washington, DC, 1986.

WALKER, S.; ORANGE, C.; and RACKLEY, R. "A Formidable Challenge: The Preparation of Minority Personnel." *Journal of Vocational Rehabilitation* 3 (1993):46–53.

WOO, A. H. "The Employment of Asian/Pacific Minority Persons with Disabilities." In *Future Frontiers in the Employment of Minority Persons with Disabilities*, eds. S. Walker, F. Z. Belgrave, R. W. Nicholls, and K. A. Turner. Washington, DC, 1991.

SYLVIA WALKER
REGINALD RACKLEY

MOBILITY IMPAIRMENTS

See MUSCULOSKELETAL DISORDERS; PROSTHETICS AND ORTHOTICS; SPINAL CORD INJURY; TRANSPORTATION ACCESSIBILITY; WHEELCHAIRS

MOOD DISORDERS

Mood (affective) disorders (depression or mania) include some of the most common and serious of psychiatric conditions and are grouped together because of a similar constellation of signs and symptoms, such as a sad affect, disrupted sleep and appetite, and suicidal thoughts.

What possible biological malfunction of the body might result in a mood disorder? Several hypotheses of biological mechanisms underlie such disorders and are not mutually exclusive. Thus a genetically determined nerve cell (neuron) membrane defect could produce a dysregulation in various neurotransmitter-receptor interactions. This in turn may affect the second messenger systems of neurons within their specific brain circuits, resulting in a disturbance of biological rhythms, such as neuroendocrine function (e.g., cortisol secretion; thyroid status). In addition, an individual's life experiences (stresses) can affect some or all of these systems. The signs and symptoms may be subtle at first, so the person may not be aware of them, but they may eventually develop into a major mood disruption with such serious consequences as suicide if left untreated.

While the focus of this entry will be on biological therapies, no illness occurs in a vacuum, and medication should never be the sole treatment. This is especially important in psychiatric disorders because of the difficulty patients have in separating themselves from the illness and its associated social stigma. Mood disorders often involve feelings of guilt, worthlessness, low self-esteem, helplessness, and hopelessness. These symptoms, coupled with the delayed onset of currently available drug treatment, make patient education, supportive counseling, and psychotherapy imperative.

A series of outpatient studies using control groups has compared treatment results of psychotherapy alone and antidepressants with psychotherapy (Klerman et al., 1974; Klerman et al., 1984; Weissman et al., 1974; Weissman, Jarrett, and Rush, 1987). The combined therapies were more efficacious in certain respects than either treatment by itself, appearing to augment each other, although other studies found a clear therapeutic effect from antidepressants but failed to find group therapy very helpful (Coui et al., 1974). Advocates have argued that some psychotherapies are also effective when used alone for treatment of major depression. The best-supported psychotherapeutic techniques are cognitive therapy and interpersonal therapy (Beck et al., 1979; Klerman et al., 1984).

Diagnosis of Mood Disorders

Depressive Disorders. Approximately one of ten Americans will suffer a major depressive episode in his or her lifetime, and one of twenty will have recurrences, with females twice as likely as males to experience an episode. The impact on patients and their families is profound, with suicide the most severe complication. Thus untreated recurrent major episodes have a 15 percent mortality risk due to suicide. In this respect, depressive disorders are a major health care problem, contributing to 70 percent of suicide-related deaths.

A major depressive episode consists of affective changes accompanied by physical symptoms on a daily basis for at least two weeks (see Table 1). Episodes may result from a diverse group of psychiatric or nonpsychiatric conditions and differ in their natural course as well as response to treatment. For example, depression can occur secondarily to a wide variety of prescription and nonprescription drugs. Alcohol abuse is the most common cause of drug-induced depressive syndromes. After chronic, sustained exposure to alcohol, symptoms generally occur upon withdrawal and may be temporarily reversed by its reinstitution.

Dysthymia represents a chronic but less severe form of depression, consisting of mood changes and other symptoms that may persist for many years. Patients who meet criteria for both a major depressive disorder and dysthymia are diagnosed as having a "double" or "dual" depression. Distinguishing between depressive and anxiety disorders is often difficult because patients present with a mixture of these symptoms. This issue has gained considerable attention given the large proportion of patients who present with a combination of anxiety and depressive symptoms. There are, however, many unanswered questions about the validity of a separate diagnostic category—that is, mixed anxiety and depression (Preskorn & Fast, 1993).

Bipolar Disorder. Bipolar disorder (manic-depressive illness) represents one of the most dramatic presentations in all of medicine and is characterized by mania (and/or hypomania, which is a milder form of mania) alternating irregularly with episodes of depression. A much smaller group—about 1 percent—experience only recurrent manic episodes. The estimated risk of developing this disorder is 0.5 to 1 percent, and the incidence of new cases per year ranges from 0.01 percent for males to 0.01 to 0.03 percent for females (Weissman & Boyd, 1983). While onset usually occurs in the third decade, the disorder can develop later in life and may

Table 1. Signs and symptoms of a major depressive episode

A major depressive episode representing a change from previous functioning is indicated by at least five of the following symptoms during the same two-week period; at least one symptom indicates either depressed mood or loss of interest or pleasure (anhedonia).

- Depressed mood (irritable mood in children and adolescents)
- Markedly diminished interest or pleasure in almost all activities
- Significant weight loss or gain (failure to attain expected weight gain in children)
- Insomnia or hypersomnia
- Observable psychomotor agitation or retardation
- Fatigue or loss of energy
- Feelings of worthlessness or excessive or inappropriate guilt (which may be delusional)
- Diminished ability to think or concentrate, or indecisiveness
- Recurrent thoughts of death; recurrent suicidal ideation, plans, or attempts

---

be more prevalent than previously believed in children and adolescents (Joyce, 1984). It is estimated that 80 percent of bipolar patients who have a manic episode will have one or more recurrences. These episodes are disruptive, life-threatening, and often have a progressive deteriorating effect on one's capacity to function.

The essential feature of mania is a distinct period of elevated, expansive, or irritable mood accompanied by several other symptoms, including:

- hyperactivity;
- pressure of speech;
- flight of ideas;
- inflated self-esteem;
- decreased need for sleep;
- distractibility;
- excessive involvement in activities that have a high potential for painful consequences (Altman, Janicak, and Davis, 1989; Tyrer & Shopsin, 1982).

Psychotic symptoms, such as delusions or hallucinations, may be present in more severe episodes and usually are consistent with one's mood (i.e., mood-congruent). The delusions seen in mania often have a religious, sexual, or persecutory theme.

Coexistent substance and alcohol abuse is much higher in bipolar patients than in the general population (Regier et al., 1990). Thus it is often necessary to clarify whether:

- an episode of mania/depression is drug- or alcohol-induced;
- concurrent drug or alcohol use is an attempt to self-medicate;
- such activity is unrelated to the present exacerbation.

Further, as with depressive disorders, concurrent substance abuse may complicate interpretation of the presenting symptoms, adversely affect the long-term course, and undermine the beneficial effects of treatment.

Treatment of Depressive Disorders

Acute Therapy. Since the early 1950s, certain drugs have been known to possess antidepressant properties and to alleviate severe depressions. Newer medications that are effective but with fewer adverse effects have been developed recently.

1. Heterocyclic Antidepressants (HCAs): HCAs adjusted by clinically determined dose titration will produce a partial response in 60 to 70 percent of depressed patients and a full remission in 30 to 40 percent. When the dose is adjusted using therapeutic drug monitoring (i.e., the measurement of drug blood concentrations), particularly with the antidepressant nortriptyline (Pamelor and others), the full remission rate may be as high as 70 percent (Perry, Pfohl, and Holstad, 1987).

The elderly, the medically compromised, those hypersensitive to side effects, or those with associated anxiety disorders may require lower doses and more gradual increases. The dose of most HCAs may be increased until there is adequate response, usually to a maximum of 300 mg per day. The ultimate total daily dose can vary dramatically, however, with some patients requiring as little as 50 mg per day.

2. Serotonin Reuptake Inhibitors (SRIs): These medications are relatively new but widely used due to their efficacy and better tolerated side effects. Fluoxetine (Prozac) is the most commonly prescribed SRI, but sertraline (Zoloft) and paroxetine (Paxil) have also been recently approved by the FDA. Controlled studies have found these agents to be superior to placebos and comparable to earlier antidepressants.

3. Monoamine Oxidase Inhibitors (MAOIs): MAOIs may be the treatment of choice for atypical (or nonclassic) depressive disorders. Features of this subgroup usually include:

- mood worse in the afternoon or evening;
- variability in the same depressive episode, from irritability to mild unhappiness to severe depression;
- sleeping or eating more than usual;
- physical complaints or prominent anxiety; "leaden paralysis" (i.e., anergic immobility);
- increased sensitivity to real or perceived rejection.

4. Other Agents: Although used less often, trazodone (Desyrel), bupropion (Wellbutrin), and buspirone (Buspar) have demonstrated antidepressant properties and may occasionally benefit those unable to achieve relief from the standard HCAs, SRIs, or MAOIs.

5. Electroconvulsive Therapy (ECT): This therapeutic modality is typically utilized in patients who present with acute, life-threatening symptoms; are truly refractory to drug therapies or intolerant to their side effects; or have a past history of good response to this approach (Janicak, Comatry, and Dowd, 1993). It is especially beneficial for psychotic depressions. Ignorance of its appropriate uses and benefits may cause needless suffering due to reluctance by patients, their families, and even clinicians to employ this therapy (Janicak et al., 1985).

Issues Complicating Treatment. Two major problems complicating the question of treatment-resistant depression are inaccurate diagnosis and inadequate therapy. In a recent study, only 3.5 percent of more than 6,000 depressed patients had received appropriate antidepressant treatment—that is, adequate dose and duration (McCombs et al., 1990). There are several options available with true treatment nonresponse (Nemeroff, 1991):

- When there has been no benefit, stop the current antidepressant and try an unrelated agent (e.g., switch from an HCA to an SRI or an MAOI).
- When there has been partial response:
  1. potentiate the effects of the current agent with lithium, thyroid hormone (e.g., T_3), or an anticonvulsant mood stabilizer (e.g., carbamazepine or valproic acid);

     or
  2. augment with the concurrent use of two different classes of antidepressants (e.g., HCA plus MAOI).

If a patient is to be switched from an MAOI to an HCA, the former drug should be discontinued for at least two weeks before beginning the HCA. At least five weeks should elapse after discontinuing fluoxetine before initiating an MAOI (Feighner et al., 1990). Some also recommend checking for measurable blood levels of fluoxetine (Prozac) or norfluoxetine (its metabolite) before initiating an MAOI. When severe anxiety and/or associated panic at-

tacks accompany a depressed episode, patients may benefit from the combination of an HCA plus an antianxiety agent or the use of an SRI, which may also have antipanic properties separate from its antidepressant effects.

Persons suffering from a psychotic depression do not benefit from an antidepressant alone and often require the combination of an antidepressant and antipsychotic or electroconvulsive therapy (ECT).

Maintenance/Prophylactic Therapy. Preventing early relapse is of critical importance in the life course of a major depressive disorder, and every effort should be made to ensure the patient's compliance. Maintenance therapy should be continued for at least six to twelve months after an acute episode, and indefinitely in those with a history of severe episodes or multiple recurrences (Frank et al., 1990; Kupfer et al., 1992).

The decision to employ ongoing prophylactic therapy should be based on the:

- severity of the depressive episode;
- frequency of past depressions;
- risk of suicide;
- risk of potential adverse drug effects.

Treatment of Bipolar Disorder

It has been estimated that one of every four or five untreated or inadequately treated patients commits suicide during the course of this illness. Further, an increase in deaths secondary to accidents or intercurrent illnesses contributes to the greater mortality rate seen in this disorder. Unfortunately, recent studies have indicated that only one-third of bipolar patients are in active treatment despite the availability of effective therapies.

Acute Therapy

A. Approximately 60 percent of all acutely ill bipolar manic patients benefit from lithium, whose efficacy has been established within a well-defined therapeutic blood level range (0.5 to 1.5 mEq/liter) for optimal benefit and minimal adverse or toxic reactions.

In a highly disturbed hospitalized patient, lithium may be supplemented with an adjunctive sedative. An antipsychotic is added only if necessary, and at the lowest dose possible for the shortest time (Janicak et al., 1988). After a stabilization period, the adjunctive medication or medications may then be gradually withdrawn and the patient often manages successfully with lithium alone. For persons who fail to respond, assuring an adequate lithium blood level and duration; discontinuing concurrent antidepressants; and use of supplemental thyroid medication may all improve outcome.

B. While use of lithium has been a major advance in the pharmacotherapy of severe mood disorders, a number of problems (e.g., slow onset; adverse effects) limit its usefulness. Further, some bipolar patients may be less likely to benefit from lithium (e.g., those who cycle rapidly between mania and depression; those with a mixture of both manic and depressive symptoms during the same episode). As a result, alternate strategies are needed (Janicak, Newman, and Davis, 1992):

- Electroconvulsive therapy (ECT) is the only truly bimodal therapy, being equally effective for both the acute depressed and manic phases of the disorder. While the primary indication for ECT is a severe, unremitting, or drug-nonresponsive depressive episode, data support its use for the treatment of acute mania, particularly manic delirium (Thorpe, 1947).
- Divalproex sodium (Depakote) is at present the best-studied of the anticonvulsant mood stabilizers and appears to be a highly effective alternative to lithium for acute mania (Janicak et al., 1993). It has a favorable and relatively safe side-effect profile compared to other agents and can be combined with commonly employed psychotropics without significantly altering their metabolism or compromising adequacy of blood levels.
- The spectrum of efficacy of carbamazepine (Tegretol and others) appears similar to that of lithium. It may be superior to lithium in mixed or dysphoric mania, rapid cyclers, and more severe episodes (Post, 1990). Its multiple and potentially deleterious drug-drug interactions make management more difficult, however, when other medications are used concurrently.
- Other agents such as calcium antagonists—for example, verapamil (Calan); noradrenergic agents—for example, clonidine (Catapres); and cholinomimetics—for example, lecithin—are

among several other classes of drugs that have been proposed as alternatives but await confirmation with definitive studies.

Maintenance/Prophylactic Therapy

It is becoming increasingly evident that prevention of relapse and adequate prophylactic strategies are much more complicated than were originally assumed.

The maintenance properties of lithium have been verified in a large number of random-assignment, double-blind studies comparing this agent to a placebo. There are little data on the maintenance/prophylactic properties of divalproex sodium or carbamazepine, but these are important issues to confirm, given the evidence supporting their acute antimanic effects (Prien & Galenberg, 1989).

Antidepressants do not prevent relapses into mania, perhaps even precipitating a manic phase. Thus lithium (with or without concomitant antidepressants) is the prophylaxis of choice for bipolar-related depressions. Carbamazepine and divalproex sodium may also be useful in the prevention of recurrent depressive episodes.

In summary, there is evidence for a higher relapse rate in patients not maintained on adequate levels of lithium, the potential for concurrent drugs to exacerbate the disorder, a more rapid recurrence with abrupt discontinuation, and possible compromised future lithium responsiveness after it is stopped (Post & Weiss, 1989). Unfortunately, patient noncompliance may be as high as 50 percent within the first year of treatment, posing a serious public health issue (Shaw, 1986). Strategies to improve compliance include:

- intensive educational efforts at the start of therapy;
- dose reduction when feasible to minimize drug adverse effects;
- supportive, individual, family, and, when indicated, drug/alcohol abuse counseling;
- aggressive treatment interventions with early signs of relapse.

Since lithium and perhaps other mood stabilizers favorably alter the longitudinal course of a bipolar disorder, which may otherwise follow a steadily progressive course, efforts to enhance long-term compliance are a necessary part of any therapeutic strategy.

Rehabilitation in Patients with Mood Disorders

Affective disorders have traditionally been viewed as episodic in course, with return to premorbid functioning following resolution of an acute exacerbation. Longitudinal studies have challenged this view, since many people with pure depression, and an even higher percentage of patients with bipolar disorder, have a poor outcome. In terms of rehabilitation, this means that while some patients are able to return to baseline functioning with minimal outside intervention, others require long-term assistance with housing, socialization, vocational training, recreation, education, crisis intervention, family counseling, and advocacy to maintain their maximal level of functioning.

Definition of Rehabilitation. Ideas about psychosocial rehabilitation are often vague and inaccurate. Leona Bachrach defines it as "a therapeutic approach to the care of mentally ill individuals that encourages each patient to develop his or her fullest capacities through learning procedures and environmental supports" and details eight fundamentals of psychosocial rehabilitation (Bachrach, 1992). The central tenet is to enable individuals to develop to the fullest extent possible. Psychosocial rehabilitation stresses the importance of environmental factors in the care of individuals with mental disabilities; it is oriented toward the development of strengths, and aims to restore hope to those suffering setbacks in functional capacity and self-esteem. It seeks to maximize vocational potential while also attending to social and recreational needs. It is essential that the individual be actively involved in all aspects of his or her care and that rehabilitation be an ongoing process rather than a single-effort intervention.

The general framework of psychiatric rehabilitation includes three steps. It begins with a comprehensive assessment of assets, impairments, and psychosocial context, involving diagnostic and functional evaluation. Careful diagnostic assessment and ongoing monitoring of symptoms are necessary initial steps, contributing significantly to the quality and effectiveness of care received. Functional assessment identifies behavioral strengths and deficits influencing role performance and is key to the appropriate provision of psychosocial services. The focus should be on activities of daily living, social skills, psychological profile, occupational functioning, behavioral impairments, and environmental factors. Particular attention must be paid to impairments most often associated with affective syndromes: alterations in mood, social withdrawal, anhedonia (the inability to experience pleasure), sleep disturbances, motor agitation or retardation, loss of energy, impaired reality testing, altered self-esteem, diminished concentration, suicidal ideation, thought disorder, distractibility, impulsivity, and decreased self-care.

Accurate assessment is the basis for the second step of rehabilitation, which is planning. Identification of areas of vulnerability permits formulation of specific goals, prioritization, and organization of treatment and rehabilitation plans. Objectives must reflect assets, impairments, and the environment. Mentally ill individuals often have many different types of difficulties (interpersonal, economic, etc.) necessitating prioritization based on urgency, motivation, and potential for success. Once realistic and limited goals are delineated, a detailed treatment plan can be designed specifying how each goal is to be met.

The final step of rehabilitation utilizes a biopsychosocial approach to put the treatment plan into action. Effective pharmacologic and nonpharmacologic therapies, as described above, are essential to maximizing functioning by diminishing primary symptoms and allowing interventions at other levels. These other strategies enable development of the patient's skills and environment. Such techniques are based on the complementary findings that training with specific objectives and techniques improves skill levels independent of symptomatology, and that rehabilitation outcomes are more strongly related to these skills than to symptoms (Anthony, Cohen, and Cohen, 1978).

It is important to distinguish between nonspecific group socialization and methods that deliberately and systematically use behavioral learning techniques in a structured approach to skills building.

Training techniques are active and directive and include:

- didactics;
- feedback;
- modeling;
- practice;
- role play;
- reinforcement;
- coaching.

Skills to be developed include social, vocational, attention-focusing, and problem-solving. Development not only improves mastery over stress and enhances social adjustment but also is associated with a lower rate of treatment noncompliance (Bellack, Hersen, and Himmelhoch, 1983).

Resource development interventions engineer environmental change. They alter people, places, and objects to assist the patient in attaining goals and support the current level of functioning. The basic intent is to aid the patient in using, modifying, and creating supportive environments, since studies show a consistently positive correlation between level of support and long-term improvements in functioning (Anthony, Cohen, and Cohen, 1978). Among the possible interventions are teaching significant others to encourage desired behavior; matching activities to the person's skill level; and finding appropriate residential facilities.

The Role of Various Professionals in the Rehabilitation Process. It must be stressed that rehabilitation is not a static process but involves regular assessment and monitoring of progress and modification of the treatment plan, with interventions as necessary. This long-term intervention requires the participation of a variety of professionals in an integrated, multidisciplinary team approach. Contributors include educators, nurses, occupational therapists, psychiatrists, psychologists, recreational therapists, rehabilitation counselors, social workers, vocational counselors, and mental health paraprofessionals. Natural caregivers, such as relatives and friends, should not be overlooked in the rehabilitation plan, nor should affiliations with residential facilities, welfare agencies, clergy, schools, family agencies, and human services groups.

The Role of Research. The psychiatric rehabilitation movement has been hindered historically in that researchers and clinicians have focused on the diagnosis and treatment of acute episodes of major mental disorders. Effective treatment of acute relapses and exacerbations is crucial but ignores the reality that many of these conditions, including mood disorders, are chronic in course, with cyclical episodes and prolonged periods of impairment. Comprehensive treatment and rehabilitation strategies are essential in meeting long-term needs for adaptation, restoration of function, and maintenance of well-being in the population.

A major obstacle in furthering the cause of psychiatric rehabilitation is the paucity of empirical research documenting effective strategies, models, and techniques. Unfortunately, much of what now passes for rehabilitation is misdirected and inadequate. The British psychiatrist Sir Aubry Lewis noted, "A great deal of rehabilitation is built upon faith, hope, and rule of thumb. We could do better than that. We could plan our programs so that they may disclose principles governing successful rehabilitation and the factors that restrict it" (Lewis, 1995). The lack of scientifically grounded research on effective psychosocial programs for people with chronic mental illness is highlighted by R. P. Liberman and C. C. Phipps's literature review on the subject (1987). They found only three pre-1970 programs with reliable and valid data supporting their efficacy, and from 1978 to 1984 only nine articles that documented effective psychosocial treatments for people with chronic mental illness.

Even with more relevant data, there remains the task of translating research findings into clinical practice. The practice of psychosocial rehabilitation requires learning concepts and skills not routinely taught in mental health professional training programs. It is up to practitioners to make themselves aware of the current state of the art and to integrate this knowledge into their repertoires of therapeutic techniques. Recent studies have noted that mood disorders are associated with global impairment and pose a significant burden on the community. This finding has led to the suggestion of broadening the scope of these disorders to include psychosocial disabilities in addition to mood symptoms (Klerman &

Weissman, 1992). Failure to utilize rehabilitation interventions amounts to treating only part of the illness.

Conclusion

There are currently effective drug treatments for both the acute and maintenance stages of mood disorders (see preceding paragraphs). The future of rehabilitation efforts for these disorders, however, will require further research on productive techniques and a plan to institute those programs shown to be useful. Less clear is how these changes will be effected, for they require a significant investment of resources; however, patients and their families can realize significant benefits from such programs. Thus practitioners and researchers must demonstrate to both public and private providers of mental health services that funding only treatment limited to acute episodes is, in the long run, more costly than underwriting comprehensive treatment and rehabilitation.

(See also: ANXIETY DISORDERS; BEHAVIOR THERAPY; PHARMACOLOGY; PSYCHIATRIC REHABILITATION; PSYCHIATRY; PSYCHOLOGY)

BIBLIOGRAPHY

ALTMAN, E.; JANICAK, P. G.; and DAVIS, J. M. "Mania: Clinical Manifestations and Assessment." In Modern Perspectives in the Psychiatry of Mood Disorders, ed. J. G. Howells. New York, 1989.

ANTHONY, W. A.; COHEN, M. R.; and COHEN, B. F. "Psychiatric Rehabilitation." In The Chronic Mental Patient, ed. J. A. Talbott. New York, 1978.

BACHRACH, L. L. "Psychosocial Rehabilitation and Psychiatry in the Care of Long-Term Patients." American Journal of Psychiatry 149 (1992):1455–1463.

BECK, A. T.; RUSH, A. J.; SHAW, B. F., and EMERY, G. Cognitive Therapy for Depression: A Treatment Manual. New York, 1979.

BELLACK, A. S.; HERSEN, M.; and HIMMELHOCH, J. M. "A Comparison of Social Skills Training, Pharmacotherapy, and Psychotherapy for Depression." Behavior Research and Therapy 21 (1983):101–107.

COVI, L.; LIPMAN, R. S.; DEROGATIS, L. R.; SMITH, J. E. III; and PATTISON, J. H. "Drugs and Group Psychotherapy in Neurotic Depression." American Journal of Psychiatry 131 (1974):191–198.

FEIGHNER, J. P.; BOYER, W. F.; TYLER, D. L.; and

NEBROSKY, R. J. "Adverse Consequences of Fluoxetine-MAOI Combination Therapy." Journal of Clinical Psychiatry 51 (1990):222–225.

FRANK, E.; KUPFER, D. J.; PEREL, J. M. "Three-Year Outcomes for Maintenance Therapies in Recurrent Depression." Archives of General Psychiatry 47 (1990):1093–1099.

JANICAK, P. G.; BRESNAHAN, D. B.; SHARMA, R. P.; and DAVIS, J. M. "A Comparison of Thiothixene with Chlorpromazine in the Treatment of Mania." Journal of Clinical Psychopharmacology 8 (1988):33–37.

JANICAK, P. G.; COMATRY, J. E.; and DOWD, S. "Electroconvulsive Therapy for Depression." In Psychiatry: Diagnosis and Therapy, 2nd ed. Flaherty, Davis, and Janicak, eds. Norwalk, CT., 1993.

JANICAK, P. G.; DAVIS, J. M.; PRESKORN, S. H.; and AYD, F. J. Principles and Practice of Psychopharmacotherapy. Baltimore, 1993.

JANICAK, P. G.; MASK, J.; TRIMAKAS, K. A.; and GIBBONS, R. "ECT: An Assessment of Mental Health Professionals' Knowledge and Attitudes." Journal of Clinical Psychiatry 46 (1985):262–266.

JANICAK, P. G.; NEWMAN, R.; and DAVIS, J. M. "Advances in the Treatment of Mania and Related Disorders: A Reappraisal." Psychiatric Annals 22 (1992):92–103.

JOYCE, P. R. "Age of Onset in Bipolar Affective Disorder and Misdiagnosis as Schizophrenia." Psychological Medicine 14 (1984):145–149.

KLERMAN, G. L.; DIMASCIO, A.; WEISSMAN, M.; PRUSOFF, B.; and PAYKEL, E. S. "Treatment of Depression by Drugs and Psychotherapy." American Journal of Psychiatry 131 (1974):186–191.

KLERMAN, G. L., and WEISSMAN, M. M. "The Course, Morbidity, and Costs of Depression." Archives of General Psychiatry 49 (1992):831–834.

KLERMAN, G. L.; WEISSMAN, M. M.; ROUNSAVILLE, B. J.; and CHEVRON, E. S. Interpersonal Psychotherapy of Depression. New York, 1984.

KUPFER, D. J.; FRANK, E.; PEREL, J. M. "Five-year Outcomes for Maintenance Therapies in Recurrent Depression." Archives of General Psychiatry 49 (1992):769–773.

LEWIS, A. J. "Rehabilitation Programs in England." Proceedings of Millbank Memorial Fund Annual Conference (1995):196–206.

LIBERMAN, R. P., and PHIPPS, C. C. "Innovative Treatment and Rehabilitation Techniques." In The Chronic Mental Patient II, ed. W. W. Menninger and G. Hannah. Washington, DC, 1987.

McCombs, J. S.; Nichol, M. B.; Stimmel, G. L.; Sclar, D. A.; Beasley, C. M., Jr.; and Gross, L. S. "The Cost of Antidepressant Drug Therapy Failure: A Study of Antidepressant Use Patterns in a Medicaid Population." *Journal of Clinical Psychiatry* 51 (1990):60–69.

Nemeroff, C. B. "Augmentation Regimens for Depression." *Journal of Clinical Psychiatry* 52 (1991): 21–27.

Perry, P. J.; Pfohl, B. M.; and Holstad, S. G. "The Relationship Between Antidepressant Response and TCA Plasma Concentrations." *Clinical Pharmacokinetics* 13 (1987):381–392.

Post, R. M. "Nonlithium Treatment for Bipolar Disorder." *Journal of Clinical Psychiatry* 51 (1990): 9–16.

Post, R. M., and Weiss, S. R. B. "Sensitization, Kindling, and Anticonvulsants in Mania." *Journal of Clinical Psychiatry* 50 (1989):23–30.

Preskorn, S., and Fast, G. "Beyond Signs and Symptoms: The Case Against Mixed Anxiety and Depression Category." *Journal of Clinical Psychiatry* 54 (1993):23–32.

Prien, R. F., and Gelenberg, A. "Alternatives to Lithium for Preventive Treatment of Bipolar Disorder." *American Journal of Psychiatry* 146 (1989): 840–848.

Regier, D. A.; Farmer, M. E.; Rae, D. S.; Locke, B. Z.; Keith, S. J.; Judd, L. L.; and Goodwin, F. K. "Cormobidity of Mental Disorders with Alcohol and Other Drug Abuse: Results from the Epidemiologic Catchment Area (ECA) Study." *Journal of the American Medical Association* 264 (1990):2511–2518.

Shaw, E. "Lithium Noncompliance." *Psychiatric Annals* 16 (1986):583–587.

Thorpe, F. T. "Intensive Electrical Convulsive Therapy in Acute Mania." *Journal of Mental Science* 93 (1947):89–92.

Tyrer, S., and Shopsin, B. "Symptoms and Assessment of Mania." In *Handbook of Affective Disorders*, ed. E. S. Paykel. New York, 1982.

Weissman, M., and Boyd, J. "The Epidemiology of Affective Disorders: Rate and Risk Factor." *Psychiatric Update* 2 (1983):406–426.

Weissman, M. M.; Jarrett, R. B.; and Rush, J. A. "Psychotherapy and Its Relevance to the Pharmacotherapy of Major Depression: A Decade Later (1976–1985)." In *Psychopharmacology: The Third Generation of Progress*, ed. H. V. Meltzer. New York, 1987.

Weissman, M. M.; Klerman, G. L.; Paykel, E. S.; Prusoff, B.; and Hanson, B. "Treatment Effects on the Social Adjustment of Depressed Patients." *Archives of General Psychiatry* 30 (1974):771–778.

Philip G. Janicak
Anne M. Leach

MULTICULTURAL ISSUES

See minorities

MULTIPLE DISABILITIES

"Multiple disabilities" is an umbrella term under which various educational, rehabilitation, government, and advocacy groups include differing combinations of disabilities. While there is no unified definition of the term, typically it refers to an individual who has two or more disabilities that significantly affect the person's ability to function in educational, vocational, and community environments without use of supportive adaptations. The combination of disabilities usually creates an interactional, multiplicative effect rather than a simple, additive effect (Hart, 1988).

There are four categories of disorders in which multiple disabilities often occur. These include cognitive disabilities, physical disabilities, sensory disabilities, and behavioral/psychiatric disorders. An individual with multiple disabilities has two or more disabilities between or among categories or within the same category. The most frequently encountered combinations are those of cognitive and physical disabilities (e.g., mental retardation and cerebral palsy; learning disability and spina bifida), cognitive and sensory disabilities (e.g., mental retardation and deafness), cognitive disability and behavioral disorder (e.g., mental retardation and hyperactivity), physical and sensory disabilities (e.g., cerebral palsy and blindness), physical disability and behavioral disorder (e.g., spinal cord injury and emotional disturbance), and sensory disability and behavioral disorder (e.g., hearing impairment and autism). The most common multiple disabilities within the same category are those with dual sensory impairments (e.g., deaf-blind), dual physical impairments (e.g., paraplegia and arm amputation), or dual behavioral impairments (e.g., emotional disturbance and substance abuse).

Autism and traumatic brain injury have been recognized as separate disability categories as of 1991. Autism may have multiple disabilities, as in a person with autism and mental retardation. Traumatic brain injury may result in a combination of cognitive, physical, sensory, and behavioral impairments.

Etiology

Multiple disabilities can occur prenatally as developmental disorders or postnatally as acquired impairments. Prenatally, genetic or chromosomal abnormalities may result in syndromes (a group of symptoms that occur together and characterize a particular abnormality—e.g., Down syndrome) with multiple disabilities. Also, fetal exposure to drugs, chemicals, maternal infections, maternal disease, or environmental agents may cause multiple cognitive, physical, sensory, or behavioral abnormalities (Pueschel & Mulick, 1990). Postnatally, a child may have a serious infection (e.g., meningitis) or an accident (e.g., near drowning) that results in physical and cognitive impairments. Other postnatal causes include substance abuse, physical abuse, lead poisoning, and malnutrition.

Diagnosis

Multiple disabilities may be diagnosed through medical examinations and diagnostic testing. Some multiple disabilities, such as those resulting from syndromes, may be diagnosed before birth through such procedures as amniocentesis and ultrasound. Other types of disabilities, such as cerebral palsy, sensory impairment, and mental retardation, may not be diagnosed until infancy or childhood, using a variety of evaluations (e.g., neurologic exams, vision and hearing tests, blood tests, X rays, brain imaging scans, developmental exams, psychological testing, and psychiatric examination). Multiple disabilities occurring after birth are usually diagnosed shortly after the accident or infection.

Prevention

There are no standard measures that can assure the prevention of multiple disabilities. However, certain preventive measures can decrease the risk of occurrence. Before conception, genetic screening and counseling may decrease the risk of syndromes, and information on parenthood may eliminate unwanted pregnancies that may result in abuse. During pregnancy, multiple disabilities may be decreased by good obstetrical care, proper nutrition, and by not taking illegal drugs or alcohol. After the child is born, proper nutrition and proper care of the child (including no abusive behavior and prevention of accidents) will decrease the risk of multiple disabilities.

Functional Limitations

Depending on the types of multiple disabilities, several functional limitations may interfere with independent functioning in school, employment, and community living. Multiple disabilities with physical and sensory impairments may result in problems accessing materials, information, and environments. An individual who has cerebral palsy and blindness, for example, may encounter difficulty locating academic, work, or household materials; accessing printed material; or moving from one area of a building to another. Interpersonal skills may be affected by a lack of knowledge of social skills (and self-confidence) due to restricted experience resulting from the physical and sensory disabilities. Multiple disabilities with a cognitive impairment may result in impaired learning in educational, vocational, and community living tasks. An individual with severe mental retardation and cerebral palsy, for example, may need additional time, strategies, and support to learn a skill. Social skills may also be affected by an inability to make judgments about the behavior of others. Multiple disabilities with a behavioral/psychiatric impairment may result in difficulty learning a task due to interfering maladaptive behavior as well as poor social skills resulting from an inability to control one's own behavior.

Treatment and Rehabilitation

The degree of independent performance in school, employment, and community living is mitigated by medical, educational, and rehabilitative efforts. Medical interventions may include medications, surgery (for physical and sensory impairments), adaptive devices, and therapy (occupational, physical, or speech). Educational efforts may include use of special education in which systematic strategies, adaptations, and adaptive devices (e.g., Braille, mobility techniques, social skill training, functional curriculum, and modified instructional strategies) would be used to teach the student to function as independently as possible. Rehabilitative techniques may include supportive employment using job coaches and environmental adaptations in the work settings. In community living, rehabilitative techniques may include supportive living with use of house parents and adaptations in the living environment. Psychological counseling and drug and alcohol rehabilitation would be part of rehabilitative efforts as needed.

Organizations

No single organization is specific to multiple disabilities. However, individual disability groups do provide services and support for individuals who have one of their named disabilities. Such groups include consumer groups (e.g., National Association of the Deaf, American Association for the Deaf-Blind, National Federation of the Blind, United Cerebral Palsy Association), family groups (e.g., The Arc, Learning Disabilities Association, Autism Society of America), advocacy groups (e.g., Congress of Organizations of the Physically Handicapped, The Association for Persons with Severe Handicaps), and professional organizations (e.g., Council for Exceptional Children, American Academy of Child and Adolescent Psychiatry, American Association on Mental Retardation). These groups assist individuals with multiple disabilities in self-advocacy, equal access with reasonable accommodations within the general community, access to government programs, and generation and dissemination of information. Organizations such as these have advocated for legislation concerning the rights of individuals in school (Individuals with Disabilities Education Act), work (Rehabilitation Act), and community (Americans with Disabilities Act).

(*See also:* DEVELOPMENTAL DISABILITIES)

RESOURCES

American Academy of Child and Adolescent Psychiatry, 3615 Wisconsin Ave., NW, Washington, DC 20016

American Association for the Deaf-Blind, 814 Thayer Ave., Silver Springs, MD 20910

American Association on Mental Retardation, 1719 Kalorama Road, NW, Washington, DC 20009

Autism Society of America, 7910 Woodmont Ave., Suite 650, Bethesda, MD 20814

Congress of Organizations of the Physically Handicapped, 16630 Beverly Ave., Tinley Park, IL 60477

Council for Exceptional Children, 1920 Association Drive, Reston, VA 22091

Learning Disabilities Association, 4156 Library Rd., Pittsburgh, PA 15234

National Association of the Deaf, 814 Thayer Ave., Silver Springs, MD 20910

National Federation of the Blind, 1800 Johnson St., Baltimore, MD 21230

The Association for Persons with Severe Handicaps, 11201 Greenwood Ave., N., Seattle, WA 98133

The Arc, 500 E. Border St., Suite 300, Arlington, TX 76010

United Cerebral Palsy Association, 1522 K St., Suite 1112, Washington, DC 20005

BIBLIOGRAPHY

HART, VERNA. "Multiply Disabled Children." In *Handbook of Developmental and Physical Disabilities,* ed. Vincent Hasselt, Phillip Strain, and Michael Hersen. New York, 1988.

PUESCHEL, SIEGFRIED, M., and MULICK, JAMES A., eds. *Prevention of Developmental Disabilities.* Baltimore, 1990.

PAUL A. ALBERTO
KATHRYN WOLFF HELLER

MULTIPLE SCLEROSIS

See NEUROLOGICAL DISORDERS; NEUROMUSCULAR DISORDERS; ORGANIC MENTAL SYNDROMES

MUSCULAR DYSTROPHY

See DEVELOPMENTAL DISABILITIES; NEUROLOGICAL DISORDERS; NEUROMUSCULAR DISORDERS

MUSCULOSKELETAL DISORDERS

Musculoskeletal disorders (MSD) constitute a broad spectrum of conditions that affect multiple soft tissues and bone, causing alterations in structural integrity and resulting in pain, altered function, and disability. Numerous etiologic factors necessitate accurate clinical diagnosis, and early treatment intervention maximizes optimal functional outcome and disability prevention.

Epidemiology and Disability Impact of MSD

Musculoskeletal disorders occur at the same rate in both men and women (124 per 1,000 population). The MSD rate is 26 percent higher for European Americans than for African Americans. The incidence increases with age. It is 140 per 1,000 for ages eighteen to forty-four and 200 per 1,000 for those over age eighty-five. MSD account for 12.8 percent of all hospitalizations, the incidence of hospitalization increasing with age.

As a whole, MSD cause activity limitations in 8.5 percent of individuals seventeen to forty-four years old and 60 percent in the seventy-four or older age group. In 1988 there were 382 million restricted activity days, 48.5 percent of which resulted from back and spine impairments and 38.5 percent from lower extremity or hip impairments. The most common activity of daily living skill that people with MSD have difficulty with is walking (20% for ages sixty-five to seventy-four and 46% for those over age eighty-five). Other reported difficult tasks include bathing and getting up and down from chairs. The most common symptoms of MSD that cause activity limitation are pain (40%), aches (13%), and weakness (2%).

These activity limitations, or restrictions in the ability of the individual to function, often cause disability. Musculoskeletal disorders are the most frequent cause of disability in the United States. The mean disability rate is 53 per 1,000 population. It increases with age. In the age group eighteen to forty-four years it is 30 per 1,000; in the age group fifty-five to sixty-four years it is 110 per 1,000.

The extent to which MSD cause disability depends on the nature and severity of the disorder, the physical impairment it causes, the duration of the disorder, and the presence of other comorbid diseases. Other factors include personal, environmental, and economic conditions, such as age, educational level, and motivation. People vary in their ability to cope with disabilities. Some people with major disabilities are able to function at a high level, while others with lesser disabilities are unable to cope at similar levels.

Musculoskeletal disorders cause disability in the following forms: work and role, leisure, economic, family, and psychological. Work disability is an important consequence of MSD, since substantial economic losses can occur. MSD rank only second to cardiovascular disease (CVD) in causing long-term work disability. Seventeen percent of all workers with disability have MSD. A study indicates that labor force participation among persons with musculoskeletal disease is declining at a greater rate than those with other chronic diseases (Yelin & Katz, 1991). The greatest work force decline for MSD is in the fifty-five to sixty-four-year age group. The overall participation in the work force by persons with MSD in 1987 was 57 percent, and for those with activity limitations it was 44 percent. In the fifty-five to sixty-four age group with activity limitation, participation was only 26 percent.

Four common musculoskeletal problems causing work disability include osteoarthritis (OA), rheumatoid arthritis (RA), tendinitis, and lower back pain (LBP). One study revealed that 29 percent of RA patients continue to work, 26 percent with OA and 59 percent with tendinitis or low back pain (Krammer, Yelin, Epstein et al., 1993). A greater percentage of RA and OA patients continued to do housework (43% and 48%, respectively). In relation to symptoms, 54 percent of RA patients, 44 percent of OA patients, and 11 percent of tendinitis patients are always symptomatic. Sixty-four percent of RA patients, 50 percent with OA, and 36 percent with tendinitis report extensive symptoms. Physician visits average 7.1 yearly for RA, 3.5 for OA, and 1.5 for tendinitis. The mean number of bed days per year for RA was 22.9, for OA 14.2, for LBP 8.3, and for tendinitis 1.1. Since OA is more prevalent than RA, the total number of days lost from work was 67 million yearly for OA and 2.2 million for RA (Yelin, Meenan, Newitt et al., 1980).

Disability tends to be more common with such severe MSD as RA, which affects many soft tissues and joint structures. It is also a systemic inflammatory disease, causing acute joint swelling, pain, and involvement of other organ systems and overall fatigue. Fifty percent of patients with RA are expected to be work-disabled ten years after their disease onset. In RA, the stage of the disease has an impact on disability. In stages I and II of the disease there is a 44 percent probability of disability, whereas in more severe stages III and IV there is a 72 percent probability. Chronicity of the disease also has an impact. In stages I and II disease of fewer than five years' duration there is 30 percent probability of disability; for more than five years it is 76 percent. Control over the work environment is important. The self-employed RA patient has a 28 percent probability of disability; if working for another, it is 62 percent. If you can control your pace of work it is 44 percent, whereas if someone else controls the pace, it is 66 percent (Yelin, Meenan, Newitt et al., 1980).

Some arthritic disorders, such as osteoarthritis (OA), are noninflammatory, have no systemic involvement, and affect only local musculoskeletal structures. In this instance, the location of the structure involved affects the degree of limitation of function. In OA, involvement of the knee, the hip, or both causes significantly more limitation of function than hand involvement of the thumb and distal finger joints primarily because hip and knee pain affects weight bearing and limits mobility.

More than 32 million musculoskeletal injuries occur yearly. In addition, there are 6,500 fractures and 14,700 sprains and dislocations. The workplace is a significant source of injury, including cumulative trauma disorders. There were 1.8 million disabling work injuries in the United States in 1990. Strains and sprains are the most frequent injuries, causing work loss and accounting for 43 percent of all occupational illness/injury work loss (others include fractures, 9.6%; inflammation of joints, tendons, and muscles, 1.1%) (Vital and Health Statistics, 1992).

Musculoskeletal disorders caused by trauma and affecting tendons, ligaments, and bursa begin as an acute focal problem. If treatment affects a resolution of the problem, the impact on function is time-limited. However, these problems may become chronic or resolve and recur and may be associated with long-term disabilities. Preventive strategies and early treatment play a major role in reducing the incidence of disability.

Low back pain is the most common cause of work disability in the United States. In those individuals who have more than six months of persistent back pain, there is a 50 percent permanent disability rate. Eighty percent of the general population have an acute episode of low back pain sometime in their life, but the likelihood of disability is low.

Prevention of work disability depends on a number of factors: job change, workplace adaptation (ergonomic interventions, altering tasks), introducing energy conservation techniques, and vocational retraining.

Diagnosis, treatment, determination, and prevention of disability associated with musculoskeletal disorders require the involvement and interaction of multiple disciplines. Orthopedists, physiatrists (physicians of rehabilitation medicine), rheumatologists, and family practitioners are typically called on. A useful model addressing the scope of this topic involves understanding the structure, function, and pathophysiology of related tissue types. This provides a basis for systematic evaluation and ultimately for principles regarding treatment and rehabilitation. For example, understanding the general approach to the patient with tendinitis should prove more meaningful than the mere description of a limited number of inflammatory tendon conditions. A model of rehabilitation principles is clearly invaluable when faced with a new but related clinical solution.

Classification of Major Musculoskeletal Disorders

Tendons and Ligaments. Tendons and ligaments, although functionally different, share structural characteristics. Tendons attach muscle to bone; ligaments connect two or more bones, cartilage, or other structures. Both are made of dense, organized connective tissue, of which 70 percent is collagen. Tendons are comprised of linearly aligned collagen fibrils that form fascicles surrounded by a fibrous sheath called an epitenon (Figure 1). Tendons functioning in straight lines are surrounded by an outer sheath called paratenon, whereas those that take an angular course are covered by a synovial sheath, which produces fluid to improve tendon glide. The blood supply to the tendon originates at musculotendinous and bone-tendon junctions. Ligaments are

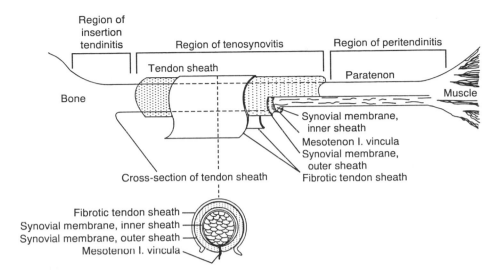

Figure 1. The muscle-tendon unit

SOURCE: Kurppa, K; Waris, P; Rokkanen, P.: Peritendinitis and Synovitis. *Scandinavian Journal of Work, Environment and Health* 5, Supplement 3 (1979): 19–24

classified according to their shape, bony attachment, function, and joint structure relationship. Their collagen bundles organize according to biomechanical stresses. Ligaments are relatively avascular, and areas of friction, compression, or torsion may further compromise vascularity.

Tendons primarily function to transmit force from muscle to bone and can withstand great tensile stresses. The tensile strength of a healthy tendon can be more than double the strength of its attached muscle. The most common site of tendon injury is the insertion site to bone (enthesis).

Ligaments impart strength and stability to their attached structures. They are weakest at or near their attachment to bone.

The mechanical properties of tendon and ligament are influenced by factors including age, sex, temperature, activity, drugs, and disease. Exercise stimulates collagen synthesis and alignment, increasing tendon strength and stiffness. Alternatively, inactivity or immobilization results in increased collagen breakdown and decreased strength.

Tendon injuries can be classified from a pathological or a functional standpoint. At least three overlapping pathological conditions exist: inflammation, degeneration, and rupture. Inflammation of paratenon alone is called paratenonitis, whereas involvement of paratenon lined with a fluid producing synovial membrane is tenosynovitis. The term "tendinitis" is reserved for injuries and inflammation specifically involving the tendon. Tendinosis is a condition describing intratendinous degeneration and atrophy with relatively little inflammation. Chronic inflammation often leads to tendinosis and may ultimately be associated with structural weakening and tendon rupture. Rupture can be partial or complete. Acute injuries have a sudden onset, subjecting the tendon to large stress. Repair and healing may be prolonged, but they follow a predictable course. Chronic injuries have an insidious onset. Improper treatment leads to chronic inflammation, prolonged pain, poor tendon repair, shortening of the muscle tendon unit, and reinjury vulnerability. Common tendon injury sites and classifications are provided in Table 1.

A functional classification of traumatic tendinitis is particularly useful in that the degree of disability correlates well with the extent of injury (Table 2). This grading system also provides objective parameters for following treatment and rehabilitation.

Inflammation, degeneration, and sometimes rupture of tendon can occur with many other inflammatory MSD, such as RA and systemic lupus erythematosus.

Ligament injury or sprains are divided into three degrees, based on the amount of ligament tearing

Table 1. Common tendon injuries

Involved Tendon	Injury Classification
Achilles	Achilles tendinitis, paratenonitis, rupture
Patella	Patella tendinitis (jumper's knee), paratenonitis, rupture
Hamstring (semimembranosus)	Hamstring tendinitis, tenosynovitis
Abductor pollicis longus; extensor pollicis brevis	DeQuervain's tenosynovitis
Common wrist extensors (extensor carpi radialis brevis)	Lateral epicondylitis, insertion tendinitis (tennis elbow)
Common wrist flexor	Medial epicondylitis, insertion tendinitis (golfer's elbow)
Rotator cuff (supraspinatus, infraspinatus teres minor, subscapularis)	Rotator cuff tendinitis, paratenonitis, (impingement syndrome), rupture
Biceps brachii	Bicipital tendinitis

(Table 3). First-degree injuries are painful but result in minimal fiber tearing and little functional loss. Second-degree tears are associated with significant bruising, swelling, and structural weakness. These are often the most challenging to assess accurately and tend to recur if improperly managed. Third-degree injuries represent complete rupture of the ligament with marked bruising, swelling, and significant functional loss. Surgical intervention is not uncommon, and prolonged immobilization is required. Failure to treat these injuries adequately may result in persistent instability of a related joint structure, leading to degenerative joint changes. Ligament sprains are commonly seen throughout the axial and appendicular skeleton (Table 4).

Table 2. Functional scale of tendinitis

Grade	Symptoms
I	Mild pain after exercise, resolving within twenty-four hours
II	Minimal pain with exercise, not interfering with activity
III	Pain that interferes with exercise
IV	Pain caused by activities of daily living
V	Constant rest pain that interferes with sleep

Ligaments become chronically stretched in many MSD, contributing to joint deformity and pain.

Muscle. Muscle is a specialized organ, made up of contractile and noncontractile elements. The basic contractile unit, the sarcomere, is composed of actin and myosin myofilaments arranged in parallel bundles of myofibrils, which constitute the muscle (Figure 2). Fibers and fiber groups make up a fasciculum. The noncontractile elements consist of connective tissue surrounding each fiber (endomysium), fiber bundles (perimysium), and entire muscle (epimysium). Most muscles attach to bone by tendons, constituting the musculotendinous unit. Tendon, being stronger than muscle, is better suited to transmit force to bone. Muscles differ in length, fiber orientation, and cross-sectional area, influencing the degree of joint movement and force generation.

Muscle contraction is an energy-dependent process requiring precise neurological control and feedback. If a contraction shortens the muscle, it is described as concentric. If muscle lengthening occurs, the contraction is eccentric. Isometric contractions are associated with no change in muscle length. Eccentric contractions are associated with the greatest overall force production.

Muscle injuries encompass a spectrum of pathological conditions varying considerably in the

Table 3. Classification of ligament injuries

Grade	Physical Signs	Functional Implications
First degree (mild)	• Local tenderness • Minimal bruising, swelling • Minimal structural loss	• Minimal transient loss of function
Second degree (moderate)	• Significant pain, bruising, and swelling • Clear structural weakness	• Requires relative rest and protective movement • Recurrence is likely
Third degree (complete)	• Significant abnormal motion and loss of structural integrity • Bruising, swelling, and pain	• Surgery not uncommon • Prolonged protected movement • Instability often persists

SOURCE: Adapted from David C. Reid, ed., *Sports Injury Assessment and Rehabilitation.* New York, 1992

amount of functional disability and treatment requirements. A general classification should include muscle strains, contusions, avulsions, and exercise-induced muscle injury (Table 5). Muscle strains range from minimal muscle damage to complete tears. Good prognostic signs for quick healing and minimal functional loss include mild to moderate strains of the muscle belly, with minimal bleeding, as opposed to the musculotendinous junction injury. Severe reinjuries with significant pain, bleeding, and loss of range and function have an increased risk of prolonged disability and complications.

Contusions, or perimuscular bleeding, overlap pathologically with strains and are divided into intermuscular and intramuscular injuries. The thigh is commonly involved in contact sports. Intermuscular lesions occur along muscle borders or fascia, where bleeding tracks, resulting in less inflammation, quicker resolution, and more rapid return of function. Intramuscular bleeding often causes a localized accumulation of blood, significant inflammation, intense pain, and marked loss of joint motion. There is an increased risk of pressure-induced tissue damage (compartment syndrome) and local connective tissue ossification (myositis ossificans). Healing is often prolonged.

Avulsions typically include the traumatic separation or tearing of bony or musculotendinous structures. Common examples include the ischial tuberosity with the hamstring muscle, the olecranon with the triceps, and the patella with the quadriceps tendon. In the skeletally immature teenager separation of an open apophysis may occur.

Exercise-induced muscle injury or delayed-onset muscle soreness (DOMS) consists of muscle pain and inflammation twenty-four to forty-eight hours after intense exercise that often includes eccentric activity. Direct muscle fiber damage has been observed. Treatment is controversial but often includes anti-inflammatory medication, stretching, and light intensity exercise. Complete recovery usually ensues.

Musculoskeletal disorders that cause joint degeneration or inflammation have a significant impact on muscle function. Muscle around these joint does not

Table 4. Common ligament sprains

Location	Involved Ligament
Shoulder	Glenohumeral ligaments; acromioclavicular ligament; medial collateral ligament
Elbow	Medial collateral ligament
Wrist	Ulnar collateral ligament (skier's thumb)
Knee	Anterior cruciate ligament; medial collateral ligament
Ankle	Anterior talofibular ligament
Pelvis	Sacroiliac, iliolumbar ligament
Spine	Interspinous, anterior, and posterior longitudinal ligaments

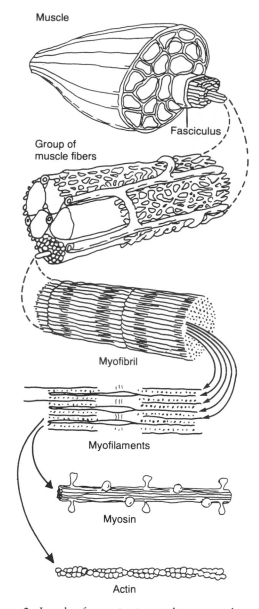

Muscle

Group of
muscle fibers

Fasciculus

Myofibril

Myofilaments

Myosin

Actin

Figure 2. Levels of organization within a muscle

SOURCE: David C. Reid, ed., *Sports Injury Assessment and Rehabilitation*. New York, 1992

contract normally and often becomes weak and atrophied. Appropriate exercise is necessary to help maintain normal muscle strength and function.

Bursae. Bursae are protective, fluid-filled synovial sacs located between tendons, tendons and bony prominences, and bone and overlying skin and tendons. By lying between structures, they reduce friction caused by motion of one tissue over another.

Bursae problems are classified into four areas: traumatic, infectious, arthritic, and neoplastic. For common areas and types of bursitis see Table 6.

Traumatic Bursitis. Trauma to the bursa from direct injury, athletic event, or overuse is common. Superficially located bursae (elbow-olecranon, hip-trochanteric, and knee-prepatellar) are frequently exposed to injury. As a result of trauma or overuse, inflammation of the synovial bursal lining occurs, producing an increased amount of fluid. In addition, direct trauma can cause bleeding into the bursal sac. Repeated trauma or misuse often results in chronic inflammation and pain, with thickening of the synovial bursal wall. Bursitis can be seen in association with tendinitis.

Infectious Bursitis. Infection of bursae can occur from a puncture wound, extension of a skin infection, or as a complication of a corticosteroid injection into the bursa to suppress inflammation. Individuals taking systemic corticosteroids or other immunosuppressive medications or who have diseases that suppress the immune system are more susceptible to infections. Bursal infections are associated with redness, intense pain aggravated by motion, surrounding muscle spasm, and fever, and should be treated promptly with appropriate drainage and antibiotics to prevent sepsis (blood poisoning). Common infecting agents are staphylococci and streptococci. Tuberculosis and fungal bursitis also may occur. Elbow, knee, and ankle bursae are superficial and particularly susceptible to infection.

Bursitis and Arthritis. It is not uncommon to see associated bursitis around an acutely inflamed arthritic joint. Bursae, particularly some of those around the knee, communicate with the joint. When the joint becomes inflamed, the bursa follows suit. The shoulder subdeltoid bursa, elbow olecranon bursa, and knee and ankle bursae are commonly involved in rheumatoid arthritis. Gouty arthritis is often associated with crystal deposits in the joints and bursae, causing intense pain and inflammation (Table 7).

Neoplastic Bursitis. Involvement of the bursa by tumor may occur. The popliteal bursa behind the knee is a common site.

Cartilage. Cartilage consists of fibrous connective tissue that is more homogeneous, stronger, and resilient than ordinary fibrous tissue. Hyaline carti-

Table 5. Classification of muscle injuries

Type		Associated Features
A.	Strains	
	First degree (mild)	Minimal bleeding, pain, and structural damage; quick resolution
	Second degree (moderate)	Partial tear; significant pain, spasm, hemorrhage, and functional impairment
	Third degree (severe)	Complete tear; severe pain, bleeding, spasm; prolonged functional loss and decreased range of motion; may require surgery
B.	Contusions	
	Intermuscular	Tracking of hematoma along muscle fascia; minimal inflammation and quick resolution
	Intramuscular	Confined bleeding; more intense inflammation and loss of range of motion; increased risk of compartment syndrome, prolonged recovery
C.	Avulsions	
	Bony	Common sites
	Apophyseal	Occurring in skeletally immature
	Muscle	Often associated with steroid injection or connective tissue disorders
D.	Exercise-induced muscle injury	Eccentric activity; delayed onset twenty-four to forty-eight hours after activity; variable pain and inflammation; limited functional loss

SOURCE: Adapted from David C. Reid, ed., *Sports Injury Assessment and Rehabilitation.* New York, 1992

lage is the most common type, often seen between adjacent weight-bearing bones. It serves as a supporting framework for softer tissues, cushions joint surfaces, and aids in diffusing joint forces. Degeneration of articular cartilage is relatively common and is associated with traumatic joint injuries and overuse injuries.

Fibrocartilage contains more dense collagen fibers and is found in areas subjected to great forces. An example is the menisci of the knee, which, in addition to transmitting joint forces, protect the articular cartilage and impart some stability to the joint. Meniscal injuries are common, occurring in at least 50 percent of sports-related knee injuries. The

Table 6. Etiology of bursitis

Type	Common Site
Traumatic	Olecranon, trochanteric, prepatellar
Infectious	Olecranon, prepatellar, malleolar
Associated with arthritis	knee bursae, olecranon
Associated with neoplasia (popliteal)	

Table 7. Bursitis—anatomical classification

Location	Type of Bursa
Shoulder	Subacromial; subdeltoid
Elbow	Olecranon
Hip	Ischiogluteal; subgluteal maximus; subgluteal medius; trochanteric
Knee	Prepatellar (housemaid's knee); suprapatellar, infrapatellar (parson's knee, carpet layer's knee)
Ankle	Anserine; popliteal, pre-Achilles; malleolar

485

mechanism of injury usually involves torsional as well as direct-impact stress on the knee. Patients typically describe pain, occasional swelling, clicking or locking of the knee, limited range of motion, and joint instability. A thorough history and physical exam, including provocative testing (e.g., McMurray test), often establishes the diagnosis. Magnetic resonance imaging (MRI) is often useful in establishing the severity of meniscal injury in addition to the integrity of the articular cartilage. Conservative versus surgical treatment of these injuries is dependent on the extent of meniscal and articular cartilage damage, pain, and the functional requirements of the patient.

Cartilage may also be worn down in degenerative arthritis (OA) or become eroded and fragmented in inflammatory arthritis (RA). This destruction of cartilage by an arthritic process results in narrowing of the joint space. In some cases the cartilage is completely destroyed and the bones rub against each other during joint motion, causing pain, wearing down of the bony joint surface, and deformity. Joints often become unstable.

Bone. Bone is the hardest of the connective tissues forming most of the skeleton. It protects vulnerable internal structures, provides attachment for muscles and ligaments, and allows for locomotion through expanded joints.

Adult bone consists of 30 percent organic material, primarily collagen, and 70 percent mineral, primarily calcium hydroxyapatite. Skeletally immature bone has a higher percentage of organic material and is, therefore, more flexible and easily influenced by joint stress. Bone mass typically peaks in the fourth decade. With advancing age, particularly in females, bone becomes less resilient as the organic matrix water is replaced by calcium hydroxyapatite, causing loss of bone volume and increased fracture risk.

The typical long bone consists of an outer shell of cortical or compact bone contributing to its strength (Figure 3). Long bone ends (epiphyses) have a thinner shell of compact bone filled by spongy bone organized into thin plates of bone, or trabeculae. Trabeculae afford a structural role, augmenting the shock-absorbing properties of the articular cartilage. The bone body or diaphysis contains the marrow cavity, responsible for blood cell production. The

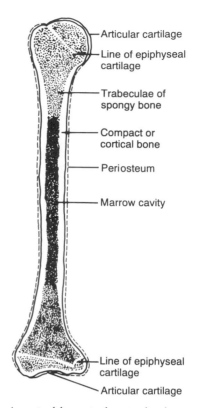

Figure 3. A typical bone in longitudinal section

SOURCE: David B. Jenkins, ed., *Hollinshead's Functional Anatomy of the Limbs and Back*, 6th ed. Philadelphia, 1991

growth plate, or epiphyseal cartilage, is responsible for the longitudinal growth of long bones. Each bone closes its growth plate at a characteristic age (girls earlier than boys). A number of factors influence the growth of the epiphyseal plates, including hormonal, mechanical, and nutritional.

Joints are the union between two bones and are classified into fibrous, cartilaginous, and synovial. The most common is cartilaginous, with fibrocartilage uniting the bone, allowing for limited movement. Belonging to this class are the intervertebral disks. Synovial joints, by contrast, allow for considerable movement. They are classified according to the shapes of the articulating surfaces. The shoulder joint represents a ball-and-socket joint in which one end of the articular surface is round and the other concave (Figure 4). This joint allows for range of motion in six planes. The knee and elbow exemplify a hinge joint, limited to back-and-forth motion. Other joint types include planar and ellipsoid (wrist)

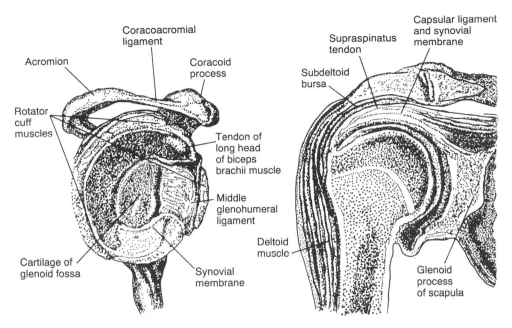

Figure 4. The shoulder joint, a typical ball-and-socket synovial joint

SOURCE: Frank H. Netter. *The Ciba Collection and Musculoskeletal System.* CIBA-GEIGY Corporation, Summit, NJ, 1987.

and condylar (knuckles). The synovial joint has a consistent structure, with cartilage lining the articular surfaces. An articular capsule adjoins the bones and is composed of both an outer fibroid membrane and an inner synovial lining that produces fluid providing joint lubrication and articular cartilage nourishment for the joint. Ligaments joining to the articular capsule provide strength and stability.

The spine or vertebral column is responsible for trunk stability and movement, head and axial skeleton support, and spinal cord protection. It consists of thirty-three vertebrae—seven cervical, twelve thoracic, five lumbar, five sacral, and four coccygeal (Figures 5 and 6).

In general, a vertebra consists of an anterior body of mainly spongy bone covered by a thin layer of cortical bone. The pedicle and lamina form the vertebral arch onto which the spinous process attaches posteriorly. Articular processes extend both inferiorly and superiorly from the junction of the pedicle and lamina. These have smooth facets, which form synovial joints allowing for articulation with vertebrae above and below. Also from this junction, transverse processes extend laterally, allowing for

the attachment of muscles and thoracic region ribs. The vertebral canal contains the spinal cord and nerve roots. Regional anatomical and functional differences exist between vertebrae. The intervertebral disks, which pad adjacent vertebrae along the spinal column, account for approximately one-fourth of the height of the spine. Each disk consists of an outer fibrocartilage layer, the annulus, and a gelatinous center, the nucleus pulposus. In addition to binding vertebrae together, the disks function as shock absorbers and allow limited movement between vertebrae.

An integrated system of muscles and ligaments maintains the structural alignment of the spine and contributes to its movement and stability.

A comprehensive discussion of bone disease is beyond the scope of this entry. A broad classification is illustrated in Table 8. The most common overuse syndrome of bone is a fatigue or stress fracture. This is distinguished from acute traumatic and pathological fractures as complications of concurrent illnesses (osteoporosis, rheumatoid arthritis, malignancy). Stress fractures are particularly common in running or jumping athletes, with the tibia and fibula being the most common fracture sites in

487

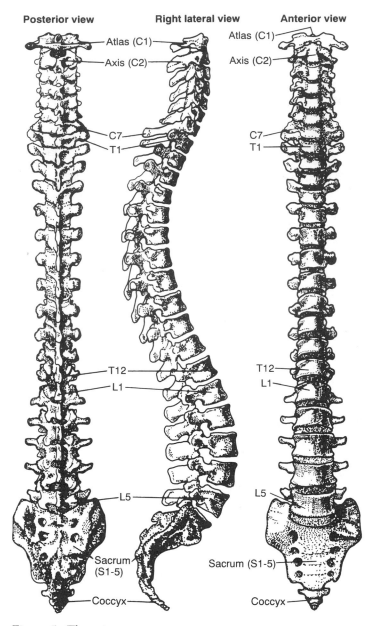

Figure 5. The spine

SOURCE: Frank H. Netter. *The Ciba Collection and Musculoskeletal System.* CIBA-GEIGY Corporation, Summit, NJ, 1987

runners. In the upper extremities, ulnar and humeral stress fractures predominate in activities such as tennis, throwing, gymnastics, and weight training. Trunk and rib fractures may be seen from lifting activities or contact sports. Vertebral stress fractures involving the pars interarticularis (spondylolysis) occur in activities such as gymnastics, requiring excessive back extension. Spondylolisthesis is a slipping of one vertebra forward on another due to bilateral spondylosis. Proposed etiologic factors for stress fractures include muscle fatigue, strong muscular contraction pulling on periosteum, or direct injury from repetitive impact. Patients complain of activity-induced point tenderness, impaired performance, and local swelling. Diagnosis can be made relatively early with radionuclide bone scanning.

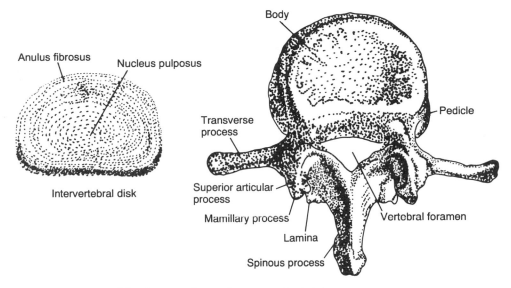

Figure 6. A typical lumbar vertebra and intervertebral disk

SOURCE: Frank H. Netter. *The Ciba Collection and Musculoskeletal System*. CIBA-GEIGY Corporation, Summit, NJ, 1987

As previously noted, loss of ligamentous integrity may result in joint subluxation or dislocation. A subluxed joint demonstrates displacement but continuity of joint surfaces as opposed to a dislocated joint in which there is complete joint separation. The articulations between the clavicle and scapula (acromioclavicular joint) and the humerus and scapula (glenohumeral joint) are particularly susceptible to acute injuries involving direct blows to the shoulder or falls on an outstretched arm. Anterior dislocation of the glenohumeral joint is by far the most common. Patients present with pain, variable swelling, restricted joint range of motion, and structural malalignment, depending on the severity of the injury. Joint subluxation may also occur due to stretching of ligaments, which occurs in many inflammatory diseases, such as RA and systemic lupus erythematosus.

Various systemic illnesses manifest with bone-related symptoms or complications, the most common being inflammatory joint arthritis. Inflammation of the joint (as in RA, gout, juvenile RA, and psoriatic arthritis) may be so intense that the bone, as well as cartilage and tendon, becomes eroded. There may be complete loss of joint space, and the bones of the joint may fuse together (ankylose). Noninflammatory arthritis such as OA may cause ex-

tra bone formation (spurs), and in addition cartilage becomes worn and the joint space reduced. The ends of the bone may begin to wear down unevenly, causing deformity.

Bone disorders with decreased mineralization of bone, such as osteoporosis, may cause considerable weakening of the bony structure and lead to easy bone fractures or to painful spontaneous fractures in the long bones (commonly hip and wrist) and in the vertebrae (compression fractures).

Bone tumors, such as osteogenic and Ewing's sarcoma, occur in a younger age group (ten to thirteen years). They initially present with bone pain that is often mistaken for muscle strain. However, the pain persists, and as the tumor grows, the bone cortex weakens and bony fracture may occur, particularly during sports events. These tumors commonly occur around the hip, knee, and shoulder areas.

Nerve. The classification of problems associated with nerves can be seen in Table 9. Compression of single or multiple nerves by soft tissue swelling, direct or repetitive trauma, or bony deformity can result in pain, paresthesis, and sensory and motor loss.

Carpal tunnel syndrome is one of the most common compression neuropathies. The median nerve at the wrist travels through a narrow tunnel before giving off branches to some of the hand muscles.

Table 8. Classification of bone disorders

Fractures

- Stress
- Epiphyseal
- Compression
- Pathologic

Joint Dislocations

- Temporomandibular
- Shoulder-glenohumeral
- Acromioclavicular
- Hip

Arthritis

- Noninflammatory degenerative joint disease
- Inflammatory:
  rheumatoid; Reiter's; ankylosing spondylitis

Infectious

- Osteomyelitis
- Diskitis

Metabolic

- Osteoporosis
- Paget's disease
- Primary hyperparathyroidism

Tumors

- Osteogenic sarcoma
- Ewing's sarcoma
- Benign cysts

Structural

- Scoliosis
- Spondylolisthesis
- Transitional vertebrae

Swelling of the tissues around the carpal tunnel, secondary to repeated trauma, diabetes or arthritis, narrows the tunnel and compresses the nerve, causing painful paresthesias in the hand and forearm and weakness and atrophy of the thumb muscles. Nerves in many other body areas may undergo similar compressive problems (Table 9).

Table 9. Common nerve syndromes

Entrapment	Location
Carpal tunnel	Wrist
Ulnar nerve	Elbow
Thoracic outlet	Clavicle
Pyriformis	
Spinal stenosis	Lumbar
Radiculopathies	Cervical; lumbar
Reflex sympathetic dystrophy	Arm; leg

Myofascial. A myofascial compartment consists of groups of muscles; a major artery; nerve; and fascia, which is a sheath of thick connective tissue often dividing adjacent muscles or existing between muscles or tendon and bone. The compartment is quite inelastic and is susceptible to increased pressure due to a variety of factors.

Fibromyalgia (fibrositis) is an example of a common myofascial pain syndrome. It includes pain and tenderness of focal muscle areas (trigger points), general body aches, and often sleep disturbance. Painful trigger point areas can be found in the neck, back, shoulder, hip, and even in the calf area. The actual trigger sites show no inflammation on tissue biopsy. Abnormal brain beta waves have been confirmed by electroencephalogram (EEG). Persons with this disorder also have decreased aerobic conditioning. The disease may occur as a primary disorder; may be precipitated by trauma or illness; or may be associated with other processes, such as cervical and lumbar discogenic disease or various types of arthritis. Other myofascial problems are noted in Table 10.

Soft-Tissue Inflammation and Repair

The treatment of musculoskeletal injuries requires an understanding of the tissue response to trauma. Among connective tissues, tendon and ligament healing can be divided into three phases: the inflammatory or cellular phase, the regeneration phase, and the remodeling phase.

The acute inflammatory response usually lasts about five to seven days and is associated with increased regional blood flow, swelling, redness, and

Table 10. Other musculoskeletal syndromes

Diffuse

- Fibrositis
- Polymyalgia rheumatica (PMR)
- Psychogenic

Myofascial

- Neck pain
- Back pain
- Trapezius pain
- Plantar fasciitis

pain. This response appears to be necessary during the first forty-eight hours as cellular debris is removed from the area and as collagen-producing cells are stimulated to initiate the healing process. Prolonged inflammation, however, may be detrimental to surrounding tissue, resulting in persistent vascular compromise, and decreased tissue oxygenation and protein production.

The repair process begins at forty-eight hours and may last from four to eight weeks. This phase is characterized by continued elimination of tissue debris, the revascularization of devitalized tissue, and the ultimate organization of newly formed collagen fibers.

The remodeling phase is most pronounced at twelve to twenty-eight days after injury and is associated with further maturation and organization of collagen; this process may continue for years. Longitudinal tension seems to play an important role in collagen fiber production, orientation, and ultimately in the flexibility and strength of the healing scar.

Inflammation of soft tissues and joints caused by arthritis occurs in three phases: acute, subacute, and chronic. Acute inflammation can occur at any time and requires treatment with anti-inflammatory medication and cold modalities. During the subacute phase, inflammatory cells and substances decrease and finally resolve in the chronic stage, which most often leaves permanent tissue damage.

Healing of muscle after trauma follows a pattern similar to that of connective tissue; however, the inability of muscle to regenerate fully without pro-

ducing scar tissue highlights the importance of limiting tissue injury. The initial phase is marked by localized bleeding around the site of muscle damage, followed by inflammation and removal of cellular debris within the first thirty-six hours. During this stage the muscle seems weakened and susceptible to further injury. At three to six days collagen-forming cells proliferate and early signs of muscle regeneration appear. Between one and two weeks the tensile strength of the healing tissue is approximately 50 percent, with further increases related to collagen maturation and rehabilitation interventions.

Understanding the processes of fracture healing in bone is clearly important but beyond the scope of this entry.

Etiology of Musculoskeletal Disorders

The causes and mechanisms of MSD are numerous but can be viewed under a general classification (Table 11). The majority of sport and occupational-related injuries are referred to as overuse syndromes or cumulative trauma disorders. These result from either tissue overload or repetitive overuse, leading to cumulative structural trauma, setting the stage for inflammation, pain, and disability. Typical examples include stress fractures of bone, tendinitis, bursitis, and recurrent ligament sprains. Runners are particularly vulnerable to medial tibial stress fractures, Achilles tendinitis, plantar fasciitis, and knee and ankle ligament sprains. Office employees engaged in prolonged deskwork often present with neck and shoulder symptoms. Both intrinsic and extrinsic factors may contribute to the onset of overuse injuries (Table 12). Age, muscle imbalance, weakness, poor flexibility, and nutrition are examples of intrinsic variables, whereas equipment, environmental conditions, and training or technique errors

Table 11. Etiology of musculoskeletal disorders

- Overuse syndromes/cumulative trauma disorders
- Direct trauma
- Structural failure
- Rheumatologic
- Metabolic
- Infectious
- Tumor

Table 12. Etiology of overuse syndromes

Intrinsic Variables

- Age
- Genetic predisposition
- Muscle imbalance/weakness
- Poor flexibility
- Anatomic malalignment
- Nutrition

Extrinsic Variables

- Improper training
- Improper equipment
- Poor technique
- Environmental conditions

exemplify extrinsic factors. Poor training is probably the leading cause of overuse injuries in the athletic population.

Direct trauma is a relatively common cause of injury. Examples include glenohumeral or acromioclavicular separation from forceful injury to the shoulder girdle, and muscular strains from direct contact. Soft tissue structures are also vulnerable to failure from forceful muscular contractions, particularly when weakened due to concurrent illness (connective tissue disorders) or medications (steroids). Examples include Achilles and patella tendon ruptures, and complete ligament tears (e.g., anterior cruciate ligament).

Musculoskeletal conditions are often seen in association with other medical disorders. The articular and extra-articular manifestations of systemic rheumatic diseases such as RA, SLE, polymyositis-dermatomyositis, the spondylo-arthropathies, and the articular problems of noninflammatory OA often lead to significant functional disability. Tendinitis, bursitis, synovitis, ligamentous laxity and rupture, muscle weakness, articular cartilage damage, and joint instability contribute to the pain, fatigue, impaired mobility, and self-care and psychosocial challenges facing this patient population.

Metabolic (e.g., osteoporosis), infectious (e.g., osteomyelitis), and endocrinologic (e.g., hyperparathyroidism, Cushing's disease) disorders may all manifest musculoskeletal abnormalities. Soft tissue

and bony tumors should always be a consideration, particularly in the young patient with musculoskeletal symptoms refractory to conventional therapies.

Clinical Evaluation

The clinical evaluation of musculoskeletal injuries is based on common principles, including a comprehensive health history, a directed physical examination, the judicious use of diagnostic tests, and an assessment of specific disability.

Pain is the most common presenting symptom for the majority of patients. A detailed pain history not only provides diagnostic information but also establishes a baseline to compare treatment outcomes. Relevant questions pertain to the intensity, quality, location, and duration of pain. Familiarity with pain referral patterns from joints, nerves, and myofascial structures is critical to accurate diagnosis. For example, the hip joint typically refers to the groin, and lumbosacral nerve root compromise (radiculopathy), related to spinal stenosis or intervertebral disc herniation, often results in lower extremity discomfort. Factors that alleviate or aggravate symptoms should be established as well as details of all failed and successful treatments, including all diagnostic procedures and pain medications.

The perception of pain and pain behavior is influenced by gender, age, psychosocial variables, and cultural norms. With this understanding the clinician may better be able to quantify the extent of pain and make a better estimate of the overall related disability.

In overuse syndromes associated with activity or occupation, specific historical information may suggest etiologic factors. Not uncommonly patients recall an acute inciting event, such as a motor vehicle accident resulting in neck pain, twisting an ankle while running, or experiencing acute back discomfort upon lifting a heavy object at work. More often symptoms present insidiously due to cumulative injury. Details with respect to exercise or occupational routines often elicit training or biomechanical errors. Examples include knee pain in the runner who has increased the frequency and intensity of training, and shoulder discomfort in the secretary entering computer data six hours per day.

The physical examination begins with inspection,

observing the patient for obvious pain, abnormal posturing or malalignments, and splinting of painful areas. Patients with cervical neck strains often present with acquired torticollis or head tilting due to muscle pain. Those with plantar fasciitis may demonstrate an antalgic or painful gait. Painful regions are examined for erythema, swelling, or edema. Range of motion testing assesses the integrity of joints and related soft tissues. Impaired range may occur secondary to pain, articular damage (RA, OA), injuries to ligaments or musculotendinous units (anterior cruciate ligament tear, Achilles tendon rupture), structural malalignments (scoliosis), or general inflexibilities (tight hamstrings in runners).

Palpation may reveal muscle spasm, taut bands, or trigger points suggestive of myofascial-related pain. Discontinuity of soft tissue can often be felt after trauma and may indicate rupture (Achilles/patella tendons, gastrocnemius muscle). Provocative testing is an essential component in diagnosing musculoskeletal problems. Testing is typically geared toward the reproduction of symptoms or accentuating physical impairments (Table 13). Functional testing is often more helpful in eliciting performance-related symptoms. Having a tennis player demonstrate painful strokes or observing the seating posture of a secretary are particular examples. Clearly a thorough neurological examination may demonstrate focal sensory deficits, muscle weakness or imbalances, reflex asymmetries, and problems with coordination.

Diagnostic testing should be used sparingly for the majority of musculoskeletal injuries in which the diagnosis is often clear after a detailed history and physical examination. Laboratory evaluations, however, are often necessary to help confirm the presence of rheumatic disease, metabolic disturbance, chronic infection, or malignancy. Radiologic studies usually are unnecessary for overuse syndrome unless symptoms are refractory to conservative management. Routine radiographs have little diagnostic yield in evaluating soft tissue but can indicate bony fractures, dislocations, osteoporosis, articular manifestations of rheumatic and metabolic diseases, and malignancy. Magnetic resonance imaging (MRI) is expensive but best able to detect soft tissue pathology such as tendon or ligament tears, muscle contusions, inflammation, and intervertebral disk

Table 13. Provocative testing in musculoskeletal injuries

Test	Diagnosis
Spurling	Cervical radiculopathy
Neer's impingement	Rotator cuff tendinitis
Yergason	Bicipital tendinitis
Adson's	Thoracic outlet syndrome
Resisted wrist extension	Lateral epicondylitis (tennis elbow)
Finkelstein	DeQuervain's tenosynovitis
Phalen's	Carpal tunnel syndrome
Straight leg raise	Lumbosacral radiculopathy
Thomas	Hip flexor tightness
Faber	Sacroiliac dysfunction
Ober	Iliotibial band tightness
Anterior drawer	Anterior cruciate ligament tear
McMurray	Meniscal damage of the knee

herniations. MRI is associated with appreciable false-positive results and should therefore be used selectively. Ultrasonography is a less expensive method of assessing soft tissue but is less sensitive and technically difficult. Computerized tomography (CT) best defines the bony skeleton and is particularly useful in assessing spine disease (spinal stenosis, vertebral metastases, osteomyelitis). Bone scans offer little structural detail but are helpful in the early detection of stress fractures, avascular necrosis of bone, and infectious processes. Finally, electromyography (EMG) and nerve conduction studies assist in the diagnosis of peripheral nervous system injuries, such as those involving the spinal nerve roots (radiculopathy), interjoining networks of nerves (pletopathy), or specific nerve regions (entrapment neuropathy).

Assessment of Function

Before treating the patient with musculoskeletal disease it is important to assess their function. This can be done with measurement assessment tools. Important areas to evaluate by means of these tools are: physical measures (joint motion muscle strength); symptoms (pain and fatigue levels); activity level (mobility, daily living, socialization); and psychological adjustment (anxiety, depression levels). Assessments are repeated during treatment programs to determine the outcome of the treatment.

Treatment and Rehabilitation of Musculoskeletal Disorders

The treatment approach to MSD is dependent on the type, location, and severity of the process. General principles do apply, however, particularly with respect to soft tissue, overuse syndromes. The vast majority of injuries and musculoskeletal problems can be treated nonsurgically, with the ultimate goal to decrease pain, restore general fitness, and improve function to the most optimal level. This becomes a more significant challenge when a musculoskeletal problem manifests as a complication of systemic illness, as in the rheumatic, metabolic, endocrine, or infectious diseases, and especially malignant tumors. In these conditions, function is often compromised due to complications of treatment (medications, surgery, chemotherapy, radiation therapy) and related systemic symptoms (fatigue, pain, weakness, weight loss/gain, fever, anemia, and depression). Understanding the limitations placed on a patient with chronic or systemic disease permits a safer and more appropriate rehabilitation prescription, reducing the chance of further injury, frustration, and anxiety.

The rehabilitation of soft tissue injuries can be divided into a number of stages (Table 14). Defining the specific anatomical and functional deficits is a critical first step. Identifying the source of shoulder pain, for example, is often a challenge, given the proximity of various structures. "Shoulder tendinitis" is nondescriptive and should be avoided. Supraspinatus or bicipital tendinitis, and subacromial bursitis are specific diagnoses allowing for more directed treatment.

Table 14. Rehabilitation of musculoskeletal disorders

- Establish the correct diagnosis
- Control inflammation and pain
- Promote healing of the involved tissue
- Improve flexibility, strength, and general conditioning
- Sport/occupation-specific retraining prior to resumption of activity

Pain and inflammation are appropriately dealt with through use of activity modification, anti-inflammatory medications, therapeutic modalities, and protective bracing. The extent of injury and inflammation dictates the amount of required rest. Grade 1 ankle sprains may necessitate brief partial weight bearing on the extremity, whereas grade 3 sprains often require nonweight bearing and splinting. Prolonged bed rest should be avoided if possible to prevent deleterious effects, including decreases in muscle strength, endurance, and general flexibility. Early protected motion helps to promote the growth, alignment, and strength of newly formed collagen in healing tissues.

Nonsteroidal anti-inflammatory medications (NSAIDS) are commonly used to control pain, curtail inflammation, and promote healing. These medications should be used cautiously as they are not without side effects, particularly with prolonged use. Corticosteroids may be injected into the inflamed peritendinous region, bursa, or synovial-lined joint. This is particularly useful for symptoms that are refractory to more conservative treatment. Intratendinous injections should be avoided because they weaken tendons and may predispose to rupture. Injections of local anesthetic with or without corticosteroids are also used to treat myofascial trigger points and inflammation related to ligament injury, particularly in the sacroiliac region.

Therapeutic modalities are commonly used as adjuncts in controlling symptoms, reducing inflammation, and promoting tissue repair. Both superficial and deep heat are commonly used, although not in the acute phase, when heat may actually increase inflammation. They can reduce pain and muscle spasm and increase collagen extensibility. Ultrasound has both thermal and nonthermal effects on healing tissue. As a deep heating modality it encourages increased local blood flow. Ultrasound can penetrate into joints and deep structures. It is often used prior to stretching exercise for joint contracture. Although not clearly understood, it likely stimulates fibroblast activity in the synthesis of reparative tissue. It may also be used in combination with topical medications such as corticosteroids, salicylates, and local anesthetics in an attempt to encourage transdermal penetration of these compounds. This modality is termed phonophoresis. Transcutaneous electrical nerve stimulation (TENS) and high-voltage galvanic stimulation have both been advocated for pain. Cryotherapy (which is the therapeutic use of cold) is a valuable modality in the treatment of musculoskeletal injuries. Used acutely, cold can reduce pain, swelling, and muscle spasm, thereby facilitating motion during active therapy. Manual therapy techniques, such as friction massage and joint mobilization, have been used, with poorly defined results.

Bracing, splinting, taping, and other assistive devices can provide joint stability, limit motion, or deweight an injured area or inflamed joint, contributing to pain relief. Braces can be described as preventive or rehabilitative and may restrict joint function completely or partially or allow it fully. Ankle braces or taping are common practice following acute ligament injuries. A forearm or counterforce brace is often used for the symptoms of tennis elbow as a way to redistribute forces about the elbow. A variety of knee braces are commercially available to counteract ligament instability of the knee. Wrist and finger splints are often prescribed in rheumatoid arthritis to relieve painful joints. Non-functional wrist-hand splints are used at night for acutely inflamed joints. Functional wrist splints that immobilize a painful wrist but allow for finger function can be used for daily activities. Foot orthotics (both shoes and inserts) provide support, correct malalignments, and relieve pain—for example, in the pronated or flat foot. Pain related to osteoarthritis of the hip responds remarkably well to deweighting by use of a straight cane used on the opposite side during ambulation.

The next phase of therapy focuses on the promotion of healing and creating a stronger, more flexible tissue. It is crucial to begin early stretching exercises to prevent soft tissue or joint restriction, encourage healthy scar formation, and prepare for progressive strengthening. A variety of range-of-motion programs are available, and under the guidance of a physical therapist, patients are instructed in progressive home exercise. Prestretch heating and post-stretch icing are key components to this type of program. Associated weaknesses and inflexibilities should also be addressed—for example, tight hamstrings or hip flexors, and abdominal weakness in patients with low back pain. For most MSD the goal

of this stage is to achieve full, pain-free range of motion. Patients with chronic arthritis often are not able to achieve normal motion. The goal in this instance is to achieve at least a motion level that will allow them to perform most of their ADLs.

The common types of exercises include isometric, isotonic (concentric and eccentric), and isokinetic. Isometrics, which require no joint motion, impose the fewest demands on healing structures and are typically begun early. Progressive resistive exercises, initially described by DeLorme, are a critical step in rehabilitating soft tissue injuries. These exercises are performed using progressively higher weights. They strengthen and hypertrophy muscles. Persons with arthritis should use only isotonic exercise with one-to two-pound weights. A stronger, more flexible musculotendinous unit is better able to withstand the demands of exercise or occupation. Exercising a muscle eccentricity may ultimately allow it to withstand greater resistance and prevent recurrence of injury. There are various types of exercise equipment for isotonic strengthening, including free weights, elastic bands, Universal machines, and Nautilus. Elastic bands come in varying tensions, are transported easily, and can be used to perform both isometric and isotonic exercise. Hydrotherapy has gained popularity, especially for arthritic conditions requiring restricted weight bearing. The gravity-eliminated water setting places less stress across painful joints. Ankle sprains, low back pain related to intervertebral disk herniation, and arthritis are three conditions in which strength and endurance can safely be increased in the water. Stretching is always recommended prior to strengthening, as is icing afterward. It is also important to focus on weaknesses or muscle imbalances distant to the site of injury. For example, strengthening the periscapular muscles is often critical in the rehabilitation of supraspinatus tendinitis.

Maintaining general aerobic fitness is particularly important for competitive athletes training to return to sport. Stationary bicycles, rowing machines, cross-country ski machines, and swimming are safe and effective alternatives. Aerobic exercise has also proven to increase aerobic capacity in persons with arthritis (RA, OA, SLE, and spondylitis).

Sport or occupation-specific training may be considered as the final phase of functional rehabilitation. Assuming the patient is pain-free and attempts have been made to create a strong, flexible muscle-tendon unit, it is imperative to minimize or eliminate potentially abusive forces that present during sport, work, or activities of daily living. For athletes it often involves changes in equipment, training schedule, and technique. Occupational or industrial rehabilitation includes work site modifications and job-specific training to prevent reinjury. Functional adaptations to the home, such as bathroom grab bars, raised toilet seats, and entrance ramps, are particularly useful in creating a safer, more functional home for those with MSD that limit functional activities.

Future Issues

Exciting advances in musculoskeletal medicine and rehabilitation should be expected. As we understand better the mechanisms of tissue injury, inflammation, and repair, treatment interventions should continue to improve. More comprehensive injury tracking systems are required to establish better epidemiological data on musculoskeletal injuries. Prevention should continue to be the focus of interest, with emphasis on risk reduction, appropriate exercise strategies, and better public awareness of rehabilitation principles. Continued efforts by employees to understand and accommodate for disability in the workplace are essential.

(*See also:* ARTHRITIS; BACK DISORDERS; DISABILITY; DISABILITY MANAGEMENT; ERGONOMICS; MASSAGE THERAPY; PAIN; PHYSICAL THERAPY; PHYSICIAN)

RESOURCES

National Rehabilitation Information Center, 8455 Colesville Road, Suite 935, Silver Spring, MD 20910-3319

The American College of Sports Medicine, 401 W. Michigan St., Indianapolis, IN 46202-3233

The American Academy of Physical Medicine and Rehabilitation, 122 South Michigan Ave., Suite 1300, Chicago, IL 60603-6107

The American College of Rheumatology, 60 Executive Park S., Suite 150, Atlanta, GA 30329

The American Academy of Sports Physicians, 17113 Gledhill St., Northridge, CA 91325

The American Physical Therapy Association, 1111 N. Fairfax St., Alexandria, VA 22314

The Physiatric Association of Spine, Sports, and Occupational Rehabilitation, 2884 Sand Hill Road, Suite 110, Menlo Park, CA 94025

The Arthritis Foundation, 1314 Spring St., NW, Atlanta, GA 30309

BIBLIOGRAPHY

AMERICAN MEDICAL ASSOCIATION. *Guides to the Evaluation of Permanent Impairment*, 4th ed. Chicago, 1993.

BASMAJIAN, JOHN V., and WOLF, STEVEN L. *Therapeutic Exercise*. Baltimore, 1990.

BEJJANI, FADI J. "Performing Artists' Occupational Disorders." *Rehabilitation Medicine: Principles and Practice*, ed. J. A. Delisa. Philadelphia, 1993.

BUSCHBACHER, RALPH M. *Musculoskeletal Disorders: A Practical Guide for Diagnosis and Rehabilitation*. Boston, 1994.

CURWIN, SANDRA, and STANISH, WILLIAM. *Tendinitis: Its Etiology and Treatment*. Lexington, MA, 1984.

DeLORME, THOMAS L. "Restoration of Muscle Power by Heavy Resistance Exercises." *Journal of Bone and Joint Surgery* 27 (1945):645–667.

DREZ, DAVID, ed. *Therapeutic Modalities for Sports Injuries*. Chicago, 1989.

FRYMOYER, JOHN W., ed. *The Adult Spine*. New York, 1991.

HABER, LAWRENCE D. "Disabling Effects of Chronic Disease and Impairment." *Journal of Chronic Disorders* 24 (1971):469–487.

HADLER, NORTIN M. "Cumulative Trauma Disorders." *Journal of Occupational Medicine* 32 (1990):38–42.

HICKS, JEANNE E., and GERBER, LYNN H. "Rehabilitation of the Patient with Arthritis and Connective Tissue Disease." In *Rehabilitation Medicine: Principles and Practice*, ed. J. A. Delisa. Philadelphia, 1993.

HICKS, JEANNE E.; NICHOLAS, JOHN J.; and SWEZEY, ROBERT L. *Handbook of Rehabilitative Rheumatology*. Atlanta, 1988.

HOLBROOK, TROY L.; GRAZIER, KYLE.; KELSEY, JENNIFER L.; and STAUFFER, RICHARD N. *The Frequency of Occurrence, Impact, and Cost of Selective Musculoskeletal Conditions in the United States*. St. Louis, 1984.

KASDAN, MORTON L. *Occupational Hand and Upper Extremity Injuries and Diseases*. St. Louis, 1991.

KIRKALDY-WILLIS, WILLIAM H., and BURTON, CHARLES V. *Managing Low Back Pain*. New York, 1992.

KRAMMER, JANE S.; YELIN, EDWARD H.; and EPSTEIN,

WALLACE V. "Social and Economic Impacts of Four Musculoskeletal Conditions." *Arthritis & Rheumatism* 26 (1983):901–907.

LEADBETTER, WAYNE B.; BUCKWALTER, JOSEPH A.; and GORDON, STEPHEN L., eds. *Sports-Induced Inflammation: Clinical and Basic Science Concepts.* Park Ridge, IL, 1990.

LEHMAN, JUSTUS F., ed. *Therapeutic Heat and Cold*, 4th ed. Baltimore, 1990.

MÜLLER, ERICH A. "Influence of Training and Inactivity on Muscle Strength." *Archives of Physical Medicine and Rehabilitation* 51 (1970):449–462.

POPE, MALCOLM H.; ANDERSON, GUNNAR B. H.; FRYMOYER, JOHN W.; and CHAFFIN, DON B. *Occupational Low Back Pain: Assessment, Treatment, and Prevention.* St. Louis, 1991.

PRAEMER, ALLAN; FURNER, SYLVIA; and RICE, DOROTHY P. *Musculoskeletal Conditions in the United States.* Park Ridge, IL, 1992.

PRESS, JOEL M., ed. *Sports Medicine: Physical Medicine and Rehabilitation Clinics of North America.* Philadelphia, 1994.

REID, DAVID C. *Sports Injury Assessment and Rehabilitation.* New York, 1992.

RENSTROM, PER, and JOHNSON, ROBERT J. "Overuse Injuries in Sports: A Review." *Sports Medicine* 2 (1985):316–333.

RENSTROM, PER, and LEADBETTER, WAYNE B. *Clinics in Sports Medicine: Tendinitis I: Basic Concepts.* Philadelphia, 1992.

———. *Clinics in Sports Medicine: Tendinitis II: Clinical Considerations.* Philadelphia, 1992.

SAAL, JEFFREY A. "Rehabilitation of the Injured Athlete." In *Rehabilitation Medicine: Principles and Practice*, ed. J. A. Delisa. Philadelphia, 1993.

SCHWAB, CONSTANCE D., ed. "Musculoskeletal Pain." In *Physical Medicine and Rehabilitation: State of the Art Reviews.* Philadelphia, 1991.

SPITZER, WALTER O.; HARTH, M.; GOLDSMITH, CHARLES H.; NORMAN, GEOFFREY R.; DICKIE, GORDON L.; BASS, MARTIN J.; and NEWELL, PAUL J. "The Arthritic Complaint in Primary Care: Prevalence, Related Disability, and Costs." *Journal of Rheumatology* 3 (1976):88–99.

TRAVELL, G., and SIMONS, D. G. *Myofascial Pain and Dysfunction: The Trigger Point Manual*, Vols. 1 and 2. Baltimore, 1983.

NATIONAL CENTER FOR HEALTH STATISTICS. *Vital and Health Statistics: Health Data on Older Americans: United States, 1992.* Hyattsville, MD, 1993.

YELIN, EDWARD H., and KATZ, PATRICIA P. "Labor Force Participation Among Persons with Musculoskeletal Conditions." *Arthritis and Rheumatism* 34 (1991):1361–1370.

YELIN, EDWARD; MEENAN, ROBERT; NEWITT, MARK; and EPSTEIN, WALLACE. "Work Disability in Rheumatoid Arthritis: Effects of Disease, Social and Work Factors." *Annals of Internal Medicine* 93 (1980):551–556.

MARK KLAIMAN
JEANNE HICKS

MUSIC THERAPY

Music therapy is the use of music and sound in the treatment of illness and the maintenance of good health. Music contains emotional value and physical properties that bring about desirable changes in physical and mental well-being. Those changes are measurable and progressive. Knowledge about music, creativity, and the liberal arts gives music therapists the tools to achieve the goals of rehabilitation in health management and care giving.

Physical disabilities range from that of not being able to speak, see, or hear, to neurological problems or brain disorders. Performing and listening to music function as aural-physical guides during rehabilitation. Adaptive music instruments and electronic equipment serve as prostheses for patients with little or no mobility. Movement of hands, feet, and facial expressions signal sound sources from which music is performed. Listening skills are enhanced through guided music sessions. Music therapy supports physical, occupational, and movement therapies and is adjunctive to medical treatments. If directed within a complete plan of care, it can give persons with physical disabilities the energy, balance, and control needed to live a rewarding life.

Mental disabilities caused by psychological, physical, or neurological disruptions range from that of not being able to communicate, emote, realize, or discriminate to severe levels of psychoses or schizophrenia. Communication through music (the act of creating music between the therapist and client or clients) is nonverbal and nonthreatening. It is a form of expressive language that is healing. Feelings such as anger, frustration, fear, and anxiety are improvised upon instruments and the voice. Those feelings are observed by the music therapist and are used as motives for musical improvisation. Improvisational music therapy is an effective means of treatment for persons with mental disabilities.

Music therapy methods consist of:

1. Improvisational music therapy—the process of inventing music between the client or clients and the therapist, as the therapist observes them. Voice, instruments, and electronic media are used in musical improvisation.
2. Vocal music therapy—evoking specific vocal responses from the client or clients through song. Those responses form opera and drama scripts that are used in music therapy. Original compositions and published song materials are available for this purpose.
3. Adaptive music therapy—the use of music to condition or educate clients for cognitive, physical, and psychological rehabilitation. Observation of physiological responses of clients during addiction and stress reduction programs is included in this method.
4. Multimodal music therapy—the use of combined methods of music therapy to achieve treatment goals and objectives for specific clients.

Professional music therapists practice in the United States, Canada, and abroad. Having fulfilled requirements and standards, they receive their credentials from the following organizations: the National Association for Music Therapy (NAMT), the American Association for Music Therapy (AAMT), or the Canadian Association for Music Therapy. Many receive board certification from the Certification Board for Music Therapists. Others practice abroad, earning this privilege by completing curricular or degree requirements from music schools that are associated with hospitals or other institutions. Some colleges and universities offer degree programs in music therapy in the United States and are accredited by the NAMT and/or the AAMT. Most are full members of the National Association of Schools of Music.

The preparation of music therapists consists of:

1. Education leading to a baccalaureate degree in music or its equivalent—completion of general studies; knowledge of music theory, history, performance, analysis, arranging, and composition.
2. Music therapy foundations and methods—knowledge of the history, processes, and practices of music therapy; performance on guitar, piano, and voice; skill in improvisation.
3. Psychological, clinical, and rehabilitative management skills—knowledge of general psychology and interpersonal relations; abnormal psychology and psychopathology; biology, anatomy (or other life sciences); human resources and case management; public relations and administration.
4. Field and internship training—completion of supervised practica and internships in compliance with a credential-granting music therapy association that the candidate selects.
5. Advanced education—completion of master's or doctoral-level degree programs in music therapy or allied disciplines; advanced development of clinical and/or research skills; publication and dissemination of music therapy findings to scholars, clinicians, and the general public.

The profession of music therapy will continue to develop its methods of practice and research. Technological advancements, however, will improve those methods to a degree that self-access to music therapy will be available to all people with disabilities and to persons in health management programs. Clinical access to music and creative arts therapies under qualified personnel will establish independence for persons with disabilities and an avenue through which use of the arts, both recreational and expressive, will be enjoyed.

Unlike the entertainment industry, self-access music and arts therapies will emphasize availability of specific treatments for persons with disabilities in which they may control their own therapy environment. Personal attention to clients, with care given to little or no restriction on time, place, and type of disability, will be a priority for therapists practicing this method. Homebound persons will be able to communicate over modems, Picturephone lines, and virtual computer networks with little or no difficulty. Equipment will be adapted to meet their needs. Clients will be able to communicate with other persons with disabilities or with nondisabled persons living abroad or within their geographic location. It will be possible for an international group music therapy session to occur.

Self-access music therapy will not replace traditional music therapy but will reinforce and enhance it. Consideration of limitations of people with disabilities and their incapacity to contact therapists regularly will be an important part of this therapy.

Music therapists, then, will practice in a manner that combines clinical, personal, and professional skills, emphasizing music as rehabilitative management for the well-being of persons with disabilities.

To maintain standards in professional practice and research, the future music therapist will continue his or her education in data management, human resources, research, development, and electronic music and recording. The future availability of music and creative arts therapies for people with disabilities will be both in and out of institutionalized life. Funding and authorized legislation will be required for such implementation.

(*See also:* ART THERAPY; DANCE/MOVEMENT THERAPY; OCCUPATIONAL THERAPY; RECREATION)

RESOURCES

American Association for Music Therapy, P.O. Box 80012, Valley Forge, PA 19484.

Canadian Association for Music Therapy, Wilfrid Laurier University, Room 238, 202 Regina St., Waterloo, Ontario N2L 3C5, Canada.

Certification Board for Music Therapists, Suite 326, Box 345, 6336 North Oracle Road, Tucson, AZ 85704-5457.

Institute for Music and Healing, P.O. 697, Immaculata College, Immaculata, PA 19345.

National Association for Music Therapy, 8455 Colesville Road, Suite 930, Silver Spring, MD 20910.

Notable Software, P.O. 1166, Dept. CSMT, Philadelphia, PA 19105.

BIBLIOGRAPHY

BRUSCIA, KENNETH. *Improvisational Models of Music Therapy.* Springfield, IL, 1987.

BRUSCIA, KENNETH, and HESSER, BARBARA. "Essential Competencies for the Practice of Music Therapy." *Music Therapy: The Journal of the American Association for Music Therapy* 1 (1981):44–48.

CLYNES, MANFRED, ed. *Music, Mind, and Brain.* New York, 1982.

HANSER, SUZANNE. "Music Therapy and Stress Reduction Research." *Journal of Music Therapy* 22 (1985):193–206.

LEE, MATHEW H. M. *Rehabilitation, Music, and Human Well-Being.* St. Louis, MO, 1989.

NORDOFF, PAUL, and ROBBINS, CLIVE. *Creative Music Therapy.* New York, 1977.

PETERS, JACQUELINE SCHMIDT. *Music Therapy: An Introduction.* Springfield, IL, 1987.

SCARTELLI, JOSEPH P. *Music and Self-Management Methods.* St. Louis, MO, 1989.

SPINTEGE, RALPH, and DROH, ROLAND, eds. *Music-Medicine.* St. Louis, MO, 1992.

WIGRAM, ANTHONY, and HEAL, MARGARET. *Music Therapy in Health and Education.* Philadelphia, 1993.

JEAN ANTHONY GILENO

MYASTHENIA GRAVIS (MG)

See NEUROMUSCULAR DISORDERS

N

NATIVE AMERICANS

See MINORITIES

NERVOUS SYSTEM

See NEUROLOGICAL DISORDERS; NEUROMUSCULAR DISORDERS

NEUROLOGICAL DISORDERS

Neurological diseases have a prevalence of 4 percent to 9 percent in the general population. Because of the high level of specialization in the nervous system, there are more than 100 disabling neurological symptoms, directly impairing almost every individual human function. Neurological disabilities are usually multifold, and combinations vary widely from patient to patient. The poor capability for regeneration by the central nervous system leads to rarely curable and often progressive disabilities.

Therefore, neurological diseases represent a tremendous challenge for rehabilitation. The following overview concerns the common neurological disorders producing disability. It is beyond the scope of this entry to provide specific details and nuances of these disorders, in which variability is commonplace.

Stroke

Stroke results from local thrombosis, embolism, or hemorrhage. The main etiologies are microangiopathies (slowly progressive lesions of the very small blood vessels), large-vessel arteriosclerosis, and cardiac embolism. The common mechanism is local interruption of blood supply leading to neuronal death.

Stroke sequelae represent the most common cause of neurological disability over age fifty. The yearly incidence of stroke in the general population is about 0.2 percent. One-third of stroke patients die within three weeks, and one-third are expected to recover fully, giving an incidence of disability of about 0.08 percent per year and a prevalence of 0.5 percent.

Extreme sensitivity of the central nervous system to ischemia, or deficiency in blood supply (i.e., neuronal death within five to ten minutes of complete ischemia) limits the practical application of potentially useful treatments to the central core of an ischemic area. Therefore, acute treatments aim at reducing the extension of stroke by optimizing blood supply (hemodilution), restoring it (thrombolysis), or supporting or rescuing the endangered tissue around the already dying ischemic epicenter (calcium antagonists, lazaroids). These treatments need to be introduced within at least six hours of the beginning of ischemia to prevent irreversible damage.

Progress in stroke research has led to the determination of risk factors: smoking, hypercholesterolemia, hypertension, diabetes, and cardiac anomalies. Such determinations allow the development of primary prevention targeted at the general population (e.g., smoking cessation, changing dietary and lifestyle habits). More specific prevention is targeted at subpopulations with an increased risk to develop a stroke. Secondary prevention aims at reducing the incidence of stroke recurrence by introducing specific treatments (e.g., antiaggregation, anticoagulation, carotid surgery, or angioplasty). Seventy-five percent of strokes due to arteriosclerosis have been preceded by transient ischemic attacks (TIA—neurological deficit completely improving within 24 hours, and usually within 30 minutes). Rapid assessment and treatment of patients with TIAs reduce their risk to develop subsequently definitive dysfunction. TIA with ipsilateral severe carotid stenosis (a reduction of 70% or more of the carotid lumen [cavity] on the same side) has been shown to be an indication for surgery (endarterectomy: surgical removal of the partial obstruction of an artery). These measures have led to an observed decrease in stroke incidence and mortality in Western countries (there has been a 20% to 50% decrease from the 1950s).

Prognosis is variable, and no good predictive index is available. As a general rule, the more severe the initial impairment, the slower the subsequent improvement during the first two weeks following the stroke, and the more severe the disability at six months. Severe sensory loss, severe paresis (paralysis), trunk balance loss, hemineglect, confusion episodes, and initial urinary incontinence usually carry poor prognoses. Stroke may herald other forms of cardiovascular disease: Myocardial infarction represents the main cause of death in stroke survivors.

In the acute phase, patients may require particular care of skin, eye, mouth, bladder, and bowel, and monitoring of cardiac and respiratory functions, especially when consciousness is impaired. They also require early mobilization of joints to prevent contracture. These management points improve long-term outcome. Initial care is usually best provided in a specialized neurological intensive care unit.

Rehabilitation represents an important part of treatment following a stroke, though few appropriate studies are available. Regarding motor function, no particular rehabilitative method has been proved to be more effective than others, but final outcomes seem better when patients are treated by rehabilitation "specialists." The intensity of the rehabilitation may have a greater impact on the speed of recovery than on the long-term result. Concerning cognitive functions, a specific evaluation is warranted for each patient to determine the type and extent of impairment. This approach allows appropriate stimulation of these patients by providing pertinent advice to caregivers and relatives. Specialized training does not appear to improve long-term outcome compared to regular stimulation by adequately informed caregivers.

Epilepsy

Seizures result from the sudden disorderly discharges of cerebral, usually cortical, neurons. Various clinical manifestations may be induced, depending on the localization and extent of the discharge. Localized seizures can mimic any single central nervous system function and are called focal or partial seizures. Generalized seizures involve the entire cortex, leading to loss of consciousness, with (grand mal) or without (petit mal) generalized tonic-clonic (firm and violent muscle contraction that is sustained [tonic] and then alternating with muscle relaxation [clonic] as motor manifestation of a seizure) seizures. Partial seizures may become secondarily generalized. The term "epilepsy" is used to denote recurrent seizures. *Status epilepticus* is a life-threatening condition defined as seizures repeating themselves continuously or frequently enough to prevent the subject from regaining consciousness.

Single or brief outbursts of seizures represent a common situation in the general population, with a lifetime prevalence of 2 percent to 5 percent and a population prevalence of 2 percent. Seizures are indicative of central nervous system involvement in numerous illnesses. If single seizures are excluded, prevalence of epilepsy is evaluated between 0.5 percent and 1 percent. Epilepsy represents the single most common serious neurological condition in children and the second most common in adults (second to cerebrovascular disease).

Though numerous etiologies exist, in most cases no cause can be demonstrated (primary or idiopathic epilepsy). The major causes of symptomatic (secondary) epilepsies are: brain trauma, congenital malformations, tumors, metabolic disturbances, drugs and toxins (e.g., alcohol), and cerebrovascular diseases and infections (meningitis, encephalitis, and abscess). Heredity is an important factor. The order of frequency of causes depends on the age of epilepsy onset. Some of the primary epilepsies, particularly during childhood and adolescence, share particularities in symptoms and prognoses, allowing grouping into syndromes: for example, Lennox-Gastaut (atonic seizures—characterized by a loss of the normal muscular tonus—with progressive intellectual impairment, and particularly resistant to current treatments); and petit mal (frequent brief and subtle consciousness suspension, often mistaken for periods of inattention, usually totally improving with anticonvulsant therapy). Classifications of epilepsy are usually based on the aforementioned characteristics: symptoms, etiology, localization, and age at onset.

Beside the potential removal of the underlying cause (when defined), treatment of epilepsy is mainly based on regular anticonvulsant drug therapy associated with physical and mental hygiene. Avoiding sleep deprivation, alcohol, and drug consumption is essential in reducing the frequency of seizures. Alterations in lifestyle may impose social or employment restriction (e.g., no "shift work").

Fortunately, in about 60 to 70 percent of patients developing epilepsy, the condition will remit and only 4 to 7 per thousand will have one or more seizures per week. When epilepsy is under control, the physical restrictions are usually minimal, and most physical activities may be allowed (e.g., driving a car is usually allowed when the patient is treated and has been seizure-free for at least six to twelve months). In contrast, when epilepsy is not controlled, and especially when seizures are not preceded by a premonition (aura), caution is essential, and many activities must be avoided (e.g., swimming, ladder climbing, and driving).

The physical problems encountered in association with epilepsy are limited (only 10% of epileptics will have an associated physical impairment). Epilepsy rehabilitation mainly faces problems of psychological support, social isolation, and employment repercussions.

Cognitive deficits are frequent. Their causes may be multiple, and a specific workup is often useful to identify and differentiate the effect of the underlying pathology from repeated minimal craniocerebral trauma due to seizures or side effects of anticonvulsant medications. A cognitive assessment may be particularly useful for the young patient making employment decisions.

Psychological and psychiatric disturbances represent a major aspect of the rehabilitation of persons with epilepsy. Anxiety and depression are common, and both can prevent the individual from being appropriately active. Aggressive and psychotic behavior may also appear, especially in association with temporal lobe epilepsy. When related to the seizure, these behavioral changes are usually stereotyped (a persistent maintaining of a bodily attitude and/or a repetition of senseless movements), and electroencephalographic discharges (EEG seizure patterns) may be recorded. These behavioral symptoms may be prolonged during the postictal (following the seizure) period and last for hours. Abnormal behavior may also be associated with the underlying condition or a maladaptive rehabilitation program. Psychiatric advice is often valuable in this context.

Neurodegenerative Disorders

Neurodegenerative disorders include Alzheimer's disease (AD), Parkinson's disease (PD), motoneuron diseases (MND), and related diseases. AD is characterized by progressive loss of cortical neurons leading to dementia. PD is due to the degeneration of the nigrostriatal dopaminergic neurons (neurons projecting from one of the deep brain nuclei to another and using the dopamine as neurotransmitter) and is clinically diagnosed on the basis of the association of two of the following: Rigidity tremor, bradykinesia (slowness of movement), and impaired postural balance. MND consists of a combination of progressive upper and lower motor neuron dysfunction, leading to paralysis.

Because the population is aging, neurodegenerative diseases will represent the second cause of mortality by the beginning of the twenty-first century (second to cardiovascular disease and surpassing cancer). Their increasing prevalence is also due to an increasing incidence in all age groups. Figures as of 1994 are: AD, incidence of 25 to 50 per 100,000 per year, with prevalence reaching 10 percent above age sixty-five; PD, respectively 15 to 20 per 100,000 per year and about 200 per 100,000; MND, 1 to 2 per 100,000 per year and 4 to 10 per 100,000.

Each of these neurodegenerative entities includes in its differential diagnosis a substantial number of treatable causes. They need to be ruled out or treated as a first priority. The actual etiologies and pathological mechanisms of the neurodegenerative diseases are unknown. Various potential causes include: environmental toxin exposure, infection, autoimmunity, heredity, and combinations of these factors. The possibility of various etiologies leading to similar clinical manifestations is certainly conceivable. Neurodegenerative diseases are characterized by relentless progression, and symptoms typically appear only after substantial irreversible neuronal loss has occurred. There is no treatment yet proven to be significantly effective in slowing down the progression of any of these diseases.

Rehabilitation of patients with neurodegenerative diseases faces the prospect of worsening disability in older patients. Long-term programs aimed at preventing function loss and maintaining independence are more appropriate than time-limited interventions. Regular reassessments may prevent detrimental over- or understimulation. Over the years, care giving often depends on substantial involvement of family and relatives. Support and appropriate information for these nonprofessional caregivers help them face the increasing workload added to the depressing reality of progressive disability in their affected relative. These carers also require occasional respite from the great strain of their long-term work (day care, short stay in hospital or home, etc.). Realistic attitudes will help avoid rapid institutionalization of patients. Following is a brief review of some peculiarities of the three major neurodegenerative disorders, keeping in mind that their features commonly overlap.

In AD there is a progressive impairment in cognitive function, leading to loss of memory, orientation, ability to solve day-to-day problems, self-care, emotional control, and judgment. The ability to learn, to adapt to new situations, or to generalize new acquisitions is progressively lost. The majority of rehabilitation techniques rely on enhancement of the less impaired functions by positive reinforcement, and on a progressive adaptation of the environment. Neuroleptics may be useful if behavior becomes aggressive.

In PD, the relative restriction of degeneration to a particular neuronal subpopulation has allowed introduction of symptomatic treatments. These treatments aim at improving dysfunctional neurotransmission, resulting in a temporary reduction in physical impairment. Controversies exist over the potential effects of these treatments on the underlying cause and course of the disease. Techniques to replace or support damaged neurons (fetal mesencephalic graft [transplantation of part of the fetal brain], neurotrophic factors—substances contributing to neuronal thriving) are currently being evaluated. Symptomatic treatments usually postpone disability effectively. This "honeymoon" interval can be used to prepare and plan for the future, when further progression will lead to reappearance of symptoms and potentially disabling side effects requiring increased drug dosages. Physiotherapy (with moderate physical training) and occupational therapy with education of patient and relatives have been proven to be beneficial.

In contrast with the two former entities, MND has a very poor prognosis, with survival from time of diagnosis ranging from one to fifteen years in amyotrophic lateral sclerosis and about five months to seven years in the bulbar form. Cognitive functions are usually preserved until death, allowing full participation of the patient in critical decisions. When the diagnosis is established, the patient needs truthful information to allow planning for the future. Moderately active and passive physiotherapy is beneficial. It optimizes the function of preserved musculature and avoids contractures. Antispasmodic medication may be beneficial when spasticity is severe. With progressing disability, orthopedic and other mechanical devices are needed to assist patients in using their limbs. To preserve maximal autonomy and communication, environmental adjustment, speech therapies, and, later, various computerized devices are needed. Difficulties swallowing leading to choking are reduced by a nasogastric tube or gastrostomy. Death, usually following bronchoaspiration and pneumonia, is often accepted by the patient as a relief. The rapid evolution of symptoms may not permit progressive adjustment by uninformed relatives. Professionals can help to avoid unrealistic procedures or expenses during the progression and any feelings of guilt coincident with impending death.

Multiple Sclerosis

Multiple sclerosis (MS) is a disease of the central nervous system white matter. The etiology is unknown, but the mechanism likely involves major participation of the immune system. MS may induce lesions in any part of the central nervous system, leading to an extremely variable clinical presentation and evolution. Clinical diagnosis is based on evidence for at least two central nervous system lesions distinct in location and in time of onset. Magnetic resonance imaging and cerebrospinal fluid examination allow earlier and more accurate diagnosis.

MS is the most common neurological cause of chronic physical disability in young adults. Its prevalence increases with latitude from the equator. The incidence of MS in the United States is estimated at 3 to 4 per 100,000 per year, and the prevalence at 60 per 100,000. In two-thirds of patients the course of the disease is remitting-relapsing, while 15 percent will have a progressive form with superimposed exacerbation. The remainder have a continuously progressive form. The ratio of continuous progressive

forms increases with length of disease, reaching 65 percent after twenty-five years of evolution.

A positive familial history increases the overall risk of having the disease about tenfold. Controversies exist concerning the roles of stress and trauma on the disease. Infection may trigger relapses, but vaccination is not detrimental. Pregnancy seems to have a "protective effect," but delivery may be followed by three to six months of a slightly increased risk of relapse.

Current treatments target the immune system. Short courses of high-dose corticosteroids have a significant beneficial impact on the acute relapse and are broadly accepted, as indicated in this context. They have no proven beneficial effect on long-term prognosis. Immunosuppression with azathioprine, cyclophosphamide, or cyclosporine has yielded minimal benefit, although side effects may be substantial. Copolymer 1 may reduce the number of relapses, as shown by a double-blind study. Similarly, treatment with beta interferon has been shown recently by a multicentric double-blind study to reduce the number of relapses. Further studies are needed to confirm these promising results. It also has to be determined if these two treatments will reduce the progression of the disability.

Prognosis is variable and difficult to predict: Monosymptomatic onset with visual and sensory symptoms appears to have a better long-term prognosis than polysymptomatic onset with motor involvement and early continuous progression. Disability increases with disease duration, reaching a significant level of impairment of 80 percent of patients after 20 years of evolution.

Motor impairment, particularly difficulty in walking, is probably the most common disabling symptom encountered in MS patients. It results from any combination of motor weakness, spasticity, cerebellar ataxia (failure of muscular coordination resulting from damage to the pathways allowing cerebellar control on the movements), and sensory dysfunction. Regular active and passive physical therapy is beneficial in increasing strength and avoiding disabling spastic contractures. Spasticity management also includes proper limb positioning, reduction of external stimuli (e.g., skin lesions and catheters), proper use of orthotics and casting, pharmacological management (general or intrathecal—delivered directly within the spinal canal), nerve or neuromuscular junction blocks, and orthopedic and neurosurgical procedures (in severe cases).

Cerebellar ataxia is particularly resistant to rehabilitation and often requires adaptive equipment. Use of intact vision may compensate for sensory loss. Impaired urinary continence is also extremely common and has important psychological effects. Treatments include medication, catheterization, and surgical procedures. Proper treatment is frequently optimized by initial urodynamic examination. Sexual dysfunction is another distressing symptom, although fertility is usually not impaired. Appropriate physical and psychological counseling is warranted in the face of various related symptoms, such as fatigue, decreased libido, and orgasm or erectile dysfunction. Pain is frequent during the course of the disease but may often be unrecognized by caregivers. Acute paroxysmal pain (neuralgia, Lhermitte's phenomenon—pain resembling an electrical shock and produced by the flexion of the neck) usually improves with carbamazepine, whereas chronic pain is more complex to treat. Fatigue is probably the most common symptom. It is not due to disability or depression, although the latter is also common in MS. Amantadine may help in severe cases of fatigue. Cognitive dysfunction has often been overlooked in the past and deserves appropriate evaluation.

Muscular Dystrophies

Muscular dystrophies are inheritable diseases leading to progressive muscular weakness and atrophy. Inheritance may be linked to the sex chromosome—for example, Duchenne's dystrophy (DD), Becker's dystrophy (BD): Females are asymptomatic carriers, transmitting the gene to half their daughters and the disease to all their sons. Linkage to autosomal chromosomes (i.e., not linked to sexual differentiation) produces various rates of transmission, depending on the dominance and penetrance of the gene. The commonest autosomal muscular dystrophies—fascio-scapulo-humeral dystrophy (FSH—dystrophy involving the muscles of the face and shoulders), and myotonic dystrophy (dystrophy characterized by the presence of sustained muscle contractions) are autosomal-dominant. Advances in genetic and mo-

lecular biology have allowed localization of the gene and, in some, identification of its defective product (e.g., the membrane-bound protein "dystrophin" in DD and BD). These advances permit prenatal diagnosis. The possibility of treatment with genetic engineering has led to significant controversy over important ethical issues.

The various dystrophies are clinically characterized by age of onset, particular distribution of the most impaired muscles, and various participation of other organs (e.g., heart, eye, brain). Spinal muscular atrophies (autosomal-recessive diseases of the motoneurons), polymyositis (inflammatory muscular diseases), and other congenital myopathies are among the principal differential diagnoses. Electromyography, biopsy of a mildly affected muscle, and blood elevation of the muscular enzyme creatine phosphokinase usually allow diagnostic confirmation.

Incidence and prevalence of DD are: 0.5 percent of male birth, 3 per 100,000. The related BD is less frequent. MD has a prevalence of 5 per 100,000.

The prognosis of these currently untreatable diseases varies from significant disability during the first decade and death at about the end of the second one in DD, to appearance of the initial signs during adolescence and almost normal life expectancy in FSH.

Rehabilitation faces three main goals: promotion of muscular function, prevention of deformities, and prevention of pulmonary complications. Muscular exercise has to be regular and prolonged rest avoided or reduced (e.g., postsurgery). Stretching may delay the appearance of atrophic contractures. Tenotomies (surgical sections of a tendon) allow compensation for the muscular shortening. Progressive introduction of orthotics may prolong independence and slow down development of contractures and deformities. Adequate regimens avoid excessive weight gain. Environmental adaptation may improve independence and help mobilization by caregivers. Orthopedic procedures may be necessary to avoid development of deformities (e.g., scoliosis), especially in the growing child or adolescent. Respiratory complications are one of the major problems encountered during the evolution of these diseases. They are due to the combination of respiratory musculature weakness, restrictive syndrome (scoliosis), and silent bronchoaspiration (pharyngeal musculature weakness). Avoiding a supine position during sleep reduces abdominal pressure on the diaphragm and risk of bronchoaspiration. Regular physiotherapy and, if necessary, assisted ventilation reduce formation of lung atelectasis (a collapsed lung) and the appearance of nocturnal hypoxia (oxygen deficiency). When cardiopathies (cardiac lesions) are associated, conduction impairment may necessitate introduction of a pacemaker.

In addition to genetic counseling, families need information and support to face these dramatic diseases, which progressively become more psychologically and physically demanding.

(*See also:* ALZHEIMER'S DISEASE; GENETIC DISORDERS; HEAD INJURY; NEUROLOGY; NEUROMUSCULAR DISORDERS; ORGANIC MENTAL DISORDERS; SPINAL CORD INJURY; STROKE)

RESOURCES

American Academy of Neurology, 2221 University Ave., SE, Suite 335, Minneapolis, MN 55414

American Congress of Rehabilitation Medicine, 5700 Old Orchard Road, 1st Floor, Skokie, IL 60077–1057

American Society of Neurorehabilitation, 2221 University Ave., SE, Suite 360, Minneapolis, MN 55414

BIBLIOGRAPHY

ADAMS, RAYMOND D., and VICTOR, MAURICE. *Principles of Neurology*, 5th ed. New York, 1993.

ASBURY, ARTHUR K.; MCKHANN, GUY M.; and MCDONALD, W. IAN. *Diseases of the Nervous System: Clinical Neurobiology*, 2nd ed. Philadelphia, 1993.

BOGOUSSLAVSKY, JULIEN, and CAPLAN, LOUIS R. *Stroke Syndromes*. Cambridge, Eng., 1995.

CALNE, DONALD B. *Neurodegenerative Diseases*. Philadelphia, 1994.

ENGEL, ANDREW G., and BANKER, BETTY Q. *Myology*. New York, 1986.

GREENWOOD, RICHARD; BARNES, MICHAEL P.; MCMILLAN, THOMAS M.; and WARD, CHRISTOPHER D. *Neurological Rehabilitation*. London, 1993.

PORTER, ROGER J., and MORSELLI, PAOLO L. *The Epilepsies*. London, 1985.

FRANÇOIS VINGERHOETS
JULIEN BOGOUSSLAVSKY

NEUROLOGY

Neurology is a medical specialty dealing with illnesses and injuries affecting the brain, spinal cord, peripheral nerves, and muscle. Examples of conditions treated by neurologists include epilepsy, headache, stroke, multiple sclerosis, cerebral palsy, dementia, disorders of the peripheral nerves, and muscular disorders. Many neurological conditions cause long-term disability and require rehabilitation. Fifty percent to 65 percent of patients in inpatient rehabilitation hospitals or units have neurological causes for their disabilities (Selzer, 1992). Training programs for neurologists must include the basic principles of rehabilitation, and some neurologists specialize in the rehabilitative aspects of neurological diseases. Neurologists sometimes serve as medical directors of rehabilitation programs.

In 1990 more than 8,000 physicians in the United States listed neurology as their primary specialty (Ringel, 1991). Physicians specializing in adult neurology are required to take at least one year of general residency training following graduation from medical school. This year must include at least six months' experience in internal medicine. Future neurologists then enter an intensive three-year residency program devoted to neurological disease. In 1992 there were 121 adult neurology training programs in the United States (JAMA, 1993), almost all affiliated with medical schools and their teaching hospitals and clinics. In addition to adult neurology, residents must have experience in psychiatry, rehabilitation, pediatric neurology, and the radiological and pathological correlates of neurological disease (AMA, 1993). Residents also receive training in electroencephalography (EEG), electromyography (EMG) and nerve conduction studies, evoked potentials, and other diagnostic procedures. In 1992 there were sixty-nine child neurology training programs in the United States. Prior training in general pediatrics is required. The three-year pediatric neurology residency curriculum is similar to that of adult neurology training programs but emphasizes pediatric neurological conditions.

Board certification in either neurology or child neurology is granted by the American Board of Psychiatry and Neurology (ABPN). Most American neurologists have attained certification (*JAMA*, 1993; Kurtzke, Murphy, and Smith, 1991). To become board-certified, candidates must successfully complete an accredited residency program and then pass rigorous written and oral examinations (ABPN, 1992). Many neurologists elect to receive additional fellowship training in one or more neurology subspecialty areas. This requires an additional one or two years of training and may result in subspecialty certification. The American Board of Psychiatry and Neurology and the American Board of Physical Medicine and Rehabilitation offer dual certification for physicians who have completed thirty months of an accredited residency program in each discipline and successfully complete the board certification examinations in both.

Most neurologists belong to one or more professional societies. Each society has certain membership benefits, holds an annual meeting, and sponsors a scientific journal. The largest organization is the American Academy of Neurology (AAN) with approximately 12,000 members in 1994. Members of the AAN who have a special interest in rehabilitation may join the Neurorehabilitation Section, currently the largest section in the AAN. Other national neurological societies include the American Neurological Association and the Child Neurology Society.

Neurologists with a special interest in rehabilitation also may join rehabilitation societies open to a variety of professional disciplines, including the American Congress of Rehabilitation Medicine (ACRM) and the American Society of Neurorehabilitation (ASNR). The ASNR offers a certified membership to physicians who are board eligible or certified in a medical specialty, who have at least one year of full-time postresidency training or experience in diagnosing and managing patients with chronic neurological disabilities, and pass the society's certifying examination.

To diagnose neurological conditions, neurologists primarily rely on the patient's medical history, general physical examination, and a special neurological examination. In addition, a variety of diagnostic tests may be ordered, depending on the nature of the patient's problem. Standardized pen and paper or computerized tests are commonly used to test cognitive abilities or intellectual functions. Other studies directly visualize the anatomy of the brain, spinal cord, or surrounding structures, and may demonstrate structural abnormalities. Examples include computerized axial tomography (CAT scans) or magnetic resonance imaging (MRI). Other tests reflect the functional abilities or metabolic activity of the brain or spinal cord. A few examples include electroencephalography (EEG), single photon emission computerized tomography (SPECT scans), and evoked potentials (EP). Other studies evaluate the function of the peripheral nerves and muscles—for example, electromyography (EMG) and nerve conduction velocities. Still other tests measure chemical, enzymatic, immunological, or inflammatory processes related to neurological disease. Included here are a variety of blood tests and evaluation of cerebrospinal fluid obtained via a lumbar puncture (spinal tap). Finally, other tests evaluate the blood supply of the brain. A variety of techniques are used depending on the specific situation, including injection of X-ray contrast dye directly into arteries (conventional X-ray angiography), and less invasive procedures such as magnetic resonance angiography (MRA), ultrasound, or Doppler studies.

After a diagnosis is established, an appropriate treatment plan is developed. Treatment is often directed both toward curing or ameliorating the underlying illness or injury and improving the functional abilities of the patient through rehabilitation. The involvement of neurologists in the rehabilitation of their patients provides continuity of care. Rehabilitation programs are an integral part of the treatment of many neurological conditions, including stroke, multiple sclerosis, cerebral palsy, muscular dystrophy, and brain injury.

The neurologist works with many traditional rehabilitation disciplines in an effort to promote functional recovery, including rehabilitation nursing, physical therapy, occupational therapy, speech/language pathology, rehabilitation psychology, recreational therapy, nutrition, and others. Services are often provided by an interdisciplinary team, of which the physician is a key member. Goals are individualized according to the needs of each person served, and a host of individual treatment strategies are employed. The physician's role is to oversee and coordinate these services in light of the person's overall medical condition so that appropriate efficacious strategies are employed and strategies that may be medically harmful to the patient are avoided.

Preventive measures for medical problems that may complicate rehabilitation should be prescribed. For example, complications such as venous thrombosis in the legs, pressure sores, contractures, and pneumonia are often preventable, and if they occur despite preventive efforts, must be promptly identified and treated. Other medical complications include seizures, depression, muscle spasticity, pain syndromes, bladder dysfunction, and urinary tract infections. Depending on the problem, treatment may include medications, orthoses (braces), or physical measures such as stretching or exercise. The neurologist should also be certain that medications are not causing detrimental side effects such as confusion, depression, or weakness, which might affect rehabilitation.

The neurologist also serves as an educational resource for the patient, family, and rehabilitation team. For example, the neurologist may explain how a neurological condition may be causing symptoms or problems that interfere with the patient's rehabilitation and suggest strategies to overcome these difficulties.

Finally, the role of neurology in advancing understanding of the basic scientific mechanisms of disease and recovery must be stressed (Selzer, 1992). The basic neurosciences consist of an extensive body of knowledge in physiology, molecular biology, and pharmacology. New knowledge regarding how the nervous system reorganizes its function after illness or injury will likely lead to new strategies to enhance recovery.

(See also: NEUROLOGICAL DISORDERS; PSYCHIATRY)

RESOURCES

American Academy of Neurology, 2221 University Ave., SE, Suite 335, Minneapolis, MN 55414

American Board of Physical Medicine and Rehabilitation, Norwest Center, Suite 674, 21 First St., SW, Rochester, MN 55902

American Board of Psychiatry and Neurology, 500 Lake Cook Road, Ste. 335, Deerfield, IL 60015

American Congress of Rehabilitation Medicine, 5700 Old Orchard Road, 1st Floor, Skokie, IL 60077-1057

American Medical Association, 515 N. State St., Chicago, IL 60610

Child Neurology Society, 475 Cleveland Ave., N, Suite 220, St. Paul, MN 55104-5051

American Society of Neurorehabilitation, 2221 University Ave., SE, Suite 360, Minneapolis, MN 55414

BIBLIOGRAPHY

AMERICAN BOARD OF PSYCHIATRY AND NEUROLOGY. "Information for Applicants." Deerfield, IL, 1992.

AMERICAN MEDICAL ASSOCIATION. "Special Requirements for Residency Training in Neurology." Graduate Medical Education Directory 1993–1994. Chicago, 1993.

Journal of the American Medical Association (JAMA). "Graduate Medical Education." JAMA 270 (1993):1116–1122

KURTZKE, JOHN F.; MURPHY, FRANCES M.; and SMITH, MELINDA A. "On the Production of Neurologists in the United States: An Update." Neurology 41 (1991):1–9.

RINGEL, STEVEN P. "Neurologists—1990." Neurology 41 (1991):1863–1866.

SELZER, MICHAEL E. "Neurological Rehabilitation." Annals of Neurology 32 (1992):695–699.

DAVID C. GOOD

NEUROMUSCULAR DISORDERS

Neuromuscular disorders (NMDs) involve the nerves (motor neurons) that connect the brain and spinal cord to muscles, the junction of these nerves and muscles (neuromuscular junction), or the muscles themselves. Since motor neurons provide both control and growth regulation for muscles, any disorder that damages these nerves will impair the muscles as well. Disorders that strike nerves primarily are known as neuropathies and may involve sensory as well as motor nerves. Disorders that attack muscle directly are known as myopathies. Disorders that affect the connection between nerve and muscle are known as neuromuscular junction disorders.

The etiology of the majority of NMDs is unknown; however, breakthroughs are occurring rapidly. There are no known preventive measures and, with the rare exception of viral diseases such as polio, they are not contagious. Further, despite vast improvements in the medical and physical management of NMDs, there are no known true cures. However, great advances have been made in understanding the genetic basis that underlies the physiological aberrations associated with many of the NMDs.

The neural circuitry that underlies the movements of our bodies is an intricate system of feedback loops and control mechanisms that result in smooth, coordinated movement. A breakdown in any part of this system may result in weakness. Motor neurons, a major part of this system, are specialized cells that receive information generated in the motor cortex of the brain and transmit it to muscles. Upper motor neurons connect the brain to the spinal cord, while lower motor neurons connect the spinal cord to the muscles. The cell body of a lower motor neuron is called an anterior horn cell. From this cell arises a massive tangle of nerve branches, called dendrites, that spread out through the spinal cord to receive messages from the brain and other nerve cells. Also arising from the anterior horn cell is the axon, a long, thin nerve "cable" that carries information out to the muscle. At its terminal end in muscle, a motor neuron axon will branch out to innervate many muscle fibers. A single motor neuron and the muscle fibers to which it is connected form the elemental unit of motor design known as the motor unit. Information in motor neurons is carried in small bursts of electrical signals known as action potentials. To generate more strength, neighboring motor neurons are recruited to help out. Sensory feedback coming back to the brain and spinal cord from the muscle fine-tunes motor unit recruitment so that strength is generated appropriately for the movement required.

The ultimate mover of the body is muscle, accounting for 45 percent of the weight of an average person. Each muscle is made up of thousands of muscle fibers. Muscle uses fats or sugars as fuel. It can function with oxygen (aerobically) or without oxygen (anaerobically) and perform work at 40 percent efficiency (about the same as a diesel engine). A fundamental property of muscle is contractility, or the ability to produce tension. Muscular tension is a direct function of the number of operating sarcomeres within muscle fibers. Sarcomeres are the basic protein structures responsible for contraction. Activation of the sarcomeres and the subsequent contraction of muscle fibers is triggered by electrical signals received from the motor neuron.

The neuromuscular junction is a distinct area at the terminal end of a motor neuron axon where it hooks up with a muscle fiber. The action potentials traveling down the motor neuron trigger the release of a chemical neurotransmitter, acetylcholine, from the tip of the neuron. This chemical, released in packets called quanta, diffuses across a small cleft and attaches to a receptor on the receiving end of a muscle fiber in an area known as the end plate. This is where the electrical signal from the motor neuron is transmitted to muscle and initiates contraction.

Diagnosis

Neuromuscular disorders can affect people of all ages. The initial symptoms usually noted are fatigue and muscular weakness. (With the exception of polio, pain is generally not an initial symptom.) This is followed by signs of muscle wasting or atrophy. For further evaluation and diagnosis, most family physicians refer the affected person to a specialist. Specialists who diagnose and treat NMDs include neurologists, physiatrists (physicians specializing in physical medicine and rehabilitation), and orthopedic surgeons. The diagnosis of NMDs is based on: (1) complete history and physical examination; (2) electrodiagnostic studies; (3) muscle biopsy; and (4) DNA analysis, usually done on blood cells.

During the physical exam, the physician completes a check of the neurological system as well as the other major organ systems. Many other diseases, including cardiac and respiratory problems, can cause weakness and fatigue and must be considered. If the physical examination is consistent with an NMD, then the physician may obtain electrodiagnostic studies. These consist of two parts: (1) nerve conduction studies, which assess electrical conductivity along the nerve and across the neuromuscular junction, and (2) electromyography, in which a needle electrode is inserted into the muscle to assess function directly. A muscle biopsy may then be performed. A small piece of muscle tissue is removed from an affected area (determined by the electrodiagnostic studies) and carefully examined under light and electron microscopes. Special stains are used to prepare the muscle. Biochemical analysis is also performed to look for metabolic problems and abnormal or missing proteins. If necessary, the nerve can be biopsied and examined.

Many of the NMDs are inheritable traits and may be passed along in a family line. NMDs that are not inherited are referred to as acquired. Transmission of inherited disease is due to a specific defect in a section of DNA (the genetic makeup of our chromosomes), which is transferred to offspring through parental sperm or egg. Every cell in our body contains twenty-three pairs of chromosomes, with both parents contributing one-half of each pair. One pair is the sex-determining (XX for female, XY for male) chromosomes. The disease traits can be dominant (need only one copy of the abnormal gene to express the trait), recessive (need two copies, one from each parent), or X-linked (disease appears predominantly in males; females may be carriers). A carrier is someone who is not affected by the disease but may pass it along to an offspring. The carrier has only one copy of the abnormal gene, and the disease is not expressed physically. In autosomal (not sex-linked) recessive disorders, a carrier must mate with another carrier to produce an affected offspring. In autosomal dominant conditions, either affected parent may transmit the condition to the offspring. In X-linked disorders, a female carrier may give birth to an affected male or a carrier female. By examining portions of DNA obtained from tissue (usually blood), scientists can detect deletions (missing segments) or mutations (abnormal segments). Disease diagnosis and carrier detection using these techniques are quite accurate. The accurate detection of a carrier allows potential parents to be informed about the risks of transmitting a disease to their offspring. Unfortunately, in many NMDs a high percentage of the cases arise in families with no history of the disease in their lineage. This happens because of a high mutation rate, which represents a genetic error arising at the time of fertilization. Thus, even with accurate carrier detection and thorough genetic counseling, many of these diseases will still occur in the population. Nevertheless, after the diagnosis of an inheritable NMD is confirmed, any affected person, and blood relatives who are considering having children, should be counseled by a geneticist or ge-

netic counselor, who explains the risks of transmitting the trait to future offspring.

Physical and Medical Complications Associated with NMDs

A common complication in NMDs, particularly the muscular dystrophies, occurs when, due to severe weakness and immobility, the joints become stiff and develop contractures. A contracture is a joint that has lost part of its normal range of motion and may become "stuck" in a certain position. Contractures may occur in any process where the joints are immobilized for a long time. This also includes the joints of the spine. Spinal deformities are also frequently seen in NMDs. Joint contractures and spinal deformities can cause difficulty with seating and positioning and can significantly impair mobility.

Breathing occurs as a result of the contraction and relaxation of the respiratory muscles, which allows inflation and deflation of the lungs. As the respiratory muscles become impaired, the patient may develop "weak bellows," referred to as restrictive lung disease. Despite this term, there is nothing wrong with the lung itself, just the muscles that bring air into the lung. Respiratory complications such as pneumonia and ventilatory failure are the most common causes of death in rapidly progressive NMDs.

The heart is generally not affected by neuropathies. However, in many of the myopathies, the heart muscle itself (myocardium) may be directly involved in the disease process. This may result in a cardiomyopathy, in which the myocardium is weak and pumps poorly, and can cause heart failure. Further, the electrical system of the heart may be involved, resulting in conduction defects and arrhythmias. Like restrictive lung disease, cardiac complications are also frequent causes of death in many of the NMDs.

Overview of the Major Neuromuscular Disorders

Neuropathies. Charcot-Marie-Tooth(CMT)disease is usually a dominant trait that attacks both motor and sensory nerves as early as the first decade of life. It is associated with abnormalities on chromosome 1, 17, and, rarely, on the X chromosome. There is no gender predilection. It is a slowly progressive disease that causes weakness and loss of sensation in the distal extremities (feet, legs, hands, forearms) and generally spares the proximal areas (shoulders, hips, and trunk). However, the phrenic nerve, which controls breathing, may also be affected, and some individuals with CMT have suffered respiratory failure. The heart is not involved. CMT is also called hereditary motor and sensory neuropathy, and there are at least three different forms of the disease. There may be variability in the severity of the diseases, even within a family line. In its mildest form, the disease causes a *pes cavus*, or high-arched foot. More advanced forms require leg braces to maintain ambulation, and sometimes a wheelchair is needed. Other problems associated with CMT include skin ulcerations, spine deformity, and progressive arthritis leading to the development of Charcot joint.

A subset of neuropathies are known more specifically as motor neuron diseases, and they include poliomyelitis, spinal muscular atrophy (SMA), and amyotrophic lateral sclerosis (ALS). ALS is also commonly known as Lou Gehrig's disease. In all three of these disorders the primary problems are caused by death of anterior horn cells and the subsequent degeneration of motor neurons. There is no gender predilection in any of the motor neuron diseases. Although the heart is not involved, mechanical ventilation may be needed to assist breathing. Wheelchairs may be required for locomotion as these disorders progress.

Poliomyelitis was one of the first NMDs whose fundamental cause was clearly delineated. The polio virus directly attacks and kills anterior horn cells, causing subsequent deterioration of motor neurons. The area of the spinal cord invaded by virus determines where the weakness occurs. Patients may suffer respiratory failure as well as arm and leg weakness. Although the exact prevalence rate of poliomyelitis is not known, it is likely the most common worldwide NMD. It remains a significant health problem in many developing countries, despite having been nearly eradicated in the industrialized countries by effective vaccinations. Postpolio syndrome is a term used to describe people who have recovered from prior poliomyelitis but experience progressive neuromuscular weakness later in life for reasons that are not clear.

SMA, of which there are at least five different types, is a recessive trait that appears to be related to an abnormality on chromosome 5. It occurs in about 1 in 20,000 live births. One form of SMA usually results in death before age one year. In milder forms of SMA, the life span may be near normal. If the affected person survives the initial loss of motor neurons, the disease may progress slowly due to an overburdening of the remaining neurons, which appear to burn out over time.

ALS is a rapidly progressive disease that causes severe muscle weakness and wasting, breathing and swallowing problems, and is uniformly fatal. Approximately 5 to 10 percent of ALS is a familial trait that is related to a specific gene defect on chromosome 21. However, most often it is an acquired disorder, striking people between forty and sixty years of age. The overall prevalence rate in the population is 5 to 7 per 100,000, making it the most common NMD in the industrialized countries. Population studies suggest that the incidence of ALS is increasing, although the reasons remain unknown.

Myopathies. Polymyositis is an acquired inflammatory myopathy that can affect any age group or sex. There are many different forms of this disease, but all involve cellular components of the immune system that mistakenly attack and destroy muscle fibers. Diseases of this nature are referred to as autoimmune disorders. As with other autoimmune disorders, polymyositis may respond dramatically to corticosteroids. This disease is one of the few NMDs that responds to a specific treatment. Severe cases may be fatal, particularly if the heart is involved.

The muscular dystrophies are inherited myopathies recognized by characteristic findings on muscle biopsy. The most widely known of the dystrophies, although not the most common, is Duchenne muscular dystrophy (DMD). Many people mistakenly think that DMD is the only form of muscular dystrophy. In fact, there are many different muscular dystrophies. The prevalence rate of DMD in the population is about 3 per 100,000. DMD is a sex-linked, recessive disorder, usually affecting only males. It is caused by a specific gene deletion on the X chromosome that codes for the production of a structural protein known as dystrophin. In the absence of dystrophin, muscle cell membranes are leaky, allowing calcium to accumulate within the cell. This accumulation triggers a cascade of events that lead to cell necrosis and death. Affected boys will show physical signs around the time they begin to stand upright and attempt walking. A waddling or clumsy walk may be the first sign, along with marked enlargement of calf muscles. Approximately one-third of boys with DMD show early impairment of verbal intelligence, which may be due to absent dystrophin in brain tissue. By age ten years, 50 percent of the boys will be using wheelchairs. Life span is limited to twenty to twenty-five years. Cardiac and respiratory problems are frequent and are usually the cause of death.

Myotonic muscular dystrophy (MMD) is the most common of the dystrophies, with a prevalence rate of 5 per 100,000 in the population. The disease is a dominant trait associated with abnormalities on chromosome 19. Both sexes are affected equally. MMD is characterized by weak muscles that relax slowly, with symptoms usually appearing in adolescence or early adulthood. Distal muscles, such as the hands, may be severely affected, making this potentially a very disabling condition. A higher incidence of cognitive and intellectual impairment has been reported in individuals with myotonic muscular dystrophy than in those with the other dystrophies, although some studies have refuted this finding. The heart is commonly involved, with arrhythmias being a frequent problem. Respiratory problems are also frequent. The severity of the disease can vary significantly, even in the same family. Ambulation is usually maintained, although bracing of the legs may be required. If cardiac and pulmonary complications are managed aggressively, life span may be near normal.

Limb girdle (LG) and fascio-scapulo-humeral (FSH) syndromes represent a family of rare, slowly progressive, myopathic disorders that may be very disabling but generally do not shorten life span. FSH appears to be linked to abnormalities on chromosome 4. Chromosomal linkages with LG syndromes have not yet been determined. Onset can vary from late childhood to adulthood, depending on the type. There is no gender predilection. Weakness tends to be proximal, involving shoulders and pelvis predominantly. Respiratory and cardiac problems are not usually seen; however, contractures and spine deformity are frequently present.

Neuromuscular Junction Disorders. Although there are several neuromuscular junction disorders, myasthenia gravis (MG) is the most common, with a prevalence rate of 3 to 5 per 100,000 population. Like polymyositis, MG is an autoimmune disorder in which antibodies mistakenly attack and destroy acetylcholine receptors on the muscle end plate, thus partially or completely blocking transmission of signals from motor neurons to muscle. Age of onset varies considerably, and the disease is three times more common in women under age forty. In older people there is no gender predilection. Weakness can occur anywhere in the body. Again, like polymyositis, it is one of the few NMDs that responds well to medical treatment. Drugs that block the breakdown of acetylcholine—along with plasmapheresis, a technique of purifying the blood—can relieve symptoms substantially. Removal of the thymus gland along with agents that suppress the immune system may inhibit the course of the disease. With appropriate medical management, life span may be normal.

Rehabilitation of NMDs

The goals of rehabilitation in patients with NMDs are to maximize functional capacities, prolong independent ambulation or locomotion, inhibit physical deformity, and provide access to full integration into society. Management is best carried out by a multidisciplinary team consisting of doctors; physical, occupational, and speech therapists; social and vocational counselors; and psychologists, among others. Treatment is goal-oriented, using various modalities. Stretching and range of motion exercises combined with supportive bracing may improve or prolong ambulation as well as enhance functional use of the extremities. Early surgical correction of spinal deformities and contractures may improve seating and positioning. For people with breathing difficulties, portable mechanical ventilators may improve respiration and comfort.

Moderate-resistance (submaximal) weight lifting and aerobic exercise may improve strength and cardiovascular performance in slowly progressive NMDs. Water exercises are well suited for people with NMDs and can be done wearing an "aqua-aerobic" type of flotation vest. Exercise programs should not be started without evaluation by a physician who has cleared the patient to participate. Cardiac and respiratory complications may be contraindications to certain exercise programs. Further, there is no substantial evidence to support exercise therapy in the rapidly progressive NMDs.

Psychosocial and Vocational Impact of NMDs

Except for Duchenne and possibly myotonic muscular dystrophy, the majority of people with NMDs show intellectual levels within the normal range. Nonetheless, in a major study a large percentage of patients with NMDs exhibited elevated scores for hypochondriasis, depression, and hysteria on the Minnesota Multiphasic Personality Inventory (MMPI) test. These indicators of emotional pathology were associated with unemployment, whereas loss of ambulation and arm function was not. Overall, employment rates for people with NMDs are substantially lower than for able-bodied persons. Despite this, a higher level of education correlated with higher employment rate and improved self-esteem in this group (Fowler, 1992). This research indicates that altered personality profiles in people with NMDs substantially affect social integration and employment rates, and, indeed, may be as important as physical abilities. Education appears to be a very important factor in employability and self-esteem and should be emphasized in people with NMDs.

Future Research

The most promising areas of research for the treatment of NMDs center around genetic manipulation to correct errors in DNA that are responsible for numerous NMDs. As our understanding of the genetic defects that underlay many NMDs increases, so does the potential to correct these defects.

Myoblast transfer, which is the technique of injecting healthy muscle cells from a donor into diseased muscle, has met with limited success. Except in the case of autoimmune NMDs, drug trials have also failed to demonstrate any unequivocally effective compounds. Nonetheless, trials with myoblast

transfers and various drugs are ongoing. Biomedical engineers continue to devise new ways for assistive mechanical devices to take over the functions of weakened muscles. Additional work is needed to study the effects of various exercise regimens on regeneration of diseased muscle. The impact of altered personality profiles on social integration and employment in NMDs warrants further investigation as well.

Governmental and Consumer Organizations

Governmental agencies that support research in NMDs include the National Institute on Disability and Rehabilitation Research (NIDRR), which is a division of the Department of Education, as well as the National Institutes of Health (NIH). Both of these organizations are based in Washington, DC.

The most prominent consumer-driven organization supporting research and clinical care for people with NMDs is the Muscular Dystrophy Association (MDA), whose central office is in Tucson, Arizona. Other major groups include Charcot-Marie-Tooth International, the ALS society, and FlaSHLiGht, a support group for people with fascio-scapulo-humeral (FSM) and limb girdle (LG) syndromes.

(*See also:* GENETIC DISORDERS; NEUROLOGICAL DISORDERS; RESPIRATORY DISEASE)

RESOURCES

Charcot-Marie-Tooth (CMT) International, 1 Springbank Dr., St. Catharines, ON, Canada L2S2K1

Muscular Dystrophy Association (MDA), 3300 East Sunrise Dr., Tucson, AZ 85718

The Amyotrophic Lateral Sclerosis Association (ALSA), 21021 Ventura Blvd., Suite 321, Woodland Hills, CA 91364

BIBLIOGRAPHY

BROOKE, MICHAEL H. *A Clinician's View of Neuromuscular Diseases*, 2nd ed. Baltimore, 1986.

ENGEL, ANDREW G., and BANKER, BETTY Q., eds. *Myology.* New York, 1986.

———. "Advances in the Rehabilitation of Neuromuscular Diseases." In *State of the Art Reviews: Physical Medicine and Rehabilitation.* Philadelphia, 1988.

FOWLER, WILLIAM M., JR. "Comprehensive Rehabilitation Management of Neuromuscular Diseases." Project H133B80016-03, National Institute on Disability and Rehabilitation Research, Progress Report, Yr. 05. Washington, DC, 1992.

FOWLER, WILLIAM M., JR., and GOODGOLD, JOSEPH. "Rehabilitation Management of Neuromuscular Diseases." In *Rehabilitation Medicine*, ed. Joseph Goodgold. St. Louis, 1988.

MUSCULAR DYSTROPHY ASSOCIATION RESEARCH BULLETINS. Tucson, AZ, 1991–1992.

RINGEL, STEVEN P. *Neuromuscular Disorders: A Guide for Patient and Family.* New York, 1987.

SCHOCK, NANCY C., and COLBERT, AGATHA P. *Ventilators and Muscular Dystrophy.* St. Louis, 1987.

SIEGEL, IRWIN M. *Muscle and Its Diseases.* Chicago, 1986.

WALTON, JOHN. *Disorders of Voluntary Muscle,* 5th ed. New York, 1988.

GREGORY T. CARTER

NEUROPSYCHOLOGY

See ASSESSMENT; HEAD INJURY; PSYCHOLOGY

NONDISCRIMINATION

See CIVIL RIGHTS

NORMALIZATION AND SOCIAL ROLE VALORIZATION

A 1991 panel of 178 experts in the field of mental retardation identified Wolf Wolfensberger's 1972 book *The Principle of Normalization in Human Services* as the most important "classic" work in mental retardation, of a possible 11,300 articles and books published over roughly 50 years (Heller et al., 1991). Most professionals in the field of human services have heard of the principle of normalization or have, at least, some idea of what it suggests. However, their views concerning normalization are often based on misunderstandings rather than on an actual reading of basic normalization literature (Wolfensberger, 1980).

The Scandinavian Formulations

One could possibly trace the roots of normalization back to the eighteenth century concept of moral treatment, especially as it was practiced and ex-

plained by William Tuke. But it was after World War II, in Scandinavian countries, particularly Denmark and Sweden, that service attitudes and principles were developed that were eventually called normalization. Niels Eric Bank-Mikkelsen, as head of the Danish Mental Retardation Service, was instrumental in having this principle written into the 1959 Danish law governing services to persons with mental retardation. Neils Eric Bank-Mikkelsen (1969) spoke in terms of letting "the mentally retarded obtain an existence as close to the normal as possible," and this idea also had an impact on the writing of a law governing services to mental retardation in 1967 in Sweden. It was, however, Bengt Nirje, then executive director of the Swedish Association for Retarded Children, who first systematically stated and elaborated the principle of normalization in human service literature, and popularized its name. Bengt Nirje (1969) stated the principle as follows: "Making available to the mentally retarded patterns and conditions of everyday life that are as close as possible to the norms and patterns of the mainstream of society."

The Scandinavian origins of normalization can be understood as a natural extension of the Nordic social-welfare experiment to its citizens with mental retardation. As it was stated by Bank-Mikkelsen and then by Nirje, normalization was and still is in Scandinavia an expression of a sociopolitical program of immense importance.

The Scandinavian formulation continued to evolve, with Nirje (1992) providing the following updated version: "The normalization principle means that you act right when making available to all persons with intellectual or other impairments or disabilities patterns of life and conditions of everyday living that are as close as possible to or indeed the same as the regular circumstances and ways of life of their communities."

Normalization in North America

Wolf Wolfensberger was instrumental in transferring the principle of normalization to North America. He reformulated the principle "for purposes of a North American audience and for broadest adaptability to human management in general" (Wolfensberger, 1972). His refinements to the principle were

515

aimed at marrying the formulations by Bank-Mikkelsen and Nirje to social science, and generalizing their applicability to all socially devalued classes. Though the Scandinavians had framed normalization primarily for persons with mental retardation, from the beginning Wolfensberger argued that the principle of normalization should be applied to all human service sectors and for all socially devalued groups (Wolfensberger, 1970). He thus framed the definition into a scientific statement that called into play a synthesis of psychological and sociological work. Early North American dissemination and training events highlighted deviancy, the developmental model, imagery, social integration, and valued social participation as fundamental concepts. The emphasis on social integration was an important difference between the Scandinavian and North American formulations, with the Scandinavians, for instance, being comfortable with people living in institutions as long as these were "normalized." For Wolfensberger, valued social participation was both a means and an end of normalization. In *The Principle of Normalization in Human Services,* Wolfensberger (1972) proposed as the first North American formulation "the utilization of means that are as culturally normative as possible in order to establish and/or maintain personal behaviors and characteristics that are as culturally normative as possible." Wolfensberger and Tullman (1982) further refined the definition: "Normalization implies, as much as possible, the use of culturally valued means in order to enable, establish, and/or maintain valued social roles for people." This set the stage for the formulation of social role valorization.

As Wolfensberger indicated, the normalization principle is deceptively simple. By and large, most people will agree to it wholeheartedly while often lacking awareness of even the most immediate of its major corollaries and implications, and while engaging in practices quite opposed to it. Wolfensberger's insight was that the elegant and parsimonious normalization principle has a myriad of implications, and it has evolved over the years as these implications have become more evident and explicated. At the outset, Wolfensberger's aim was quite ambitious: the formulation of a complete human management model, including tools of analysis, implementation, training, and evaluation. Moreover, he suggested

that the framework of service no longer be the medical model but rather something he then called the developmental model, suggesting that developmental potential rather than sickness was the proper perspective for human service management.

In North America, the first widespread practical applications of the normalization principle occurred in Nebraska and especially in the ENCOR regional service system around Omaha, where Wolfensberger then worked. The National Institute on Mental Retardation of the Canadian Association for the Mentally Retarded (now called the Canadian Association for Community Living) took up the gauntlet when it brought Wolfensberger to Canada (1971–1973) and published his book *The Principle of Normalization in Human Services* in 1972. G. Allan Roeher, then director of the National Institute on Mental Retardation, developed with Wolfensberger an impressive method of dissemination that was tied to staff training, program evaluation, and pilot projects throughout Canada. Over the years a great number of groups have taken up systematic normalization training, a discipline that has now spread to England, Australia, New Zealand, France, and Switzerland. In North America alone since 1971, tens of thousands of human service workers have attended courses or workshops of one to seven days' duration on normalization, or later on social role valorization.

Over the years, the training materials that were developed by Wolfensberger and his associates continued to evolve, as did the concept and definition itself. The refinements were aimed at capturing the richness of the principle as well as attempting to lay to rest some misunderstandings or objections.

There has been an ongoing dialogue among the theorists of the normalization principle. Gunnar Dybwad (1982), Bengt Nirje (1992), and Burt Perrin and Bengt Nirje (1985) have expressed disagreement with Wolfensberger's formulation, exchanging clarifications, and proposing different emphases. In fact, in Scandinavia, Wolfensberger's formulation has never been widely accepted because it was felt that it tried to make normalization too much of a social science and was unnecessarily complicated.

The principle of normalization has become an easily recognized and almost pervasive notion of immense importance in the evolution of human services, especially for persons with mental retardation. It has been invoked in the framing of public policy and laws and as a basis for litigation. However, one of the reasons why other fields have been reluctant to embrace either the normalization principle (or later social role valorization or SRV), or to acknowledge their debt to these ideas, is almost certainly that the field of mental retardation did so first. Also, important misunderstandings continue to exist (Nirje, 1985; Wolfensberger, 1980, 1983), which has led Wolfensberger to propose a new term and a new and still evolving formulation.

Social Role Valorization

In 1983, Wolfensberger reconceptualized the normalization formulation, and, in part to lay to rest much terminological confusion, renamed it social role valorization (SRV). In 1991 Wolfensberger published a monograph, now in its second edition (Wolfensberger, 1992), in which he gives a brief overview of this important concept, which has had a tremendous impact on the conceptualization of human services and legislation in North America.

The genesis of the new concept of SRV can be briefly sketched as follows. In 1979, Wolfensberger and his associates changed the focus of the principle of normalization, leaving behind its reliance on the sociological concept of deviancy, and turning to the concept of social devaluation, which they married to a compelling phenomenological view of the life experiences of societally devalued people and service recipients. In the late 1960s Wolfensberger had written extensively on the historical deviancy roles of socially rejected persons (Wolfensberger, 1969). With Steve Tullman (Wolfensberger & Tullman, 1982), he returned to the concept of roles and proposed that positive social roles were fundamental to counter social devaluation; and this led to his most recent revision of the normalization principle.

In 1981 and 1982, while translating some of his writings into French, Wolfensberger found that his French associates used the term *dévalorisation* to translate the word devaluation. In French, the positive of *dévalorisation*, *valorisation*, is readily used to express positive valuation. In 1983, in Paris, he suggested that the French not translate literally the word "normalization" as it had been adopted from the Scandinavians. Rather, he proposed that the French term should suggest a system for the improvement of the social roles of persons who are at risk of devaluation. Later in 1983 he proposed the term *social role valorization* (SRV) for what had become a new concept that subsumed normalization.

SRV's starting point is the socially devalued person, and it provides a compelling phenomenological view of this person, whether a service recipient or not. In Wolfensberger's three-day introductory workshops on SRV, trainers spend close to five hours, of a total of twenty-four, reviewing the typical experiences of socially devalued people, which includes almost all clients in several major service sectors. For Wolfensberger, devaluation is the hallmark of society's response to people with certain characteristics and identities (including impairments), and as a result, being "wounded" in various ways is their common, pervasive, and often lifelong experience. A person perceived by society to be of low value is apt to be treated in ways that reflect this perception: low-quality housing, poor schooling or no education at all, low-paying and low-prestige employment (if any employment at all), poverty, and poor-quality health care. The devalued person will be rejected, separated, and excluded, and the good things in life, which are taken for granted by valued persons, will be denied or taken from a devalued person, including supportive relationships, respect, autonomy, and participation in the activities of valued persons.

Thus a service system that merely occupies itself with "rehabilitation" rather than addressing devaluation and its impacts is, at least to a significant degree, doomed to failure, and can possibly even be a tool of oppression (Wolfensberger, 1987). For Wolfensberger, social devaluation and the needs of devalued people are not simple problems, and SRV is therefore a complex and broad response strategy.

Wolfensberger has defined social role valorization as "the enablement, establishment, enhancement, maintenance, and/or defense of valued social roles for people, particularly for those at value risk, by using as much as possible culturally valued means" (1991, 1992). This definition is written with Occam's razor in mind: a brief statement to convey a clear, practicable message. The emphasis on roles is probably new to many, and in it are contained the seeds of a radically different phenomenological understanding of many people of devalued identity and clienthood, and a new perspective on the means and ends of human service. Social role valorization is useful because its theory is well supported and validated by research. One major difference between SRV and normalization, in addition to SRV's emphasis on social roles, is that SRV is much more of a social science than normalization. Normalization was a combination of social science elements with ideology, but SRV is essentially pure social science, even though it is concordant with many positive ideologies and beliefs (e.g., about the value of all people). An example of social science grounding is that it presents what has to be done or avoided to achieve a goal (such as improvement of attitudes, or enhancement of a particular competency) for a devalued person or group, laying out action decisions on the basis of what is known to be likely to work or not to work, not on the basis of what one wants or feels or would like to be true.

Also, there is a package of evaluation and teaching tools: *PASS* (Wolfensberger & Glenn, 1975) and *PASSING* (Wolfensberger & Thomas, 1983) are both well-documented, validated, and reliable tools for program evaluation (e.g., Flynn et al., 1991) that are also intended and widely used for teaching people about normalization and SRV. Therefore it is a relatively comprehensive program that can cover the total spectrum of human service. Its emphasis on using "culturally valued" means implies capitalizing on positive familiarity with, and expectations upon, the means, and avoiding measures that strike most members of a culture—including clients—as alien and dubious. This approach should more readily elicit both public support and a client's engagement. In its emphasis on choosing "valued" activities, roles, and so on for persons at value risk, we find another important difference from at least the Scandinavian formulations of the normalization principle, where what is "normative" is seen to be sufficient. SRV proposes that to defend and even enhance the status of devalued persons and groups, one must often employ those alternatives that are on the more valued end of a continuum.

In the creation of SRV, Wolfensberger has drawn widely on the corpus of social science. Upon reading the 1991–1992 monograph, for instance, one will be reassured by many well-known concepts. New theoretical implications and new practical uses have been found for many concepts that have otherwise been well researched but little used or pulled together into a single framework for practical application. Thus work on expectations and self-fulfilling prophecy finds new life in SRV, as well as research in areas such as social perception, semiotics, and labeling theory. The developmental model and the issue of personal competency enhancement are given fresh new meaning within this metatheory.

Social Roles

A good example of Wolfensberger's integration of diverse elements of social science comes in his treatment of the concept of roles and his utilization of role theory. "A social role may be defined as a socially expected pattern of behaviors, responsibilities, expectations, and privileges" (Wolfensberger, 1992). Social role theory, sometimes referred to as the nexus between sociology and psychology, is of great importance to both fields, but few practitioners have garnered much practical use from it. Yet roles are pervasive, with people going from one role to the next, and generally filling many roles at the same time. "For instance, in any single day, a person may be in roles such as 'customer,' 'shopper,' 'teacher,' 'voter,' 'driver,' 'wife' or 'husband,' 'mother' or 'father,' 'daughter' or 'son,' 'sister' or 'brother,' 'friend,' 'neighbor,' etc." (Wolfensberger, 1992). SRV provides an understanding of how roles are shaped; how they are attributed; and, most important, how they can be used to counteract devaluation.

SRV is a tool of both social analysis and intervention. Wolfensberger's insight is that the devalued person would not be in difficulty (or at least would be in less difficulty) if he or she had access to valued roles, for then that person would be afforded many of the positive expectations and circumstances that, on the one hand, would improve his or her competencies, and on the other would either support or compensate for his or her deficiencies. The good things in life, which most people take for granted but are so widely missing from the life experience of a devalued person, become available in connection with incumbency in positive social roles.

For SRV, roles and competencies are not the

same thing but also are not altogether independent. Roles are signaled or evoked by many indicators: behavior, dress, the immediate physical and social context, and so on. Thus a person can claim many roles, or have them attributed to him or her, irrespective of that person's competencies, as long as the trappings of the roles are associated with him or her. The opposite is also true: People will not be willing to attribute a particular role to a person, even though he or she has the competencies necessary to fulfill it, if the indicators are not there to confirm that the person in fact "has" the role. For instance, the fact that we are willing to trust a medical practitioner who is otherwise unknown to us is based on where we meet him or her; the person's demeanor, and, of course, what he or she wears. SRV proposes that having positive social roles can minimize or even overcome the negative social and practical effects of an impairment, even though the impairment is real, perhaps even severe, and continues to exist. Thus SRV is not simply "taking away" or relabeling a devalued condition.

Moreover, SRV recognizes that the major tool of the multibillion-dollar advertising industry in normative culture also has applicability to the creation of positive images of people at risk of social devaluation, by constructing positive juxtapositions to build up their image in the eyes of others. This strategy will go a long way in facilitating the attribution of valued social roles to persons who are at value risk, or their actual insertion into such roles (Thomas & Wolfensberger, 1982). It is therefore not surprising that SRV proposes that to achieve valued social roles for people, image enhancement is at least as important as competency enhancement. After all, the mental representations we have of people are constructed by how they look and act, their appearance and behavior, what the observer is told about a person or the class to which the person is seen to belong, the language used to describe and refer to that group, and miscellaneous other symbols that are associated with it. Because these mental images also structure our expectations, and our expectations direct our behavior, they can have a direct impact on the competencies that persons develop. If, for instance, the images we hold of a person or group have convinced us of their worthlessness or their incapacity to achieve certain com-

petencies, we will not provide that party with the opportunities to learn and master them.

SRV proposes that the ways services are organized and set up can have a major impact on the images associated with the persons who are served. Thus the service setting (location, external and internal facility features, etc.); the social contacts provided to a client; the activities, routines, and rhythms of a service; the language and labels applied to and about people served and their service; and the funding sources and the fund-raising appeals that support a service—all these generate images that can be positive or destructive for the people served.

If image enhancement would be for most people a novel insight into the structure of human service, competency enhancement should be more readily understandable. But here again, SRV charts new ground. First and foremost, competency is highly valued in our society. Our Western cultural value tradition prizes individual self-sufficiency and productivity, and many positive images attach themselves to people who are highly competent. Some roles can be held only if one possesses certain competencies. To address the issue of personal competencies, a human service must select strategies that have both "relevance" and "potency." To be relevant to the needs of the people it serves, a service must identify and prioritize their needs very precisely. For many services this seems to be very difficult because so many human services do not give people what they really need, but rather what the servers like to do, what the founders demand be done, or what the government will fund. All of this is often not at all what the people being served need, or need most of all. In terms of potency, SRV introduces the concept with a sobering proposal ". . . that there be an appreciation of the sacredness of each person's lifetime, and that therefore, the person's time not be wasted in irrelevance or even inactivity, but instead, that effective and intense use be made of the time the person spends in a service" (Wolfensberger, 1992).

Nothing Less Will Do

Social role valorization may also be understood as an ecological theory that proposes the addressing of image and competency enhancement vis-à-vis the individual person; the person's primary and intermediate social systems (the latter including agencies that provide service to the person); and finally, on community and societal levels. It is important to attend not only to the individual at risk but also to all surrounding social systems. SRV emphasizes that action must include doing things to and with devalued parties, to help them more easily fill valued roles and to help members of society to value them more positively; however, surrounding social systems (including services and even society as a whole) must also be accommodating and more tolerant of differences and weakness.

If implemented, SRV would have a dramatic impact on service provision. For instance, its emphasis on what is culturally valued means that at least generally, informal structures that are valued in a culture, and applied to valued people, are to be preferred as the first avenue of recourse. Among other things, this means that when a person needs help or a service, SRV would give primacy to traditional informal helping and serving roles and relationships, rather than professionalized or formalized ones.

It is sometimes suggested that valuing the person "as he or she is" is a morally superior strategy to social role and competency enhancement. This approach is something of a defiant challenge to the world to value the person irrespective of his or her condition or identity. But an unbiased reading of history shows the inadequacy of this approach unaided by other means: Historically, those who strive to value persons "as they are" commonly still engage (often quite unconsciously) in role degrading behavior that is eventually injurious to the persons at issue because yet other people who encounter these role degradations are negatively affected by them in their attitudes, and hence act in ways that confirm the person's role-degraded identity. Social devaluation and divisiveness are part and parcel of the human condition, and people need all the help they can get to overcome their baser inclinations along these lines. SRV theory, being strongly grounded in empiricism, provides effective ways and means for pursuing more valued social roles for people at value risk. Attributing valued roles to otherwise devalued persons, valorizing the roles they already hold, or

crafting new valued roles for them, can go a long way toward facilitating the valuing of such persons.

When using the right means is already a good part of the end (as it is in SRV), then many of the ethical problems associated with the means in other systems (e.g., aversive procedures in behavior modification) are resolved. Further, the means sought by SRV are not only culturally valued but also well researched and well validated. In contrast to many present technologies and approaches that are embedded in the medical-curative paradigm, and where anything but client change in the direction of rehabilitation is deemed a failure, SRV can enhance the social roles and life conditions even of people who do not change, or cannot be rehabilitated, or where the rehabilitation efforts are still taking place and their outcomes are unknown.

(See also: ATTITUDES; CIVIL RIGHTS; CONSUMERS; DEINSTITUTIONALIZATION; INDEPENDENT LIVING; INTERNATIONAL REHABILITATION; PHILOSOPHY OF REHABILITATION; SOCIOLOGY)

BIBLIOGRAPHY

BANK-MIKKELSEN, NIELS E. "A Metropolitan Area in Denmark: Copenhagen." In *Changing Patterns in Residential Services for the Mentally Retarded*, eds. R. Kugel and Wolf Wolfensberger, Washington, DC, 1969.

DYBWAD, GUNNAR. "Normalization and Its Impact on Social and Public Policy." In *Advancing Your Citizenship: Normalization Reexamined*. Eugene, OR, 1982.

FLYNN, ROBERT J.; LAPOINTE, N.; WOLFENSBERGER, WOLF; and THOMAS, SUSAN. "Quality of Institutional and Community Human Service Programs in Canada and the United States." *Journal of Psychiatry and Neuroscience* 16 (1991):146–153.

HELLER, H. W.; SPOONER, F.; ENRIGHT, B. E.; HANEY, K.; and SCHILIT, J. "Classic Articles: A Reflection into the Field of Mental Retardation." *Education and Training in Mental Retardation* 26 (1991):202–206.

NIRJE, BENGT. "The Normalization Principle and Its Human Management Implications." In *Changing Patterns in Residential Services for the Mentally Retarded*, eds. R. Kugel and Wolf Wolfensberger. Washington, DC, 1969.

———. "The Basis and Logic of the Normalization

Principle." *Australia and New Zealand Journal of Developmental Disabilities* 11 (1985):65–68.

———. *The Normalization Principle Papers.* Uppsala, Sweden, 1992.

PERRIN, BURT, and NIRJE, BENGT. "Setting the Record Straight: A Critique of Some Frequent Misconceptions of the Normalization Principle." *Australia and New Zealand Journal of Developmental Disabilities* 11 (1985):69–74.

THOMAS, SUSAN, and WOLFENSBERGER, WOLF. "The Importance of Social Imagery in Interpreting Societally Devalued People to the Public." *Rehabilitation Literature* 43 (1982):356–358.

WOLFENSBERGER, WOLF. "The Origin and Nature of our Institutional Models." *Changing Patterns in Residential Services for the Mentally Retarded,* eds. R. Kugel and Wolf Wolfensberger. Washington, DC, 1969.

———. "The Principle of Normalization and Its Implications to Psychiatric Services." *American Journal of Psychiatry* 127 (1970):291–297.

———. *"The Principle of Normalization in Human Services.* Toronto, Canada, 1972.

———. "The Definition of Normalization: Update, Problems, Disagreements and Misunderstandings." In *Normalization, Social Integration, and Community Services,* eds. Robert J. Flynn and K. E. Nitsch. Baltimore, 1980.

———. "Social Role Valorization: A Proposed New Term for the Principle of Normalization." *Mental Retardation* 21 (1983):234–239.

———. *The New Genocide of Handicapped and Afflicted People.* Syracuse, NY, 1987.

———. *A Brief Introduction to Social Role Valorization as a High-Order Concept for Structuring Human Services.* Syracuse, NY, 1991.

———. *A Brief Introduction to Social Role Valorization as a High-Order Concept for Structuring Human Services,* 2nd rev. ed. Syracuse, NY, 1992.

WOLFENSBERGER, WOLF, and GLENN, L. *Program Analysis of Service Systems (PASS): A Method for the Quantitative Evaluation of Human Services,* 3rd ed. Toronto, 1975.

WOLFENSBERGER, WOLF, and THOMAS, SUSAN. *Program Analysis of Service Systems' Implementation of Normalization Goals (PASSING): Normalization Criteria and Ratings Manual.* Toronto, 1983.

WOLFENSBERGER, WOLF, and TULLMAN, STEVEN. "A Brief Outline of the Principle of Normalization" *Rehabilitation Psychology* 27 (1982):131–145.

RAYMOND A. LEMAY

NURSING, REHABILITATION

Nursing is defined by the American Nurses' Association as "the diagnosis and treatment of human responses to actual or potential health problems." The Association of Rehabilitation Nurses (ARN) has described rehabilitation nursing as a specialty area of nursing practice in which nurses diagnose and treat disability-related human responses that interrupt or alter function and life satisfaction. Accordingly, the goal of rehabilitation nursing is to facilitate the achievement and maintenance of a maximum level of functioning for individuals or groups with disabilities. Rehabilitation nursing has grown concurrently with the field of rehabilitation. Rehabilitation nurses contribute their specialized knowledge and clinical skills to the overall rehabilitation effort as caregivers, teachers, client/family advocates, consultants, and researchers. As key members of the interdisciplinary rehabilitation team, rehabilitation nurses collaborate with physicians, physical therapists, occupational therapists, social service workers, dietitians, rehabilitation counselors, and other health care providers.

The various types of rehabilitation nurses may be differentiated in terms of their educational preparation. The generalist rehabilitation nurse is a registered nurse who has graduated from a basic nursing education program. This individual may be a graduate of a hospital-based program, a two-year community college associate degree nursing program, or a four-year college bachelor's degree nursing program. Generalists usually provide direct patient care and perform the familiar nursing procedures shown in Table 1. However, many rehabilitation nurses have become involved in expanded role activities, such as those also shown in Table 1, and now perform a myriad of functions. Specialized rehabilitation nursing knowledge is obtained by the generalist through self-study, on-the-job training programs, and attendance at workshops and professional conferences.

The advanced practice rehabilitation nurse has earned a master's degree with a focus on rehabilitation nursing. In addition to specialized rehabilitation nursing knowledge learned in the classroom and

Table 1. The scope of rehabilitation nursing practice

Familiar Rehabilitation Nursing Procedures

- Improving hydration and nutrition
- Maintaining physical mobility
- Strengthening respiratory function
- Establishing effective patterns of elimination
- Preserving body tissue integrity
- Responding to psychosocial issues
- Promoting comfort
- Managing pain

Expanded Rehabilitation Nursing Roles

- Providing primary care to individuals with disabilities
- Serving as rehabilitation consultants in various health care settings
- Coordinating the interdisciplinary rehabilitation team
- Planning for patient discharge from the hospital
- Obtaining services and resources as a case manager
- Advocating for disabled individuals
- Functioning as a vocational rehabilitation liaison
- Securing third-party payment for rehabilitation services
- Working with the insurance industry as a certified insurance rehabilitation specialist (CIRS)
- Influencing health policy and legislation

SOURCES: Familiar rehabilitation nursing procedures adapted from Rehabilitation Institute of Chicago, Division of Nursing, *Rehabilitation Nursing Procedures Manual*, Rockville, MD, 1990. Expanded rehabilitation nursing roles adapted from Pamela G. Watson, "Components of Rehabilitation Nursing Practice Advancement," *Rehabilitation Nursing* 10 (1985): 28–31.

in clinical settings, the advanced practice nurse has formal education in pathophysiology, theory development, research methods, ethics, health policy, rehabilitation principles, and interdisciplinary team functioning (Watson, 1985). Advanced practice rehabilitation nurses usually function as clinical nurse specialists, administrators, or teachers.

Clinical nurse specialists are considered experts in a specific area of disability or rehabilitation. Clinical nurse specialists provide, direct, manage, and influence patient care when advanced nursing knowledge and skills are needed. These nurses provide expert consultation in many situations (Derstine, 1992). Clinical nurse specialists work closely with nursing staff members and other health care providers to assure that high-quality care is provided and that the highest possible level of functioning is achieved by patients and families.

Advanced practice rehabilitation nurses are often also found in administrative positions in rehabilitation settings. These nurses have additional formal education in organizational behavior, management, and rehabilitation program planning and evaluation. Some advanced practice nurses become members of nursing faculty. As faculty members, they endeavor to integrate rehabilitation philosophy and principles into undergraduate nursing curricula (Edwards & Kittler, 1991). Some advanced practice rehabilitation nurses continue their education and earn doctoral degrees in nursing or a related field. Those who do so usually serve as university faculty members and conduct clinical research to advance nursing knowledge and the scientific basis for practice. These individuals also assume leadership roles in professional associations and contribute research findings to the literature.

Generalist and advanced practice rehabilitation nurses can become certified by taking a written examination offered by the Certified Rehabilitation Registered Nurse (CRRN) program of the Association of Rehabilitation Nurses. The certification process validates the acquisition of the specialized knowledge and skills required to work with patients who have disabilities and their families. Some rehabilitation nurses elect to become certified as insurance rehabilitation specialists (CIRS). This option is available through testing by the Certification of Insurance Rehabilitation Specialists Commission.

Scope of Practice

Because of the complexities of health problems presented by individuals with disabilities, generalist and advanced practice rehabilitation nurses tend to delineate their practices by client age and type of disability. Thus they will work with either children or adults or the elderly. Common types of populations with disabilities served by rehabilitation nurses include children with developmental disabilities and individuals with spinal cord injury, head injury, major multiple trauma, burns, orthopedic conditions, stroke, cardiac disease, pulmonary disorders, cancer,

Table 2. Rehabilitation nursing practice guidelines

The rehabilitation nurse:

1. Collects comprehensive and accurate patient assessment data in an ongoing manner.
2. Analyzes patient assessment data and makes appropriate nursing diagnoses.
3. Collaborates with the patient, significant others, and various disciplines to formulate a realistic rehabilitation plan that includes specific goals, nursing procedures, and resources to meet individual needs.
4. Intervenes to prevent complications and promote optimal physical and psychosocial functioning.
5. Evaluates the patient's responses to nursing interventions, and revises the rehabilitation plan accordingly.
6. Assumes responsibility for continuing education and career development and contributes to the professional growth of others.
7. Works with the interdisciplinary team on all activities related to the rehabilitation process.
8. Participates in peer review and interdisciplinary program evaluation to assure that high-quality nursing care is provided to patients in rehabilitation settings.
9. Contributes to the scientific base of rehabilitation nursing practice through the application of research findings.

SOURCE: Adapted from American Nurses' Association and Association of Rehabilitation Nurses, *Standards of Rehabilitation Nursing Practice.* Kansas City, MO, 1986

collagen diseases, or neurologic conditions. Some rehabilitation nurses work with individuals with mental impairments or substance abuse problems, but these are not typical areas of practice.

Most rehabilitation nurses practice on rehabilitation units in tertiary care settings or in rehabilitation hospitals (Meyer, 1993). For the future, it is expected that more advanced practice rehabilitation nurses will be found practicing in the community, particularly in home health care settings. These nurses will increasingly become involved in case management (Biller, 1992; McBride, 1992) and providing primary care to persons with disabilities in their homes (Buchanan, 1992).

Direct patient care given by rehabilitation nurses

is intended to promote adaptation to disability, prevent complications of disability, and help patients achieve optimal functioning. Rehabilitation nurses are guided in their practice by the standards of care shown in Table 2. In addition, the Association of Rehabilitation Nurses has developed and published a core curriculum that is a comprehensive resource for practice (Association of Rehabilitation Nurses, 1993). The core curriculum includes extensive information on functional health patterns and nursing diagnoses used as a basis for rehabilitation nursing interventions (Table 3). Consistent with its empha-

Table 3. Functional health pattern–based nursing diagnoses frequently used by rehabilitation nurses

Functional Health Pattern	Nursing Diagnosis
Health management	Health maintenance alteration Increased injury potential
Nutrition	Alteration in nutrition Swallowing impairment Fluid volume imbalance
Elimination	Bowel incontinence Urinary retention
Activity/exercise	Activity intolerance Impaired mobility Self-care deficits
Cognition/perception	Alteration in comfort Perception deficit Memory deficit
Self-perception	Fear/anxiety Powerlessness Body image disturbance
Roles/relationships	Social isolation Family process alteration Withdrawal
Sexuality/reproduction pattern	Sexual dysfunction
Coping/stress tolerance pattern	Ineffective individual or family coping

SOURCE: Adapted from Christine Mumma, ed., *Rehabilitation Nursing: Concepts and Practice, a Core Curriculum.* Skokie, IL, 1987

sis on outcomes, ARN has published a document titled *Rehabilitation Nursing Scope of Practice: Process and Outcome Criteria for Selected Diagnoses* to help nurses identify appropriate patient outcomes.

Unique Contributions of Rehabilitation Nurses

As noted, rehabilitation nurses have specialized knowledge and skills, but to grasp the full extent of their contribution to rehabilitation one must consider the nurse-patient relationship. Many health care providers become involved when an individual acquires a disability. These professionals treat, or counsel, the person with the disability for specified periods of time, each of which rarely exceeds an hour per day. In contrast, rehabilitation nurses intervene on a twenty-four-hour basis, seven days a week. Rehabilitation nurses have the most sustained contact with patients and families. In fact, rehabilitation nurses play a major role in reinforcing and following through with the treatment plans and recommendations of the other rehabilitation practitioners. Rehabilitation nurses see patients through the most difficult times. Unlike the other practitioners, nurses can't "come back another time" when patients are unreceptive or stop interventions with patients who don't have rehabilitation potential. Instead, rehabilitation nurses must draw on attributes of endurance, compassion, and optimism and always keep trying on behalf of individuals with disabilities and their families.

(*See also:* ALLIED HEALTH PROFESSIONS; DISABILITY MANAGEMENT; HOSPITAL, REHABILITATION; PRIVATE SECTOR REHABILITATION)

RESOURCES

Rehabilitation Nursing, 5700 Old Orchard Road, Skokie, IL 60077-1057

Rehabilitation Nursing Research, 5700 Old Orchard Road, Skokie, IL 60077-1057

Archives of Physical Medicine and Rehabilitation, Suite 1310, 78 East Adams St., Chicago, IL 60603-6103

BIBLIOGRAPHY

AMERICAN NURSES' ASSOCIATION AND ASSOCIATION OF REHABILITATION NURSES. *Standards of Rehabilitation Nursing Practice.* Kansas City, MO, 1986.

ASSOCIATION OF REHABILITATION NURSES. *Rehabilitation Nursing Scope of Practice: Process and Outcome Criteria for Selected Diagnosis.* Skokie, IL, 1993.

BILLER, ANGELA MARINA. "Implementing Nursing Care Management." *Rehabilitation Nursing* 17 (1992):144–147.

BUCHANAN, LISA CYR. "A Rehabilitation Clinical Nurse Specialist: Evaluation of the Role in a Home Health Care Setting." *Holistic Nursing Practice* 6 (1992):42–50.

DERSTINE, JILL B. "The Rehabilitation Clinical Nurse Specialist of the 90s: Role Assumed by Recent Graduates." *Rehabilitation Nursing* 17 (1992):139–140.

EDWARDS, PATRICIA A., and KITTLER, ANN W. "Integrating Rehabilitation Content in Nursing Curricula." *Rehabilitation Nursing* 16 (1991):70–73.

McBRIDE, SUSAN M. "Rehabilitation Case Managers: Ahead of Their Time." *Holistic Nursing* 6 (1992):67–75.

MEYER, CHARLES. "The Changing Face of Rehabilitation Nursing." *American Journal of Nursing* 93 (1993):76–79.

MUMMA, CHRISTINE, ed. *Rehabilitation Nursing: Concepts and Practice, a Core Curriculum.* Skokie, IL, 1987.

REHABILITATION INSTITUTE OF CHICAGO, DIVISION OF NURSING. *Rehabilitation Nursing Procedures Manual.* Rockville, MD, 1990.

WATSON, PAMELA G. "Components of Rehabilitation Nursing Practice Advancement." *Rehabilitation Nursing* 10 (1985):28–31.

PAMELA G. WATSON

NUTRITION

See EATING DISORDERS; WELLNESS

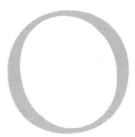

OBSESSIVE-COMPULSIVE DISORDERS (OCD)

See ANXIETY DISORDERS; EATING DISORDERS; PERSONALITY DISORDERS

OCCUPATIONAL INFORMATION

The use of occupational information has been a very important part of the vocational rehabilitation process since its inception as a formalized discipline of a "special" kind of career guidance process in the mid-1950s. While the medium that transmits the information has changed over time (from hard copy to computerized technology), such mainstays of occupational information as the *Occupational Outlook Handbook* (OOH) and the *Dictionary of Occupational Titles* (DOT), both published by the U.S. Department of Labor, have been reliable references to counselors in the United States, including those who work with persons with disabilities.

The *Occupational Outlook Handbook* has been available in various forms since 1950. The latest edition is 1994–1995. It is compiled and revitalized every two years to give information about selected occupations in the United States. The *Dictionary of Occupational Titles* was first formulated in 1939, and the revised fourth edition came out in 1991. It is a description of more than 12,000 jobs in the United States. Along with its supplements, which give expanded characteristics about jobs, it is most useful in a variety of ways in career counseling for all persons, with or without disabilities.

The DOT describes jobs presented by title, with a coded arrangement for occupational classifications. Jobs are assigned a nine-digit code, which places them in an occupational group and indicates whether the job is skilled, semiskilled, or unskilled, and which worker-functions the job involves. Since the mid-1980s there has been an increasing tendency to use the DOT and its supplements in computerized form; it is often available in computerized software.

Another significant government reference is the *Guide to Occupational Exploration* (GOE). It is published by the U.S. Department of Labor's Employment and Training Administration. The U.S. Government Printing Office has a variety of other pieces of occupational information, such as business patterns by county and state. State departments of labor have descriptions of the labor market, often including growth patterns, in states, counties, and regions. Occupational information can be helpful in describing the job market in the United States in a given state or region.

In addition to standard materials from federal, state, and local governments, a number of special packages have been developed, such as the Occupational Access Systems (OASYS). OASYS (1991) is published by Vertek and is a job-search source that uses DOT codes as a basis for evaluating transferable skills. A listing of previous jobs held by a client can be entered into the system, disability can be factored in, and the residual functional capacity can be determined via computer. The OASYS system can then generate information on jobs available at the person's current residual functional capacity, and depending on the state the client is in, can describe the current job market by zip code.

Other computerized systems that do this include VDARE (Vocational Diagnosis and Assessment of Residual Employability) and RAVE (Realistic Assessment of Vocational Experiences).

Sometimes the evaluation system is also fully or partially computerized. Evaluation helps to establish residual functional capacity of a client. Such computerized evaluation systems, most notably the VALPAR system 2000 (1995) of VALPAR, Inc., generate job titles after the evaluation screenings, which are based on the DOT.

Resources for occupational information seem to be abundant, but more important is what the client and counselor do with the occupational information once it has been obtained. When the rehabilitationist has the residual functional capacity described through an evaluation as part of the vocational rehabilitation process, these computerized searches can be very helpful in generating job possibilities, especially when they are connected to an actual labor market pool, as OASYS is in certain states. The rehabilitationist can list for the rehabilitation client, as part of the career guidance activity, the jobs the person can do, based on an estimate of current functional capacities. The rehabilitationist either can guide the person to explore these occupations or can be more directive in searching out career information and training options as well as using job-seeking skills techniques to get interviews for his or her client.

The job market is dynamic: information gathered at one time may not be relevant shortly thereafter. The OOH is published every other year, and listings in the DOT are updated periodically, although a small percentage of the job titles are updated annually. The information, while interesting and generic and having some long-standing value in career guidance, may not be relevant to a particular location and may not be relevant at all to a particular client.

Some of the job titles and job descriptions are not current because of the changing technologies. For example, the job title screen printer (any industry), 979.684-034, originally was for a job that could be done by someone with limited manual dexterity and required fairly low educational training and specific vocational preparation as well as some physical agility. The way the job currently is done is more mechanized and requires less physical ability but higher intellectual capacity. Originally the worker physically painted emblems on shirts or posters; this is now done in a mechanized fashion by "pushing buttons." However, the client needs to know exactly what buttons to push, and when.

The problem with occupational information is that it is gathered at a specific point in time. However, the world at work may change very dramatically, with increases in technology, decreases in technology in certain areas, shifting of populations, shifting of priorities, and other external variables that can't be easily controlled, such as recessions and labor market trends.

In conclusion, occupational information has its place in the world of rehabilitation, but it should be appreciated for what it is and not made into something it isn't. It gives trends and information at a particular point in time. It can be helpful in describing a job market. It can be helpful in doing a job analysis, but in reality the rehabilitationist must be sensitive to and aware of the realities of the world of work in the communities in which he or she functions with clients who have disabilities. No occupational information system is going to take the place of a rehabilitationist who knows how to do a good labor market survey or a good job analysis on jobs that really exist in the community. Sensitivity to the positive interaction of the rehabilitationist, his or her own skill level, and the availability of occupational information is something to strive for.

(See also: CAREER COUNSELING; JOB PLACEMENT; VOCATIONAL EVALUATION)

BIBLIOGRAPHY

U.S. DEPARTMENT OF LABOR, BUREAU OF LABOR STATISTICS. *Occupational Outlook Handbook*. Indianapolis, IN, 1994.

U.S. DEPARTMENT OF LABOR, EMPLOYMENT AND TRAINING ADMINISTRATION. *Dictionary of Occupational Titles*, 4th ed., rev. Indianapolis, IN, 1991.

———. *Guide for Occupational Exploration*. Indianapolis, IN, 1991.

VALPAR INTERNATIONAL CORPORATION. "*VALPAR System 2000.*" Tucson, AZ, 1995.

VERTEK, INC. OASYS: *The Occupational Access System Matching People's Abilities to Employer Needs*. Bellevue, WA, 1991.

CHRISANN SCHIRO-GEIST

OCCUPATIONAL THERAPY

Occupational therapy is a unique health and rehabilitation service. Its goal is to aid individuals with disabling conditions to become as independent as possible in carrying out the tasks of their daily lives.

Occupational therapy is beneficial to people of all ages with a wide variety of physical, mental, or developmental problems. Premature infants may require the help of occupational therapy to develop the sucking and swallowing reflexes necessary for feeding. Youngsters with birth injuries such as cerebral palsy often need occupational therapy to learn basic tasks of development, such as the reaching and grasping needed for play.

Occupational therapy also plays an important role in helping parents and teachers of schoolchildren to adapt physical surroundings and learning tasks to promote independence for a child with a disability. This may include providing a desk that positions a child for handwriting, consulting with parents about home tasks for a youngster with a learning disability, or aiding a teacher in choosing the proper behavior management of a child with an emotional problem.

When auto accidents and sports injuries cause temporary or permanent disability for young adults, occupational therapy is there with the tools and techniques necessary for independence. For the individual with a spinal cord injury, occupational ther-

apy may include techniques for eating, bathing, dressing, preparing meals, caring for home tasks, or even operating an adapted automobile. In cases where the person has very limited ability to move, the occupational therapy practitioner recommends and teaches the use of such sophisticated technology as a wheelchair with controls so sensitive they can be operated with a breath of air blown into a plastic straw connected to a computer.

When mental health problems prevent a person of any age from functioning in the community, there is help available through occupational therapy. As part of the treatment team in both hospital- and community-based programs, occupational therapy uses practical, everyday tasks to help people to learn and practice such skills as planning use of leisure time, completing work tasks, and caring for personal needs.

Occupational therapy is an essential service for those health problems occurring in or affecting the workplace. In industrial rehabilitation, occupational therapists may be working directly with employees at the work site, simulating work environments in the clinic, or employing technology, such as work simulators and simulated work environment, that can mimic the functional demands of nearly any job. A person's capacity to perform can be measured safely and effectively, and practice activities can be initiated and gradually increased in frequency, duration, or difficulty.

Treatment for work-related problems includes prevention of injuries, such as hand and wrist pain associated with word processing, and back pain from improper lifting, twisting, or sitting. Stress and mental health problems on the job are addressed through adjusting work tasks and interpersonal contacts to promote the greatest possible function.

Often problems associated with aging interfere with a person's ability to manage life independently. People recovering from stroke or those with chronic health problems benefit from the tools and techniques occupational therapy offers to compensate for functional limitations. Rearranging kitchen equipment and providing items requiring use of only one hand often make it possible for a stroke survivor to plan and prepare simple meals. Adaptations to clothing and bathroom equipment also make it possible for those with arthritis or limited hand strength to manage bathing, dressing, and other personal needs.

Occupational therapy is based on the tenet that the individual who is productively "occupied" in meeting the needs of his or her life can be said to be enjoying health. This basic principle was noted in the writings of physicians dating back to the Greek and Roman periods.

In the 1400s, physicians treating the "insane" in a hospital in Spain noted that the charity patients who performed household tasks to earn their keep recovered faster than those whose wealth kept them in more luxurious style.

Early occupational therapy in the United States was provided primarily to mental health and tuberculosis patients who underwent prolonged periods of hospitalization. World War I accelerated the expansion of treatment into the area of physical disabilities. World War II created a major demand for occupational therapy, and by the end of the war some 2,200 individuals were practicing in the profession.

The American Occupational Therapy Association (AOTA) reports a membership of more than 48,500 occupational therapists and occupational therapy assistants, while close to 200 colleges and universities offer training in the field. The World Federation of Occupational Therapy has a membership of 44 countries and recognizes more than 281 education programs worldwide.

In the United States, the registered occupational therapist has completed either a bachelor's or a master's degree program that includes six to nine months of supervised clinical experience. Upon completion of the education program, the individual is eligible to take a national certification examination. The certified occupational therapy assistant has completed an associate degree program, a period of supervised clinical experience, and has successfully passed a national examination. All but two states regulate the practice of occupational therapy.

As of 1994, the demand for occupational therapists and occupational therapy assistants far outstrips the number of qualified practitioners. The U.S. Bureau of Labor Statistics predicts that the shortage will continue at least through the year 2005, primarily because of the survival rate of premature infants, accident victims, and individuals with chronic illness as well as the rapidly increasing numbers of people dealing with functional limitations related to aging.

Occupational therapy is well positioned to respond to the changes taking place in the health care system because of its focus on consumer-oriented, community-based primary service. Working directly with individuals in the home, workplace, and community and using everyday activities as treatment, occupational therapy contains costs while advancing human potential.

The reasons for occupational therapy's effectiveness continue to be validated through outcome studies, and research information is being communicated widely to consumer and professional audiences. Current data provide continued rationale for occupational therapy's emphasis on patient and family motivation as critical elements in the achievement of treatment goals.

Leaders in the field of occupational therapy predict that the changing health care marketplace will redefine the model of the individual occupational therapist as a primary provider of direct intervention to individuals on a one-to-one basis. Tomorrow's occupational therapist is likely to be a manager of interventions and services administered by a variety of service providers who possess differing levels of professional preparation.

(*See also:* ALLIED HEALTH PROFESSIONS; PEDIATRIC REHABILITATION; PHYSICAL THERAPY; PSYCHIATRIC REHABILITATION)

RESOURCES

The AOTA office will provide a list of currently accredited schools:

American Occupational Therapy Association, 1383 Piccard Dr., P.O. Box 1725, Rockville, MD 20850–4375

MARY M. EVERT

OPHTHALMOLOGIST

See BLINDNESS AND VISION DISORDERS

ORGANIC MENTAL SYNDROMES

"Organic mental syndrome" is a term used to describe a group of psychological or behavioral signs and symptoms referable to dysfunction of the brain.

DSM-III-R (American Psychiatric Association, 1987) recognized six categories of organic mental syndromes: (1) delirium and dementia; (2) amnestic syndrome and organic hallucinosis; (3) organic delusional, mood, or anxiety syndromes; (4) organic personality syndromes; (5) intoxication and withdrawal; and (6) organic mental syndromes not otherwise specified. The conceptual basis of this breakdown is questionable in that the syndromes share no common cause apart from brain dysfunction, and the symptoms are quite variable. Although the term "organic mental syndrome" is well established, its usage is likely to decline since its removal from diagnostic standard DSM-IV (American Psychiatric Association, 1994).

Delirium, also known as acute confusional state, is characterized by a disorder of arousal and attention. Consciousness is disturbed, and delirious individuals may be either hyperactive or lethargic. The cause of delirium is most often an acute metabolic disturbance or illness. Common contributors include fever, dehydration, and medication side effects. Delirium occurs most often in the elderly and children. Diagnosis is based on identification of the underlying causes, and treatment focuses on supportive care and correction of causative factors. Delirium is most often a time-limited process without prolonged disability, but it often occurs in a setting of chronic disease, where it can be mistaken for dementia.

Dementia is the most prevalent chronic organic mental syndrome and is caused by many illnesses. Dementia affects memory and other aspects of cognition to a degree that interferes with previously achieved function in work, social activities, or relationships with others. The primary degenerative neurologic diseases, especially Alzheimer's disease, are most common, representing a contributing factor in up to 70 percent of all cases. No diagnostic tests are available for the degenerative dementias that offer specificity better than careful clinical evaluation. Cerebrovascular disease contributes to perhaps half of all cases of dementia and frequently co-occurs with the degenerative diseases. Some dementia results from such reversible causes as depression, hypothyroidism, and vitamin B_{12} deficiency. The evaluation of the demented individual should include appropriate tests to exclude these treatable conditions. For the degenerative dementias, there is

no known prevention or cure, and treatment focuses on symptoms. Dementia is associated with major functional impairments, including performance of activities of daily living (ADL), such as bathing and toileting, and instrumental ADLs, such as cooking and driving. For all dementia types the treatment should focus on reduction of excess disability due to medical complications and behavioral disturbances. Progressive dementia leads to loss of ability to work, live independently, and maintain social relationships. Many dementia patients require extensive community services and eventually nursing home care in the advanced stages of their illness. A multidisciplinary approach to care, involving physician, nurse, social worker, and other disciplines as required by the patient's needs, is ideal. Community-based advocacy and support agencies such as The Alzheimer's Disease and Related Disorders Association are also of great value to caregivers. An active international research effort is directed at the identification of the causes of Alzheimer's disease and therapies to prevent it or slow its progression. In 1994 the available treatments (only tacrine in the United States) offered modest symptomatic benefit to some individuals.

Organic amnestic syndromes are characterized by impairment in memory function unassociated with the more global impairments found in delirium and dementia. There is an isolated loss in short- and long-term memory, which is commonly associated with disorientation and confabulation (the substitution of imaginary events in place of actual memory). On testing, these individuals demonstrate an inability to learn new information. The most common cause is Korsakoff's syndrome (alcohol amnestic disorder), a late complication of a deficiency of the nutrient thiamine. Herpes simplex virus infection of the brain, ruptured aneurysm of the anterior cerebral artery, and head trauma are other common causes, and individuals with these illnesses may benefit from cognitive rehabilitation programs. Prevention of alcohol-related cases depends on adequate nutrition and thiamine supplementation. The deficits tend to be stable once acquired and lead to major disability, including inability to live independently or function in normal employment.

Organic hallucinatory, delusional, mood, anxiety, and personality syndromes are illness states resembling primary psychiatric illness but are more directly attributable to brain dysfunction. They may occur following any brain insult, and common causes include stroke, trauma, epilepsy, and inflammatory syndromes such as systemic lupus erythematosus. One of the most common of these conditions is the mood disorder known as poststroke depression. Other common causes of the mood and anxiety syndromes include drug effects (including alcohol and cocaine) and hormonal disorders. The onset of these conditions is unpredictable, and given their relationship with disabling illnesses, it may be difficult to distinguish these syndromes from adjustment disorders. Treatment is symptomatic and supportive. The organic personality syndromes are frequently characterized by irritability, mood swings, behavioral outbursts, impairments in social judgment, and suspiciousness. A characteristic personality disturbance involving verbosity, religious excess, and sometimes aggression has been associated with persons having "temporal lobe" epilepsy. Illness states affecting the frontal lobes of the brain may cause personality changes, including apathy and indifference, or disinhibition with socially inappropriate behavior. The nature of these syndromes can lead to alienation of previous social support networks, such as friends and family, and may be associated with an inability to maintain employment. The prognosis is variable, depending on the course of the underlying cause. Some cases may be transient or gradually disappear with recovery or treatment of the causative factors, but most are chronic.

Drug intoxication and withdrawal effects are most often of short duration. The diagnosis of intoxication requires the presence of maladaptive behaviors associated with ingestion of psychoactive substances. DSM-IV distinguishes between a state of physiologic intoxication and the associated behavioral syndrome by the presence of maladaptive behaviors such as impaired occupational and social function, impaired judgment, or aggression. The nature of the behavioral disturbances depends entirely on the physiologic effects of the ingested substance and can range from stupor to dangerous hyperactive states, such as with cocaine and phencyclidine (PCP) intoxication. Withdrawal is a behavioral syndrome caused by the cessation or reduction of intake of a regularly used psychoactive substance. Its manifestations are generally similar to intoxication.

Behavioral abnormalities associated with general medical illnesses, such as diabetes mellitus, may not meet criteria for any of the above conditions. These illnesses account for the category of "not otherwise specified."

Because of the diversity of these syndromes, in both cause and duration, the approach to rehabilitation is problematic. Rehabilitation plans must take into account the time course of the illness state (i.e., transient in delirium, progressive in dementia, chronic in personality disorders) and work toward enhancing functional capability while reducing excess disability resulting from the behavioral abnormalities typical of these syndromes.

(See also: ALCOHOL REHABILITATION; ALZHEIMER'S DISEASE; DRUG REHABILITATION; NEUROLOGICAL DISABILITIES; PSYCHIATRIC REHABILITATION; PSYCHIATRY; PSYCHOLOGY; STROKE)

RESOURCE

Alzheimer's Disease and Related Disorders Association, National Headquarters, 919 North Michigan Ave., Suite 1000, Chicago, IL 60611-1676

BIBLIOGRAPHY

AMERICAN PSYCHIATRIC ASSOCIATION. *Diagnosis and Statistical Manual of Mental Disorders (DSM-III-R)*, 3rd ed., rev. Washington, DC, 1987.
———. *Diagnostic and Statistical Manual of Mental Disorders (DSM-IV)*, 4th ed. Washington, DC, 1994.

DAVID S. GELDMACHER
PETER J. WHITEHOUSE

ORTHOPEDICS

See MUSCULOSKELETAL DISORDERS

ORTHOTICS

See PROSTHETICS AND ORTHOTICS

OSTEOARTHRITIS

See ARTHRITIS; MUSCULOSKELETAL DISORDERS

P

PAIN

Acute and chronic pain remain vexing problems for society, and their understanding and effective management have often been elusive. The socioeconomic costs of pain are staggering:

- One-half billion workdays are lost per year due to pain, with the highest frequency of missed workdays due to low back pain or headaches.
- 20,000 tons of aspirin are consumed in this country per year, a number that likely will continue to increase (Koenig, 1973; Turk, Meichenbaum, and Genst, 1983).
- Thirty percent of households contain chronic, nonmalignant pain sufferers (Crook, Rideout, and Browne, 1984).
- Ninety billion dollars per year is spent on chronic pain, and the amount is increasing (Morris, 1991).

Chronic malignant or cancer pain has failed to receive sufficient attention in the past; 25 percent of patients report receiving inadequate pain relief with standard medical treatment (Moulin, 1991). Further, pediatric pain has historically been undertreated because health care professionals often have underestimated the level of pain experienced by children undergoing surgical or rehabilitative procedures.

Defining Pain

The International Task Force on Acute Pain (Ready & Edwards, 1992) has developed the following definition of pain:

> Acute Pain: "Pain of recent onset and probable limited duration. It usually has an identifiable temporal and causal relationship to injury or disease. This is in distinction to chronic pain, which is defined as a pain lasting for long periods of time. Chronic pain commonly persists beyond the time of healing of an injury and frequently there may not be any clearly identifiable cause."

Examples of acute pain are pain due to a broken bone, inflammation from a disease process, or post-surgical pain. Acute pain may also be classified as acute recurrent, as in migraine headache or pancreatitis. Acute pain is also subclassified into somatic, with pain originating from the musculoskeletal system, or visceral, where the pain may have a primary autonomic response (Gildenberg & DeVaul, 1985).

In contrast to acute pain, chronic nonmalignant pain develops in a time frame of three months or longer. Chronic pain syndrome can also evolve. In this syndrome, the symptoms show increased severity with perceived marked physical disability, somatic focus, depression, social and family maladjustment, multiple trials of ineffective treatment, and vocational impairment. At this chronic phase, overt pain behavior, such as limping, grimacing, or inappropriate medication use, may develop. Pain behavior may initially be reinforced by a reduction in pain, although external psychosocial or financial consequences may also serve to maintain the disability. While pain behavior may be functional in the case of acute pain, because it allows the individual to avoid a potentially damaging noxious stimulus, pain behavior in the chronic pain patient becomes dysfunctional and the ultimate focus of a rehabilitation intervention.

Chronic malignant pain usually refers to cancer pain, with the pain representing ongoing tissue damage and active disease process. With cancer pain there are generally few inappropriate pain behaviors, and the goals are pain relief and treatment of the underlying disease process.

Pain Physiology

A classic work published in 1965 by Ronald Melzack and Patrick Wall provided the basis for an understanding of pain as a dynamic rather than static experience. Since that date the details of this dynamic process have slowly been elucidated. We now recognize that the response characteristics of pain receptors (nociceptors) fluctuate widely in response to chemical influence from the peripheral nerves, surrounding tissue, and the blood elements. This process explains, for example, why sunburned skin hurts when it is touched. Peripheral stimulation may even block or "turn off" the system by activation of inhibiting fibers. Hence there remains a rationale for the comment "if you rub it, it feels better . . ."

This complex process continues in the central nervous system, with damping signals sent back down the spinal cord. The process is also chemical in nature. The brain produces its own endogenous chemicals, such as serotonin, and these also have a related role in cases of depression and sleep disorder. In fact, antidepressant medications appear to have an effect on the serotonergic system and have been used in the treatment of both pain and depression. Pain is not a simple linear communication from a noxious stimulus to the brain, even in cases of acute injury. A number of investigations have shown that there is no absolute link between peripheral stimulation and the perception of pain. The use of neurosurgical techniques to treat certain types of chronic nonmalignant pain has thus declined, because simply cutting the nerves at the periphery does not necessarily resolve the problem on a long-term basis.

Psychosocial Factors

Pain is an unpleasant sensory and emotional experience; suffering is the reaction of an organism to the experience of pain. With the onset of acute pain, suffering can also be manifest by physiological and cognitive symptoms of anxiety, with concomitants such as increased perspiration, heart palpitations, and muscle contraction. These symptoms generally disappear as the acute pain subsides and the individual perceives control. Pharmacological and behavioral treatments have been used to manage anxiety symptoms, thereby reducing suffering and pain.

When pain persists, depression may ensue, because the neurochemistry of affective disorder is closely linked to that of chronic pain. It has been reported that 80 percent of patients suffering from chronic nonmalignant pain also display depression, and cognitive-behavioral as well as pharmacologic treatments for depression necessarily are included in multidisciplinary pain clinics. Results have shown a reduction in disability behavior (Sullivan et al., 1992; Turner & Jensen, 1993).

Personality variables have been implicated as factors influencing the perception of pain. However, investigators have argued that the presence of chronic pain and the social and financial consequences of an injury often *cause* psychological symptoms such as depression and anxiety (Gamsa, 1990).

Expectancy and suggestion are also powerful factors that influence pain. Placebos are about half as effective as active analgesics. However, a placebo cannot distinguish "real" from "psychological" pain, and placebo use without the patient's knowledge is generally considered an unethical practice (Gildenberg & DeVaul, 1985).

Treatment

Given the difference in the etiology of acute and chronic pain, different treatments are required. Acute pain is a symptom, not a disease or syndrome. Hence the underlying cause must be addressed. Analgesics often are the mainstay of acute pain treatment, with medications prescribed on a fixed interval schedule to provide the patient with relief and facilitate the rehabilitation process. To avoid "learning" inappropriate pain behavior, the patient with acute pain should not have to experience pain and display pain behavior to obtain relief.

Similarly, some pain conditions, such as acute low back pain, also show reduced recurrence with a structured behavioral treatment approach that focuses on aggressive management at the earliest onset of injury (Fordyce et al., 1988). Attention to vocational factors at this stage also may prevent chronicity. For example, dissatisfaction with one's supervisor has been shown to be the best predictor of acute back pain recurrence, controlling more variance than medical diagnostic predictors.

While chronic malignant pain should be treated with adequate analgesia, there has been a growing but controversial acceptance of narcotic maintenance therapy for nonmalignant chronic pain. This approach, however, may not alter the level of physical disability.

Nerve blocks have also been used with some success for diagnostic and treatment purposes. Additionally, surgical procedures have been attempted for some types of chronic pain, although results from this approach have been disappointing. Surgery or nerve blocks may be more effective with chronic malignant pain. Other invasive procedures such as spinal column stimulators and narcotic pump implantation also have been tried with some success for cancer and neuropathic pain. However, results have been less promising with nonmalignant pain when

investigators failed to screen adequately psychological and medical variables.

The management of chronic nonmalignant pain has focused on rehabilitative approaches aimed at improving function rather than reducing underlying tissue pathology. "Work-hardening" programs have gained popularity for treating patients when an acute injury fails to resolve adequately, there is no active disease process, and return to work is the primary goal. However, no controlled studies support the effectiveness of work-hardening programs.

Chronic pain patients with more severe disabilities may benefit by functional restoration or multidisciplinary pain rehabilitation programs. Studies report a return-to-work rate of 60 to 80 percent with these approaches, depending on pain severity and the program structure (Flor, Fydrich, and Turk, 1992; Mayer et al., 1987). Finally, single-discipline "pain relief" treatments such as biofeedback and relaxation, acupuncture, TENS, or cognitive behavior therapies have been used for treating specific chronic pain states such as headache or phantom limb pain. These treatments have proven less effective with chronic pain syndrome when used outside a multidisciplinary setting.

Future Directions

National and international organizations focusing on the study of pain have evolved since the late 1960s. These include the American Pain Society (APS) and the International Association for the Study of Pain, both of which have regional professional societies throughout the world. In 1994 the APS established quality improvement standards for acute and cancer pain. The American Chronic Pain Association, developed by pain patients as a support group system, now includes more than six hundred chapters worldwide. Self-help manuals have also proliferated (Rapoport & Sheftel, 1992; Sternbach, 1988).

The quality of pain services remains an issue, and formal accreditation of treatment programs have advanced as a result. Another major problem is access to treatment in that health care cost containment efforts continually restrict reimbursement.

Efforts to address quality and cost have been varied. Some health care providers have reworked their treatment structure and eliminated the term "pain management" in an effort to provide patients with access to services. Others have returned to controversial focus on using narcotic analgesics as the first line of treatment for chronic nonmalignant pain, a less expensive and possibly questionable alternative to rehabilitation.

RESOURCES

American Chronic Pain Association, P.O. Box 850, Rocklin, CA 95677

American Pain Society, 5700 Old Orchard Rd, 1st Floor, Skokie, IL 60077–1057

BIBLIOGRAPHY

CROOK, JEAN; RIDEOUT, ELIZABETH; and BROWNE, GINA. "The Prevalence of Pain Complaints in the General Population." *Pain* (1984):299–314.

FLOR, HERI; FYDRICH, THOMAS; and TURK, DENNIS C. "Efficacy of Multidisciplinary Pain Treatment Centers: A Meta-analystic Review." *Pain* 49 (1992): 221–230.

FORDYCE, WILBERT; BROCKNAY, JOHN; BERGMAN, JAMES; and SPANGLER, DANIEL. "A Control Group Comparison of Behavioral Versus Traditional Methods of Acute Back Pain." *Journal of Behavioral Medicine* 9 (1988):127–140.

GAMSA, ANNE. "Is Emotional Disturbance a Preceptor or a Consequence of Chronic Pain?" *Pain* 42 (1990):183–195.

GILDENBERG, P. L., and DeVAUL, R. A. "The Chronic Pain Patient." In *Pain and Headache*, ed. P. L. Gildenberg. New York, 1985.

JENSEN, MARK; TURNER, JUDITH; ROMANO, JOHN; and KAROLY, PAUL. "Coping with Chronic Pain: A Critical Review of the Literature." *Pain* 47 (1991):249–283.

KOENIG, P. "The Placebo Effect in Patient Medicine." *Psychology Today* 4 (1973):7–60.

KULICH, RONALD J., and WARFIELD, CAROL A. "Relaxation in the Management of Pain." *Hospital Practice* 2 (1985).

MAYER, T. G.; GATCHEL, R. J.; MAYER, H.; KISHINO, N. D.; KEELEY, J.; and MOONEY, V. "A Prospective Two-Year Study of Functional Restoration in Industrial Low Back Injury." *Journal of the American Medical Association* 258 (1987).

MELZACK, RICHARD, and WALL, PATRICK. "Pain Mechanisms: a New Theory." *Science* 50 (1965): 971–979.

MORRIS, DAVID B. *The Culture of Pain*. Berkeley, CA 1991.

MOULIN, DWIGHT E. "Treatment Outcome in a Multidisciplinary Cancer Pain Clinic by Banning et al." *Pain* 47 (1991):127–128.

RAPOPORT, ALLAN, and SHEFTEL, FRED D. *Headache Relief: A Comprehensive, Up-to-Date, Medically Proven Program That Can Control and Ease Headache Pain.* New York, 1992.

READY, BRIAN, and EDWARDS, THOMAS. *Management of Acute Pain: A Practical Guide.* Seattle, 1992.

STERNBACH, RICHARD A. *Mastering Pain. A Twelve-Step Program for Coping with Chronic Pain.* 1988.

SULLIVAN, MICHAEL; REESOR, KENNETH; MIKAIL, SAMUEL; and FISCHER, RONALD. "The Treatment of Depression in Chronic Low Back Pain: Review and Recommendations." *Pain* 5 (1992):5–13.

TURK, DENNIS; MEICHENBAUM, DONALD; and GENEST, MICHAEL. *Pain and Behavioral Medicine: A Cognitive-Behavioral Approach.* New York, 1983.

TURNER, JUDITH A., and JENSEN, MICHEL P. "Efficacy of Cognitive Therapy for Chronic Low Back Pain." *Pain* 52 (1993):169–177.

RONALD J. KULICH

PANIC DISORDER

See ANXIETY DISORDERS; PHARMACOLOGY; PSYCHIATRY

PARALYSIS

See NEUROLOGICAL DISORDERS; NEUROMUSCULAR DISORDERS; SPINAL CORD INJURY; STROKE

PEDIATRIC REHABILITATION

Advances in emergency medical services and trauma care have resulted in increasing survival rates of children with injuries; however, the severity of their injuries and consequent disabilities have also increased. This entry describes pediatric rehabilitation as more than a short-term medical intervention. It is presented as a comprehensive and multifaceted system that includes medical, rehabilitation, educational, and prevocational components. The special needs of children who have been disabled by traumatic injuries are presented. Sections include the incidence and causes of traumatic injuries; the emotional impact of hospitalization; transfer to rehabilitation programs; and transitions to early intervention programs, special education, and prevocational services. Brain injury is the diagnosis most frequently recorded in the National Pediatric Trauma Registry. It is also the diagnosis that results in the highest proportion of children who are expected to have multiple long-term impairments, especially in behavior and cognition. Therefore, the needs of children with brain injuries are given special attention in this entry.

Incidence and Causes of Injuries to Children

Injuries are the leading cause of death and disability among children. Injuries are not random events but occur in predictable patterns to children. Among infants and toddlers, injuries result from falls from furniture, down stairs, or out of windows. Tragically, physical abuse is a major cause of serious brain injuries among very young children, especially infants. Another cause is the failure to use protective automotive safety seats while transporting infants and toddlers. This lack of protection increases their risk of serious injury during a collision.

As children become more active and mobile, they leave their homes to engage in activities outside direct parental supervision. Injuries occur when children are hit by motor vehicles while playing, bicycling, crossing, or darting into the street. They are also injured as passengers in motor vehicle collisions and too often are unrestrained by seat belts. The incidence of injuries involving all-terrain vehicles, mopeds, and motorcycles increases. Sports-related injuries involving boating, diving, sledding, and skiing fluctuate with seasonal activities. As older children approach adolescence, they are more prone to injuries from violence, including gunshot wounds and stabbings. Motor vehicles continue to be major mechanisms of injuries among adolescents as experimentation with drugs and alcohol increases.

Tragically, most injuries can be prevented through improved safety programs and the use of protective devices or restraints. In contrast to the decrease in children's death from disease, including cancer and birth-related disorders, the percentage of children's deaths from injury has steadily increased

(Children's Safety Network, 1991). Injuries account for almost 40 percent of deaths among children aged one to four years and 70 percent of all deaths among children and adolescents aged five to nineteen years. Each year an estimated 600,000 children are hospitalized as a result of injuries. Injuries lead to more hospital days, cause the highest proportion of discharges to long-term care facilities, and result in the highest proportions of children requiring home health care after hospital discharge than any disease (Division of Injury Control, CDC, 1990).

Pediatric rehabilitation is based on the fundamental premise that children have different needs than adults. They are not simply little adults. Just as their medical needs require specialized pediatric services, so their emotional, social, educational, and prevocational needs require programs that are appropriate and responsive to their ages and stages of development. The needs and reactions of infants differ from those of toddlers, who differ from school-age children, who differ from adolescents. Unlike parents' prior experience with routine childhood illnesses, rehabilitation for childhood injuries is a long-term process that is not synonymous with recovery.

Predicting the outcome of rehabilitation for children is even more complex than for adults because children are constantly growing and changing. Adults have an intact base of learning, knowledge, skills, experience, and achievements to draw on when their lives change due to the onset of an injury. However, the interruption of a child's development by the onset of an injury threatens not only the child's current level of functioning and skills but his or her mastery of future goals as well. Consequently, families and rehabilitation experts need to distinguish between progress that is due to the child's normal growth and maturation, and changes that are results of treatment and interventions.

Every parent fears that a child may be born with some type of disorder or disease. The birth of a healthy infant signals joy and relief to parents. A parent's primary role is to provide the physical care and emotional support that are essential for a child's development and maturation. Parents act as caregivers, supervisors, teachers, and disciplinarians for their children. However, it is their role as protectors that is critical to ensuring the child's safety. Young children who have not yet mastered the physical skills required for independence and the judgment needed to monitor their behaviors require the guidance of an adult to protect them from harm. Consequently, when a previously healthy and able-bodied child is seriously injured and faces the possibility of a lifelong disability as a result, the stability of the family is shaken at its core. The statement "An injured child is an injured family" is not an oversimplification but an accurate reflection of the far-reaching effects of childhood injuries (Doelp, 1989).

Hospital-Based Rehabilitation

Hospitalization separates the child from the security of home and family. The child whose hospital admission is anticipated by scheduled treatment or surgery, such as a tonsillectomy or appendectomy, can be prepared for the new and strange hospital environment by visits, pictures, and explanations beforehand. Children's anxieties may be lessened by educational and orientation programs that allow them to try out hospital gowns and masks or hold tools such as stethoscopes, needle plungers, and tongue depressors. The impact of the child's separation from the security and familiarity of home is also lessened by hospital policies that allow parents to "room in."

Such preparatory strategies are not available to the child who is suddenly injured and hospitalized. Diminished levels of consciousness may further distort the child's memory and perceptions of events, surroundings, and explanations. Children with brain injuries may lose consciousness and become comatose for periods ranging from minutes to days, weeks, or months. Brain injuries may result in posttraumatic amnesia so that the child doesn't remember the accident and following events. Memory difficulties, confusion about time and place, and the effects of physical and emotional shock can further disorient the child.

Injuries are not necessarily isolated events. Other family members may be injured and parents or siblings hospitalized as well; this commonly occurs in motor vehicle collisions and fires. Family members may die at the scene or after hospital admission. Just as the injured child most needs the presence and comfort of parents, they may be separated due to their medical conditions and even treated at different hospitals. A parent who has been severely injured may be unaware of, or be unable to respond to, an injured child. The other parent may have to choose between hospital visits to a spouse or child. There may be other children still at home who also need information and attention.

Emotional Impact of Injury and Hospitalization. To understand the emotional impact of a child's injury on a family, one must look at the cause of injury. In cases of birth-related disorders, physicians are often able to alleviate parents' guilt by assuring them that nothing they did during the child's pregnancy caused the abnormality. However, more injuries are preventable. Failure to use a child safety seat in the car, failure to require that a child use a seat belt or wear a bicycle helmet increases the child's risk for serious injury. Likewise, when a child is injured while in the care of a parent, sibling, or other relative, that person is responsible for the child's safety. A fall down the stairs, a near drowning in the backyard wading pool, a spilled pan of boiling water from the stove, or an attack by an unleashed dog—they all are preventable.

The initial shock of a child's injury is compounded by the guilt parents experience over their failure to protect their child from harm. The anger that accompanies this guilt may be directed at oneself, a spouse, a sibling, or a stranger whose actions endangered a child. There is no logical, orderly path and timetable for the emotions that parents experience following a child's injury. Rather, parents go through an intense emotional seesaw of hopes and fears with an uncertain outcome. The initial shock usually passes into a feeling of, "It can't be true" or ". . . as bad as they say" as parents struggle to come to grips with the possibility that their child will never be the same as before the injury.

The vigil that many parents hold at their child's bedside, particularly for children who are comatose following injuries to the brain and central nervous system, is emotionally as well as physically exhausting. The depth and duration of a coma following a brain injury is directly related to the likelihood that long-term disabilities in physical, sensory, communication, or cognitive skills will result. Since many children who are seriously injured are transferred from local hospitals to pediatric trauma centers in urban areas, parents may lose the immediate contact and support of relatives and friends in their communities. Both children and parents are removed from all that is familiar as they enter a world of medical specialties and technologies.

The support that parents and relatives expect to receive from each other is often thwarted by the different reactions and coping styles among family members. Following the initial relief that a child will survive the injuries, parents face the consequences of survival. The news that a child's mobility, visual, hearing, speech, memory, or breathing has been permanently damaged raises frightening possibilities. Paralysis, muscle weakness, and balance difficulties are conditions that are visible. More difficult to measure, understand, and predict are changes from brain injuries that result in problems with memory, learning, organizing information, controlling impulses, and monitoring behaviors.

As the impact and consequences of an injury become known and the initial emotional shock passes, many parents question whether death might be preferable to their child's survival with a severe and permanent disability. Too often, however, parents are ashamed to think such thoughts and do not even share them with spouses. This "death wish" is a common reaction to a severe injury to a child. Losses are more than physical changes. Families also grieve the loss of the child's potential and the lost hopes and dreams for the future.

"Acceptance" is a word that is readily used but hard to define. The process and timing vary for each family. It is not an end point that parents reach, but rather a balance between hopes and disappointment, expectations and limitations. It is a time when the central focus of a family's life is no longer the child who has been injured, but instead a time when the needs of the injured child are balanced with the needs of all others in the family. There will always be periodic and often unexpected reminders that stir sadness for what has been lost. However, gradually the emphasis shifts from past to present, and the future begins to seem possible.

Transfer to Rehabilitation Programs. The peak incidence of spinal cord injuries and brain injuries occurs in young adults between ages fifteen and thirty. Rehabilitation programs have concentrated on this population. There are few specialized inpatient rehabilitation programs exclusively for children

with traumatic injuries in the United States. A study by the National Pediatric Trauma Registry found that 93.3 percent of children admitted with injuries go directly home upon discharge from the trauma center. More children with four or more impairments as a result of injuries were discharged directly home (44%) then were transferred to rehabilitation hospitals (40%) (DiScala, 1993).

Most inpatient pediatric rehabilitation programs are for children with a range of developmental disabilities that include children with multiple disorders, birth defects, mental retardation, and those dependent on medical technology. Visiting such hospital-based programs for pediatric rehabilitation can be emotionally traumatic for parents who have no prior experience or exposure to these programs or populations. Transferring a child who has been recently injured to such programs confronts parents with the reality of disability at a time when they are just realizing the long-term implications of their child's condition.

Because of the lighter size and weight of children who have been injured, their parents have options for home care that relatives of adults do not have. Following weeks or months of hospitalization, often distant from home, parents and children are anxious to return to familiar surroundings. Children's emotional needs for support and reunification with their families may contribute to the families' choice of rehabilitation services on an outpatient basis closer to home. Another factor that may influence the family's decision is their insurance coverage.

Community-Based Services

Rehabilitation does not end with a child's discharge from the hospital. A new phase begins in the community, and parents become the central planners and coordinators of services.

Early Intervention Programs. In 1983, amendments to the Education of the Handicapped Act were passed. The Early Intervention Program for Infants and Toddlers with Disabilities was established. It was reauthorized in 1991 under the Individuals with Disabilities Education Act. This law applies to infants and toddlers who have identified disabilities or are at high risk for a disability. The purpose of this federal legislation was to set up statewide systems of services to families of infants and toddlers through center-based or home-based programs. Commonly known as "early intervention programs," they are based on the premise that early treatment of a disabling condition enhances the child's potential for developing skills and strengths, maximizes long-term gains, and prevents complications. Most importantly, the family is a critical and essential partner with professionals in the child's care. This family-centered philosophy recognizes that families need emotional and social supports as well as clinical expertise to care for a child with a disability. The Individualized Family Service Plan (IFSP) is the central tool for assessing, planning, delivering, and evaluating services. Many early intervention programs prepare families for the future by providing informational materials and training programs that emphasize the advocacy skills needed to access local, state, and federal programs.

Physical abuse is a major cause of injuries to infants and toddlers. It can result in serious brain damage, multiple bone fractures, burns or scalds, and/or internal injuries. Many children with serious or repeated injuries are discharged from trauma units to foster parents or guardians to protect them from further harm (DiScala, 1993). The immediate and long-term effects of child abuse can be devastating. Beating, battering, or shaking a young child can seriously injure the brain and result in damaged sight or hearing. Paralysis, muscle weakness, and nerve damage may affect a child's ability to walk, to control balance, and to coordinate fine motor movements using hands and fingers. Damage to facial muscles, tongue control, and swallowing reflexes may affect the production or clarity of speech. In addition to the physical damage, a child who has been abused is emotionally traumatized and may need long-term counseling. Many children injured from abuse are placed in multiple foster homes, because their physical and emotional needs for care and attention can quickly exhaust caregivers.

Because the brains of infants and toddlers are still developing, many subtle and long-term effects of injuries may not appear for years. As their brains are challenged with increasingly complex tasks as they enter and progress in school, they may have difficulties in learning and concentration that are di-

rectly related to the injuries sustained as infants or toddlers.

Falls are another major cause of injury among young children. Many are injured in motor vehicle collisions because they are not restrained in protective child safety seats or because seat belts are used improperly. Those held in an adult's arms or lap can hit the windshield or be thrown from the car in a collision or abrupt stop. A young child's head is larger in proportion to overall body size than an adult's and consequently is more vulnerable to injury, especially during falls or collisions. The phrase "if only" is heard often as parents relive the events preceding their child's injury.

Parents of infants and toddlers who have been injured are likely to have no prior knowledge of or experience with early intervention programs. They may believe that such programs are only for children who have been born with disabilities or injured via abuse. Visiting early intervention programs may expose parents of recently injured children to those with multiple and severe disabilities for the first time. If this occurs just as they are learning about the medical consequences of their child's injury, such programs may arouse painful conflicts of denial, hope, and despair. For parents to agree to early intervention services, they may need supportive counseling to deal with the emotional impact of their child's injuries.

Special Education. The Individuals with Disabilities Education Act (IDEA) of 1991 specifically recognizes that children with traumatic brain injuries have unique needs for special education and related services. By creating a separate category for children with traumatic brain injuries, states are obligated to provide services that are appropriate and responsive to their unique needs. Previously, many children with traumatic brain injuries who applied for special education services in public schools were inappropriately classified as having a learning disability, emotional disorder, mental retardation, or were placed in a generic category labeled "other health impairment."

The child's entry or return to school following a disabling injury represents the next stage in his or her rehabilitation. It also presents a host of new challenges and difficulties for the child who has been injured, for classmates and peers, for educators and school staff, and for family members. Prolonged absences, multiple hospitalizations, outpatient rehabilitation programs, and home-based tutors further separate and distance the child from the local school. A child's education is much more than an intellectual process. School is an arena where children develop social skills and learn how to become independent and self-reliant. It represents a major step in his or her ability to function outside the protection and guidance of parents and beyond the familiarity of home.

It is critical that families consult with teachers to prepare school staff and classmates for changes in the child's appearance and functioning. Young classmates may be afraid of "catching it" when an injury is confused with illness or disease. Descriptions and pictures of the child while hospitalized can help classmates understand the consequences of injuries and prepare them for physical changes. Visits to the child's home can help classmates reestablish contact more informally and reduce the injured child's anxiety about returning to school and fears about classmates' reactions.

The child who returns to school following a severe injury may have physical changes that restrict mobility and activities. Special equipment, such as wheelchairs, crutches, braces, or canes, may require that the classroom or child's desk area be rearranged or modified. Stairs, hallways, and bathrooms may create barriers or hazards that require structural modifications such as ramps, handrails, or safety devices. Fatigue and side effects from medications may affect the child's endurance and concentration so that shortened schedules or intermittent rest periods are needed. Changes in sight, hearing, and speech may necessitate seating rearrangements. Changes in appearance, such as scarring, facial disfigurements or amputated limbs, may make the child self-conscious and fearful of ridicule or rejection by peers.

Whereas physical changes are often visible, other changes may be more subtle and harder for school staff and peers to understand. Injuries, particularly those involving the brain, typically affect children's ability to learn, concentrate, and recall information. Children may have trouble controlling impulsive behaviors. Emotions may fluctuate from erratic temper outbursts to silliness or alternate with uncontrollable laughter and crying. The consequences

of brain injuries are frequently misunderstood by classmates and teachers, and these children may be accused of being lazy, stubborn, or delinquent. This perception is reinforced when children with brain injuries are evaluated using standard intelligence tests. When the results produce scores in the normative range, problematic behaviors, poor attention, and lowered grades may be attributed to poor attitudes or emotional difficulties. The child's self-esteem and confidence are further jeopardized. These results may be in sharp contrast to performance prior to the injury.

It is critical that students with brain injuries be evaluated by a neuropsychologist experienced in brain injuries to children. The IQ tests commonly used by schools in evaluations for special education are not always helpful in evaluating a student with a brain injury because they tend to measure what the child has learned in the past. Many children who experience brain injury do not lose the academic knowledge they gained before the injury. Thus their test scores on IQ tests may show little change and give a misleading picture of the child's ability to function in the classroom. The ability to learn *new* information may have been damaged by the injury. A neuropsychologist specializes in evaluating how the brain injury has affected the child's ability to learn, communicate, plan, and organize time, to do schoolwork, participate in play, and relate to others. Neuropsychological evaluations focus on the relationships among the various parts of the brain and the child's abilities and behaviors. Children's brains change rapidly during the twelve to eighteen months after an injury, so it is critical that neuropsychological evaluations be an integral part of the child's educational planning upon return to school and thereafter as difficulties are identified and new questions arise (Lash & Wolcott, 1992).

A skilled neuropsychologist can guide teachers and parents in designing educational strategies and plans to enable the child to learn effectively and function in a classroom setting, with peers and at home. Specific suggestions and techniques should include classroom strategies for completing assignments, methods to improve new learning, effective ways to prompt or redirect the student, and guidelines for managing inappropriate behavior. Methods for learning in various settings should include one-to-one instruction as well as learning in small groups. Use of adaptive devices for memory, communication, and organization should be specific. Alternative methods of student evaluation may include open-book tests, untimed tests, oral instead of written responses, pictures rather than words, multiple-choice rather than essay tests, and silent or auditory techniques for reading (Lash & Wolcott, 1992).

It is critical, however, for families and educators not to be deceived by the emphasis on the child's initial return to school. Rehabilitation and education are long-term processes. The transitions of the injured child from hospital to home to school are only two of many. They are only the first links in a long chain. Children will have many changes in school that require careful and integrated planning for consistency and continuity in their recovery and rehabilitation. Transitional planning is required for children as they move from class to class, teacher to teacher, and school to school. Since the education law explicitly states that parents hold the final authority to approve or reject the educational plan proposed by the school, they are ultimately in the best position to ensure that schools communicate information and techniques to various teachers and settings. Only parents have the long-range view of a child's progress following an injury as well as the comparison of pre- and postinjury skills and performance.

Prevocational Needs. The transition from childhood to adulthood is signified by the student's graduation from high school. However, the high unemployment rate of persons with disabilities is a symbol of the difficulties and challenges ahead. The following tips are designed to help prepare the child for adulthood during the final stages of pediatric rehabilitation.

1. *Start Early.* The federal education law (IDEA) contains an important provision that, upon reaching age fourteen, the transitional needs of students with disabilities must be included in their educational plans. The success of pediatric rehabilitation programs, including special education, may be best measured by the child's skills and abilities to live as an adult.

As the end of high school approaches, adolescents are expected, and often pressured, to define their interests and goals. Finding a job, entering a training program, going to college, or moving away from home are options. An injury can jeopardize these plans. Many high-school students take part-time jobs, join various clubs, or are active in sports; these opportunities may be lost or limited if a student is seriously injured and requires extensive time out of school for hospitalization and ongoing treatment.

All young people have to figure out what they want, gather and sort through information about jobs, gain experience, and develop their academic and interpersonal skills. Young people who have been injured or have disabilities must do the same. The job found or career held is not determined by the person's injury or disability, but by their abilities, qualifications, and experience. It is critical to begin the process of exploring job options, career interests, and additional school or training as early as possible while still in school.

2. *Avoid Premature Graduation.* Students with disabilities may be eligible for special education services until they are twenty-one years old. Some states provide these services until age twenty-two. However, once a student accepts a high-school diploma, eligibility for these services ends. By delaying graduation, students with disabilities may receive several more years of education and training that can help prepare them for employment and independent living.

However, many students who are injured, particularly in their latter years of high school, are upset to see their classmates graduating and do not want to be left behind. Schools may waive attendance, course, or grade requirements for a recently injured student out of sympathy or to reward their hard work despite extended absences during hospitalization. Families should consult carefully with special education staff and disability advocates before accepting a diploma. Unlike the laws that ensure a child's right to education, there is no comparable guarantee of a job or training once a student leaves school.

3. *Work Experience Is Important.* The Americans with Disabilities Act was passed in 1990. It grants civil rights protection to individuals with disabilities by guaranteeing equal opportunity in employment, public places, transportation, state and local government services, and telecommunications. Despite this protection there are many ways that employers can and *do* discriminate regarding hiring people with disabilities. The law does not guarantee that a person with a disability will be hired. To be hired, the person must *first* be qualified.

Training and experience are the two major items that employers look for. Adolescents and young adults who have been injured or have disabilities often are at a disadvantage when applying for jobs because they have less work experience than other applicants. Setting educational goals with the school or building work experience through volunteer positions and part-time jobs are methods of improving the future employability of a student who has a disability. Educational plans must include functional skills as well as academic knowledge if young adults with disabilities are to compete successfully for jobs.

4. *Choosing Priorities and Finding a Balance in Life.* Becoming an adult is a long and complicated process for anyone and is filled with hopes and dreams, setbacks and disappointments. The basic elements by which an adult's success and independence are traditionally measured are the ability to hold a job, earn money, live safely and comfortably, establish a network of friends, and pursue special interests. Perhaps the most persistent fear of a parent for a child who has been injured or is disabled is the unknown future. The fear that a disabled child raised at home will end up in an institution as an adult still haunts many parents. This need not and should not happen.

Adulthood requires balancing many facets of life. A job is only one of many elements that determine an individual's achievements and satisfaction. The logistics of living independently, finding accessible transportation, a job, and affording housing, receiving sufficient income, and becoming part of a community may be more complicated for a person with a disability. The art of finding a balance between one's abilities and needs requires careful judgment and understanding of oneself

(*See also:* ADOLESCENTS, REHABILITATION OF; CHILD-HOOD DISABILITIES; CHILDHOOD PSYCHIATRIC DISORDERS; DEVELOPMENTAL DISABILITIES; FAMILY; GENETIC DISORDERS; GROWTH DISORDERS; HEAD INJURY; MULTIPLE DISABILITIES; PSYCHOSOCIAL ADJUSTMENT; SPECIAL EDUCATION; VIOLENCE)

RESOURCES

Children's Safety Network, Education Development Center, Inc., 55 Chapel St., Newton, MA 02160

Federation for Children with Special Needs, 95 Berkeley St., Boston, MA 02116

National Center for Education in Maternal and Child Health, 38th and R St., NW, Washington, DC 20057

National Head Injury Foundation, 1776 Massachusetts Ave., NW, Suite 100, Washington, DC 20036

National Information Center for Children and Youth with Disabilities, P.O. Box 1492, Washington, DC 20013–1492

National Spinal Cord Injury Association, In Touch with Kids Program, 545 Concord Ave., Cambridge, MA 02138

Research and Training Center in Rehabilitation and Childhood Trauma, Tufts-New England Medical Center, 750 Washington St., #75K-R, Boston, MA 02111

BIBLIOGRAPHY

CHILDREN'S SAFETY NETWORK. *A Data Book of Child and Adolescent Injury.* Washington, DC, 1991.

DISCALA, CARLA. *National Pediatric Trauma Registry Biannual Report.* Boston, 1993.

DIVISION OF INJURY CONTROL, CDC. "Childhood Injuries in the United States." *American Journal of Diseases of Children* 144 (1990):627–646.

DOELP, ALLEN. *In the Blink of an Eye: Inside a Children's Trauma Center.* New York, 1989.

KREMENTZ, JILL. *How It Feels to Fight for Your Life.* Boston, 1989.

LASH, MARILYN. *When Your Child Is Seriously Injured: The Emotional Impact on Families.* Boston, 1991.

———. *When Your Child Goes to School After an Injury.* Boston, 1992.

———. and WOLCOTT, GARY. *Educating Children with Traumatic Brain Injuries.* Weston, MA, 1992.

MIRA, MARY; TUCKER, BONNIE; and TYLER, JANET. *Traumatic Brain Injury in Children and Adolescents.* Austin, TX, 1992.

PORTER, S.; BURKLEY, J.; BIERLE, T.; LOWCOCK, J.; HAYNIE, M.; and PALFREY, J. *Working Toward a Balance in Our Lives.* Boston, 1992.

WILLIAMS, JANET, and KAY, THOMAS, eds. *Head Injury: A Family Matter.* Baltimore, 1991.

MARILYN H. LASH

541

PERSONAL ASSISTANCE SERVICES

Personal Assistance Services (PAS) are key services for the approximately 25 to 30 percent of Americans with disabilities who have the most significant levels of disability (Litvak & Kennedy, 1993). These are people, of all ages and with all types of disabilities, living in the community and in institutions, who need assistance of another person for personal maintenance, hygiene, household and child maintenance, and work-related and community interaction tasks. This assistance can be hands-on, cuing, or standby. Not having this assistance is a major barrier to full participation for many persons with disabilities (Louis Harris & Associates, 1986).

For people with significant disabilities, personal assistants can literally mean the difference between life and death, because they help people with survival needs, such as getting into and out of bed, using the toilet, and eating. For others, the assistance, while less linked to survival, is equally crucial to health, well-being, and interaction in the community. To be able to live in the community as opposed to an institution, for example, people with psychiatric disabilities may need a live-in attendant to ensure their safety or periodic cuing regarding proper nutrition and medication. People with cognitive disabilities use assistants to help them plan their day, remember tasks, deal with legal and fiscal matters, and make decisions. People with sensory disabilities use readers, drivers, personal shoppers, and interpreters in their daily lives.

The Role of Personal Assistants

Many persons with disabilities explain the attendant's role as being an extension of the body of the person with disability, providing what that person's body cannot do, whether it involves moving, thinking, remembering, learning, or judging. This is the independent living model of service, which is based on the assumption that the individual with a disability knows best when, where, how, and by whom the assistance needs to be provided (DeJong & Wenker, 1979; DeJong, Batavia, and McKnew, 1992). Early conceptions of this model called for PAS users to train, supervise, select, hire, fire, and pay their attendant or attendants in order to be in full control

of the service. In contrast, most older PAS programs and many providers have operated under a medical model, which views PAS as taking care of patients who are sick. In this model people need a doctor's prescription for services, oversight by a nurse who monitors the service, which is provided by a home-care agency, which decides who the provider is and the tasks that person will perform.

More recently there has been discussion of the need for choice and flexibility so that consumers get what they need on an individual basis (GAO/Kaiser Family Foundation, 1993; Litvak, 1991). In this way all the PAS management tasks, including recruitment, hiring, payment, firing, training, supervising, and advocating, are available on an as-needed basis. This lessens the need for more expensive service models and is more acceptable to some PAS users.

Recruitment and Training

Turnover is a major problem (Litvak, et al., 1990). Provider wages hover around the minimum wage and can be even lower for live-in providers. Benefits, particularly for individual providers hired directly by the individual with a disability, tend to be limited to Social Security and workers' compensation (if they exist at all). Wages and benefits for agency providers have improved somewhat (Litvak & Kennedy, 1991a).

In some states, agency providers must be trained by the agencies, and minimum hours and even training content are specified. A number of independent living centers provide training for attendants and/or people with disabilities that underscores the independent living philosophy and teaches people with disabilities how to manage an attendant.

The notable Pennsylvania Attendant Care Program for people under sixty-five years old has built a menu of support services that consumers can choose from as needed to help them with the full range of management tasks. In other areas some of these tasks, such as recruitment, screening, and tax withholding may be available through a local aging agency or independent living center.

Personal Issues

Providers and users, especially those who work together many hours per week, talk about forming close relationships. Recent research has shown that for many users being able to choose one's providers is key to satisfaction with the services (Commonwealth Commission, 1991).

Involved in the personal assistant/individual with disability dyad are many issues involving mutual respect, respect for privacy, and certain rights, including the right not to be abused (DeGraff, 1988; Litvak, Heumann, and Zukas, 1987). Abuse can be active as well as passive, including not showing up on time (or at all) and other forms of neglect by the attendant.

Ethical Issues

In addition to more obvious ethical issues, such as maintaining privacy and respecting the rights of the assistant and the person with disability, there are also issues of how much one can ask an attendant to do. Can an attendant refuse to assist the individual with a disability in performing tasks the attendant views as harmful? Under what circumstances should an attendant step over the line and limit consumer choice?

There are many issues surrounding our society's obligation to provide services. Many in the disability movement argue that PAS is a right. When does the quality of life of the individual supersede the fiscal and liability concerns of the state? Do people with disabilities have the right to remain in the community even in the rare cases when it is cheaper or less risky to institutionalize them? Can we withhold payment for an assistant when we know that services lessen the abuse suffered by elderly people and decrease the incidence of pressure sores (GAO, 1991; Nosek, 1990).

Finally, in recent years there has been great concern that judges are sanctioning assisted suicide for individuals with disabilities who are not fully aware that they can have a high quality of life in the community with personal assistance, but this service is either not available at an affordable price to the individual or is completely unknown (Shapiro, 1993).

Economic Issues

Only two million of the almost 8 million living in the community who need PAS received some or all PAS services from publicly funded programs in 1988

(Litvak & Kennedy, 1991a). People who need PAS have substantially lower personal incomes than the general population and a sharply lower probability of working. No private insurance coverage exists for long-term PAS. Consequently, most PAS users who live in the community live with relatives and rely on them to meet their PAS needs. Few programs reimburse family members who serve as attendants. Many do not allow people who have nondisabled spouses or other family members living in the home to become eligible for service. Consequently, people with little informal/volunteer support and high PAS needs are very likely to end up in nursing homes. Older people without family support, most of whom are women, make up 90 percent of nursing home residents. The degree of disability is not the key factor determining nursing home residency. There are more people with significant disabilities living in the community than in nursing homes (Pepper Commission, 1990).

The low income eligibility requirements of PAS programs create penalties for employment and marriage among those needing PAS. Only a handful of programs provide PAS to people who work, and even these do not allow the attendant to assist the individual with a disability on the job. Most programs do not allow the attendant to provide PAS outside the home except for medically related trips.

Role of Legislation in Development of These Issues

The main sources of funding for PAS are Medicaid, Social Service block grants, state funds, and Title III of the Older Americans Act. The majority of these programs were not designed to provide PAS. They were designed to provide medical care or minimal assistance to low-income families in distress.

In the late 1970s, state-level independent living advocates pushed for programs geared to the needs of people with significant disabilities who wanted to work, and Congress initiated the Medicaid waivers. These waivers were to demonstrate the cost-effectiveness of community-based programs in keeping persons with significant disabilities out of nursing homes and/or institutions for people with mental retardation. To counteract the tendency for waiver monies to go to group homes for people with developmental disabilities, the Community Supported Living Arrangements Act was established to provide PAS in people's own homes. Other legislation has reversed the medical orientation of the Medicaid Personal Care Optional Benefit, the largest federal source of PAS funds.

President Clinton's health care reform proposal in 1993 called for a new program of community-based personal assistance that would allow choice of agency or independent providers who could be paid through cash allowances or vouchers, at state discretion. This proposal also presumes a model in which a package of long-term services could be designed to suit the needs of each person with a disability. Many aspects of this proposal appear to reflect the wave of the future. These aspects include flexible services, individualized service plans, direct pay, elimination of penalties for working and marriage, coverage for people with all types of disability, and eligibility for services regardless of income with a sliding-fee scale. All of these innovations have been tried successfully in pockets of reform around the country and the world.

Current Application and Future Directions

Though most users rely on family volunteers for assistance, family providers are often unsatisfactory (Nosek, 1990). Use of family providers can severely limit the personal and financial independence of both recipients and providers, and the stress on family relationships may increase the potential for abuse or neglect. Shifting family structures and increasing numbers of women entering the workforce mean that traditional family supports will become less available over time (Etheredge, 1987). Parents may die or become unable to assist their child with a disability. In addition, it may be feasible for family to assist at home, but it is quite awkward and often inconvenient for family to come to the work site or accompany a child to college.

Even if more people were served by the public system, their accommodation problems would not be solved because publicly funded personal assistance services are inadequate to meet the needs of people with significant disabilities. Services are inequitably distributed around the United States (Litvak, Heumann, and Zukas, 1987). The system

is fragmented, complex, and lacks a comprehensive, coordinated policy framework. Programs have developed in response to state and local needs, priorities, and advocacy efforts, and were designed to target particular populations. State funding sources vary from state to state. As a result, programs differ in age and groups with disability served, and not all groups with disability are served in every state. Most programs will serve people with physical disabilities, but far fewer will serve people with either cognitive or psychiatric disabilities. States vary considerably in the percentage of their population served by PAS programs.

Most programs are inadequate to meet the needs of consumers. They do not deliver enough hours of service, a broad enough range of services, or a comprehensive PAS package, including paramedical services such as catheter assistance. The decision as to what type of provider and system are best for the consumer is not dictated by the consumer's capacity for or interests in self-direction and management of their own service, nor by the volatility of their particular condition. What type of PAS program a particular individual is referred to depends on the range of choices available in a particular community or within a particular program (Kimmick & Godfrey, 1991). Suitable program fit is both a quality-of-life and an economic question. Concerns regarding liability and quality monitoring have dictated choices regarding the mode of service delivery and the design of provider training programs and have limited consumer control. Generally, policymakers have designed programs without attempting to differentiate among consumers in their ability to manage all or part of their PAS (Kapp, 1990).

Major Organizations Involved in This Area

State agencies that deliver PAS include those for health, social services, and aging. The National Governors' Association, the National Medicaid Directors' Association, and the National Association of State Units on Aging are key players in PAS policy development.

Provider agencies, some of which are multistate and linked largely to state Medicaid programs, are represented by trade associations.

Consumer-based advocacy organizations that play

a role on state and national levels include independent living centers and the National Council on Independent Living (NCIL); ADAPT (American Disabled for Attendant Programs Today); the PAS Committee of the Consortium for Citizens with Disabilities (CCD), led by the United Cerebral Palsy Association (UCPA), The Arc, and the World Institute on Disability; the Older Women's League (OWL); the Alzheimer's Association; and the American Association of Retired Persons (AARP).

Several public policy institutes and foundations, including The Brookings Institution, Families USA, and the Commonwealth Fund, have funded research and campaigns regarding these services.

Research has been carried out by the World Institute on Disability and its Research and Training Centers on PAS and Public Policy in Independent Living, Independent Living Research Utilization (ILRU) at Baylor University, Human Services Research Institute (HSRI), United Seniors Health Cooperative, and the National Rehabilitation Hospital. Funding for research and demonstrations has come from the Charles Stewart Mott Foundation, the Retirement Research Foundation, the Commonwealth Fund, the U.S. Department of Health and Human Services, and the National Institute on Disability and Rehabilitation Research (NIDRR). Data on PAS utilization have been collected in several national surveys, the Survey of Income and Program Participation (SIPP), the National Medical Expenditure Survey (NMES), the disability supplement to the National Health Interview Survey (NHIS), and the National Long-Term-Care Survey.

(See also: AGING; CAREGIVING; CIVIL RIGHTS; CONSUMERS; FAMILY; INDEPENDENT LIVING; PSYCHIATRIC REHABILITATION; PSYCHOSOCIAL ADJUSTMENT; QUALITY OF LIFE; RESPITE CARE)

RESOURCES

For the names and basic information on PAS programs in your state contact:

The World Institute on Disability, 510 16th St., Oakland, CA 94612

For assistance with accessing PAS programs, contact your local Center for Independent Living (CIL). To find out the name and number of your CIL, contact:

Independent Living Research Utilization (ILRU), 2323 S. Shepherd #1000, Houston, TX 77019

The National Council on Independent Living, 2111 Wilson Blvd., Suite 405, Arlington, VA 22201

To find out what organizing around PAS is occurring in your state, call several of the following organizations in your area:

Local Center for Independent Living; State Independent Living Council (SILC) c/o your State Government's Agency on Vocational Rehabilitation; Local United Cerebral Palsy Association (UCPA); Local chapter of The Arc; Local chapter of the American Association of Retired Persons (AARP), Older Women's League (OWL) or Grey Panthers

BIBLIOGRAPHY

COMMONWEALTH COMMISSION ON ELDERLY LIVING ALONE. *The Importance of Choice in Medicaid Home Care Programs: Maryland, Michigan, and Texas.* New York, 1991.

DEGRAFF, ALFRED H. *Home Health Aides: How to Manage the People Who Help You.* Clifton Park, NY, 1988.

DEJONG, GERBEN; BATAVIA, ANDREW I.; and MCKNEW, LOUISE BOUSCAREN. "The Independent Living Model of Personal Assistance in National Long-Term-Care Policy: Why Has This Approach Been Largely Overlooked?" *Generations* 16 (1992).

DEJONG, GERBEN, and WENKER, TEG. "Attendant Care as a Prototype Independent Living Service." *Archives of Physical Medicine and Rehabilitation* 60 (1979):477–482.

ETHEREDGE, LYNN. "Private Foundations and Social Change: Home- and Community-Based Care for the Elderly." *Health Affairs* 6 (1987):176–189.

GOVERNMENT ACCOUNTING OFFICE (GAO). *Elder Abuse: Effectiveness of Reporting Laws and Other Factors.* Washington, DC, 1991.

GOVERNMENT ACCOUNTING OFFICE (GAO)/KAISER FAMILY FOUNDATION. *Long-Term-Care Forum Discussion Paper.* Washington, DC, 1993.

KAPP, MARSHAL B. "Improving the Choices Regarding Home Care Services: Legal Impediments and Empowerment." Dayton, OH, 1990.

KIMMICK, MADDY, and GODFREY, TERESA. *New Models for the Provision of Personal Assistance Services: Final Report.* Bethesda, MD, 1991.

LITVAK, SIMI. "A Yardstick for System Reform: The Choice Model of Personal Assistance Services." In

Personal Assistance Services: A Guide to Policy and Action, ed. World Institute on Disability. Oakland, CA, 1991.

LITVAK, SIMI; HEUMANN, JUDY; and ZUKAS, HALE. *Attending to America: Personal Assistance for Independent Living.* Berkeley, CA, 1987.

LITVAK, SIMI, and KENNEDY, JAE. *Policy Issues Affecting the Medicaid Personal Care Services Optional Benefit: Appendices A Through E.* Oakland, CA, 1991a.

———. *Policy Issues and Questions Affecting the Medicaid Personal Care Services Optional Benefit.* Oakland, CA, 1991b.

———. "The Status of Personal Assistance Services in the United States." In *Personal Assistance Services in Europe and North America: Report of an International Symposium,* eds. Barbara Duncan and Susan Brown. New York, 1993.

LITVAK, SIMI; ZUKAS, HALE; LIEBER, ELLEN; BREWSTER, LARRY; ANDRAE, ROBIN; and KENNEDY, JAE. *Source Book of Personal Assistance Program Case Study Information, Appendix C: New Models for the Provision of Personal Assistance Services.* Oakland, CA, 1990.

LOUIS HARRIS & ASSOCIATES. *The ICD Survey of Disabled Americans: Bringing Disabled Americans into the Mainstream.* New York, 1986.

NOSEK, MARGARET. "Presentation of Initial Results of Current NIDRR Funded Research." Bethesda, MD, 1990.

PEPPER COMMISSION. *A Call for Action: Final Report for Bipartisan Committee on Comprehensive Health Care.* Washington, DC, 1990.

SHAPIRO, JOHN. *No Pity: People with Disabilities Forging a New Civil Rights Movement.* New York, 1993.

WORLD INSTITUTE ON DISABILITY and RUTGERS UNIVERSITY BUREAU OF ECONOMIC RESEARCH. *The Need for Personal Assistance.* New Brunswick, NJ, 1990.

SIMI LITVAK

PERSONALITY DISORDERS

Personality disorders are primarily characterized by a disturbance in interpersonal relationships. They are reflected through personality characteristics that are enduring ways an individual thinks about his or her relationships, environment, and self. These characteristics are displayed in social, personal, and occupational settings. They are maladaptive and cause subjective distress and significant functional impairment. These characteristics refer to behaviors or personality traits that reflect functioning in the past year as well as long-term functioning since early adulthood. Personality disorders are grouped clinically into three major clusters. Cluster A includes paranoid, schizoid, and schizotypal personality disorders. Cluster A generally describes a group of individuals whose behavior appears odd, eccentric, or bizarre. Cluster B includes antisocial, borderline, histrionic, and narcissistic personality disorders. These individuals may appear impulsive, emotional, and unpredictable. Cluster C includes avoidant, dependent, and obsessive-compulsive personality disorders. These individuals are characterized by excessive fearfulness or anxiety.

Diagnosing Personality Disorders

Personality disorders are diagnosed on Axis II of the Diagnostic and Statistical Manual of Mental Disorders (DSM-IV), with Axis I diagnosing clinical syndromes (e.g., schizophrenia), Axis III describing physical disorders (e.g., diabetes), Axis IV addressing psychosocial problems, and Axis V giving a global assessment of functioning. Disorders diagnosed on Axis I are not interchangeable with Axis II disorders, although both may occur.

Substantial overlap occurs among diagnoses of personality disorders. It is as yet uncertain whether this pattern is due to coexisting disorders, association among certain personality disorder groups, imprecise definitions of criteria, or heterogeneity among members of each diagnostic category. The DSM-IV uses a categorical method of diagnosis, and it may be that personality disorders should be seen along dimensions of psychopathology rather than as discrete independent entities. The presence of an Axis I disorder may complicate and make it more difficult to assess the presence of an Axis II disorder.

Paranoid personality disorder is identified by a pattern of interpreting the actions of others as deliberately demeaning or threatening. This type of individual generally expects exploitation and harm. In a work environment, she or he questions the intentions of colleagues and supervisors and tries to find hidden meanings in remarks, assigned tasks, or responsibilities. They question the loyalty and trustworthiness of friends and intimates without justification. They hold grudges, look for malevolence in new situations, and are easily slighted and quick to respond angrily.

Individuals diagnosed with schizoid personality disorder prefer to be alone. They display an indifference to social relationships with no desire to have close friends or be in a family. Consequently, they choose solitary activities. In the workplace they may have difficulty if interpersonal involvement is necessary. However, they also may excel in work performance that needs to be done in social isolation.

The criteria for schizotypal personality disorder reflect persistent disturbances in perception/cognition as it relates to self and others. These disturbances may include referential ideation, magical thinking, perceptual distortions, and impoverished interpersonal relationships. Some studies suggest a relationship with schizophrenia for this disorder suggesting a biologic, familial/genetic association. This information might also suggest that among clients with schizotypal personality disorder there exists a subgroup that may be genetically related to schizophrenia. Therefore, neuroleptics might benefit the person who experiences psychotic-like symptoms.

Antisocial personality disorder is identified by patterns of social irresponsibility, criminal activity, and impulsive/aggressive behaviors preceded by adolescent antisocial behavior. There is a clear connection between conduct disorder in childhood and antisocial personality disorder in adulthood; thus these two disorders share common psychosocial roots. For a diagnosis of antisocial personality disorder, the current age must be eighteen or older. Antisocial behaviors fail to conform to the social norms of adulthood (e.g., stealing, property destruction, reckless behavior).

Borderline personality disorder is defined by a pattern of instability in self-image, interpersonal relationships, and mood. These are manifested by intolerance of aloneness, intense inappropriate anger, impulsivity, rapid shifts in affective states, and disturbed interpersonal relations as central dysfunctions. These symptoms may be expressed as recurrent suicidal/self-damaging behaviors, exaggerated affective responses, and substance abuse. This disorder has been shown to overlap extensively with other Axis II disorders and is prevalent in individuals who report a history of trauma or sexual abuse as children. Caution must be used in making this diagnosis with survivors of sexual victimization because symptom constellation is similar to that of posttraumatic stress disorder.

Histrionic personality disorder can be traced to Freud's work with hysterical personality features. Thus there is a question whether this diagnostic category is prejudicial against women. The criteria include excessive emotionality and attention-seeking behaviors. These individuals constantly seek reassurance, need to be the center of attention, have little tolerance for frustration or delayed gratification, and are overly concerned with physical attractiveness. Their intimate relationships can be stormy.

Narcissistic personality disorder may have had its beginnings with Freud's use of the term "narcissism." This disorder may manifest itself through grandiosity, entitlement, lack of empathy, and the need for constant attention and admiration. These individuals are overly reactive to criticism and respond with rage. Their occupational endeavors may be striving for success or filled with depression and conflicted superior/subordinate relationships.

Individuals with avoidant personality disorder experience low self-esteem and broad-ranging fears of relating to others. They appear socially distant, which is due to interpersonal anxiety rather than interpersonal indifference, as in schizoid personality disorder. They have few close relationships, although there is a desire for them. They may resist promotions at work if it involves social demands and are hypersensitive to negative evaluation.

Dependent personality disorder is characterized by an excessive need for attachment, which elicits fears of separation, submissive, and clinging behavior. These individuals are unable to make everyday decisions without advice and reassurance from others. In fact, they let others make important decisions and have difficulty with initiative in life. They are intent on getting others to like them so that they may take on unpleasant tasks or agree with people even though they think the person is wrong. Since more women than men are diagnosed with this disorder, the issue of gender bias needs further investigation.

Obsessive-compulsive personality disorder is broadly defined by patterns of perfectionism and inflexibility. Individuals are so preoccupied with details, rules, and order that they often do not complete tasks at hand. They require that others do it their way. Work takes priority to the exclusion of pleasure and interpersonal relationships. Decisions are avoided for fear of a mistake. These people tend to be conscientious, moralistic, and judgmental of themselves and others. They withhold their feelings and are stingy about material possessions.

Treatment of Personality Disorders

Treatment approaches that have been useful for personality disorders include psychodynamic, interpersonal, behavioral, and cognitive therapies. Behavioral treatment has successfully been used for treatment of avoidant and borderline personality disorders. There is some evidence that psychodynamic therapy might be helpful in treating clients with coexisting disorders. For those individuals who display acting-out behaviors, hospitalization may be necessary to aid in behavioral containment. Professionals must be eclectic and flexible in their approach, since the etiology, course, and outcome of the different disorders are not yet fully understood.

As individuals experience alleviation of distress and are more able to turn their attention to, for example, employment or educational concerns, professionals within the mental health and rehabilitation settings will encounter these individuals. Given the trouble manifested in interpersonal relationships, as attention is focused on anxiety-producing changes, reeruption of symptoms may occur. This may be reflected in not keeping appointments, manipulative or dependent behaviors, or self-defeating, acting-out behaviors.

The model of psychiatric rehabilitation (Anthony, Cohen, and Farkas, 1990) that uses a cognitive, goal-setting process that develops deficit skills divorces itself from the often tumultuous emotional interplay. This client-centered approach enables the person to set his or her own goals. Problems in relationships are dealt with through interpersonal skills teaching. The focus is on how to help people achieve their goals, with particular attention paid to behaviors that interfere with the desired outcome. It is time- and labor-intensive; thus there is a high staff-to-client ratio.

The psychiatric rehabilitation model based on the notion of relationship-building presents a problem in the two-tiered system that now exists. Success for those individuals who can afford to pay for treatment, medication, and carefully managed relationships will be higher than for those not as advantaged, who must rely on public care in a system that is overworked, underpaid, and does not give high rewards for keeping problematic clients in services. There still exists a major need for more psychiatric rehabilitation services that target a personality-disordered population as well as those individuals who also have comorbid Axis I disorders.

Future research must focus on biological correlates and pharmacological interventions, outcome studies from different theoretical orientations of psychotherapy, rehabilitation outcomes on the different groups of personality disorders, and cleaner delineation of symptoms among personality disorders as well as between Axis I and Axis II disorders.

(*See also:* MOOD DISORDERS; PHARMACOLOGY; PSYCHIATRIC REHABILITATION; PSYCHIATRY; PSYCHOLOGY; SCHIZOPHRENIA)

BIBLIOGRAPHY

AMERICAN PSYCHIATRIC ASSOCIATION (APA). *Diagnostic and Statistical Manual of Mental Disorders*, 4th ed. (*DSM-IV*). Washington, DC, 1994.

ANTHONY, WILLIAM A.; COHEN, MIKAL; and FARKAS, MARIANNE M. *Psychiatric Rehabilitation*. Boston, 1990.

COOPER, ARNOLD; FRANCES, ALLEN; and SACKS, MICHAEL, eds. *The Personality Disorders and Neuroses*. Philadelphia, 1988.

HARTOCOLLIS, PETER, ed. *Borderline Personality Disorder*. New York, 1977.

OLDHAM, JOHN M., ed. *Personality Disorders: New Perspectives on Diagnostic Validity*. Washington, DC, 1991.

SUSAN J. LEWIS

PHARMACOLOGY

Pharmacology is that branch of science concerned with interactions between biochemical agents and living organisms. The term "pharmacology" is derived from the Greek word *pharmakon*, which means "drug, medicinal agent, remedy, or magic potion." Pharmacotherapeutic agents (e.g., drugs or medications) play an essential role in reducing the effects of disease and disability and improving the functioning of persons with physical or mental disabilities.

Pharmacokinetics deals with the absorption, distribution, biotransformation, and excretion of drugs (what the body does to the drug). Pharmacodynamics deals with the biochemical and physiological effects of drugs and their mechanisms of action (what the drug does to the body). Pharmacotherapeutics deals with the prevention and treatment of disease and disability. Toxicology deals with the adverse effects of drugs (Gilman et al., 1990).

For a medication to exert its intended therapeutic effect, it must first be introduced into the body of the person being treated. Directions for the exact usage of a given medication are specified in the prescription, which contains instructions for the type, form (e.g., tablet, capsule, solution), and strength of medication, the number of medication units, and the precise dosing regimen (e.g., dosage frequency and duration of the course of treatment). In addition, it is both ethically and legally necessary for the prescribing physician to obtain the person's informed consent before the treatment is initiated. This protocol requires the physician to explain to the person the nature of the prescribed medication, the anticipated beneficial effects, the possible side effects and adverse effects (including complications) associated with the medication, treatment alternatives, and the person's right to refuse or discontinue treatment. Following this discussion the person typically authorizes the physician to implement treatment.

The medication may be delivered into the person's body in a variety of ways, using oral, nasal, dermal, rectal, vaginal, subcutaneous, intramuscular, intravenous, intraspinal, or peritoneal (intraabdominal) routes. The route of administration is usually determined by factors pertinent to the specific treatment situation. After the medication enters the body, it is absorbed into the bloodstream, following which it is distributed throughout the body and the action of the drug is typically manifested. Ultimately the medication undegoes biotransformation, usually in the liver, which results in its biological alteration and deactivation. It is finally eliminated from the body via excretory mechanisms.

Because of these pharmacokinetic considerations, persons with impaired absorption (e.g., due to stom-

ach or duodenal disease), distribution (e.g., cardiovascular disease), biotransformation (e.g., hepatic disease) or elimination (e.g., renal disease) are at increased risk for treatment complications and/or failure. For example, a person who has undergone partial or total gastrectomy (removal of the stomach) for alcohol-related ulcer disease or stomach cancer would have difficulty benefiting from oral medications because of impairment of gastric absorption and resultant undermedication. Similarly, a person with atherosclerosis (arteriosclerosis, pathological hardening and narrowing of arteries) would be at risk for undermedication because of impairment of drug distribution mechanisms. In contrast, a person with alcohol-related cirrhosis of the liver or liver cancer would be at risk for overmedication and/or toxicity because of impairment of hepatic biotransformation. And a person with diabetes-related kidney disease or cancer would also be at risk for overmedication and/or toxicity (especially with lithium) because of impairment of renal elimination.

With regard to the mechanisms of drug action, two basic types exist: those associated with structurally nonspecific drugs, and those associated with structurally specific drugs (Carroll, 1993). Structurally nonspecific drug actions involve a generalized effect on a mass of body cells and are typically observed with anesthetic agents, ethyl alcohol, and antiseptic preparations. In contrast, structurally specific drug actions result from a unique interaction, known as "binding," between the chemical agent, or drug, and a designated component of the cellular structure of the organism, or receptor. The resultant drug-induced effect involves modification of ongoing cellular/bodily function; however, a drug cannot induce new or novel function. And if there is no drug-receptor binding interaction, then there is no observable drug action or effect.

The body produces its own natural chemical substances, known as neurotransmitters, which also bind to designated cellular receptor sites and produce specific cellular responses. Drugs that bind to the same site as a particular endogenous neurotransmitter and mimic or enhance its effects are termed "agonists". Other drugs, which are themselves devoid of intrinsic regulatory activity, bind to a particular receptor and, in so doing, prevent endogenous neurotransmitters and exogenous agonists from binding to that receptor site. As a consequence, these drugs, termed "antagonists," induce effects by inhibiting or blocking a particular cellular response.

The majority of pharmacological agents used in clinical medicine, psychiatry, and rehabilitation are structurally specific, and they modify cellular function by one or more of the following methods:

1. Stimulation: an increase in the rate of functional activity—epinephrine, phenylephrine (Neo-Synephrine), ephedrine, amphetamine, methylphenidate (Ritalin), caffeine, nicotine, albuterol (Ventolin), levothyroxin (Synthroid), digitalis, antidepressant agents (Elavil, Norpramin, Trazodone, Prozac, Paxil, Parnate), thrombolytic agents (TPA, streptokinase), diuretics (Diuril, Lasix), Interleukin-2.

2. Depression: a reduction in the rate of functional activity—barbiturates, benzodiazepines (Valium, Librium, Xanax, Ativan, Dalmane), ethanol, morphine, meperidine (Demerol), anticonvulsants (Dilantin, Tegretol, Depakote), phenothiazines and other antipsychotic agents (Thorazine, Navane, Prolixin, Haldol, Clozaril, Risperdal).

3. Blocking or inhibition: an obstruction that effectively prevents a particular action or response—neostigmine, atropine, propanolol (Inderal), atenolol (Tenormin), angiotensin converting enzyme (ACE) inhibitors (Capoten, Vasotec), calcium-channel blockers (Verapamil, Cardizem), cholesterol lowering (hypolipidemic) agents (Mevacor, Colestid), cortisone, prednisone, antihistamines (Benadryl, Dramamine, Antivert), anti-inflammatory agents (aspirin, ibuprofen, naproxen), antineoplastic (anticancer) agents (tamoxifen, cyclophosphamide [Cytoxan], methotrexate), immunosuppressive agents (cyclosporine, interferon), anticoagulants (Heparin, Coumadin), narcotic antagonists (naloxone, naltrexone), phenothiazines and other antipsychotic agents.

4. Replacement: the provision of a substitute or equivalent substance to restore an optimal condition—insulin, thyroid, levodopa, estrogen, ACTH.

5. Killing or inactivating organisms: the destruction or prevention of the growth of disease-causing organisms—antibiotics and antiviral agents, including AZT.

6. Irritation: the abnormal excitement of some body part or function—laxatives.

Additional factors influencing drug actions include diagnostic accuracy, prescribing methodology, patient compliance, presence and degree of adverse and/or side effects, duration of medication exposure, age, body weight, gender, attitudinal considerations, and the existence of comorbid features, including additional disease states and/or disabling conditions, and associated concurrent pharmacotherapy (polypharmacy).

The rehabilitation practitioner will encounter pharmacologic issues in a wide variety of contexts. This entry focuses on three primary areas: (1) persons who are exposed to the adverse consequences of prolonged bed rest; (2) persons with severe physical disabilities; and (3) persons with severe mental disabilities.

Individuals who are recovering from traumatic brain injuries, including strokes, as well as individuals with progressive neurodegenerative diseases (multiple sclerosis, amyotrophic lateral sclerosis, Parkinson's disease), cardiovascular diseases (atherosclerosis, diabetes), rheumatoid arthritis, muscular dystrophy, or spinal cord injury may be confined to bed for extended periods of time. Such persons are at increased risk for infection, including pneumonia and urinary tract infections, and often require antibiotic treatment. In addition, the risk of vascular complications such as thrombophlebitis and pulmonary embolus may warrant the use of anticoagulants such as Heparin or Coumadin. Finally, the risk of cardiac complications, such as heart failure and associated arrhythmias, and embolic stroke may require the use of digitalis and/or diuretics.

Ideally, the person with physical or mental disabilities receives the array of treatments necessary to promote symptom stability prior to his or her engagement in the rehabilitation process. Therapeutic pharmacology, typically a primary component of the initial stage of treatment, is designed to reduce or eliminate the disease process in some cases (infections, certain malignancies). More often, however, it is designed to reduce the degree of disabling symptomatology and promote a period of symptom stability, during which requisite rehabilitative interventions are designed and implemented.

Individuals with nonprogressive conditions such as traumatic brain injury, stroke, spinal cord injury, epilepsy, and polio will require an initial period of treatment during which their acute condition will be stabilized. For certain patients who have suffered stroke this treatment will include thrombolytic agents (TPA, streptokinase) to minimize infarction-related deficits, as well as steroidal medication to reduce cerebral edema. The person with epilepsy will be evaluated and treated with anticonvulsants such as Dilantin or Tegretol to suppress seizure activity. The goals of pharmacotherapy in these cases are to minimize the degree of deficit, to reduce the disabling symptomatology, and to prevent or reduce the development of secondary complications.

Individuals with progressive conditions such as multiple sclerosis, Parkinson's disease, Huntington's disease, Alzheimer's disease, amyotrophic lateral sclerosis, muscular dystrophy, myasthenia gravis, atherosclerosis, emphysema, cystic fibrosis, diabetes, rheumatoid arthritis, lupus erythematosus, acquired immunodeficiency syndrome, or certain malignancies, also require an initial therapeutic pharmacological regimen designed to promote symptom stabilization. The person with multiple sclerosis may present initially with motor symptomatology such as weakness, spasticity, or gait impairment. Pharmacological treatment might commence with methylprednisolone, which appears to reduce motor deficit symptoms, and Valium for muscle spasticity. The person with atherosclerosis may present with coronary and hypertensive symptomatology and might receive nitroglycerine, Cardizem and/or Mevacor to reduce coronary ischemia (angina pectoris), hypertension, and blood cholesterol levels. And the person with rheumatoid arthritis may present with inflamed, swollen, and painful joints, for which a nonsteroidal anti-inflammatory agent such as aspirin or Naprosyn might be prescribed. In each case, the initial pharmacotherapeutic goal is to promote clinical stability by reducing the degree of acute, disabling symptomatology.

The first goal of pharmacotherapy has been achieved when the acute, initial symptomatology has been eliminated, reduced, or stabilized. Individuals with some conditions (e.g., infections, certain malignancies, stroke, traumatic brain injury, spinal cord injury) may require no further pharmacotherapy unless case-specific circumstances dictate otherwise (e.g., recurrence of infection or malignancy, occurrence of depression, seizure). In other individuals with nonprogressive conditions, long-term maintenance pharmacotherapy may be indicated. For example, an individual with epilepsy may require continuing treatment with anticonvulsant medication to prevent seizure recurrence; and an individual who has undergone mitral valve replacement may require continuing treatment with anticoagulant medication to prevent thromboembolic complications such as stroke. In each of these cases, however, the primary goal of maintenance pharmacotherapy is to prevent or reduce the likelihood of the occurrence of complications.

In contrast, maintenance pharmacotherapy for individuals with progressive conditions is designed to achieve two goals: reduction or stabilization of primary disease-related symptomatology, and prevention or minimization of complications. Accordingly, the individual with multiple sclerosis who had been stabilized on methylprednisolone may exhibit an exacerbation or reemergence of disease-related symptomatology. This development may, in turn, necessitate redesign of the pharmacological regimen (e.g., the addition of Cytoxan or a switch to beta interferon therapy) to effect another clinical remission. This same individual may also develop complications such as seizure disorder, depression, or urinary tract infections that would necessitate additional appropriate pharmacotherapy regimens. The individual with progressive rheumatoid arthritis may require a switch to a pharmacotherapy regimen that is both more effective and, in many instances, more toxic (methotrexate, cyclosporine). And the individual with progressive diabetes may require not only more aggressive treatment with insulin, strict dietary regulation, and strict monitoring, but also treatment for complicating conditions such as hypertension, coronary artery disease, glaucoma, peripheral neuropathy, and infection.

It is also true that many severely disabling physical conditions are complicated by the appearance and often the persistence of chronic pain. Pain is a prominent feature in rheumatoid arthritis, osteoarthritis, degenerative disc disease, and many forms of malignancy. Narcotic analgesics such as morphine and Demerol, which are often required by those persons in severe pain, are associated with problematic pharmacological effects such as sedation and respiratory depression. These considerations, along with physician concerns that patients would be more likely to become addicted to narcotics if doses were increased, have contributed to a tendency to undermedicate patients in chronic pain in many instances. The recent advent of patient-controlled analgesia (PCA) has been salutary in this regard. Contrary to the predictions of many medical experts, patients who were given responsibility for managing their own pain medication regimens demonstrated enhancement of pain relief without any indications of overmedication or addiction (Graves et al., 1983). Nonetheless, self-medication with narcotic analgesics by some persons with chronic pain disabilities, with consequences ranging from dependency to overdose, continues to be a problem in pharmacotherapeutic management and must be aggressively assessed.

Psychopharmacology, the specialized branch of pharmacology that deals with the variety of medications used in the treatment of mental disorders, essentially came into being in 1952 with the discovery that Thorazine acted to reduce the psychotic symptomatology associated with schizophrenia (Laborit, Huguenard, and Alluaume, 1952). Since the early 1950s additional medications have been developed for the treatment of a variety of mental disorders including schizophrenia, bipolar disorder, depression, anxiety disorders (including panic, phobic, obsessive-compulsive, and stress-related disorders), and, more recently, certain personality disorders and chemical-dependency disorders.

The pharmacodynamic operations of psychoactive drugs are closely linked to five principal endogenous neurotransmitter substances: dopamine, norepinephrine, serotonin, gamma-aminobutyric acid (GABA), and acetylcholine. Although lithium's mechanism of action remains to be elucidated definitively, it has been demonstrated that many of the medications used in psychopharmacotherapy produce many of their effects by interacting selectively and specifically with these neurotransmitters and/or their receptor sites.

The observation that Thorazine was beneficial in the treatment of patients with schizophrenia stimulated research into the pharmacodynamics of Thorazine and related compounds. It was first suggested in 1963 that antipsychotic drugs acted by blocking dopamine receptors (Carlsson & Lindqvist, 1963). This work stimulated the formulation of the dopamine hypothesis, which suggested that schizophrenic symptomatology was a consequence of hyperactivity of brain dopamine receptors. In support of this hypothesis is the fact that amphetamine, a drug capable of producing a psychosis that is clinically indistinguishable from schizophrenia, appears to act by potentiating dopamine receptors. Recent advances in the pharmacotherapy of schizophrenia have resulted in the development of more effective "atypical" antipsychotic medications such as clozapine (Clozaril) and risperidone (Risperdal) and in a clearer understanding of neurotransmitter receptor site phenomena (Breier et al., 1994; Lieberman et al., 1994; Lindenmayer, 1993; and Marder & Meibach, 1994).

Joseph Schildkraut (1965) proposed the bioamine hypothesis of affective disorders, which postulated a causal association between depression and norepinephrine depletion states. This hypothesis was supported by the observation that imipramine, a tricyclic compound that had shown efficacy in the treatment of depression (Kuhn, 1958), acted to increase brain levels of norepinephrine by blocking its synaptic reuptake and biodegradation. Subsequent work has also established a causal association between depression and serotonin depletion states (Leonard, 1993), and the "new" antidepressants such as Prozac, Zoloft, and Paxil are known as "selective serotonin reuptake inhibitors."

Although the therapeutic effect of lithium in manic patients was first described in 1949 (Cade), the toxicity and morbidity associated with lithium treatment trials delayed its use in the United States until 1970. Research suggests that lithium influences a number of neurotransmitters (e.g., norepinephrine, dopamine, serotonin, acetylcholine) in diverse ways. Experience has established the mood-stabilizing efficacy of some anticonvulsants (e.g., Tegretol and valproic acid) in the treatment of some persons with bipolar disorder (Schaff, Fawcett, and Zajecka, 1993).

The pharmacotherapy of anxiety disorders consists, in the main, of benzodiazepine agents such as Valium and Xanax, which appear to exert their anxiolytic (antianxiety) effect by their potentiating interaction with the inhibitory neurotransmitter gamma-aminobutyric acid (GABA). Moreover, "benzodiazepine receptors" have been found in the brain's limbic system, and these appear to play a fundamental role in the modulation of limbic alert, arousal, and behavioral-inhibition mechanisms. This discovery of neuronal receptors for which benzodiazepines have a high affinity suggests the existence of endogenous anxiolytic substances, an idea that is conceptually supported by the earlier discovery of endogenous morphine substances, or endorphins.

Research has suggested a relationship between serotonin deficit states and a variety of clinical manifestations including impulsivity, aggressivity, suicidality, and possibly panic disorders, obsessive-compulsive disorders, eating disorders, and addictive disorders (Fuller, 1992). Such studies have stimulated clinical trials of serotonin-enhancing drugs in the treatment of at-risk individuals, including arsonists, violent offenders, addicted individuals, and individuals with personality disorders (e.g., borderline, antisocial).

The pharmacotherapy of persons with alcoholism and/or drug abuse involves the prescription of medications for both the psychological and medical components of the particular disability. For example, treatment of alcohol-related delirium tremens (DTs) requires a medical intensive-care approach incorporating intravenous fluids, thiamine, antibiotics, benzodiazepines, and, if indicated, anticonvulsant medication. For the person who is dependent on heroin who presents with a drug overdose, Narcan, a narcotic antagonist that blockades endorphin receptors, may be life-saving. Anxiolytic and/or antipsychotic medications may be indicated in the treatment of persons presenting with alcohol- and/or drug-induced psychotic states. Benzodiazepines, clonidine (Catapres), lithium, imipramine, and Prozac have all shown some efficacy in the management of alcohol and drug withdrawal states, and, in combination with other relapse prevention components, Norpramin, clonidine, and Prozac have been associated with decreased drug craving and preservation of sobriety and abstinence in some individuals.

As is the case with medical pharmacology, psychopharmacology consists of an acute, "therapeutic" phase during which disabling symptomatology is targeted and reduced if not eliminated. After functional stability has been achieved, many individuals can undergo a gradual reduction in the dose of their medication during the "maintenance" phase, and some individuals can discontinue their medications entirely. However, persons with psychiatric disability are challenged during their recovery phase by a return to their families, social support systems, jobs, and educational pursuits, and the psychiatrist must carefully and continually assess the person's ability to cope with the vicissitudes of life. A flexible psychopharmacological treatment regimen that is congruent with the person's shifting functional capacities is desirable in this regard. In some cases, recurrence of symptomatology will necessitate periodic, or even continual psychopharmacotherapy.

While antipsychotic, antidepressant, antimanic, and anxiolytic medications have all demonstrated efficacy in selected populations of individuals with disabilities, there are nonetheless salient toxicological concerns in that all of these medications are associated with adverse effects and, in some cases, potential morbidity and even fatality. With the possible exceptions of the new "atypical" drugs (e.g., clozapine and risperidone), the antipsychotics are frequently associated with a variety of neurological and endocrinological side effects, some of which (e.g., tardive dyskinesia) may be permanent. As a consequence, these drugs may induce "secondary" impairments that compromise an individual's ability to function adequately in social, vocational, and educational spheres of activity. Of even greater concern is the inherent toxicity of lithium and many of the older (tricyclic) antidepressants. When ingested in accidental or intentional overdose amounts, or in combination with alcohol and/or substances of abuse, these drugs can produce highly toxic conditions characterized by extreme cognitive impairment, cardiorespiratory depression, and even death. Fortunately, the newer antidepressants, such as Trazodone, Prozac, Zoloft, Paxil, and venlafaxine, appear to be safer in these respects. And the major risk associated with the use of benzodiazepines in both the treatment of anxiety disorders and sleep disorders is their high potential for abuse and dependence, as well as their toxicity when combined with alcohol and/or drugs.

During the course of their pharmacotherapy, many individuals receive more than one medication in their treatment regimens. This "drug-drug" combinative therapy, known as polypharmacy, imposes additional risks: the risks inherent to each individual drug, as well as a multiplicity of risks due to the additive, potentiating, synergistic, antagonistic, and/or inhibitory effects that result from the ingestion of a combination of drugs. For example, many individuals receive both antipsychotic and antidepressant medications simultaneously. Pharmacokinetic mechanisms may raise blood levels of both drugs higher than if either had been administered alone. As a consequence, additive sedative, anticholinergic, and cardiovascular effects, including malignant ventricular arrhythmias and cardiac arrest, may occur (Gelenberg, Bassuk, and Schoonover, 1991). Furthermore, psychoactive medications can also interact adversely with drugs used to treat nonpsychiatric conditions. The combination of certain antipsychotic and antihypertensive drugs has resulted in dangerous decreases in blood pressure and toxic delirium. Antidepressant drugs may lower blood Dilantin levels, thereby increasing the risk of seizure. And lithium may elevate blood digitalis levels, causing life-threatening cardiac arrhythmias. Finally, because smoking induces increased production of liver enzymes associated with drug metabolism, it causes reduction in plasma levels of drugs such as antipsychotics, antidepressants, and anxiolytics that undergo hepatic biotransformation (Ciraulo et al., 1989).

Medical consumerism and advocacy by patients' rights groups and other interest groups have resulted in increased awareness of the benefits as well as the possible liabilities associated with medical and psychiatric pharmacological agents. The right of an individual to refuse medical and/or psychiatric treatment has now been legally codified (Gutheil, 1986) and has posed new and important questions. Is it ethical to permit a person with psychosis to decline treatment that could ameliorate that psychotic state, when the persistence of the psychosis excludes that individual from his or her family, social network, and workforce? Is it ethical to permit a person with epilepsy to refuse anticonvulsant medication? Is it ethical to permit a person to refuse "life-saving" medication, or to grant a person's request for "life-ending" medication?

The trend in pharmacology is to develop newer medications that are associated with more precisely focused biochemical activity and fewer side effects (e.g., Cardizem, Corgard, Prozac, Risperdal)—that is, drugs that are both more therapeutically effective and safer. In this regard, continuing problems are the mounting cost of medications, proprietary laws pertaining to the manufacture of "brand" drugs, and quality assurance concerns related to the manufacture of "generic" drugs. The Food and Drug Administration (FDA) is the governmental agency charged with the responsibility for overseeing drug development and manufacture and for ensuring some degree of efficacy and safety in marketed medicinal agents. The Drug Enforcement Administration (DEA) regulates the prescription and medical use of "controlled substances" such as narcotics, amphetamines, and benzodiazepines.

Only physicians and osteopaths may prescribe medications in most jurisdictions. However, there are expanding efforts to enact legislation that would permit psychologists, chiropractors, nurses, nurse practitioners, and physician's assistants to prescribe medications. While it is true that some psychiatrists develop special expertise in psychopharmacology, any duly licensed physician may prescribe any legal medication. Prescriptions are typically filled by pharmacists who have completed master's or doctorate-level studies in pharmacy. Drug companies employ research chemists and pharmacologists in the development and manufacture of medicinal agents.

(*See also:* DRUG REHABILITATION; ETHICS; MOOD DISORDERS; MUSCULOSKELETAL DISORDERS; NEUROMUSCULAR DISORDERS; PERSONALITY DISORDERS; PSYCHIATRIC REHABILITATION; PSYCHIATRY; REHABILITATION MEDICINE; SCHIZOPHRENIA)

RESOURCES

American Association of Health Systems Pharmacists, 7272 Wisconsin Ave., Bethesda, MD 20814

American Medical Association, 515 N. State St., Chicago, IL 60610

American Pharmaceutical Association, 2215 Constitution Ave., NW, Washington, DC 20037

American Psychiatric Association, 1400 K. St., NW, Washington, DC 20005

BIBLIOGRAPHY

BREIER, ALAN; BUCHANAN, ROBERT W.; KIRKPATRICK, BRIAN, et al. "Effects of Clozapine on Positive and Negative Symptoms in Outpatients with Schizophrenia." *American Journal of Psychiatry* 151 (1994):20–26.

CADE, JOHN F. J. "Lithium Salts in the Treatment of Psychotic Excitement." *Medical Journal of Australia* 11 (1949):349–352.

CARLSSON, A., and LINDQVIST, M. "Effect of Chlorpromazine or Haloperidol on Formation of 3-Methoxytyramine and Normetanephrine in Mouse Brain." *Acta Pharmacologia* 20 (1963):140–144.

CARROLL, CHARLES R. *Drugs in Modern Society.* Madison, WI, 1993.

CIRAULO, DOMENIC A.; SHADER, RICHARD I.; GREENBLATT, DAVID I.; and CREELMAN, W., eds. *Drug Interactions in Psychiatry.* Baltimore, 1989.

FULLER, RAY W. "Basic Advances in Serotonin Pharmacology." *Journal of Clinical Psychiatry* 53 (1992):36–45.

GELENBERG, ALAN J.; BASSUK, ELLEN L.; and SCHOONOVER, STEPHEN C., eds. *The Practitioner's Guide to Psychoactive Drugs.* New York, 1991.

GILMAN, ALFRED G., RALL, THEODORE W.; NIES, ALAN S.; and TAYLOR, P., eds. *The Pharmacological Basis of Therapeutics.* New York, 1990.

GRAVES, D.; FOSTER, T.; BATENHORST, R.; et al. "Patient Controlled Analgesia." *Annals of Internal Medicine* 99 (1983):360–366.

GUTHEIL, THOMAS G. "The Right to Refuse Treatment: Paradox, Pendulum and Quality of Care." *Behavioral Science Law* 4 (1986):265–277.

KUHN, ROLAND. "The Treatment of Depressive States with G22355 (Imipramine Hydrochloride)." *American Journal of Psychiatry* 115 (1958):459–464.

LABORIT, HENRI; HUGUENARD, P.; and ALLUAUME, R. "Un nouveau stabilisateur végétatif, le 4560 RP." *Presse Médecin* 60 (1952):206–208.

LEONARD, BRIAN E. "The Comparative Pharmacology of New Antidepressants." *Journal of Clinical Psychiatry* 54 (1993):3–15.

LIEBERMAN, JEFFREY A.; SAFFERMAN, ALAN Z.; POLLACK, SIMCHA; et al. "Clinical Effects of Clozapine in Chronic Schizophrenia: Response to Treatment and Predictors of Outcome." *American Journal of Psychiatry* 151 (1994):1744–1752.

LINDENMAYER, JEAN-PIERRE. "Recent Advances in Pharmacotherapy of Schizophrenia." *Psychiatric Annals* 23 (1993):201–208.

MARDER, STEPHEN R., and MEIBACH, RICHARD C. "Risperidone in the Treatment of Schizophrenia." *American Journal of Psychiatry* 151 (1994):825–835.

SCHAFF, MARY R.; FAWCETT, JAN; and ZAJECKA, JOHN M. "Divalproex Sodium in the Treatment of Refractory Affective Disorders." *Journal of Clinical Psychiatry* 54 (1993):380–384.

SCHILDKRAUT, JOSEPH J. "The Catecholamine Hypothesis of Affective Disorders: A Review of Supporting Evidence." *American Journal of Psychiatry* 122 (1965):509–522.

DAVID E. CREASEY

PHILOSOPHY OF REHABILITATION

The history of rehabilitation is replete with examples of those individuals who have overcome the social and personal barriers that exist for many persons with disabilities (Maki, 1986; Wright, 1980). The richness of the rehabilitation effort is reflected not only in these examples of success but also in the voluminous legislation that stands ready, as a result of that effort, to serve all individuals with disabilities (Meyen & Skrtic, 1988; Wehman, 1993; Wright, 1980). Additionally, numerous principles exist to guide and support the rehabilitation effort (Wright, 1981). If one were to attempt to describe rehabilitation in two words, those two words would be, simply, "equal opportunity" (Maki, 1986).

Rehabilitation professionals at every level strive to emphasize the uniqueness of each individual involved in the rehabilitation process, with a goal of normalizing (Wolfensberger, 1972) their lives through greater individual self-awareness and a sense of community participation and citizenship (Emener, 1991; Maki, 1986; Wehman, 1993).

Thus the philosophy of rehabilitation values freedom, equality, individuality, and—most important—functional ability (Dougherty, 1991; Emener, 1991; Riggar, Maki, and Wolf, 1986; Wright, 1980; Wright, 1981). Further, these values exist in the context of multicultural (Ivey, 1987; Speight et al., 1991) and ethical (Callahan, 1988; Kitchener, 1984; Rest, 1984; Tarvydas & Cottone, 1991) considerations. Rehabilitation, then, is the process of maximizing the correspondence between ability and opportunity with the assistance of rehabilitation clinicians (Dawis, 1986;

Maki, 1986; Whitehouse, 1975), consistent with the wishes of the individual to be served (Emener, 1991; Maki, 1986; Maki et al., 1978; Scofield et al., 1980). These efforts are guided by both philosophy (Dougherty, 1991; Maki, 1986; Wright, 1980; Wright, 1981) and theory (Hardy, 1971; Hershenson, 1990; Maki et al., 1978). Philosophically, the goal of any rehabilitation effort is always maximum functional independence, to the greatest extent possible, for the person who is served (Maki, 1986; Meyen & Skrtic, 1988; Wright, 1980).

Additionally, interdependence among the various service components involved (Cottone & Emener, 1990; Maki, 1986; Maki et al., 1978), as well as interaction between the individual and his or her environment (Condeluci, 1991; Maki, 1986; Maki et al., 1978; Nadolsky, 1969), serve to define this philosophy as one that is systemic (Chubon, 1992; Cottone, 1987; de Shazer, 1985; O'Hanlon & Weiner-Davis, 1988) and existential (Nadolsky, 1969).

Thus the central issue involved in the philosophy of rehabilitation "is based on a fundamental belief in the worth and dignity of each individual" (Maki et al., 1978, p. 27). Further, the individual ideally guides the rehabilitation process, from beginning to a functional ending of the service component, with an overall focus on adaptation from an ecological perspective (Scofield et al., 1980). This entire process serves to minimize the difference between what is "ideal" (Wright, 1981)—that is, the person's dreams—and what is "real" (Wright, 1981), or the actual potential outcomes as a result of intervention.

Finally, an evolution of paradigm shifts (Cottone & Emener, 1990; Kuhn, 1970) now places the rehabilitation clinicians' focus (Whitehouse, 1975) on interpretation of the individuals' wishes across a variety of life areas (Maki, 1986), broadly subsumed under the categories of vocational (Cottone, 1987; Maki, 1986; Maki et al., 1978; Wright, 1980), social (Myers, 1992; Rusch, 1990; Witmer & Sweeney, 1992), and independent living (Crewe & Zola, 1983; Maki, 1986; Wright, 1980) outcomes.

Components and Related Issues

The philosophy of rehabilitation is holistic (Maki, 1986; Vash, 1981, 1992; Wright, 1980; Wright, 1981), such that an individual cannot be divided into discrete parts. Rather, each individual is unique, and aspects within each individual contribute to form a unique entity (Jacques, 1970). Dennis R. Maki (1986) further describes these holistic components as "elements [necessary in] understanding the concept of rehabilitation" (p. 4), summarized as follows: "Rehabilitation is an individualized process that is comprehensive in scope and prescriptive in nature that serves to develop or restore capacity with a goal of functional independence." Thus rehabilitation assessment and subsequent interventions encompass many operational constructs of the individual, with the belief that all of these components contribute, in some meaningful way, to a person's ability to perform, to the extent possible, as a fully functioning member of society.

While the overriding belief lies in the right of the individual to contribute in a citizen capacity (Maki, 1986; Wright, 1981), it is both necessary and wise that rehabilitative efforts are prescriptive (Maki, 1986). Thus some assessment of both interest and ability, at a minimum, across several functional domains is generally recommended (Wright, 1980). However, all measurement contains some error (Thorndike et al., 1991), and there is always the chance, however minimal, of over- or underestimating ability or interest (Thorndike et al., 1991; Wright, 1980). Further, due to prior segregated policies and procedures related to intervention (Wright, 1980), there is the issue of the experiential ability level of persons with disabilities, such that inventories may not accurately reflect genuine individual interest due to lack of exposure to normalized environments. As such, ecological assessment procedures (Maki et al., 1978; Scofield et al., 1980) are a viable alternative and may yield valuable information, although results may not be reliable across environments and may have limited application.

These issues do not preclude the prescriptive intention of assessment procedures (Maki, 1986), but ideally should be taken into consideration prior to implementation of results. Additionally, these issues take on particular importance when considering the increased emphasis, in general, on testing in our society (Thorndike et al., 1991). In the context of this increased emphasis, the Minnesota Theory of Work Adjustment model (Dawis, 1986) reflects these holistic and correspondent theoretical beliefs, on a vocational level, involved in the philosophy of rehabilitation (Maki, 1986; Maki et al., 1978).

Finally, such a holistic philosophy engenders several paradigm shifts, specifically from problem-solving (Maki et al., 1978) to solution-focused outcomes (de Shazer, 1985; O'Hanlon & Weiner-Davis, 1988); from charity (Wright, 1980) to community participation (Maki, 1986); from segregated (traditional) vocational training models to supported employment (Berg, Wacker, and Flynn, 1990; Rusch, 1990; Wacker, Berg and Flynn, 1990; Wehman & Kregel, 1985); and from illness and disablement (Cottone & Emener, 1990) to wellness over all developmental life stages (Myers, 1992; Witmer & Sweeney, 1992), with the inclusion of spirituality as a "fundamental life task" (Witmer & Sweeney, 1992, p. 140).

Philosophical Tenets

The philosophy of rehabilitation advocates for consumer choice and empowerment, issues that stand at the threshold of a renewed service delivery system for persons with disabilities (Campbell, 1991; Gould, 1986; Rhodes, Browning, & Thorin, 1986; Wacker, Berg & Flynn, 1990). These issues are further reinforced by legislation designed to place persons with disabilities in control of their own lives to the greatest extent possible (Wehman, 1993). While consumer choice and empowerment are laudable outcomes of the rehabilitation philosophy, they are not without criticism. In a discussion of internal and external considerations of empowerment, William G. Emener (1991) notes, with some irony, that systemic implementation of the Individual Written Rehabilitation Plan (IWRP), mandated by the Rehabilitation Act of 1973, had a disempowering effect on rehabilitation counselors. Emener goes on to address the need for professionals, nevertheless, to assure that they are "not externally impeded from having self-management and self-regulatory controls, and that they have the external empowerment necessary to advance and enhance their professionalism." (p. 9). Further, issues related to agency relationships, when viewed from a systemic perspective, may negatively affect consumer choice and empowerment, and ultimately outcomes, in the delivery of rehabilitation services (Chubon, 1992;

Cottone, 1987). Another issue related to consumer choice and empowerment is that of informed consent (Callahan, 1988). The question here is whether there is actually freedom to choose, since choice is a function of knowledge of the available alternatives. Such may not be the case, for example, with persons experiencing cognitive and/or emotional impairments. Thus, while the philosophy of rehabilitation holds consumer choice and empowerment at the core of individuality, knowledge of these related and critical issues is needed (Tarvydas & Cottone, 1991).

The philosophy of rehabilitation values integration (Maki, 1986; Maki et al., 1978). Consistent with the "equal access" intent of the Americans with Disabilities Act (ADA) and the mandate for social change (Wehman, 1993), this philosophy reflects an emerging trend of integrated, community-based employment for persons with varying levels of ability (Fabian, 1972; Fabian, Edelman, and Leedy, 1993; Nietupski et al., 1993; Stevens, Curl, and Rule, 1993; Wehman & Kregel, 1985; West & Parent, 1992). Integration of persons with disabilities into community jobs occurs at all levels of rehabilitation service systems, from transitioning students directly from school to work (Nietupski et al, 1993; Wehman & Kregel, 1985) to developing accommodation and support systems in the workplace for all persons with disabilities (Fabian, Edelman, and Leedy, 1993; Stevens, Curl, and Rule, 1993). Integrated employment options are believed to enable consumers to access complementary community amenities and benefits, with the intention of greater integration at all levels of society for persons with disabilities (Wacker, Berg, and Flynn, 1990). Such an ambitious effort, however, includes risk to the individual. Assessment of potential risk mandates consideration of ethical principles and issues, once again, related to informed consent (Callahan, 1988). Decisions related to potential risk require, consistent with the philosophy of rehabilitation, implementation of an ethical decision-making model that facilitates a moral course of action consistent with the rights and best interests of the individual (Rest, 1984; Tarvydas & Cottone, 1991). Full consideration must be given to all pertinent ethical principles involved (Kitchener, 1984), with consideration given to the individuals' right to fail as one potential outcome involved with the element of risk. More specifically, this involves *any* risk taken or assumed by *any* person.

Generally speaking, any change in any component of a service delivery package will, more often than not, necessitate further changes in complementary services. Thus persons in integrated employment settings may, for example, as a result of this intervention, decide to choose integration at other levels of community involvement. Thus an integrated job may influence a person's wishes for involvement with persons without disabilities (Rusch, 1990), a less restrictive residential setting or independent living status (Crewe & Zola, 1983), or a greater demand for more freedom and privacy. While the philosophy of rehabilitation embraces greater community involvement at all levels for persons with disabilities (Maki, 1986; Maki et al., 1978), controversial issues may arise out of these new choices; the most notable of these involve issues related to sexuality. Intimacy and sexuality (Vash, 1981) are of such a nature that "the urge for pairing is almost ubiquitous . . . and does not disappear when disability intervenes" (p. 70). Even beyond consideration of the Human Immunodeficiency Virus (HIV) or Acquired Immune Deficiency Syndrome (AIDS) (Bartlett & Finkbeiner, 1991; Hoffman, 1991), a more basic consideration challenges the philosophy of rehabilitation. That is, what opportunities related to sexual involvement exist for persons with disabilities, and is individual choice-making involved concerning access to these opportunities? Clearly, Carolyn Vash (1981) affirms that this should be so, and so do many others. The philosophy of rehabilitation embraces a person's right to choose relationships. Related issues naturally develop as a result of participation in a sexually active relationship or sexually active behavior outside the context of a specific relationship per se. Mentioned above is the critical nature of potential harm as a result of a pernicious sexually transmitted disease; however, a more practical application of this area of concern includes issues related to sterilization (Elkins & Andersen, 1992).

While the debate over the rights and responsibilities of sexually intimate behavior is far from over, it is important to recognize, consistent with the philosophy of rehabilitation, that such a philosophy is dynamic and evolving, and at the core of the philosophy is the individual's right to choose consistent with the ability to do so (Callahan, 1988; Rest, 1984; Tarvydas & Cottone, 1991) in consideration of maximum empowerment (Emener, 1991), in a least restrictive environment (Meyen & Skrtic, 1988). Certainly the issue of intimacy potentially places the greatest demand on ethical considerations and principles (Kitchener, 1984), with special consideration given to the principle of autonomy and nonmaleficence.

R. Rocco Cottone (1987) addresses a systemic approach to vocational rehabilitation, and a systemic approach from additional authors (Chubon, 1992; Gilbride, 1993) also includes family considerations. The philosophy of rehabilitation includes discussion of necessary and natural support systems, and parents of children may be critical to such a support system. Dennis Gilbride (1993) suggests that parents with more positive attitudes related to their children with disabilities were found to have higher vocational and social expectations for their children. Such a finding is consistent with maximizing the functional abilities that all persons with disabilities have (Maki, 1986) and contributes to the prescriptive nature of rehabilitation interventions. Similarly, such positive attitudes seem likely to facilitate removal of a "fundamental negative bias" (Wright, 1988, p. 8) that is often reported as a stereotypical measure of persons with disabilities; any conceptualization such as this fundamental negative bias detracts from expectations of functional abilities. Thus societal attitudes represent yet another paradigm shift necessary for full community participation to occur for persons with disabilities (Wehman, 1993).

Finally, a trend consistent with the philosophy of rehabilitation is that of quality of life, referred to by some authors as "personal ecology" (Peterson, 1993, p. 5). Since a universally accepted definition of quality of life does not exist, perhaps one that embraces the philosophy of rehabilitation most accurately is taken from Harvey Schipper, Jennifer Clinch, and Valerie Powell (1990), and is summarized as follows, with particular consideration given to related operational domains outlined by these authors: "Quality of life emphasizes the daily comings and goings of a free, living individual across four broad domains, which contribute to the overall effect: physical and occupational function, psychologic state and social interaction." Such a construct definition clearly relates to all aforementioned material and is totally consistent with aspects of freedom (Vash, 1981, 1992), domains (Maki, 1986; Wright, 1980; Wright, 1981), and integration and full inclusion (Emener, 1991; Jacques, 1970; Meyen & Skrtic, 1988; Nietupski et al, 1993; Wehman, 1993; Wehman & Kregel, 1985; Wright, 1981). Clearly, such a free, living individual may indeed exercise individual, inalienable rights to community and citizenship.

(*See also:* CIVIL RIGHTS; CONSUMERS; DISABILITY LAW AND SOCIAL POLICY; ETHICS; FORENSIC REHABILITATION; HISTORY OF REHABILITATION; NORMALIZATION AND SOCIAL ROLE VALORIZATION; QUALITY OF LIFE; SEXUALITY AND DISABILITY; WELLNESS; WORK)

BIBLIOGRAPHY

BARTLETT, JOHN, and FINKBEINER, ANN. *The Guide to Living with HIV Infection.* Baltimore, 1991.

BERG, WENDY; WACKER, DAVID; and FLYNN, THOMAS. "Teaching Generalization and Maintenance of Work Behavior." In *Supported Employment: Models, Methods, and Issues,* ed. F. Rusch. Sycamore, IL, 1990.

CALLAHAN, JOAN, ed. *Ethical Issues in Professional Life.* New York, 1988.

CAMPBELL, JOSEPH F. "The Consumer Movement and Implications for Vocational Rehabilitation Services." *Journal of Vocational Rehabilitation* 57 (1991):67–75.

CHUBON, ROBERT. "Defining Rehabilitation from a Systems Perspective: Critical Implications." *Journal of Applied Rehabilitation Counseling* 23 (1992):27–32.

CONDELUCI, AL. *Interdependence: The Route to Community.* Orlando, FL, 1991.

COTTONE, R. ROCCO. "A Systemic Theory of Vocational Rehabilitation." *Rehabilitation Counseling Bulletin* 30 (1987):167–176.

COTTONE, R. ROCCO, and EMENER, W. G. "The Psychomedical Paradigm of Vocational Rehabilitation and Its Alternatives." *Rehabilitation Counseling Bulletin* 34 (1990):91–102.

CREWE, NANCY M., and ZOLA, IRVING K. *Independent Living for Physically Disabled People.* San Francisco, 1983.

DAWIS, RENE V. "The Minnesota Theory of Work Adjustment." In *Handbook of Measurement and Evaluation in Rehabilitation,* ed. B. Bolton. Baltimore, 1986.

DE SHAZER, STEVE. *Keys to Solution in Brief Therapy.* New York, 1985.

DOUGHERTY, CHARLES J. "Values in Rehabilitation: Happiness, Freedom, and Fairness." *Journal of Rehabilitation* 57-1 (1991):7–12.

ELKINS, THOMAS, and ANDERSEN, H. FRANK. "Sterilization of Persons with Mental Retardation." *The Journal of the Association for Persons with Severe Handicaps* 17 (1992):19–26.

EMENER, WILLIAM G. "Empowerment in Rehabilitation: An Empowerment Philosophy for Rehabilitation in the 20th Century." *Journal of Rehabilitation* 57-4 (1991):7–12.

FABIAN, ELLEN S. "Supported Employment and the Quality of Life: Does a Job Make a Difference? *Rehabilitation Counseling Bulletin* 36 (1992):84–97.

FABIAN, ELLEN S.; EDELMAN, ANDREA; and LEEDY, MARGARET. "Linking Workers with Severe Disabilities to Social Supports in the Workplace: Strategies for Addressing Barriers." *Journal of Rehabilitation* 59 (1993):29–34.

GILBRIDE, DENNIS. "Parental Attitudes Toward Their Child with a Disability: Implications for Rehabilitation Counselors." *Rehabilitation Counseling Bulletin* 36 (1993):139–150.

GOULD, MARTIN. "Self-Advocacy: Consumer Leadership for the Transition Years." *Journal of Rehabilitation* 52 (1986):39–42.

HARDY, RICHARD. "The Issue of Theory in Rehabilitation." *Rehabilitation Literature* 32 (1971):19–21.

HERSHENSON, DAVID. "A Theoretical Model for Rehabilitation Counseling." *Rehabilitation Counseling Bulletin* 33 (1990):268–279.

HOFFMAN, MARY A. "Counseling the HIV-Infected Client: A Psychosocial Model for Assessment and Intervention." *The Counseling Psychologist* 19 (1991):467–542.

IVEY, ALLEN. "Reaction: Cultural Intentionality: The Core of Effective Helping." *Counselor Education and Supervision* 26 (1987):168–171.

JACQUES, MARCELINE. *Rehabilitation Counseling: Scope and Services.* Boston, 1970.

KITCHENER, KAREN. "Intuition, Critical Evaluation, and Ethical Principles: The Foundation for Ethical Decisions in Counseling Psychology." *The Counseling Psychologist* 12 (1984):43–55.

KUHN, THOMAS. *The Structure of Scientific Revolutions,* 2nd ed. Chicago, 1970.

MAKI, DENNIS R. "Foundations of Applied Rehabilitation Counseling." In *Applied Rehabilitation Counseling*, ed. T. F. Riggar, D. R. Maki, and A. W. Wolf. New York, 1986.

MAKI, DENNIS R.; McCRACKEN, NANCY A.; PAPE, DEBORAH A.; and SCHOFIELD, MICHAEL E. "The Theoretical Model of Vocational Rehabilitation." *Journal of Rehabilitation* 44 (1978):26–28.

MEYEN, EDWARD, and SKRTIC, T., eds. *Exceptional Children and Youth: An Introduction*, 3rd ed. Denver, 1988.

MYERS, JANE E. "Wellness, Prevention, Development: The Cornerstone of the Profession." *Journal of Counseling and Development* 71 (1992):136–139.

NADOLSKY, JULIAN N. "The Existential in Vocational Counseling." *Journal of Rehabilitation* 35 (1969):22–24.

NIETUPSKI, JOHN; MURRAY, GERALD C.; CHAPPELLE, SANDRA; STRANG, LYNN; STEELE, PAT; and EGLI, JULIE. "Dispersed Heterogeneous Placement: A Model for Transitioning Students with a Wide Range of Abilities to Supported Employment." *Journal of Vocational Rehabilitation* 3 (1993):43–52.

O'HANLON, WILLIAM H., and WEINER-DAVIS, MICHELE. *In Search of Solutions: Creating a Context for Change*. New York, 1988.

PETERSON, LIZETTE. "Behavior Therapy: The Long and Winding Road." *Behavior Therapy* 24 (1993):1–5.

REST, JAMES. "Research on Moral Development: Implications for Training Counseling Psychologists." *The Counseling Psychologist* 12 (1984):19–29.

RHODES, CINDY M.; BROWNING, PHILIP L.; and THORIN, ELIZABETH J. "Self-Help Advocacy Movement: A Promising Peer-Support System for People with Mental Disabilities." *Rehabilitation Literature* 47 (1986):2–7.

RIGGAR, T.; MAKI, DENNIS; and WOLF, ARNOLD, eds. *Applied Rehabilitation Counseling*. New York, 1986.

RUSCH, FRANK, ed. *Supported Employment: Models, Methods, and Issues*. Sycamore, IL, 1990.

SCHALOCK, ROBERT L.; KEITH, KENNETH D.; HOFFMAN, KAREN; and KARAN, ORO C. "Quality of Life: Its Measurement and Use." *Mental Retardation* 27 (1989):25–31.

SCHIPPER, HARVEY; CLINCH, JENNIFER; and POWELL, VALERIE. "Definitions and Conceptual Issues." In *Quality of Life Assessment in Clinical Trials*, ed. B. Spilker. New York, 1990.

SCOFIELD, MICHAEL; PAPE, DEBORAH; McCRACKEN, NANCY; and MAKI, DENNIS. "An Ecological Model for Promoting Acceptance of Disability." *Journal of Applied Rehabilitation Counseling* 11 (1980):183–186.

SPEIGHT, SUZETTE L.; MYERS, LINDA J.; COX, CHIKAKO I.; and HIGHLEN, PAMELA S. "A Redefinition of Multicultural Counseling." *Journal of Counseling and Development* 70 (1991):29–36.

STEVENS, MARGO L.; CURL, RITA; and RULE, SARAH. "From Protection to Independence: Utilizing Intersector Cooperation to Ensure Consumer Options." *Journal of Rehabilitation* 59 (1993):35–39.

TARVYDAS, VILIA, and COTTONE, R. ROCCO. "Ethical Responses to Legislative, Organizational, and Economic Dynamics: A Four-Level Model of Ethical Practice." *Journal of Applied Rehabilitation Counseling* 22 (1991):11–18.

THORNDIKE, ROBERT M.; CUNNINGHAM, GEORGE K.; THORNDIKE, ROBERT L.; and HAGEN, ELIZABETH P. *Measurement and Evaluation in Psychology and Education*. New York, 1991.

VASH, CAROLYN. *The Psychology of Disability*. New York, 1981.

———. "The Freedom-Protection Continuum: A Personal Perspective." *Journal of Applied Rehabilitation Counseling* 23 (1992):59–61.

WACKER, DAVID P.; BERG, WENDY; and FLYNN, THOMAS H. "Promoting Competitive Employment Services for Persons with Severe Handicaps Through a Coordinated Longitudinal Model." In *Supported Employment: Models, Methods and Issues*, ed. F. Rusch. Sycamore, IL, 1990.

WEHMAN, PAUL. Review of *The ADA Mandate for Social Change*. In *The Journal of the Association for Persons with Severe Handicaps* 18 (1993):304–305.

WEHMAN, PAUL, and KREGEL, JOHN. "A Supported Work Approach to Competitive Employment of Individuals with Moderate and Severe Handicaps." *The Journal of the Association for Persons with Severe Handicaps* 10 (1985):3–11.

WEST, MICHAEL D., and PARENT, WENDY S. "Consumer Choice and Empowerment in Supported Employment Services: Issues and Strategies." *The Journal of the Association for Persons with Severe Handicaps* 17 (1992):47–52.

WHITEHOUSE, FREDERICK A. "Rehabilitation Clinician." *Journal of Rehabilitation* 41 (1975):24–26.

WITMER, J. MELVIN, and SWEENEY, THOMAS J. "A Holistic Model for Wellness and Prevention Over the Life Span." *Journal of Counseling and Development* 71 (1992):140–148.

WOLFENSBERGER, WOLF. *Citizen Advocacy for the Handicapped: A Review of Selected Research and Development*. Washington, DC, 1972.

WRIGHT, BEATRICE A. "Value-Laden Beliefs and Principles for Rehabilitation." *Rehabilitation Literature* 42 (1981):113–116.

———. "Attitudes and the Fundamental Negative Bias: Conditions and Corrections." In *Attitudes Toward Persons and Disabilities*, ed. H. Yuker. New York, 1988.

WRIGHT, GEORGE. *Total Rehabilitation.* Boston, 1980.

DENNIS R. MAKI

GERALD C. MURRAY

PHYSICAL MEDICINE

See HOSPITAL, REHABILITATION; PHYSICIAN

PHYSICAL THERAPY

Physical therapy is an allied health profession that provides services in the areas of development, restoration, and preservation of physical function. The basic goals of a physical therapist include but are not limited to the following: relief of pain, restoration of functional movement, promotion of healing, motivation of individuals toward goals of optimal recovery, and assistance with the adaptation to permanent physical disability.

Physical therapy means the examination, treatment, and instruction of human beings to detect, assess, prevent, correct, alleviate, and limit physical disability, movement dysfunction, bodily malfunction, and pain from injury, disease, and any other physical or mental condition. It includes the administration, interpretation, and evaluation of tests and measurements of bodily functions and structures. The physical therapist is primarily responsible for the planning, administration, evaluation, and modification of treatment. The patient plan often includes instruction in the use of physical modalities, activities, and exercises for preventive and therapeutic purposes. Physical therapy also provides consultation, education, and other advisory services for the purpose of reducing the incidence and severity of physical disability, movement dysfunction, bodily malfunction, and pain (model definition of physical therapy adopted by the American Physical Therapy Association [APTA] Board of Directors, March 1986).

Since the 1980s, physical therapists have become more involved in the development of health care policy and the facilitation of quality health services that are accessible, available, and cost-effective. Within the spectrum of clinical practice, the therapist must assess, identify problems or determine if the diagnosis is a physical therapy diagnosis, then set goals, provide treatment services, evaluate effectiveness, and modify treatment to optimize the desired outcome (APTA House of Delegates, 1992).

The consumer of physical therapy services has myriad problems and limitations resulting from injury, disease, disability, or other health-related conditions. Those individuals commonly benefiting from physical therapy intervention may be individuals who have survived an accident; people who have cancer; athletes; burn victims; newborns, including premature infants; children with muscular dystrophy or cerebral palsy; individuals with arthritis, amputations, stroke, or heart disease; pre- or postoperative individuals; and people who have spinal cord injury or head injury.

Physical therapy intervention starts with an initial evaluation. A typical initial evaluation by the physical therapist includes the following:

- A background interview. This involves the taking of a medical, familial, social, and occupational history. The presenting problem and the events related to it are explored.
- Observation of the client. This may involve observation of posture, range of motion, and ability to move, walk, dress, or perform activities associated with job performance that may be of concern.
- Performance and interpretation of tests and measurements. To establish a physical therapy diagnosis, treatment, prognosis, and options for prevention, a battery of tests is performed. Some examples of these are a manual muscle test, which measures voluntary muscle function to determine muscle strength or weakness, and goniometry, in which the therapist measures joint movement or lack thereof using a goniometer.

After a review of the information gained from the initial evaluation, the therapist designs a plan of treatment. These therapeutic interventions may include, but are not limited to, the use of therapeutic exercise with or without assistive devices; modalities such as: heat, cold, light, air, water, sound, electricity; mobilization technique, bronchopulmonary hygiene, and muscle training or conditioning. In addition, the therapist may provide consultative, educational, or other advisory services.

Physical therapists work closely with the other medical professionals who help make up the rehabilitation team. These medical professionals include physicians, nurses, occupational therapists, speech pathologists, orthotists, prosthetists, and exercise physiologists. Other members of the rehabilitation team may include mental health professionals, rehabilitation counselors, and medical social workers. A key member of the team is the client, because the effort the client puts into recovery can often influence the outcome of physical therapy.

To become a physical therapist, an individual must earn a bachelor's degree in physical therapy or an entry-level physical therapy master's degree from one of the 130 accredited physical therapy programs in the United States. The accreditation of education programs for the physical therapist assures that programs prepare graduates who will be effective in contemporary practice. An accredited program is acknowledged to have the right to establish objectives in addition to those outlined in the Standards for Accreditation of Education Programs for Preparation of Physical Therapists (Commission on accreditation for APTA).

These standards encourage diversity, innovation, and uniqueness in education programs. Upon completion of all academic requirements a graduate must submit application for licensure. All states require physical therapists to pass a licensing examination prior to beginning clinical practice.

As the profession of physical therapy has expanded and the demands for services have increased, the areas of practice also have grown. Hospital physical therapy departments have traditionally been the primary area of practice. Because of changes in health care and practice without physician referral in some states, physical therapists now practice in many diverse settings. While the hospital remains the most popular place of practice for new graduates, some other settings include:

- Private physical therapy practices. Physical therapists in many states have their own private practices, offering physical therapy services without a physician's referral.
- Home care physical therapy services. Physical therapists travel to patient homes to assist with rehabilitation programs.
- Academic institutions. Many physical therapists hold advanced master's degrees and/or doctorates. These individuals teach and conduct research aimed at developing more effective evaluation and intervention strategies.

Physical therapists also work in public schools, long-term-care facilities, and adult day-care centers.

The APTA is a national organization dedicated to meet the physical therapy needs of society, address the needs and interests of its members, and develop and improve the art and science of physical therapy, including practice, education, and research.

Because physical therapy services offer people with disabilities the opportunity to lead more active and independent lives, the demand for them has grown rapidly. Although the profession has become more diverse and complex, the need for services has outpaced the number of physical therapists available to meet the demand. Surveys suggest that physical therapy is one of the fastest-growing professions, and it offers diverse career paths and strong job security. For all of these reasons, the profession faces challenges and choices unique among the health care professions.

(See also: ALLIED HEALTH PROFESSIONS; MASSAGE THERAPY; MUSCULOSKELETAL DISORDERS; OCCUPATIONAL THERAPY)

RESOURCES

American Physical Therapy Association (APTA), 1111 North Fairfax St., Alexandria, VA 22314

CATHERINE CERTO

PHYSICIAN

The overall goal of medical rehabilitation is to minimize the disability and handicap of persons with congenital or acquired physical impairments (World Health Organization, 1980). This goal basically requires a team effort, often prolonged, in which the physician plays a crucial leadership role. Medical rehabilitation takes place in a variety of settings, including general hospitals, independent (freestanding) rehabilitation hospitals (IRH), outpatient departments, skilled nursing facilities, day programs, and home care. The specific physical impairments that are dealt with in medical rehabilitation are principally spinal cord injury, traumatic brain injury, major multiple trauma, stroke, amputations, neurological disorders, polyarthritis, hip fractures, burns, and congenital deformities. In all cases, the medical rehabilitation goal is to bring the individual with physical impairment to the highest level of functional performance (least disability) and the lowest degree of handicap (reduced social role and poor quality of life) of which he or she is capable.

Obviously, the care of such complicated cases requires the cooperation of many kinds of physicians, nurses, and other associated health practitioners. The physician group that is particularly relevant includes orthopedists, neurosurgeons, general surgeons, emergency physicians (and paramedics), urologists, neurologists, and rheumatologists. Others, such as infectious disease specialists, ophthalmologists, otolaryngologists, nephrologists, and hematologists, are major contributors in particular cases. This entry will concentrate on the role of the rehabilitation physician and describe his or her background, training, and relationship to the classic rehabilitation team of associated health professionals.

Increasingly, the rehabilitation physician is a physiatrist. Physiatrists are trained in special residency programs consisting of one year of general medicine and three years of physical medicine and rehabilitation (PM&R) (De Lisa & Bans, 1993; Goodgold, 1988; Kottke & Lehman, 1990). There are seventy-three accredited PM&R training programs in the United States and approximately four hundred physiatrists (Lee & Clark, 1993). In addition to the regular four-year programs in PM&R, there are now, in some institutions, five-year programs that combine PM&R with pediatrics, neurology, or internal medicine. Certification in the specialty of PM&R is given by the American Board of Physical Medicine and Rehabilitation after a two-part examination. As the number of physiatrists grows, there are progressively fewer physicians from other specialties practicing medical rehabilitation.

In the United States, the formal practice of rehabilitation medicine is performed by a rehabilitation team. This consists of physiatrists; rehabilitation nurses (often with a master's degree in rehabilitation nursing) (Dittmar, 1989), including nurse practitioners and physician's assistants; physical therapists (entry-level bachelor's degree); occupational therapists (entry-level bachelor's degree); speech pathologists (entry-level master's degree); and a variety of psychosocial professionals, including psychologists (Ph.D.), social workers (M.S.W.), and rehabilitation counselors (entry-level master's degree). This rehabilitation team is not only traditional but also is required for accreditation by the Joint Commission for the Accreditation of Health Organizations (JCAHO, 1992) and the Commission for the Accreditation of Rehabilitation Facilities (CARF, 1994). Reimbursement for medical rehabilitation comes from Medicare, Medicaid, no-fault insurance, and a variety of private insurance carriers. Under Medicare, rehabilitation medicine is exempt from the diagnostic related groups (DRG) system and is reimbursed by a special formula established by the Tax Equity and Fiscal Responsibility Act of 1982 (TEFRA). This system may change with new health care policies.

While each of the associated health professionals in the rehabilitation team has its own identity, organizations, and journals, in the rehabilitation setting all work together to bring each individual patient to the highest functional level of which he or she is capable.

The role of the physiatrist in medical rehabilitation begins with assuring, as an early consultant, that the acute care being received by the patient is not only medically optimal but also that adequate nursing, physical, occupational, and other therapy is provided to reduce the frequency of preventable disabilities when the patient finally comes to rehabilitation. An example would be the acute stroke patient who needs special positioning, bowel and bladder management, and range of motion exercises from the very beginning of hospitalization (Gresham, 1992). Close cooperation with the neurologist, neurosurgeon, orthopedist, or other acute care physician, is vital.

The next role is to select patients who can benefit

from the rehabilitation process in terms of enhanced function and to direct them to the most appropriate setting (hospital, skilled nursing facility, day care, outpatient department, or home care) to receive these services. In all instances, the goal is to minimize physical disability and maximize physical independence and overall quality of life.

The process of selecting appropriate candidates for medical rehabilitation and designating the most appropriate setting requires great clinical judgment and experience. The physiatrist must perform a functional evaluation, as well as a physical examination, and ascertain the cognitive level of the patient. He or she must also assess how the acute or concurrent medical problems will affect the clinical course of the patient and medical rehabilitation efforts. For example, a spinal cord injury patient with concurrent head injury and impaired cognitive function presents a much more complicated challenge and will require much more time to complete the rehabilitation process than an individual with spinal cord injury alone.

Most spinal cord injury patients will be transferred to inpatient rehabilitation centers for an intensive program emphasizing maximal independence. For patients with complete lesions, the functional potential is relatively clear-cut: paraplegics (both legs paralyzed) should become independent at the wheelchair level, and quadriplegics (with higher levels of paralysis) up to the fifth cervical spinal cord level should be able to be largely independent with proper assistance and appropriate mechanized equipment. Fourth cervical spinal cord level patients will require facial control power wheelchairs or else be bed bound; third cervical spinal cord and higher level patients will be respirator-dependent. For the physiatrist, the decision must be made as to when and where to transfer the patient and to manage not only the rehabilitation services but intercurrent medical problems as well. For example, the rehabilitation nurse will develop the patient's bowel and bladder program, the physical therapist will work toward maximum mobility, the occupational therapist will emphasize maximal independence in activities of daily living, and counselors will work with psychosocial problems; but the physiatrist, in addition to coordinating these rehabilitative services, must manage intercurrent problems such as urinary

tract infections and take measures to prevent deep venous thrombosis and other possible complications (De Lisa & Bans, 1993; Goodgold, 1988; Kottke & Lehman, 1990).

The steadily increasing number of traumatic brain injury (TBI) patients presents a great challenge to the judgment of the physiatrist. The clinical manifestations can be almost anything, due to the diffuse nature of brain injuries, and cognitive and behavioral dysfunction are present in varying degrees in most conscious patients. In general, the physical problems of the TBI patient will resolve long before the cognitive and affective ones. Extremely prolonged treatment, especially with a behavioral emphasis, may be required, and some patients will remain in a coma for years. Therefore it is obvious that the TBI patient presents a formidable challenge to the rehabilitation team, but the physiatrist must choose carefully the level and place of care and modify these as the situation changes. In these cases, new imaging techniques, such as computerized axial tomography and magnetic resonance imaging, are very helpful in localizing the specific areas of the brain that have been damaged.

Stroke rehabilitation can be carried out in a variety of settings. The physiatrist must designate hospital, skilled nursing facility, or home care and keep track of the patient or transfer him or her to another competent physician. Stroke patients receive all the therapies, including speech pathology, if they manifest any kind of speech or swallowing disorder. Stroke patients progress rapidly due to both spontaneous neural recovery and rehabilitation, and the average length of stay in U.S. rehabilitation units is fewer than thirty days (Granger, Hamilton, and Fiedler, 1992). Stroke patients usually manifest a single major brain lesion, due to specific loss of vascular supply, as opposed to the highly diffuse group of deficits seen in TBI patients.

Stroke and other types of patients often require bracing, and most patients with amputations need artificial limbs. Therefore, the physiatrist must be expert in the prescription of both orthotics and prosthetics. Much of this work is done on an outpatient basis and requires close cooperation with the physical therapists, occupational therapists, orthotists, and prosthetists. Walking aids and extensive adaptive equipment may also be required. Environmental control systems, when appropriate, can also increase the independence of many patients.

Multiple trauma (two or more limbs fractured) and hip fracture patients comprise a large group of medical rehabilitation patients. Here the physiatrist must work closely with the orthopedists and surgeons, be highly knowledgeable about the clinical problems involved, and provide expert guidance to the physical therapists, who will actually mobilize the patient. Elective total joint replacements also require close cooperation between the orthopedic surgeon and the rehabilitation team that will prepare the patient for surgery as well as provide rehabilitative aftercare.

Various neurologic disorders, such as multiple sclerosis, Guillain-Barré syndrome, congenital deformities (such as spina bifida), and burn rehabilitation, require specialized team efforts characterized by a high degree of knowledge and interaction between the rehabilitation team and the neurologist, developmental pediatrician, and surgeon, respectively. Some physiatrists limit their work entirely to the pediatric setting, where they work with children who have cerebral palsy, congenital diseases, and malformations as well as acquired injuries. Here, again, close cooperation with the developmental pediatrician is mandatory.

Finally, the physiatrist deals with a multitude of neurologic and musculoskeletal disorders in patients who are not candidates for surgery. This work includes many types of low back problems, such as herniated disks; neck and shoulder problems; and all types of weakness or paralysis, whether due to neurologic causes or intrinsic muscle disease.

This broad spectrum of clinical responsibilities and skills requires that the well-trained physiatrist possesses extensive knowledge and procedure skills. Mastery of anatomy, especially neuroanatomy and musculoskeletal anatomy; clinical skill in all nervous and musculoskeletal diseases; competence in electrodiagnosis (electromyography, nerve conduction studies, and somatosensory evoked potentials); familiarity with the injections of muscles, tendons, and other structures; a thorough understanding of exercise and biomechanics; expertise in functional assessment; and a thorough knowledge of what each of the therapies has to offer, are all examples of the knowledge base required by the well-trained physiatrist.

The professional organizations of physiatrists are the American Academy of Physical Medicine and Rehabilitation (membership limited to physicians certified by the American Board of Physical Medicine and Rehabilitation), the American Association of Electrodiagnostic Medicine (admission by examination), the Association of Academic Physiatrists, and numerous local and medical-society-related subgroups. Physiatrists are also a major component of the American Congress of Rehabilitation Medicine, which is a national organization open by election to all rehabilitation professionals.

In addition to these organizations, each component profession of the rehabilitation team has its own national organization and its own credentialing and licensure requirements. Among the major professional organizations are the American Physical Therapy Association, the American Occupational Therapy Association, the American Speech-Hearing-Language Association, the Association of Rehabilitation Nurses, and others.

A unique facet of rehabilitation medicine is its long-term commitment to the patient with physical impairment. Because it is often difficult to find general physicians with the expertise and interest in caring for them, many such patients will continue to receive care from physiatrists and other members of the rehabilitation team for years.

Another important role of physiatrists and rehabilitation team members is patient advocacy, especially providing support and encouragement for initiatives by the population with disabilities itself. The numerous federal and state laws enacted to meet the needs of persons with disabilities are excellent examples of what the mobilized political power of this population and their advocates can accomplish. Independent living centers are also increasing in number and are enormously helpful.

As mentioned above, the process of medical rehabilitation takes place in a variety of settings. The specialized rehabilitation unit or independent rehabilitation hospital (IRF) is still the most prominent setting, but skilled nursing facilities, day care, and home care programs are growing rapidly. In addition to meeting specific accreditation requirements (CARF, 1994; JCAHO, 1992), these facilities must be prepared for possible changes in reimbursement policies, particularly prospective payment, which is very likely to occur by the end of the decade. Active in these discussions, which also include government agencies and many private organizations, is the American Rehabilitation Association (formerly the National Association of Rehabilitation Facilities, NARF).

Still another role of the rehabilitation physician is to decide, in concert with the rehabilitation team, when specific rehabilitation services should be terminated. This is often a very difficult decision, but the classic thinking in IRFs is failure to document any further functional improvement after a two-

week period. A part of this activity, of course, is the decision as to where the patient should go to live. Again with the help of the rehabilitation team, the patient returns home (if a supportive family is available or the patient can manage safely on his or her own) or to a protected environment. Rehabilitation services, if needed, can be continued in any setting; the emphasis on discharge is safety and the least restrictive environment.

The focal role of the rehabilitation physician at this time is to assess the outcome of the rehabilitation of each patient to make sure that nothing has

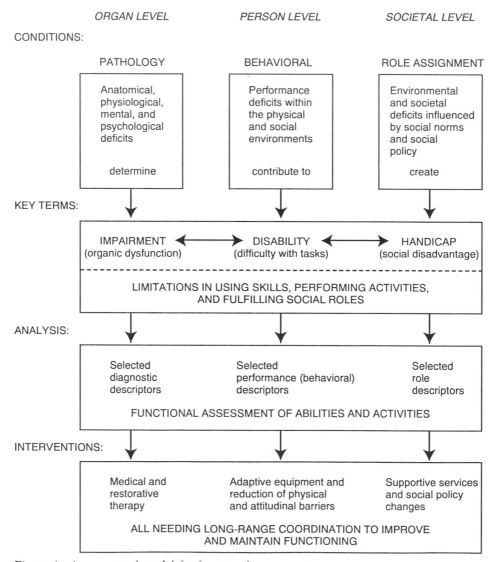

Figure 1. A conceptual model for functional assessment

SOURCE: Graphic formulation of the ICIDH developed by Philip H. N. Wood (World Health Organization, 1980) and from the concepts of Saad Z. Nagi (Granger & Gresham, 1984)

been missed and that the patient has been made optimally independent in an appropriate environment. In addition, adequate follow-up services, if needed, must be arranged.

The unique common language of rehabilitation professionals is functional assessment (Granger & Gresham, 1984). The term "functional assessment" refers to a system of numerous parameters used by rehabilitation professionals to classify rehabilitation patients, monitor their progress, and promote communication among professional staff, program monitoring, and research.

Functional assessment is based on the International Classification of Impairments, Disabilities, and Handicaps (ICIDH) model (Figure 1), as devised by Granger in 1984.

Among the many instruments used in functional assessment are the following:

1. Global scales, which give an overall rating of the patient's functional status. The Rankin Scale is the most venerable of these (Rankin, 1957).

2. Cognitive function measurements, of which the most common is the Folstein Mini-Mental Scale (Folstein, Folstein, and McHugh, 1975), although more in-depth study by neuropsychologists is also of great help, especially in TBI cases.

3. Scales measuring competence in activities of daily living, which include mobility, eating, grooming, personal hygiene, dressing, and all the skills required for independent personal function. The most widely used ADL scales are the Barthel Index (Mahoney & Barthel, 1965) and the Functional Independence Measure (Granger et al., 1986).

4. Other functional domains that must be addressed are motor function, speech, swallowing, hand function, instrumental ADL, quality of life, and family support systems. Multiple techniques for assessing these can be obtained from the literature (Granger & Gresham, 1984).

Functional assessment also provides proof of rehabilitation outcomes. It is of growing importance to physiatrists and all rehabilitation professionals. Functional assessment, as a concept and technique, should be familiar to all physicians and health care professionals who deal with patients with disabling problems.

In summary, the role of the physician in medical rehabilitation is a complex one, requiring not only multiple clinical skills and specific knowledge but also that both physician and allied health professionals emphasize a functionally oriented approach to the entire process.

(*See also:* ALLIED HEALTH PROFESSIONS; HEAD INJURY; HOSPITAL, REHABILITATION; MULTIPLE DISABILITIES; NURSING, REHABILITATION; OCCUPATIONAL THERAPY; PHYSICAL THERAPY; REHABILITATION CENTER; HOSPITAL, REHABILITATION; SPINAL CORD INJURY; STROKE; SURGERY)

RESOURCES

American Academy of Physical Medicine and Rehabilitation, 78 East Adams St., Suite 310, Chicago, IL 60603–6103

American Association of Electrodiagnostic Medicine; 21 Second St., SW, Suite 103, Rochester, MN 55902

American Board of Physical Medicine and Rehabilitation, Northwest Center, Suite 674, 21 First St., SW, Rochester, MN 55902

American Congress of Rehabilitation Medicine, 5700 Old Orchard Rd, 1st floor, Skokie, IL 60077–1057

American Occupational Therapy Association, P.O. Box 1725, Rockville, MD 20849–1725

American Physical Therapy Association, 1111 North Fairfax St., Alexandria, VA 22314–1488

American Speech-Language-Hearing Association, 10801 Rockville Pike, Rockville, MD 20852–3279

Association of Academic Physiatrists, 7100 Lakewood Building, Suite 112, 5987 East 71st St., Indianapolis, IN 46220

Association of Rehabilitation Nurses, 5700 Old Orchard Rd, 1st floor, Skokie, IL 60077–1057

National Association of Rehabilitation Facilities (NARF), P.O. Box 17675, Washington, DC 20041

BIBLIOGRAPHY

COMMISSION FOR THE ACCREDITATION OF REHABILITATION FACILITIES (CARF). *Standards Manual for Organizations Serving People with Disabilities.* Tucson, 1994.

DE LISA, JOEL A., and BANS, BRUCE M., eds. *Rehabilitation Medicine: Principles and Practice,* 4th ed. Philadelphia, 1993.

DITTMAR, SHARON S. *Rehabilitation Nursing: Process and Application.* St. Louis, 1989.

FOLSTEIN, MARSHALL F.; FOLSTEIN, SUSAN; and

McHugh, Paul R. "Mini-Mental State Exam: A Practical Method for Grading the Cognitive State of Patients for Clinicians." *Journal of Psychiatric Research* 12 (1975):189–198.

Goodgold, Joseph G., ed. *Rehabilitation Medicine.* St. Louis, 1988.

Granger, Carl V., and Gresham, Glen E., eds. *Functional Assessment in Rehabilitation Medicine.* Baltimore, 1984.

Granger, Carl V.; Hamilton, Byron B.; and Fiedler, Roger C. "Discharge Outcome After Stroke Rehabilitation." *Stroke* 23 (1992):978–982.

Granger, Carl V.; Hamilton, Byron B.; Keith, Robert A.; Zieliezny, Maria; and Sherwin, Frances S. "Advances in Functional Assessment for Medical Rehabilitation." *Topics in Geriatric Rehabilitation* 1 (1986):59–74.

Gresham, Glen E. "Rehabilitation of the Stroke Survivor." In *Stroke: Pathophysiology, Diagnosis, and Management,* eds. Henry J. M. Barnett, J. P. Mohr, Bennett M. Stein, and Frank M. Yatsu. 2nd ed. New York, 1992.

Joint Commission on Accreditation for Healthcare Organizations (JCAHO). *1993 Accreditation Manual for Hospitals.* Oakbrook Terrace, IL, 1992.

Kottke, Frederic J., and Lehman, Justus F., eds. *Krusen's Handbook of Physical Medicine and Rehabilitation.* 4th ed. Philadelphia, 1990.

Lee, Kyu-Ha, and Clark, Gary S. Personal communication, 1993.

Mahoney, Florence J., and Barthel, Dorothea W. "Functional Evaluation: The Barthel Index." *Maryland Medical Journal* 14 (1965):61–65.

Rankin, John. "Cerebral Vascular Accidents in Patients over the Age of 60: II. Prognosis." *Scottish Medical Journal* 2 (1957):200–215.

World Health Organization: *International Classification of Impairments, Disabilities, and Handicaps.* Geneva, 1980.

Glen E. Gresham

POLICY

See DISABILITY LAW AND SOCIAL POLICY; STATE–FEDERAL REHABILITATION PROGRAM

POLIO

See NEUROMUSCULAR DISORDERS

PREJUDICE

See ATTITUDES

PRESIDENT'S COMMITTEE ON EMPLOYMENT OF PEOPLE WITH DISABILITIES

When the noted disability rights leader Justin Dart sat on the platform with President Bush for the July 26, 1990, signing of the Americans with Disabilities Act, a historic milestone in American civil rights was marked. Dart, a former businessman and person with a disability for more than forty years, through his work unifying Americans with disabilities to fight for their rights and the new law, created a grassroots movement of empowerment that has changed the roles of people with disabilities in the United States. As Dart was also chairman of the President's Committee on Employment of People with Disabilities, the history of this small federal agency with an unusual public-private structure was equally marked. In many ways the change in focus and objectives of the president's committee reflects commensurate changes in what is now called the disability rights movement.

The President's Committee on Employment of People with Disabilities was created through a 1947 executive order signed by President Harry S Truman. Its original intent was to assist in the employment of returning World War II veterans. An example of the original focus is symbolized through its chairman for many years, Harold Russell, who portrayed the issues of returning veterans through his Academy Award-winning performance in the film *The Best Years of Our Lives.* Russell himself had lost both hands in a World War II training accident. His character outlined the pity and stereotyping faced by returning disabled veterans. By the late 1980s, Russell and his small staff at the committee had worked for more than three decades to address attitudinal and other employment barriers and began to address more specifically worker preparation, vocational rehabilitation, legislative concerns, minority issues, veterans' issues, medical and insurance concerns, the role of government agencies, job accommodation, media handling of disability issues, and particularly the role of business as employer of people with disabilities.

As time went on, it became clear to leaders at the President's Committee and to those emerging as leaders of the "disability community" that results were not forthcoming. By 1989 it was estimated that there were more than 43 million Americans with disabilities, and yet close to 70 percent of those of working age were not working, and the percentage of unemployed among them was still growing.

Statistics indicated the cost to the nation of those with disabilities not working totaled $200 billion yearly in public and private benefits. Surveys indicated that individuals with disabilities wanted to work but found discrimination in the workplace so prevalent and disheartening that most gave up, and those who did work reported frequent unemployment or underemployment.

Under Chairman Justin Dart's leadership, beginning in 1989, the committee began to refocus its energies around the key publics and issues that were believed to be the clues to a productive and participating disability community. Dart's philosophies had been developed for more than twenty years as an international businessman, government leader, and advocate with a civil rights background as well as his personal experience as a wheelchair user since contracting polio while in college.

In 1991, Rick Douglas was named executive director of the committee. He is the first person with a disability to serve in this capacity in the organization's history. Douglas is a former businessman, wheelchair-using disability advocate, and trained rehabilitation professional. He came to the President's Committee with more than twenty years' experience in these fields, most notably as British Airways' U.S. advertising director and Vermont's director of vocational rehabilitation. Together with an increasing professional staff, Douglas, with Justin Dart's leadership, worked to direct the agenda of the President's Committee, focusing on three key agendas.

Empowerment of people with disabilities is the first activity of the President's Committee. Although this word is used in many contexts, empowerment implies to people with disabilities an involvement at the grassroots level with issues that affect their lives. Drafting the Americans with Disabilities Act and then providing information to assure its passage were the first efforts of disability community leaders working together in harmony rather than squabbling for a larger share of a small pie for their specific disability group. The lessons learned during the experience were similar to those of other civil rights groups. Sharing information, technology, focusing on equal rights, working for legislation to achieve those rights, and finally exercising responsibility are the goals of this emerging constituency. In responding to this public, the President's Committee has created a disability community leadership network of more than 6,000 leaders and communicates with them to identify and eliminate the key disability barriers to employment and community life. Those barriers have been identified through meetings in every state as being health insurance, implementation and enforcement of the Americans with Disabilities Act (ADA), education and training, personal assistance services, Social Security barriers, transportation, and housing. The President's Committee will continue this communication and assure that other key public entities, such as business, federal and state government, and rehabilitation and other professionals are aware of these issues for the future and for the continuing empowerment of the disability community.

There are fifty state governors' committees and more than eight hundred mayors' committees representing significant additional grassroots communication. These state committees replicate in many ways the President's Committee's functions by working also with business and government. Local committees provide a means to bring the disability community and the business community together to work jointly on employment issues and to provide communication and advice to the President's Committee.

Employment is the next main organizational thrust of the President's Committee. The role of the employer and the needs of business are paramount here, and the committee has a traditional focus toward providing a forum for business and representation for employers' interests. In the environment of the ADA, this role has sharpened and become more necessary as business determines its new responsibilities under the ADA.

The committee has long established a separate subcommittee of employer representatives from the business community. Over the years this group has provided much valuable direction and guidance. The most recognized accomplishment was the establishment of the Job Accommodation Network (JAN) in the mid-1980s. JAN operates as an arm of the President's Committee on Employment of People with Disabilities at West Virginia University and handles more than 4,000 requests monthly for job accommodation and ADA-related information. JAN is reached through a toll-free number: 800-ADA-WORK.

The Business Leadership Network is being established by the committee. The purpose is to identify business leaders who are advanced in implementing the ADA, particularly when it comes to inclusion of people with disabilities in their workforce. A second criterion is to find those businesses who have also addressed the market potential of people with disabilities as a customer market. Business leaders will be identified in each state, and they in turn will work with disability community leaders to determine how to educate and communicate with other businesses.

An important role of the President's Committee and its state partners is to serve as a facilitator for the disability community and the business community to work out issues together.

Communications in the news, entertainment, and advertising media have profound effects on public perception of people with disabilities and how they view themselves. As the third major thrust of the mission of empowerment of people with disabilities through employment, the President's Committee has created a communications unit and a Communications Committee. In the short term the focus is to provide quality information to constituents and a press release program on disability issues and employment. In the long term the goal is to develop an educational plan to change gradually portrayals of people with disabilities within the communications industries toward independence and self-determination and away from the pity, charity, paternalistic, or heroic approaches.

In overall operating structure, the President's Committee will continue to serve as a facilitator and leader, working through collaborative relationships with others. The committee is headed by a volunteer chair who is appointed by the president and guided by four vice chairs and an executive committee of thirty members representing key constituency groups, including business and labor, the disability community, government, technology, rehabilitation professionals, minorities, disabled veterans, and state leaders. As the key barriers relative to employment are addressed, other public entities will be included, such as those representing current issues around health insurance reform.

The President's Committee on Employment of People with Disabilities reports directly to the president of the United States and is responsible for communicating about and advocating for employment policies relative to people with disabilities that support individual empowerment, inclusion, and independence. Working with and through others, the committee will continue to sharpen the focus toward the most significant issues that prevent employment or provide access to it for people with disabilities.

(*See also:* AMERICANS WITH DISABILITIES ACT; CIVIL RIGHTS; CONSUMERS; DISABILITY LAW AND SOCIAL POLICY; JOB PLACEMENT; WORK)

RESOURCE

President's Committee on Employment of People with Disabilities, 1331 F St., NW, Washington, DC 20004–1107

RICK DOUGLAS

PRIVATE SECTOR REHABILITATION

Private (or proprietary) rehabilitation refers to the provision of vocational and related services within a for-profit setting. These services are usually reimbursed through private funding sources—typically insurance carriers or self-insured employers.

Recipients of Private Rehabilitation Services

Typically (though not always) the recipient of services is an individual with a disability originating in adulthood, through an accident or illness covered by some form of insurance. Most recipients of private-sector rehabilitation services are injured workers covered by workers' compensation insurance, though long-term disability and casualty insurance also pay for substantial portions of the private rehabilitation services delivered. Therefore, by comparison to individuals being served in the public rehabilitation system, the typical individual receiving private rehabilitation services is one who is more likely to have:

- a recent work history;
- a disability resulting from trauma rather than congenital or gradual onset, and thus a need for services to help with adjusting to a physical or mental limitation;
- cumulative trauma/repetitive motion disorder;
- motivational concerns due to burnout;
- ongoing pain.

Development of Private Rehabilitation

Since the early 1970s private rehabilitation activity has increased, as has the emphasis on return to work for injured workers. In the late 1960s, insurance companies began to use private rehabilitation companies to help with medical case management (containing the cost of claims) and preparing injured workers to get back to work.

In 1970 the federal Occupational Safety and Health Act called for creation of the National Commission on State Workers' Compensation and the passage of supporting laws. A federal interdepartmental task force studied the recommendations and emphasized the provision of vocational rehabilitation services. Other factors contributing to the growth of private rehabilitation have been:

- skyrocketing medical and compensation costs to injured workers and accident victims;
- mandatory rehabilitation provisions in the worker's compensation laws of a growing number of states;
- an increasing emphasis in publicly funded programs on meeting the needs of individuals with the most severe disabilities, with a shift in caseloads to more individuals with developmental disabilities, and more widespread provision for school-to-work transition and independent living services.

Services and Goals in Private Rehabilitation

Private rehabilitation emphasizes return to the same (preinjury) job, or at least to the same employer, as the preferable outcome. If that goal proves infeasible, short-term retraining is undertaken, building on the worker's transferable skills, followed by job placement, or as a last resort, self-employment. Only very rarely does private rehabilitation provide—or do third-party payers authorize—the types of long-term training plans undertaken more frequently by publicly funded rehabilitation programs. The length of training commitment is typically capped. A related distinction between public and private rehabilitation is that public providers have a mandate to help the individual receiving services to attain his or her maximum vocational potential, while the most private providers are expected to do is restore the individual to his or her preinjury level of functioning. Many public sector rehabilitation clients have no work history.

The services provided by private sector rehabilitation professionals include:

- medical care coordination, case management, and health care cost containment;
- vocational evaluation, assessment of skills and interests, assessment or testing of physical and/or mental abilities, vocational counseling, transferable skills analysis, and functional capacity evaluation;
- provision or coordination of formal training, vocational training, work hardening, and job seeking skills training;
- job development, placement, and postplacement follow-up;
- job analysis, labor market surveying, work site modification, job modification consultation, and testimony and analysis of a vocational expert.

The Professionals in Private Rehabilitation

Professionals in the private rehabilitation field typically have academic training, sometimes masters' degrees, in fields such as rehabilitation counseling or vocational evaluation; others are nurses or have other specialized training. Many professionals become certified as insurance rehabilitation specialists

(CIRS), as certified rehabilitation counselors (CRC), or in another specialty area by boards of certification or review, in areas such as case management certification. Continuing education is seen as an important part of expected professional development. Many of these professionals have experience working in the state–federal rehabilitation system or in the nonprofit sector prior to working in the private-for-profit sector.

Numerous professional organizations have been formed within the world of private rehabilitation for ongoing education and other member services, legislative advocacy, and gathering and distributing information. Some of the largest such organizations are the National Association of Rehabilitation Professionals in the Private Sector (NARPPS); state-specific associations of rehabilitation professionals; the National Association of Service Providers in Private Rehabilitation, a division within the National Rehabilitation Association; and the Case Management Society of America.

Issues and Trends

Professionals in the private rehabilitation field see, as possible future developments:

- the blurring of the distinctions between public and private rehabilitation, possibly related to insurance reform that places all medical coverage and related services under a single umbrella;
- an increase in emphasis on disability management in the workplace, including prevention of lost time by efforts to accommodate work limitations, as well as access to rehabilitation services that are not linked to a specific insurance claim;
- a continuation of the trend within long-term disability insurance to include rehabilitation as a benefit;
- changes in the Social Security Disability Insurance program to increase return-to-work incentives (or to mitigate work disincentives), such as a combined compensation-and-support-services strategy that allows productive work without loss of benefits;
- a blurring of the distinctions between medical care and rehabilitation services, including in-creased communications and even a team approach to restoration of functioning;
- advances in technology and rehabilitation engineering that will increase the options available to recipients of rehabilitation services and allow more independent functioning;
- increasing involvement of rehabilitation professionals in litigation-related settings, whether related to disputed workers' compensation claims or to complaints under the Americans with Disabilities Act;
- increasing importance of program evaluation.

One of the recurring issues in private rehabilitation, and a frequent focus of discussion at workshops and conferences, is the ethical dilemma often faced by professionals in the field. The key question is: "Who is the client?" Public rehabilitation providers have an unambiguous responsibility to view as primary the needs and interests of the individual receiving services. Private rehabilitation professionals, by contrast, often feel a dual obligation: one to the individual they are serving, and another to the organization paying for the services or the individual authorizing those services, and it is worth emphasizing that the interests of the two sides may differ. Different professional organizations have adopted different approaches to this ethical issue. NARPPS has a code of ethics for members that states: "When there is a conflict of interest between the disabled client and the NARPPS member's employing party, the member must clarify the nature and direction of his/her loyalty and responsibilities and keep all parties informed of that commitment." Others, including the CRC code of ethics, insist that the interests of the individual with a disability always come first.

(*See also:* CAREER COUNSELING; DISABILITY MANAGEMENT; ETHICS; FORENSIC REHABILITATION; JOB PLACEMENT; LIFE CARE PLANNING; STATE–FEDERAL REHABILITATION PROGRAM; VOCATIONAL EVALUATION; WORK)

RESOURCES

National Association of Service Providers in Private Rehabilitation, National Rehabilitation Association, National Office, 633 South Washington St., Alexandria, VA 22314

National Association of Rehabilitation Professionals in the Private Sector, 313 Washington St., Suite 302, Newton, MA 02158

BIBLIOGRAPHY

COLLIGNON, FREDERICK C.; BARKER, LINDA TOMS; and VENCILL, MARY P. "The Growth and Structure of the Proprietary Rehabilitation Sector." In *American Rehabilitation* 18 (1992):7–10.

EMENER, WILLIAM G. "Future Perspectives on Rehabilitation in America." In *Journal of Private Sector Rehabilitation* 1 (1986):59–70.

GARDNER, JOHN A. "Early Referral and Other Factors Affecting Vocational Rehabilitation Outcome for the Workers' Compensation Client." In *Rehabilitation Counseling Bulletin, Special Issue, Disability Management and Industrial Rehabilitation* 34 (1991):197–209.

LUI, JOHN W. "Trends and Innovations in Private Sector Rehabilitation in the 21st Century." In *Private Sector Rehabilitation: Insurance, Trends and Issues for the 21st Century, A Summary of the 17th Mary E. Switzer Memorial Seminar,* ed. Carl E. Hansen, and Leonard G. Perlman. Washington, DC, 1993.

PIMENTAL, RICHARD; BISSONNETTE, DENISE; and WRIGHT, ANITA LEE. *Job Placement for the Industrially Injured Worker.* Northridge, CA, 1987.

TAYLOR, L. J.; GOLTER, M.; GOLTER, GARY; and BACKER, THOMAS E., eds. *Handbook of Private Sector Rehabilitation.* New York, 1985.

MARY VENCILL

PROGRAM EVALUATION

See EVALUATION OF REHABILITATION PROGRAMS

PROSTHETICS AND ORTHOTICS

Prosthetists and orthotists are professionals associated with the fields of prosthetics and orthotics. Historically these fields have been closely associated with the medical specialties of physical medicine and rehabilitation and orthopedic surgery—medical specialties particularly involved with preservation and/or the restoration of function of the musculoskeletal and neuromuscular systems. The classical fields of prosthetics and orthotics use external devices to accomplish rehabilitation and orthopedic goals. These goals mainly have to do with fitting artificial limb replacements (limb prosthetics) or fitting external structures (orthotics) to assist or to support body parts that are limited in function because of injury, pain, or disease. The initial five letters of orthopedics and orthotics come from the Greek root *ortho*, which means "straight" or to "make right or correct." The word "prosthesis" comes from a Greek root meaning to "add to." A prosthesis is a replacement limb that is "added to" or "placed before" the residual limb after amputation.

Prosthetic and orthotic concepts have existed since antiquity. Images exist from Egyptian, Greek, and Roman cultures that illustrate the use of simple artificial limbs (prostheses) and crutches (orthoses). Armor makers are often considered to be the persons who first developed the craft of making prostheses and orthoses through the skills they developed in making armor for knights during the fourteenth and fifteenth centuries. Wars have frequently been a stimulus for the development of the prosthetics and orthotics fields. To a great extent, the practice of limb prosthetics in the United States emerged as a significant area of activity because of the Civil War, whereas the Napoleonic wars were influential in this way in Europe. Orthotics probably got its greatest impetus with the treatment of disabilities resulting from polio. Orthoses are commonly used by persons with injuries, diseases, or conditions that result in hemiplegia (e.g., stroke), paraplegia, or quadriplegia (e.g., spinal injury or cerebral palsy).

The words "prosthetics" and "orthotics" are often used in wider contexts than has classically been the case. Any replacement organ (e.g., artificial hip or knee joint, heart valve, etc.) may be called a prosthesis. Eyeglasses, hearing aids, or pacemakers could be thought of as orthoses, because they assist weakened organs, but by a quirk of language they are often referred to as prostheses. Another anomaly of daily language is that the word "orthotics" is often used not as a field of endeavor but as a name for various kinds of inserts for shoes. In this entry the words are used in their classical sense.

Role of the Orthotist and Prosthetist. The general role of the orthotist is to work with a medical team to help "make right" a person with disability due to injury, disease, or pain. The general role of the prosthetist is to work with a medical team in the care of people who have lost limbs and in many cases to fit them with artificial limbs. The prosthetist and the orthotist are members of the rehabilitation team and need to work closely with physical and occupational therapists, with rehabilitation psychologists, social workers, and other rehabilitation specialists—as well as physicians—to assist disabled people in the achievement of the maximal functional abilities of which they are capable.

Orthotists are concerned with evaluation of disabled persons, with recommendation of orthoses, with fabrication and fitting of orthoses, and with follow-up orthotics care. Orthoses are external supports (braces) especially designed to correct or prevent deformities of the limbs and spine, to limit range of motion, to relieve pain or avoid additional injury, to provide support, and to help improve function (e.g., walking). Prosthetists are concerned with the evaluation of persons with limb loss, with recommendations for limb replacement, with fabrication and fitting of prostheses, and with follow-up care. Prosthetics is therefore the field involved with provision for limb replacement and care for the person with an amputation. Prosthetists and orthotists are the professionals involved with the care of persons with disabilities who have need of prostheses or orthoses.

Orthoses and Prostheses. In the context used here, prostheses and orthoses serve the purpose of improving function, comfort, protection, and appearance of persons with orthopedic deformities, amputations, or other disabilities. Function for individuals with upper-limb disabilities involves their ability to manipulate objects in their environment to be able to provide for self-care (e.g., grooming, hygiene, eating), activities that are often called activities of daily living (ADL). Occupational therapists frequently work with the patient and with the prosthetist or orthotist in improving functional skills of the upper limb. Persons with arm amputations, even some with loss of both hands, can drive cars, fly airplanes, work as machinists or in other occupations, and generally lead a productive and independent life. Hooklike prehensors are very functional, but some persons find electric-powered hands, which produce pinch forces as high as 25 lbf (pounds force), to be very practical. Electric hands may be controlled by using muscle electricity (myoelectricity) that is created when muscles remaining in the residual limb are contracted. Hand or finger replacement that do not have active inner

mechanisms but that are crafted to be life-like in appearance can provide the important function of "acceptable social presentation."

Function for individuals with lower-limb disabilities may include standing, walking, and running. It may involve only the ability to move or transfer oneself from bed to chair or wheelchair, or to enable a person to bathe or use the toilet. Physical therapists help people with leg amputations and persons with leg orthoses to learn to walk safely and efficiently. A person with one leg missing below the knee can usually walk on an artificial leg in such a natural way that others are not aware the leg is missing. Many young people with amputations below the knee jog and run. In 1993 the world record in the 100-meter dash for people with below-knee amputations was 11.65 seconds. Persons with paraplegia (paralysis of the lower limbs) or quadriplegia (paralysis in all four limbs) often use wheelchairs for mobility. Rehabilitation engineers may customize wheelchair seats and provide them with electronic control systems and environmental access that allows for great independence in living. Wheelchair racers with paraplegia can cover the marathon distance quicker than all but world-class runners. Some persons with paraplegia walk on forearm crutches using braces on their legs (knee-ankle-foot orthoses).

The spine supports the body's upright position, protects the spinal cord, and supports the ribs, which protect vital organs. The spine often needs support to stabilize its position, to protect it, to relieve pain, to avoid or reduce deformities (e.g., scoliosis—bending of the spine), or to enable the limbs to function well. Spinal orthotics influence general well-being and can play a key role in rehabilitation.

Successful orthotic-prosthetic management returns function, protects the body, relieves pain, promotes an improved appearance, and in so doing helps people to enhance their self-image and to improve the quality of their life. These results cannot be accomplished without a positive attitude by the recipient of the prosthesis or orthosis. The person receiving a prosthesis or orthosis ultimately determines its success or failure, no matter how good the device is intrinsically. Consequently, psychology plays an important part in successful rehabilitation, and a positive approach by the prosthetist or orthotist can be critical to successful fittings.

Orthotic Procedures

In-depth treatment of orthotic procedures may be found in the *Atlas of Orthotics* (American Academy of Orthopaedic Surgeons, 1985).

Evaluation. Orthotists begin their treatment of orthopedic or rehabilitation patients with an evaluation. Information is supplied by the physician, physical therapist, other health-related professionals treating the patient, and from diagnostic testing such as X rays. The orthotist evaluates the limbs and spine for bone, joint, muscle, and neurological problems. The limbs are examined by range of motion and by manual testing of muscle strength. The orthotist needs to be aware of the typical ranges of motion and muscle strengths for persons without injury, disease, or pain. Orthotists are trained to observe normal and pathologic movements, including normal and pathologic walking patterns. Video recordings of walking can augment the visual system's ability to see what is happening in "real time." Gait analysis systems can also be useful, but as of 1995 they were mainly used in research laboratories. They are used clinically to help physicians plan surgical procedures and orthotic management for the improvement of walking by persons with cerebral palsy.

Patient information and medical history are recorded. It is very important for the orthotist to listen carefully to what the patient says. The patient needs to be thought of as one of the members (the most important member) of the team associated with the rehabilitation process. The patient is interviewed regarding his or her goals for orthotic management, and an attempt should be made to match the patient's goals with the physician's goals and the orthotist's ability to achieve these goals. The *Atlas of Orthotics* defines the ideal orthosis as one that controls only those motions that are abnormal or absent and permits unrestricted motion in regions where normal function remains. From the patient's standpoint the ideal orthosis is also invisible and weightless.

Measurement. The orthotist measures the circumference of the patient's limb at several levels. The outline of the patient's limb is also drawn by tracing. A plaster impression of the involved limb or spine is taken if a plastic orthosis is to be fabricated.

Metal orthoses are fabricated from measurements and from the drawing of the limb's shape.

Fabrication. There are basically two kinds of orthosis fabrication materials: metal and plastic. For a plastic orthosis, the plaster impression is filled with plaster to create a cast or positive mold of the patient's limb. The casting is then modified according to the measurements of the patient and according to established practice for the orthosis being made. For a static plastic orthosis, thermoplastic is cut to size, heated, and thermoformed over the casting. This plastic is trimmed to prescribed trimlines and polished. The finished static plastic orthosis has straps that hold it in place on the limb. An example of a static plastic orthosis is a plastic resting wrist-hand orthosis (Figure 1).

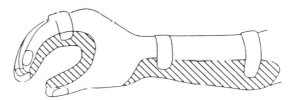

Figure 1. Plastic resting wrist hand orthosis

A metal orthosis is fabricated by contouring metal to the prescribed measurements and the outline of the patient's limb or spine. Tracings of the contour silhouette of the limb are also termed delineations in the orthotics field. The metal components are bent to follow the patient's body contour to provide stability and a nice appearance. Bridging body contours may be used to provide correction of deformities. For example, a spinal orthosis may have metal bars that bridge the contour of the patient's lumbar curvature to correct it as the orthosis is worn. Another example of contouring is a metal ankle-foot orthosis (Figure 2, p. 576).

A dynamic plastic orthosis is made from the modified casting in a different way. Metal bars with joints or hinges for the prescribed motion are placed over the casting in the area meant to articulate. The plastic is vacuum-formed over or under the joints so that the finished orthosis is a combination of metal and plastic. The metal portions provide the mobility of the orthosis, and the plastic portions provide the

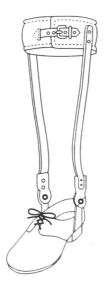

Figure 2. Metal and leather ankle foot orthosis

stability. An example is a plastic knee-ankle-foot orthosis (Figure 3).

Fitting. Orthoses are fitted according to pre-scribed guidelines associated with the objective of the orthosis. The orthotist checks the orthosis for smooth trimlines that will not irritate the soft tissues. The degree to which correction or accommodation of the deformity is accomplished is examined. Fit of the orthosis is checked. Total contact of the orthosis is usually desirable, but it must not cause excessive pressure. Finally, the orthotist evaluates the orthosis for its practical function during use.

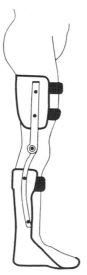

Figure 3. Plastic and metal knee ankle foot orthosis

Prosthetic Procedures

An in-depth view of prosthetics procedures may be found in the *Atlas of Limb Prosthetics* (American Academy of Orthopaedic Surgeons, 1992).

Evaluation. An evaluation of a person with an amputation begins with a review of the patient's medical history, physical condition, range of joint motion, and muscle strength. The patient's vocation and avocations, as well as goals and expectations, are thoroughly discussed. Elderly persons with poor circulation, low physical strength, and complicated medical conditions (e.g., a heart condition) cannot be expected to do as well as a younger individual in excellent health.

The process of being fitted with a prosthesis may take several months, depending on the condition of the limb and whether amputation was a result of disease, trauma, or birth anomaly. A limb that has been amputated must be well healed and free from edema or swelling before a permanent fitting is attempted. The prosthetist can accelerate the process by using techniques to control swelling and by shaping the limb prior to fitting the prosthesis. When working with a well-trained rehabilitation team, the individual with a lower limb amputation can be successfully treated with an immediate or early postsurgical prosthesis. This prosthesis is applied soon after surgery—sometimes even in the recovery room. It is made from plaster bandage and may have a pylon and foot attached to it. This technique allows the person with a lower limb amputation to begin walking, under supervision, soon after the amputation, and this can speed up the rehabilitation process. Not all persons can use this approach. When healing problems or other medical complications prohibit this procedure, more conservative techniques must be employed. Elastic bandages, compression socks, or rigid dressings can also be used to control post-surgical swelling while monitoring the limb for proper healing. Once the limb has healed and swelling has been reduced, a preparatory or temporary prosthesis can be designed.

Measurement. The fitting process begins with making a plaster cast of the person's amputated limb. Measurements of limb size are made using a tape measure. The impression should duplicate the shape of the person's limb as much as possible. To ensure

576

proper measurements and a good fitting, the prosthetist will often fit an evaluation interface (socket, the part of the prosthesis that fits intimately with the residual limb). This interface shape is normally fabricated from a transparent kind of plastic material and fit over the person's limb for evaluation. Any necessary changes in the shape of this interface will be noted and incorporated. The development of computer-aided design and computer-aided manufacturing (CAD/CAM) in prosthetics can improve the fit and evaluation of interfaces. The prosthetist relies on experience and training to mold and modify an impression to achieve the optimal fit. CAD/CAM will likely alter all aspects of prosthetics—as well as orthotics—greatly during the early years of the twenty-first century.

Fabrication. Prostheses are made from a variety of materials. The most common materials used are plastics. These materials allow prosthetists to fabricate a prosthesis that is both strong, to resist the forces involved with walking or running, and light in weight, to decrease the effort needed to use it. Two basic designs are used in lower limb prosthetics: exoskeletal and endoskeletal. The exoskeletal design is comprised of a rigid plastic shell that encompasses the entire prosthesis to provide a durable outer surface for strength (Figure 4). This design may not provide the kind of appearance some individuals desire in a prosthesis. The endoskeletal design is comprised of a soft foam cover that hides the supporting pylon of the prosthesis (Figure 5). While this design

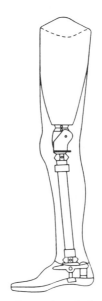

Figure 5. Transfemoral endoskeletal prosthesis

may have a better appearance and feel (soft), it may not be as durable as the exoskeletal design.

Fitting. The goals in fitting a prosthesis can be summarized by four words: comfort, function, appearance, and safety. When evaluating the fit (i.e., comfort) of a prosthesis, the prosthetist must take into account the means by which the person will bear weight between the body and the prosthesis. Comfort is normally accomplished by shaping the prosthetic interface (socket) to allow the transfer of weight through the soft tissues and bony structures to occur without excessive pressure on any tissues. If the load is properly distributed, the prosthesis will allow the person to walk without discomfort. For a prosthesis to function properly, it must be aligned correctly on the person. Correct alignment means that the foot must be placed in the proper position with respect to the limb and the body. Proper alignment allows for smooth, comfortable, economic walking. Prosthetists achieve appropriate alignment through empirical knowledge and through the use of adjustable foot components in the prosthesis so that "optimal" alignment can be achieved, partially by trial-and-adjust procedures. The person walks, and the prosthetist observes the gait. Adjustments are then made to correct observed walking deviations

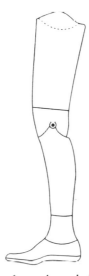

Figure 4. Transfemoral exoskeletal prosthesis

and to satisfy the subjective indications of the wearer. Appearance may involve how a prosthesis moves dynamically as well as how it appears statically. Safety requires a prosthesis or orthosis to function without failure, enduring the often high cyclical and static loads of everyday usage. When comfort, appropriate function, a nice appearance, and safety are achieved, a positive outcome usually results.

Education and Certification of Prosthetists and Orthotists, and Professional Organizations

There are two education tracks through which one can obtain the educational background needed to become a professional clinician in orthotics or prosthetics. One approach is to attend a college or university that has an undergraduate program of study that leads to a baccalaureate-level degree in prosthetics and orthotics. An alternative track for persons who already possess a bachelor's degree is to attend a postgraduate certificate program in either prosthetics or orthotics. These postgraduate programs have course prerequisites to assure that entering students will possess basic knowledge in biology, anatomy, biomechanics, mathematics, chemistry, and other sciences.

Educational programs also exist so that students can study to become a prosthetic/orthotic technician. Technician programs require a high school education. These are associate degree, vocational programs. Technicians are trained in the methods used to make orthoses and prostheses. Upon completion of any of the above programs, graduates can procure positions within private prosthetics/orthotics facilities, within major medical and rehabilitation centers, or within educational and research institutions.

Certification. Orthotists and prosthetists in the United States are certified by the American Board for Certification in Orthotics and Prosthetics, Inc. (ABC). The certification process is to ensure that adequate training and educational requirements are met by those seeking certification. To become certified as an orthotist or prosthetist, one must have completed a board-approved educational program, as already described. After completing the educational requirement, the prospective practitioner must complete a period of clinical practice (patient management and laboratory work). When this requirement has been met, the prospective practitioner is board-eligible and can take the ABC certification exams. These exams consist of written, clinical, and practical sections to test the potential practitioner's ability effectively to care for and fit persons who need orthoses or prostheses. The practitioner's certification is time-limited. He or she must reapply for renewal of certification every five years, during which time continuing education requirements must be met.

Technicians are also registered with ABC. The registration procedure for technician includes successful completion of a board-approved educational program as well as passing written and technical examinations.

The American Board for Certification in Orthotics and Prosthetics certifies (recognizes) orthotics and prosthetics facilities where prosthetists and orthotists work with technicians in the provision of prostheses and orthoses for patients. Specific requirements for good clinical practice must be met. Although certification of individuals and facilities does not guarantee successful treatment for persons who require prosthetics or orthotics services, it is generally in the best interest of persons with disabilities to be treated by certified practitioners in certified laboratories. ABC publishes a listing of certified practitioners and of certified facilities. This listing is available to interested persons by contacting the ABC at 1650 King Street, Suite 500, Alexandria, VA 22314.

Professional Organizations. Certified practitioners in orthotics and prosthetics can belong to a variety of professional organizations. Besides the required membership in the American Board for Certification, there are both scientific and business organizations. The American Academy of Orthotists and Prosthetists (AAOP) is the national scientific organization of certified practitioners dedicated to continuing education, research, and clinical service. The Academy holds an annual national meeting. Regional chapters of AAOP are comprised of volunteers who conduct local scientific seminars and meetings. These seminars, along with the national meetings, are one avenue open to practitioners to receive continuing education credits necessary for continued certification. AAOP also has societies, small groups of practitioners who focus their efforts on specific areas of orthotic/prosthetic care (e.g., upper-limb prosthetics, gait analysis). These groups work at improving patient management in this specific area, advancing technology and educating practitioners.

The American Orthotic and Prosthetic Association (AOPA) is the business branch of the prosthetics and orthotics field in the United States. This organization is divided into regions, which are comprised of volunteer practitioners and business owners who represent their constituencies for business issues both nationally and locally. AOPA holds an annual national meeting and combines with local chapters of AOPA for regional meetings where practitioners gather for business and scientific presentations as well as trade shows of manufacturers' products.

There are many other professional organizations to which practitioners belong. The International Society for Prosthetics and Orthotics (ISPO) is a worldwide scientific organization that includes in its membership not only prosthetists and orthotists but also therapists, physicians, engineers, and others engaged in prosthetics and orthotics care. The focus of this group is dissemination of orthotic and prosthetic knowledge on an international scale. The Society holds congresses every three years at different locations around the world. The Association of Children's Prosthetic-Orthotic Clinics is comprised of many physicians and related health professionals who staff the many pediatric clinics around the country. This association holds seminars in conjunction with other groups, including AAOP and the American Academy of Cerebral Palsy and Developmental Medicine (AACPDM).

(*See also:* AMPUTATION; ASSISTIVE TECHNOLOGY; ENGINEERING; PHYSICIAN; PSYCHOSOCIAL ADJUSTMENT; WHEELCHAIRS)

RESOURCES

American Board for Certification in Orthotics and Prosthetics, 1650 King St., Alexandria, VA 22314

International Society of Prosthetics & Orthotics (ISPO), Attention: ISPO Secretariat, Borgervoenget 5, 2100 Copenhagen 0, Denmark

Orthotics & Prosthetics National Office, 1650 King St., Suite 500, Alexandria, VA 22314

BIBLIOGRAPHY

AMERICAN ACADEMY OF ORTHOPAEDIC SURGEONS. *Atlas of Limb Prosthetics: Surgical, Prosthetic, and Rehabilitation Principles,* 2nd ed. St. Louis, 1992.

———. *Atlas of Orthotics: Biomechanical Principles and Application,* 2nd ed. St. Louis, 1985.

DUDLEY S. CHILDRESS
LAURA FENWICK
MARK EDWARDS

PSYCHIATRIC REHABILITATION

Psychiatric rehabilitation has been defined as "giving people with psychiatric disabilities the opportunity to work, live in the community, and enjoy a social life, at their own pace, through planned experiences in a respectful, supportive, and realistic atmosphere" (Hilburger, 1993). The overall goal of psychiatric rehabilitation is to help individuals to be successful and satisfied in their daily living (Anthony, 1980). Rehabilitation typically involves helping people gain or improve the skills and obtain the resources and support they need to achieve their goals.

Persons Served by Psychiatric Rehabilitation

Psychiatric disabilities span a wide range of disorders. In contrast to physical disabilities, which often have easily quantified measures of impairment (e.g., hearing loss, reduced range of motion), psychiatric disabilities are more difficult to measure. They are no less real, however. To have a psychiatric disability, a person must first have a psychiatric diagnosis. These diagnoses include schizophrenia, affective disorders (such as major depression and manic-depressive disorder), and anxiety disorders (such as posttraumatic stress disorder). However, not everybody with a psychiatric diagnosis has a psychiatric disability. For example, schizophrenia, regarded as the most disabling of all psychiatric disorders, does not affect everyone in the same way. One-third or more of persons diagnosed with schizophrenia completely recover after a single episode (McGlashan, 1988). Also, some disorders are highly disabling, but only within specific situations. Phobias are a good example: A woman may have a paralyzing fear of heights, yet function normally as long as she avoids situations that challenge her phobia. If avoiding heights does not interfere with working or with her lifestyle, then she would not need rehabilitation. Generally speaking, some psychiatric disorders, while they are unpleasant and inconvenient, do not interfere significantly in major life roles.

As a practical matter, most psychiatric rehabilitation programs limit their services to persons with the most disabling conditions. Ordinarily, program admission requires that clients have a serious mental illness (SMI). Serious mental illness also referred to as "chronic mental illness," "serious and persistent mental illness," and various other terms, is defined by three general criteria: diagnosis, disability, and duration (Goldman, 1984). The application of these criteria varies somewhat from state to state, although the general definition is widely accepted. To meet the diagnostic criteria, an individual must have a major mental disorder, as indicated by the *Diagnostic and Statistical Manual of Mental Disorders* (APA, 1994). Most persons with SMI have a diagnosis of schizophrenia, and a sizable minority have affective disorders. Other psychiatric disorders also qualify if the symptoms are severe enough. Disability is defined by impairment in such areas of functioning as self-care, self-direction, interpersonal relationships, learning and recreation, independent living, and economic self-sufficiency. Typically the duration criterion is met when an individual has at least one admission to a psychiatric hospital or other restrictive setting (e.g., a group home) within a five-year period.

Some common limitations in everyday functioning experienced by persons with SMI comprise difficulties with interpersonal situations, including the most basic ones (greeting a friend on the street, paying for a purchase in a store); problems coping with stress (including minor hassles, such as finding an item in a store); difficulty concentrating; and lack of energy or initiative. Because of the severity of impairment in many persons with SMI, psychiatric rehabilitation programs face a challenging task. The community employment rate among persons with SMI is less than 20 percent (Anthony, 1980). Even when they seek vocational services, persons with psychiatric disabilities have success rates only about half those of persons with physical disabilities (Marshak, Bostick, & Turton, 1990). Many persons

with psychiatric disabilities are not living independently. Perhaps one-third of former patients live with their family of origin (Goldman, 1982), and significant proportions of the remainder live periodically in shelters for the homeless, in single-room-occupancy hotels, or in supervised housing. Three-fourths of persons with SMI are moderately to very isolated (Minkoff, 1978). The effectiveness of psychiatric rehabilitation should be judged against the severity of disability suggested by these statistics.

Types of Services Provided

A possible misconception about psychiatric rehabilitation services is that they are highly structured procedures provided solely within mental health centers, sheltered workshops, group homes, hospitals, and other such settings. Only some of the services fit this description. In fact, services often involve learning experiences in informal, seemingly routine activities. The locations where rehabilitation may take place are endless: They include community settings such as clients' homes, their places of employment, grocery stores, Laundromats, and parks.

Psychiatric rehabilitation services are offered both individually and in groups. Formats range from a single rehabilitation professional training a group of clients to a team of professionals meeting with an individual client. Services also involve assisting, training, and consulting with others besides the client, including family members, other professionals, other agencies (such as the Social Security office), and members of the community (such as landlords and employers). Especially during the planning process, rehabilitation may entail meetings involving a group of individuals concerned with the welfare of the client, such as those just mentioned. Some psychiatric rehabilitation services are provided by individuals who themselves are or have been rehabilitation clients. Recently there has been increasing use of "natural supports"—that is, involving "ordinary people"—to help in the rehabilitation process. So, for example, a coworker might be designated as the key person to assist in the rehabilitation plan for a client who is learning a new job.

Psychiatric rehabilitation is usually provided through programs. Programs may offer either a single service or a range of services. Services most frequently offered relate to employment, housing, and case management. Other services include assistance in education, socializing, and recreational services. Psychiatric rehabilitation programs help clients with every aspect of everyday living (e.g., use of public transportation, personal hygiene, exercising, and dieting).

To be effective, psychiatric rehabilitation must be closely coordinated with management of psychiatric medications. Clients benefit most when they take medications, with careful monitoring by psychiatrists, while they are receiving rehabilitation services (Hogarty, Goldberg, and the Collaborative Group, 1973).

Professionals Involved

In terms of academic preparation, psychiatric rehabilitation professionals come from a variety of backgrounds, including social work, rehabilitation counseling, psychiatric nursing, psychiatry, and clinical psychology. Because most university programs do not provide adequate training in psychiatric rehabilitation, staff learn most of their skills on the job and through in-service training. As of 1993, no accrediting body had developed a description of competencies defining a specialization in psychiatric rehabilitation.

Some psychiatric rehabilitation programs use multidisciplinary teams, with staff who have different areas of expertise (Test, 1992). More commonly, however, psychiatric rehabilitation staff consist of "generalists" without regard to academic training (Dincin, 1975). In most programs, the majority of staff workers have no academic degree beyond a bachelor's degree.

History and Models of Psychiatric Rehabilitation

Historical Trends. The roots of current rehabilitation practices can be traced to the development of "moral treatment" in France and the United States at the end of the eighteenth century. The prevailing attitude at the time was that patients with mental disabilities were dangerous and subhuman. They were confined to mental asylums, where they often were chained to the walls. In 1793 Pinel, a French

physician, was put in charge of a large asylum. Appalled by the conditions, he ordered the chains removed. In their place he instructed staff to treat patients with dignity and compassion, which he believed would restore patients to more normal behavior. In the United States, Tuke, a Quaker businessman, converted a country estate into a retreat for patients with mental disabilities. Tuke believed that removal from the stresses of the everyday world, combined with hard work, were therapeutic.

Contemporary approaches to psychiatric rehabilitation date to the post–World War II period. Previously, formal rehabilitation services in the United States were limited to physical disability, according to federal legislation. In 1943, the Barden-La Follette Act passed by Congress extended the range of disabilities eligible for rehabilitation services to mental disabilities, including psychiatric disorders. However, the commitment of the federal-state vocational rehabilitation (VR) system to the psychiatric population has never been complete, even with later legislation (e.g., the Rehabilitation Act of 1973) intended to make this mandate for services clearer.

There have been four major themes in the treatment and rehabilitation of persons with SMI during the last half of the twentieth century: institutionalization, transitionalism, community support, and consumer empowerment. Each of these themes (or philosophies) has been especially popular during a particular decade, although all four approaches are still influential today.

1. Institutionalization. Until the late 1950s, rehabilitation for persons with mental illness was not considered possible except within hospitals. During this era it was not uncommon to expect individuals committed to mental hospitals to remain there for the rest of their lives. The only method considered for helping patients prepare for employment was in hospital-based programs. Patients often worked without pay, performing chores necessary for the operation of the hospital (in kitchens, laundry rooms, and the like). In some cases these activities had a rehabilitative intent, but sometimes patients were exploited. A court case in 1973 (*Souder* v. *Brennan*) finally made such practices illegal.

In the 1960s many experts were optimistic that sheltered workshops would successfully prepare persons with SMI to work in community jobs (Black, 1988). In a fairly brief time, however, most administrators concluded that persons with SMI generally were not suited for workshops. Sheltered workshops, which usually are as segregated from normal society as hospitals, typically require that clients complete factory work for low wages determined by their productivity. Individuals with psychiatric disabilities often failed because of the unpredictable course of their illness, lack of stamina, and lack of "motivation." For their part, clients with SMI were frequently unhappy in workshops, finding them stigmatizing and demeaning (Estroff, 1981).

Institutional approaches, usually centering around skills training, continue in many psychiatric hospitals and sheltered workshops. A typical skills training program is led by a trainer in a classroom setting. The trainer might teach a skill such as "starting up a conversation." The trainer first explains the skill and why it is important to use, next demonstrates the use of the skill, and then structures an exercise in which clients themselves practice using the skill. There have been hundreds of studies showing that persons with SMI can learn skills in this format (Wallace et al., 1980). Unfortunately, however, many skills learned in this fashion do not generalize well outside the classroom (Test & Stein, 1978). For example, teaching patients to cook in a hospital kitchen may not lead to their applying these skills in a community setting with a different type of stove. Studies have also found that participation in hospital work programs does not result in better community employment outcomes when patients are discharged. Further, providing rehabilitation in sheltered settings actually may be counterproductive in that clients may develop an "institutional dependency" that inhibits their motivation to seek out "normal" environments such as community employment (Bond, 1992).

2. Transitionalism. The next phase can best be understood in the context of "deinstitutionalization" (the movement of mental patients from psychiatric hospitals into the community). Between 1950 and 1985 the number of residents in state mental hospitals in the United States declined from more than 550,000 to fewer than 120,000. During this time there was a twelvefold increase in outpatient services (Goldman & Morrissey, 1985).

Deinstitutionalization was prompted by several factors. These included humanitarian concerns about the barbaric conditions in many overcrowded hospitals. A second factor was the discovery of a new drug, chlorpromazine, which had a dramatic calming effect on persons with schizophrenia. It rapidly became the main treatment for persons with schizophrenia in mental hospitals. This development in turn changed expectations about the possibility of discharging patients who before were seen as too unstable to leave the close supervision of the hospital. A third factor was economic. State departments of mental health capitalized on the opportunity to shift the costs of care for discharged patients to federal sources. This cost-shifting was made possible by federal legislation passed between 1956 and 1972. It included amendments extending Social Security benefits to persons with disabilities and the creation of Medicare and Medicaid in 1965.

Another important development at the federal level was the passage of the Community Mental Health Center Act of 1963, which authorized creation of a network of community mental health centers (CMHCs) with a broad mission to address the mental health needs of the nation, including the care and treatment of discharged patients with mental disorders. However, vocational rehabilitation has never been mandated as a CMHC service. Nor were residential services mandated until 1975. Because their rehabilitation needs were ignored, discharged patients were poorly served by CMHCs.

During the 1960s, transitionalism emerged as the prevailing rehabilitation model. The concept of the "halfway house" became popular, the idea being that a discharged patient would "transition" to a group home outside the hospital setting but continue to receive close supervision and training. After a period of adjustment the patient would then move to a less supervised setting, eventually leading to independent housing.

In the employment arena, transitionalism is expressed in the philosophy that clients improve their work habits and job performance through meeting expectations in successively more demanding work environments, beginning with relatively low-demand environments (Dincin, 1975). Eventually, as clients move through a rehabilitation continuum, their behaviors are "shaped" to satisfy community employment standards.

The clubhouse model, first developed by Fountain House in New York (Beard, Propst, and Malamud, 1982), and the Fairweather Lodge, in California (Fairweather et al., 1969), are examples of program models emerging out of this tradition. The historical importance of these approaches is that they offered former mental patients hope and professional help with employment, housing, and recreational activities during an era when most mental health programs ignored these needs.

Transitional approaches continue to be a popular rehabilitation philosophy in many mental health systems. The underlying assumptions of transitionalism have been questioned, however. Paul J. Carling (1993), for example, has criticized transitional housing. He notes that requiring individuals to complete a series of residential moves is often quite stressful. In addition, many surveys have shown that persons with psychiatric disabilities generally do not like transitional housing. Carling suggested an alternative approach: Helping clients from the outset find permanent housing while acknowledging that they will likely need continuing attention, depending on their individual circumstances.

3. Community support. The failure of deinstitutionalization has been widely documented (e.g., Goldman & Morrissey, 1985). Most patients were discharged from mental hospitals with little attention to rehabilitation needs. Because they lacked the skills and resources to cope with community living, many returned to the hospital. Over half of all psychiatric patients released from state hospitals returned within two years (Anthony, 1980). Some returned repeatedly, leading to the label of "revolving door" clients.

In reaction to the failure of CMHCs to address the needs of persons with SMI, the National Institute of Mental Health (NIMH) sponsored a national conference to develop a set of principles necessary for the successful treatment and rehabilitation of persons with SMI. A program using these principles was called a "community support program" (CSP) (Turner & TenHoor, 1978). The CSP approach insists that in intervening with this population, many nontraditional mental health roles are necessary. These include outreach to clients not receiving services, assistance in housing and other basic needs, development of permanent supportive networks, vocational rehabilitation, and advocacy.

Independent of these developments within the psychiatric field, advocates for persons with developmental disabilities began seeking alternatives to sheltered workshops, which they concluded were ineffective (Wehman & Moon, 1988). They noticed that individuals with severe disabilities had difficulty applying training received in sheltered workshops to new settings. This is, of course, the same conclusion that Mary A. Test and Leonard I. Stein (1978) reached in their work with psychiatric inpatients. Paul Wehman and his colleagues developed a new approach known as "supported employment." Its underlying philosophy is that individuals with severe disabilities are more likely to succeed if they are trained *after* they are placed on a community job. Another key principle is that clients receive assistance on a time-unlimited basis, in contrast to the time-limited services traditionally offered under state-federal VR program funding guidelines. By the late 1980s this new vocational training model was being adapted for other disability groups, including persons with psychiatric disabilities. Through the efforts of Wehman and other advocates, the 1987 amendments to the Rehabilitation Act included new regulations stating that supported employment was a defined service eligible for VR funding.

Before the 1980s, persons with psychiatric disabilities who had educational aspirations were usually discouraged by mental health and rehabilitation professionals from pursuing such goals (Shepard, 1993). In the 1980s Boston University's Center for Psychiatric Rehabilitation first developed and tested the concept of supported education (Unger et al., 1987). Three types of supported education approaches have been identified: the self-contained classroom, on-site support, and mobile support. As developed by Boston University, the self-contained classroom is tailor-made to help consumers define academic goals, to familiarize them with the college environment, and to teach study skills and other survival skills. On-site support typically is offered through a college office of student counseling services or services for persons with disabilities. Mobile support services consists of an outreach worker from a mental health program who makes contact with consumers on campus. Judith A. Cook and Mardi L. Solomon (1993) found that clients receiving mobile support while attending college or technical school increased in self-esteem without suffering greater anxiety.

4. Consumer empowerment. Self-help groups for former psychiatric patients—or "consumers," as they now commonly describe themselves—have been forming since at least the 1940s. These groups have been active in developing drop-in centers and in providing friendship, social and recreational activities as well as concrete assistance. Carol T. Mowbray, Richard Wellwood, and Phil Chamberlain (1988) have described an exemplary consumer-run support service to help others find housing, income assistance, and other such resources.

It was not until the 1980s that mental health self-help activities started to form into a national movement. Beginning in 1985, a series of national conferences was held. In that same year, an informal network of self-help groups throughout the United States formed the National Mental Health Consumers' Association. Judi Chamberlin, Joseph A. Rogers, and Caroline S. Sneed (1989) reported 500 different groups with a total of 5,000 members.

Starting in the late 1980s, the concept of consumers working as mental staff workers side by side with professionals began to be tried on a wide scale. Projects in Philadelphia and Denver received national attention for their case management training programs and subsequent employment of consumers. In the Denver program, consumers were successfully employed by local mental health centers in positions as case manager aides (Sherman & Porter, 1991). These projects have challenged deeply held assumptions by many professionals about the capabilities of individuals with psychiatric disabilities.

Family members of persons with mental illness increasingly have played a direct role in lobbying for better mental health services. Since its formation in 1979, the National Alliance for the Mentally Ill (NAMI), an organization for families, had grown to a membership of 130,000 with 1,050 local chapters by 1992. NAMI has advocated for more federal money for research and has fought against stigmatizing stereotypes of mental illness in the mass media. A few NAMI chapters also have provided direct services by developing and supervising housing programs and other rehabilitation programs.

The Americans with Disabilities Act (ADA) of 1990 promised to expand the emphasis on consumer empowerment in this decade. Among the provisions of this legislation is the requirement that most employers make "reasonable accommodation" in the workplace for persons with disabilities. Impairments often requiring accommodation among persons with SMI relate to difficulties in concentrating, dealing with stress, and interacting with other people. The ADA also makes it illegal to ask prospective employees about their psychiatric history. This proviso is an important change because of the stigma of mental illness, which is a barrier to employment. One national survey found that only 19 percent of those polled said they were "very comfortable" with people with mental illness, compared to 59 percent who were very comfortable with people in wheelchairs (NOD, 1991).

Models. Among the many psychiatric rehabilitation models in current practice, two—the clubhouse model and assertive community treatment—merit special attention because of their influence on current thinking.

1. The clubhouse model. The clubhouse model is a comprehensive group approach that focuses on practical issues in informal settings. Clubhouses offer vocational opportunities, housing, problem-solving groups, case management, recreational activities, and academic preparation. As the name suggests, this approach always has a central meeting place. Persons attending clubhouse programs are referred to as "members." Professional staff have supportive roles and serve as role models. The clubhouse philosophy differs greatly from the hierarchical, organizational structure of a medical setting. The daily routine in a clubhouse finds members involved in activities necessary for the clubhouse to function—answering the phone, cleaning the building, and cooking the lunchtime meal.

Transitional employment is the centerpiece of the clubhouse model. Transitional employment positions are entry-level jobs. The rehabilitation staff locate these jobs by contacting employers in the community. Members work part-time in these positions, usually for three to nine months. Over time, different members are rotated through each transitional employment position.

The clubhouse model is a well-defined model with a strong national network. Only a few studies have examined the effectiveness of clubhouse approaches, but research suggests that it is an effective approach, especially for individuals who are motivated to pursue community employment and who enjoy group activities.

2. Assertive community treatment (ACT) is an approach that works with clients on an individual basis, mostly in the clients' homes and neighborhood rather than agency offices. ACT programs are staffed by a group of professionals who work as a team. The ACT team keeps in frequent contact with clients, typically averaging two visits per week. The nature of the contacts depends on the needs of a client on a given day. ACT teams help in such things as budgeting money, shopping, finding housing, taking medication, finding jobs, and problem-solving difficulties on the job. Some visits are "friendly visits" in which the staff checks the client's progress. ACT teams attempt to anticipate crises— for example, by paying attention to the warning signs of a relapse. ACT programs are very accessible: Clients can call staff workers and receive help quickly in emergency situations.

Several features make the ACT approach distinctive. ACT programs exemplify assertive outreach in that staff initiate contacts with clients rather than depending on clients to keep appointments. For this reason, the dropout rate from ACT is much lower than in most other approaches. A second feature of ACT is its emphasis on continuity and consistency. Clients are not discharged from ACT teams but continue to receive services on a time-unlimited basis. The importance of this feature is the research finding that clients often function poorly once they leave psychiatric rehabilitation programs. Another characteristic is that ACT programs combine treatment and rehabilitation in a comprehensive approach. For example, the psychiatrist works closely with other staff to identify medication problems. Staff members hold daily team meetings to discuss each client's treatment plan and how it may affect rehabilitation goals, and vice versa. For example, if a client shows an increase in symptoms, the team would review the client's housing arrangements and

vocational activities to see if adjustments are needed to reduce the stress.

Leonard I. Stein and Mary A. Test (1980) developed the ACT model in Madison, Wisconsin, in the 1970s. Its effectiveness in helping clients has been shown by a growing number of researchers (Test, 1992). It has been widely adopted in programs across the United States, especially for revolving-door clients.

Outcomes from Psychiatric Rehabilitation. Because of the many psychiatric rehabilitation approaches, it is difficult to draw general conclusions about their impact. Psychiatric rehabilitation programs reduce hospital use and increase independent living (Dion & Anthony, 1987). There is relatively little research on whether programs have achieved the goal of integrating clients into everyday society. Until 1990, research on vocational approaches did not show much of an impact in helping clients maintain permanent jobs (Bond, 1992). Several supported employment studies completed since then, however, have been quite positive. The costs of psychiatric rehabilitation programs, relative to their benefits, have not been widely studied.

Major Governmental, Professional, and Related Organizations. At the federal level, NIMH, since its creation in 1946, has been the agency responsible for providing national leadership in services for persons with mental illness. Among NIMH activities are funding of research projects relating to mental illness, management of the development of CMHCs, distributing publications, and sponsoring conferences. Historically, CSP has been the single office at NIMH that has consistently encouraged innovative psychiatric rehabilitation programs. CSP has funded many demonstration projects throughout the United States. It has been particularly instrumental in nurturing the consumer self-help movement. In 1992, in a major reorganization, most of NIMH was shifted to the National Institutes of Health, while CSP moved to a newly formed agency called the Substance Abuse and Mental Health Services Administration.

Two other federal agencies also affect psychiatric rehabilitation services. Within the Department of Education, the Rehabilitation Services Administration (RSA) and the National Institute of Disability and Rehabilitation Research fund training and research projects related to rehabilitation. RSA also directs the federal-state VR program. Other federal agencies responsible for programs serving persons with psychiatric disabilities include the Social Security Administration and the Department of Housing and Urban Development. The number of other participating agencies is extensive. Indeed, the large number of agencies involved, each with its own rules and eligibility criteria, makes the understanding of them complicated at both the federal and the local levels. This fragmentation is a huge problem for clients trying to obtain benefits.

As of 1995 there were three federally funded Research and Training Centers on Psychiatric Rehabilitation: at Boston University, at Thresholds (in Chicago), and at Matrix Research Institute (in Philadelphia). All three have been active in producing written materials, sponsoring conferences, and offering technical assistance. The work of William A. Anthony and his colleagues at Boston University was especially important in helping gain acceptance of the concept of psychiatric rehabilitation during the 1980s. This center has defined basic concepts and showed the relationship between psychiatric rehabilitation and the larger rehabilitation field (Anthony, 1980).

The International Association of Psychosocial Rehabilitation Services is an organization of psychiatric rehabilitation agencies, practitioners, and others dedicated to promoting, supporting, and strengthening community-oriented rehabilitation services. As of 1995 its membership numbered more than 500 organizations in addition to approximately 1,200 individual members.

Future Trends

Recent trends in health care financing are likely to have both positive and negative impacts on rehabilitation services. Increasing numbers of states are capitalizing on the rehabilitation option within the federal Medicaid program to fund case management and other services to persons with SMI; in some states this apparently has increased access to services. This funding source has been a mixed blessing, however. Services eligible for Medicaid reimbursement are encouraged through this system, while ineligible services are discouraged. In most states, vocational rehabilitation services cannot be billed through Medicaid. This is unfortunate because it makes sense for treatment teams to provide mental health and vocational services together. Programs depending on Medicaid funding have usually ignored vocational needs.

Throughout the United States there is a movement toward the adoption of "managed care." Under this financial system, instead of reimbursing programs on the basis of units of service provided, programs are paid a flat rate for the care of a fixed number of individuals. The amount paid depends on estimates of client need for services. Theoretically this method should ensure that clients will not be ignored even if they require many services. No one knows how or how well managed care will work on a broad scale.

Managed care is intended to increase attention to outcomes of services and to consumer satisfaction with services—a healthy development for the mental health field. The values of psychiatric rehabilitation, with its practical orientation and focus on quality of life, are consistent with this value orientation.

We live in an era with a substantial body of knowledge about the needs of consumers and about what is effective. William A. Anthony and Marianne D. Farkas (1989) have suggested that we have left the deinstitutionalization era behind and moved into the "rehabilitation era." They believe that we now have a coherent technology to provide high-quality services, should we have the commitment to doing so.

Another source of major change may be in the directives and funding policies of the VR system. In the early 1990s the General Accounting Office produced a report indicating a lack of long-term effects for traditional time-limited VR service system (GAO, 1993). If this report is used by legislators, it will reinforce some policies already in place to foster supported employment at the expense of sheltered programs.

Consumers have a large stake in their own future. Self-help groups have the advantage that they are inexpensive and are not beholden to the medical establishment. The amount of consumer influence and the effectiveness of consumer-run alternatives were hard to estimate as of 1995, but some visions of the future presume consumer empowerment to be the key.

The family movement has already had a huge impact on setting the agenda for mental health research and service delivery. With its exponential growth, NAMI can be predicted to have an increasing influence. NAMI has emphasized the search for more effective medications that are also affordable, attention to quality assurance in the public mental health system on a state-by-state basis, reduction of stigma, and the development of housing options for mental health consumers. We can expect these themes to continue.

Medical technology may eventually revolutionize psychiatric rehabilitation. Clozapine, a medication for schizophrenia introduced in the United States in the late 1980s, has already been reported as opening up possibilities for rehabilitation of persons for whom it previously was not thought feasible.

Beyond these influences, however, the single most important factor will be the efficacy of psychiatric rehabilitation approaches as reflected in high-quality research and confirmed in actual practice. It is unlikely that a single model will emerge as best for all clients. On the other hand, it is essential to discard ineffective models. The evidence in favor of sheltered and institutional approaches (e.g., hospital-based programs, partial hospitalization programs, sheltered workshops, and prevocational programs) is weak. Based on evidence available in 1995, such approaches should decline. Correspondingly, individualized approaches emphasizing high levels of support when necessary, and training and assessment in natural settings, should increase in importance.

(*See also:* CONSUMERS; DEINSTITUTIONALIZATION; FAMILY; MOOD DISORDERS; PERSONALITY DISORDERS; PHARMACOLOGY; PHILOSOPHY OF REHABILITATION; PSYCHIATRY; PSYCHOLOGY, REHABILITATION; SUPPORTED EMPLOYMENT; WELLNESS)

RESOURCES

Center for Psychiatric Rehabilitation, Boston University, 930 Commonwealth Ave., Boston, MA 02215

Community Support Programs Section, Center for Mental Health Services, Substance Abuse and Mental Health Services Administration, 5600 Fishers Lane, Room 11C-22, Rockville, MD 20857

International Association of Psychosocial Rehabilitation Services, 10025 Governor Warfield Parkway #301, Columbia, MD 21044–3357

Matrix Research Institute, 6008 Wayne Ave., Philadelphia, PA 19144

National Alliance for the Mentally Ill, 2101 Wilson Blvd., Suite 302, Arlington, VA 22201

National Institute of Mental Health, Parklawn Building, 5600 Fishers Lane, Rockville, MD 20857

Program of Assertive Community Treatment, 108 S. Webster, Madison, WI 53703

Rehabilitation Services Administration, U.S. Department of Education, 400 Maryland Ave., SW, Washington, DC 20202–4275

Thresholds National Research and Training Center on Rehabilitation and Mental Illness, 2001 North Clybourn Ave., #302, Chicago, IL 60614–4036

BIBLIOGRAPHY

AMERICAN PSYCHIATRIC ASSOCIATION (APA). *Diagnostic and Statistical Manual of Mental Disorders*, 4th ed., Washington, DC, 1994.

ANTHONY, WILLIAM A. *The Principles of Psychiatric Rehabilitation*. Baltimore, 1980.

ANTHONY, WILLIAM A., and FARKAS, MARIANNE D. "The Future of Psychiatric Rehabilitation." In *Psychiatric Rehabilitation Programs: Putting Theory into Practice*, eds. William A. Anthony and Marianne D. Farkas. Baltimore, 1989.

BEARD, JOHN H.; PROPST, RUDYARD N.; and MALAMUD, THOMAS J. "The Fountain House Model of Rehabilitation." *Psychosocial Rehabilitation Journal* 5 (1982):47–53.

BLACK, BERTRAM J. *Work and Mental Illness: Transitions to Employment*. Baltimore, 1988.

BOND, GARY R. "Vocational Rehabilitation." In *Handbook of Psychiatric Rehabilitation*, ed. Robert P. Liberman. New York, 1992.

CARLING, PAUL J. "Housing and Supports for Persons with Mental Illness: Emerging Approaches to Research and Practice." *Hospital and Community Psychiatry* 44 (1993):439–449.

CHAMBERLIN, JUDI; ROGERS, JOSEPH A.; and SNEED, CAROLINE S. "Consumers, Families, and Community Support Systems." *Psychosocial Rehabilitation Journal* 12 (1989):93–106.

COOK, JUDITH A., and SOLOMON, MARDI L. "The Community Scholar Program: An Outcome Study of Supported Education for Students with Severe Mental Illness." *Psychosocial Rehabilitation Journal* 17 (1993):83–97.

DINCIN, JERRY. "Psychiatric Rehabilitation." *Schizophrenia Bulletin* 1 (1975):131–148.

DION, GEORGE L., and ANTHONY, WILLIAM A. "Research in Psychiatric Rehabilitation: A Review of Experimental and Quasi-Experimental Studies." *Rehabilitation Counseling Bulletin* 30 (1987):177–203.

ESTROFF, SUE. *Making It Crazy.* Berkeley, CA, 1981.

FAIRWEATHER, GEORGE W.; SANDERS, DAVID H.; MAYNARD, HUGO; CRESSLER, DAVID L.; and BLECK, DOROTHY S. *Community Life for the Mentally Ill: An Alternative to Institutional Care.* Chicago, 1969.

GENERAL ACCOUNTING OFFICE (GAO). *Vocational Rehabilitation: Evidence for Federal Program's Effectiveness Is Mixed.* Washington, DC. 1993.

GOLDMAN, HOWARD H. "Mental Illness and Family Burden: A Public Health Perspective." *Hospital and Community Psychiatry* 33 (1982):557–559.

———."Epidemiology." In *The Chronic Mental Patient: Five Years Later*, ed. John A. Talbott. Orlando, FL, 1984.

GOLDMAN, HOWARD H., and MORRISSEY, JOSEPH P. "The Alchemy of Mental Health Policy: Homelessness and the Fourth Cycle of Reform." *American Journal of Public Policy* 75 (1985):727–731.

HILBURGER, JOHN. "Editorial." *Psychosocial Rehabilitation Journal* 16 (1993):1.

HOGARTY, GERALD E.; GOLDBERG, SOLOMON C.; and THE COLLABORATIVE GROUP. "Drug and Sociotherapy in the Aftercare of Schizophrenia Patients: One-Year Relapse Rates." *Archives of General Psychiatry* 28 (1973):54–64.

MARSHAK, LAURA E.; BOSTICK, DAVID; and TURTON, LAWRENCE J. "Closure Outcomes for Clients with Psychiatric Disabilities Served by the Vocational Rehabilitation System." *Rehabilitation Counseling Bulletin* 33 (1990):247–250.

McGLASHAN, THOMAS H. "A Selective Review of Recent North American Long-Term Follow-up Studies of Schizophrenia." *Schizophrenia Bulletin* 14 (1988):515–542.

MINKOFF, KENNETH. "A Map of Chronic Mental Patients." In *The Chronic Mental Patient*, ed. John A. Talbott. Washington, DC, 1978.

MOWBRAY, CAROL T.; WELLWOOD, RICHARD; and CHAMBERLAIN, PHIL. "Project Stay: A Consumer-Run Support Service." *Psychosocial Rehabilitation Journal* 12 (1988):33–42.

NATIONAL ORGANIZATION ON DISABILITY (NOD). "Public Attitudes Toward People with Disabilities." Survey conducted by Louis Harris and Associates, Inc. 1991.

SHEPARD, LORI. "School Daze." *Psychosocial Rehabilitation Journal* 17 (1993):7–10.

SHERMAN, PAUL S., and PORTER, RUSSELL. "Mental Health Consumers as Case Management Aides." *Hospital and Community Psychiatry* 42 (1991):494–498.

STEIN, LEONARD I., and TEST, MARY A. "Alternative to Mental Hospital Treatment, I: Conceptual Model, Treatment Program, and Clinical Evaluation." *Archives of General Psychiatry* 37 (1980):392–397.

TEST, MARY A. "Training in Community Living." In *Handbook of Psychiatric Rehabilitation*, ed. Robert P. Liberman. New York, 1992.

TEST, MARY A., and STEIN, LEONARD I. "Community Treatment of the Chronic Patient: Research Overview." *Schizophrenia Bulletin* 4 (1978):350–364.

TURNER, JUDITH C., and TENHOOR, WILLIAM J. "The NIMH Community Support Program: Pilot Approach to a Needed Social Reform." *Schizophrenia Bulletin* 4 (1978):319–348.

UNGER, KAREN V.; DANLEY, KAREN S.; KOHN, LARRY; and HUTCHINSON, DORI. "Rehabilitation Through Education: A University-Based Continuing Education Program for Young Adults with Psychiatric Disabilities on a University Campus." *Psychosocial Rehabilitation Journal* 10 (1987):35–49.

WALLACE, CHARLES J.; NELSON, CONNIE J.; LIBERMAN, ROBERT P.; AITCHISON, ROBERT A.; LUKOFF, DAVID; ELDER, J. P.; and FERRIS, CHRIS. "A Review and Critique of Social Skills Training with Schizophrenic Patients." *Schizophrenia Bulletin* 6 (1980):42–63.

WEHMAN, PAUL, and MOON, M. SHERRIL, eds. *Vocational Rehabilitation and Supported Employment.* Baltimore, 1988.

GARY R. BOND

PSYCHIATRY

Psychiatry plays an important role in reducing the effects of disability and improving the functional capacity of persons with mental or physical disabilities. A psychiatrist is a physician who has completed three to four years of postmedical school training during which he or she learns how to evaluate, diagnose, and treat individuals with mental disorders. Following residency, the American Board of Psychiatry and Neurology certifies candidates who successfully complete qualifying examinations. The psychiatrist typically treats two groups of individuals who have a disability: those with primary mental disorders, and those with psychological problems arising out of a physical disorder.

If the psychiatrist is to reduce the effects of disability and improve the functional capacity of persons with physical or mental disabilities, he or she must follow an established set of guidelines and procedures. All physicians are bound by this principal rule of medicine: "First, do no harm." Since a physician cannot remedy a condition until he or she understands it, the essential task is the formulation of the correct diagnosis. Because the diagnosis is a conclusion arrived at after a careful and thorough analysis of the facts of the case, or data, the psychiatrist must first obtain a history of the disorder from the patient and/or anyone else who may have relevant information. The psychiatrist inquires about both the nature and timing of symptoms, predispositions in the patient (genetics, past illnesses, traumas), and possible contributing, or even precipitating, events. The psychiatrist also inquires about medical conditions and about the use of prescribed and nonprescribed medications. The psychiatrist performs both a physical examination and a mental status examination on the patient and will also order laboratory tests, psychological testing, X rays, and, frequently, a neurological examination. The psychiatrist may also prescribe medication as indicated. Ideally, this assembly of data tends to suggest a specific mental illness or psychiatric disorder.

In particular, the mental status examination is the means by which the psychiatrist examines the patient's mind. A number of elements are included in this examination, including the patient's appearance, behavior, attitude, level of consciousness, affect and prevailing mood, thought processes and associations, thought content and mental trend, perceptual experiences, memory, general knowledge, judgment, insight, and level of personality development. Throughout the course of this process, the patient's conduct and responses are observed and carefully noted so the functional capacity of his or her mind can be assessed.

The American Psychiatric Association has developed the *Diagnostic and Statistical Manual IV* (DSM-IV), which is a guideline for diagnostic evaluation. The DSM-IV emphasizes the importance of considering a number of factors, including symptoms, character or personality organization, medical status, drug and medication history, life events (stresses, changes, losses, traumata), and ability to function in psychological, social, vocational, and leisure-time spheres of activity. When the diagnosis is determined, the appropriate treatment plan is instituted. For many psychiatric disorders, including schizophrenia, depression, manic-depressive illness (also known as bipolar disorder), and some anxiety disorders, treatment typically involves a combination of verbal psychotherapy, psychopharmacotherapy (use of psychiatric medications), and rehabilitative therapies, including occupational therapy, social work, psychiatric rehabilitation, vocational rehabilitation counseling, and social skills training. As the patient's symptoms are reduced in the earlier phase of therapy, he or she is encouraged to reengage with the real world, including family, social, school, and work environments. The goal is to assist the person to adapt to the stresses and demands of a physical and/or mental disability in order to achieve maximum independence and rehabilitative success, and thereby to facilitate the transformation of the disabled "patient" into the functioning "person" he or she now has the capacity and potential to become.

Mental Disabilities

Perhaps the most challenging psychiatric disorder is schizophrenia, the essential features of which are characteristic psychotic symptoms, such as hallucinations and delusions; disturbances in affect, or emotional expression; disturbances in behavior, including disorganized and inappropriate conduct; and failure to develop interpersonal, social, and vocational skills and abilities (American Psychiatric Association, 1994). During the active phases of this disorder, the person is "out of touch with reality" —he or she manifests impaired judgment and reasoning abilities and poor coping skills. The first goal of the psychiatrist in treating schizophrenia is to achieve stabilization of the patient. Medication and hospitalization are usually necessary to suppress the psychosis and restore the patient's ability to participate in reality. After stabilization is achieved, ideally within days to several weeks, a plan is developed that will include methods to teach the patient how to cope better with both the psychological vulnerabilities associated with schizophrenia and the pressures of the real world. For example, many people with schizophrenia begin to decompensate and become symptomatic because they cannot cope with and manage anxiety. Therefore, medication that reduces the degree of anxiety, together with training in stress reduction and access to individual and group treatment supports, serves to increase the patient's ability to cope with and learn to tolerate degrees of anxiety. During this process, the patient also learns the importance of applying these skills to social and vocational environments, where change, pressures, and stresses often exist. Indeed, advocacy groups such as the National Alliance for the Mentally Ill promote the idea that persons with disabilities are in essence consumers of mental health and rehabilitative services, and as such they must contribute to the development and disposition of these restorative resources.

In the case of schizophrenia, the psychiatrist directs the treatment plan first to symptom management and restoration of reality testing. The second phase, following stabilization of the patient, is devoted to the education of the patient about his or her condition, what benefits and sustains stability and what disrupts and undermines stability. During this phase of the psychotherapy the patient begins to learn and thereby to gain some control or mastery of the disorder. As discussed above, if anxiety precipitates a psychotic episode, then both anticipating and reducing anxiety may prevent a recurrence of the active schizophrenic state. The third and essentially rehabilitative phase of treatment involves working with allied health professionals, especially social, psychiatric, and vocational rehabilitation counselors, to support the patient's reentry into social and vocational environments. During this phase the patient continues to learn how to manage the psychiatric disorder and also learns new skills that will fortify his or her functional abilities in social and vocational environments. For some persons with schizophrenia, because of the long-term nature of their illness, medication, individual and group therapy, and skill-building and maintenance achieved through rehabilitative programming continue to be necessary for many years.

Patients with other primary psychiatric disorders, such as manic-depressive illness, depression, and anxiety disorders (including phobias and panic disorders), tend to do much better in psychotherapy (Nicholi, 1988). These conditions all result from the inability of the patient to cope with intense emotions, but these conditions, except in severe cases of mania and depression, are not typically associated with psychotic symptoms. Therefore, in each case the individual is stabilized, often with medication and occasionally with hospitalization, a process that usually requires less time than is necessary in treating schizophrenia. Stabilization is again followed by patient education so that he or she can understand some of the elements associated with the disorder. For example, patients with recurrent depression tend to be vulnerable during periods of stress or change and especially after losses. Knowing this, an individual may seek out treatment in advance or alert his or her psychiatrist that events capable of provoking depression are anticipated. Such preparation tends to reduce the debilitating impact of negative influences on mental health and stability. Success has also been achieved in the treatment of phobias and panic states. Treatment typically includes both medication to reduce the disabling impact of the emotion, such as severe anxiety and/or fear, and cognitive-behavioral techniques, which provide the patient with new ways of thinking about and dealing with anxiety-provoking situations. For these patients as well, rehabilitative interventions often provide the means by which the coping and mastery achieved in psychotherapy are applied to real-world situations.

Psychiatric impairments can produce severe mental disabilities that may constitute incapacitating handicaps. An anecdote about Sigmund Freud describes his belief that mental health depends upon *Lieben und Arbeiten*; that is, a person's ability to love and to work. Mental illness limits and, in some cases, eclipses both an individual's ability to participate in loving relationships and his or her capacity to work, which in turn has a major impact on the rehabilitation process. Since many people tend to define themselves according to what they do (doing equals being), then a person who cannot *do* because of a disability may therefore cease to *be* that person because of that same disability. The psychiatrist is devoted to the promotion of mental wellness, a condition of being in which both mind and body function according to their optimal capabilities. Abraham Maslow called such persons "self-actualized" in that they are able to express their potential abilities fully (Maslow, 1968). Indeed, many psychiatrists believe that mental health is much more than the absence of symptoms—it must also include the ability of a person to participate actively, effectively, and enthusiastically in the process of living.

Physical Disabilities

Psychiatrists are afforded another opportunity to intervene when individuals with primary medical and/or physical disabilities develop psychological disorders. Because of the intimate interrelationships between doing and being, a change or loss in functional capacity challenges the very nature of one's self-concept. For example, a psychiatrist may be called upon to evaluate and treat an athlete who has been severely injured, such as a swimmer who has been paralyzed following a diving injury. After the individual, who was an "athlete" and now is a "quadriplegic," is medically stabilized, he or she begins to appreciate the nature of the injury and the resultant disability. It is only natural that such devastating loss in functional capacity will evoke feelings of mourning for the death of the athlete self, and sometimes a clinical depression arises. In such a case, the psychiatrist must understand the difference between adaptive grieving, on the one hand, and pathological depression, on the other. Until the patient has accepted the reality of the loss, grieving cannot occur; and until grieving occurs, the patient cannot direct his or her energies to the considerable work of redefining the self. The psychiatrist, therefore, must intervene with medication and/or suicidal precautions if and when these modalities are deemed necessary; otherwise the work of therapy here is to promote and facilitate the grieving process, to foster the redefinition and emergence of an alternate self, and to help the individual access other allied health professionals who will assist in the achievement of these goals. The former swimmer may reemerge as a consultant to the swimming team, or perhaps as a teacher, or therapist, or computer programmer. What is most important is the ability of the individual to accomplish this transformation in a way that ensures survival of self-esteem, dignity, and integrity.

In another example, a person who is employed as a construction worker sustains a broken back in a work-related injury. This "construction worker" who is now a "paraplegic" is similarly challenged to accomplish the transformation of his worker self into a redefined self who will prove to be capable of maximal adaptive functioning, perhaps as a dispatcher or a flight controller. Similarly, a psychiatrist may be consulted to assist a person with AIDS who is overwhelmed with anxiety, despair, and anger. In each case, the individual is evaluated to determine the nature of the problem and the necessary treatment. The designated patient is not the only affected person; family members and loved ones are also involved in the consequences of disability, and effort must be directed to understanding and addressing their needs as well.

Many psychiatrists now believe that symptom reduction, while very important, is but one of an array of essential elements in an effective and truly restorative treatment plan. The patient's ability to commence participation in the rehabilitative therapies marks a vital point in the recovery process because it indicates that the patient is now sufficiently in control of those operations involving thinking, emotionality, and behavior to allow him or her to concentrate on the challenges and opportunities that are involved in the program for recovery. As noted above, mental health is much more than the absence of pain or symptoms; it also entails the lifelong availability of and access to the essential elements of the rehabilitation process, including specific supports and resources that serve to reinvest the former patient in the activities and experiences of living that make the struggle to maintain wellness worthwhile: to be able to work, to be able to participate in loving and supportive relationships, to value one's self and one's capabilities, and thereby to become the embodiment and expression of one's fullest potential.

(See also: ANXIETY DISORDERS; ASSESSMENT; MOOD DISORDERS; PERSONALITY DISORDERS; PHARMACOLOGY; PSYCHIATRIC REHABILITATION; PSYCHOLOGY; SCHIZOPHRENIA)

RESOURCES

American Board of Psychiatry and Neurology, 500 Lake Cook Road, Deerfield, IL 60015

American Psychiatric Association, 1400 K St., NW, Washington, DC 20005

BIBLIOGRAPHY

AMERICAN PSYCHIATRIC ASSOCIATION (APA). *Diagnostic and Statistical Manual of Mental Disorders*, 4th ed. Washington, DC, 1994.
MASLOW, ABRAHAM H. *Toward a Psychology of Being.* New York, 1968.
NICHOLI, ARMAND M., ed. *The New Harvard Guide to Psychiatry.* Cambridge, MA 1988.

DAVID E. CREASEY

PSYCHOLOGY

Psychology is the branch of science concerned with the mind and behavior of individuals. Since it is such a broad science, many specialties have developed within psychology (e.g., clinical, community, developmental, rehabilitation). Thus the practice of psychology as a profession involves numerous and varying roles, depending on the context in which the credentialed psychologist works. Because disabilities are largely defined on the basis of their effect on the mind and behavior of the person, the science of psychology is fundamental to the assessment and treatment of disabilities and to the design and implementation of rehabilitation strategies. The focus of this entry will be to examine the role of the psychologist in reducing the effects of disability and in improving the functional capacity of persons with physical and mental disabilities. To accomplish this task it will be necessary to delineate (1) how these individuals receive the appropriate credentials that demonstrate expertise in working with persons with disabilities; (2) what general procedures are used by psychologists in the diagnosis, treatment, and rehabilitation of persons who have major functional limitations as a result of a disabling condition; and (3) what impact psychologists may have on quality of life issues among persons with disabilities.

Educational Background and Qualifications

Considerable debate exists over the appropriate academic doctoral training for psychologists, especially for those who wish to specialize in disabilities and rehabilitation (Elliott & Gramling, 1990). Of those psychologists who belonged to Division 22 (Rehabilitation Psychology) of the American Psychological Association (APA) in 1982, 32 percent held a degree in clinical psychology, 19 percent held a degree in counseling psychology, 18 percent held a degree in rehabilitation counseling, and 17 percent held a degree in another area of psychology (Jansen & Fulcher, 1982). In a more recent survey, Harry J. Parker and Fong Chan (1990) reported on the credentials held by heads of more than two hundred "psychology services" in major rehabilitation service settings across the country; 60 percent of the doctoral specialties were in clinical psychology; 21 percent were in counseling psychology; and the remainder were scattered among rehabilitation, education, industrial/organizational psychology, and other disciplines.

Actual academic credentials vary for specialties within psychology. For example, clinical and counseling psychologists are expected to graduate from an APA-approved training program with an APA-approved clinical internship. Other specialties, such as school psychology or rehabilitation psychology, do not make such specific demands. In terms of actual work experience and postdoctoral training, however, most programs that result in official certification or licensing have similar requirements (Kemp, 1992).

Considerable debate continues within APA-approved training programs regarding which psychology specialties are most appropriate to function within the general realm of rehabilitation psychology. For example, neuropsychology, the subdiscipline responsible for testing and assessment of cognitive and behavioral deficiencies, is a well-established part of clinical psychology but is only beginning to be incorporated into counseling psychology curricula. Numerous counseling psychology educators see neuropsychology as a specialty for which their graduates may also be well suited to practice (Kemp, 1992). However, persons who practice neuropsychology and are recognized experts in the field, often are graduates of experimental and developmental psychology programs that are not required to meet APA guidelines for predoctoral internship experience, for example. A large number of persons who now identify themselves as neuropsychologists obtained their clinical training at the postdoctoral level. This training was accomplished by enrollment in a highly specialized postdoctoral program in clinical neuropsychology or through an apprenticeship with a practicing, recognized expert in the field. Thus there is a vested interest by professionals in the field as to who is appropriately credentialed as a neuropsychologist in the clinical arena.

Most psychologists, regardless of their original academic training, seek further knowledge and training through postdoctoral fieldwork and additional specialized courses. This practice appears to be especially true of psychologists who work specifically with persons who have physical impairments and disabilities. As disability has become more broadly defined by the influx of sports medicine and wellness programs, the practice of psychologists in these areas has taken on a specific flavor in light of the individuals and impairments with which they are concerned. Such professionals often define themselves as behavioral health psychologists.

Professional psychologists are expected to become affiliated with one or more professional organization. The American Psychological Association represents psychologists of all persuasions and is the preeminent professional psychological organization; most psychologists belong at least to the APA. Among the professional organizations to which psychologists who work in the field of disabilities commonly belong are the American Rehabilitation Counseling Association, the National Academy of Neuropsychology, the American Counseling Association, the International Association of Psychosocial Rehabilitation, the National Rehabilitation Association, and the American Congress of Rehabilitation Medicine.

Psychological Procedures Utilized in Diagnosis, Treatment, and Rehabilitation

Those interventions used by psychologists in working with persons whose impairments have resulted in functional limitations involve various forms of assessments and treatment strategies based on the results of assessment findings. For example, in working with individuals who suffer from the effects of traumatic brain injury, the importance of establishing the cognitive and behavioral consequences of such injuries is essential before any effective treatment or rehabilitation strategy can be initiated. Thus the psychologist working with persons impaired by a brain injury will most likely employ a battery of tests designed to assess cognitive functioning. The most commonly used neuropsychological assessment series of tests is known as the Halstead-Reitan Neuropsychological Battery. This battery is concerned with assessing how input from the external environment is processed by the individual in light of his or her impairment and how this information is acted on cognitively, affectively, and behaviorally. Measures assessing tactile, visual, auditory, kinesthetic, and verbal encoding (the process of attending to stimuli and sending coded information to the brain for interpretation and storage) is used specifically. However, this specific battery of tests will often be supplemented by other neuropsychological measures, depending on the specific hypotheses the psychologist has formulated and wishes to verify or disprove. In addition to measures aimed at how information is processed via the senses, the psychologist also needs to establish how the individual solves problems, abstracts from specific circumstances to understand common elements among novel situations, how the individual processes information that involves visuospatial reasoning versus verbal (linguistically based) reasoning, and whether the individual can comprehend a set of events in terms of an overriding concept or theme. In this regard he or she will use tests of intelligence such as the Wechsler Adult Intelligence Scale; the Raven's Progressive Matrices; the Wisconsin Card Sorting Test; or the Category Test, which is a component of the Halstead-Reitan Battery. At other times the psychologist is interested in specific aspects of cognitive behavior, such as memory or attention. In those instances, he or she will use tests that have been shown to measure these processes reliably and validly.

Once assessment data are analyzed, the psychologist will proceed to use the results to formulate recommendations regarding treatment and rehabilitation strategies. With acute impairments, often these recommendations involve remedial strategies. Once the impairment is judged to be chronic or nonremitting in nature, the psychologist will be concerned with compensatory strategies. For example, if an individual is left with a memory impairment that prevents him or her from learning new ways of doing things or new sets of information because that person has an anterograde memory loss (memory for present and future learning), he or she will be taught how to keep a daily log, or a memory calendar of tasks to be accomplished, appointments to keep, important telephone numbers to retrieve, and other significant data. Specific training in how to remember may not be appropriate if the cognitive processes necessary to be employed in the learning process are no longer accessible to the individual. If the attentional component of memory is impaired, other cues from the environment will play critical roles in enabling that individual to sustain independent functioning in his or her own home. The use of buzzers to signal that a burner has been left on or a faucet has been left running in the bathtub longer than a designated period of time, or a red light in the bathroom to signal time for bedtime medications are examples of such compensatory strategies.

In addition to the use of formal psychometric procedures (tests and measurements based on standardized testing procedures and comparison groups), the psychologist will also use a variety of other assessment procedures that contribute to an understanding of an individual's functional capacities and limitations. These include observations of the individual's behavior or activities in a given situation, or having the individual keep a log of behaviors, including antecedent and consequent circumstances that may interfere with the learning of a new task or the extinction of a habitual but dysfunctional behavior. Individuals who during the course of a given day experience a tremendous amount of anxiety that renders them unable to sustain employment, for example, may upon interview not be able to recall the specific circumstances that have led to their current state of anxiety. However, when specifically focused on the advent of such emotional states because they are to record their frequency and intensity, they can provide vital assessment data not otherwise available to the psychologist for treatment or rehabilitation planning.

Finally, the psychologist will often find the work and findings of other professionals of vital importance in the work of accurately assessing functional capacities. Data available through various neuroimaging techniques such as computerized axial tomography (CAT scan), positron emission tomography (PET scan), and magnetic resonance imaging (MRI), to name the most well known, are most helpful in working with persons with neurological and neuromuscular disorders, such as multiple sclerosis, or other diseases that have a degenerative course. While these devices can pinpoint lesions in the central nervous system and the brain, they cannot predict functional capacities for any given individual. It is the work of the psychologist to evaluate organic impairments as they relate to residual capacities in any given individual and to work with those remaining functional capacities in the rehabilitation process.

While we have focused on rehabilitation strategies such as those employed with persons with memory, attentional, cognitive, or neurological impairments, there are also long-standing complications of injury or disease that require rehabilitation interventions as well. Here one thinks of the use of hypnosis and biofeedback with individuals who suffer chronic pain. There is exciting work done by psychologists in extending range of motion, for example, through the use of hypnosis and teaching self-hypnosis techniques (Appel, 1992). Myron G. Eisenberg and Mary A. Jansen (1987) provide an excellent overview of the roles assumed by rehabilitation psychologists in medical settings. They describe psychologists' use of behavioral strategies in the treatment of otherwise difficult conditions such as chronic pain, voluntary control of blood pressure, and reinstatement of bladder control in patients with spinal cord injury with neurogenic bladders. In other settings, many of the strategies employed by sports medicine psychologists are being adapted for persons who have debilitating physical impairments.

Specific Roles for Psychologists: Impacts on Quality of Life

While the preceding discussion has focused on those psychologists' interventions in the assessment and treatment process, there is also a role for psychologists in the overall adjustment to disability and in the quality of life that a person with a physical or mental impairment may experience. Oftentimes the "glamor of being a psychologist" is associated with the acute adjustment of an individual to a particular life trauma, whether that be a physical illness, a reaction to stress, or a major life crisis. However, not all persons with disabilities acquire their impairment in later life; many individuals are born with a serious and functionally limiting disability. Others are subject to a slowly progressive and/or deteriorating condition, or are simply disabled by virtue of old age. Individuals with disabilities are also members of society in the broadest sense, and in the narrowest sense are members of a family. Functional limitations and functional capacities cannot be defined outside of the life circumstances specific to an individual. Socioeconomic status, race, culture, gender, level of education, income level, and source of income all define the effects of disability on any given individual (Albrecht, 1992).

Given the nature of disability and its resultant impact on functional capacities in an individual, quality of life considerations define a major role for the psychologist. There is accumulating evidence that mortality itself is affected as much by quality of life factors as by the severity and nature of the disability (Krause & Kjorsvig, 1992). What does this mean for the psychologist? Broadly speaking, the psychologist becomes defined as an educator, an advocate, and a collaborator. The needs of family members, coworkers, and peer group members for information regarding various disabilities are enormous. The current effort to mainstream children with severe impairments and disabilities into regular education (a process known as inclusion), and resistance to these efforts by educationally related professionals in particular, speak eloquently to the real need for an "educated" professional with people skills, hopefully embodied by someone with psychological training and expertise.

Mitchell Rosenthal and Kenneth I. Kolpan (1986) note an increasingly heavy emphasis on the use of the psychologist as an "expert witness" in litigation involving injuries and resultant impairment. They emphasize the variety of "legal" roles and responsibilities that the rehabilitation psychologist may be called on to fill. These include submitting psychological reports and treatment summaries; providing expert witness testimony in court; appearing at SSDI appeal hearings; providing specific information to third-party payers as to the extent, duration, and permanence of disability; directing family members to the appropriate agencies or community resources that will best meet their needs; and consulting with attorneys. They conclude that "the rehabilitation psychologist may be the most important professional involved in the seemingly interminable struggle to regain independence and some measure of productivity and life satisfaction."

Psychologists are also employed by government agencies concerned with disability determination and the payment of workers' compensation or various disability funds. Equally important is the role the psychologist can play as an advocate, helping to ensure access to appropriate social benefits as well as facilitating the exercise of rights among persons with disabilities in the workplace, the educational institution, community recreational facilities, and health care resources.

Two additional seemingly diverse roles for psychologists that have an impact on quality of life for persons with disabilities are those involving career/vocational counseling and the role of family consultant for persons with severe mental illness. While vocational counseling has been a major and traditional component of rehabilitation counseling programs whose target population for service delivery is persons with disabilities, there is renewed interest in counseling psychology in this area, although of much more recent origin (Blustein, 1992). Interactions among career choice, vocational opportunities, and work-related problems and mental health in general are major moderators of quality of life parameters in all persons and certainly in those with severe disabilities in particular.

The second role is discussed specifically by Kayla F. Bernheim (1989). She has designated this role "family consultation," with particular focus on families of persons who have severe mental illness. Her position is further validated by Dale L. Johnson (1989), who represents the opinion held by the National Alliance for the Mentally Ill (NAMI) with respect to the need for communication between psychologist and family members. He emphasizes that this communication can be relevant only if the two parties are able to "speak the same language" in terms of the latest theories and research regarding the etiology, assessment, and treatment of persons with severe disabilities, including the schizophrenias. Bernheim points out, in addition, that psychologists have special expertise that lends itself to working with families of persons with severe mental illness. Expertise in behavioral management, skills training, and stress management skills are given as examples. However, she points out that psychologists in public service have ethical and moral obligations to widen their perspectives to include attention to the "tasks and burdens of relatives of patients and to recognize that part of [our] job is to make their jobs easier" (p. 563). She also emphasizes the need for curricular revisions in the training of next generation psychologists, which will include focused attention on the biological aspects of mental illness, among other issues. "Those of a more creative frame of mind might even wish to consider including families in the development of new curricula" (p. 563).

This entry would not be complete if the issue of the HIV epidemic and its implications for psychology were not addressed. Anthony R. D'Augelli (1990) presents roles for community psychologists and includes specific steps to be taken in establishing a community-oriented network for AIDS issues by these psychologists. These steps include intervention strategies as well as network planning goals. D'Augelli suggests that the HIV epidemic provides "unprecedented opportunities for professional and personal commitment to social change." That psychologists, particularly rehabilitation psychologists, become involved in the policymaking process was addressed by Andrea L. Solarz (1990), and in a parallel vein reinforces the role for psychologists in general in the process of social change that was raised by D'Augelli with respect to community psychologists.

In conclusion, the field of disabilities is such that no one professional can deliver appropriate and needed services in a vacuum. To do so is to short-change the person who needs access to individualized, comprehensive, relevant, systematic, and ongoing assessment, treatment, and rehabilitation services. Psychologists must function as members of a team with many players, the most important of whom is the individual with the disabling condition. Often in the establishment of turf by various professional groups, the professionals lose sight of the purpose for their very discipline or professional practice. Psy-

chologists, like other health professionals, are members of a service industry—in this case, services for individuals with disabilities. For appropriate and necessary services to be delivered, whose efficacy can be measured, collaboration among all players is essential. Just as no quarterback makes a very effective defensive tackle, so no one health care professional can assure "quality of life" without the benefit of collaboration among his or her peers and, most important, without active participation of the individual in need of rehabilitation services.

(See also: ASSESSMENT; BEHAVIOR THERAPY; FAMILY; FORENSIC REHABILITATION; NEUROLOGICAL DISORDERS; NEUROLOGY; PSYCHIATRIC REHABILITATION; PSYCHIATRY; PSYCHOLOGY, REHABILITATION; PSYCHOSOCIAL ADJUSTMENT; QUALITY OF LIFE)

RESOURCES

American Psychological Association, Division 22, Rehabilitation Psychology, 750 First St., NE, Washington, DC 20002–4242

American Rehabilitation Counseling Association, a division of the American Counseling Association, 5999 Stevenson Ave., Alexandria, VA 22304–3300

National Academy of Neuropsychology. Contact the Executive Secretary for information: see recent issue of Archives of Clinical Neuropsychology for address of current officers.

National Alliance for the Mentally Ill, 2101 Wilson Blvd., Suite 302, Arlington, VA 22201

BIBLIOGRAPHY

ALBRECHT, GARY L. The Disability Business, Newbury Park, IL, 1992.

APPEL, PHILIP R. "The Use of Hypnosis in Physical Medicine and Rehabilitation." Physical Medicine and Rehabilitation 10 (1992):133–148.

BERNHEIM, KAYLA F. "Psychologists and Families of the Severely Mentally Ill: The Role of Family Consultation." American Psychologist 44 (1989):561–564.

BLUSTEIN, DAVID L. "Toward the Reinvigoration of the Vocational Realm of Counseling Psychology." Counseling Psychologist 20 (1992):712–723.

D'AUGELLI, ANTHONY R. "Community Psychology and the HIV Epidemic: The Development of Helping Communities." Journal of Community Psychology 18 (1990):337–346.

EISENBERG, MYRON G., and JANSEN, MARY A. "Rehabilitation Psychologists in Medical Settings: A Unique Subspecialty or a Redundant One?" *Professional Psychology: Research and Practice* 18 (1987):475–478.

ELLIOTT, TIMOTHY R., and GRAMLING, SANDY E. "Psychologists and Rehabilitation: New Roles and Old Training Models." *American Psychologist* 45 (1990):762–765.

JANSEN, MARY A., and FULCHER, ROBERT. "Rehabilitation Psychologists: Characteristics and Scope of Practice." *American Psychologist* 39 (1982):1282–1283.

JOHNSON, DALE L. "Schizophrenia as a Brain Disease: Implications for Psychologists and Families." *American Psychologist* 44 (1989):553–555.

KEMP, ARTHUR D. "Counseling Center Psychologists in Neuropsychology: Counseling Neuropsychology." *Counseling Psychologist* 20 (1992):571–604.

KRAUSE, JAMES S., and KJORSVIG, JOAN M. "Mortality After Spinal Cord Injury: A Four-Year Prospective Study." *Archives of Physical Medicine and Rehabilitation* 73 (1992):558–563.

PARKER, HARRY J., and CHAN, FONG. "Psychologists in Rehabilitation: Preparation and Experience." *Rehabilitation Psychology* 35 (1990):239–248.

ROSENTHAL, MITCHELL, and KOLPAN, KENNETH I. "Head Injury Rehabilitation: Psycholegal Issues and Roles for the Rehabilitation Psychologist." *Rehabilitation Psychology* 31 (1986):37–46.

SOLARZ, ANDREA L. "Rehabilitation Psychologists: A Place in the Policy Process?" *American Psychologist* 45 (1990):766–770.

LYNDA J. KATZ

PSYCHOLOGY, REHABILITATION

Rehabilitation psychology is a specialized area of study and practice within the larger discipline of psychology, involving the application of psychology to persons with physical, cognitive, emotional, or developmental disabilities and their rehabilitation. Rehabilitation psychology's primary objective is to reduce the effects of disability and to improve the functional capacity of persons with disabilities.

Much of the early research and practice of rehabilitation psychology emphasized the adjustment process of persons to traumatic injury and chronic illness as well as attitudes toward persons with disabilities. The initial theoretical foundation of somatopsychology, which evolved into rehabilitation psychology, was the field theory model of Kurt Lewin. Perhaps the most accurate characterization of current rehabilitation psychology is its psychosocioecological emphasis. The psychosocioecological approach involves not only a focus on the person but also recognizes the importance of factors outside the person that may bring about disability. Disability in this approach is seen as not only involving the individual, the traditional domain of psychology, but also as broader in scope, including attention to the social and environmental barriers faced by persons with disabilities. In this model, the rehabilitation psychologist works with persons having disabilities to identify and eliminate barriers in their interpersonal or physical environment that interfere with their full participation in society.

Roles and Functions

Recognizing that rehabilitation psychologists must do more than just work with the person with the disability, rehabilitation psychologists have multiple roles and functions. Some of these roles are dependent on the particular work setting, which varies considerably. For example, rehabilitation psychologists work in acute medical rehabilitation settings in hospitals or rehabilitation centers; subacute rehabilitation programs, including specialized community reintegration programs for persons with traumatic brain injury; pain centers; vocational rehabilitation; veterans' programs; workmen's compensation; independent living settings; private practice; mental health agencies; and academic research and educational institutions.

Within these settings, rehabilitation psychologists may be involved with assessment, intervention, or consultation. Assessment may involve traditional intellectual and personality evaluations but with emphasis on the implications of these assessments on activities of daily life and vocational potential. Assessments include evaluation of environmental and situation factors, and rehabilitation psychologists often adapt traditional psychological instruments and procedures to specific populations, such as persons who have sensory impairments or who have chronic illnesses. Some rehabilitation psychologists are also trained to provide neuropsychological evaluations to assess cognitive disabilities to assist in the planning of rehabilitation programming, while other rehabilitation psychologists have special expertise to assess and evaluate change during the rehabilitation process.

Intervention and consultation by rehabilitation psychologists include a wide variety of treatment modalities. These may involve individual or group counseling or psychotherapy, psychological support, stress and anxiety reduction, social skills, and/or assertiveness training. Other therapies employed by rehabilitation psychologists include biofeedback, behavioral technology, and hypnotherapy. In addition, rehabilitation psychologists work with persons with disabilities in acquiring, feeling comfortable with, and using assistive technology. An increasingly important role of rehabilitation psychologists is to serve as consultants in working with rehabilitation team members, school systems, vocational rehabilitation, and community rehabilitation programs related not only to the rehabilitation process and disability concerns but to enhance team and organizational function as well.

Rehabilitation psychologists who do research investigate areas unique to rehabilitation settings, such as motivation and rehabilitation, the impact of cultural values on rehabilitation, the role of social support and rehabilitation, and depression and its influence on rehabilitation, as well as broader questions related to rehabilitation outcomes and the impact of assistive technology. Other rehabilitation psychology researchers concentrate on the modalities used in rehabilitation intervention as well as on the evolution of attitudes, myths, and stigmata associated with persons with disabilities.

The passage of the Americans with Disabilities Act in 1990 further expanded the potential role of rehabilitation psychologists in employment and workplace settings. Rehabilitation psychology will have an increasing role, especially with persons with severe and persistent mental illness, in the identification of reasonable accommodations. Advocacy with and on behalf of persons with disabilities has always been an inherent part of rehabilitation psychology, not only in their own communities but at state and federal levels as well.

While many of these functions may be similar to all psychologists, a primary distinction is not only the setting or the populations that rehabilitation psychologists serve but also the recognition that many of the barriers that persons with disabilities face are in the social environment. A hallmark of rehabilitation psychology has always been the emphasis on the full participation of the person with the disability in the planning and implementation of his or her rehabilitation.

Preparation/Credentials

As with the discipline of psychology, practicing rehabilitation psychologists must have a doctoral degree in a program of studies that is primarily psychological and be licensed by the state in which they practice. A majority of rehabilitation psychologists have a doctoral degree in clinical or counseling psychology, with increasing numbers having specialized training in rehabilitation of persons with disabilities. There has been considerable discussion related to what should be included in a curriculum of studies in rehabilitation psychology at the doctoral level. Many rehabilitation psychologists believe that specific specialty education is necessary, while others believe that rehabilitation psychologists have more in common with specialties such as clinical and counseling psychology, and that specialty training can be accomplished through the practicum and internship process.

Division 22, Rehabilitation Psychology, of the American Psychological Association (APA), adopted a postdoctoral sequence in 1992 containing content areas in which a well-trained rehabilitation psychologist should have exposure. Examples of content areas include sexual functioning and disability, psychosocial models of disability and chronic illness, ergonomics and barrier removal, and behavioral applications in assessment and treatment. In 1993 Division 22 also initiated an application toward specialty diplomate status for rehabilitation psychologists under the American Board of Professional Psychology.

Professional Organizations

The primary organization to which rehabilitation psychologists belong is Division 22, Rehabilitation Psychology, of the APA. Initially formed as a special interest group of the APA, the National Council on Psychological Aspects of Disabilities was organized in 1949. APA sponsored the first formal conference related to rehabilitation psychology in 1958, and in the same year the national council was granted divisional status. The division changed its name in 1960 to Psychological Aspects of Disability and again in 1972 to the Division of Rehabilitation Psychology. Approximately 1,400 psychologists were members of the division in 1995. Division 22 publishes the journal *Rehabilitation Psychology* and a quarterly newsletter. Members also adhere to the ethical standards promulgated by the APA.

Other organizations to which rehabilitation psychologists belong include those specific to different disabilities, such as the Head Injury Foundation or the Arthritis Foundation, and to rehabilitation-oriented organizations such as the American Congress of Rehabilitation Medicine and the National Rehabilitation Association. Rehabilitation psychologists also belong to groups with specific psychological focus in areas of neuropsychology, substance abuse, and mental retardation.

(*See also*: ASSESSMENT; CREDENTIALS; DISABILITY; DISABILITY MANAGEMENT; PSYCHIATRY; PSYCHOLOGY; PSYCHOSOCIAL ADJUSTMENT)

RESOURCE

American Psychological Association, Division 22, Rehabilitation Psychology, 750 First St., NE, Washington, DC 20002–4242

BIBLIOGRAPHY

EISENBERG, MYRON G., and JANSEN, MARY A. "Rehabilitation Psychology: State of the Art." In *Annual Review of Rehabilitation*, vol. 3, ed. E. L. Pan, T. Backer, and C. Vash. New York, 1983.

ELLIOTT, TIMOTHY R., and GRAMLING, S. "Psychologists and Rehabilitation: New Roles and Old Training Models." *American Psychologist* 45 (1990):762–765.

FRANK, R. G.; GLUCK, J.; and BUCKELEW, S. "Rehabilitation: Psychology's Greatest Opportunity?" *American Psychologist* (1990):757–761.

GOLDEN, C., ed. *Current Topics in Rehabilitation Psychology.* Orlando, FL, 1984.

NEFF, WALTER S., ed. *Rehabilitation Psychology.* Washington, DC, 1971.

WRIGHT, BEATRICE, ed. *Psychology and Rehabilitation.* Washington, DC, 1959.

PAUL LEUNG

PSYCHOSOCIAL ADJUSTMENT

Disability due to injury, chronic illness, or genetic or congenital conditions can have a major impact on an individual's social, psychological, physical, and economic status. Although a number of factors influence the extent of the impact, the onset of disability, regardless of the cause, necessitates some alteration in the person's life. Individuals encountering disability may be faced with a number of losses, including changes of body image, social status, and earning capacity. These changes may be accompanied by any number of psychological reactions, including grief, anger, and anxiety. The process that persons undergo in trying to cope with the psychological stress of disability is known as adjustment. During this time individuals attempt to cope, understand, and come to terms with their disability as well as try to learn new skills and plan for the future.

Adjustment is complex and highly individual and is influenced by a number of intervening variables. Rather than a stable state, adjustment is a process that evolves over time. Determining when a person has completed the process is nebulous, and definitions of adjustment vary. Adjustment may be viewed as individuals' response and ability to cope with their disability, as their ability to problem-solve, or as their ability to regain control and self-determination over events that affect their life. Commonly, some version of productivity, either in the form of activities of daily living or of employment, is used to assess the level of adjustment an individual has reached.

The process of adjustment has been studied from the perspective of a number of academic disciplines, from the viewpoint of a number of theories, and in the context of a variety of disabling conditions. Despite the attempts to understand adjustment, there is no universal consensus concerning the nature of the process of adjustment to severe disability, although a variety of theories and models have been proposed to explain and describe it.

Stage Theory

The view that persons go through various stages in attempting to adjust to disability is well documented. Stage theorists postulate that with the onset of disability individuals experience a given sequence of psychological reactions, which they move through to reach the final stage of adjustment (Crewe & Krause, 1987). Although emotional reactions to disability vary, reactions typically described in the literature include depression, anxiety, denial, anger, guilt, and grief (Falvo, 1991).

Stage theory is a way of describing reactions in the context of specific stages of adjustment. Placing reactions into stages provides a basis for categorizing behavior and reactions of the individual, thus designating a means for monitoring progress in the adjustment process. Although there are a number of different stage theories, most of them contain the similar premise that persons move from the initial shock of the disability through a series of stages until adjustment is achieved. Most stage theorists recognize that stages of adjustment are points on a continuum rather than discrete categories and that not all individuals progress through each stage in sequence, with the same intensity, or at the same rate.

One example of stage theory was proposed by Franklin C. Shontz (1965, 1982). His initial model (1965) contained five phases of adjustment: shock, realization, defensive retreat, acknowledgment, and adaptation. The shock phase is designated as the initial stage of adjustment in which the individual experiences blunted emotional responses and shows minimal feelings and reactions. During the next stage, the stage of realization, Shontz proposed that individuals begin to approach and recognize the implications of their condition. As they come to acknowledge the reality and seriousness of their situation they react with anxiety, fear, depression, or anger. As a way of coping with the stress of this realization, the person moves into the next stage of adjustment, defensive retreat, when he or she denies the existence of the disability or minimizes its seriousness as a means to combat fear and anxiety. When the reality of the situation becomes more apparent, and as individuals begin to find mechanisms to cope with anxiety, they move into the next phase of Shontz's model, called acknowledgment. This stage is described as a phase when the person reaches an understanding of the nature of the disability and its accompanying limitations. The final stage of this model of adjustment is adaptation. During this stage, individuals have psychologically worked through their reaction to the disability and realistically accept their limitations. Individuals begin to plan for the future and focus on their abilities to reach their maximum potential.

Although most stage theories describe similar reactions, phases characterizing different stages of adjustment are not universal and have not been validated empirically. Individuals may not progress through all phases, nor experience all reactions described in each phase. For example, depression is a common feature noted in many stage theories. Depression in many instances is viewed as a predictable and time-limited phenomenon and necessary for psychological recovery. However, many personal and environmental variables have been found to moderate the presence of depression. Consequently, although some persons with disability may experience depression, empirical evidence does not suggest that it is a necessary component of adjustment (Shontz, 1975).

Developmental Perspectives

Adjustment to disability has also been viewed in the context of the age at which the disability occurs. Individual adjustment to the consequences of congenital disability or one that is experienced in early childhood may differ from adjustment to a disability manifested after the person is an adult (Sutkin, 1984). Needs, responsibilities, and resources differ at varying stages of life and consequently can influence the adjustment process. Each stage of life has its own particular stresses or demands apart from those experienced as a result of disability. In spite of the disability, individuals must also accomplish developmental tasks that enable them to make the transition from one life stage to the other.

From a developmental perspective, adjustment to disability is considered in the context of individuals' particular life stage and the way demands during that time, in association with changes and limitations of the disability, influence their attitudes, perceptions, actions, behavior, and adjustment.

Research findings regarding the relationship between age at time of disability and adjustment have been inconclusive. While it has been suggested that adjustment may be facilitated when disability occurs in adult years after a number of skills have been learned and incorporated into one's self-concept, it is also thought that persons who experience disability in childhood, or who have a congenital disability, incorporate the disability into their self-concept earlier, consequently facilitating adjustment. The exact mechanism, or the extent to which age affects adjustment to disability in either a positive or a negative way, has not been established (Wright, 1983).

Social Support

The influence of social interactions on individual adjustment to disability is well documented (Shontz, 1975; Wright, 1983). Many of the psychological effects of disability result from social implications in terms of acceptance or nonacceptance, and integration or reintegration into a larger society. Persons within society are ascribed certain social roles, which include various rights and responsibilities as well as expectations of behavior in those roles. Adjustment to disability in this context focuses on individuals' ability to negotiate or renegotiate their identities and roles within a variety of social groups.

When individuals experience disability, adjustment may be affected by how society perceives the role of individuals with disability, or by the individual's own expectations of that role (English, 1977). Much may also depend on the social role the individual filled prior to the disability, and the extent to which the role has changed. There is some indication that continued membership in highly valued groups increases the person's ability to cope with disability, while when membership is restricted, a loss of social value and importance can occur, which in turn can influence adjustment. Reassurance of worth and social integration appear to be mediating factors in facilitating adjustment and have been associated with lower levels of depression in individuals with disability.

The degree of social support, and especially intrafamilial support, has been demonstrated as contributing to the adjustment process (Power, 1985; Steward et al., 1992). Chronic illness or disability may disrupt performance and role expectations within the family and may have behavioral consequences related to adjustment. Family, friends, and other social contacts who interact with the person with disability can have a powerful influence over the individual's sense of value and worth and subsequent adjustment. Overprotectiveness of family members toward the individual with disability may diminish confidence and result in dependence and passivity. However, positive family support can enhance adjustment (Dell Orto & Power, 1994; Kelley & Lambert, 1992; Power & Dell Orto, 1986; Power, Dell Orto, and Gibbons, 1988).

Stigma

Individual adjustment may be influenced by societal values and negative societal attitudes or by the degree of stigma the person with disability experiences or perceives. Stigma associated with disability can serve as a barrier to social integration and alter or disrupt social relationships. Chronic illness or disability are stigmatizing to the extent that they are viewed as deviations from what is normally expected in everyday social interchanges. When discrepancy exists between the reality of the disability and the societal value of physical or mental perfection, persons with disability can become devalued, ostracized, or may be barred from full integration into society. Consequently, negative social interactions can shape the individual's self image and influence adjustment.

Minority Status

From a social perspective an analogy has been drawn between the social position of persons with disability and that of members of underprivileged minorities (Braithwaite, 1988). Individuals with disability, like traditional minority groups, may be subject to group stereotypes, role conflict between acting normal versus disabled, and underprivileged social status. Like members of other minority groups, the person with disability faces the task of overcoming many social barriers to reach the quality of life enjoyed by most. The process of adjustment in this model necessitates social adjustments and changes in interpersonal communication to be used in becoming assimilated into a culture of disability. Using this model, adjustment is defined by the degree to which individuals are able to learn the physical and social skills that enable them to reintegrate into the community as persons of independence and worth.

Race, ethnicity, and gender contribute to an individual's self-definition and may also influence adjustment to disability. Persons may experience difficulties due to disparities in values orientation, and discrimination, stereotyping, and prejudice due to race, ethnicity, or gender in addition to societal attitudes related to their disability.

Other Variables Influencing Adjustment

Research has shown that a number of factors play an important part in an individual's ability to adjust to his or her disability. Among the variables influencing adjustment, attribution, self-concept, and nature of disability will be discussed here.

Attribution. Attribution refers to assigning responsibility or blame for an event. Attribution theory has been applied to the adjustment to a variety of life events (Miller & Porter, 1983; Westbrook & Nordholm, 1986; Wortman, 1983), although most of these theoretical models have focused on how individuals react to the experiences of others rather than to their own life events (Bulman & Wortman, 1977). Contradictory findings exist in the few empirical studies that have dealt directly with how attribution theory may influence the adjustment of persons with disability (Bordieri, Comninel, and Drehmer, 1989; Wortman, 1976). While some studies conclude that there is a negative correlation between adjustment and the degree to which individuals blame another for their injury (Bulman & Wortman, 1977), other studies have indicated that blaming another for disability may be adaptive.

Body Image and Self-Concept. The impact of disability on an individual's body image and self-concept has been well documented. Self-concept is the individual's perception of self and moderates the individual's reactions and interactions with others. The concept of body image encompasses more than a perception of physical appearance; it also includes perception of function, sensation, feelings, and thought. The terms "self-concept" and "body image" are often used interchangeably, and they are

inextricably interwoven (Lubin, 1986). Both are related to an individual's experiences with others and to his or her view of self in terms of self-esteem and identity. Individuals' perception of self is influenced by their perception of how others perceive them. Likewise, individuals act in accordance with expectations projected to others. The impact of disability on self-concept and body image is related to environmental and social consequences as well as premorbid personality characteristics and can influence adjustment.

Nature of Disability. Adjustment related to the disability type, its manifestations, and its limitations have been studied extensively. Findings are inconsistent regarding the impact of different disabling conditions on adjustment and the degree to which adjustment is uniform across all types of disability. Individuals' adaptation to their condition may or may not be related to the type of disability. In some instances it has been suggested that different norms for psychosocial adjustment may exist across types of disability, making such comparisons difficult. In other instances, adjustment may be more affected by variables, such as uncertainty and control, rather than the degree of disability itself (Christman, 1990; Falvo, Allen, and Maki, 1982; Ozer, 1987; McClelland, 1988).

In many instances it has been suggested that the extent of the disability, whether extreme or minor, may not be as crucial as the person's perception of it. Adjustment may also be mediated by the individual's appraisal of the disability and his or her perceived resources for dealing with it (Lazarus & Folkman, 1984). Resources in this sense refers not only to tangible resources but also to the person's belief that he or she can cope with the stress the disability produces. There is limited research available that examines the role of appraisal or coping in adjusting to disability, except as it relates to premorbid personality characteristics.

Facilitation of Positive Adjustment

The rehabilitation process is designed to assist persons with disabilities attain physical and psychological adjustment, to overcome barriers, and to learn skills and attitudes that enhance their reintegration into society. One objective is to assist individuals with disability to appraise the disability realistically, to recognize limitations but not exaggerate them, and to use their assets to live as fully as possible.

One of the major tasks of the rehabilitation professional is to identify positive coping strategies that will augment and enhance rehabilitation and to identify maladaptive coping strategies that can then be redirected. While dealing with psychological issues is essential, environmental factors are also important in helping persons adjust to disability. Consequently, in the rehabilitation process focus is also placed on alterable conditions within the environment in which changes can be made. Examples of more concrete environmental factors are architectural barriers, housing, transportation, assistive devices, and training or education. More abstract issues within the environment that must also be addressed to facilitate positive adjustment are discriminatory practices, stereotypes and prejudice, lack of employment opportunities, and family or relationship problems.

A variety of theoretical viewpoints have been used in helping individuals through the adjustment process. The types of therapeutic measures are endless; however, no specific therapy has been found to be beneficial for all. A variety of strategies, including group techniques and peer counseling (Lasky, Dell Orto, and Marinelli, 1984), individual counseling, family counseling, educational counseling, and behavioral management techniques have been used to facilitate adjustment (Marinelli & Dell Orto, 1991).

Quantifying and Qualifying Adjustment

Although the issue of adjustment to disability has been studied from the perspectives of different academic disciplines, from the viewpoint of a number of theories, and from the context of different disabling conditions, there are few consistent findings regarding the nature of the adjustment process or effective indicators of when adjustment has been achieved. In part such inconsistencies are attributable to a variety of clinical and methodological difficulties associated with studying adjustment and how it is attained.

Much information gained about adjustment to disability has come from clinical impressions rather than empirical studies (Crewe & Krause, 1987), and many of these studies have been retrospective rather than longitudinal. Data that demonstrate clinically

observed phases of adaptation originated from only a few studies, which used a limited number of measuring instruments.

Measurement of adjustment has also been impeded by a number of factors. Not all psychosocial assessment instruments are appropriate for use with all disabling conditions. Some instruments that have been used have few validity and reliability studies. Utilization of standard instruments with persons with disability involves additional limitations. Some individuals may have emotional impairment or impairment of cognitive function as a result of their disability, which may confound accurate measurement of psychosocial adjustment. Likewise, without predisability information it is difficult to assess the extent to which any instrument is measuring adjustment or personality variables that existed before the disability.

The term "disability" is also not precise, nor has it been used consistently. Consequently, comparisons of adjustment across different disabling conditions, or among individuals with the same condition, are difficult. In addition, no clear distinction is systematically made between features of the disability itself and whether it is acquired or congenital, terminal or chronic, visible or invisible. Such diversity makes generalizations about adjustment as a process difficult.

Much research has also been flawed by researchers' erroneous hypotheses about the meaning of disability to individuals who have varying conditions and factors that contribute to their adjustment (Myerson, 1988). Defining adjustment alone has its limitations. Defining adjustment in terms of productivity or integration into a societal group may impose value judgments and may not be applicable to all individuals. Productivity can be defined in a number of ways. Persons who are disabled and appear productive by societal terms may be employed but poorly adjusted psychologically or socially, while other individuals who appear nonproductive as typically defined may still be well adjusted.

Summary

A number of theories have been proposed to describe and predict the adjustment process. However, most approaches emphasize adjustment as a continuous process of coping. Adjustment can be a lengthy process, sometimes lasting for years. In the case of progressive disability, new adjustments may be needed with each subsequent loss of function. Although the onset of disability causes disruption in the individual's psychological equilibrium, it does not uniformly cause disturbing psychological reactions in all persons with disability (Shontz, 1982). Reactions, whether favorable or unfavorable, are not necessarily directly related to the physical parameters of the individual's disability. Many other factors in the person's life may be more responsible for his or her reaction than the disability itself.

The process of psychological adjustment to disability is highly individual and dependent on a number of intervening variables. Although persons with disability appear to experience similar reactions during the adjustment process, no consistent order or universal pattern has been empirically documented across disabilities. Although emphasis on achieving vocational goals and other measures of productivity may be one measure of adjustment, productivity may be defined differently by different individuals. The best measure of adjustment may be self-esteem and the ability to maintain satisfying relationships as well as productivity (Crewe & Krause, 1987).

(*See also:* ABILITY; ATTITUDES; CONSUMERS; DISABILITY; DISABILITY MANAGEMENT; FAMILY; LOSS AND GRIEF; MINORITIES; SELF-CONCEPT; SEXUALITY)

BIBLIOGRAPHY

BORDIERI, JAMES E.; COMNINEL, MARY E.; and DREHMER, DAVID E. "Client Attributions for Disability: Perceived Accuracy, Adjustment, and Coping." *Rehabilitation Psychology* 34 (1989):271–278.

BRAITHWAITE, DAWN O. "Viewing Persons with Disabilities as a Culture." In *Intercultural Communication: A Reader,* eds. Larry Samovar and Richard Porter. 5th ed. Belmont, CA, 1988.

BULMAN, RONNIE JANOFF, and WORTMAN, CAMILLE B. "Attributions of Blame and Coping in the 'Real World': Severe Accident Victims React to Their Lot." *Journal of Personality and Social Psychology* 35 (1977):351–363.

CHRISTMAN, NORMA J. "Uncertainty and Adjustment During Radiotherapy." *Nursing Research* 39 (1990): 17–20.

CREWE, NANCY M., and KRAUSE, JAMES S. "Spinal Cord Injury: Psychological Aspects." In *Rehabilita-*tion Psychology Desk Reference, ed. Bruce Caplan. Rockville, MD, 1987.

DELL ORTO, ARTHUR E., and POWER, PAUL W. *Head Injury and the Family.* Winter Park, FL, 1994.

ENGLISH, R. WILLIAM. "The Application of Personality Theory to Explain Psychological Reactions to Physical Disability." In *The Psychological and Social Impact of Physical Disability,* eds. Robert Marinelli and Arthur E. Dell Orto. New York, 1977.

FALVO, DONNA R. *Medical and Psychosocial Aspects of Chronic Illness and Disability.* Gaithersburg, MD, 1991.

FALVO, DONNA R.; ALLEN, HARRY; and MAKI, DENNIS. "Psychosocial Aspects of Invisible Disability." *Rehabilitation Literature* 43 (1982):1–2, 26.

KELLEY, SUSAN D., and LAMBERT, SELDEN S. "Family Support in Rehabilitation: A Review of Research 1980–1990." *Rehabilitation Counseling Bulletin* 36 (1992):98–119.

LASKY, ROBERT G.; DELL ORTO, ARTHUR E.; and MARINELLI, ROBERT P. "Structured Experiential Therapy: A Group Approach to Rehabilitation." In *The Psychological and Social Impact of Physical Disability,* eds. Robert Marinelli and Arthur E. Dell Orto. New York, 1984.

LAZARUS, R. S., and FOLKMAN, S. *Stress Appraisal and Coping.* New York, 1984.

LUBIN, ILENE MOROF. *Chronic Illness: Impact and Interventions.* Boston, 1986.

MARINELLI, ROBERT P., and DELL ORTO, ARTHUR E. *The Psychological and Social Impact of Disability,* 3rd ed. New York, 1991.

McCLELLAND, R. J. "Psychosocial Sequelae of Head Injury: Anatomy of a Relationship." *British Journal of Psychiatry* 153 (1988):141–146.

MILLER, DALE T., and PORTER, CAROL A. "Self-Blame in Victims of Violence." *Journal of Social Issues* 39 (1983):141–154.

MYERSON, LEE. The Social Psychology of Physical Disability." *Journal of Social Issues* 44 (1988):173–188.

OZER, LYNNIE. "Hidden Disability." *Journal of Rehabilitation,* vol. 63,1(1987):67–69.

POWER, PAUL W. "Family Coping Behaviors in Chronic Illness: A Rehabilitation Perspective." *Rehabilitation Literature* 46 (1985):78–83.

POWER, PAUL W.; and DELL ORTO, ARTHUR E. "Families, Illness, and Disability: The Roles of the Rehabilitation Counselor." *Journal of Rehabilitation* 17 (1986):40–41.

POWER, PAUL W.; DELL ORTO, ARTHUR E.; and GIBBONS, MARTHA. *Family Interventions Throughout Chronic Illness and Disability.* New York, 1988.

SHONTZ, FRANKLIN C. "Reactions of Crisis." *Volta Review* 67 (1965):364–370.

———. *The Psychological Aspects of Physical Illness and Disability.* New York, 1975.

———. "Adaptation to Chronic Illness and Disability." In *Handbook of Clinical Health Psychology*, eds. Theodore Millon, C. Green, and R. Meagher. New York, 1982.

STEWARD D. A.; STEIN, A.; FORREST, G. C.; and CLARK, D. M. "Psychosocial Adjustment in Siblings of Children with Chronic Life-Threatening Illness: A Research Note." *Journal of Child Psychology and Psychiatry* 33 (1992):779–784.

SUTKIN, LaFAYE C. "Introduction." In *Chronic Illness and Disability Through the Life Span: Effects on Self and Family*, eds. Myron G. Eisenberg, LaFaye C. Sutkin, and Mary A. Jansen. New York, 1984.

WESTBROOK, MARY, and NORDHOLM, LENA. "Reactions to Patient's Self—or Chance—Blaming Attributions for Illness Having Varying Life-Style Involvement." *Journal of Applied Social Psychology* 16 (1986):428–446.

WORTMAN, CAMILLE B. "Causal Attribution and Personal Control." In *New Directions in Attribution Research*, eds. John H. Harvey, W. J. Ickes, and R. F. Kidd. Hindsdale, NJ, 1976.

———. "Coping with Victimization: Conclusions and Implications for Future Research." *Journal of Social Issues* 39 (1983):195–221.

WRIGHT, BEATRICE. *Physical Disability—A Psychosocial Approach.* New York, 1983.

DONNA R. FALVO

PSYCHOTHERAPY

See MOOD DISORDERS; PHARMACOLOGY; PSYCHIATRY; PSYCHOLOGY, REHABILITATION

PUBLIC REHABILITATION SYSTEM

See STATE–FEDERAL REHABILITATION PROGRAM

PULMONARY DISORDERS

See RESPIRATORY DISEASE

QUADRIPLEGIA

See SPINAL CORD INJURY

QUALITY OF LIFE

The quality of life (QOL) of persons with disability has been addressed in the literature since the early 1970s. Although early studies tended to focus on differences between the quality of life of persons with disability and those without disabilities, since the 1980s quality of life research in rehabilitation has examined how such research can be used to promote quality lives in the community. For example, Richard Lamb (1981), writing about persons with serious mental illness, suggested that "we need to realize that if we can 'only' improve the quality of life of these patients . . . we have taken a great step forward in making real the benefits expected of deinstitutionalization" (p. 106). A *Rehab Brief* (1988) from the National Institute on Disability and Rehabilitation Research noted that "improving the quality of life is what rehabilitation is all about."

The purpose of this entry is to review the history of QOL research, distribute definitional and measurement issues related to persons with disability, and discuss future trends.

Context of Quality of Life Research in Rehabilitation

The social policy thrust of QOL research reflects the dramatic legislative and social movements that have changed the political climate for persons with disability since the 1970s. For example, social movements such as normalization, least restrictive environment, and deinstitutionalization have characterized the shift in disability policy from powerlessness and professionalism to empowerment and consumerism. Concurrently, rehabilitation legislation has shifted from an emphasis on individual needs and functioning to a consideration of equal rights and environmental accessibility. These philosophical and legislative emphases on empowerment and consumerism are relevant to QOL research, where programs and services are evaluated from the subjective experience of how such programs improve the lives of the participants.

Another trend that has shaped the interest in QOL measures for persons with disability is the interest in holistic measures of individual growth and change (Fabian, 1990). That is, rehabilitation evaluation research has moved from unidimensional ratings of specific behavioral change toward a desire to assess outcomes using multidimensional approaches that include the unique personal and cultural perspectives of the individual (Fabian, 1993). Assessing program services and interventions from the perspective of the individual is fundamental to understanding the meaning of the disability experience and to exploring how different cultural and gender identities influence this meaning.

A third trend contributing to the interest in assessing subjective quality of life has been generated by medical advances, some of which have succeeded in prolonging life while generating numerous concerns about life quality (Hollandsworth, 1988). In physical medicine and rehabilitation, quality of life assessment may be used as an outcome indicator measuring the effectiveness of various medical interventions such as surgery, or therapeutic modalities such as nursing, or even may influence decisions concerning which particular medical intervention would make the most sense for the patient.

Definitions and Theory of Quality of Life for Persons with Disability

Although quality of life can refer to objective indicators associated with demographic and related statistics that determine how "good" a particular community, city, or country is, QOL research in the area of disability has relied primarily on subjective approaches to understanding and measuring the construct. Sometimes referred to as subjective well-being, one definition of quality of life that is frequently used for persons with disability is life satisfaction, relying on the "standards of the respondent to determine what is the good life" (Diener, 1984, p. 543). Life satisfaction definitions of quality of life are based on individual ratings or evaluations of various aspects of life. Individuals reach these evaluations of life based on such standards as needs, expectations, desires, hopes, and experiences.

However, the subjective nature of life satisfaction, together with the difficulty inherent in measuring the construct for persons with severe disabilities, led to arguments for construing quality of life as degree of adaptive or independent functioning (Baroff, 1986). Defining quality of life in terms of adaptive functioning is based on the theoretical assumption that the more individuals feel competent and the more they demonstrate mastery of themselves and their environments, the higher is their quality of life. These assumptions are also embedded in the philosophies of least restrictive environment and normalization. Although the theoretical leap from subjective well-being to adaptive functioning may appear large, empirical studies have supported the overlap between individual evaluations of life satisfaction and measures of adaptive or independent functioning (e.g., Andrews & Withey, 1976; Franklin et al., 1986).

Measurement Issues. Since quality of life definitions for persons with severe disability are frequently formulated in terms of either life satisfaction or adaptive functioning, instruments for measuring the construct represent these two distinct approaches. Quality of life as a measure of life satisfaction typically assesses both global satisfaction and life domain–specific satisfaction from the subjective perspective of the individual (Fabian, 1991). These inventories or structured interviews include scales asking respondents to evaluate how they feel about a particular aspect of their life. For individuals with severe disabilities, structured interviews with an illustration of scale points are frequently used. Although these instruments have demonstrated fairly robust reliability and validity statistics as reported in the literature (Campbell, Converse and Rogers, 1976; Lehman, 1988), authors have noted their limitations in general (Cheng, 1988), and their specific limitations when applied to individuals with disabilities (Baroff, 1986). One of the most problematic issues in using these scales for persons with severe disabilities is that restricted life experiences can constrain an individual's ability to reach evaluations of particular aspects of his or her life (Baroff, 1986). This latter issue is particularly salient when using QOL indicators to evaluate particular program effects.

As mentioned, a second way that quality of life has been measured for persons with severe disabilities is in terms of adaptive functioning or independence. In this regard, Carol Sigelman, Linda

Vengroff, and Cynthia Spanhel (1979) noted that "rehabilitation techniques may enhance life outcomes by directly improving life quality" (p. 106). Margaret Nosek, Marcus Fuhrer, and Carol Howland (1992) used quality of life scales to measure the perceived control that an individual experiences over aspects of his or her life. Alex Zautra and Darlene Goodhart (1979) noted that quality of life is related to experiences of self-mastery, and Frank Andrews and Stephen Withey (1976) suggested that self-efficacy may be the most significant predictor of life satisfaction.

Current Issues and the Future of Quality of Life Research

The use of QOL indicators to inform social policy or reach evaluations of life's meaning is controversial and requires caution. For example, quality of life indices have been used to evaluate the viability and potential of newborns with serious illnesses. Second, concerns about the validity of subjective evaluations of life for persons whose experiences have been seriously constricted, such as persons with severe developmental disabilities and mental illness, are problematic in the interpretation of outcome data (Fabian, 1991). Third, conflicting evidence regarding life satisfaction outcomes for various ethnic and racial groups suggests a need for more QOL research to understand how rehabilitation programs affect individuals from diverse backgrounds and how different people attach meaning to the disability experience (Fabian, 1993).

QOL research represents a potentially powerful method for assessing rehabilitation program outcomes and individual experiences. However, until measurement issues and theoretical models have been clarified, such research needs to be conducted with attention to its limitations and cautious interpretation of the results.

BIBLIOGRAPHY

ANDREWS, FRANK M., and WITHEY, STEPHEN B. *Social Indicators of Well-Being: Americans' Perceptions of Life Quality*. New York, 1976.

BAROFF, GARY S. "Maximal Adaptive Competency." *Mental Retardation* 24 (1986):367–368.

CAMPBELL, ANGUS; CONVERSE, PHILIP E.; and RODG-ERS, WILLARD L. *The Quality of American Life: Perceptions, Evaluations, and Satisfactions*. New York, 1976.

CHENG, STEPHEN T. "Subjective Quality of Life in the Planning and Evaluation of Programs." *Evaluation and Program Planning* 11 (1988):123–134.

DIENER, E. "Subjective Well-Being." *Psychological Bulletin* 95 (1984):542–575.

FABIAN, ELLEN. "Quality of Life Research: A Review of Theory and Practice Implications for Individuals with Long-Term Mental Illness." *Rehabilitation Psychology* 35 (1990):161–170.

———. "Using Quality of Life Indicators in Rehabilitation Program Evaluation." *Rehabilitation Counseling Bulletin* 34 (1991):344–356.

———. "Differential Effects of Race and Life Satisfaction for People with Disabilities: An Exploratory Study." Unpublished manuscript. University Park, PA, 1993.

FRANKLIN, JACK L.; SIMMONS, JANE; SOLOVITZ, BRENDA; CLEMONS, JIMMIE R.; and MILLER, GARY E. "Assessing Quality of Life of the Mentally Ill: A Three-Dimensional Model." *Evaluation and the Health Professions* 9 (1986):376–388.

HOLLANDSWORTH, JAMES G. "Evaluating the Impact of Medical Treatment on the Quality of Life: A Five-Year Update." *Social Science and Medicine* 26 (1988):425–434.

LAMB, H. RICHARD. "What Did We Really Expect from Deinstitutionalization?" *Hospital & Community Psychiatry* 32 (1981):105–109.

LEHMAN, ANTHONY F. "A Quality of Life Interview for the Chronically Mentally Ill." *Evaluation and Program Planning* 11 (1988):51–60.

NATIONAL INSTITUTE ON DISABILITY AND REHABILITATION RESEARCH, OFFICE OF SPECIAL EDUCATION AND REHABILITATION SERVICES, U.S. DEPARTMENT OF EDUCATION. "Quality of Life Research in Rehabilitation." *Rehabilitation Brief* 19 (1988).

NOSEK, MARGARET A.; FUHRER, MARCUS J.; and HOWLAND, CAROL A. "Independence among People with Disabilities: II. Personal Independence Profile." *Rehabilitation Counseling Bulletin* 36 (1992): 21–36.

SIGELMAN, CAROL K.; VENGROFF, LINDA P.; and SPANHEL, CYNTHIA L. "Disability and the Concept of Life Functions." *Rehabilitation Counseling Bulletin* 23 (1979):103–113.

ZAUTRA, ALEX, and GOODHART, DARIENE. "Quality of Life Indicators: A Review of the Literature." *Community Mental Health Review* 4 (1979):1–10.

ELLEN S. FABIAN

R

RARE DISORDERS

See DEVELOPMENTAL DISABILITIES; ENDOCRINE DISORDERS; GENETIC DISORDERS

REASONABLE ACCOMMODATION

Reasonable accommodation is a concept that drives a legally mandated practice to assure people with disabilities meaningful access and opportunity in employment. It establishes the right of qualified employees and prospective employees with disabilities to individualized adaptations or adjustments ("accommodation") within the employment environment, enabling the individual to perform the essential duties of the job applied for or held. The only mitigating ("reasonable") circumstances that limit an employer's obligation to provide an accommodation are modifications or adaptations that would either change the nature of the employer's business or impose undue hardship. Though not defined explicitly, reasonable accommodation (1) acknowledges the abilities of people with disabilities;

(2) expresses cognizance of the need to change environments, not people; and (3) affirms humankind's nearly limitless ability to discover equally effective alternative methods to participate fully in society. Although the legal term first appeared only in the nondiscrimination regulations promulgated pursuant to Section 504 of the Rehabilitation Act of 1973 (the Act), the concept of reasonable accommodation has become the cornerstone of effective implementation of all antidiscrimination statutes affording protection to people with disabilities.

With the passage of the Rehabilitation Act of 1973, Congress furnished the framework that spawned the concept of reasonable accommodation. The seemingly innocuous language contained in section 504 of the Act, saying, "No otherwise qualified individual . . . shall, solely by reason of his handicap, be excluded from participation, be denied the benefits of, or be subjected to discrimination under any program or activity receiving federal financial assistance" set into motion a radical change in national social policy regarding people with disabilities.

Before the Act, vocational rehabilitation legislation affecting people with disabilities mirrored society's dim expectations of people with disabilities in general, and no expectations for people with severe disabilities. Such laws as the National Defense Act (1916); the Smith-Hughes Act (1917); the Smith-Sears Veterans Rehabilitation Act (1918); the Smith-Fess Act (1920); the Social Security Act of 1935, as amended in 1940; the Barden-LaFollette Act (1943); and the Vocational Rehabilitation amendments of 1953, 1965, and 1968 fostered dependency and reliance on public benefit. Most important, the tacit premise of vocational rehabilitation that individuals with disabilities could somehow be "fixed" and thus made to be like everyone else, erected formidable disincentives to people with disabilities' participation in the social and economic mainstream.

The obligation to promulgate Section 504 regulations was assigned to the Office of Civil Rights (OCR) in the Department of Health, Education, and Welfare. Historically uncompromising in its approach, OCR had amassed experience with Title VI of the Civil Rights Act of 1964 and Title XI of the Education Amendments of 1972 (both had language similar to Section 504), invoking statutorily defined standards to establish administrative and legal mechanisms and deeming cost factors irrelevant in any equation guaranteeing civil rights.

In the absence of any clear sense of congressional intent—the substance of the committee report on Section 504 contained scant legislative history and no cost projections—OCR's first duty in drafting regulations was to define "handicapped individual" clearly. The Act defined "handicapped individual" as "a person having a physical or mental disability which . . . results in a substantial handicap to employment and . . . can reasonably be expected to benefit in terms of employability from vocational rehabilitation services. . . ." The definition failed to (1) address severely disabled individuals; (2) extend to people with disabilities the right of equal access and opportunity in all federally assisted programs and services; (3) encompass the full spectrum of individuals with disabilities who might be discriminated against in federally funded programs, particularly people with limited prospects for employment; and (4) recognize individuals potentially subject to discrimination either because of a history of disability or an erroneous perception about the existence of a disability.

While OCR was grappling with the regulatory process, a disability rights movement was growing outside government and bringing together, for the first time, people with different categorical disabilities. Spearheaded by people with disabilities, this movement was organized around the larger issue of civil rights as the means to achieve independence within the mainstream of society.

In 1974 Congress amended the Act and redefined "handicapped individual," for the purposes of Section 504, as an individual "who (a) has a physical or mental disability that substantially limits one or more major life activities, (b) has a record of such impairment, or (c) is regarded as having such an impairment." Having identified the individuals to be afforded protection under the Act, it was next necessary to articulate what acts of commission or omission constituted discrimination.

OCR determined that equal treatment would not necessarily constitute nondiscrimination. People with disabilities experienced similar discriminatory practices and attitudinal barriers in employment and program and service access as people afforded protection by other civil rights legislation. Even in the absence of attitudinal barriers, however, there were physical barriers that precluded people with disabilities from meaningful participation. In new construction or alterations to existing facilities, the problems of physical access were easily dealt with by requiring accessibility features be integrated into construction. However, requiring the same accessibility standards for existing structures was too costly and politically unrealistic. Thus a concept of service and program accessibility was adopted that would not necessarily require structural modifications. Access could be achieved through such accommodations as reassigning services to an accessible location, redesigning or modifying equipment, and providing auxiliary aids and equipment (e.g., interpreters, readers, and telecommunications devices).

Nondiscrimination in employment posed other problems in the regulatory process. Again, merely affording equal opportunity would not necessarily result in equal access to employment. Because of the nature of disability, no regulatory language could be

612

formulated to encompass the full spectrum of functional limitations and abilities. Consequently OCR promulgated regulations in 1977 that contained broad language effectively requiring covered entities to undertake a process that considered the functional limitations of the individual as well as the employer's particular circumstances, financial and otherwise, on a case-by-case basis.

In its evolution through court decisions and otherwise, reasonable accommodation has come to include making existing facilities accessible to people with disabilities, job restructuring, part-time or modified work schedules, providing or modifying existing equipment, auxiliary aids, adjusting or modifying examinations, training materials or policies, providing qualified interpreters or readers, and other modifications, limited only by the boundaries of imagination and creativity, and whether the accommodation constitutes an undue hardship, given the particular circumstances of the individual and the employer.

The philosophical concepts arising from the regulatory interpretation of the Act, as amended, regarding reasonable accommodation in employment and access to services and programs through accommodation have been given broader application with the implementation of the Americans with Disabilities Act of 1990. No longer are the principles solely applicable to entities receiving federal funds: They apply to any employer of fifteen or more employees; all state and local government operations; and, to a lesser extent, places of public accommodation.

Successful application of the law requires that both protected individuals and covered entities approach issue resolution in good faith. Given both the inherent ambiguity and the subjective interpretation of many terms used in the legislation, conscious and unconscious abuses may skew the process. Individuals with or without disabilities may occasionally use the law as a sword rather than a shield in an attempt to obtain a perceived right or benefit that they might not otherwise be entitled to. The perceptions and attitudes of covered entities and/or their employees, either through lack of knowledge or by design, may also make fair implementation elusive in individual cases. Regardless, the law requires that dialogue take place. Through the ex-

change, individuals on both sides of the equation will learn about the needs and limitations of the other.

(*See also:* AMERICANS WITH DISABILITIES ACT; ATTITUDES; CIVIL RIGHTS; DISABILITY LAW AND SOCIAL POLICY; ERGONOMICS; HISTORY OF REHABILITATION; JOB PLACEMENT; WORK)

RESOURCES

ABLEDATA, 8455 Colesville Rd, Suite 935, Silver Spring, MD 20910

Job Accommodation Network, West Virginia University, 918 Chestnut Ridge Rd, Suite 1, Morgantown, W.VA 26506–6123

National Council on Disability, 1331 F St., Suite 1050, NW, Washington, DC 20004

New York State Office of Advocate for Persons with Disabilities, One Empire State Plaza, Suite 1001, Albany, NY 12223–1150

President's Committee on Employment of People with Disabilities, 1331 F St., NW, Washington, DC 20004–1107

U. S. Department of Justice (USDOJ), Civil Rights Division, USDOJ Public Access Section, P.O. Box 66738, Washington, DC 22035–6738

U. S. Department of Labor, Employment Standards Administration, Office of Federal Contract Compliance Programs, 200 Constitution Ave., NW, Washington, DC 20210

U. S. Equal Employment Opportunity Commission, 1801 L St., NW, Washington, DC 20507

BIBLIOGRAPHY

BERKOWITZ, EDWARD D. *Disabled Policy: America's Programs for the Handicapped.* New York, 1987. 28 C.F.R. Part 35. 28 C.F.R. Part 39. 28 C.F.R. Part 41. 29 C.F.R. Part 1630.

SCOTCH, RICHARD K. *From Good Will to Civil Rights: Transforming Federal Disability Policy.* Philadelphia, 1984.

SHAPIRO, JOSEPH P. *No Pity.* New York, 1993. 42 U.S.C. § 1211 et seq. 42 U.S.C. § 12101 et seq. 29 U.S.C. § 706. 29 U.S.C. § 794.

U. S. COMMISSION ON CIVIL RIGHTS. *Accommodating the Spectrum of Individual Abilities.* Washington, DC, 1983.

GREGORY K. JONES
YVONNE A. WILLIAMS

RECREATION

Recreation provides important benefits for all human beings. It offers the opportunity for physical activity, emotional release, social involvement, creative expression, and development of human potential. While all recreation can thus be considered "therapeutic," recreation serves a special function in therapy and rehabilitation.

Although recreation has been used in the healing process since prehistoric times, more recent support for the use of recreation as a form of rehabilitation has come from many noted physicians who recognized its benefits. They include William C. Menninger (*Recreation and Mental Health*, 1948), Alexander Reid Martin (*Recreation and the Mentally Ill*, 1958), and Paul Haun (*Recreation: A Medical Viewpoint*, 1964).

Robert Felix wrote in the preface to *Recreation in Treatment Centers* (1962) that recreation contributes significantly to the "more rapid physical, mental, and social rehabilitation of the patient and thus has come to be recognized as a clinically oriented discipline acknowledged by other branches of medical and health professions." Howard Rusk was one of the first authorities to stress the need to provide leisure counseling as a means of promoting social integration upon return to community life. Therapeutic recreation is a significant part of the rehabilitation process.

What Is Therapeutic Recreation?

Therapeutic recreation is the use of recreation activities in the care, treatment, and rehabilitation of individuals with illnesses, disabilities, and/or limitations. It is a process that uses recreational activities as a form of goal-directed treatment to minimize symptoms and improve the physical, mental, social, and emotional well-being of the client. Therapeutic recreation, also known as recreational therapy, is a professional service that assists people with illnesses and disabilities to have a leisure lifestyle that encompasses functional independence, health, and well-being.

Therapeutic recreation includes provision of treatment services and recreation services. Treatment services, often referred to as recreational therapy, are designed to restore, remediate, or rehabilitate to improve functioning and independence as well as to reduce or eliminate the effects of an illness or disability. Recreation services are designed to provide recreation resources and opportunities to improve or maintain physical, mental, emotional, and/or social well-being. Therapeutic recreation services are provided in clinical, residential, and community settings. For services to be most effective, a continuum of services should be available, bridging the span from acute care to community living.

Comprehensive therapeutic recreation services include:

- Treatment. The use of recreation activities to remediate or rehabilitate functional abilities and to assist in diagnosis.
- Leisure education. The use of recreation activities to acquire skills, knowledge, and abilities that facilitate an independent leisure lifestyle.
- Recreation participation. Providing opportunities to engage in leisure activities that enhance health, growth, development, and well-being.

Therapeutic Recreation Services

The services provided by a therapeutic recreation specialist (TRS) are based on the client's needs and interests as well as the mandate of the agency in which services are provided. Therapeutic recreation specialists conduct assessments of physical, mental, emotional, and social functioning to determine the client's needs, interests, and abilities. They work with the client, family members, and other specialists to design and implement an individualized treatment, education, or program plan, depending on the setting. A variety of activities are employed in putting the treatment plan into operation, including fitness programs, community outings, leisure education, family leisure groups, stress management, adventure-based activities, and crafts, among others. A critical component of the treatment plan is the leisure discharge plan, which addresses the leisure needs of the client on returning to the community, and identifies the resources available.

The TRS working in a community recreation setting also conducts assessments to determine client needs and interests. In the community setting, special programs and activities are offered to meet client needs. The TRS is also responsible for adapting activities, as needed, and providing adaptive equipment to enable individuals with disabilities to participate. The TRS is involved directly or indirectly in providing such programs as adapted aquatics, a wheelchair basketball league, a social program for adults with mental retardation, a downhill skiing program for individuals with physical disabilities, integrated summer day camps, and adapted golf lessons. The TRS will generally seek to integrate clients into existing programs and classes when possible, and then provide in-service training for recreation staff who will serve individuals with disabilities.

All therapeutic recreation specialists have an ethical obligation to advocate for leisure opportunities for individuals with disabilities and/or limitations. This obligation includes addressing limited transportation resources, inaccessible facilities, and legislation that has an impact on people with disabilities. The TRS frequently serves on advisory committees and consults with outside agencies to ensure that services and resources are provided for people with disabilities.

Benefits of Therapeutic Recreation

In 1988, Temple University was awarded a three-year grant from the National Institute for Disability and Rehabilitation Research to determine the efficacy of therapeutic recreation in rehabilitation. As part of the grant, a national consensus conference was held on the benefits of therapeutic recreation in rehabilitation. Conference participants identified documented outcomes determined in research literature. The outcomes of numerous study groups were consolidated and broadly classified into the following areas:

- improving physical health and health maintenance;
- improving cognitive functioning;
- improving psychosocial health;
- improving growth and personal development;
- improving personal and life satisfaction;
- societal and health care systems outcomes.

The proceedings of the conference and a summary of the study groups were published in *Benefits of Therapeutic Recreation: A Consensus View* (1991). Therapeutic recreation, like all allied health disciplines, must demonstrate treatment outcomes to remain viable in today's health care environment.

Professional Preparation in Therapeutic Recreation

Therapeutic recreation is provided by professionals who are trained and certified, registered, and/or licensed. Professional credentialing has become essential for employment. National certification is available through the National Council for Therapeutic Recreation Certification (NCTRC), an independent credentialing body. The NCTRC awards the title of certified therapeutic recreation specialist based on prescribed education and experience requirements (e.g., successful completion of recreation coursework and therapeutic recreation coursework, and a supervised internship) and successful performance on a national examination. Some states have requirements for licensure, registration, or certification as well. Credentialing is one way to ensure that a therapeutic recreation professional has met the minimum requirements needed to provide therapeutic recreation services safely.

Career Opportunities

The U.S. Department of Labor, Bureau of Labor Statistics' 1994–1995 *Occupational Outlook Handbook* estimates that there were approximately 30,000 therapeutic recreation positions in the United States in 1992. Employment can be found in a wide variety of settings, working with individuals with varying types of disabilities. Employment of recreational therapists is expected to grow faster than the average for all occupations through the year 2005 because of the anticipated expansion in long-term care, physical and psychiatric rehabilitation, and services for individuals with disabilities.

(*See also:* ART THERAPY; DANCE/MOVEMENT THERAPY; MUSIC THERAPY; WELLNESS)

RESOURCES

American Therapeutic Recreation Association (ATRA), P.O. Box 15215, Hattiesburg, MS 39404–5215

National Therapeutic Recreation Society (NTRS), 2775 S. Quincy St., Suite 300, Arlington, VA 22206–2204

Credentialing information may be obtained from: National Council for Therapeutic Recreation Certification (NCTRC), P.O. Box 479, Thiells, NY 10984–0479

BIBLIOGRAPHY

COYLE, CATHERINE P.; KINNEY, W. B.; RILEY, BOB; and SHANK, JOHN W., eds. *Benefits of Therapeutic Recreation: A Consensus View.* Washington, DC, 1991.

FELIX, ROBERT H. Preface to *Recreation in Treatment Centers.* Washington, DC, 1962.

HAUN, PAUL. *Recreation: A Medical Viewpoint.* Arlington, VA, 1964.

KRAUS, RICHARD. *Therapeutic Recreation Service: Principles and Practices,* 3rd ed. Philadelphia, 1978.

MARTIN, ALEXANDER REID. "Professional Attitudes and Practices." *Recreation and the Mentally Ill.* Washington, DC, 1958.

MENNINGER, WILLIAM C. "Recreation and Mental Health." *Recreation* 42(1948) 340–346.

O'MORROW, GERALD S., and REYNOLDS, RON P. *Therapeutic Recreation: A Helping Profession,* 3rd ed. Englewood Cliffs, NJ, 1989.

PETERSON, CAROL A., and GUNN, SCOUT L. *Therapeutic Recreation Program Design: Principles and Procedures,* 2nd ed. Englewood Cliffs, NJ, 1984.

RUSK, HOWARD. "Therapeutic Recreation." *Hospital Management* 89 (1960):35–36.

U.S. DEPARTMENT OF LABOR, BUREAU OF LABOR STATISTICS. *Occupational Outlook Handbook 1994–1995 Edition.* Washington, DC.

WOLFFE, JOSEPH B. *The Doctors and Recreation in the Medical Setting.* Raleigh, NC, 1962.

KAREN C. WENZEL

REHABILITATION

For discussion of the rehabilitation of specific disabilities, disorders, or impairments, see: ALZHEIMER'S DISEASE; AMPUTATION; ANXIETY DISORDERS; APHASIA; ARTHRITIS; AUTISM; BACK DISORDERS; BLINDNESS AND VISION DISORDERS; BLOOD DISORDERS; BURNS; CANCER REHABILITATION; CHILDHOOD DISABILITIES; CHILDHOOD PSYCHIATRIC DISORDERS; CHRONIC FATIGUE SYNDROME; COMMUNICATION DISABILITIES; CORONARY ARTERY DISEASE; DEAF-BLINDNESS; DEAFNESS AND HEARING IMPAIRMENT; DEVELOPMENTAL DISABILITIES; EATING DISORDERS; ENDOCRINE DISORDERS; GASTROINTESTINAL DISORDERS; GENETIC DISORDERS; GROWTH DISORDERS; HEAD INJURY; HUMAN IMMUNODEFICIENCY VIRUS DISEASE AND ACQUIRED IMMUNODEFICIENCY SYNDROME; KIDNEY DISORDERS; LEARNING DISABILITIES; MENTAL RETARDATION; MOOD DISORDERS; MULTIPLE DISABILITIES; MUSCULOSKELETAL DISORDERS; NEUROLOGICAL DISORDERS; ORGANIC MENTAL SYNDROMES; PAIN; PERSONALITY DISORDERS; RESPIRATORY DISEASE; SCHIZOPHRENIA; SICKLE CELL ANEMIA AND THALASSEMIA (HEMOGLOBINOPATHIES); SPINAL CORD INJURY; STROKE. *For discussion of specific rehabilitation issues and procedures, see:* ADOLESCENTS, REHABILITATION OF; ALCOHOL REHABILITATION; CANCER REHABILITATION; CORRECTIONAL REHABILITATION; DRUG REHABILITATION; EDUCATION, REHABILITATION; ENGINEERING, REHABILITATION; EVALUATION OF REHABILITATION PROGRAMS; FORENSIC REHABILITATION; FUTURE OF REHABILITATION; HOSPITAL, REHABILITATION; INTERNATIONAL REHABILITATION; NURSING, REHABILITATION; PEDIATRIC REHABILITATION; PHILOSOPHY OF REHABILITATION; PRIVATE SECTOR REHABILITATION; PSYCHIATRIC REHABILITATION; PSYCHOLOGY, REHABILITATION; REHABILITATION CENTER; REHABILITATION COUNSELING; RURAL REHABILITATION; STATE–FEDERAL REHABILITATION PROGRAM; VETERAN VOCATIONAL REHABILITATION IN THE U.S. DEPARTMENT OF VETERANS AFFAIRS; VETERANS' MEDICAL REHABILITATION IN THE U.S. DEPARTMENT OF VETERANS AFFAIRS; WOMEN IN REHABILITATION

REHABILITATION CENTER

A rehabilitation center is an organization of professional and paraprofessional staff interacting as a team in a facility designed to help people with physical and/or psychosocial disabilities to acquire the skills necessary to become functionally independent and enjoy a greater quality of life. Professional staff may include physicians, nurses, social workers, speech and language pathologists, physical therapists, occupational therapists, psychologists and rehabilitation counselors, recreation therapists, music therapists, orthotists, and prosthetists as well as a host of other supporting staff such as dieticians, dentists, vocational specialists, pastoral counselors, and rehabilitation engineers.

The rehabilitation center is an important place for clients with disabilities and their families to begin the development of functional skills that lessen the impact of disability. Another important function of the rehabilitation center is to provide education regarding disability, available community resources, and adaptive devices and leisure activities that help improve the quality of life. However, not all rehabilitation should occur in a rehabilitation center.

Successful reentry to home or the community requires gradual and supervised transition out of the rehabilitation center while progress toward greater independence is carefully monitored. The rehabilitation team must continually interact with family and client, setting and reaching toward greater functional goals and finally moving the client beyond the rehabilitation center toward a discharge goal. Integrating rehabilitation skills into a functional lifestyle can take a lifetime and begins upon discharge from the rehabilitation center.

Disability can occur as the result of an accident, illness, drug or alcohol addiction, or disease that causes physical dysfunction as well as psychiatric illnesses requiring rehabilitation. In physical rehabilitation centers, the treatment team assists the patient disabled by stroke, spinal cord injury, brain injury, or other neurological or orthopedic impairment to become as functional and independent as possible by using therapies and assistive devices. In psychiatric rehabilitation centers, therapists assist clients in overcoming emotional disabilities that have prevented them from functioning fully. Drug and alcohol rehabilitation centers provide therapy that helps clients overcome drug and alcohol dependencies and move on to productive and healthy lives.

Rehabilitation centers are guided by standards of care authorized by accreditation organizations. Physical rehabilitation, psychiatric, and drug and alcohol centers follow standards of care developed by the Commission on Accreditation of Rehabilitation Facilities (CARF) and the Joint Commission on Accreditation of Healthcare Organizations (JCAHO). In addition, state licensures may be required by a health facilities commission and department of mental health and mental retardation. Various state, federal, and advocacy organizations are available to assist rehabilitation centers respond to issues and problems. Lists of these resources are available at libraries, government offices, and at the rehabilitation centers.

States also require licensure of various professional staff. Physicians, nurses, psychologists, physical therapists, occupational therapists, social workers, and other rehabilitation professional staff must fulfill state requirements for licensure by passing professional board examinations and applying for state licensure. Professional staff may not practice legally until credentialed with the appropriate state licensure. Each state has a licensing board regulating the practice of each discipline in that state. In addition to professional licensure, many staff members also belong to national professional advocacy organizations representing their specific disciplines. These organizations offer continuing education, lobby for important discipline causes, and help regulate the discipline practice. Each state usually has a chapter of the national organization. Membership is voluntary.

Although rehabilitation centers provide an invaluable resource to persons with disabilities, some problems exist. First, there is a growing demand for rehabilitation services and an insufficient supply of resources to meet those needs. Driving the demand is a rapidly growing population of persons with disabilities. Science saves more patients from catastrophic injuries and diseases than ever before, adding thousands of surviving people with severe disabilities each year. In addition, with better education and medical management, persons with disabilities are living longer. Also adding to the numbers is an expanding definition of disability to include those functionally impaired with cancer, AIDS, and work-related injuries. Yet, as the demand grows, professional staff members and the treatment dollars do not grow proportionately.

Fewer students are entering the allied health fields, and those who do often choose a highly specialized area in a private rehabilitation practice or a private clinic practice rather than a rehabilitation center. Also, as the demand exceeds the amount of money available for services, more persons with disabilities are left untreated or undertreated. As this problem grows, ethical issues will arise around who should receive that level of rehabilitation, and ultimately who has the greatest chance of recovery.

Another problem relates to the documentation of the value of rehabilitation. Rehabilitation success is measured in the degree of functional improvement a patient makes and the costs incurred in producing that improvement. Unfortunately, there is no reliable standard measurement of improvement or outcome by diagnosis from one rehabilitation center to another and no definition of cost for producing measures of functional improvement. Payers are thus unable to determine if one rehabilitation center can provide a more efficient and effective service than another. Standard measures of improvements with known costs might produce greater competition among rehabilitation centers as well as greater efficiency and effectiveness.

Rehabilitation centers serve a vital role in assisting persons with disabilities to recover from their physical and emotional limitations, become more functionally independent, and enjoy a better quality of life. Also important are the savings in long-term costs associated with the person with a disability becoming more self-caring rather than medically dependent for a lifetime. Often the person may become employed, furthering the payback as a taxpaying citizen.

The future of the rehabilitation center and rehabilitation professionals is bright. The growing population of people with disabilities will require independence-producing services. The cost for services provided will be justified by decreases in long-term medical expense as the person with disability becomes independent and productive. These centers will become more competitive and efficient as well as provide services on an increasingly specialized basis to persons with complex and severe disabilities. Expanding opportunities will be available for work at all levels in the rehabilitation center.

(*See also:* ALLIED HEALTH PROFESSIONS; DISABILITY MANAGEMENT; FACILITIES; HOSPITAL, REHABILITATION; PSYCHOSOCIAL ADJUSTMENT; REHABILITATION COUNSELING)

RESOURCES

Commission on Accreditation Facilities (CARF), 101 N. Wilmot Road, Suite 500, Tucson, AZ 85711

Joint Commission on Accreditation of Healthcare Organizations (JCAHO), One Renaissance Blvd., Oakbrook Terrace, IL 60181

GREGORY L. THOMSEN

REHABILITATION COUNSELING

Rehabilitation counseling began to emerge as a profession in 1954 when federal funds were first allocated for training rehabilitation counselors at the master's degree level. Rehabilitation counseling is directed toward job placement and personal adjustment of persons with severe disabilities. Numerous role and function studies have been conducted to describe the nature and scope of rehabilitation counseling. Whether rehabilitation counselors work in educational, medical, correctional, or mental health settings, they involve clients in making vocational choices and coordinate plans and services to assist clients in meeting their goals.

Preparation of Rehabilitation Counselors

Rehabilitation counseling students accumulate specialized knowledge of disabilities in graduate-level coursework. The majority of programs including such coursework are located within colleges of education, while others are found in allied health or psychology departments. Several rehabilitation counseling programs are part of independent institutes that house other rehabilitation specialties. The implications for work and independent living of a wide range of physical, intellectual, and emotional disabilities are studied. The students also learn that the planning and coordination of rehabilitation services uses medical, psychological, or educational information received from other professionals.

Counseling skills are the basis for rehabilitation counseling, and students learn to interact with persons who have disabilities through practicum experiences and supervised internships. Students develop a relationship with persons who have disabilities and attempt to create opportunities for fulfilling their goals.

Knowledge of the world of work, of the laws that prohibit discrimination against persons with disabilities and provide rehabilitation services, of vocational assessment and career development is also gained through graduate study. A look at any rehabilitation counselor education curriculum accredited by the Council on Rehabilitation Education (CORE) reflects the three dimensions of rehabilitation counseling suggested by Jerome Bozarth (1981): a rehabilitation counseling professional is a therapeutic responder, a vocational diagnostician, and a community facilitator.

CORE revised its standards in 1991 to require 48 semester hours or 72 quarter hours of graduate study within seven major areas. The seven study areas include the foundations of rehabilitation counseling (history, philosophy, laws, ethics, organizational structure of rehabilitation, and societal issues); counseling services (theory and practice, multicultural and gender issues); case management (planning and coordination of independent living and vocational rehabilitation services, use of community resources, computer tools used in case management); vocational and career development (theories and occupational and labor market information); assessment (medical and psychosocial aspects of disabilities, evaluation approaches); job development and placement (employer contacts, application of appropriate technology, supported employment); and research (research design, analyses, literature). The CORE standards also call for clinical experience totaling 100 hours of supervised practicum and 600 hours of supervised internship experience in rehabilitation settings.

Procedures Used by Rehabilitation Counselors

Rehabilitation counselors involve clients in the planning of their rehabilitation programs. The counseling skills learned in their graduate preparation are the tools they use to understand the client's perspective and to form a working alliance. Clients may need to express the feelings brought on by a disability, others' responses to the disability, or environmental barriers. Clients may also need information about medical or psychological treatment or the financial implications of their treatment decisions. By providing information and respecting the views of the client and family members, the rehabilitation counselor builds a relationship of mutual trust and conjointly constructs a rehabilitation plan.

Rehabilitation counselors also discuss (with the permission of the client) the medical, psychological, and educational aspects of a client's disability with all involved parties, including physicians, psychologists, other health care professionals, and employers. Often, the rehabilitation counselor becomes a client advocate in the health care system. When the relevant information is shared by all parties, understandings can be reached, such as the physician's gaining an accurate view of the physical demands of the client's environment, or the employer's acceptance of job site modifications.

Because its roots are in public rehabilitation, the rehabilitation process has been closely tied to federal and state vocational rehabilitation policy. Changes in the Rehabilitation Act have altered the traditional rehabilitation process, which originally emphasized the proving of eligibility. Before 1993, rehabilitation counselors employed by state vocational rehabilitation agencies were required to follow a substantial process of initial interview, evaluation of rehabilitation potential, eligibility determination, development of an individually written rehabilitation plan, provision of services, job placement, and follow-up. Rehabilitation counselors employed in the private sector follow a similar process, with more emphasis on return to work in the most expedient fashion. For the private sector rehabilitation counselor, negotiation of differences among the client, employers, attorneys, claims adjusters, and physicians is an essential skill (Lynch & Beck, 1987).

The Rehabilitation Act Amendments of 1992 changed the public sector rehabilitation counselor's responsibility from one of establishing client eligibility to one of proving that an individual is incapable of benefiting from vocational rehabilitation services. All people with disabilities are presumed to have employment potential, and an extended evaluation period is required before any applicant for vocational rehabilitation services can be determined ineligible due to the severity of disability. For the vocational assessment to be valid, factors in the client's environment must be considered in the extended evaluation. Rehabilitation counselors are responsible for assembling data related to the unique strengths, resources, priorities, interests, and needs of the client as well as the provision of rehabilitation technology required for the client to perform in a work environment.

The 1992 amendments to the Rehabilitation Act also increase the control of the client or consumer in the decision-making process. Clients now write a statement that will be included in the individually written rehabilitation plan, describing their involvement in choosing among goals and services. Consumers are also policymakers, serving on state and federal advisory councils that monitor service provision and service providers. While the rehabilitation process has at its heart respect for the client, many service providers have not had the formal training in counseling and rehabilitation philosophy/ethics needed to enable them to establish reciprocal relationships with their clients. Recognition of the importance of the client's involvement in the process became a practice standard with the enactment of the 1992 amendments.

Despite the important changes contained in the 1992 amendments to the Rehabilitation Act that will affect rehabilitation counselors working in public vocational rehabilitation agencies, the orderly sequence of events that characterizes the rehabilitation process continues to shape the actions of rehabilitation counselors working in any setting. Any service that facilitates a client's movement toward employment and community integration is considered. Rehabilitation counselors, using client and family information, ask: "What will it take?" The comprehensiveness of a rehabilitation plan is clear from the scope of services that must be considered. Such services include counseling and guidance; physical and mental restoration services; vocational and training services; the payment of living expenses during the rehabilitation process; transportation; interpreter or note-taking services; reader, telecommunications, or other assistive devices; placement and postemployment services; license or permits to enter a trade or profession; and personal assistance with daily living activities.

While rehabilitation counselors do not provide all the possible services, they may evaluate, counsel for career development, develop jobs, and place and follow up clients in jobs. Increasingly, natural work settings are being used to assess work habits, physical tolerance, and social skills. The purpose of the evaluation is to identify possible alternatives. Next, the rehabilitation counselor and the client discuss local labor market information and the client's personal preferences. A plan is jointly developed that will meet the client's career and placement goals. Knowledge of community resources and skill in identifying any additional information that might affect the desired goals is useful at this stage of career and job development. The rehabilitation counselor reviews several important criteria for job placement as a job search develops: compatibility with the client's capabilities, working conditions that will not jeopardize the safety of the client or others, employment that is reasonably permanent with reasonable pay, and opportunity for advancement within a reasonable period of time (Vandergoot, 1987).

Similar procedures are used by rehabilitation counselors working with clients in the private rehabilitation sector, where clients covered by insurance compensation systems are served. Four additional areas of expertise are needed in private rehabilitation: knowledge of benefits contained in various disability insurance compensation systems, legal and insurance terminology, forensic applications, and cost containment through negotiation of fees (Matkin, 1987).

New Roles for the Rehabilitation Counselor

As rehabilitation counselors developed the knowledge and skills needed to enable them to function in state vocational rehabilitation agencies and private rehabilitation settings, changes within other human service systems increased the demand for their skills in other state agencies. Deinstitutionalization was undertaken within every state agency bearing responsibility for services to specific populations. Mental health, mental retardation, aging, corrections, and education programs adopted policies that necessitated transition experts. The skills of rehabilitation counselors in returning persons with disabilities to communities to live, work, recreate, learn, and function actively as citizens, rather than as patients or inmates, are transferable to all human-service systems.

The change in philosophy resulted in rehabilitation counselors being hired in community mental health programs, where they instituted case management and vocational programs for clients discharged from psychiatric hospitals. As large institutions for mentally retarded adults were emptied, local facilities employed rehabilitation counselors in workshops and, subsequently, in community-based vocational programs. State programs for older citizens found the case management and independent living technology developed in rehabilitation to be instrumental in supporting elders who wished to work and live in their own homes. Correctional institutions were decentralized to allow work-release and early probation programs. Schools began to emphasize the transition to work for youth with disabilities. Wherever community integration became the goal of a human service system, rehabilitation counselors were called on as experts in ascertaining client needs, mobilizing community resources, and monitoring the adjustment of clients to new circumstances.

Economic forces have also affected the job market for rehabilitation counselors. Hospitals must now compete for patients, and many institutions have increased the range of outpatient services offered to the community. Rehabilitation units have been established in general hospitals throughout the country, with rehabilitation counselors providing assessment and placement services to patients who need assistance in preserving their jobs or finding new ones.

The newest employer of rehabilitation counselors is the corporation. Disability management is an approach that emerged in the 1980s to minimize the impact of disability on the individual and the workplace and to encourage return to work for employees with disabilities. Escalating health care costs have prompted employers to control and manage health care costs through early intervention, rapid return-to-work initiatives, and case management (Schwartz et al., 1989). Rehabilitation counselors are equipped to function within corporations or as consultants to corporations interested in disability management. The Americans with Disabilities Act also created a need for rehabilitation counselors within corporations seeking to comply with employment and public access regulations.

Rehabilitation counseling, because of its breadth, can be likened to a liberal arts education at a graduate level. Graduate programs accredited by CORE prepare a generalist, although some students choose, at the time of their internship, to specialize in a setting where a specific disability group is served. The benefit of such broad training is that graduates can move literally between service systems and settings, decreasing the risk of burnout. The cost of generalist training is that the amount of material that might be included in the rehabilitation counseling curriculum increases daily, as does pressure from various constituencies for the curriculum to emphasize specific types of disabilities, service settings, or functions (Patterson, 1992).

Specialization is possible not only for specific disability groups but also for employment settings (e.g., public or private rehabilitation), job functions (e.g., vocational assessment or job placement), and counseling emphasis (e.g., marriage and family or vocational counseling). Rehabilitation counselors who work with state vocational rehabilitation agencies are typically generalists, although in some states counselors have specialized caseloads (e.g., people with visual impairment, hearing impairment, or mental illness). Rehabilitation counselors who work in community rehabilitation programs may specialize in the disability group they serve or in the function they most frequently perform (e.g., assessment, case management, job placement). Some rehabilitation counselors prefer the variety of a general caseload; others enjoy increasing their knowledge and skill to work with specific disability groups who require specialized rehabilitation technologies and counseling competencies.

Rehabilitation Counseling Credentials

The Commission on Rehabilitation Counselor Certification was created by two professional organizations in the hope of setting national standards for the profession of rehabilitation counseling. The National Rehabilitation Counseling Association and the American Rehabilitation Counseling Association established this joint commission, which began a program of rehabilitation counselor certification in 1974. The goal of initiating a credentialing procedure was to ensure quality in the practice of rehabilitation counseling (Wright, 1980). The new credential was named certified rehabilitation counselor (CRC).

Certification of rehabilitation counselors was closely tied to their formal preparation. Accreditation standards were developed during the same period when rehabilitation counselor certification emerged. The Council on Rehabilitation Education, established in 1974, consists of representatives from five associations who review the standards regularly and rule on accreditation applications submitted by rehabilitation counseling programs. By beginning the arduous process of defining educational outcomes in 1974, rehabilitation counselors pioneered standard development for all other counseling groups.

Students enrolled in a CORE-accredited program may take the certification examination when they have completed 75 percent of their coursework. They are not required to have CRC-supervised work experience if their internship was supervised by a CRC. In 1995 a master's degree was required for applicants taking the CRC exam. In 1995 approximately 13,000 persons were certified rehabilitation counselors. To maintain certification, rehabilitation counselors must participate in continuing education programs and notify the commission of their efforts.

A separate credential sometimes pursued by rehabilitation counselors is also administered by the Board of Rehabilitation Certification (BRC). The certified insurance rehabilitation specialist (CIRS) is viewed as meeting a minimum standard for service providers in the private sector. A different examination is required for CIRS, emphasizing workers' compensation legislation, transferable skill assessment, functional limitations of disability, and vocational testimony. While CRCs are eligible to take the CIRS examination, many CIRS are not eligible to take the CRC examination; for example, many nurses without counseling degrees are certified insurance rehabilitation specialists.

Other credentials in the rehabilitation field include those for certified vocational evaluator (CVE) and certified work adjustment specialist (CWAS). Individuals who have training in vocational evaluation and work adjustment and have passed the appropriate certification examination are certified in these areas. CRCs are eligible for these certifications; however, many certified vocational evaluators and certified work adjustment specialists are not eligible for the CRC examination. Vocational experts recognized by the legal system include CRCs.

Certification differs from licensure, which is the most restrictive form of occupational regulation. Certification is a national, voluntary effort to identify practitioners who meet a standard well above that required for licensure. Licensure restricts persons from practicing a specific occupation in which they do not have recognized training and experience. Counselors are licensed in most states, but while rehabilitation counseling is considered a specialty of counseling, few states license rehabilitation counselors. Each state purchases the examination of its choice to license counselors, and rehabilitation counselors completing a CORE-accredited program more than meet the requirements to take the licensure examination. In states where counselors are licensed, most rehabilitation counselors take both the state counselor licensing examination and the CRC examination.

Professional Organizations

There are three major professional rehabilitation counseling organizations: the American Rehabilitation Counseling Association (ARCA), the National Rehabilitation Counseling Association (NRCA), and Division 22 of the American Psychological Association (APA). Each of these organizations is a division of a larger professional organization, with ARCA representing professional counseling as a division of the American Counseling Association, NRCA the broader field of rehabilitation as a division of the National Rehabilitation Association, and APA rehabilitation psychologists specializing in the psychological aspects of disability. ARCA requires a master's degree in rehabilitation counseling for membership; NRCA includes persons with bachelor's degrees and work experience; and APA requires a doctorate in psychology for full membership but accepts associate members with master's degrees. Each professional rehabilitation counseling organization publishes a journal as does its parent organization (i.e., the American Counseling Association publishes the *Journal of Counseling and Development;* the American Rehabilitation Counseling Association publishes the *Rehabilitation Counseling Bulletin;* the National Rehabilitation Association publishes the *Journal of Rehabilitation;* the National Rehabilitation Counseling Association publishes the *Journal of Applied Rehabilitation Counseling;* the American

Psychological Association publishes the *American Psychologist*; and Division 22 of the APA publishes *Rehabilitation Psychology*).

Other professional organizations also attract rehabilitation counselors who have specific interests and work settings. The Vocational Evaluation and Work Adjustment Association (VEWAA) concentrates on the vocational aspects of rehabilitation, and the National Association of Rehabilitation Professionals in the Private Sector (NARPPS) addresses the professional needs of rehabilitation counselors working in the private sector.

The variety of specialization within rehabilitation counseling is evidenced by the professional memberships that many rehabilitation counselors also enjoy. Many rehabilitation counselors who work primarily with persons who are physically disabled join the American Academy of Physical Medicine and Rehabilitation and receive their publication, *Archives of Physical Medicine and Rehabilitation*. Rehabilitation counselors specializing in psychiatric rehabilitation join the International Association of Psychosocial Rehabilitation Services, which publishes the *Psychosocial Rehabilitation Journal*. Rehabilitation counselors who are interested in the sociological aspects of rehabilitation join the Society for Disability Studies and receive the *Disability Studies Quarterly*. Each major disability category (e.g., hearing impairment, visual impairment, head injury) has an established organization for professionals and consumers, and many rehabilitation counselors are also members of these groups and read their literature.

(*See also:* ADVOCACY; CAREER DEVELOPMENT; CONSUMERS; DISABILITY LAW AND SOCIAL POLICY; DISABILITY MANAGEMENT; FORENSIC REHABILITATION; HISTORY OF REHABILITATION; JOB PLACEMENT; PHILOSOPHY OF REHABILITATION; PRIVATE SECTOR REHABILITATION; PSYCHOSOCIAL ADJUSTMENT; STATE–FEDERAL REHABILITATION PROGRAM; VOCATIONAL EVALUATION; WORK)

RESOURCES

American Psychological Association, 750 First St., NE, Washington, DC 20002–4242

American Rehabilitation Counseling Association, 5999 Stevenson Ave., Alexandria, VA 22304–3300

National Rehabilitation Counseling Association, 633 South Washington St., Alexandria, VA 22314

BIBLIOGRAPHY

BOZARTH, JEROME. "Philosophy and Ethics in Rehabilitation Counseling." In *Rehabilitation Counseling*, eds. Randall Parker and Carl Hansen. Boston, 1981.

COUNCIL ON REHABILITATION EDUCATION. *Accreditation Manual for Rehabilitation Counselor Education Programs.* Champaign, IL, 1991.

LYNCH, ROSS, and BECK, RUTH. "Rehabilitation Counseling in the Private Sector." In *Rehabilitation Counseling: Basics and Beyond,* ed. Randall Parker. Austin, TX, 1987.

MATKIN, R. "Private Sector Rehabilitation." In *Foundations of the Vocational Rehabilitation Process,* eds. Stanford Rubin and Richard Roessler. Austin, TX, 1987.

PATTERSON, JEANNE. "Graduate Level Preparation of Rehabilitation Counselors." In *Journal of Vocational Rehabilitation* 2, pp. 28–34, eds. Paul Wehman, Susan Hasazi, and Martha Walker. Stoneham, MA, 1992.

SCHWARTZ, GAIL; WATSON, SARA; GALVIN, DONALD; and LIPOFF, ELISE. *The Disability Management Sourcebook.* Washington, DC, 1989.

VANDERGOOT, DAVID. "Placement and Career Development in Rehabilitation." In *Rehabilitation Counseling: Basics and Beyond,* ed. Randall Parker. Austin, TX, 1987.

WRIGHT, GEORGE. *Total Rehabilitation.* Boston, 1980.

MARTHA LENTZ WALKER

REHABILITATION EDUCATION

Rehabilitation education refers to the education and training of service providers involved in the vocational rehabilitation of individuals who are unable to work or live independently because of physical, mental, or emotional disabilities. Specific service providers include rehabilitation counselors, rehabilitation administrators, vocational evaluators, supported employment specialists, job placement specialists, and independent living specialists.

There are several different levels and types of rehabilitation education programs. These include preservice rehabilitation education programs in universities at the undergraduate, master's degree, and doctoral levels; in-service programs, usually associated with universities or state rehabilitation agencies; university-associated continuing education programs; and programs at university-affiliated rehabilitation research and training centers.

While undergraduate degree programs in rehabilitation services prepare individuals for technical positions in the field, the master's degree is the professional practitioner's degree, and the doctoral degree is obtained by individuals, usually with experience in the field of vocational rehabilitation, for the purpose of entering rehabilitation education, research, or administration.

Philosophy, Historical Development, and Theories/Models

Rehabilitation education programs are based on three basic philosophical principles of learning. The first principle emphasizes the importance of experiential learning. Rehabilitation education is a combination of theoretical classroom learning and practical application of theory through class projects, field placement, and internship experiences. The second principle is that rehabilitation education prepares the student to enter a career as a professional. The third principle stresses the importance of rehabilitation education's contribution to the emergence of the vocational rehabilitation professions by using research to develop a unique body of knowledge for them.

Vocational rehabilitation programs for civilians in the United States date back to the early 1920s. The 1920 Rehabilitation Act instituted a state/federal program to provide services to persons who were physically disabled but did not include funds to train the service providers (Scalia & Wolfe, 1986). Early service providers, called rehabilitation agents, were mostly individuals with bachelor's degrees with experience in education or in placing workers with disabilities in employment (Emener, 1986; Luck & Rothrock, 1984; Obermann, 1965). Only a few service providers had master's degrees, and they were primarily in guidance and counseling from schools of education (Luck & Rothrock, 1984).

During these early years, rehabilitation education was left primarily up to the state boards and departments of education in which the vocational rehabilitation programs were located (Cull & Hardy, 1972). The amendments to the Vocational Rehabilitation Act of 1943 included the authorization for

state agency administrators to train or pay for the training of personnel (Scalia & Wolfe, 1986). In the early 1940s short-term training and workshops for rehabilitation personnel were developed and offered through university extension divisions for new as well as experienced staff (Cull & Hardy, 1972). The first universities to establish and develop programs for the education of rehabilitation counselors were New York University in 1941, Ohio State in 1944, and Wayne State in 1946 (Cull & Hardy, 1972; Obermann, 1965). By 1948 the federal Office of Vocational Rehabilitation had assisted eight universities in establishing programs for the education and training of rehabilitation counselors (Obermann, 1965). Since there were no rehabilitation counselors educated at the doctoral level, the faculties of these early programs came from the fields of education, social work, special education, and psychology, and they naturally brought with them the perspectives and approaches of those disciplines.

The 1954 amendments to the Vocational Rehabilitation Act gave great impetus to the development of rehabilitation education. The amendments made available federal monies for the development of training for physicians, nurses, occupational therapists, physical therapists, and rehabilitation counselors through the awarding of training grants to universities (Scalia & Wolfe, 1986). By 1955, ninety-one universities had received grants to broaden their curricula to include rehabilitation, and by 1956, twenty-five universities had developed rehabilitation counselor education programs utilizing federal grant monies (Emener, 1986; Scalia & Wolfe, 1986).

In the years that have elapsed since the passage of the 1954 amendments, federal monies made available through the training grant program have made possible the development of university-based programs for vocational rehabilitation disciplines in addition to those for rehabilitation counseling generalists. These programs include vocational evaluators, rehabilitation administrators, supported employment specialists, independent living specialists, and job placement specialists; specialists to meet the needs of specific populations with disabilities, such as persons who are hearing-impaired (rehabilitation counselors, interpreters), persons who are visually impaired (rehabilitation counselors, mobility training specialists, teacher-counselors), and persons with severe disabilities (rehabilitation counselors, independent living specialists, rehabilitation engineers); personnel to fill staff positions in expanding work settings (rehabilitation facilities and centers); and programs to meet the need for research and continuing education (rehabilitation research and training centers, regional rehabilitation continuing education programs).

The first undergraduate program in rehabilitation services was established in the early 1960s at Pennsylvania State University, and doctoral degrees were first awarded in 1944 by New York University (Emener, 1986). By 1977–1978 there were university programs in the following areas funded in part through the federal Rehabilitation Services Administration: eight in rehabilitation of persons who are visually impaired, fifteen in regional rehabilitation continuing education, eighty in rehabilitation counseling, six in rehabilitation of persons who are hearing-impaired, sixteen in rehabilitation administration (eleven in workshop administration and five in vocational evaluation), thirty in undergraduate education in rehabilitation services, and twenty in doctoral programs (Bitter, 1979). The number of training programs at the masters level has remained relatively constant at eighty while the number of doctoral programs has increased to thirty in 1992 (Maki & Berven, 1992; National Council on Rehabilitation Education, 1992).

Two additional developments have had a considerable impact on rehabilitation education. The first was the expansion of private practice opportunities for rehabilitation professionals in the 1970s through workers' compensation rehabilitation programs and forensic rehabilitation in personal injury, Social Security disability/Supplemental Security Income hearings, and so on. This change has led to the modification of rehabilitation education curricula, especially preservice, to prepare students for these opportunities. A second major development was the publication of the journal *Rehabilitation Education* by the National Council on Rehabilitation Education (NCRE) in 1987. This publication provides a forum for specific contributions to the body of knowledge related to rehabilitation education and also furthers the professional status of vocational rehabilitation service providers and educators.

The model for the delivery of rehabilitation education is a university-based combination of theoretical and practical experiences preparing the student to enter a profession. This model is most clearly seen in the master's degree in rehabilitation counseling, which has a curriculum of two academic years consisting of a minimum of forty-eight semester hours or seventy-two quarter hours including courses in the foundations of rehabilitation counseling; counseling services; case management; vocational and career development; assessment; job development and placement, and research; and clinical experiences in the form of practicum and internship (*Council on Rehabilitation Education,* 1991).

Major Professional, Governmental, and Other Significant Organizations

In the years immediately following the passage of the 1954 amendments to the Vocational Rehabilitation Act, a series of meetings was held between coordinators of rehabilitation education programs and representatives of the Office of Vocational Rehabilitation (now the Rehabilitation Services Administration), the governmental organization administering the training grant program (Miller, 1980). Attending these meetings were representatives of the Committee on Training of the Council of State Administrators of Vocational Rehabilitation (CSAVR). These interactions led to the formation of the Joint Liaison Committee in 1962 (Miller, 1980). The termination of the Joint Liaison Committee in 1967, primarily for financial reasons, led to the formation of the Council of Rehabilitation Counselor Education (CRCE). CRCE continued to serve as a vehicle for rehabilitation educators to formulate ideas for improvement of rehabilitation counselor education (Johnson, 1980) until 1976, when the organization's name was changed to the National Council on Rehabilitation Education (NCRE), and membership was broadened to include all rehabilitation educators and researchers. The NCRE's *1992–93 Membership Directory* (1992) lists seventy-seven university/institutional members and thirty-four undergraduate degree programs, sixty-nine master's degree programs, twenty-five doctoral degree programs, three rehabilitation research and training centers, and nine regional rehabilitation continuing education programs.

As the professional association for rehabilitation educators, NCRE has a partnership with the Rehabilitation Services Administration (RSA) and the CSAVR at the federal level. For several years these three groups have cosponsored a national education conference for the evaluation and discussion of mutual concerns. NCRE was a founding member of the Foundation for Rehabilitation Education and Research, which includes the Commission of Rehabilitation Counselor Certification (CRCC), the Certification of Insurance Rehabilitation Specialist Commission (CIRSC), and the Commission on Certification of Work Adjustment and Vocational Evaluation Specialists (CCWAVES), organizations that graduates of rehabilitation education programs apply to for national certification. NCRE was also instrumental in the founding of the Council on Rehabilitation Education (CORE), which has been the accrediting body for rehabilitation counselor education programs since 1974. NCRE continues to have a close relationship with professional organizations for rehabilitation counselors and other rehabilitation professionals, such as the American Rehabilitation Counseling Association (ARCA), the National Rehabilitation Counseling Association (NRCA), the National Association for Rehabilitation Professionals in the Private Sector (NARPPS), the Vocational Evaluation and Work Adjustment Association (VEWAA), and Division 22 (Rehabilitation Psychology) of the American Psychological Association. All of these professional organizations include rehabilitation educators as active members and officers.

Significant Issues and Concerns

Several issues and concerns that developed during the early days of rehabilitation education and more recently continue to be debated and discussed. Among these is the concern regarding for whom rehabilitation education programs are providing graduates—public or private delivery systems. The history of rehabilitation education is closely related to the development of the state/federal vocational rehabilitation system in the United States. For many years, the major employer of rehabilitation educa-

tion graduates was state vocational rehabilitation agencies. A large number of the university programs offering graduate education at the master's level in rehabilitation counseling and other disciplines were started with training grant funds from the Rehabilitation Services Administration. Stipend awards to students under the RSA training grants include a payback clause if the recipient has not been employed after ten years in a state vocational rehabilitation agency or related agency as defined by the grant regulations. The problem is that state vocational rehabilitation agencies, because of a scarcity of rehabilitation counselors with master's degrees or because of state personnel board regulations, financial concerns, or a feeling that master's-educated counselors do not perform as well as nonmaster's-level personnel, have tended not to hire graduates of rehabilitation education programs. In many states, large numbers of rehabilitation education graduates have gone to work for private, for-profit vocational rehabilitation firms. Rehabilitation education programs have the sometimes difficult task of preparing graduates on a broad basis for employment in a number of different work settings serving a diverse group of employers.

The 1992 amendments to the Rehabilitation Act contain a definition of qualified personnel requiring that state vocational rehabilitation agencies establish procedures for hiring individuals who meet state or national certification, registry, or licensure standards applicable to that discipline. This means that state agencies will need to hire counselors who meet the standards of certified rehabilitation counselors. Certification requirements include a master's degree in rehabilitation counseling or a closely related area. As a result, rehabilitation education programs will be called on to produce more graduates than ever before to meet state agency needs.

The role of the counselor has been debated in rehabilitation education since the beginning of the public vocational rehabilitation program. Does the rehabilitation counselor function as a counselor or coordinator, generalist or specialist? Are rehabilitation personnel best prepared at the undergraduate or graduate level? Does the person with a disability receive better services from an individual who has a disability (a peer counselor), or are education and training sufficient to enable the counselor to be sensitive to and able to meet the vocational needs of clients and consumers? These questions continue to be discussed and debated.

Another issue that rehabilitation education programs face is the task of keeping the curricula both current and manageable. Rehabilitation education programs, through grant application emphases, accreditation requirements, and a desire to offer the most up-to-date curriculum, have had to add courses and emphases to programs while maintaining core preparation courses and keeping the length, requirements, and number of units within reason. This delicate balance has led to much discussion and differing points of view over the years.

The Future of Rehabilitation Education

As has been indicated by a review of the history of rehabilitation education, much has been accomplished since it began in the 1940s. Although the issues and concerns mentioned above need to be addressed, several trends make the future of rehabilitation education look promising overall.

Advances in technology both in terms of assistive devices for persons with disabilities and in the areas of education and learning will need to be assimilated into rehabilitation education programs so that they can produce personnel qualified to assist clients in accessing this new technology and reach students who would otherwise be deprived of the opportunity for professional education. The use of distance-learning technology (satellite television transmission), computer-based learning, computer-assisted instruction, and interactive television marks the beginning of an explosion in new technologies. Rehabilitation education programs will have to update facilities and faculty skills to be able to take advantage of these advances.

Since the late 1960s clients/consumers with disabilities have become increasingly vocal and involved in seeing that their rehabilitation and community-accessibility needs are met. The 1990 Americans with Disabilities Act has given great impetus to the integration of persons with disabilities into American society. This activism and involvement has appropriately been extended into rehabilitation education as well. Universities will need to increase the opportunities for input and active involvement in the education process by the individuals whom the vocational rehabilitation delivery systems, both public and private, are designed to serve.

Finally, there is a distinct trend toward individual states passing licensing laws for counselors. Many of these laws cover rehabilitation counselors. Rehabilitation education programs and rehabilitation educators will need to become more active within the professional organizations that are developing these laws. This effort will ensure that their graduates will be able to meet requirements to practice that reflect the educational goals and processes already in place for rehabilitation personnel in both the public and private vocational rehabilitation delivery systems.

(*See also:* CREDENTIALS; HISTORY OF REHABILITATION; REHABILITATION COUNSELING)

RESOURCES

American Rehabilitation Counseling Association (ARCA), 5999 Stevenson Ave., Alexandria, VA 22304–3300

Certified Insurance Rehabilitation Specialists Commission (CIRSC), 1835 Rohlwing Rd, Suite E, Rolling Meadows, IL 60008

Council on Rehabilitation Education Inc., 1835 Rohlwing Rd, Suite E, Rolling Meadows, IL 60008

Commission on Certification of Work Adjustment and Vocational Evaluation Specialists (CCWAVES), 7910 Woodmont Ave., Suite 1430, Bethesda, MD 20814–3015

Commission on Rehabilitation Counselor Certification (CRCC), 1835 Rohlwing Rd, Suite E, Rolling Meadows, IL 60008

Council of State Administrators of Vocational Rehabilitation (CSAVR), P.O. Box 3776, Washington, DC 20007

Division 22 Rehabilitation Psychology, American Psychological Association, 750 First St., NE, Washington, DC 20002–4242

Foundation for Rehabilitation Education and Research, 1835 Rohlwing Rd, Suite E, Rolling Meadows, IL 60008

National Association of Rehabilitation Professionals in the Private Sector (NARPPS), 313 Washington St., Suite 302, Newton, MA 02158

National Council on Rehabilitation Education (NCRE), Administrative Services Office, Department of Special Education, Utah State University, Logan, UT 84322–2870

National Rehabilitation Counseling Association (NRCA), 8807 Sudley Rd, Suite 102, Manassas, VA 22110–4719

Rehabilitation Education, Elliott & Fitzpatrick, Inc., 1135 Cedar Shoals Drive, Athens, GA 30605

Rehabilitation Services Administration, United States Department of Education, Office of Special Education and Rehabilitation Services, 400 Maryland Ave., SW, Washington, DC 20202

Vocational Evaluation and Work Adjustment Association (VEWAA), 202 East Cheyenne Mountain Blvd., Colorado Springs, CO 80906

BIBLIOGRAPHY

BITTER, JAMES A. *Introduction to Rehabilitation*. St. Louis, 1979.

COUNCIL ON REHABILITATION EDUCATION. *Accreditation Manual for Rehabilitation Counselor Education Programs*, Champaign, IL, 1991.

CULL, JOHN G., and HARDY, RICHARD E. *Vocational Rehabilitation: Profession and Process*. Springfield, IL, 1972.

EMENER, WILLIAM G., ed. *Rehabilitation Counselor Preparation and Development: Selected Critical Issues*. Springfield, IL, 1986.

EMENER, WILLIAM G.; PATRICK, ADELE; and HOLLINGSWORTH, DAVID K., eds. *Critical Issues in Rehabilitation Counseling*. Springfield, IL, 1984.

JOHNSON, BOB. "CRCE—Its Development." In *The History of the National Council on Rehabilitation Education*, ed. Joseph A. Szuhay. Washington, DC, 1980.

LUCK, RICHARD S., and ROTHROCK, JAMES A. "The Education and Training of Rehabilitation Counselors." In *Critical Issues in Rehabilitation Counseling*, eds. William G. Emener, Adele Patrick, and David K. Hollingsworth. Springfield, IL, 1984.

MAKI, DENNIS R., and BERVEN, NORMAN L. *Directory of Doctoral Study in Rehabilitation*. Washington, DC, 1992.

MILLER, GREGORY A. "Early Years." In *The History of the National Council on Rehabilitation Education*, ed. Joseph A. Szuhay. Washington, DC, 1980.

NATIONAL COUNCIL ON REHABILITATION EDUCATION 1992–93 MEMBERSHIP DIRECTORY. Logan, UT, 1992.

OBERMANN, C. ESCO. *A History of Vocational Rehabilitation in America*. Minneapolis, 1965.

RIGGAR, T. F.; MAKI, DENNIS R.; and WOLF, ARNOLD W., eds. *Applied Rehabilitation Counseling*. New York, 1986.

SCALIA, VINCENT A., and WOLFE, RICHARD C. "Rehabilitation Counselor Education." In *Applied Rehabilitation Counseling*, eds. T. F. Riggar, Dennis R. Maki, and Arnold W. Wolf. New York, 1986.

E. W. (BUD) STUDE

REHABILITATION RESEARCH

See RESEARCH

RELIGION

Religion has not traditionally played a clearly defined role in meeting the needs of people with disabilities. This situation has been created by a variety of contributing factors: (1) The occurrence of disability and the need for rehabilitation have long been considered the concerns of health professionals, and the contribution of spiritual support has gone largely unrecognized; and (2) a large number of religions in the United States and Europe are based on Judeo-Christian traditions, which have been influenced by ancient perspectives of disability as sin, weakness, punishment, and a means of purification; such traditions have contributed to religion's confusion about the place of those with disabilities in the theology and practice of spirituality. This confusion is reflected in the education and training of religious professionals and in the attitudes of both professionals and laypeople toward persons with disabilities.

Fear of those who are different has hindered acceptance and inclusion of persons with disabilities as equal participants in religious observance. Persons with disabilities may be seen as threats to others, capable of "infecting," or unable to practice self-care and therefore "dirty." The ability of persons with disabilities to contribute to their religion and society has been widely held to be minimal or nonexistent.

Chaplain service began to encompass persons with disabilities and to move into rehabilitation facilities after World War II. It was then and has continued to be primarily a service of temporary intervention, available most often as long as the individual is a patient in a medical facility. A great many of these facilities have a small chaplaincy staff to serve a large community and do not require special training for work among persons with disabilities. Once released from a hospital or rehabilitation center, the person with a disability cannot automatically expect the attentions of a chaplain. Such services may have been inadequate for the needs of people with disabilities, and if the family's religious adviser is called on, the inadequacy is likely to continue unless the person has been educated in specialized ministries. The introduction and passage of the Americans with Disabilities Act (ADA) in 1990 did much to arouse the conscience and awareness of both religion and society. There has been an incomplete but still dramatic movement toward changing attitudes and improving architectural accessibility, and the effects of this movement may be expected to increase inclusion for persons with disabilities in the full participation of their religion. Perhaps its greatest impact in religious circles has been an understanding of religion's almost purely theoretical involvement in disability and rehabilitation. That relationship is being recognized as one in which talk must generate movement into a defined role and direction.

Religion's role in disability and rehabilitation will always depend to some extent on the beliefs of the individual religion. Its basic purpose, however, is guidance toward spiritual growth in a way that encourages acceptance and adjustment. If religion is to perform its role successfully and in meaningful ways, certain changes will be necessary: Expanded education and training for religious professionals in disability and rehabilitation issues is vital; no less important to a competent ministry is the education of laypeople toward greater understanding and acceptance of persons with disabilities; religious professionals will want to seek out and accept greater participation in the processes of recovery and rehabilitation from the initial time of illness/injury and disability; and the availability of religion's ministry will need to be reassessed and altered to meet the needs of different types of people.

A structured, informed ministry to persons with disabilities often involves clergy, laypeople, religious counselors, and other religious professionals in pro-viding multifaceted care. As is true in other types of ministries, the problems faced by persons with disabilities are not always visible and may have no simple solutions. The role of religion in these instances is first to incorporate awareness of disability lifestyles into flexible programs of care that can address lifestyle adjustments and problems effectively. The most effective of such ministries approach the individual holistically, as a person in need of several kinds of support. The professionals in these ministries understand the importance of communication with other caregivers who are concerned about quality of life issues. Religious professionals who can see the levels of effort involved in recovery and rehabilitation are able to bring religion into that experience as a spiritual and life-affirming ally. The ministry that is not prepared to face the reactions to loss of mobility, financial security, social acceptance, job, and perhaps even family is destined to fail the people it seeks to serve.

A number of needs assert themselves when a person with a disability faces reentry into the community, and regardless of when these needs become apparent, their resolution will call for the kind of strength and determination a spiritual perspective can provide. A need for the support of caring people is primary. Religious professionals can help provide spiritual, emotional, and psychological support by accepting the anger, depression, disbelief, and denial as natural and necessary reactions to disability and loss. There is strength and comfort to be gained in understanding divine acceptance on an equal basis for all humanity, and the religious counselor who can give support to another through times of doubt and crises of faith also serves as an example of that acceptance.

Religious professionals can also offer opportunities for self-discovery that contribute to serenity. Disability brings with it time for reflection and meditation, as a rule. The pastor's weekly visit or the counselor's hour of therapy can be times of guidance in discovering what is in the self—beliefs, fears, courage, despair, hope, rage, all valid human responses and all in need of exploration if the person with a disability is to rebuild a life of quality, empowerment, and independence. It is admittedly difficult for religious people to stand fast in the face of negative reactions to their faith, but professionals can comprehend and probably empathize: Most of the people in the world doubt divine goodness in times of loss and pain. At the very least, they wonder why they have been "chosen" to suffer. The professional's role is not that of judge but helper and guide into the self, where the ability to make changes and the faith in divine love exist. Discovering what one has been, and why, can inspire the incentive to live life differently, with greater purpose and meaning.

Another part of religion's role in serving persons with disabilities is helping to find meaning in an altered lifestyle. The tendency, after all, to feel dependent is common after disability, even among those who regain mobility, independence, and vocational skills through rehabilitation. If the religious contacts in the life of a person with a disability can encourage that person to see the Divine in their being and all of life, an empowerment to find meaning in life, no matter how able or disabled, can follow. Rather than searching for an explanation for disability, the person who has experienced a loss can feel a greater power, sustaining life for a purpose, and can search for that purpose. Biblical accounts of imperfect people serving the Supreme Being—Paul with his "thorn in the flesh" and Moses's lack of fluency, sometimes assumed to be a speech impediment—exist and show the believer the Divine's ability to use all life in positive, constructive ways.

Perhaps the greatest part religion can play in disability and rehabilitation is the twofold role of achieving acceptance and acquiring positive coping skills. "Acceptance" in this context refers to the individual's willingness to accept disability as part of the lifestyle and to use emotional energy to make the required adjustments so life still can be meaningful and have purpose. Acceptance depends on a strong external support system—family, clergy, health professionals, friends—and internal strength; it does not take place in an atmosphere of pity, dependence, rejection, self-absorption, or denial. It thrives in an atmosphere of growth where independence, empowerment, involvement, and communication are encouraged. Religious professionals can be instrumental in teaching these values from a spiritual perspective. Religion's contributions to positive coping are humane, caring, respectful philosophies that em-

phasize the value of life, harmony, and peace. Persons with disabilities may forget to live by the Golden Rule, just as people without disabilities do. Religion can teach persons with and without disabilities to cope in positive ways that express respect and regard for life. It cannot give the individual skills for coping with every situation, but the serenity and perspective of religious faith encourage introspective rational thought and action.

Religion's role in advocacy for persons with disabilities also has more than one dimension. An inclusive ministry advocates accessibility, opportunity, and acceptance, contributing to a more open world for those who have traditionally been excluded. This type of advocacy often sensitizes religious people to another issue of disability: survival of the family. Nowhere is advocacy needed more. Families having members with disabilities separate at least as often as they remain together, in part because of the demands generated by the disability and the lack of help available to families. Only limited resources exist to assist families experiencing financial and personal chaos caused by the enormous demands of disability, and families who need but cannot afford professional counseling services usually have no choice but to seek out their clergy. Religious professionals whose ministry has made a commitment to advocacy will recognize the right of each family to survive intact in a society often inclined to view the person with a disability as a burden. In this context the religious professional may be the only supporter of family adjustment and cohesion. Again, it is through religious as well as other values that people come to respect the rights and potential of each human life.

The future of religion in disability and rehabilitation is potentially one of increased involvement and advocacy. Religion has not always been in the forefront of the movement toward equality, accessibility, and acceptance, but its philosophies of love and harmony certainly embrace those concepts, and the extent of its role in the future rests primarily on the willingness of its people to commit themselves. Many of the major religions have established internal groups whose purpose is closer to advocacy than the traditional charity, and these groups can serve to enlighten and educate their respective religions into greater activity. In some instances these religions have sought to encourage their members in advocacy by sponsoring financial programs to increase accessibility, or by ecumenical conferences addressing inclusion.

The needs of those who have disabilities are, or should be, a basic issue for religion, just as poverty is—an issue of compassion that has existed for centuries and will most likely continue to exist, one that demands the interest and involvement of caring people if change is to occur. The future of religious ministries to persons with disabilities can be one that helps to improve the quality of life as it provides an example of concern and inclusion. This and much more are possible if the apathy and biases of religious people can be resolved.

The equal-access and antidiscrimination provisions of the ADA do not extend into the religious sector. The religious community's willingness to observe those provisions, even though not required to do so, will help to establish its leadership role in the future. A commitment to accepting and including persons with disabilities is vital to that role; as the commitment is made, the role will begin to take on enhanced structure and definition, and the contributions of the religious community will be expanded.

Religion is likely to find its contributions are needed (1) from the onset of disease/disability, (2) in an organized and consistent manner, and (3) in ways that enhance quality of life and promote awareness. A commitment to a ministry for persons with disabilities should recognize the value of having competent spiritual healers attending the individual as soon as possible. The person who is affected by illness or injury is usually given immediate medical care; little consideration is given, ordinarily, to the restorative powers of the spirit in such a scenario, and so it may be weeks or months before a religious professional is asked to help. That help, coming late in the process of recovery, may then be sporadic and limited, when the need is for regular, ongoing sessions of spiritual guidance. If the religious professional cannot then open the way for the type of introspection, self-awareness, and values assessment so important to acceptance and adjustment, the opportunity for improved quality of life may be lost or delayed. A religious counselor may be the only source of hope for a person with a disability and the only professional trusted by both the individual and the family to help in rebuilding life outside the caring facility; in many cases, he or she is the only professional who makes house calls, has the opportunity to help maintain the individual's place within the religious community, and can expect a long-term relationship with the person with a disability and the family. Yet the religious professional has been and is still a widely untapped resource for assisting those with disabilities.

The role of religion, then, already exists; one might say it has always existed. It waits only for more well-trained professionals, well-organized and adequately funded programs, and a commitment to acceptance and inclusion of persons with disabilities as equal participants in a divine plan. Its future involvement in the lives of people with disabilities has extraordinary potential.

(See also: ADVOCACY; ATTITUDES; DISABILITY; ETHICS; FAMILY; LOSS AND GRIEF; PHILOSOPHY OF REHABILITATION; PSYCHOSOCIAL ADJUSTMENT; QUALITY OF LIFE; RESPITE CARE)

BIBLIOGRAPHY

BLAIR, WILLIAM A., and DAVIDSON, DANA. "Pastoral Interventions with the Newly Diagnosed Multiple Sclerosis Person." *Journal of Pastoral Counseling* (Winter 1990):135–144.

———. "Accepting and Including the Handicapped." *Alert* (November 1991):2–4.

COOPER, BURTON Z. *Why, God?* Atlanta, 1988.

COX-GEDMARK, JAN. *Coping with Physical Disability.* Philadelphia, 1980.

GAEBELEIN, FRANK E., gen. ed. *The Expositor's Bible Commentary.* Grand Rapids, MI, 1979.

JUNG, CARL G. *Modern Man in Search of a Soul.* New York, 1933.

KUSHNER, HAROLD S. *When Bad Things Happen to Good People.* New York, 1981.

LAYMON, CHARLES M., ed. *The Interpreter's One-Volume Commentary on the Bible.* Nashville, TN, 1971.

LEWIS, CLIVE S. *Surprised by Joy.* London, England, 1955.

LOCKE, STEVEN, and COLLIGAN, DOUGLAS. *The Healer Within.* New York, 1986.

WILKE, HAROLD. *Strengthened with Might.* Philadelphia, 1952.

WRIGHT, BEATRICE A. "Changes in Attitudes Toward People with Handicaps." *Rehabilitation Literature* 34 (1973):354–357.

————. *Physical Disability: A Psychosocial Approach.*
New York, 1983.

WILLIAM BLAIR
DANA DAVIDSON

REPETITIVE MOTION DISORDERS

See ARTHRITIS; DISABILITY MANAGEMENT; ERGONOM-
ICS; MUSCULOSKELETAL DISORDERS

RESEARCH

As of 1995 there were approximately 48 million
Americans with disabilities. These disabilities include physical, psychiatric, and developmental disabilities and combinations thereof. Determination
of the effects of disabilities on human functioning
and the amelioration of these effects are the primary
focus of rehabilitation research. Some effects of disabilities on human functioning are due to the nature
of the disability itself; other effects are due to societal responses to persons with disabilities. These effects result in barriers to full participation in the
mainstream of life. Through rehabilitation research,
methods are discovered that improve the capacity
and opportunity for persons with disabilities to live,
learn, work, and recreate within the scope of their
personal needs and desires. A question posed by the
eminent researcher Gordon Paul summarizes the
concerns of rehabilitation research: "What treatment, by whom, is most effective for this individual,
with that specific problem, under which set of circumstances?" (Paul, 1967).

A unique characteristic of the field of rehabilitation research is its multidisciplinary nature. Rehabilitation research encompasses contributions from
medicine, bioengineering, psychology, and social
policy as well as other disciplines concerned with
human functioning. As such, rehabilitation researchers come from a wide variety of backgrounds
and experience.

The Rehabilitation Research Community

The rehabilitation research community consists of
organizations and individuals from both the public
and private sectors. In the public sector, the National Institute of Disability and Rehabilitation Research (NIDRR) in Washington, DC, coordinates
rehabilitation research efforts across the country.
Among its many responsibilities, NIDRR oversees a
network of more than forty rehabilitation research
and training centers (RRTC). The purpose of these
RRTCs is to conduct research to improve rehabilitation methodology and service delivery systems
and to promote the utilization of research findings
through dissemination and training activities. Each
center focuses on a core area of research and related
training. Examples of these core areas include spinal
cord injury, aging, children's mental health, traumatic brain injury, improving supported employment
outcomes for individuals with disabilities, and improving the management of rehabilitation information systems. NIDRR also oversees rehabilitation
engineering centers throughout the country. These
centers focus on technology development and application of engineering principles to problems of
disability. Additionally, NIDRR coordinates the
work of numerous principal investigators who have
received grants for disability-related research projects
such as research and demonstration projects, field-
initiated research projects, research training
projects, and research utilization projects.

Although NIDRR is a prominent presence in the
national rehabilitation research effort, it is by no
means the only national agency involved. For example, Public Law 101-613, National Institutes of
Health amendments of 1990, established the National Center for Medical Rehabilitation Research.
This center focuses on research concerning the rehabilitation of persons with physical disabilities
resulting from diseases of the neurological, musculoskeletal, cardiovascular, pulmonary, or other physiological systems and has a particular orientation
toward research on orthotic and prosthetic devices.

There is a substantial commitment at the federal
level for support of rehabilitation research. In addition to the above-mentioned agencies, rehabilitation-related research is supported at approximately
thirteen institutes of the National Institutes of
Health in addition to programs in the Department of
Health and Human Services, the Department of Education, and the Rehabilitation Services Administration. An important source of information on
rehabilitation research funding opportunities is the

NIH Guide for Grants and Contracts, published by the National Institutes of Health.

In addition to public sector effort in rehabilitation research, numerous national and local private foundations provide support. Examples of these foundations include the Robert Wood Johnson Foundation, the MacArthur Foundation, the Easter Seal Research Foundation, the American Heart Association, and the Foundation of Physical Therapy, among others.

Contributors to rehabilitation research come from a wide variety of settings. Universities, rehabilitation and other hospitals, and public and private human service agencies and programs have individuals who are interested and active in disability-related research. Some individuals conduct research funded by grants from national, state, or local organizations. Others rely on their own resources.

Rehabilitation Research Projects

Historically, rehabilitation research has been practice-driven. Ideas for projects come from the need to find practical solutions to problems caused by the disabling effects of certain physical and mental conditions. The underlying orientation of the field of rehabilitation research is to focus on factors that contribute to successful rehabilitation outcomes. These factors include practitioner-related variables such as practitioner skill, technological variables such as improved adaptive equipment, and process-related variables such as improved physical, vocational, and psychosocial assessment techniques.

Ideas for rehabilitation research projects come from many sources. The need for an innovative intervention with a particular disability group, follow-up or replication of previous research, and the curiosity of rehabilitation researchers are all potential sources for new projects. Perhaps the most significant source of rehabilitation research projects is in response to rehabilitation legislation. The history of rehabilitation and rehabilitation research in the United States parallels the development of legislation that has shaped disability-related social policy. The specific mandates of legislation often serve to stimulate research. Important rehabilitation legislation has led to dramatic changes in the status of persons with disabilities in the United States since the 1970s. The Rehabilitation Act of 1973 was a watershed piece of legislation. It emphasized the expansion of services for persons with severe disabilities, client participation in the rehabilitation process, the elimination of barriers to full participation in society, the development of mechanisms to determine rehabilitation effectiveness, and the protection of civil rights of persons with disabilities as outlined in sections 502, 503, and 504 of the act. This legislation unleashed a wave of research to find innovative methods for serving persons with severe disabilities and for determining the impact of the other components of the act.

Another important piece of legislation, the Americans with Disabilities Act of 1990 (ADA), has extended efforts to eliminate discrimination toward persons with disabilities. Discrimination with respect to hiring practices and access to transportation and physical facilities are the key elements in this legislation. Many years of research will be needed to determine the impact of the ADA on employers, the public, and persons with disabilities.

The Rehabilitation Act of 1992 reflects the influence of years of study concerning the most appropriate qualifications needed by persons involved in the provision of rehabilitation services in the public sector, particularly rehabilitation counselors. The act mandates appropriate training and personnel standards to ensure that service providers will be adequately qualified. In this instance, rehabilitation research influenced the development of social policy through legislation and set the stage for future research projects to determine the impact of this legislation. This process—of rehabilitation research influencing legislation and of legislation triggering new research initiatives—is a hallmark of the field of rehabilitation research.

Rehabilitation Research Methods

Although the focus of rehabilitation research is the improvement of services for persons with disabilities, the methodology of rehabilitation research is based on the scientific tradition and the scientific method. Consequently, the traditional research designs and the analytic procedures that are used in basic and applied research in the medical and social sciences are applicable to the field of rehabilitation.

An important consideration for rehabilitation researchers is the ability to determine the causal relationship between rehabilitation interventions and client outcomes. It is important for rehabilitation practitioners to know that their interventions have a high probability of success with their clients. By establishing a causal relationship between rehabilitation intervention and outcome, the demonstrated effectiveness of an intervention can be known and the potential benefit can be estimated. The determination of causality requires rigorous experimental designs. Experimental designs establish causality by ruling out alternative explanations of rehabilitation outcome other than that the rehabilitation intervention caused the outcome. Unfortunately, when research is conducted in settings other than laboratories, experimental designs are difficult to implement. These field-based studies present many challenges to the researcher, who desires to control as many aspects of the research environment as possible in order to establish a causal relationship. Much of rehabilitation research is field-based. Consequently, rehabilitation researchers must often work with research designs that do not allow the degree of scientific rigor that would be found in a laboratory. Through the creative application of research principles, the rehabilitation researcher builds a body of evidence to support particular interventions by demonstrating positive effects with different groups of disabled individuals, by comparing different interventions and their effects on outcome, and by analyzing the data from less experimentally rigorous studies in new and interesting ways. The creative application of quantitative and qualitative analyses to less experimentally rigorous research designs can often provide insight about the relationship between rehabilitation intervention and outcome.

Another important consideration for rehabilitation researchers is whether the results of these studies have relevance to groups of disabled individuals other than those in their studies. The ability to generalize results beyond the confines of a particular research study also presents significant challenges to the rehabilitation researcher, who performs a balancing act between establishing the causal relationship of rehabilitation interventions and outcomes and generalizing the results of studies.

Rehabilitation Research Information

Unless information from rehabilitation research studies is used by practitioners to improve the lives of persons with disabilities, justification for conducting rehabilitation research is limited. A necessary step to utilization of research by practitioners is access to information. The National Rehabilitation Information Center (NARIC) is a NIDRR-funded repository of data. NARIC has computerized databases such as REHABDATA that contain information from National Institute on Disability and Rehabilitation Research–funded projects, rehabilitation-related journals, and other publications. NIDRR supports the SERIES computer network at the University of Oregon, an electronic mail system that links consumers of information with information providers. NIDRR also supports *Rehab Brief* (Bringing Research into Effective Focus), a publication that summarizes the findings of selected research projects in specific topic areas. Other sources of information include published materials from rehabilitation research and training centers; rehabilitation-related journals, such as the *Rehabilitation Counseling Bulletin, Rehabilitation Psychology,* the *Journal of Rehabilitation,* and the *Journal of Applied Rehabilitation Counseling;* and publications of federal, state, and local agencies involved in the delivery of rehabilitation services.

A challenge for rehabilitation researchers is to produce reports of their research that increase the chances of access and use by rehabilitation practitioners. The ever-expanding body of rehabilitation information and the increased need to link that information to relevant users will be greatly enhanced by the continuing development of computer-based information systems.

Rehabilitation Research Ethics

Of considerable concern to rehabilitation researchers is the principle that rehabilitation research be conducted according to the highest ethical standards. Rehabilitation researchers are encouraged and expected to follow the ethical guidelines of their respective disciplines and ethics regulations of federal, state, and local agencies. In general, these codes of ethics require that the confidentiality of client data is protected, that protection of the rights of human and animal subjects is ensured, that results of studies are reported accurately, and that human subjects provide informed consent of their participation in research. Specific guidelines are found in the codes of ethics of the respective disciplines involved in rehabilitation research and in the ethics regulations of rehabilitation agencies. Sensitivity to ethical issues in research will result in increasing participation of persons with disabilities in the planning and implementation of rehabilitation research projects.

The Future

The dawn of the twenty-first century brings both challenges and opportunities to rehabilitation researchers. The challenges lie in the changing social conditions to which rehabilitation must respond. The increasing prevalence of persons with multiple disabling conditions, the increasing population of elderly persons with age-related disabilities, the effects of emerging disease conditions such as HIV/AIDS, and new environmentally related diseases will generate questions about needed rehabilitation interventions. Changes in the workplace of the future, where different skills will be needed to perform the jobs of tomorrow, will challenge rehabilitation researchers to discover new and better ways to prepare individuals with disabilities for these jobs. As the body of research knowledge about rehabilitation accumulates, this information will coalesce into new theories of how people with disabilities function in different environments. The evolution of rehabilitation theory will be an important focus of future rehabilitation research.

These future challenges will bring new opportunities to rehabilitation researchers. The further development of computer technology will create new tools for the analysis of complex research data. Developments in biomedicine, bioengineering, and biotechnology will yield potentially beneficial interventions for persons with disabilities. The evolution of enlightened social policy will increase opportunities for persons with disabilities in the mainstream of their culture. Consequently, the need for qualified rehabilitation researchers will increase as these new opportunities for rehabilitation research expand.

(*See also:* ETHICS; EVALUATION OF REHABILITATION PROGRAMS; INFORMATION RESOURCES; TECHNOLOGY)

BIBLIOGRAPHY

BOLTON, BRIAN, and PARKER, RANDALL M. "Research in Rehabilitation Counseling." In *Rehabilitation Counseling: Basics and Beyond*, eds. Randall M. Parker and Edna Syzmanski. Austin, TX, 1992.

DELLARIO, DONALD J. "Rehabilitation Research: A Need for Perspective." *Journal of Rehabilitation* 19 (1978):66–70.

NATIONAL INSTITUTE ON DISABILITY AND REHABILITATION RESEARCH. *Rehab Brief* 11 (1989):1–4.

PARKER, RANDALL M. "Science, Philosophy, and Politics in the Search for Truth in Rehabilitation Research." *Rehabilitation Counseling Bulletin* 34 (1990): 165–169.

PAUL, GORDON L. "Outcome Research in Psychotherapy." *Journal of Consulting Psychology* 31 (1967): 109–118.

RUBIN, STANFORD E., and RICE, JAMES M. "Quality and Relevance of Rehabilitation Research: A Critique and Recommendations." *Rehabilitation Counseling Bulletin* 30 (1986):33–43.

WRIGHT, GEORGE N. *Total Rehabilitation.* Boston, 1980.

DONALD J. DELLARIO

RESPIRATORY DISEASE

All diseases of the respiratory system result in primary impairment either of blood oxygenation or of lung ventilation. The former is from intrinsic lung disease; the latter, from neurologic restrictive pulmonary conditions. The diseases that produce these impairments and their treatments are distinctly different, but they are all too frequently treated the same because of the general lack of knowledge of physical medicine approaches.

Diseases with Primary Impairment of Blood Oxygenation

Individuals in this category have diseased lungs, diseased airways, or, most commonly, both. These intrinsic diseases occur either from inherited metabolic or structural abnormalities as seen in cystic fibrosis, bronchodysplasia, or certain forms of chronic obstructive pulmonary disease (COPD) such as emphysema and bronchitis, or more commonly from exposure to toxins such as cigarette smoke, asbestos, or coal dust. These toxins are the most common cause of COPD as well as of pulmonary fibrosis, a condition in which the lung is severely diseased without obstruction of airways. Asthma results from a combination of an inherited predisposition that, with exposure to allergens and emotional factors, triggers spasm of the airways. Early on, all asthmatics have reversible bronchospasm that is readily reversed by medications. With time, however, the bronchospasms may become irreversible, and the individual then has COPD.

COPD affects 10 to 40 percent of all Americans and is the fifth leading cause of death in the United States. Its incidence more than doubled from 1970 to 1994, and it is becoming increasingly prevalent. Fifty percent of patients have activity limitations and 25 percent are restricted to bed (Bach, 1993b).

Assessment. The main symptom of COPD is shortness of breath, initially with exercise, later at rest. It is diagnosed by observing a typical clinical appearance, including a "barrel" chest and the use of pulmonary function tests that, among other things, evaluate the patient's ability to create high expiratory flows during a forced (rapid) exhalation maneuver. The forced expiratory volume exhaled during the first second (FEV_1) is the most common parameter used to assess the severity of COPD. When the FEV_1 is less than 1,500 milliliters, shortness of breath develops with minimal to moderate activity; when it is less than 750 milliliters, the prognosis for five-year survival is poor. Another common test of the integrity of the lungs is diffusion capacity, which is a measure of the lungs' ability to transfer oxygen and carbon dioxide across the membranes that separate the terminal airways and their air sacs from the capillary blood. Diffusion capacity is abnormal when lung tissue is diseased but may be normal when only airway obstruction is present. Chest radiographs and other scans of the chest can also demonstrate lung disease; however, neither the extent of the anatomical aberrations nor the results of pulmonary function tests accurately assess the effects of lung disease on patient function. Clinical exercise testing is more useful in this regard.

Clinical exercise testing is the measurement of the oxygen consumed and the carbon dioxide produced during graded exercise. With exercise the COPD patient must breathe more deeply and rapidly than normal (high ventilatory requirement) to transfer oxygen into the bloodstream because oxygen diffusion is reduced. This causes shortness of breath, which limits exercise. At times, however, the shortness of breath with exercise is due not to lung disease but to heart disease. Although often missed in the clinical examination, this condition can be observed during clinical exercise testing as a decreased oxygen utilization per heartbeat. Likewise, some shortness of breath with exercise is not due to COPD but to exercise-induced bronchospasm, which can only be diagnosed during exercise testing. Clinical exercise testing provides the best estimate of the patient's exercise tolerance and general functioning capabilities. A repeat exercise test following the patient's rehabilitation program also objectively documents improvements.

Since both hypoxemia (low blood oxygen levels) and hypercapnia (high blood carbon dioxide levels) can disturb cerebral functioning, patients often present with impaired abstraction, attention, and memory. Because of the functional deficits patients also become increasingly dependent, preoccupied with their bodily functions and health, and less socially active, all of which tend to cause stress.

Candidates for Rehabilitation and Expected Rehabilitation Outcomes. Patients who are medically stable with mild COPD and shortness of breath with only moderately strenuous activities are treated in an outpatient setting. They are candidates to increase exercise tolerance; decrease shortness of breath, respiratory rate, and the risk of hospitalization; and improve their work output, activities of daily living, cognitive function, and sense of well-being and quality of life in general (Bach, 1993b). Anxiety and depression are also decreased. Patients who are recuperating from acute respiratory failure, especially when still requiring ventilatory assistance, are best treated in an acute inpatient rehabilitation setting. These individuals may be moderately to severely debilitated, but they must be able to take part in two or more hours per day of physical and occupational therapy and have potential for relatively rapid improvement. They will benefit from all of the rehabilitation outcomes expected for mildly involved patients, and in addition be weaned from ventilatory support or transferred to the use of noninvasive respiratory muscle aids (Hardy, 1994). Less cooperative or more severely debilitated individuals, who cannot take part in more than one to two hours of therapy per day and for whom progress is expected to be very slow, should be managed in a specialized chronic care institution in which the nurses are trained to help the patient set and reach rehabilitation goals and in which the patient can receive at least one hour of therapy per day.

Therapeutic Interventions and Rehabilitation. The patient's medical regimen should be optimized prior to undertaking the program. Pharmacological management may include methylxanthines, adrenergics (preferably beta 2 agonists), anticholinergics, glucocorticoids and synthetic steroids, mast-cell membrane stabilizers, and antihistaminics. Most of these medications can be delivered orally or as aerosolized solutions. Other medications, such as expectorants, mucus liquefying agents, and antibiotics may be used along with humidification, ample fluid intake, and airway secretion management as warranted. Training in the proper use of inhalers, nebulizers, and ventilatory equipment is critical; otherwise medications are often largely deposited uselessly on the tongue. Oxygen therapy should be provided whenever the blood oxygen levels are less than 55 to 60 millimeters of mercury. Oxygen therapy can decrease dyspnea (shortness of breath, air hunger), enhance performance, exert a cardioprotective effect on patients with coronary artery disease, and prolong life (Anthonisen, 1986). During respiratory tract infections early medical attention is important.

For a large comprehensive rehabilitation program the multidisciplinary team consists of a physiatrist; respiratory, physical, and occupational therapists; an exercise physiologist; a psychiatrist or psychologist; a social worker; a vocational counselor; and a dietitian. For an outpatient program, a physician, respiratory therapist, and dietitian are critical; other team members are consulted on an individual basis.

Psychosocial interventions should be integrated into a multidisciplinary rehabilitation program. Numerous strategies, including the use of nicotine-impregnated gum and programmed reduction, can be used to sustain smoking cessation (Fisher & Rost, 1986). COPD patients should be counseled on adhering to their medication regimens and on avoiding environmental pollutants and other aggravating factors such as pollen, excessive humidity, stress, and

respiratory tract pathogens. Flu and pneumococcal vaccinations are recommended. Good hydration should be maintained with ample fluid intake.

Malnourishment is very common in COPD. It can cause respiratory failure, difficulty in ventilator weaning, and infection. Short-term refeeding improves respiratory muscle endurance and, at times, respiratory muscle strength.

Dyspnea often causes fear and panic. Relaxation exercises and biofeedback may be used to decrease tension and anxiety (Kahn, 1977). Specialized diaphragmatic and pursed-lip breathing exercises also aid in relaxation. Inspiratory muscle strengthening exercises can improve the strength and endurance of respiratory muscles (Bach, 1993b).

Airway secretion clearance is crucial. The patient's cough may be weak, and with airway obstruction, attempts at coughing can cause airway collapse and fatigue. "Huffing," or frequent short expulsive bursts following a deep breath, is effective. Chest percussion and postural drainage can be useful for patients with considerable sputum production. Newer techniques to mobilize airway secretions include autogenous breathing, the use of positive expiratory pressure masks, and devices that oscillate the airway to favor expulsion of secretions (Hardy, 1994).

Hypercapnia (increases in blood carbon dioxide levels) occurs to avoid overloading inspiratory muscles, fatigue, and acute respiratory failure. Hypercapnia also weakens respiratory muscles (Stubbing et al., 1980). Relatively minor changes in breathing pattern or respiratory muscle loading, such as during a respiratory tract infection, can trigger acute respiratory muscle fatigue and failure. Interspersing periods of exercise and muscle rest is a basic principle of rehabilitation. Diaphragm rest can be achieved by assisting ventilation by using either body ventilators or mouthpiece or nasal intermittent positive pressure ventilation (IPPV) (Bach, 1993b).

Oxygen therapy can be provided only during the patient's inspiratory phase of breathing, or pulsed oxygen therapy can be given. Especially when delivered through a minitracheostomy tube, oxygen delivery is most efficient, avoids waste, and decreases the discomfort and drying of mucous membranes. Mechanical ventilation may also be beneficial for patients with concomitant carbon dioxide retention.

Although the use of exercise reconditioning may be limited by pain, fatigue, dyspnea, or light-headedness in these deconditioned individuals, the intensity of reconditioning exercises may be guided by parameters determined through clinical exercise testing—for example, 80 to 85 percent of maximum achievable heart rate, or heart rate at ventilation levels of thirty-five times FEV_1 (Jones & Campbell, 1982). Walking, stair climbing, calisthenics, bicycling, and pool activities may be pursued. Upper extremity reconditioning should be included. The patient should be made responsible for a progressive program. Purchase of a stationary bicycle for the patient's home and its use twice a day, a daily twelve-minute walk, and possibly several daily fifteen-minute sessions of inspiratory muscle training are recommended (Bach, 1993b). A daily log should be kept of these activities. The program should consist of weekly reevaluations of the logs, exercise parameters, and educational and peer groups sessions used to reinforce the activities. Such a program is inexpensive, minimally intrusive, and optimizes the chances for continued adherence to the protocol following the ten- to twelve-week program. For more severely debilitated individuals the exercise tolerance goals are more modest, but relative improvements are as significant as for more mildly affected individuals (Foster, Lopez, and Thomas, 1988).

Following the acute rehabilitation period, continued surveillance and attention to abstinence from smoking, good bronchial hygiene, breathing retraining, physical reconditioning, oxygen therapy, and airway secretion mobilization have been shown to reduce hospital admissions, the length of hospital stays, and cost (Roselle & D'Amico, 1990). The American Lung Association in New York City and the Cystic Fibrosis Association in Bethesda, Maryland, have educational literature and provide other support for individuals with lung disease.

Diseases with Primary Ventilatory Impairment

Ventilatory failure is a common cause of morbidity and mortality for individuals with generalized neurological disorders. Rehabilitation interventions are most effective for patients who can fully cooperate. Therefore, discussion will be limited to severe neurological disorders in which ventilatory but not cognitive function is severely impaired. Such disorders may be progressive, essentially static, remittent, or have intermittent exacerbations.

The progressive neuromuscular diseases include myopathies, generalized neuropathies, and motor neuron diseases. The classifications and the natural histories of these conditions have been previously described (Bach & Lieberman, 1993; Younger, 1991a, 1991b). In conditions such as postpoliomyelitis there is also evidence of increasing paralysis and general and respiratory muscle disability due to senescent loss of previously unaffected nerve cells. Likewise, patients with Guillain-Barré syndrome, polymyositis, myasthenia gravis, multiple sclerosis, or traumatic tetraplegia deteriorate with time. In a sense, virtually all paralytic syndromes are progressive.

Assessment. Often patients who can walk complain of shortness of breath; otherwise, fatigue, anxiety, and other subtle symptoms may be all that might signal chronic ventilatory insufficiency (Bach & Alba, 1990). Increased breathing rate, decreased depth, and low vocal volume are key signs. Maximum inspiratory and expiratory pressures generated at the mouth correlate best with inspiratory and expiratory muscle strength. The vital capacity (VC), or the deepest breath that one can blow through a spirometer, gives an indication of respiratory muscle strength and is simple, easy to measure, objective, and very reproducible. Since hypercapnia begins and is worse during sleep, the VC should be evaluated with the patient supine. Since expiratory (abdominal) muscle weakness causes impaired clearance of airway secretions and is the major cause of acute respiratory failure for these individuals, peak cough expiratory flows (PCEFs) should also be measured using a simple flow meter. Peak cough expiratory flows of at least 3 liters per second are necessary to mobilize secretions. Manually assisted coughing PCEFs should be determined.

Nocturnal oximetry (oxygen saturation or SaO_2 monitoring) should be performed for patients with supine VC of less than 40 to 50 percent of predicted normality, especially for those with rapidly evolving conditions and loss of VC. The oximeter must summarize the data. Any symptomatic patient with a VC of less than 50 percent of predicted normality, and a mean SaO_2 of less than 95 percent for at least one hour during sleep, has significant nocturnal hypoventilation and requires treatment. Patients with hypercapnia and a mean SaO_2 in the low nineties during much of the night should be treated even in the absence of overt symptoms.

Treatment of Paralytic/Restrictive Pulmonary Conditions and Counseling. Early and effective rehabilitation intervention is essential if hospitalizations and episodes of acute respiratory failure are to be avoided, or reversed with tracheal intubation. Counseling is similar to that for the COPD patient. In addition, the patient should be cautioned to avoid routine oxygen use and sedatives. Central ventilatory drive can be suppressed by oxygen therapy, carbon dioxide retention exacerbated, and the risk of acute respiratory failure increased (Bach & Alba, 1990). An abdominal binder may be useful to increase diaphragmatic excursion for seated spinal cord injured patients. Since treated patients with progressive neuromuscular diseases can have greatly increased life expectancies, they should also be encouraged to undertake goal-oriented activities and plan for their futures.

Respiratory muscle strengthening exercises have not been shown to delay the need for ventilator use (Bach, 1993b). Interestingly, however, interspersing respiratory muscle rest by ventilatory assistance and inspiratory muscle training has been reported to facilitate ventilator weaning (Aldrich et al., 1989).

Maximal insufflations provide range of motion for the hypomobile tissues of the lungs and chest walls. They are necessary for normal development of the rib cage and thorax (Bach, 1992), to avoid or reverse atelectasis (a collapsed or airless condition of part of the lung), to optimize cough flows, and to increase voice volume. Taking deep breaths on one's own (incentive spirometry) cannot substitute for receiving deep insufflations with the use of a ventilator or device that blows deeply into the lungs.

Glossopharyngeal breathing (GPB)—or the use of the tongue and pharyngeal muscles to project boluses of air past the vocal cords—is used to provide maximal insufflations and as a noninvasive method to support ventilation ("gulping air"). It is an excellent backup in the event of ventilator equipment failure. The patient takes a deep breath, then augments it by GPB. The vocal chords close with each

"gulp" (Bach, 1992). Six to eight gulps comprise a 600 milliliter addition to the patient's tidal volume.

Pulmonary restrictive syndrome patients are often unable to generate adequate peak cough expiratory flows (PCEF) to mobilize airway secretions. These secretions can precipitate life-threatening mucous plugging of airways and acute respiratory failure. This is also true for the intubated or tracheostomized patient who cannot close the glottis to generate expiratory pressures. Suctioning via an endotracheal tube does not mobilize deep secretions, the suction catheter usually fails to enter the left main stem bronchus, it irritates bronchial membranes, and it is uncomfortable.

Chest percussion is performed by rhythmically percussing the patient's chest with cupped hands or by applying a mechanical vibrator to the chest. By positioning the patient in nine distinct positions, gravity-assisted postural drainage can help clearing of bronchopulmonary segments. These techniques are only marginally effective. No studies demonstrate that they shorten hospital stays, reduce morbidity, lessen the number of exacerbations, or decrease mortality (Bach, 1993b).

Manually assisted coughing can usually generate adequate PCEF for neuromuscular patients to mobilize secretions (De Boek & Zinman, 1984). To be optimally effective for patients with VCs of less than 1,000 milliliters, manually assisted coughing should be preceded by a deep insufflated breath. When inadequate, mechanical insufflation-exsufflation can deliver an independently adjusted positive pressure insufflation followed by an independently adjusted negative pressure exsufflation via an anesthesia mask or, if present, an endotracheal tube (Bach, 1993a). The pressure drop is usually about 80 centimeters of water, and the negative pressure is sustained to carry secretions, mucous plugs, and other debris into the mouth and anesthesia mask, from where they can be easily suctioned. Ideally an abdominal thrust should be delivered to the patient concurrently with the exsufflation phase of insufflation-exsufflation.

The patient should learn the use of noninvasive methods of ventilatory support. Such supports can be used for up to twenty-four hours a day as alternatives to tracheostomy intermittent positive pressure ventilation (IPPV). Noninvasive IPPV is delivered via mouthpieces or nasal interfaces (Bach,

1993b). As underventilation develops during sleep, the patient tries various nasal interfaces and uses a nasal IPPV nocturnally. As ventilatory insufficiency proceeds throughout daytime hours, the patient extends the hours of use of the nasal IPPV or uses a mouthpiece IPPV in the daytime. A mouthpiece IPPV can also be used overnight with a lipseal retention system to diminish air leakage out of the mouth and firmly retain the mouthpiece (Bach, Alba, and Saporito, 1993). The placement of an indwelling tracheostomy tube is indicated *only* when use of noninvasive aids are contraindicated by the presence of depressed cognitive function, orthopedic conditions interfering with the application of IPPV interfaces, inadequate oropharyngeal muscle strength for functional speech and swallowing, severe intrinsic lung disease necessitating high levels of supplemental oxygen, uncontrolled seizures or substance abuse, or an assisted PCEF of less than 3 liters per second.

Some Community Resources. The Jerry Lewis Muscular Dystrophy Association (Tucson, Arizona) supports some of the clinical activities of clinics specializing in the diagnosis and management of individuals with progressive neuromuscular diseases. Amyotrophic lateral sclerosis patient and family support groups are often organized by local Muscular Dystrophy Association clinics. Families of Children with Spinal Muscular Atrophy is another organization devoted specifically to individuals with this condition (Highland Park, Illinois). The World Disability Fund (San Francisco, CA) supports activities of persons with disabilities. Gazette International Network Inc. in St. Louis and the National Association for Ventilator Dependent Individuals, a newly formed social service organization, also sponsor periodicals and provide considerable support services for ventilator users.

Vocational Issues

Irrespective of the extent of pulmonary or generalized disability, vocational rehabilitation specialists, with the help of the Division of Vocational Rehabilitation—a federal program that provides support for disabled individuals to return to the work force—can train individuals to use residual strength to operate the computers or the other devices necessary to return them to work. There is currently considerable incentive in the form of governmental subsidies for large companies to hire people with disabilities. When shortness of breath is the principal problem, sedentary employment is realistic. However, even when only residual eyelid movement remains, 24-hour-a-day ventilator users can earn a living as engineers, lawyers, judges, journalists, etc. Therefore, motivation, ingenuity, and a supporting environment are the major factors that limit an individual's potential for gainful employment.

(*See also:* INDEPENDENT LIVING; NEUROMUSCULAR DISORDERS; PHYSICIAN; SPINAL CORD INJURY; WELLNESS)

RESOURCES

American Lung Association, 1740 Broadway, New York, NY 10019

Amyotrophic Lateral Sclerosis Association (ALSA), 21021 Ventura Blvd., Suite 321, Woodland Hills, CA 91364

Cystic Fibrosis Foundation, 6931 Arlington Rd, Bethesda, MD 20814

Gazette International Networking Institute, 100 Oakland Ave., Suite 206, St. Louis, MO 63110

Muscular Dystrophy Association (MDA), 3300 East Sunrise Drive, Tucson, AZ 85718

BIBLIOGRAPHY

ALDRICH, TOM K.; KARPEL, JILL P.; UHRLASS, RAYMOND M.; SPARAPANI, MARK A.; ERAMO, DONNA; and FERRANTI, REDENTO. "Weaning from Mechanical Ventilation: Adjunctive Use of Inspiratory Muscle Resistive Training." *Critical Care Medicine* 17 (1989):143–147.

ANTHONISEN, N. R. "Home Oxygen Therapy in Chronic Obstructive Pulmonary Disease." *Clinics of Chest Medicine* 7 (1986):673–678.

BACH, JOHN R. "Pulmonary Rehabilitation Considerations for Duchenne Muscular Dystrophy: The Prolongation of Life by Respiratory Muscle Aids." *Critical Reviews in Physical and Rehabilitation Medicine* 3 (1992):239–269.

———. "Mechanical Insufflation-Exsufflation: Comparison of Peak Expiratory Flows with Manually Assisted and Unassisted Coughing Techniques." *Chest* 104 (1993a):1553–1562.

———. "Pulmonary Rehabilitation." In *Rehabilitation Medicine: Principles and Practice.* Philadelphia, 1993b.

BACH, JOHN R., and ALBA, AUGUSTA S. "Management of Chronic Alveolar Hypoventilation by Nasal Ventilation." *Chest* 97 (1990):52–57.

BACH, JOHN R.; ALBA, AUGUSTA S; and SAPORITO, LOU R. "Intermittent Positive Pressure Ventilation via the Mouth as an Alternative to Tracheostomy for 257 Ventilator Users." *Chest* 103 (1993):174–182.

BACH, JOHN R., and LIEBERMAN, JAMES S. "Rehabilitation of the Patient with Disease Affecting the Motor Unit." In *Rehabilitation Medicine: Principles and Practice*, ed. Joel D. Delisa. 2nd ed. Philadelphia, 1993.

CASABURI, RICHARD, and PETTY, THOMAS L., eds. *Principles and Practice of Pulmonary Rehabilitation.* Philadelphia, 1993.

DE BOECK, CHRISTIANE, and ZINMAN, RAEZELLE. "Cough versus Chest Physiotherapy: A Comparison of the Acute Effects on Pulmonary Function in Patients with Cystic Fibrosis." *American Review of Respiratory Disease* 129 (1984):182–184.

FISHER, E. B., JR., and ROST, KATHRYN. "Smoking Cessation: A Practical Guide for the Physician." *Clinics of Chest Medicine* 7 (1986):551–565.

FOSTER, STEVEN; LOPEZ, DEBORAH; and THOMAS, HENRY M. "Pulmonary Rehabilitation in COPD Patients with Elevated pCO_2." *American Review of Respiratory Disease* 138 (1988):1519–1523.

HAAS, FRANÇOIS, and AXEN, KENNETH, eds. *Pulmonary Therapy and Rehabilitation.* Baltimore, 1991.

HARDY, KAREN A. "A Review of Airway Clearance: New Techniques, Indications, and Recommendations." *Respiratory Care* 39 (1994):440–455.

HODGKIN, JOHN E.; CONNORS, GERILYNN L.; and BEL, C. WILLIAM, eds. *Pulmonary Rehabilitation: Guidelines to Success,* 2nd ed. Philadelphia, 1993.

JONES, NORMAN L., and CAMPBELL, E. J. MORAN. "Clinical Exercise Testing," 2nd ed. Philadelphia, 1982.

KAHN, AMAN U. "Effectiveness of Biofeedback and Counter-conditioning in the Treatment of Bronchial Asthma." *Journal of Psychosomatic Research* 21 (1977):97–104.

ROSELLE, SUE, and D'AMICO, FRANK J. "The Effect of Home Respiratory Therapy on Hospital Readmission Rates of Patients with Chronic Obstructive Pulmonary Disease." *Respiratory Care* 35 (1990): 1208–1213.

SNIDER, GORDON L., ed. *Clinics in Chest Medicine: Pulmonary Rehabilitation.* Philadelphia, 1986.

STUBBING, DAVID G.; PENGELLY, L. DAVID; MORSE, JOHN L. C.; and JONES, NORMAN L. "Pulmonary

Mechanics During Exercise in Subjects with Chronic Airflow Obstruction." *Journal of Applied Physiology* 49 (1980):511–515.

YOUNGER, DAVID S., ed. "Paralysis: Part I." *Seminars in Neurology* 13 (1991a):241–315.

———. "Paralytic Syndromes: Part II." *Seminars in Neurology* 13 (1991b):319–379.

JOHN R. BACH

RESPITE CARE

Since the early 1970s there has been a dramatic decrease in institutional programs for people with disabilities and a corresponding increase in community-based services (Mesibov 1990). This trend has dramatically improved the quality of life for many people with disabilities. Although the deinstitutionalization movement has dramatically increased opportunities, it has also presented new challenges for communities and families. For communities, the challenge has been to develop the full continuum of services that these clients require. For families, there has been the need to support their family member with the twenty-four-hour care formerly provided by institutions.

Although most families agree that having their member home is a great relief and a wonderful opportunity, there is also considerable stress associated with full-time care (Bristol, 1987; Schopler & Mesibov, 1983). One support service that has proven very important in helping family members to cope with that stress is called respite care. Respite care is defined as any program providing direct supervision and care of persons with disabilities so a family can be temporarily relieved of their care-giving responsibilities. Ranging from two hours to thirty days, this service has proven invaluable and is typically one of the most frequently requested when parents are asked to describe their needs (Bristol, 1987; DeMyer, 1979; Schopler & Mesibov, 1983). Shorter respite opportunities allow families time to go shopping, see a movie, have dinner, or just spend a quiet evening at home. Longer respite services provide opportunities for family vacations or extended trips. Respite care is especially helpful during family emergencies to ease the pressures of caregiving at these emotionally stressful times.

There are two basic respite care models: center-based and home-based. Center-based respite programs are similar to residential group homes. Housed in residential communities, these homes are staffed by competent and well-trained professionals. Respite programs usually have a maximum number of days per visit and per year during which families can use their services. The benefit of these center-based models is their comprehensiveness and responsiveness to a wide range of family needs. A fully trained staff is available at all times, and center-based respite care offers families the flexibility to do whatever they need while the program is caring for their child or other family member. The main disadvantage of this model is the cost; maintaining a house in a neighborhood is expensive. Another problem is the difficulty some families have in transporting their family member to the respite facility.

The home-based model is a less costly alternative and provides fully trained respite workers who go into a family's home to take care of people with special needs for short or extended periods. Although this model is not as expensive to administer as center-based care, it offers the family less flexibility because they must leave their home while using the respite service. This situation imposes a financial burden on families, some of whom do not have the resources for this. Respite workers also suffer from not having the opportunity to work together, over extended periods, in the cohesive teams that are inherent in center-based programs.

Efforts to expand the home-based model may offer greater flexibility. Some of these programs designate specific, licensed respite care providers to take people with disabilities into their homes, thus incorporating some of the advantages of the center-based programs without the expense. Two challenges that must be addressed with designated respite care homes are monitoring care providers and giving them consistent exposure to other respite care providers.

Carole C. Upshur (1982) investigated the most common kinds of respite programs and found that most are operated by respite care agencies, although nursing homes (11%) and group care programs (17%) were also administering agencies. Respite care is most often provided to clients with mental retardation (94%) and least often to people with autism (37%). The majority of programs contacted (60%) provided in-home respite care.

Darcey L. Marc and Larry MacDonald (1988) surveyed programs to see who uses respite care. They found that users of these services were more likely to have three or more children or children with severe handicaps. They were also more likely to make use of other professional services. The authors concluded that frequent respite users tend to be particularly needy families.

Outcome research from several studies shows that respite care meets important needs in families of people with developmental disabilities. Shelly Botuck and Bertrand G. Winsberg (1991) found increased feelings of well-being and less depression in mothers who took advantage of respite care for their children. A. Rimmerman (1989) also found a reduction in maternal stress associated with using respite care as well as an enhancement of mothers' coping responses. Kathleen Joyce, Mark Singer, and Richard Isralowitz (1983), collecting data from twenty-four families using in-home respite care, demonstrated that these services had a positive impact on their lives. Several families cited, along with less family stress, improved relationships among family members and with their children with disabilities. In their study, Joyce, Singer, and Isralowitz found no relationship between the number of respite hours and indices of "quality of the family's life," suggesting that the availability of respite care is more important than any specific number of hours.

Respite care programs are meeting important needs for families coping with illness or disability of a family member while remaining in the community. They are a proven way to decrease pressures on families challenged by the demands of caregiving. Because of the important role that respite care is playing in service delivery systems, more work is essential in identifying new models and evaluating their effectiveness.

(*See also:* CAREGIVING; CHILDHOOD DISABILITIES; FAMILIES; PEDIATRIC REHABILITATION; QUALITY OF LIFE)

BIBLIOGRAPHY

BOTUCK, SHELLY, and WINSBERG, BERTRAND G. "Effects of Respite on Mothers of School-Age and Adult Children with Severe Disabilities." *Mental Retardation* 29 (1991):43–47.

BRISTOL, M. "Mothers of Autistic and Communication-Impaired Children: Successful Adaptation and the Double ABCX Model." *Journal of Autism and Developmental Disorders* 17 (1987):469–486.

DeMyer, M. K. *Parents and Children in Autism.* Washington, DC, 1979.

Joyce, Kathleen; Singer, Mark; and Isralowitz, R. "Impact of Respite Care on Parents' Perceptions of Quality of Life." *Mental Retardation* 21 (1983):153–156.

Marc, Darcey L., and MacDonald, Larry. "Respite Care—Who Uses It?" *Mental Retardation* 26 (1988):93–96.

Mesibov, Gary B. "Normalization and Its Relevance Today." *Journal of Autism and Developmental Disorders* 20 (1990):379–390.

Rimmerman, A. "Provision of Respite Care for Children with Developmental Disabilities: Changes in Maternal Coping and Stress over Time." *Mental Retardation* 27 (1989):99–103.

Schopler, E., and Mesibov, Gary B., eds. *The Effects of Autism on the Family.* New York, 1983.

Upshur, Carole C. "Respite Care for Mentally Retarded and Other Disabled Populations: Program Models and Family Needs." *Mental Retardation* 20 (1982):2–6.

Gary B. Mesibov
Jemma C. Price

RURAL REHABILITATION

Rural America is a diverse and changing place. Small-town America, the family farm, and the frontier West are images that have long formed the foundation of the rural American dream. Basic rural values that are ingrained in visions of open spaces, picturesque rolling hills, rich farmsteads, patchwork waves of grain, and majestic mountains are alive and romanticized in our culture. Yet these popular images of rural America mask the reality that it is an extremely significant, diverse, and complex part of our society, with problems and needs that are extensive and largely misunderstood.

The U.S. Bureau of the Census estimates that more than 66 million Americans, or about 27 percent of the population, live in a rural environment. Although this segment of Americans is approximately equal in size to the country's central city population, its visibility to policymakers is much less salient, since it is dispersed across more than 75 percent of the landscape. Yet there is significant evidence that rural Americans experience social, health, economic, and educational disadvantages that are equal to or greater than their central city counterparts (Norton & McManus, 1989; Seekins, 1992). In fact, the highest rates of poverty in this country are found in rural areas, where more than 14 million people live below the poverty line (Rojewski, 1992).

When the rural or nonmetropolitan sectors are disaggregated from the rest of the country, the most striking characteristic is not how similar these sectors are, but the diversity that prevails in rural America (Blakely & Bradshaw, 1981; Cordes, 1989). For example, the U.S. Department of Agriculture classifies six types of nonmetropolitan counties in relation to their primary economic base: agriculture; mining, oil, and energy; specialized government functions; persistent poverty; federal lands; and destination retirement.

While farm or ranch living once accounted for a substantial portion of rural residents—more than sixty percent in 1920—recent estimates indicate that fewer than 10 percent of the rural population lived on farms or ranches in the late 1980s (U.S. Bureau of the Census, 1988). Contrary to the popular myth that cowboys and farmers are the backbones of our rural society, the majority (56%) of the rural labor force over age fifteen work in service, financial, and wholesale and retail trade industries (Seekins, 1992; U.S. Bureau of the Census, 1988). Interestingly, off-farm employment is the primary source of income for the majority (53%) of families living on farmsteads. Thus, when we cast aside much of the romanticism and myth about rural Americans, we find ourselves with a population that seems invisible to modern, urban American society (Figure 1, p. 644).

Government efforts to address the broad range of conditions faced by rural society have nearly a century of history (Rasmussen, 1985). Americans living in rural areas have generally lacked equal access to important resources as well as the ability to purchase needed services (Leland & Schneider, 1982; Omohundro, et al., 1983; Page, 1989; Richards, et al., 1984; Swanson, 1990). While conventional wisdom assumes that it is less expensive to live in rural areas, the fact is that rural residents spend significantly more of their personal family income on living ex-

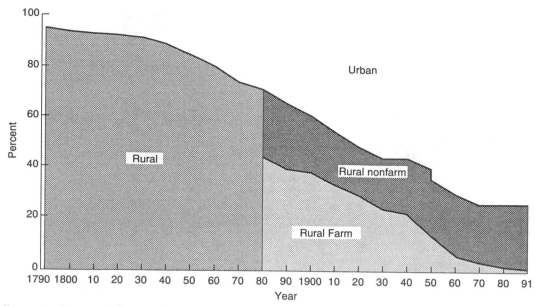

Figure 1. Percent of the population residing in urban areas and in farm and nonfarm portions of rural areas: 1790–1991

SOURCE: Dacquel, L. T. & D. C. Dahmann (1993). *Residents of Farms and Rural Areas: 1991.* Washington, DC: U.S. Bureau of the Census, Current Population Reports

penses than urban dwellers do (Seekins, 1992). For example, in 1988 urban residents spent about 90 percent of their average family income of $29,543 on living expenses (e.g., food, housing, apparel, transportation, health care, insurance), while rural residents spent 97 percent of their $22,132 average family income on living expenses. Thus urban residents generally have four times the discretionary income of their rural counterparts.

Despite these discrepancies, population-adjusted federal expenditures for human resource programs are substantially greater in metropolitan areas (Cordes, 1989). Further, inadequate rural health care has long been recognized as a national crisis. Rural hospitals have been closing at an alarming rate for several years (Moscovice, 1989; Reczynski, Tibbs, and Turk, 1987), and the proportion of physicians available to rural residents is significantly less in number and specialization than those available to urban residents (American Hospital Association, 1989; Norton & McManus, 1989). Linda Tonsing-Gonzales (1989), former president of the Association of Programs for Independent Living (APRIL), noted at the first national conference of the Research and Training Center on Rural Rehabilitation

Services in 1988, "Choosing between services or service providers [in rural areas] is a laughable concept; getting any service at all is the critical question."

As such, concern for equity and efficiency is at the heart of many of the problems identified by rural Americans (DeFriese & Ricketts, 1989). Researchers and rural advocates consistently marshal evidence that rural populations receive disproportionately less of society's resources to address problems that are often greater than those experienced in urban areas. For example, a study of hospital services for Medicare beneficiaries indicates that the average program payment per discharge was approximately 41 percent higher for beneficiaries living in urban areas than for rural residents. In general, rural areas have a more limited range of services, and their residents must use more informal and less specialized services, travel longer, use more of their income for them, and get less quality assistance than their urban counterparts (Rowland & Lyons, 1989). Sam Cordes (1989) points out that urban per capita expenditures for health and social service programs, training, and employment are twice what they are in rural areas despite the fact that rural areas contain a significantly larger proportion of economically disadvantaged people, such as those receiving SSI and food stamp payments.

Disability and Rehabilitation in Rural America

Disability and rehabilitation are a significant, though often overlooked, part of the complex rural American situation. Researchers (Coward & Cutler, 1989; DeFriese & Ricketts, 1989; Norton & McManus, 1989) point out that rural Americans account for a greater proportion of chronic disease and disability than urban populations while having fewer services or resources to address the issues.

Given a rural population base of about 66 million persons, it is likely that 13.2 million rural residents have at least one chronic or permanent impairment based on the 20 percent prevalence rate of Mathematica Policy Research, Inc. (1984). Further, Mitchell LaPlante's (1988) report of a 14.1 percent rate of activity limitation due to chronic conditions would lead to an estimated 9.6 rural residents having limitations to their daily activities. Since many chronic conditions are reported at significantly higher rates by nonmetropolitan residents (Norton & McManus, 1989), these prevalence rates may be underestimated, with estimates of the rural disabled population being as high as 15 million Americans (Rojewski, 1992).

The research and training agenda for rural rehabilitation services is broad. Such an agenda must extend to all segments of the rural population. In its total, this agenda must address the needs of people of any age or gender and with any disability. It must also include most forms of rehabilitation. Its focus should be both on programs and procedures that can solve specific problems, but that also may have general applicability.

If the rural agenda focused solely on one sector of rural residents or one type of rehabilitation, the issues of the majority of this underserved population would remain unaddressed. Accordingly, the state-of-the-art of rural rehabilitation parallels the issues people with disabilities who live in rural areas encounter. Richard Offner (1990) has suggested that:

"While developments in modern society have reduced the pronounced rural-urban differences that classical sociologists wrote about, rural-urban locality-based differences do exist. Thus, social science fact supports the case that we need different rural service models. Importantly, the divergent factors and/or barriers that affect the ability of rural clients to live independently require rehabilitation personnel and services capable of providing innovative and often untraditional service approaches."

Some Promising Examples of Innovations from Rural America

Given the breadth of issues involved in rural rehabilitation, it is impossible to summarize the range of innovative approaches taken in rural education, rural early intervention, rural services to the aging, and rural mental health services. Yet a sample of some programs helps to convey the quality of rural rehabilitation and the approaches that have emerged. They also suggest issues and approaches that are likely to emerge in the future. Some of them contain lessons for those addressing issues of importance to populations other than those directly concerned, including those faced by people with disabilities and living in urban areas.

Transportation. The lack of transportation is one of the most frequently reported problems facing rehabilitation providers in rural areas (Kidder, 1989; Page, 1989; Tonsing-Gonzales, 1989; Nosek, Zhu, and Howland, 1992). The most widely promoted model for rural transportation services involves developing cooperatives between existing human service agencies that own and operate vans (Kidder, 1989). Unfortunately, these programs often require a relatively dense rural population—sufficient to support the location of several agencies serving diverse populations—and rarely address the needs of people in smaller rural or remote areas.

In response, a handful of voluntary transportation programs have emerged to address the transportation needs of individuals with disabilities living in sparsely populated rural areas (e.g., Mathews, 1992). These programs range from agencies that coordinate volunteer rides to those that administer funds to subsidize individuals who seek their own transportation. They include organizations operated by statewide support groups for visually impaired adults (e.g., Visions Northwest, in Oregon) and local independent living centers (e.g., Summit, Inc., in Montana). These systems vary in their structure and operation but share the characteristic that transportation is provided by volunteers using their personal vehicles.

These programs offer a new alternative to rural transportation for people with disabilities: namely, to examine ways to employ natural community supports and to get resources for transportation directly to consumers. One model being explored by Brad Bernier, Steve Dalin, and Tom Seekins (1994) is referred to in general as Supported Voluntary Rural Transportation Systems (SVRTS). This project is evaluating the effectiveness of a rural transportation voucher system. Three sites in Alaska, South Dakota, and Montana are implementing such a voucher system to explore its utility, limitations, and costs.

Surprisingly, however, adults with physical disabilities living in rural areas do not rate transportation as being as much of a problem as other issues. Respondents to a national survey of adults with disabilities and living in rural areas rated the ability to get to where they were going as the forty-fifth problem of sixty-eight issues (Seekins, Jackson, and Dingman, 1991). Rehabilitation and consumer leaders have suggested that the relatively low rating accorded transportation problems is a function of consumers simply concluding that since nothing has been done and there are no clear solutions, nothing can be done. Others have pointed out that per capita ownership of personal vehicles is much higher in rural areas than in urban areas (Kidder, 1989). However, this is true only for those who can afford it, as 57 percent of rural poor families do not own a car (Gillis, 1989). The underlying assumption is that individuals who choose to reside in rural areas accept personal responsibility for transportation. Based on this perspective, a future direction will undoubtedly involve examining how personal transportation options can fill the gap.

Health and Medical Rehabilitation in Rural Areas. People with disabilities are at risk for a variety of secondary conditions (Marge, 1988; Pope & Tarlov, 1991). Many of these conditions are preventable or might be managed to maintain health and independence. Such efforts have become part of a national agenda for disability prevention.

Research suggests that adults with physical disabilities and living in rural areas may be particularly at risk for secondary complications. Rural service providers working with this population have rated access to support services and to health care providers knowledgeable about disabilities as a leading rural rehabilitation problem (Jackson et al., 1990; Seekins et al., 1990). Further, research has shown that adults with physical disabilities in Montana rate their overall health and independence as fair to poor, and experience limitations in daily activities due to an average of fourteen secondary conditions a year (e.g., Clay, Seekins, and Cowie, 1992; Seekins, Clay, and Ravesloot, 1994; Seekins, et al., 1991).

Gerbon DeJong (1979) argues that self-care is a primary foundation of independent living philosophy, yet there has been little systematic attention paid to health promotion for consumers. While adults with physical disabilities may be in the best situation to manage their own health, they may require access to specialized information and support services to do so efficiently. Such services and supports may include training in the use of cognitive strategies and behavioral practices that promote health and independence. In rural areas, however, consumers may be particularly isolated from such information and support. There is a need to develop mechanisms to support the efforts of adults with physical disabilities living in rural areas to prevent and manage secondary conditions.

One approach to such an effort is to build on the rural tradition of self-care. Tom Seekins (1992) reported that a simple workshop model for teaching consumers basic self-care and health management practices—delivered by independent living center staff in cooperation with local public health providers and other experts—was somewhat effective in reducing the severity of reported secondary conditions. Further, these services were provided at a cost of $15 per person per session that even included transportation to and from the workshops. Such self-help approaches to health promotion for people with disabilities may hold particular promise for those living in rural areas.

Other approaches focus on improving the transition from in-patient rehabilitation to home communities and improving the skills of local health care providers. For example, Summit, Inc., a rural independent living center, and Community Medical Center, a comprehensive in-patient rehab hospital, have developed a comprehensive transition planning process for rural patients that incorporates greater communication with hometown service providers prior to discharge and the establishment of a home-care program upon discharge.

The Center for Disability Policy and Research (1994) at the University of Washington is investigating access to primary health care services by people with disabilities and living in rural America. In a program focusing on one condition, dysphagia, Elizabeth Kohler (1991) reports on the development of a rural referral network that relies on direct care providers learning to identify symptoms of dysphagia risk, with referral to a trained network of consulting therapists. These two projects focus on building capacity among existing local providers who are generalists or paraprofessionals. It is unclear how pressures for insurance reform will affect rural Americans with disabilities.

Employment and Vocational Rehabilitation Approaches. Adults with work disabilities and living in nonmetropolitan areas of the United States are less likely to be in the workforce, more likely to be unemployed, and likely to earn less and have a smaller disposable income than their urban counterparts (Seekins, 1992). Importantly, those with disabilities appear to have less access to vocational rehabilitation service than their urban counterparts (Jackson, 1994).

While various rural economic development strategies are debated (Miller, 1985), entrepreneurial approaches, including self-employment, are advocated as an option of particular utility in rural areas (Malecki, 1988). Interestingly, the U.S. Bureau of the Census (1983) reports that people who report a work disability are nearly twice as likely to be self-employed (14.7%) as the general population (8%). While self-employment is used as a vocational rehabilitation closure more frequently in rural than in urban states, nationally it accounts for no more than 2.6 percent of closures annually.

Several innovative approaches using this strategy have recently emerged. Nancy Arnold and Thomas Seekins (1994) found that many state vocational rehabilitation policies hinder the use of self-employment and propose a policy framework intended to facilitate the use of self-employment. Thomas Seekins (1994) also suggests that sheltered

workshops in rural communities might "convert" portions of their programs to local business incubators serving the entire community. In a particularly innovative approach, Randall Brown (Verstegen & Nietupski, 1994) has used vocational rehabilitation resources to invest in businesses in their area. This has led to the initiation of several new businesses, the expansion of others, and the employment of vocational rehabilitation clients as business owners or employees. Further, it has made vocational rehabilitation one of the largest investors in business in the area and immensely improved its status within the business community. Such approaches, emerging from rural areas, may also have significant implications for urban areas.

Independent Living. Independent living centers (ILC) are community-based, nonprofit, nonresidential programs that are controlled by the consumers with disabilities they serve (Frieden, Richards, and Cole, 1979). These programs provide a wide range of services directly or through referral, including personal assistance services, peer counseling, independent living skills training, housing and transportation assistance, public and community education, rights and benefits counseling, social and recreational activities, and organized consumer advocacy.

Since their establishment in the Rehabilitation Act, more than 400 have emerged across the country. While most urban areas are served by an ILC, residents in fewer than 30 percent of the nation's 2,400 rural counties have even basic access to ILCs (Seekins, Ravesloot, and Maffit, 1992). Approximately 98 rural centers serve 44,000 people annually. Expanding services to all rural counties using this same model would reach approximately 150,000 individuals with severe disabilities who have access to few other services (Rural Institute on Disabilities, 1993). Such universal access to ILC services would also provide a broad infrastructure for involvement in rural community development by people with disabilities.

Technology. Assistive technology is sometimes the only need a person with a disability has. Unfortunately, it is often the most difficult service to acquire. For the broad population of rural residents with disabilities, the Technology Related Assistance for Individuals with Disabilities Act of 1988 specifies that rural and underserved areas are to receive special attention. One of the more innovative approaches followed in several states involves the development of local circles of support and ingenuity networks (Leech, 1993). Generally, these involve organizing local community resources to provide low-tech support to individuals rather than relying solely on high-tech support offered by medical suppliers.

A program of particular note serving rural areas is Breaking New Ground at Purdue University (Breaking New Ground Resource Center, 1991). Originally the program focused on developing equipment modifications for farmers with disabilities so they could continue to run their operations. The work of this group has led to extensive technical information about modifying agricultural tools and equipment for farmers with disabilities. It has also served as a model for the development of the AgrAbility Program sponsored by the U.S. Department of Agriculture. These programs, operated by the department's Extension Service in fourteen states, provide a wide range of education and support services to agricultural workers with disabilities and their families (U.S. Department of Agriculture, undated).

Housing. A major problem in rural areas is the availability of affordable, accessible housing. Since nearly 80 percent of the nation's manufactured housing stock is in rural America, several rehabilitation researchers are exploring issues of accessibility and ownership of both existing and new manufactured housing (Czerniak, 1988; Davidson, 1991). More importantly, disability advocates have worked with housing manufacturers to begin designing and providing manufactured housing that is accessible or that can be easily modified.

Native American Rehabilitation. Native Americans represent a significant minority population in the United States, especially in the twenty-six mainly western states (Clay, 1993). Although the smallest of the major American population groups, it is also perhaps the most diverse, with about 1.6 million Native Americans distributed among about 500 tribes and village units. Approximately 46 percent of the Native American population live on the 278 designated reservations, all but 2 with populations of fewer than 10,000 and often located in remote areas (U.S. Department of Education, 1987). Of those living on reservations, Julie Clay (1993)

estimates that as many as 105,000 have one or more chronic or permanent impairment.

Recognizing the cultural diversity between these tribal members and the majority culture, and the diversity of cultures among tribes, the Rehabilitation Services Administration has established tribal-controlled vocational rehabilitation programs, referred to as Section 130 Programs. Twenty-five tribal vocational rehabilitation programs are in operation. These programs typically operate close to their consumers, employ Native American staff of the same tribe, and recognize more traditional means of economic activity (e.g., self-sufficiency, hunting, etc.).

Of particular note, despite the fact that Native Americans have the highest rates of disability of any population group, tribal governments and reservations are specifically excluded from application of the Americans with Disabilities Act (Bazan, 1991). Julie Clay and her colleagues (1993), in collaboration with the National Congress of American Indians, have initiated a project to explore the development of a process that respects tribal sovereignty and cultural diversity, but that will allow tribal governments to consider their laws in relation to disability issues.

Trends in Rural Rehabilitation

Historically, rural advocates have strived for justice by advocating for the extension of the same benefits and services as urban advocates. The examples cited above and other efforts in rural disability and rehabilitation have begun to emphasize community development approaches. Rather than focus exclusively on trying to extend urban-based programs into rural areas, this new trend involves building on existing rural resources to develop contextually appropriate services and supports (e.g., Fawcett, Mathews, and Fletcher, 1980). One such approach, a resource management strategy (Jackson, Seekins, and Offner, 1992), assumes that it is unlikely (and perhaps undesirable) that there will ever be enough resources allocated to rural rehabilitation services to solve all problems using urban models. Rather, in the rural tradition, this approach asks how available resources can be redefined, redistributed, enhanced, extended, or supplemented to support the efforts of people with disabilities to live independent lives in their rural communities. Importantly, this approach often involves horizontal integration of community structures rather than the creation of separate or segregated programs—that is, redefining existing services (e.g., libraries) to provide support to people with disabilities in their communities. This trend exemplifies the spirit of the intent of the Americans with Disabilities Act.

(*See also:* ASSISTIVE TECHNOLOGY; CONSUMERS; HOUSING; INDEPENDENT LIVING; QUALITY OF LIFE; TECHNOLOGY; TRANSPORTATION ACCESSIBILITY)

RESOURCES

AgrAbility Projects, USDA Extension Service, Room 3346 South Building, Washington, DC 20250–0900

American Council on Rural Special Education (ACRES), 221 Milton Bennion Hall, Department of Special Education, University of Utah, Salt Lake City, UT 88412

American Hospital Association, Section for Small or Rural Hospitals, 840 North Lake Shore Drive, 5 East, Chicago, IL 60611

Association of Programs for Rural Independent Living (APRIL), Summit ILC, 1900 Brooks St., Suite 120, Missoula, MT 59801

Community Transportation Association of America, 1440 New York Ave., NW, Suite 440, Washington, DC 20005

Indiana Breaking New Ground Resource Center, Perdue University, 1146 Department of Agricultural Engineering, West Lafayette, IN 47907–1146

Montana University Affiliated Rural Institute on Disabilities, 52 Corbin Hall, University of Montana, Missoula, MT 59812

National Association for Rural Mental Health, P.O. Box 570, Wood River, IL 62095

National Council on the Aging, 600 Maryland Ave., SW, W. Wing, Washington, DC 20024

National Rural Health Association, One West Amour Blvd., Suite 301, Kansas City, MO 64111

RESNA Rural Technology Special Interest Group, 1700 North Moore St., Suite 1540, Arlington, VA 22209–1903

Rural Information Center, Room 304, National Agricultural Library, USDA, Beltsville, MD 20705

BIBLIOGRAPHY

AMERICAN HOSPITAL ASSOCIATION. *AHA Guide to the Health Care Field.* Chicago, 1989.

ARNOLD, NANCY, and SEEKINS, TOM. "Self-Employment as a Vocational Rehabilitation Closure: An Examination of State Policies." *Journal of Disability Policy Studies* 5 (1994):65–80.

BAZAN, ELIZABETH. *CRS Report for Congress: The Possible Applicability of the Americans with Disabilities Act to Indian Tribes.* Washington, DC, 1991.

BERNIER, BRAD; DALIN, STEVE; and SEEKINS, TOM. *Supported Volunteer Rural Transportation System.* Missoula, MT, 1994.

BLAKELY, EDWARD D., and BRADSHAW, TED K. "Implications of Social and Economic Changes on Rural Areas." *Human Services in the Rural Environment* 6 (1981):11–21.

BREAKING NEW GROUND RESEARCH CENTER. *Agricultural Tools, Equipment, Machinery, and Buildings for Farmers and Ranchers with Physical Disabilities.* West Lafayette, IN, 1991.

CENTER FOR DISABILITY POLICY AND RESEARCH. *Access to Primary Health Care Among Persons with Disabilities in Rural Areas: A Summary of the Literature.* Seattle, WA, 1994.

CLAY, JULIE. "Native American Independent Living." *Rural Special Education Quarterly* 11 (1992):41–50.

———. *American Indian Disability Legislation: Toward the Development of a Process that Respects Sovereignty and Cultural Diversity.* Missoula, MT, 1993.

CLAY, JULIE; SEEKINS, TOM; and COWIE, CECILIA. "Secondary Disabilities Among American Indians on Three Reservations in Montana." *Rural Special Education Quarterly* 11 (1992):20–25.

CORDES, SAM. "The Changing Rural Environment and the Relationship Between Health Services and Rural Development." *Health Services Research* 23 (1989):757–784.

COWARD, RAYMOND T., and CUTLER, STEPHEN A. "Informal and Formal Health Care Systems for the Rural Elderly." *Health Services Research* 23 (1989):785–806.

CZERNIAK, R. "Manufactured Homes as Affordable Housing in Rural Areas." Beltsville, MD, 1988.

DAVIDSON, CASEY. "Affordable Accessible Housing?" *Paraplegia News* (Aug. 1991) pp. 41–42.

DeFRIESE, GORDON, and RICKETTS, THOMAS. "Primary Health Care in Rural Areas: An Agenda for Research." *Health Services Research* 23 (1989):931–974.

DeJONG, GERBON. "Independent Living: From Social Movement to Analytic Paradigm." *Archives of Physical Medicine and Rehabilitation* 60 (1989):435–446.

FAWCETT, STEPHEN B.; MATHEWS, R. MARK; and FLETCHER, R. KAY. "Some Promising Dimensions for Behavioral Community Technology." *Journal of Applied Behavior Analysis* 13 (1980):505–518.

FRIEDEN, LEX.; RICHARDS, LAUREL.; and COLE, JEAN. *ILRU Sourcebook: A Technical Assistance Manual on Independent Living Research Utilization.* Houston, TX, 1979.

GILLIS, WILLIAM R. "Introduction: The Relevance of Rural Transportation." *Profitability and Mobility in Rural America,* ed. William R. Gillis. University Park, PA, 1989.

JACKSON, KATHLEEN O. *Vocational Rehabilitation: The Challenge of Equity in Rural Service Delivery.* Missoula, MT, 1994.

JACKSON, KATHLEEN, O.; SEEKINS, TOM; DINGMAN, SHERRI; and RAVESLOOT, CRAIG. *Rural Transition Issues: Report of the Rehabilitation Facility Survey.* Missoula, MT, 1990.

JACKSON, KATHLEEN O.; SEEKINS, TOM; and OFFNER, RICHARD. "Involving Consumers and Service Providers in Shaping Rural Rehabilitation Agenda." *American Rehabilitation* 18 (1992):23–29, 48.

KIDDER, ALICE. "Passenger Transportation Problems in Rural Areas." *Profitability and Mobility in Rural America,* ed. William R. Gillis. University Park, PA, 1989.

KOHLER, ELISABETH S. "A Dysphagia Management Model for Rural Elderly." *Physical and Occupational Therapy in Geriatrics* 10 (1991):81–95.

LAPLANTE, MITCHELL. *Data on Disability from the National Health Interview Survey, 1983–85: An InfoUse Report.* Washington, DC, 1988.

LEECH, PETER. "Assistive Tools for Independent Living: Developing Local Circles of Support." *Proceedings of the 1993 Common Threads Conference,* eds. Kathy Dwyer, Diana Spas, and Susan Duffy. Missoula, MT, 1993.

LELAND, MICHAEL, and SCHNEIDER, MARY JO. *Rural Rehabilitation: A State of the Art.* Fayetteville, AR, 1982.

MALECKI, EDWARD J. "New Firm Startups: Key to Rural Growth." *Rural Development Perspectives* 4 (1988):18–23.

MARGE, MICHAEL. "Health Promotion for Persons with Disabilities: Moving Beyond Rehabilitation." *American Journal of Health Promotion* 2 (1988):29–44.

MATHEMATICA POLICY RESEARCH, INC. *Digest of Data on Persons with Disabilities.* Washington, DC, 1984.

MATHEWS, R. MARK. "Innovations in Rural Independent Living." *American Rehabilitation* 18 (1992):11–13.

MILLER, JAMES P. "Rethinking Small Business as the Best Way to Create Rural Jobs." *Rural Development Perspective* 1 (1985):9–12.

MOSCOVICE, IRA. "Rural Hospitals: A Literature Synthesis and Health Services Research Agenda." *Health Services Research* 23 (1989):891–930.

NORTON, CATHERINE, and MCMANUS, MARGARET. "Background Tables on Demographic Characteristics, Health Status, and Health Services Utilization." *Health Services Research* 23 (1989):725–756.

NOSEK, MARGARET; ZHU, YILIN; and HOWLAND, CAROL. "The Evolution of Independent Living Programs." *Rehabilitation Counseling Bulletin* 35 (1992):174–189.

OFFNER, RICHARD. "The Challenge of Rural Rehabilitation Services in the 90s." *Journal of Rehabilitation Administration* (1990):97–98, 122.

OMOHUNDRO, JULIE; SCHNEIDER, MARY JO; MARR, JOHN, N.; and GRANNEMANN, BRUCE D. "A Four County Needs Assessment of Rural Disabled People." *Journal of Rehabilitation* (1983):19–24.

PAGE, CHARLES. "Rural Rehabilitation: It's Time Now." In *Meeting the Rehabilitation Needs of Rural America,* ed. Gill Foss. Missoula, MT, 1989.

POPE, ANDREW M., and TARLOV, ALVIN R. *Disability in America: Toward a National Agenda for Prevention.* Washington, DC, 1991.

RASMUSSEN, WAYNE D. "90 Years of Rural Development Programs." *Rural Development Perspectives* 2 (1985):2–9.

RECZYNSKI, DEBORAH; TIBBS, BELZA; and TURK, LORI. *Environmental Assessment for Rural Hospitals 1988.* Chicago, 1987.

RICHARDS, LAUREL. *Independent Living in Rural America: The Real Frontier.* Houston, TX, 1984.

ROJEWSKI, JAY. "Vocational Rehabilitation in Rural America: Challenges and Opportunities." *American Rehabilitation* 18 (1992):39–44.

ROWLAND, DIANE, and LYONS, BARBARA. "Triple Jeopardy: Rural, Poor, and Uninsured." *Health Services Research* 23 (1989):975–1004.

RURAL INSTITUTE ON DISABILITIES. *Universal Access to Independent Living Services: Estimating Federal Costs in Rural Areas.* Missoula, MT, 1993.

SEEKINS, TOM. *Rural and Urban Employment Patterns: Self-Employment as a Metaphor for Rural Vocational Rehabilitation.* Missoula, MT, 1992.

———. "From Sheltered Workshop to Business Incubator: A Rural Economic Development Model." *Goodwill Forum* 8 (1994):10–12.

SEEKINS, TOM; CLAY, JULIE; and RAVESLOOT, CRAIG. "A Descriptive Study of Secondary Conditions Reported by a Population of Adults with Physical Disabilities Served by Three Independent Living Centers in a Rural State." *Journal of Rehabilitation* 60 (1994):47–51.

SEEKINS, TOM; JACKSON, KATHLEEN O.; and DINGMAN, SHERRI. *Rural Rehabilitation Issues from the Consumers Perspective.* Missoula, MT, 1991.

SEEKINS, TOM; JACKSON, KATHLEEN O.; and OFFNER, RICHARD. *Demography of Rural Disability.* Missoula, MT, 1991.

SEEKINS, TOM; RAVESLOOT, CRAIG; JACKSON, KATHLEEN. O.; and DINGMAN, SHERRI. *Transitions from Rehabilitation Hospital to Rural Independent Living: Survey Results from Rural Independent Living Centers.* Missoula, MT, 1990.

SEEKINS, TOM; RAVESLOOT, CRAIG; and MAFFIT, BOB. "Extending the Independent Living Center Model to Rural Areas: Expanding Services Through State and Local Efforts." *Rural Special Education Quarterly* 11 (1992):11–15.

SEEKINS, TOM; SMITH, NAOMI; McCLEARY, TIM; CLAY, JULIE; and WALSH, JAMES. "Secondary Disability Prevention: Involving Consumers in the Development of Policy and Program Options." *Journal of Disability Policy Studies* 1 (1991):21–35.

TONSING-GONZALES, LINDA. "Rural Independent Living: Conquering the Final Frontier." *Meeting the Rehabilitation Needs of Rural Americans*, ed. Gilbert Foss, Missoula, MT, 1989.

U.S. BUREAU OF THE CENSUS. *Rural and Rural Farm Population: 1988.* Washington, DC, 1988.

———. *Labor Force Status and Other Characteristics of Persons with a Work Disability: 1982.* Washington, DC, 1983.

U.S. CONGRESS. *The Rehabilitation Act of 1973.* Washington, DC, 1973.

———. *Technology Related Assistance for Individuals with Disabilities Act of 1988.* Washington, DC, 1988.

U.S. DEPARTMENT OF AGRICULTURE. *AgrAbility Project: Promoting Access in Agriculture for People with Disabilities and Their Families.* Washington, DC, undated.

U.S. DEPARTMENT OF EDUCATION. *A Report of the Special Problems and Needs of American Indians with Handicaps Both on and off the Reservation.* Washington, DC, 1987.

VERSTEGEN, DALE, and NIETUPSKI, JOHN. *Increasing Employment Opportunities for Individuals with Disabilities Through Economic Development: Creating Business and Corporate Initiatives.* Richmond, VA, 1994.

THOMAS W. SEEKINS

RUSK, HOWARD A.

In 1946, a genial, strapping physician from Missouri brought to New York University (NYU) Medical Center his experiences in wartime injury rehabilitation techniques. Against conventional wisdom and at considerable personal sacrifice, Dr. Howard Archibald Rusk (1901–1989) undertook what was to become a lifelong mission—the development of rehabilitation procedures that would become part of standard medical practice throughout the world.

Before his death from stroke at age eighty-eight, Dr. Rusk became known as the father of rehabilitation medicine and saw one of the world's foremost institutions of rehabilitation medicine—NYU Medical Center's Howard A. Rusk Institute of Rehabilitation Medicine—named in his honor.

For five decades, Dr. Rusk's concern was "what happens to people after the stitches are out and the fever is down." Then, he said in a 1982 interview, "the crucial task is to take them back into the best lives they can live with what they have left."

At the heart of Dr. Rusk's approach to rehabilitation medicine is the concept that it should focus on the whole patient, including emotional, psychological, vocational, and other behavioral needs associated with the patient's disability.

Because of Dr. Rusk's concept, millions of persons with disabilities who would have become forgotten members of society are leading better-quality and more productive lives today than anyone would have thought possible just a few generations ago.

Dr. Rusk was born April 9, 1901, in Brookfield, Missouri, the son of Michael and Augusta Rusk. He graduated from Brookfield High School, earned a bachelor's degree from the University of Missouri, and received his medical degree in 1925 from the University of Pennsylvania Medical School.

From 1926 to 1942 he practiced as a specialist in internal medicine in St. Louis and served as associate chief of staff at St. Luke's Hospital there. He later joined the medical school faculty at Washington University in St. Louis.

Dr. Rusk's ideas about rehabilitation medicine began taking shape while he was serving in the Army Air Force Medical Corps during World War II. His work with people with disabilities was spurred by the anguish he said he felt when "wounded boys from the battlefield began being packed into hospitals by the planeload. Suddenly we were faced with men with broken bodies and, all too often, broken spirits," he wrote in his 1977 autobiography *A World to Care For.*

One of his early projects was a "training in bed" program designed to occupy wounded soldiers productively as they recuperated from war injuries. From their beds, mechanics were soon repairing altimeters and radio operators were practicing coded messages. Eventually, similar methods were introduced at twelve special military centers for people with severe wounds—people with paraplegia, amputations, and visual impairments.

Dr. Rusk went on to revolutionize the training of physicians and other health professionals, developed innovative techniques in rehabilitation medicine, and established the field internationally as an important new medical specialty.

From 1946 to 1969 Dr. Rusk propounded many of his ideas on rehabilitation and other medical topics as a weekly columnist for the *New York Times.* In 1946 he founded the world's first comprehensive medical training program in rehabilitation medicine: the Department of Rehabilitation at the New York University School of Medicine.

Two years later, with the help of more than $1 million donated by financier Bernard Baruch, Dr. Rusk founded the Institute of Physical Medicine and Rehabilitation at NYU Medical Center and served as its director until 1978.

The institute, now named the Howard A. Rusk Institute of Rehabilitation Medicine, works with both inpatients and outpatients with disabilities and sends a high percentage of patients on to school or gainful employment.

Dr. Rusk also served as president of the World Rehabilitation Fund, which he founded in 1955. Through the fund, the Rusk Institute has drawn up programs for professionals in more than 150 countries and has trained several thousand physicians, psychologists, and other specialists in advanced rehabilitation techniques.

Over the years Dr. Rusk was variously a consultant on rehabilitation to the Veterans Administration, the U.N. Secretariat, and the New York City Department of Hospitals; president of the International Society for the Rehabilitation of the Disabled; and an adviser to seven presidents.

In his work, Dr. Rusk truly was a world citizen. He directed refugee and health programs during the conflicts in Korea and Vietnam and established a cooperative Israel–Egypt program of care for people with brain damage. In 1967 he was sent to Vietnam by President Lyndon Johnson to help in coordinating relief projects.

During his long tenure as a physician, Dr. Rusk had a number of famous patients, including Joseph P. Kennedy, the father of President John F. Kennedy; the baseball player Roy Campanella; bandleader Vincent Lopez; and U.S. Supreme Court justice William O. Douglas.

Outside the realm of rehabilitation, Dr. Rusk was an early advocate of enlarging public health programs for the growing number of elderly people, including those affected by dementia.

An articulate and eloquent spokesman for rehabilitation medicine, he wrote six books and more than 500 articles on the subject. His more than 200 awards included twenty-three honorary university degrees, the French Legion of Honor, America's Distinguished Service Medal, and three separate Albert Lasker Foundation awards, one for work in the public health field and two for services to persons with physical disabilities.

Dr. Rusk often said that it was the incredible force of hope among persons with disabilities that enabled rehabilitation medicine to harness their latent abilities, and that it was persons with disabilities who "produced their own miracles."

But it took Dr. Rusk to recognize that force and to find ways to make those miracles possible.

RESOURCE

Rusk Institute of Rehabilitation Medicine, 400 East 34th St., New York, NY 10016

BIBLIOGRAPHY

RUSK, HOWARD A. *A World to Care For.* New York, 1977.

DAN PERKES

S

SCHIZOPHRENIA

Schizophrenia is arguably the most chronic and severe of the mental illnesses. Frequently mistaken for multiple or split personality by the general public, it remains an illness shrouded in mystery and fear. All too often, the public's first glimpse of this illness comes from a tabloid headline such as "Paranoid Schizophrenic Runs Amok." Yet, most people suffering from schizophrenia are not violent; rather, they are confused, lonely, and in despair. Data suggest that they are much more likely to be victims of crime and violence rather than perpetrators (Teplin, 1991).

Although some would argue that the illness is a derivative of recent times, most are willing to accept ancient writings that describe conditions like schizophrenia going back several millennia. First conceptualized in 1919 by Emil Kraepelin (1971) and called dementia praecox, the condition was described as the early onset of a dementing illness. Kraepelin further concluded that if a person recovered from this condition, it was highly unlikely that the diagnosis was correct. In his original sample only 12 percent returned to baseline functioning. The name "schizophrenia" was applied to this condition by Eugen Bleuler (1950). While Kraepelin took a descriptive or phenomenologic approach to the illness, Bleuler focused on underlying dynamic processes and deficits—the "four a's"—ambivalence, autistic behavior, affect that was limited or flat, and associations that were loose. He departed from the Kraepelinian concept by pointing out that it was not necessarily either an illness that began early, nor one that had a dementing or uniformly poor outcome. Until the 1970s Bleuler's concept was far more influential in the United States than in most of Europe, where Kraepelinian concepts achieved primacy. Since the 1970s, as a direct result of cross-national studies of schizophrenia and influential studies done in the United States, American psychiatry has taken a more descriptive or phenomenological approach to diagnosis than had been the case earlier.

The term "schizophrenia" is derived from the Greek meaning "split mind." This definition engenders the incorrect image of "split personality" noted above. What is split in schizophrenia, however, is the mind's capacity to determine what is real from what is not. The mind begins to misinterpret both internal and external stimuli. Internal thoughts become "heard" as voices—hallucinations. External images—a stranger smiling—become distorted into unshakable beliefs—delusions. The basic fabric of a person's life disintegrates with the loss of will, pleasure, emotional range, and spontaneity.

Definitions of Schizophrenia

Unlike many other areas of medicine, there are no laboratory tests or pathognomonic symptoms that can make the diagnosis of schizophrenia with certainty. The current convention relies on symptoms that can be reliably defined and that represent the best fit of research on nosology (the classification of diseases), genetics, treatment, and clinical course. The diagnosis was revised three times from 1974 to 1994, and in 1994 the version in the *Diagnostic and Statistical Manual* (DSM-IV) of the American Psychiatric Association became the standard (Andreasen & Carpenter, 1993). The following are the symptoms from DSM-IV that define schizophrenia:

A. *Characteristic Symptoms: At least two of the following, each present for a significant length of time during a one-month period (or less if successfully treated):*

1. Delusions
2. Hallucinations
3. Disorganized speech
4. Grossly disorganized or catatonic behavior
5. Negative symptoms, i.e., affective flattening, alogia (impoverished thinking and cognition), or avolition (lack of drive, interest, or energy)

[Note: only one "A" symptom is required if delusions are bizarre or hallucinations consist of a voice keeping up a running commentary on the person's behavior or thought, or two or more voices conversing with each other.]

B. *Social/Occupational Dysfunction*

C. *Duration: Continuous signs of the disturbance persist for at least six months.*

In addition, there are several exclusion criteria—schizoaffective and mood disorder, and substance-related/general medical conditions.

In summary, the illness as currently defined pre-sents with psychotic symptoms (hallucinations or delusions); thought disorder as manifested through disorganized speech; and negative symptoms of affective flattening, alogia, or avolition. It requires a period of social or occupational dysfunction and must last in either the fully manifest condition or an attenuated form for at least six months. The major change between the earlier DSM-III and DSM-III-R versions and DSM-IV was the requirement that the characteristic "A" symptoms last for one month instead of one week. It was felt that this increase in duration would eliminate "false positives" (those given the diagnosis who did not actually have it) and therefore the accompanying potential stigmatizing impact of the label of schizophrenia. For those whose characteristic symptoms lasted less than one month, the diagnosis would most likely be brief psychotic disorder. For those whose characteristic symptoms lasted one month or longer but who recovered fully before six months, the diagnosis would be schizophreniform disorder. And for delusional disorder, the essential feature is the presence of a persistent, nonbizarre delusion.

Epidemiology and Course

Schizophrenia (combined with schizophreniform disorder) affects 1.5 percent of the U.S. population (Keith, Regier, and Rae, 1991). This fact makes schizophrenia six times more common than muscular dystrophy, eighty times more common than Huntington's disease, and slightly more common than severe diabetes (as defined by requiring hospitalization). The illness spares no single group of people. It occurs equally in men and women, although the onset of the illness is three to four years earlier in men, and they are more likely to have a poorer long-term outcome than women. Comparing socioeducational status (SES) shows an eightfold increase for the lowest when compared to the highest social class (Keith, Regier, and Rae, 1991). In terms of outcome, however, the poorest outcomes are seen in the lowest and the highest social classes, with better outcomes for those in between. If SES status is controlled, there is no difference in prevalence among African Americans, Hispanics, and Caucasians. People suffering from schizophrenia are less likely to be married, less likely to have completed a college education, and have a high suicide rate—among males approaching 10 percent in the first ten years of the illness.

Its onset may be relatively sudden, over a period of a few days, or, more common, insidiously over an extended period of time. Two common developmental patterns exemplify these patterns of onset. The first would be college students who may have been overachievers in high school, but to their friends and family, may have seemed destined for a life of full productivity. At some time in their first year of college, during what for many may be their first extended time away from home, their behavior begins to alter, sleep patterns may be disrupted, and finally their thinking becomes confused, and they become delusional or may begin to hallucinate. The insidious onset course of illness often begins in childhood with missed developmental milestones, odd behavior, and social isolation. At some point in adolescence, the transition toward frank hallucinations or delusions may occur and the diagnosis of schizophrenia can be made. Early diagnosis is often difficult in the adolescent age group, as this developmental period is often fraught with behavior that may be erratic and difficult, and problems with identity are quite common. Alternative or rapidly changing diagnoses are common, and it is not until the person begins to add the characteristic "A" symptoms that the diagnosis becomes more clear. Even here, however, the use of alcohol and drugs can complicate the diagnosis. Studies have indicated that almost 50 percent of those with a diagnosis of schizophrenia will also have a substance use disorder (Regier et al., 1993).

Fewer than 20 percent to 25 percent of those suffering from schizophrenia will have a full recovery. An equal percent will have a steadily deteriorating course, refractory to most therapeutic interventions. The remaining 50 percent will have an intermittent course of the illness, interrupting development, education, careers, and repeatedly destroying attempts to carry on a life once filled with such promise. The course of this illness spawns additional health problems, making the person with schizophrenia twice as likely to die at any age from medical causes as the general population.

Etiology and Pathophysiology

Although for descriptive purposes we refer to schizophrenia as though it were a single illness, it would probably be more accurate to refer to it etiologically and pathophysiologically as the schizophrenias. Because the underlying causes and processes that bring about the symptoms of schizophrenia are most likely heterogeneous, and the brain is such a difficult organ to access, the etiology and pathophysiology have remained elusive. Just as a symptom such as shortness of breath may have as its underlying cause heart or lung disease, but may have as the causal agent a bacteria, virus, cigarette smoke, or congenital malformations, and may have environmental contributors such as altitude or exercise, so schizophrenic symptomatology may come from a diverse constellation of causality.

We have strong evidence that some elements of this illness are genetic. As noted above, the prevalence of schizophrenia in the general population is 1.5 percent. If one has a parent with schizophrenia, the risk is 10 percent. If one has two parents with schizophrenia, the risk is 40 percent. And if one's identical twin has schizophrenia, the risk is 50 percent. While this is impressive evidence that genetics are involved, it also points out that there may be more than genetics operating, for if it were purely a genetic disorder, one would expect 100 percent risk for identical twins, one of whom developed schizophrenia. In a creative exploration of just this situation, a group led by Dr. E. Fuller Torrey examined identical twins in which only one twin had schizophrenia (Suddath et al., 1990). In comparing the affected with the unaffected twin, they found neurophysiological and anatomical differences with the affected twin more severely involved. The explanation for these biological changes remains elusive, but possible causes including neonatal hypoxia, intrauterine infection, or viral infection at a critical developmental period early in life are all being considered.

On a neurochemical basis, neurotransmitter studies have been major contributors to our potential understanding of underlying mechanisms of schizophrenia and, perhaps even more significantly, to development of new pharmacological treatments. For many years, one neurotransmitter (the chemical messengers that conduct impulses from one nerve cell to another), dopamine, has been the major focus of investigation. Although antipsychotic medication was introduced in the early 1950s, it was not until ten years later that Arvid Carlsson and M. Lindqvist presented a potential mechanism of action for these drugs: They all caused a dopamine receptor blockade. From this observation Carlsson and Lindqvist developed the "dopamine hypothesis" of schizophrenia that has dominated the field since the middle to late 1960s. We know, however, that these drugs do more than operate on the dopamine system and that the dopamine system itself is not as simple as we once thought, with, at the present time, five distinct dopamine receptors having been cloned. Further, the impact of a new generation of antipsychotics would seem to cover the serotonin system, alpha receptors, and sigma receptors. The future is bright for the development of a rational pharmacology looking at various combinations of multiple receptor activity for providing improved responsiveness to the various forms of schizophrenia.

Although their contribution to the understanding of schizophrenia is just beginning, new "windows" into the human brain hold much promise for the further delineation of schizophrenia. Magnetic resonance imaging, spectroscopy, positron emission tomography, and other developing technologies are beginning to shed new light on underlying causes and mechanisms of this illness.

Of the potential elements that contribute to the etiologies of schizophrenia, the era of blaming families or interactions within families seems to have passed. Few if any clinicians hold to this particularly painful era of psychiatry, when families were blamed for causing the illness, excluded from its treatment, and yet expected to support this sometimes financially ruinous condition. Families are now looked on as being important clinical allies in the treatment of schizophrenia, as will be discussed below.

Treatment

The available treatments for schizophrenia can be grouped as follows: medication, psychosocial treatment, and the combination of the two.

In the medication arena, antipsychotic medica-tions, also referred to as neuroleptics, are typically prescribed to treat the positive or psychotic symptoms of schizophrenia. Some of the better-known ones include chlorpromazine (Thorazine), haloperidol (Haldol), fluphenzine (Prolixin), and thioridazine (Mellaril). The choice of medication may vary from one patient to another, dependent on a patient's previous response to a particular medication, family history of response, and side effects. The more common side effects include drowsiness, shakiness, muscle stiffness, and restlessness, most of which are generally mild and can be controlled by adjusting the medication dosage or by addition of an ancillary medication. However, tardive dyskinesia (TD)—a neurological syndrome of movements often in the lips, jaw, or tongue, and sometimes involving the legs, feet, hands, or even in severe cases the entire body—can be a severe side effect associated with neuroleptic treatment. Dilip V. Jeste and Michael P. Caligiuri (1993) report that the overall mean prevalence rate of TD is approximately 24 percent for patients treated over several years, with the rate being higher in older patients. The risk of such side effects must be weighed against their well-documented efficacy. Controlled clinical trials conducted from the mid-1950s to the mid-1990s support standard antipsychotic medications as being effective in reducing the acute psychotic symptoms associated with schizophrenia in about 60 percent of patients (Schooler & Keith, 1993), with the success rate even higher (70% to 85%) in patients experiencing psychotic symptoms for the first time (Lieberman et al., 1992). However, a majority of patients (60%) will experience subsequent relapse, even when antipsychotic medication is maintained. This finding holds true even for patients who are experiencing their first episode of illness. Although some studies of maintenance antipsychotic treatment for first-episode patients have been able to demonstrate efficacy in the first year—relapse rate of 41 percent for patients on placebo versus none on continued medication (Kane et al., 1985)—by two years, even first-episode patients show the all-too-frequent relapse patterns—62 percent for placebo versus 46 percent for active medication (Crow et al., 1986). Armed with the recognition that antipsychotic medication does not eliminate the risk of relapse for schizophrenia, researchers have examined strategies to maximize the benefits of medication while reducing the unwanted side effects by trying to find the lowest possible dose of medication that effectively protects against relapse. As might be anticipated, medication affords protection from periods of symptom exacerbation, and the greater the reduction in dosage, the more necessary it is that this strategy be embedded in a system that can carefully monitor and respond to patients' clinical needs. Finally, new medications have been introduced—risperidone, a first-line medication, and clozapine, for patients who are consistently nonresponsive to traditional antipsychotic treatment. Although clozapine has shown beneficial results (effective in about one-third of patients previously unresponsive to all treatments), it requires close patient monitoring for potentially life-threatening side effects (e.g., agranulocytosis—a marked decrease in the number of granulocytes). Experience with its use in more than 25,000 patients in the United States shows the cumulative risk of agranulocytosis after 1½ years of treatment to be 0.91 percent (Lieberman & Alvir, 1992).

In the psychosocial area, treatments that have been systematically explored include individual, group, and family treatments. Although the results of research investigations have found some limited support for the value of individual and group therapies in enhancing patient outcome, when used in an intensive manner their role in good patient supportive care is important. Family treatment has been an area of most intense investigation, showing promising results.

Many people with schizophrenia are discharged from treatment facilities to the care of their families. Thus the family is a natural resource for providing treatment. It is important to realize that modern family treatment of schizophrenia focuses on the positive aspects of including families in the care of family members with schizophrenia. Older theories implicating the family in causing schizophrenia are no longer accepted by most mental health professionals. A body of research has accumulated on effective family treatment strategies that may provide additional protection from relapse through stress reduction, and address the often enduring negative symptoms of schizophrenia, including impairments in social, work, and general community functioning. Although the specifics of family treatment interventions have varied, the following principles are common among reported studies:

1. engagement of the family in a positive therapeutic alliance;
2. provision of psychoeducational material about schizophrenia;
3. introduction of social learning principles of problem-solving and interpersonal communication skills to the family to enhance management of everyday stresses and major life events;
4. enhancement of family social networks, particularly through mutual support groups.

Data from extant studies show that family treatment offers substantial benefit to patients, especially when combined with optimal medication treatment. For example, Ian R. H. Falloon, Jeffrey L. Boyd, and Christine W. McGill (1984) reported that providing families with a home-based behavior family therapy was superior to routine clinical supportive care in preventing major symptomatic exacerbations (6% versus 44%), symptom remission (56% versus 22%), and community tenure (e.g., readmission in 11% of cases versus 50%). In a study by Michael Goldstein and colleagues (1978) using brief (six-week), crisis-oriented family sessions, no patients receiving both family therapy and a standard dose of medication relapsed, compared to 9 percent for those on low dose and family therapy, 10 percent for standard dose and no family therapy, and 24 percent for low dose and no family therapy. Overall, 4.5 percent of patients receiving family therapy relapsed, compared to 17 percent of those not receiving family therapy; and 5 percent of patients receiving standard dose versus 16.5 percent on low dose relapsed. At six months, the same pattern of relapse was reported. Consistent across these studies and others is the finding that family treatment can be implemented in a variety of settings (clinic, home) and that the influence of patient and family participation on treatment may significantly enhance patient outcome.

Rehabilitation

Rehabilitation of people with schizophrenia is an important aspect of their long-term management. Persons with schizophrenia typically experience the disorder during a period when they were trying to complete important developmental tasks, such as completing an education or initiating a career. Rehabilitation focuses on the person's functional status and quality of life, with the goal to provide individuals with the skills and support needed to function in their environment. As with impairments produced by physical illnesses, those produced by schizophrenia may require extended rehabilitation. Additionally, a majority of patients desire rehabilitation in one form or another, with employment and vocational rehabilitation most often sought after (Nagaswami et al., 1985), underscoring the importance of including rehabilitation in the overall scheme of providing comprehensive treatment for patients.

In a review of psychiatric rehabilitation by Charles Wallace (1993), the ability of patients to learn new skills and to transfer these skills to new settings was described, although patients tend to perform better in their teaching environments. Comprehensive, intensive social skills training can significantly lower symptoms and delay relapse (Liberman et al., 1986). However, as noted by Robert Liberman and Michael Green (1992), rehabilitation efforts should be congruent with laboratory findings of specific cognitive and information processing deficits often found in schizophrenia. These deficits (e.g., misinterpretation of social interactions) may endure beyond the period of acute psychotic symptomatology and must be considered when designing rehabilitation programs. Several rehabilitation paradigms—for example, UCLA Social and Independent Living Skills Program (Liberman et al., 1986)—have been proposed to address these deficits and incorporate cognitive and behavioral methods in the teaching of skills. The findings have been positive (Eckman et al., 1992), with patients making significant gains in each of the areas taught. But, as noted by Charles Wallace (1993), "These positive outcomes, however, are conditional. They are achieved when the methods of teaching role skills are tailored to individuals' cognitive impairments and disabilities; when there is a partnership between the teaching and the environment so that the one supports the other; and when the full range of clinical services are provided on a schedule and with an intensity that fit the ongoing course of each individual's illness" (p. 220).

While complex and difficult to implement, it is critical that comprehensive treatment and rehabilitation programs be established to meet the myriad of needs for patients with schizophrenia. Leonard Stein and Mary Ann Test (1980) developed an effective model program, the Training in Community Living (TCL) program, which has been replicated in twenty states. The program provides comprehensive care and includes the following factors, which Stein and Test believe to be critical for effective community adjustment:

1. material resources, such as food, shelter, clothing, and medical care;
2. coping skills to meet the demands of community life;
3. motivation to persevere and remain involved with life;
4. freedom from pathologically dependent relationships;
5. support and education of community members who are involved with patients;
6. a supportive system that assertively helps the patient with the previous five requirements.

The results have been quite positive (reduced hospitalization, enhanced community tenure, and patient adjustment); however, the positive impact of the program does not extend beyond a patient's actual participation in the program. Thus rehabilitation cannot be a short-term effort but rather has been shown to be effective when provided in an ongoing manner (congruent with the ongoing nature of schizophrenia as described above).

Schizophrenia is indeed a complex illness, causing disruption in the major areas of a person's life: cognition, affect, and behavior. The effects tend to be enduring, often leading to a life of ongoing disability. Treatments are effective in providing symptomatic relief, but in many instances the empty, joyless existence continues. It becomes particularly important then to look at those psychosocial treatments that can be delivered through and in the environment in which the patient lives— family treatment and rehabilitation. The value of comprehensive treatment programs cannot be underestimated. We may not have all the answers we need, but we must not fail to apply the ones we have.

(*See also:* FAMILY; PHARMACOLOGY; PSYCHIATRIC REHABILITATION; PSYCHIATRY; PSYCHOLOGY)

BIBLIOGRAPHY

ANDREASEN, NANCY C., and CARPENTER, WILLIAM T. "Diagnosis and Classification of Schizophrenia." *Schizophrenia Bulletin* 19 (1993):199–214.

BLEULER, EUGEN. *Dementia Praecox or the Group of Schizophrenias,* trans. Joseph Zinkin. New York, 1950.

CARLSSON, ARVID, and LINDQVIST, M. "Effect of Chlorpromazine or Haloperidol on Formation of 3-Methoxytyramine and Normetanephrine in Mouse Brain." *Acta Pharmacologica* 20 (1963):140–144.

CROW, THOMAS J.; MACMILLAN, J. F.; JOHNSON, A. L.; and JOHNSTONE, E. C. "The Northwick Park Study of First Episodes of Schizophrenia. II. A Randomized Clinical Trial of Prophylactic Neuroleptic Treatment." *British Journal of Psychiatry* 148 (1986):120–127.

ECKMAN, THAD; WIRSHING, WILLIAM; MARDER, STEPHEN; LIBERMAN, ROBERT; JOHNSTON-CRONK, KATHLEEN; ZIMMERMAN, KARIN; and MINTZ, JIM. "Technique for Training Schizophrenic Patients in Illness Self-Management: A Controlled Trial." *American Journal of Psychiatry* 149 (1992):1549–1555.

FALLOON, IAN R. H.; BOYD, JEFFREY L.; and McGILL, CHRISTINE W. *Family Care of Schizophrenia.* New York, 1984.

GOLDSTEIN, MICHAEL; RODNICK, ELIOT; EVANS, JEROME; MAY, PHILIP; and STEINBERG, MARK. "Drug and Family Therapy in the Aftercare of Acute Schizophrenics." *Archives of General Psychiatry* 35 (1978):1169–1177.

JESTE, DILIP V., and CALIGIURI, MICHAEL P. "Tardive Dyskinesia." *Schizophrenia Bulletin* 19 (1993):303–315.

KANE, JOHN M.; RIFKIN, ARTHUR; WOERNER, MARGARET; REARDON, GERALD; KREISMAN, DELORES; BLUMENTHAL, RICHARD; and BORENSTEIN, MICHAEL. "High Dose vs. Low Dose Strategies in the Treatment of Schizophrenia." *Psychopharmacology Bulletin* (1985):533–537.

KEITH, SAMUEL J.; REGIER, DARREL A.; and RAE, DONALD S. "Schizophrenic Disorders." In *Psychiatric Disorders in America,* eds. Lee N. Robbins and Darrel A. Regier. New York, 1991.

KRAEPELIN, EMIL. *Dementia Praecox and Paraphrenia,* trans. and ed. R. Mary Barclay and George M. Robertson. Huntington, NY, 1971.

LIEBERMAN, JEFFREY A., and ALVIR, JOSÉ M. J. "A Report of Clozapine-Induced Agranulocytosis in the United States." *Drug Safety* 7 (1992):1–2.

LIEBERMAN, JEFFREY A.; ALVIR, JOSÉ M. J.; WOERNER, MARGARET; DEGREEF, GUSTAV; BILDER, ROBERT; ASHARI, MANGAR; BOGERTS, BERNHARD; MAYERHOFF, DAVID; GEISLEY, STEPHEN; LOEBEL, ANTONY; LEVY, DEBORAH; HINRICHSEN, GREGORY; SZYMANSKI, SALLY; CHAKOS, MIRANDA; KOREEN, AMY; BORENSTEIN, MICHAEL; and KANE, JOHN. "Prospective Study of Psychobiology in First-Episode Schizophrenia at Hillside Hospital." *Schizophrenia Bulletin* 18 (1992):351–371.

LIBERMAN, ROBERT, and GREEN, MICHAEL. "Whither Cognitive-Behavioral Therapy for Schizophrenia?" *Schizophrenia Bulletin* 18 (1992):27–35.

LIBERMAN, ROBERT; MUESER, KIM; WALLACE, CHARLES; JACOBS, HARVEY; ECKMAN, THAD; and MASSEL, H. KEITH. "Training Skills in the Severely Psychiatrically Disabled: Learning Coping and Competence." *Schizophrenia Bulletin* 12 (1986):631–647.

NAGASWAMI, VIGAY; VALECHA, VIJAYALAKSHUMI; THARA, R.; RAJKUMAR, S.; and MENON, M. SARADA. "Rehabilitation Needs of Schizophrenic Patients: A Preliminary Report." *Indian Journal of Psychiatry* 27 (1985):213–220.

REGIER, DARREL A.; NARROW, WILLIAM E.; RAE, DONALD; MANDERSCHEID, RONALD W.; LOCKE, BEN Z; and GOODWIN, FREDERICK K. "The De Facto US Mental and Addictive Disorders Service System." *Archives of General Psychiatry* 50 (1993):85–94.

SCHOOLER, NINA R., and KEITH, SAMUEL J. "The Clinical Base for the Treatment of Schizophrenia." *Psychopharmacology Bulletin* 29 (1993).

STEIN, LEONARD, and TEST, MARY ANN. "Alternative to Mental Hospital Treatment. I. Conceptual Model, Treatment Program, and Clinical Evaluation." *Archives of General Psychiatry* 37 (1980):392–397.

SUDDATH, R. L.; CHRISTISON, G. W.; TORREY, E. FULLER; CASANOVA, M. F.; and WEINBERGER, DANIEL R. "Anatomical Abnormalities in the Brains of Monozygotic Twins Discordant for Schizophrenia." *New England Journal of Medicine* 322 (1990):789–794.

TEPLIN, LINDA A. "The Criminalization Hypothesis: Myth, Misnomer, or Management Strategy." In *Law and Mental Health: Major Developments and Research Needs,* eds. Saleem Shah and Bruce Sales. Rockville, MD, 1991.

WALLACE, CHARLES. "Psychiatric Rehabilitation." *Psychopharmacology Bulletin* 29 (1993).

SUSAN S. MATTHEWS
SAMUEL J. KEITH

SCHOOL

See LEARNING DISABILITIES; SPECIAL EDUCATION

SELF-CONCEPT

Self-concept is an image an individual has of himself or herself (Burns, 1982). It is formed by a conceptualization process (Kelly, 1955) that is informed by a generalized view of others' perceptions. Much of the psychological development of a person is bound up with the emerging sense of self. In spite of its importance, the phenomenon of the self is one of the most difficult to explain. Physical ability as well as emotional and intellectual resources are important to the way an individual becomes conscious of and develops a unique, separate identity. These resources are important in the area of general mobility, maintaining body functions, and enhancing the whole early learning processes of social interaction, the building of self-esteem, and the achievement of life goals. Other people's perceptions of an individual, and that individual's perception of himself or herself, can be greatly affected by physical appearance as well as by other personal characteristics. Therefore, because the physical component is such an important factor in the development of the individual (Cohen, 1977), it could be argued that physical disability probably affects the formation of self-concept.

Since the primary means of learning in the first two years of life is action (Cohen, 1977), limited physical functioning can influence self-concept formation (Dunn, McCartan, and Fugua, 1988).

In the process of gaining independence and managing the stigma of disability, the person with a disability will face a number of environmental constraints. Herbert Blumer (1962), however, argues that there is an element of choice in the process of self-conceptualization, and he speaks of "role-making" (a form of empowerment) rather than "role-taking," which is determined by the role expectations others might have. Labels, both positive and negative, used to describe persons with a disability can influence their self-concept and how others react to them; for example, applying a disability label to a person may cause the person to behave in a more disabled fashion because of increased self-consciousness. Procedures for decreasing the negative effects of labeling by making others more aware of the individuality and positive attributes of persons with disabilities are now available (Yuker, 1987). This process has been further facilitated by the more positive portrayal in the media of the accomplishments of many very able people with disabilities. The need for achievement in some sphere of life is very important (Super & Block, 1992) and can have a positive impact on the overall development process.

Children with a disability may encounter difficulties in growing up with the same expectations as their peers without disabilities. The former have had fewer norms to guide them, and there is the possibility of an unclear and confused self-concept, with unrealistic goals and aspirations (Shakespeare, 1975). There is also the additional possibility of negative labeling resulting in the stigmas of "incompetent" and "unproductive."

The first crisis of the developmental process may well arise when children with a disability start school. Tension between the child's actual and ideal self-image and the resources of peers may lead to feelings of inadequacy, low self-esteem, and anxiety. These feelings may result in poor adjustment, depression, and a negative self-concept. This may also occur during adolescence—a time when secondary sex characteristics and physical prowess are significant. The individual's emotional stability can be threatened when the superego experiences more punishment than reward, and feelings of uncertainty, inadequacy, and inferiority are engendered along with social unacceptability. Account must also be taken of gender differences in the developmental process. Some research suggests that females with disabilities have relatively lower levels of participation in the sociocultural system and poorer limiting self-concepts (Blackbourn & Blackbourn, 1987; Hanna & Rogorsky, 1991). Other findings buttress the paradigm in which disability is viewed as a response to the individual as well as to societal circumstances (Mudrick, 1989).

In the process of forming the self-concept, inferiority and anxiety may create a devaluing effect, and there may be at least three adverse responses to this. The first is "mourning," which refers to sadness, and results from the lack of functional skills; the second is "devaluation," when persons with disabilities see themselves as more handicapped than they really are; and the last is "spreading," which refers to those who see their disability expanding from the original source to the whole body. All or any one of these responses may lead to an underestimation of oneself, and the self-concept formed is therefore not appropriate to the "real self" (Tweed, Shern, and Ciarlo, 1988).

However, most people with a disability are well adjusted individuals with a positive self-image, and struggle for recognition as competent and productive people, just like individuals without disabilities. The possibility of success depends also on consistent support, positive encouragement, empowerment, and relevant role models. Another consideration is the severity of the disability: Self-directed change of the physical environment becomes more difficult the more severe the disability, and the self-concept may be lower as a result. However, the options and empowerment resulting from increased accessibility, visionary legislation, and assistive technology have created more opportunities for people with disabilities. These new possibilities in turn can provide an environment favorable to the emergence and growth of a sense of control and competence that can have a positive effect on the self-concept.

A generalized view of others' perceptions and attitudes toward disability can be very influential in formation of the self-concept. In the past, the mistaken belief that persons with a disability were hopeless often resulted in denying accessibility to social, educational, and vocational opportunities; this circumstance often was more performance-limiting than the disability. Many agencies and services are designed to help people with disabilities live more independently and contribute to their communities, where they have greater control over the choice of goals and solutions to problems, use of peer role models, and encouragement toward self-help approaches. The success of persons with disabilities in competing favorably with their peers without disabilities in certain spheres of society has been well publicized (Black & Kahan, 1989; Tindall & Gugerty, 1987). Role models who help raise the expectations and aspirations of people with disabilities and positive promotion by educators and counselors are all important factors in building a positive self-concept.

Community agencies are encouraged to integrate people with disabilities fully by providing training to help attitude change and personal and professional consciousness-raising (Marks & Rousso, 1991). Group-, peer-, and student-centered counseling programs that focus on topics such as self-perception, assertiveness, familial relationships, and independent living can significantly cultivate and improve the self-concept (Johnson & Johnson, 1991; Mayberry, 1990). Programs designed to enhance self-esteem, taking into account the cognitive, emotional, and behavioral aspects of individuals with a disability, can lead through progressive dynamics and intervention to the development of a positive self-image (Frey & Carlock, 1989). Achievement motivation promotes a positive self-concept, especially in children with disabilities (Obiakor & Stile, 1990).

Educators differ on how best to enhance the self-concept of students with disabilities; the debate rages on the merits of integration in the mainstream or the need for special school placement. Many and varied programs and manuals assist teachers and counselors to ensure that students who have disabilities integrate and succeed in classrooms and in sports, meet the requirements of new competency-based school standards educationally and vocationally, and enjoy leisure pursuits (Bullock, 1991). At all times, teachers, counselors, parents, and siblings should strive for a sensitive awareness of the possible self-perceptions of the individual, and therefore each student should be closely evaluated to determine whether integrated education is the best option in a particular instance for a particular disability. Two of the most important considerations are teacher expectation and attitude, which have significant influence on the development of a positive self-concept (Tuttle, 1987).

A number of developments will potentially enhance the social position, empowerment, independence, and the self-concept of people with disabilities. Legislation and advances in technology have ameliorated the negative consequences of disability, as have innovations in education and counseling. These changes seek to enhance and improve self-concept in a more direct manner, making operative the notion of "empowerment." Important elements here are self-evaluation and the clarification of values of self and of others through a number of techniques such as group work and counseling. Awareness of one's strengths and weaknesses, and the role of others in the individual's perceptions and self-evaluation, are important steps in accepting constraints and using possibilities. Positive social awareness, legislation, and technological advances will potentially enhance strengths, reduce limitations, and further build independence and a sense of individuality and worth.

(*See also:* ABILITY; ATTITUDES; CONSUMERS; DISABILITY; PSYCHOSOCIAL ADJUSTMENT; SPECIAL EDUCATION)

BIBLIOGRAPHY

ANDERSON, ELIZABETH M., and CLARKE, LYNDA. *Disability in Adolescence.* London, 1982.

BLACK, C., and KAHAN. *Return on Equity: A Resource Guide for the "Science Abled" Video Program.* Washington, DC, 1989.

BLACKBOURN, JOE M., and BLACKBOURN, VONDA. "Self-Concepts of Young Handicapped Children: An Analysis of Race and Sex." *Perceptual and Motor-Skills* 65 (1987):626.

BLUMER, HERBERT. "Society as Symbolic Interaction." In *Human Behavior and Social Processes,* ed. Arnold M. Rose. Boston, 1962.

BULLOCK, C. *The Wake Leisure Program: An Integral Part of Special Education: A Facilitator's Manual Containing Field-Tested Leisure Education Curriculum Materials.* Chapel Hill, NC, 1991.

BURNS, ROBERT. *Self-Concept Development and Education.* London, 1982.

COHEN, S. *Special People.* Englewood Cliffs, NJ, 1977.

DUNN, NANCY L.; MCCARTAN, KATHLEEN W.; and FUGUA, ROBERT W. "Young Children with Orthopaedic Handicaps: Self-Knowledge About Their Disability." *Exceptional Children* 55 (1988):249–252.

FREY, DIANE, and CARLOCK, C. JESSE. *Enhancing Self-Esteem,* 2nd ed. Muncie, IN, 1989.

GOFFMAN, ERVING. *Stigma.* London, 1978.

HANNA, WILLIAM J., and ROGORSKY, BETSY. "Women with Disabilities: Two Handicaps Plus." *Disability, Handicap and Society* 6 (1991):49–63.

IOWA STATE DEPARTMENT OF EDUCATION. *Core Competency Modification: A Manual for Working with at-Risk/Special Needs Students.* Des Moines, IA, 1991.

JOHNSON, CHARLES L., and JOHNSON, JANET A. "Using Short-Term Group Counseling with Visually Impaired Adolescents." *Journal of Visual Impairment and Blindness* 85 (1991):166–170.

KELLY, GEORGE A. *The Psychology of Personal Constructs,* vols. 1 and 2. New York, 1955.

MARKS, L., and ROUSSO, H. *Barrier-Free: Serving Young Women with Disabilities.* Washington, DC, 1991.

MAYBERRY, WANDA. "Self-Esteem in Children: Considerations for Measurement and Intervention." *American Journal of Occupational Therapy* 44 (1990):729–734.

MUDRICK, NANCY R. "The Association of Roles and Attitudes and Disability Among Midlife Women and Men." *Journal of Aging and Health* 1 (1989):306–326.

NATIONAL COUNCIL ON VOCATIONAL EDUCATION. *America's Hidden Treasure: The Urgent Need to Recognize and Promote the Nation's Vocational-Technical Education System: A Report to the American People.* Washington, DC, 1989.

OBIAKOR, FESTUS E., and STILE, STEPHEN W. "The Self-Concepts of Visually Impaired and Normally Sighted Middle School Children." *Journal of Psychology* 124(1990):199–206.

SHAKESPEARE, ROSEMARY. *The Psychology of Handicap.* London, 1975.

SHERRILL, CLAUDINE; HINSON, MARILYN; GENCH, BARBARA; and KENNEDY, SUSAN O. "Self-Concepts of Disabled Youth Athletes." *Perceptual and Motor Skills* 70 (1990):1093–1098.

SUPER, JOHN T., and BLOCK, J. R. "Self-Concept and Need for Achievement of Men with Physical Disabilities." *Journal of General Psychology* 119 (1992): 73–80.

THOMAS, R. M. *Body Image and Body Language. The International Encyclopedia of Education.* Oxford, 1985.

TINDALL, LLOYD W., and GUGERTY, JOHN J. "Careers for Persons with Disabilities." *Journal of Career Development* 13 (1987):5–13.

TUTTLE, DEAN W. "The Role of the Special Educational Teacher-Counsellor in Meeting Students' Self-Esteem Needs." *Journal of Visual Impairment and Blindness* 81 (1987):156–161.

TWEED, DAN L.; SHERN, DAVID L.; and CIARLO, JAMES A. "Disability, Dependency, and Demoralization." *Rehabilitation Psychology* 33 (1988):143–154.

WRIGHT, BEATRICE A. *Physical Disability: A Psychological Approach.* New York, 1960.

YUKER, HAROLD E. "Labels Can Hurt People with Disabilities." In *et cetera* 44 (1987):16–22.

B. G. LAWRENCE
S. G. BENNETT

SELF-HELP IN DISABILITY

Self-help has become a vital agent of health care services in this country. In response to decreasing mortality rates, increased costs of medical care, limited access to medical treatment, and limited resources to pay for it, self-help organizations have arisen to bridge the widening gaps in treatment and medical technology. By 1989 there were estimated to be 6 million to 15 million members of self-help support groups in the United States (Jacobs & Goodman, 1989). Their substantial popularity led the former surgeon general of the United States, C. Everett Koop, to convene a workshop in 1987 to help define the self-help movement and promote self-help initiatives in physical and mental health care (U.S. Department of Health and Human Services, 1987). This workshop was a landmark of a remarkable grassroots movement that has grown rapidly in the United States since the late 1960s. Although self-help organizations have flourished with little professional assistance, the surgeon general's workshop represented a recognition by the professional community of the substantial value of mutual aid organizations. Indeed, the very inclusion of this entry in this encyclopedia is evidence of the value of self-help in medical care and rehabilitation.

There are a multitude of self-help organizations, with widely disparate missions, populations, ideologies, and operations. The exponential growth and diversity of this movement have created considerable difficulty in formulating a uniform terminology and conceptual framework (Katz & Bender, 1976b; Lieberman, 1986; Schubert & Borkman, 1990). There are self-help groups for every major physical and mental health problem, disabling condition, or behavior or lifestyle problem. This entry does not attempt to be comprehensive in scope but to focus on the salient aspects of self-help organizations pertinent to physical disability and rehabilitation. For this purpose, Alfred Katz and Eugene Bender (1976b) offer the following definition:

> Self-help groups are voluntary, small group structures for mutual aid and the accomplishment of a special purpose. They are usually formed by peers who have come together for mutual assistance in . . . overcoming a common handicap or life-disrupting problem, and bringing about desired social and/or personal change. . . . They often provide material assistance, as well as emotional support; they are frequently "cause"-oriented, and promulgate an ideology or values through which members may attain an enhanced sense of personal identity (p. 9).

This definition clearly distinguishes self-help from professional help. For the purpose of this entry, self-help is not considered an "alternative" to traditional medicine as much as it is a complementary form of treatment within the larger context of total health care, of which self-help and professional help are but two different aspects. Unfortunately, self-help is frequently relegated to second-class status by the professional community (Chesler, 1990). It is this author's position, however, that not only is self-help a principal element of health care in the United States today, but it will continue to increase in significance as the gaps in traditional health care widen.

History

The underlying premise of self-help is endemic to social survival, according to Peter Kropotkin, a late-nineteenth-century writer. In his classic work *Mutual Aid* (reprint, 1972), Kropotkin refuted the predatory theory of social Darwinism and claimed that mutual assistance and collective efforts for protection and sustenance were critical to the development of social structures and evolution. Throughout the history of civilization, mutual assistance among peers has been able to stabilize communities and manage the struggles of the common citizens in the absence of authoritative or administrative methods. The Middle Ages saw the first craft guilds, organizations that provided sustenance and some vocational security for its members. An outgrowth of the guilds, the Friendly Societies were established during the industrial revolution in England to help their constituents deal with the overcrowded and unsanitary conditions of the burgeoning cities. The preambles of many of these societies referred to Christian charity, the social being of humans, and the ongoing need for mutual assistance and support (Katz & Bender, 1976a).

In the United States, various cooperatives and mutual aid organizations grew and perished, but eventually some craft and trade unions held a place and were able to amass economic independence and viability, provide cooperative housing, purchase banks, and establish their own schools (Katz & Bender, 1976a). Many ethnic groups also formed their own self-help organizations to assist their fellow immigrants, who were frequently discriminated against by the public, social services, and charitable organizations. A few of these fraternal organizations still exist today.

Following World War II there was a subtle and persistent growth of self-help groups consisting of people who were disaffected, afflicted, or stigmatized by a rapidly evolving society. In Veterans Administration hospitals, veterans with quadriplegia formed their own informal support groups, which helped them cope with their disability and thrive more successfully outside the hospital. Parents of children with physical and mental disabilities petitioned the government for aid and organized self-help groups to help them cope with the medical, personal, and social problems associated with their children's conditions. These parents formed organizations such as the Association for Retarded Children and the National Hemophilia Foundation and sought public and professional assistance with their problems.

Advances in medical research and technology, surgical and treatment techniques, pharmacology, and other related fields vastly decreased mortality rates. Rehabilitation centers were built to restore to the community the increasing number of individuals who would have perished years earlier. In the 1950s and 1960s, federal agencies recognized the needs of people with chronic illness and disability and increased support for rehabilitation programs. Awareness of the social and psychological needs of people with newly acquired disabilities—and the scarce resources available to help them—grew along with the rehabilitation movement.

The self-help movement was another face of a massive social transformation in the United States in which the socially stigmatized were becoming empowered. Although overshadowed by the civil rights and women's movements, the self-help movement reflected the shared themes of social liberation, self-determination, personal responsibility, and social tolerance. The increased attention to the needs of the socially neglected culminated in the passage of the Americans with Disabilities Act (1990), which many people call the civil rights or the equal rights amendment for people with disabilities.

Self-Help Benefits

Although self-help organizations for people with physical disabilities are diverse, they share certain characteristics, among them, the providing of support for their members and the encouragement of advocacy. Most local support groups are associated with national organizations. For example, the Better Breathers Club is supported by the American Lung Association; Reach to Recovery, the Lost Chord Club, and Living Today by the American Cancer Society; many local ostomy groups by the United Ostomy Association; and local family support groups by the National Alliance for the Mentally Ill (NAMI). Most public libraries carry comprehensive lists of self-help groups and other organizations providing support services. On the national level these organizations raise funding for research and treatment, promote legislative change, and increase public awareness through the media.

On the local level self-help organizations have a direct and immediate influence on their members. Phyllis Silverman (1992) maintains that people see self-help groups during periods of critical change in their lives, when old coping methods are not effective. This situation is the one faced by people with newly acquired disabilities. Their transition involves giving up a way of life, and the personal meaning of that lifestyle, and trying to come to grips with an altered identity. Self-help groups not only facilitate their members' finding of a new meaning and perspective on life but also teach pragmatic behavior changes consistent with the new identity. This transformation process involves the following elements, which are found in most self-help organizations for people with physical disabilities.

Emotional and Social Support. The personal benefit received from experiential sharing is one of the most salient aspects of a self-help support group and the most readily identified by its members (Borkman, 1990; Hedrick, Isenberg, and Martini, 1992; Katz, 1993; Mullan, 1992). As opposed to professional services, which some consider to be scientific, unidirectional, and emotionally distant, the subjective value of self-help group membership presents a participatory, personal experience that is validating and frequently comforting during the painful adjustments that people with newly acquired disabilities must make (Borkman, 1990; Bryant, 1990). This support is vital to successful adjustments to new body images and lifestyle changes. Through formal support group meetings and classes and through informal telephone contact and gatherings, the new members of a support group are sustained by peers and provided with role models for healthy adjustment and identity change.

Not only does the new member benefit from the personal acceptance and emotional support of the older members, but the "veterans" of the group receive self-satisfaction from caring for others and fulfilling a specialized need as well. What was once considered an impediment (e.g., paraplegia, chronic obstructive pulmonary disease) becomes a vital resource to the group. The older members gain interpersonal competence and support from others. As role models, they are reinforced by their own messages according to the old adage "The best way to learn is to teach" (Comstock & Mohamoud, 1990). The relationships that develop among the veterans, the rookies, and those in between are meaningful and important in making difficult personal transformations from loss and grieving to an active, healthy, and fulfilling lifestyle.

Education. A major component of successful adaptation to disease or disability involves new learning, which is a primary goal of most self-help organizations. As opposed to scientific information, mutual aid groups communicate a knowledge base that is unique to the members. Thomasina Borkman (1990) refers to "experiential learning communities" in which self-help groups "create, test, use, and disseminate a body of experiential knowledge about their shared problem, and workable resolutions" (p. 21). Information on how to choose a physician or therapist, which appliances or devices are most effective, what the side effects of medications are, and which restaurants are wheelchair-accessible are examples of knowledge that a peer with a disability could best communicate. It is probably this single feature, more than any other, that sets self-help groups apart from other lay and professional helpers.

Self-help groups usually distribute factual information through newsletters, brochures, lectures, and workshops. Topics may include finances, legal issues, medical services, insurance, Medicare, political ac-

tion, and so on. Local and national clearinghouses are frequently established to collect and distribute information about specific conditions (Wollert, 1990). The rapid increase in the number of clearinghouses represents its own "movement" within the self-help community. Finally, self-help groups seek to educate the lay public and professional communities through newspaper and magazine articles, TV and radio interviews, and presentations to civic, government, and business groups.

Advocacy. Advocacy is a form of education, perhaps in a more assertive format, in which self-help groups participate to varying degrees. To be active advocates for a disability or illness, Frank Mullan (1992) states that individuals must have their "act together," that is, they must have made some positive adjustment to their condition. It requires great self-confidence to petition legislators, insurance companies, hospitals, businesses, and universities because of the public attention these activities tend to draw. Advocates must have some comfort with their disability to take such action, which is why advocacy activities usually are conducted by more veteran self-helpers.

Some self-help groups are politically active by charter, such as the Americans Disabled for Attendant Programs Today (ADAPT), which actively solicits local governments, businesses, and community leaders to improve the "civil rights, life opportunities, and self-images of people with disabilities" (Mental Health Association of Memphis and Shelby County, 1992, p. 1). In Memphis, Tennessee, some ADAPT members and other individuals in wheelchairs were arrested for conducting a "sit-in" at a local movie theater to protest the inadequate wheelchair accessibility to the company's theaters. They not only received media exposure for their issues but also achieved their purpose—getting the company's commitment to improve the theaters. Additionally, the local police became "enlightened" to the difficulties of arresting and confining individuals who use electric wheelchairs, which are exceptionally heavy.

Most advocacy, however, is of a less dramatic nature. The mother of a child with a head injury who is returning to school meets with administrators and teachers to tell them about special problems they may encounter and the solutions. An individual in a wheelchair may point out to a store manager the barriers to his store and merchandise inaccessibility. An individual with a hearing impairment may assert his or her employability during a job interview. All of these forms of advocacy are supported and instructed by most self-help groups.

Empowerment. This term has become rather a cliché, arising out of the various "rights" and broader self-help movements, but it is an appropriate descriptor of the process by which those who were once powerless and alienated by their disability are transformed into powerful or empowered individuals. Empowerment is less a direct result of participation in self-help groups than a product of successful change and adaptation to a new lifestyle (Hedrick, Isenberg, and Martini, 1992).

The collective power of the group is imparted to the individual through participatory identification and support. Empowered individuals assume responsibility for themselves, as opposed to blaming others for their shortcomings, and are assertive in taking care of their own needs. They are responsible for their health care and lifestyle, minimizing their dependency on others while appropriately using medical services and self-help groups (Katz, 1993). They portray the role of "prosumer," a self-help consumer who is "empowered" by his or her unique condition and experiential knowledge and who assists others in ways different from the traditional forms of help provided by the community or professionals (Hedrick, Isenberg, and Martini, 1992).

Independent Living Movement

The independent living (IL) movement presents an approach to services for people with disabilities unlike other self-help organizations. Created by and for people with disabilities, IL organizations seek to encourage "people with disabilities to live as they choose in their communities rather than confining them in institutions" (Crewe & Zola, 1983, p. ix). As opposed to self-help groups that address a single disease or disability, the centers for independent living (CILs) were created to assist those with a variety of disabling conditions. For instance, CILs may serve individuals with spinal cord injury, multiple sclerosis, head injury, cerebral palsy, rheumatoid arthritis, or post-poliomyelitis syndrome. A variety of services are offered by CILs, including transitional or residential housing; contracting for services by community providers; classes, groups, counseling, and training; and funding for ramps and assistive devices for individuals with disabilities. Services are provided with an overriding ideology in mind—to promote the highest level of functional independence for individuals in their community. CILs seek to educate the lay and professional public on issues neglected by traditional medical care, such as sexuality, and are frequently active in social action and advocacy, seeking to obtain barrier-free community access and community changes in architecture and services for people with disabilities (DeLoach, Wilkins, and Walker, 1983).

The IL movement has explicit legislative mandates and strong grassroots imperatives. Following a series of state amendments activated by parents of children who had been excluded from school because of their disabilities, the first legal precedent for IL was the passage of Title V of the federal Rehabilitation Act of 1973. This amendment extended statutory rights to people with disabilities, declared that people with the most severe disabilities were to receive priority services, and mandated affirmative-action programs for employment of people with disabilities within agencies receiving federal funds. Establishing the basic rights of people with disabilities, section 504 of this act prohibits discrimination against "otherwise qualified handicapped individuals under any program or activity receiving federal financial assistance." Finally, legitimacy for the IL movement came with the passage of Title VII of the Rehabilitation, Comprehensive Services, and Developmental Disabilities Act of 1978, which provided for federal funding for IL centers.

The grassroots aspect of the IL movement probably began at the University of Illinois in 1948. The university offered special services for World War II veterans with disabilities, then later expanded the program to include civilians. Designed to enhance the independence of people with moderate disabilities, their programs offered a variety of services, including wheelchair-accessible housing and transportation, specialized medical care, peer counseling, and training in daily hygiene and housekeeping skills. One of the first CILs was established by a group of students with disabilities at the University of California at Berkeley in the early 1970s. These students labored successfully for architectural changes at the university to obtain access and mancuverability in buildings and facilities that were previously inaccessible to wheelchairs. Working diligently to obtain grants and contracts, they were able to apply what they had learned at Berkeley and develop a wide range of services in the San Francisco Bay area. The Berkeley center became the prototype for centers across the country, and it truly embodies the concept of empowerment of those with disabilities (Crewe & Zola, 1983; DeLoach, Wilkins, and Walker, 1983; Katz & Bender, 1976a).

Other CILs appeared in the 1970s: the Boston Center for Independent Living, New Options in Houston, Texas, and Timbers in Wichita, Kansas, each with a different program model but each "intent on reshaping the thinking of disability professionals and researchers, on promoting new forms of service delivery, and on encouraging new direction in research" (DeJong, 1983, p. 5). This expansion of services in many CILs has also included the provision of services to people with mental or emotional disabilities.

The IL movement as embodied in the CILs across the country owes allegiance and thanks to movements in civil rights, consumerism, self-help, demedicalization/self-care, and deinstitutionalization. In addition to providing for the immediate needs of people with disabilities through support groups, educational programs, and service provision, as do most other disease-specific self-help organizations, CILs help people with disabilities gain access to their broader political and cultural rights (Katz & Maida, 1990). The attitudes engendered by the IL movement achieved fruition in the Americans with Disabilities Act of 1990, the culmination of years of struggle by people with disabilities to attain the full range of opportunities of citizenship in this country.

Conclusion

To appreciate the self-help movement adequately, one must take in the full panoply of health care in our nation. Traditional medicine is but part of a continuum of health services, along with holistic medicine, preventive care, community services, and self-help. Self-help groups have grown to fill in the gaps in this picture, and to address the personal and subjective aspects of health care that other means have failed to do. This situation is not necessarily the fault of the other treatment systems, but a reflection of the enormous complexity of health care and the inadequacy of any single system to provide total care. As Kropotkin's theory of mutual aid predicts, people come together to take care of those needs not met by existing social systems.

The relationship between the self-help community and the professional community has historically been uncertain, occasionally antagonistic, and frequently ambivalent or indifferent. This relationship is complex and multidimensional, with areas of overlap and congruence and areas of divergence and dissension. It is also a relationship that has been improving with the continuing acceptance of self-help by professionals (Katz, 1992).

Although progress has been made, there is still much to be done. The shrinking medical dollar creates an ongoing imperative to find new solutions but also creates a threat to professionals, who face a loss of income and diminished prominence in medical care. In the face of this threat, territoriality and conflict will only serve to diminish health services, both self-help and professional. Clearly, new areas of rapprochement are necessary to improve the total health care continuum. To improve this hesitant affiliation between self-help and professional help, it is strongly recommended that education in self-help benefits, and particularly involvement in self-help groups, be a required part of professional training. Professionals are encouraged to participate and contribute to self-help growth, but not to control or dominate the organizations. Also, more education for self-help group members about professional issues, limitations, and practices is needed. Finally, much more research is needed to answer questions about self-help, such as which kind of groups are best for particular problems; who is most likely to benefit from self-help groups; how professionals can best work with self-help groups; and how self-help groups can maintain and monitor appropriate, quality service.

The growth of self-help organizations appears inexorable. We only stand to gain—and have practically nothing to lose—if we enhance the progress and application of self-help in disability and chronic illness.

(*See also:* ADVOCACY; CIVIL RIGHTS; CONSUMERS; INDEPENDENT LIVING; PSYCHOSOCIAL ADJUSTMENT)

RESOURCES

National Alliance for the Mentally Ill (NAMI), 2101 Wilson Blvd., Suite 302, Arlington, VA 22201

National Multiple Sclerosis Society, 733 Third Ave., New York, NY 10017–3288

National Spinal Cord Injury Association, 545 Concord Ave., Cambridge, MA 02138

Independent Living Research and Utilization, 2323 South Shepherd St., Suite 1000, Houston, TX 77019

BIBLIOGRAPHY

BORKMAN, THOMASINA J. "Experiential, Professional, and Lay Frames of Reference." In *Working with Self-Help*, ed. Thomas J. Powell. Silver Spring, MD, 1990.

BRYANT, N. "Self-Help Groups and Professionals: Cooperation or Conflict." In *Helping One Another: Self-Help Groups in a Changing World*, eds. A. H. Katz and Eugene Bender. Oakland, CA, 1990.

CHESLER, MARK A. "The 'Dangers' of Self-Help Groups: Understanding and Challenging Professionals' Views." In *Working with Self-Help*, ed. Thomas J. Powell. Silver Spring, MD, 1990.

COMSTOCK, CHRISTINE M., and MOHAMOUD, JOYCE L. "Professionally Facilitated Self-Help Groups: Benefits for Professionals and Members." In *Working with Self-Help*, ed. Thomas J. Powell. Silver Spring, MD, 1990.

CREWE, NANCY M., and ZOLA, IRVING K. *Independent Living for Physically Disabled People*. San Francisco, 1983.

DEJONG, GERBEN. "Defining and Implementing the Independent Living Concept." In *Independent Living for Physically Disabled People*, eds. Nancy M. Crewe and Irving K. Zola. San Francisco, 1983.

DELOACH, CHARLENE P.; WILKINS, RONALD D.; and WALKER, G. W. *Independent Living: Philosophy, Process, and Services*. Baltimore, 1983.

HEDRICK, H. L.; ISENBERG, D. H.; and MARTINI, C.J.M. "Self-Help Groups: Empowerment Through Policy and Partnerships." In *Self-Help: Concepts and Applications*, ed. Alfred H. Katz. Philadelphia, 1992.

JACOBS, M. K., and GOODMAN, G. "Psychology and Self-Help Groups: Predictions on a Partnership." *American Psychologist* 44 (1989):536–545.

KATZ, ALFRED H. "Professional/Self-Help Group Relationships: General Issues." In *Self-Help: Concepts and Applications*, ed. Alfred H. Katz. Philadelphia, 1992.

———. *Self-Help in America: A Social Movement Perspective*. Boston, 1993.

KATZ, ALFRED H., and BENDER, EUGENE I. "Self-Help Groups in Western Society: History and Prospects." *Journal of Applied Behavioral Science* 12 (1976a): 265–282.

———, eds. *The Strength in Us: Self-Help Groups in the Modern World*. New York, 1976b.

———, eds. *Helping One Another: Self-Help Groups in a Changing World*. Oakland, CA, 1990.

KATZ, ALFRED H., and MAIDA, C. A. "Health and Disability Self-Help Organizations." In *Working with Self-Help*, ed. Thomas J. Powell. Silver Spring, MD, 1990.

KROPOTKIN, PETER. *Mutual Aid: A Factor of Evolution*. Reprint. New York, 1972.

LIEBERMAN, M. A. "Self-Help Groups and Psychiatry." *American Psychiatric Association Annual Review* 5 (1986):744–760.

MENTAL HEALTH ASSOCIATION OF MEMPHIS AND SHELBY COUNTY. *Self-Help Support Group Directory*. Memphis, TN, 1992.

MULLAN, FRANK "Rewriting the Social Contract in Health." In *Self-Help: Concepts and Applications*, ed. Alfred H. Katz. Philadelphia, 1992.

SCHUBERT, M. A., and BORKMAN, T. J. "An Organizational Typology for Self-Help Groups." *American Journal of Community Psychology* 19 (1990):769–787.

SILVERMAN, P. R. "Critical Aspects of the Mutual Help Experience." In *Self-Help: Concepts and Applications*, ed. Alfred H. Katz. Philadelphia, 1992.

U.S. DEPARTMENT OF HEALTH AND HUMAN SERVICES. *The Surgeon General Workshop on Self-Help and Public Health*. Washington, DC, 1987.

WOLLERT, R. "Self-Help Clearinghouses: An Overview of an Emergent System for Promoting Mutual Aid." In *Working with Self-Help*, ed. Thomas J. Powell. Silver Spring, MD, 1990.

C. KIRVEN WEEKLEY

SEXUALITY AND DISABILITY

The medical interest in sexuality and sex therapy that intensified in the 1980s has its roots in the pioneering work of Masters and Johnson. The work in human sexual response they completed in the late 1960s marked a new era in which sexuality became a legitimate area of clinical work and investigation (Masters & Johnson, 1966). This work was an important component of the sexual revolution of the 1960s. Since that time, the field of sex therapy has undergone a tremendous explosion as new advances in medicine and psychology have expanded the understanding of human sexual activity and behavior. Moreover, research and clinical practice in sexuality have now become an interdisciplinary activity that spans a broad range of theoretical approaches and medical treatment.

For people with disabilities, the acceptance of sexuality as a justifiable and sanctioned area of rehabilitation has been much more controversial. Not surprisingly, people with disabilities often received little or no information in the area of sexuality. In fact, they have generally been perceived as being nonsexual and incapable of achieving an intimate and sexual relationship with another person. Unfortunately, this misperception not only has persisted in the general population but has been prevalent in the medical community as well.

The history of sexuality services for people with disabilities dates back only to the mid-1970s, when Theodore and Sandra Cole began their Sexual Attitude Reassessment Seminars at the University of Minnesota (Cole, Chilgren, and Rosenberg, 1973). The focus of these early workshops was on values clarification and communication. Their purpose was to increase the practitioner's level of comfort and awareness of sexual issues among people with disabilities. To some extent the idea of sexual education for people with disabilities was academic. People in rehabilitation were beginning to recognize the need for sexuality services, but there was little agreement as to how and when these services should be provided.

In many ways, the sexual functioning of people with disabilities is not so different than it is among people without disabilities. However, sexuality is a complex phenomenon, and a number of important variables should be considered in a comprehensive discussion of the topic. These include developmental aspects of sexuality, adjustment and psychological issues, physical functioning, and issues of staff training and education.

Sexuality as a Developmental Issue

As the individual moves through life, he or she encounters a number of tasks set by the cultural milieu and by himself or herself as a biological entity. These developmental tasks are particularly critical because they must be mastered if the individual is to develop more mature social and interpersonal skills. When disability occurs, not only are the current developmental tasks threatened, but the person, at least temporarily, regresses to an earlier stage of development. This has broad implications for the individual's psychological and sexual adjustment. Because the person's sense of masculinity or femininity is an integral part of these developmental milestones, disability can create confusion and conflict in both gender identity and gender role, identity and role being different aspects of the same process. Gender identity is the inner experience of oneself as male or female; role is the outward expression of that identity. Without resolution of these conflicts, more complex tasks such as the development of relationships, and the achievement of a positive self-esteem, may never occur (Ducharme & Ducharme, 1983). Thus for a person with a disability, a healthy sexual adjustment and the ability to achieve intimacy depend on successful resolution of the developmental tasks at the time of injury or onset of illness.

The theory of developmental tasks was originally discussed by the psychologist Erik Erikson (1953). The developmental stages Erikson identified represent the critical periods of development from birth to death. The first three stages of development occur in infancy and childhood. They reflect the achievement of trust, autonomy through mobility, and the ability to explore the environment. Even at these early stages in life, sexual behaviors and curiosity are quite typical and expected. This is true for children with and without disabilities.

Congenital disabilities often prevent the child from gaining essential information about the body. Overprotection by parents, discouragement of sexual exploration, and lack of adequate socialization often increase confusion about male and female roles. Since identity is formulated before the age of three years, confusion regarding sexuality lends itself to later feelings of inferiority and difficulty relating to members of the opposite sex. The child with a disability is often isolated from peers and may regard himself or herself as "not equal" to his or her playmates. These deficits in the sexual education of a child can easily become more difficult to manage later in life.

During puberty and adolescence, the achievement of sexual identity and acceptance in peer group relationships are the goals to be accomplished. As the adolescent grows and enters young adulthood, one of the primary developmental tasks is the development of intimacy and the concurrent strivings toward independence. Traumatic injury at this time threatens these important peer relationships and fosters dependency on the family unit. Adolescents with a disability often feel unattractive and ashamed of their bodies. Subsequently they feel unwanted by the opposite sex and incapable of establishing a meaningful relationship. Without a sense of sexual identity, even late adolescents can lack the ability to make vocational and educational decisions or to assume responsibility for their own behavior. Thus future emotional growth is threatened.

Sexual Adjustment

Adjustment to a physical disability or illness is a gradual process that occurs over an extended period of time. The individual must mourn the losses and ultimately develop coping strategies that will validate the meaningfulness of the new postinjury life. Successful adjustment depends on the recognition that choice is still available and is influenced by many factors, such as age at onset, quality of social supports, physical health, gender, and type of illness or injury.

Successful sexual adjustment also requires the same gradual and painful emotional process. Losses need to be grieved so the remaining strengths can be developed and nurtured. Because of different personality styles, however, not everyone completes this difficult adjustment. Everyone, though, regardless of disability, has the ability to function sexually and enjoy the closeness of an intimate relationship. Frequently individuals, after a traumatic disability, go through a period of reduced sexual drive or performance. Others go through a period of sexual acting out, presumably to validate their survival and sexual identity. However, substantial numbers of people fail to resume an active sex life after injury due to misinformation, problems of adjustment, or shame regarding body image and functioning. Those who do assume an active sex life after injury are often advised by rehabilitation staff members to keep

separate the roles of sexual partner and care provider. Mixing these roles often places one member in a needy, helpless position while the other member is perceived as powerful and giving. Such an unequal balance of power in a relationship tends to dilute feelings of intimacy and to be the source of feelings of resentment and anger.

To the extent that the person with the disability can learn to value his or her new sexual abilities and establish a positive level of communication as opposed to trying to gain the same sexual expressions as before injury, the person will achieve a satisfying sexual adjustment. Those people with disabilities who achieve success in their sexual functioning often do so because of increased communication and a willingness to experiment with developing romance and intimacy as well as technique. They are secure enough to realize that not every experiment will work, and they value nongenital erogenous zones. They are typically more comfortable with their own bodies and continue to feel a sense of self-worth and self-respect. As a result, partners also feel validated and perceive the sexual relationship to be warm, caring, and a mutually enjoyable experience.

As discussed above, the importance of communication cannot be overstated. The development of skills in communication about sexual topics and methods of pleasure is the single most critical aspect of successful sexual adjustment. Specific and immediate communication between partners can relieve intense feelings of anxiety, fears of rejection, and concerns about physical safety. For this reason, psychological counseling and education about sexuality during rehabilitation must emphasize these areas and provide individuals with the opportunity to develop and strengthen these skills.

Although psychological considerations need to be addressed in all discussions regarding sexuality, physical functioning is equally important. Often in rehabilitation, it can be extremely supportive and helpful to patients if a sensitive discussion regarding physical capabilities is provided as soon as the individual is ready. Usually people will indicate their readiness by asking questions regarding attractiveness, dating, relationships, and intimacy. Even if the individual does not raise these concerns during hospitalization, it is usually appropriate for staff members to offer information if the patient seems interested and curious. Such topics as erections, lubrications, fertility, mobility, sensation, and bladder functioning are all relevant to the sexual functioning of people with disabilities.

Male Sexual Functioning

The capacity to achieve psychogenic erections is usually altered in most men who sustain damage to the central nervous system. This typically includes injuries such as spinal cord injury and stroke as well as progressive disabilities such as multiple sclerosis and diabetes. Interestingly, men with head injury do not report similar impairments but often note changes in sexual desire and libido. Men with congenital disabilities such as cerebral palsy or muscular dystrophy often retain the ability to achieve erections but more often report difficulties in mobility, positioning, and communication. If erections are altered, such as with spinal cord injury, the man may still be capable of reflexogenic erections. Although these may not be suitable for intercourse, they can usually be achieved and sustained by ongoing manual stimulation of the genital area.

Sensory disturbances are also a prominent symptom in many of the disabilities that affect erectile functioning. For example, a man may be capable of a psychogenic or reflex erection but may be unable to feel his penis in his partner's vagina. Other men may experience some sparing of sensation in the genital area, although these areas may not be as sensitive as prior to the injury. For example, the man may be able to differentiate hard touch but unable to experience soft touch or stroking. Areas of intact sensation, usually above the level of injury, are often hypersensitive and another source of erotic pleasure. These areas may be at the nipple line, for example, or in the vicinity of the ears, scalp, and neck.

Since the 1980s treatments such as penile injections, implants, vacuum constrictive devices (which fit over the penis), and various surgical procedures have gained increased popularity among men with neurogenic erectile difficulties. One of the most promising forms of treatment was the subject of a study completed in Denmark in 1992 in which nitroglycerin plasters were applied directly to the penile shaft and enabled men with spinal injuries to achieve erections sufficient for intercourse (Sonksen & Biering-Sorenson, 1992). Such noninvasive techniques represent a new wave of thinking in which medical science is offering a great deal of encouragement to men with disabilities.

In the field of male fertility, the ability to diagnose and treat infertility is another area that continues to improve. For men with disabilities of the central nervous system, fertility rates have generally ranged from 1 to 10 percent. Reports of pregnancies were typically undocumented and anecdotal. Problems were due either to difficulties of sperm retrieval or to poor sperm quality. In the 1990s, however, newer methods of retrieving sperm through electroejaculation and vibratory stimulation are demonstrating very positive results. In other cases, surgical sperm aspiration coupled with *in vitro* fertilization is offering new hope for couples wishing to have children. Techniques to reduce testicular temperatures are also having positive results on spermatogenesis and sperm production.

Female Sexual Functioning

The literature on the sexuality of women with disabilities is minimal compared to that on male issues. Although a number of hypotheses have been made to explain this substantial difference, the best answer may lie in the fact that most of the research in sexuality is conducted by male researchers who are more interested in men's issues. Thus there are still many unanswered questions, including how female genital responses change at different levels of spinal cord trauma and specific questions regarding pregnancy and childbirth.

For the most part, changes in the female genital tract are most common after neurologic trauma or disease. These changes may affect vaginal lubrication, labial swelling, clitoral swelling and regression, and a sequence of events at the time of orgasm that is similar to that occurring in men. Many aspects of a woman's sexuality may be altered after a traumatic injury, including libido or desire, arousal, response, and specific sexual behaviors. Complications that face women with traumatic disabilities include management of autonomic hyperreflexia (drastic changes in blood pressure), management of bowel and bladder continence, and management of spasticity. In some women with multiple sclerosis or spinal injury, lubrication may become reflexogenic, allowing penile entry to the vagina. Changes in desire and arousal may result from the impact of changes in her physical status on her perception of herself, from role changes that may occur as a result of injury, or from the anger and depression that often accompany the onset of a disability (Gill & Ducharme, 1992). Women tend to remain fertile after disability, although it may take up to six months following trauma for menstruation to resume.

Research on female sexuality being conducted in the 1990s is exploring issues related to vaginal contractions, intensifying perception of orgasm, and stimulating vasodilation of the pelvic region. All of these areas require further investigation, but the fact that the research is being pursued indicates a renewed interest in the field and a commitment to understanding female sexuality and disability. Most important, such research is providing a renewed sense of hope for women with disabilities and has important applications for clinical practice (Leyson, 1991).

Staff Training and Education

Staff training in sexuality is a critical feature of any worthwhile rehabilitation program. This training must include programs aimed at values clarification as well as those that provide specific information on disability and sexuality. In addition to the training curriculum, administrative support of the sexuality program must be evident to staff members, families, and patients alike. This administrative approval establishes a positive therapeutic environment where openness, empowerment, and caring are the foundations of the rehabilitation process.

Although not all staff members need be sex counselors, all should feel comfortable with the topic of sexuality and communicate a sense of openness about it. This necessitates an awareness of one's own values and reactions to sexually related issues. Generally, anxiety, shame, or discomfort about sexuality are common among most people. Putting such feelings aside and becoming aware of one's personal reactions to sexual issues is a long process that requires sensitization, education, and practice. Often a first step in reducing this tension is acknowledging one's

feelings to another person. In a work setting, a peer support group or discussion with a colleague can be especially helpful in overcoming personal barriers about sexuality.

In addition to processing personal feelings about sexuality, staff members must also master specific information on sexuality and disability. Without correct, up-to-date information about sexuality, staff members will only add confusion to an already difficult topic. Even worse, the patient and partner could be given incorrect information that will have a negative effect on their overall adjustment and relationship. An ongoing lecture series is often helpful in this regard. Typical issues addressed in such a program include sexual anatomy and physiology, effects of medications, physical functioning, treatment options such as penile injections and implants, counseling techniques, and professional roles.

In-service education programs provide an opportunity for discussion of staff-patient interactions. This is usually the primary area of staff anxiety, and sensitive discussion of it is most often welcomed and appreciated. In addition, the presentation of an overview of behavior modification techniques can be helpful. This overview should be geared around sexual issues and combined with theoretical discussions of reinforcement schedules and behavioral contingencies. Finally, the importance of limit setting and professional boundaries should be discussed and emphasized.

The development of a sexuality committee within a facility is often the method of choice in addressing ongoing sexual issues and problems. Ideally, a member of the administration should serve on the committee. This person validates the committee's function and provides a sense of security, safety, and recognition to its members. The development of institutional guidelines and procedures is usually the first task of the committee and often its most important function. It is essential that the committee establish guidelines for some of the most sensitive interactions that occur in the day-to-day functioning of the institution. Issues to be addressed typically include such matters as whether to establish a privacy room, public versus private masturbation, partner sexual activity, dissemination of birth control information and supplies, prevention of sexual assault, prevention of sexually transmitted diseases, and policies concerning the relationships between patients and staff members.

Conclusion

There are multiple restrictions on the expression of sexuality by people with disabilities. These restrictions originate from cultural biases, social ignorance, and unfounded fears regarding people with disabilities. The responsibility of health professionals is to achieve a balance between protecting the rights and privacy of hospitalized patients and providing a safe and enriching environment. As the emphasis of staff training shifts away from the imposition of control and restrictive values, a therapeutic environment that fosters self-esteem and sexual growth will emerge in the rehabilitation setting.

The 1980s and early 1990s were a time of tremendous progress in the area of sexuality and disability. What began as a passing fad outside mainstream rehabilitation became an accepted standard of practice for the rehabilitation team. Education about sexuality is now a critical component of the rehabilitation process. More important, people with disabilities are now recognized as having the same rights, needs, and desires as people without disabilities.

(*See also:* ADOLESCENTS, REHABILITATION OF; CONSUMERS; FAMILY; NEUROMUSCULAR DISORDERS; PSYCHOSOCIAL ADJUSTMENT; QUALITY OF LIFE; SPINAL CORD INJURY; STROKE)

RESOURCES

American Association of Sex Educators, Counselors, and Therapists, 435 North Michigan Ave., Suite 1717, Chicago, IL 60611

Journal of Sexuality and Disability, Human Sciences Press, 233 Spring St., New York, NY 10013

The National Task Force on Sexuality and Disability, American Congress of Rehabilitation Medicine, 5700 Old Orchard Road, Skokie, IL 60077

Sexuality and Disability Training Center, Boston University Medical Center, 88 East Newton St., Boston, MA 02118

Sexuality and Disability Training Center, University of Michigan Medical Center, 1500 East Medical Center Drive, Ann Arbor, MI 48109

BIBLIOGRAPHY

COLE, THEODORE M.; CHILGREN, RICHARD; and ROSENBERG, PAUL. "A New Program of Sex Educa-

tion and Counseling for Spinal Injured Adults and Health Care Professionals." *International Journal of Paraplegia* (Aug. 1973):111–124.

DUCHARME, STANLEY, and DUCHARME, JACQUELINE. "Sexual Adaptation." *Seminars in Neurology* 3 (1983):135–140.

ERIKSON, ERIK. *Childhood and Society.* New York, 1953.

GILL, KATHLEEN, and DUCHARME, STANLEY. "Female Sexual Functioning." In *Handbook of Clinical Neurology: Spinal Cord Trauma,* ed. H. Frankel. Amsterdam, 1992.

LEYSON, JOSE F. "Controversies and Research in Female Sexuality." In *Sexual Rehabilitation of the Spinal Cord Injured Patient,* ed. Jose F. Leyson. Clifton, NJ, 1991.

MASTERS, WILLIAM H., and JOHNSON, VIRGINIA E. *Human Sexual Response.* Boston, 1966.

SONKSEN, J., and BIERING-SORENSEN, F. "Transcutaneous Nitroglycerin in the Treatment of Erectile Dysfunctions in Spinal Cord Injured." *Paraplegia* 30 (1992):554–557.

STANLEY H. DUCHARME

SHELTERED EMPLOYMENT

See SUPPORTED EMPLOYMENT

SICKLE CELL ANEMIA AND THALASSEMIA (HEMOGLOBINOPATHIES)

Hemoglobinopathies are blood disorders caused by a genetically determined change in the molecular structure of hemoglobin. This entry will discuss, in turn, sickle cell anemia and thalassemia.

Sickle Cell Anemia

Sickle cell anemia is inherited predominately within the black population, with approximately 10 percent carriers (sickle trait) for the gene. In Equatorial Africa, the presence of sickle trait confers better survival of malaria than having a normal hemoglobin A. When two individuals with sickle trait have children, there is a one-in-four risk for every pregnancy that the child will have it. There are other variants of sickle cell hemoglobinopathy: hemoglobin SC and S thalessemia. These combinations result from the union of a person who has sickle cell trait and one who has a trait for thalassemia or hemoglobin C.

Normal hemoglobin is made up of two alpha and two beta chains. The genetic mutation in sickle cell anemia is at the sixth amino acid of the beta chain and results in the insertion of a valine for the normal glutamic acid. A person with sickle trait carrier has one normal beta chain and one beta S chain and is asymptomatic. Carriers can be detected by a variety of solubility tests of hemoglobin and confirmed on electrophoresis because the amino chain substitution alters the charge of the molecule and its movement in an electrophoretic field.

In a person with sickle cell anemia the hemoglobin in red blood cells changes from a liquid to a solid (crystal) state when the red blood cells give up oxygen to the tissues. The red cells then get stuck in capillaries throughout the body, giving rise to a variety of problems.

At birth newborns have predominately approximately 80 percent fetal hemoglobin (Hgb FH). Screening of the newborn can identify a child with a major sickle hemoglobinopathy by finding hemoglobin S and F (or SCF) and no traces of hemoglobin A. Symptoms, however, do not begin until the fetal hemoglobin declines after birth, and begin at three to six months of age. The initial signs may be swelling of the hands and feet—dactylitis—with any combination of the extremities involved. Children develop a large spleen and pallor due to anemia. The sudden enlargement of the spleen, acute splenic sequestration, can be life-threatening, and transfusions are needed immediately. As the child grows older, other effects on the bones may be seen, such as aseptic necrosis (sterile destruction) of the hips, which leads to the need for hip replacement.

The spleen becomes congested with the sickle cells and does not function normally to remove bacteria from the blood. Children are at high risk from dying from an infection with the common pneumococcus. This situation can be prevented by taking penicillin twice a day.

As the child grows, pain crises begin to occur. "Crises" is a poor term as there is little risk of death, but certainly these incidents are painful. In infants the hands and the feet are affected; in children the arms and the thighs; and in adults the back, pelvis, and chest. There are no tests to tell whether a patient is in a pain crisis, as there are no significant changes in blood tests. A major risk is that the child will develop drug-seeking behavior as the result of exposure to narcotics.

The acute chest syndrome mimics a pneumonia because the patient has fever and an infiltrate on the chest X ray. There may be a decreased ability of the red cells to absorb oxygen from the lungs. Such patients need antibiotics and transfusions to increase the blood oxygen-carrying capacity. The patient may require therapy in intensive care units, and in severe situations, an exchange transfusion. In milder cases a transfusion of red blood cells is needed. Leukopour (white cell depleted) red blood cells should be used to decrease transfusion reactions.

The aplastic crisis is an infection with parvovirus B 19, which temporarily reduces red blood cell production in everyone. But normal people whose red cell life span is 120 days do not become anemic if they do not make red blood cells for five to seven days. However, patients with sickle cell disease make seven to fifteen times the normal number of red blood cells every day, and when they get a parvovirus B 19 infection, anemia develops very quickly and the patient may need a transfusion. This situation usually occurs only once because the child develops antibodies to the parvovirus that will prevent reinfection.

Stroke is a low-risk event, probably in fewer than 1 percent of the patients. However, it has approximately a 66 to 75 percent recurrence rate if the individual is not placed on lifelong transfusion of normal red cells and chelation therapy (see the section on thalassemia in this entry). If a child develops a transient ischemic attack, the child should be referred to a center familiar with sickle cell disease, and serious consideration should be given to chronic transfusion therapy. The stroke is caused by sickling in the capillaries of the blood vessels of the brain, which causes the wall to bulge in and thus block blood flow. How much damage depends on which blood vessel was blocked. Stroke can be seen in teenagers but more commonly in children under age ten.

Educational expectations should be that of a normal child. Children with sickle cell disease have a wide variety of interests, and the intelligence range is normal. Because of the presence of the anemia, jobs that require a great deal of stamina will not be doable. As far as physical activity is concerned, children should not be arbitrarily limited but should use exertional tolerance as the guide to which sports and activities they engage in. It is perfectly fine for patients with sickle cell disease to fly in airplanes because they are pressurized. Of only historical interest was the problem of individuals with sickle trait who during World War II flew in unpressurized airplanes over the Alps and developed a mild sickle crisis.

The life expectancy may be quite good. Deaths in infancy from streptococcal pneumonia and acute splenic sequestration have been reduced by education of the parents and by daily penicillin therapy. Women with sickle cell disease have had children, but this poses great physiological stress. Pregnant women with sickle cell disease should be under the care of a sickle cell center, and liberal indications for transfusions are indicated. As individuals with sickle cell disease become adults, they may develop leg ulcers; kidney failure, and require dialysis; heart failure; or blindness. Gallstones result from rapid red blood cell destruction. However, many people with sickle cell disease have very satisfactory lives and jobs.

Most sickle cell centers give blood transfusions to sickle cell anemia patients requiring major surgery. Experimental therapy would include bone marrow transplantation, if there is a compatible family donor. However, there is always the risk of graft-versus-host disease and death from the procedure. Drugs that increase the fetal hemoglobin in red blood cells, and therefore reduce the rate of sickling, are being administered in several centers in the United States to adults and teenagers who have frequent severe crises. These drugs have yet to be studied in infants and prepubertal children.

Thalassemia

Thalassemia major (Cooley's anemia; Mediterranean anemia) is a severe, transfusion-dependent, lifelong inherited anemia.

Thalassemia is inherited from both carrier parents, who are asymptomatic. The risk with each subsequent pregnancy is one in four, or a 25 percent chance for an additional child with thalassemia. The carrier state can be detected by the small size of the red blood cells in the parents. Red cell size is measured by mean corpuscular volume (MCV), and in the Mediterranean area an MCV of less than seventy-three in an adult is very suspicious for thalassemia trait (in the absence of iron deficiency anemia). Hemoglobin, the oxygen-carrying component of red blood cells, is not produced in adequate quantity in a person with two beta thalassemia genes. Normal hemoglobin A results from the synthesis from two normal alpha chains and two beta chains. Fetal hemoglobin in the developing child *in utero* is composed of two alpha chains and two gamma chains. In thalassemia major, the beta chains are not produced adequately, and the anemia develops after birth. The severe anemia produces extreme pallor and decreased activity. On physical examination a large liver and spleen are present, and the blood count shows a severe anemia with normal white count and platelet production.

Therapy should be at a specialized center or at least coordinated by a physician experienced in thalassemia. The child will require lifelong regular blood transfusions to keep the hemoglobin at nearly normal levels. With repeated transfusions, the child will grow and develop normally. The transfusions should always be of leukodepleted blood (white cells removed) to decrease transfusion reactions to the white cells present in the donor blood. Regular transfusions will result in a large amount of iron hemochromatosis in the patient. This excess iron needs to be removed by chelation. Hemochromatosis produces abnormalities of the pancreas, causing diabetes, liver problems, heart failure, and sterility. Patients with thalassemia receive iron chelation eight to twelve hours a day via a portable pump which infuses Desferal subcutaneously. Chelation therapy is effective but expensive. There are as yet no oral iron chelating drugs. Disability need not result from hemochromatosis as long as the chelation therapy is followed. Wearing the portable pump does not interfere with the child's attending school. The transfusions usually require an absence of a half-day to a day every three to four weeks, and accommodation needs to be made for this schooling. Transfusions are given on an outpatient basis, but transfusion clinics tend to be open from

9:00 A.M. to 5:00 P.M. Monday through Friday. Children can do schoolwork during the transfusion, but most watch TV.

The major employment problem for thalassemia patients is the expensive therapy and the repeated blood transfusions. These young adults have no other limitations regarding intellectual function, and because of their regular transfusions and chelation are not frail individuals. Many employers do not hire persons with such an expensive chronic medical problem.

With effective chelation and regular transfusion, girls affected with thalassemia grow up and have children of their own. Assuming that the partner is normal, all the children of a patient with thalassemia would be carriers but not themselves affected unless their spouse carried the trait.

Thalassemia can be cured by a bone marrow transplant, provided the child has a histocompatible sibling. The best results are obtained by transplant when the child is young, before many red blood cell transfusions. However, there is a risk for graft-versus-host disease following transplantation as well as the risk of death due to bone marrow transplantation procedure. Gene therapy has not yet been developed; the gene would need to be inserted into red blood cell-forming cells in the bone marrow. Another approach is to increase the production of the *in utero* hemoglobin F by increasing a gamma chain of production.

For parents of a child with thalassemia major who are desirous of additional children, options include artificial insemination of sperm from a donor who does not carry the thalassemia gene, or implantation in the mother's womb of an egg from a woman who does not carry the thalassemia gene, with fertilization by the husband. These options may not be acceptable to some parents.

In most large cities there are Cooley's Anemia Foundations, which provide support groups and educational materials to affected families.

(*See also:* BLOOD DISORDERS)

RESOURCES

Cooley's Anemia Foundation, 105 East 22nd St., Suite 911, New York, NY 10010
National Association for Sickle Cell Disease, Inc.,
200 Corporate Pointe, Suite 495, Culver City, CA 90010

BIBLIOGRAPHY

CHARACHE, SAMUEL; LUBIN, BERTRAM; and REID, CLARICE D. "Management and Therapy of Sickle Cell Disease." NIH Publication No. 92-2117. Washington, DC, 1992.

RUTH ANDREA SEELER

SOCIAL POLICY

See DISABILITY LAW AND SOCIAL POLICY

SOCIAL WORK PRACTICE IN REHABILITATION

Social workers can promote and enhance the quality of life of the individual with a disability and his or her family throughout the life cycle. Persons new to the challenges and demands of disability need a resource person to answer their spoken and unspoken questions about their physical, emotional, social, and sexual concerns.

Yet, the good intentions of a social worker to provide treatment may not be readily accepted by people with disabilities and their family members traumatized by the physical, medical, and economic crises associated with the disability. The social worker must first form a working alliance with the person and the family members by providing them with concrete services such as financial assistance or the acquisition of appliances or knowledge about the condition.

Often work with people with disabilities must be based on a short-term crisis-intervention model. The social worker must quickly individualize the family's ego strengths, limitations, and potentialities. Social work treatment can then mobilize the individual and family's strengths and provide support for the family's shaken self-concept, social position, and the member's individual adjustment.

For parents of a child with a disability, information on child development helps them to relate more appropriately to the child and to overcome feelings of inadequacy. The social worker can be a model of empathic care while emphasizing the child's strengths to the parents, child, other family members, the medical staff, and teachers.

In addition, the social worker can point out the child's constitutional endowments, stamina, will to survive, alertness, intellectual capacity, and fortitude in the face of illness, surgery, and hospitalizations. The social worker can emphasize that the parents' caregiving tasks are the same for the youngster with a disability as for his or her siblings without disabilities. The social worker can identify parenting skills that the parents already use and can assist them in learning new skills to address the child's special needs. The social worker can promote mutuality by reminding the parents of their strengths and their love of the child and by pointing out his or her developmental potential and achievements. As the child grows, the social worker can emphasize that there is no intrinsic ceiling on the child's ego development and that there is thus hope for an optimistic future.

Since the trauma of disability creates a crisis for the person, his or her family, and the surgical-medical team, an important function of the social worker is to facilitate an informed dialogue and working alliance between the family and staff. Informed medical staff, allied health professionals, teachers, and other persons with disabilities and their family members can be crucial sources of guidance and encouragement by helping the person and family maintain the positive attitudes and behaviors that lead to physical and developmental strides. The social worker can inform parents about these resources, bring them together, and be an advocate for the person and his or her family in obtaining the information and services they require.

The social worker must also attempt to synthesize for the person and family the many divergent medical perspectives, recommendations, and procedures necessary for the treatment of the person with multiple disabilities. Hence the social worker can be the individual's advocate and interpreter to family and medical staff of his or her experiences, thoughts, feelings, and behaviors. As advocate, the social worker may also need to comment frankly to the individual and the family about the medical staff's attitudes and feelings regarding the disability, which often affect how staff members interact with the individual and the family.

While the person with the disability and the family members need to express ambivalent feelings about the condition and its ramifications to the social worker, it should be done when they can understand and accept these feelings without being overwhelmed. The individuals who receive supportive casework services are assisted in burying, to some extent, these feelings and hence postpone confronting them and the reality of the disability. It has been found that the use of denial and avoidance to suppress these feelings may be adaptive until the shock of the condition and its manifestations can be incorporated into the person and family members' egos and self-concepts.

In the case of a child with a disability, the social worker can recommend specialized nursery programs that help prepare children for mainstreaming. When the child starts nursery school, kindergarten, and first grade, the social worker can help prepare the parents, the child, and the school personnel for the transition.

Research shows that a person of any age with a disability, as well as his or her family members, benefits from observing and identifying with individuals with disabilities who have adapted successfully. The social worker should be aware of the hope it gives the family to have these adaptive models and should facilitate the family's meetings with them. In this way the social worker can also assist in finding appropriate avenues of socialization with peers in an attempt to spur autonomous ego functioning.

Social work studies also have shown that the social worker should provide clinical services not only to the child with a disability and his or her parents but to the siblings as well. Siblings in all families feel anger, anxiety, resentment, embarrassment, jealousy, grief, and guilt. Yet to varying degrees the siblings' acceptance and support can contribute to increased levels of physical activity and social, psychological, and cognitive development on the part of the child with the disability. Since siblings' attitudes and participation can contribute to the ego development and positive self-concept of the child with the disability, it is necessary to consider their needs and concerns.

In summary, the social worker attempts to assist

the person with a disability and his or her family members to find adaptive solutions to the disability experience so the person with a disability and the family can return to their own individual and collective developmental paths.

Licensure as a social worker is granted by a state's board of registration in social work according to various levels of training and experience. Although licensure levels vary from state to state, the usual licensures are the licensed independent clinical social worker (LICSW), the licensed clinical social worker (LCSW), the licensed social worker (LSW), and the licensed social work assistant (LSWA).

There is a doctorate in social work, either a D.S.W. or a Ph.D. A master's degree in social work is required to enter doctoral programs. The doctorate prepares the professional social worker to assume advanced clinical positions and/or positions in education, research, and social policy and practices.

The master of social work degree is traditionally considered a terminal professional degree. It requires a bachelor's degree and completion of a two-year master's program at an accredited graduate school of social work. Persons with a master's in social work and two years of supervisory experience can take the LICSW exam. Persons with a master's in social work without two years' experience can take the LCSW exam.

There is also a bachelor's degree in social work, which is awarded upon completion of a five-year program that provides a basic knowledge of the field. The social worker with this degree can take the LSW exam.

Some social service agencies, such as state departments of social services, may employ persons with associate's degrees in social services or a related field. These persons can take the LSWA exam.

(See also: ADVOCACY; CHILDHOOD DISABILITY; FAMILY; LOSS AND GRIEF; PEDIATRIC REHABILITATION; PSYCHOSOCIAL ADJUSTMENT)

RESOURCES

Spina Bifida Association of America, 4590 MacArthur Blvd., NW, Suite 250, Washington, DC 20007–4226

American Association of Spinal Cord Injury Psychologists and Social Workers, 75-20 Astoria Blvd., Jackson Heights, NY 11370–1178

National Center for Social Policy and Practice, National Association of Social Workers, 750 First St., NE, Suite 800, Washington, DC 20002–4241

Society for Disability Studies, Department of Sociology, Gallaudet University, 800 Florida Ave., NE, Washington, DC 20005

TASH, 11201 Greenwood Ave. North, Seattle, WA 98133

BIBLIOGRAPHY

JOHNSON, ALLEN F. "Challenged Adolescents with Spina Bifida." In *Family Interventions Throughout Chronic Illness and Disability*, eds. Paul W. Power, Arthur E. Dell Orto, and Martha B. Gibbons. New York, 1988.

———. "Forum for the Challenged." In *SCI Psychosocial Process*. New York, 1988.

NAGLER, MARK. *Perspectives on Disability: Text and Readings on Disability*. Palo Alto, CA, 1990.

TOMASZEWSKI, EVELYN. *Disability Awareness Curriculum for Graduate Schools of Social Work*. Washington, DC, 1992.

ALLEN F. JOHNSON

SOCIOLOGY

The sociology of health provides a unique perspective to rehabilitation by situating analyses of disability within their appropriate social contexts. Sociology, as a discipline, views human behavior as largely shaped by the groups to which people belong and by the social interactions within those groups. Sociologists examine the distribution of disability in society; analyze the antecedents and consequences of disability; develop theoretical models to define disability and explain rehabilitation; sensitize observers to the social experience of persons with disabilities; and study the rehabilitation response to disability on individual, organizational, and institutional levels (Albrecht, 1992). Sociologists produce research information that alerts policymakers to the problems of persons with disabilities and suggest innovative and effective rehabilitation programs to address these issues (Taylor, 1994).

For the sociologist, disability is a gap between an individual's personal capability and environmental demand (Verbrugge & Jette, 1993). Disability is not a static condition, so thinking about the problem is best considered in a life course perspective, acknowledging that chronic conditions and activity limitations experienced at birth or early in life have different definitions and consequences than those acquired during the middle and late years. Disability typically results from a pathophysiological condition but is experienced and expressed through activity limitations and in diminished or adjusted role performance over the life course. Within the life course perspective, sociologists view chronic illness and disability as life course events that mark persons with disabilities and those around them, altering their relationships with other people (Albrecht & Levy, 1991). The onset of disability, for example, may prompt a person to acquire more education and change to a white-collar career that demands less physical exertion and pays more money. In other situations, disability can exert so much stress on a marriage that divorce results. Adjustment to disability is dependent on the time that the disability occurs in the life course, the severity and duration of the disability, and the effects that these have on other life course events, such as education, marriage, bearing and rearing children, work, and retirement.

Rehabilitation is both a philosophy and a practice designed to enable persons with disability to function at their highest possible physical, social, and psychological levels. Sociologists focus on the social factors that facilitate or impede this enablement process. Rehabilitation, for example, requires the negotiation of a series of physical and social transitions, such as moving from home to hospital and clinics to home again and from being a wage earner to being without a job and then trying to reenter the labor force. Sociologists study how these transitions are managed and how persons with disabilities become empowered. All of this activity is shaped by the physical and social environment and resources available to the person with disabilities. Integral families, adequate insurance, and rich social networks, for instance, provide a resource base that facilitates rehabilitation. Sociologists also study how disability can be moderated through prevention. Ideally, prevention forestalls what might have been, whereas rehabilitation enables people to live as full a life as possible.

Sociologists address these topics through multiple methods and procedures. In the exploratory and de-

scriptive stages of an investigation, researchers use case studies, ethnographies, participant observation, and focus groups to map the nature and extent of the problem (Denzin & Lincoln, 1994). Case studies of rehabilitation choose representative individuals with disabilities to follow closely over a period of time from disability onset through rehabilitation, or carefully describe the evolution of selected rehabilitation organizations and programs. The purpose of the case study is to provide in-depth snapshots of the rehabilitation process, which in turn will raise more formal questions to pursue. Ethnography refers to a detailed scientific description of a group of people, such as a group of persons with disabilities, or a family having a member with a disability. Ethnographies capture how others live, organize their lives, and interpret their actions. Participant observation typically involves the direct immersion of the investigator into the daily lives and world of the person with disabilities, and capturing this experience in extensive organized notes. Ethnographic and participant observation methods are frequently combined to produce elaborate descriptions and analyses of the world of persons with disabilities (Charmaz, 1991). Focus groups use group interviewing techniques where the researcher directs group members to discuss very specific questions about their experiences with disabilities and the rehabilitation process.

In more formal analyses of disability and rehabilitation, sociologists undertake large representative surveys or perform secondary data analyses of information gathered by the National Health Interview Survey, the Centers for Disease Control, the Census Bureau, the Bureau of Labor Statistics, and Lou Harris Associates to test hypotheses and develop models of rehabilitation. These surveys often concentrate on persons with disabilities, their families, work, and place in society. Questions in these surveys are designed to measure levels of functional limitation and dependency, needs, access to and costs of care, discrimination, the effect of disability across the life course, experiences with the rehabilitation system, and the effect of disability laws on those with the problems. The results are used by disability activist groups to lobby for needed system changes and by policymakers to fit programs and services better to the needs of the population.

In all of these endeavors, sociologists are deeply

concerned about the validity and reliability of their research and about policy implications of their findings. Validity refers to the accuracy with which these studies measure what they purport to measure, and reliability to the applicability of the findings to other groups. Increasingly, sociologists are undertaking evaluation research of rehabilitation policies and programs. Study design and methods are critically important here because the results will be used to modify programs and change policies. Solid and informative results will result in improved programs. Sociological research on disability and rehabilitation has enormous policy implications, because impairments and medical conditions often dramatically change people's lives, and the burden of disability on society has major social and economic consequences. Furthermore, this research is important because the way that a society treats its persons with disabilities often reflects its fundamental social values.

Sociologists of health generally spend their lives doing research and teaching in universities, health science centers, government agencies, or nonprofit research organizations. While they are trained at the bachelor's, master's, and Ph.D. levels, the vast majority of investigators have a Ph.D. degree from a research-oriented university. Their doctoral program consists of courses in sociological theory, the sociology of health and illness, disability and rehabilitation, methods, measurement, survey design, statistical analysis, and qualitative research. During their training, they assist senior faculty in research and write a thesis based on their own original work. Research-oriented sociologists belong to and are active in such organizations as the Medical Sociology Section of the American Sociological Association, the British Sociological Association, the International Sociological Association, the American Public Health Association, the American Association of Public Opinion Research, the Association for Health Services Research, and the American Congress of Rehabilitation Medicine. A few sociologists are interested in delivering direct clinical services. They are credentialed by the American Sociological Association.

Under health care reform, sociologists could play an increasingly significant role in the field of rehabilitation. Blueprints for health care reform are based on a few basic principles, including universal access, core benefits for all Americans, contained costs, increased competition among providers, shifting services to the community, and outcome orientation. Because those who are covered inadequately or not at all by the current health care system are more likely to have poorer health and to be disabled than the general population, there would be an increased demand for rehabilitation. Moreover, there would be increased pressures to make service delivery more efficient.

Sociologists possess the skills and expertise to design and evaluate service outcomes in hospital- and community-based programs. In addition, sociologists are familiar with the lives and problems of the homeless, prisoners, disenfranchised, workers in dangerous jobs, and older Americans—those most likely to acquire disabilities. Because of their knowledge and expertise, sociologists will increasingly be called on to help others understand the world of persons with disabilities, develop enriched personal and community resources, design and situate innovative programs in the community, and evaluate the results of new interventions both in medical settings and the community.

(*See also:* DISABILITY; PSYCHOSOCIAL ADJUSTMENT; RESEARCH, REHABILITATION)

RESOURCES

American Association of Public Opinion Research, P.O. Box 1248, Ann Arbor, MI 60603

American Congress of Rehabilitation Medicine, 5700 Old Orchard Rd, Skokie, IL 60077

American Public Health Association, 1015 15th St., NW, Washington, DC 20005

American Sociological Association, 1722 N St., NW, Washington, DC 20036

British Sociological Association, Unit 36, Mountjoy Research Centre, Stockton Rd, Durham DH1 3UR England

International Sociological Association, Pinar 25, E-28006 Madrid, Spain

BIBLIOGRAPHY

ALBRECHT, GARY L. *The Disability Business: Rehabilitation in America.* Newbury Park, CA, 1992.

ALBRECHT, GARY L, and LEVY, JUDITH A. "Chronic

Illness and Disability as Life Course Events." *Advances in Medical Sociology* 2 (1991):3–13.

CHARMAZ, KATHY. *Good Days, Bad Days: The Self in Chronic Illness and Time.* New Brunswick, NJ, 1991.

DENZIN, NORMAN K., and LINCOLN, YOLANDA S., eds. *Handbook of Qualitative Research.* Newbury Park, CA, 1994.

TAYLOR, HUMPHREY. *N.O.D. Survey of Americans with Disabilities.* Washington, DC, 1994.

VERBRUGGE, LOIS M., and JETTE, ALAN M. "The Disablement Process." *Social Science and Medicine* 38 (1993):1–14.

GARY L. ALBRECHT

SPECIAL EDUCATION

Legislative emphases on school-to-work transition have renewed interest in the linkage between special education and rehabilitation services (DeStefano & Wermuth, 1992; Szymanski, Hanley-Maxwell, and Asselin, 1992). Thus it is important for rehabilitation professionals to have at least cursory knowledge of special education. To this end, the purpose of this entry is to provide rehabilitation professionals with information about the following aspects of special education: recent history and legislation; theory, philosophy, and reforms; methods and techniques; the profession of special education; and major issues.

Recent History and Legislation

Special education was shaped by a wide range of social forces, legislation, and litigation. In the nineteenth century, charitable groups dominated education of people with disabilities (Liachowitz, 1988; Wright, 1980). However, by the early twentieth century, public school classes for students with mental retardation and residential programs for students with sensory impairments were well established (Liachowitz, 1988; Rubin & Roessler, 1987). Subsequently, the enforcement of compulsory education laws added momentum to the development of public special education (Hallahan & Kauffman, 1988).

The simple availability of special education in some locations did not constitute the right to education for students with disabilities. In fact, in the early decades of this century, one could be denied the opportunity for education simply due to a disability (Laski, 1985). Although the historic 1954 U.S. Supreme Court decision *Brown v. Board of Education* outlawed racial segregation in public education, students with disabilities were not given the right to education until 1975. Even then, they often were not fully included in school activities (Hahn, 1989).

The Education for All Handicapped Children Act of 1975, which was later renamed the Individuals with Disabilities Education Act (IDEA), was considered to be the landmark legislation of special education (Laski, 1985). It mandated that all students whose disabilities were determined to present special instructional needs be provided with a free and appropriate public special education in the least restrictive environment. The law also required due process considerations and the development of an individualized education program (IEP), which was to connect assessment to curriculum and provide a basis for measuring progress (Laski, 1985; Podemski et al., 1984).

Initial implementation of the IDEA legislation addressed the typical age range of school attendance. The 1986 amendments added focus on infants and toddlers, who were defined as children from birth through age two who experienced developmental delays or who were "at risk" of developing such delays without early intervention (IDEA, 1986). A central point of the amendments was the individualized family service plan, which is similar to the IEP but reflects emphasis on the family as well as the child.

The 1990 amendments to IDEA emphasized the other end of the school age continuum—the transition from school to work or postsecondary education. Transition services were defined as "a coordinate set of activities for a student, designed within an outcome-oriented process, which promotes movement from school to postschool activities . . . based upon the individual student's needs, taking into account the student's preferences and interests . . ." (IDEA, 1990). Students' IEPs were required to contain consideration of transition planning by age sixteen (IDEA, 1990).

Rehabilitation counseling was specifically added to the list of related services in the 1990 IDEA amendments. Its omission in previous years had not been intended to exclude rehabilitation counselors from consideration as related service professionals in special education. In fact, the report that accompanied passage of the amendments specifically mentioned rehabilitation counseling as an allowable related service and an important component of transition services for students with disabilities (Hanley-Maxwell & Szymanski, 1992; House of Representatives Report 101-544, 1990).

Although special education and rehabilitation services are both administered through the U.S. Department of Education's Office of Special Education and Rehabilitation Services, there are critical service delivery differences (Szymanski, Hanley-Maxwell, and Asselin, 1992). The difference that is often most confusing for rehabilitation counselors relates to financing. Specifically, special education services have a direct connection to local and/or state tax bases, whereas rehabilitation services are funded solely by federal and state subsidies (Szymanski, Hanley-Maxwell, and Asselin, 1992). As a result, rehabilitation services have funding constraints and when states cannot serve all eligible individuals, individuals with severe disabilities are accorded selection priority (Rehabilitation Services Administration, 1993). Special education services, on the other hand, have no such constraints. School districts are required to provide all eligible students with a free, appropriate, special education, including related services when necessary (IDEA, 1975, 1990).

Theory, Philosophy, and Reforms

Special education can be considered an atheoretical or applied field based on assumptions that disabilities are diagnosable individual characteristics and that a coordinated system of diagnosis and instructional interventions can benefit identified students (Skrtic, 1991). The essence of the assumptions of special education is questioned in theoretical discourse outside the discipline (e.g., Apple, 1990; Mehan, Hertweck, and Meihls, 1986; Szymanski & Trueba, 1994). However, with few notable exceptions (e.g., Amado, 1988; Meyer & Evans, 1993), this discourse remains largely outside the special education literature (Skrtic, 1991). Thus the discipline of special education is relatively insular and does not often enter into the larger philosophical and social debates that contextualize education.

Although special education may be relatively atheoretical, it has no shortage of philosophical approaches and ideologies. The IDEA legislation presented a paradoxical blend of two opposing philosophies—the medical model and normalization. On the one hand, students are required to have specified diagnoses and educational plans that address strengths and weaknesses. However, on the other hand, instructional programs are required to educate students in the least restrictive environment and integrate them to the greatest extent possible with their same-aged non-disabled peers (Podemski et al., 1984).

The complexity of the relation of the IDEA legislation to special education philosophies has led to some paradoxical situations. For example, although the legislation mandated inclusion of students with disabilities in academic activities, transportation complications often resulted in their exclusion from after-school activities such as clubs or teams, which are critical parts of the sociocultural environment of the school and community (Hahn, 1989). Further, although special education has been based on the importance of individualized plans, tendencies toward overgeneralization of specific ideologies have limited available alternatives for students (Howe & Miramontes, 1992).

The combination of the paradoxical blend of ideologies in special education and the relative paucity of theoretical discourse have led to recurring reform efforts (Skrtic, 1991). Reform movements have emerged from different constituencies and involved issues relating to both instructional strategies and the location of instruction. Critics of the existing special education system argue that evidence has not shown special education to be effective (Lipsky & Gartner, 1989) and that special education must be viewed as part of a larger system, not a separate programmatic entity (Skrtic, 1991). While some proponents of school reform have supported the need for collaboration between special education and regular education, another contingent has promoted the wholesale elimination of special education (Fuchs & Fuchs, 1991).

In the 1980s, pressure exerted by groups of special educators resulted in two educational reform movements. The regular education initiative addressed concerns relating to the integration of students with mild and high-incidence disabilities into the instructional mainstream. The full inclusion movement sought the location and instruction of students with the most severe disabilities in regular classrooms (Fuchs & Fuchs, 1994).

The Regular Education Initiative. The regular education initiative (REI) focused concern on the combination of the setting of instruction and the methods of acquiring competencies (Pugach & Sapon-Sevin, 1987; Reynolds, Wang, and Walberg, 1987; Will, 1986). Within her position at the U.S. Office of Special Education and Rehabilitative Services, Assistant Secretary Madeline Will (1986) brought discussion of the REI into public focus. Will did not specifically label this movement, but she clearly called for increased cooperation between general and special educators to decrease the "fragmented approach" to service delivery. Additionally, Will placed the responsibility for potential changes in service delivery at the school building, not the legislative level (Will, 1986). Will's report initiated and fueled ongoing discussion in the field (Lilly, 1989).

Regular educators, such as Maynard Reynolds, Margaret Wang, and Herbert Walberg (1987), and others, called for merger of special education and regular education. Suggested strategies included (1) waivers of regulations; (2) modification of the educational options; and (3) reorganization of classrooms (Fuchs & Fuchs, 1994). Examples of classroom reorganization included alternative learning environment model (Wang & Birch, 1984) and cooperative learning approaches (Slavin & Stevens, 1991). Interestingly, most proponents of REI have not supported full-scale elimination of special education but rather have advocated a shift in the roles of special educators to coteachers, consultants, and specialists (Fuchs & Fuchs, 1994).

The Full Inclusion Movement. Some people have characterized educational reform as a continual evolution toward inclusion (Reynolds, 1989). Central to the reform agenda has been a push toward deconstruction of special education and elimination of the continuum of services (Biklen, 1985; Lipsky & Gartner, 1992; Taylor, 1988). This idea is currently reflected in platforms linked to the "inclusive schools movement." Inherent to this initiative are the basic tenets of local control, teacher empowerment, and reconfiguration of professional roles (Stainback &

Stainback, 1992). The movement is further characterized by a balanced emphasis on both the academic and social aspects of school (Giangreco, 1992).

It is important to note that the full inclusion movement does not necessarily mean that students spend all their time in regular education classrooms. While a regular education classroom base in the student's home school is a necessary foundation, additional experiences (e.g., instruction in work environments) are required to prepare students with severe disabilities for valued adult roles (Brown et al., 1991).

To the supporters of full inclusion, the shift from REI to full inclusion reflects a larger change in the basic conceptualization of education (Lipsky & Gartner, 1992). From their view, a paradigm shift has occurred, representing a major change in how the education of students with disabilities is conceptualized. This new paradigm rejects the concept of education as system built on student deficits and limitations and suggests a sociocultural phenomenon focusing on individual capacities and learning as a life-span activity (Bishop, Foster, and Jubala, 1993; Stainback & Stainback, 1992).

Reform movements will no doubt continue in special education. It has been suggested that although the profession has been based on repudiation of overgeneralizations about children and education, it is nonetheless prone to overgeneralization about what works (Kauffman, 1992). For example, some members of the deaf community and some educators specializing in deafness oppose the full inclusion movement on the basis of the unique needs of children with deafness. They contend that inclusion limits development of language and social skills of children with deafness and seriously inhibits deaf culture (Lane, 1992). This contention of nonapplicability exemplifies the limitations of any one approach to meet the perceived needs of all special education stakeholders. Thus it is likely that reforms will continue as various approaches are put forth and debated.

Methods and Techniques

Instructional approaches in special education are as diverse as the needs of the students (D'Alonzo, Arnold, and Yuen, 1986). This diversity is compounded by the fact that varied philosophical approaches to instruction have evolved (Lipsky & Gartner, 1989; Stainback & Stainback, 1992). Most special education approaches can be grouped in two categories: those that teach specific skills or groups of skills to students, and those that support regular education teachers and other staff members to facilitate the integration of students with disabilities.

In the first category, systematic instruction includes a variety of behavioral approaches to address the instructional and social needs of students with disabilities. In systematic instruction, assessment and intervention are related in an ongoing fashion. Baseline data are collected; interventions are designed and implemented to address the particular learning or behavioral objective; and information from ongoing assessment is used to measure the effectiveness and to improve interventions (Snell, 1987). In direct instruction, which is one example, instructional methods are scientifically planned and evaluated (Tarver, 1992).

Also in the first category, but based on a contrasting philosophy of education, the whole language approach integrates the code of reading into the substance of what is read, thus facilitating learning in the context of social and personal meaning (Stahl & Miller, 1989). The whole language approach views the student as the center of what is meaningful in instruction.

Philosophical differences result in debates between advocates of different methods for teaching specific skills. For example, on the one hand, whole language proponents perceived direct instruction as too mechanistic and too teacher-centered (Heshusius, 1991). On the other hand, direct instruction proponents perceived whole language as ignoring the foundation strategies on which future learning can be most effectively built (Tarver, 1992).

The second category of interventions addresses the "interactive process which enables people with diverse expertise to generate creative solutions to mutually defined problems" (West & Idol, 1990). The underlying concept is that when educators unify their technical, theoretical, and material resources, both students and staff benefit from the "collective wisdom" (Thousand et al., 1992). Collaborative consultation involves the provision of skill training and support services to assist regular education teachers and others in addressing the unique needs of special education students.

Special education interventions across both categories are often applied to the context of the criterion of ultimate functioning. Specifically, the criterion suggests that all interventions should prepare students to function effectively in their current and future domestic, social, educational, and vocational environments (Brown et al., 1980). The challenges of this criterion have renewed the importance of preparing effective professionals who can design and implement meaningful educational programs for students with disabilities.

The Profession of Special Education

The profession of special education has been heavily influenced in its development by other disciplines, most notably education, psychology, medicine, and sociology. In fact, many early leaders in special education were trained in psychology (Hallahan & Kauffman, 1988). Personnel preparation in special education did not really begin to develop until the 1950s. Interestingly, "until that time the pervading philosophy in education was that any good teacher could teach any child or group of children" (Asselin, Hanley-Maxwell, and Szymanski, 1992). Since that time, however, states increasingly have based teacher certification on disability-specific course and field experience requirements, and colleges and universities developed specialized personnel preparation programs (Lilly, 1989).

Legislation during the 1950s and 1960s provided funds to train special educators. In 1958 the federal government allocated monies to train teachers of students with cognitive disabilities (Dybwad, 1980). Most states employ a licensure system that requires at least a bachelor's degree and relies on certification by a college or university that a student has completed a prescribed course of study and field experience. A variety of speciality categories and generic certifications exist, and requirements vary across states. This system has been considered by some people to restrict innovation and limit the flexibility of higher education to address areas of personnel shortages in a timely fashion. Some states (e.g.,

Oregon and California) have developed innovative approaches to teacher certification, while others (e.g., New Jersey), faced with personnel shortages, have developed alternative routes to licensure (Lilly, 1992).

While the field of special education has continued to develop, the old questions about the responsibilities of all teachers to teach all students have reemerged. The disproportionate placement of minority children in special education has been seen as evidence of the failure of regular education to meet the needs of an increasingly diverse student population (Bishop, Foster, and Jubala, 1993; Cummins, 1986; Skrtic, 1991; Trueba, 1989). And the importance of a general knowledge base for teacher education has been reasserted (Wang, Haertel, and Walberg, 1993). Thus certification and personnel preparation categories based on student difference have been called seriously into question (Pugach, 1992; Skrtic, 1991).

The body of knowledge in special education is reflected in a wide range of journals, some of which are connected to professional associations. The major association for special educators is the Council for Exceptional Children, which was founded in 1922 and has divisions for student-related specialties (e.g., learning disabilities, mental retardation, early childhood, career development) and job-related specialties (e.g., teacher education, administration, research) (Hallahan & Kauffman, 1988). Other associations of interest to special educators include the Association for Children with Learning Disabilities, which was founded in 1963 (Myers & Hammill, 1982) and the Association of Persons with Severe Handicaps, which has played a major role in the full inclusion and supported employment movements (Sailor, 1989). Significant journals include *The Journal of Learning Disabilities*, which published a classic special issue on the regular education initiative (Skrtic, 1991) and remedial and special education. Both of these journals are published by the Austin-based company Pro-Ed, which publishes a number of special education and related journals and books. Other, nonspecial education journals, such as *Harvard Educational Review* and the *American Educational Research Journal*, have periodically included articles relating to special education.

Major Issues

Although the IDEA legislation was considered by most special educators and advocates to be a major step forward, scholars have pointed to unintended negative outcomes (Skrtic, 1991). Since IDEA first took effect in 1975, there has been a 23 percent increase in students identified as having disabilities (Fuchs & Fuchs, 1994). This increase has been most pronounced in the area of learning disabilities, in which there has been a 119 percent increase (Hume, 1988b). Further, students from diverse racial and ethnic backgrounds are grossly overrepresented in special education (Harry, 1992; Hume, 1988a). In fact, it has been suggested that assessment and special education have been used to legitimize the failures of minority students (Trueba, 1989) and students with disabilities (Amado, 1988; Szymanski & Trueba, 1994).

If outcomes are considered, evidence suggests that special education is not necessarily associated with valued adult roles. Specifically, the National Longitudinal Transition Study (NLTS) found that only 46 percent of persons with disabilities who left school in 1987 were competitively employed, in comparison with 65 percent of the general youth population in 1991. Although a causal relationship cannot be established, many leaders in special education have considered these results as a call to action supporting the importance of the transition emphasis of current legislation.

Conclusion

Special education, like rehabilitation counseling, is based on the concept of disability as deviance (Szymanski & Trueba, 1994). This concept has been seriously challenged (Hahn, 1989, Higgins, 1992; Skrtic, 1991; Szymanski & Trueba, 1994). Further, it has been suggested that individual professionals, in both special education and rehabilitation, can actually contribute to the construction of deviance and thus do more damage than good (Amado, 1988; McKnight, 1977; Stubbins, 1988).

The transition from school to work poses unique challenges for students with disabilities and for the professionals who work with them. These challenges will best be met when rehabilitation professionals

685

collaborate with special education teachers to assist students with disabilities in recognizing and capitalizing on their work-related talents (Asselin, Hanley-Maxwell, & Szymanski, 1992). Without such collaboration, and without a primary focus on the needs and goals of the student and family, professionals can become agents of the status quo, limiting the full participation of persons with disabilities in society (Szymanski, 1994).

(*See also:* ADOLESCENTS, REHABILITATION OF; CHILDHOOD DISABILITIES; DEVELOPMENTAL DISABILITIES; DISABILITY LAW AND SOCIAL POLICY; FAMILY; LEARNING DISABILITIES; NORMALIZATION AND SOCIAL ROLE VALORIZATION; SUPPORTED EMPLOYMENT; TRANSITION FROM SCHOOL TO WORK)

BIBLIOGRAPHY

AMADO, A. R. NOVAK. "A Perspective on the Present and Notes for New Directions." In *Integration of Developmentally Disabled Individuals into the Community*, eds. L. W. Heal, J. I. Haney, and A. R. Novak Amado. 2nd ed. Baltimore, 1988.

APPLE, MICHAEL. *Ideology and Curriculum*, 2nd ed. New York, 1990.

ASSELIN, SUSAN; HANLEY-MAXWELL, CHERYL; and SZYMANSKI, EDNA M. "Transdisciplinary Personnel Preparation." In *Transition from School to Adult Life: Models, Linkages, and Policy*, eds. Frank R. Rusch, Lizanne DeStefano, Janice Chadsey-Rusch, L. Allen Phelps, and Edna M. Szymanski. Sycamore, IL, 1992.

BIKLEN, DOUGLAS. *Achieving the Complete School.* New York, 1985.

BISHOP, KATHRYN D.; FOSTER, WILLIAM; and JUBALA, KIMBERLEE A. "The Social Construction of Disability in Education: Organizational Considerations." In *Educational Administration in a Pluralistic Society*, ed. Colleen A. Capper. Albany, NY, 1993.

BROWN, LOU; FALVEY, MARY; PUMPIAN, IAN; BAUMGART, DIANE; NISBET, JAN; FORD, ALISON; SCHROEDER, JACK; and LOOMIS, RUTH. *Curricular Strategies for Teaching Severely Handicapped Students Functional Skills in School and Nonschool Environments.* Madison, WI, 1980.

BROWN, LOU; SCHWARZ, PATRICK; UDVARI-SOLNER, A.; KAMPSCHROER, ELISE F.; JOHNSON, FRAN; JORGENSEN, JACK; and GRUENEWALD, LEE. "How Much Time Should Students with Severe Intellectual Disabilities Spend in Regular Education Classrooms and Elsewhere?" *Journal of the Association of Persons with Severe Handicaps* 16 (1991):39–47.

CUMMINS, JIM. "Empowering Minority Students: A Framework for Intervention." *Harvard Educational Review* 56 (1986):18–36.

D'ALONZO, BRUNO J.; ARNOLD, BARBARA J.; and YUEN, PING C. "Teaching Adolescents with Learning and Behavioral Differences." In *Teaching Secondary Students with Mild Learning and Behavior Problems*, eds. Lowell F. Masters and Allen A. Mori. Rockville, MD, 1986.

DeSTEFANO, LIZANNE, and WERMUTH, THOMAS R. "IDEA (P.L. 101-476): Defining a Second Generation of Transition Services." In *Transition from School to Adult Life: Models, Linkages, and Policy*, eds. Frank R. Rusch, Lizanne DeStefano, Janis Chadsey-Rusch, L. Allen Phelps, and Edna M. Szymanski. Sycamore, IL, 1992.

DYBWAD, GUNNAR. "Avoiding Misconceptions of Mainstreaming, the Least Restrictive Environment, and Normalization." *Exceptional Children* 47 (1980):85–88.

FUCHS, DOUGLAS, and FUCHS, LYNN S. "Framing the REI Debate: Abolitionists versus Conservationists." In *The Regular Education Initiative: Alternative Perspectives on Concepts, Issues, and Models*, eds. John W. Lloyd, Nirbhay N. Singh, and Alan C. Repp. Sycamore, IL, 1991.

———. "Inclusive Schools Movement and the Radicalization of Special Education Reform." *Exceptional Children* 60 (1994):294–309.

GIANGRECO, MICHAEL R. "Curriculum in Inclusion-Oriented Schools: Trends, Issues, Challenges, and Potential Solutions." In *Curriculum Considerations in Inclusive Classrooms: Facilitating Learning for All Students*, eds. Susan Stainback and William Stainback. Baltimore, 1992.

HAHN, HARLAN. "The Politics of Special Education. In *Beyond Separate Education: Quality Education for All*, eds. Dorothy K. Lipsky and Alan Gartner. Baltimore, 1989.

HALLAHAN, DANIEL P., and KAUFFMAN, JAMES M. *Exceptional Children: Introduction to Special Education*, 4th ed. Englewood Cliffs, NJ, 1988.

HANLEY-MAXWELL, CHERYL, and SZYMANSKI, EDNA M. "Transition and Supported Employment." In *Rehabilitation Counseling: Basics and Beyond*, eds. Randall M. Parker and Edna M. Szymanski. 2nd ed. Austin, TX, 1992.

HARRY, BETH. *Cultural Diversity, Families, and the Special Education System.* New York, 1992.

HESHUSIUS, LOUIS. "Curriculum-Based Assessment and Direct Instruction: Critical Reflections on Fundamental Assumptions." *Exceptional Children* 57 (1991): 315–328.

HIGGINS, PAUL C. *Making Disability: Exploring the Social Transformation of Human Variation.* Springfield, IL, 1992.

HOUSE OF REPRESENTATIVES REPORT 101-544. "Report to Accompany HR-1013, the Individuals with Disabilities Education Act Amendments of 1990." Washington, DC, 1990.

HOWE, KENNETH R., and MIRAMONTES, OTELIA B. *The Ethics of Special Education.* New York, 1992.

HUME, MAGGIE. "OCR Data Show Minorities Overrepresented Among Disability Groups." *Education Daily,* Feb. 17, 1988a, pp. 5–6.

———. "Another Year Increases the Demands on Special Educators, Report Says." *Education Daily,* Mar. 4, 1988b, pp. 7–8.

Individuals with Disabilities Education Act (IDEA) of 1975. 20 U.S.C. 1400 (formerly titled the Education of the Handicapped Act [PL 94-142]). Washington, DC, 1975.

Individuals with Disabilities Education Act (IDEA) Amendments of 1986. 20 U.S.C. 1400 (formerly titled the Education of the Handicapped Act Amendments [PL 99-457]). Washington, DC, 1986.

Individuals with Disabilities Education Act (IDEA) Amendments of 1990. 20 U.S.C. 1400 (PL 101-476). Washington, DC, 1990.

KAUFFMAN, JAMES M. "Foreword." In *The Ethics of Special Education,* eds. Kenneth R. Howe and Otelia B. Miramontes. New York, 1992.

LANE, HARLAN. *The Mask of Benevolence: Disabling the Deaf Community.* New York, 1992.

LASKI, FRANK J. "Right to Habilitation and Right to Education: The Legal Foundation." In *Living and Learning in the Least Restrictive Environment,* eds. R. H. Bruininks and K. C. Lakin. Baltimore, 1985.

LIACHOWITZ, CLAIRE H. *Disability as a Social Construct: Legislative Roots.* Philadelphia, 1988.

LILLY, M. STEVEN. "Teacher Preparation." In *Beyond Separate Education: Quality Education for All,* eds. Dorothy K. Lipsky and Alan Gartner. Baltimore, 1989.

———. "Research on Teacher Licensure and State Approval of Teacher Education Programs." *Teacher Education and Special Education* 15 (1992):148–160.

LIPSKY, DOROTHY K., and GARTNER, ALAN. *Beyond Separate Education: Quality Education for All.* Baltimore, 1989.

———. "Achieving Full Inclusion: Placing the Student at the Center of Educational Reform." In *Controversial Issues Confronting Special Education: Divergent Perspectives,* eds. William Stainback and Susan Stainback. Boston, 1992.

McKNIGHT, JOHN. "Professionalized Service and Disabling Help." In *Disabling Professions,* eds. Ivan Illich, Irvin K. Zola, John McKnight, Jonathan Caplan, and Harley Shaiken. London, 1977.

MEHAN, HUGH; HERTWECK, ALMA; and MEIHLS, J. LEE. *Handicapping the Handicapped: Decision-Making in Students' Educational Careers.* Stanford, CA, 1986.

MEYER, LUANNA H., and EVANS, IAN M. "Science and Practice in Behavioral Intervention: Meaningful Outcomes, Research Validity, and Usable Knowledge." *The Journal of the Association of Persons with Severe Handicaps* 18 (1993):224–234.

MYERS, PATRICIA I., and HAMMILL, DONALD. *Learning Disabilities: Basic Concepts, Assessment Practices, and Instructional Strategies.* Austin, TX, 1982.

NATIONAL LONGITUDINAL TRANSITION STUDY. *Highlights.* Menlo Park, CA, 1991.

PODEMSKI, R. S.; PRICE, B. J.; SMITH, T. E. C.; and MARSH, G. E. *Comprehensive Administration of Special Education.* Rockville, MD, 1984.

PUGACH, MARLENE C. "Unifying the Preservice Preparation of Teachers." In *Controversial Issues Confronting Special Education: Divergent Perspectives,* eds. William Stainback and Susan Stainback. Boston, 1992.

PUGACH, MARLENE C., and SAPON-SEVIN, MARA. "New Agendas for Special Education Policy: What the National Reports Haven't Said." *Exceptional Children* 53 (1987):295–299.

REHABILITATION SERVICES ADMINISTRATION. *A Synopsis of the Rehabilitation Act Amendments of 1992.* Washington, DC, 1993.

REYNOLDS, MAYNARD C. "An Historical Perspective: The Delivery of Special Education to Mildly Disabled and at-Risk Students." *Remedial and Special Education* 10 (1989):7–11.

REYNOLDS, MAYNARD C.; WANG, MARGARET C.; and WALBERG, HERBERT J. "The Necessary Restructuring of Special and Regular Education." *Exceptional Children* 53 (1987):391–398.

RUBIN, STANFORD E., and ROESSLER, RICHARD T. *Foundations of the Vocational Rehabilitation Process,* 3rd ed. Austin, TX, 1987.

SAILOR, WAYNE. "The Educational, Social, and Vocational Integration of Students with the Most Severe Disabilities." In *Beyond Separate Education:*

Quality Education for All, eds. Dorothy K. Lipsky and Alan Gartner. Baltimore, 1989.

SKRTIC, THOMAS M. *Behind Special Education: A Critical Analysis of Professional Culture and School Organization.* Denver, 1991.

SLAVIN, ROBERT E., and STEVENS, ROBERT J. "Cooperative Learning and Mainstreaming." In *The Regular Education Initiative: Alternative Perspectives on Concepts, Issues, and Models,* eds. John W. Lloyd, Alan C. Repp, and Nirbhay N. Singh. Sycamore, IL, 1991.

SNELL, MARTHA. *Systematic Instruction of Persons with Severe Handicaps,* 3rd ed. Columbus, OH, 1987.

STAHL, STEVEN, and MILLER, PATRICIA. "Whole Language and Language Experience Approaches for Beginning Reading: A Quantitative Research Synthesis." *Review of Educational Research* 57 (1989):87–116.

STAINBACK, SUSAN, and STAINBACK, WILLIAM. "Schools as Inclusive Communities." In *Controversial Issues Confronting Special Education: Divergent Perspectives,* eds. William Stainback and Susan Stainback. Boston, 1992.

STUBBINS, JOSEPH. "The Politics of Disability." In *Attitudes Toward Persons with Disabilities,* ed. H. E. Yuker. New York, 1988.

SZYMANSKI, EDNA M. "Transition: Life-Span, Life-Space Considerations for Empowerment. *Exceptional Children* 60 (1994):402–410.

SZYMANSKI, EDNA M.; HANLEY-MAXWELL, CHERYL; and ASSELIN, SUSAN. "The Vocational Rehabilitation, Special Education, Vocational Education Interface." In *Transition from School to Adult Life: Models, Linkages, and Policy,* eds. Frank R. Rusch, Lizanne DeStefano, Janis Chadsey-Rusch, L. Allan Phelps, and Edna M. Szymanski. Sycamore, IL, 1992.

SZYMANSKI, EDNA M., and TRUEBA, HENRY T. "Castification of People with Disabilities: Potential Disempowering Aspects of Classification in Disability Services." *Journal of Rehabilitation* 60 (1994):12–20.

TARVER, SARA G. "Cognitive Behavior Modification, Direct Instruction, and Holistic Approaches to the Education of Students with Learning Disabilities." *Journal of Learning Disabilities* 19 (1986):368–375.

———. "Direct Instruction." In *Controversial Issues Confronting Special Education: Divergent Perspectives,* ed. William Stainback and Susan Stainback. Boston, 1992.

TAYLOR, STEVEN J. "Caught in the Continuum: A Critical Analysis of the Principle of Least Restrictive Environment." *Journal of the Association of Persons with Severe Handicaps* 13 (1988): 41–53.

THOUSAND, JACQUELINE; VILLA, RICHARD A.; PAOLUCCI-WHITCOMB, PHYLLIS; and NEVIN, ANN. "A Rationale for Collaborative Consultation." In *Controversial Issues Confronting Special Education: Divergent Perspectives,* eds. William Stainback and Susan Stainback. Boston, 1992.

TRUEBA, HENRY T. "Instruction for Linguistic Minority Students: Theoretical Principles, Curriculum Design, and Teacher Preparation." In *Raising Silent Voices: Educating Linguistic Minorities for the 21st Century,* ed. Henry Trueba. New York, 1989.

WANG, MARGARET C., and BIRCH, JANE W. "Comparison of a Full-Time Mainstreaming Program and a Resource Room Approach." *Exceptional Children* 51 (1984):33–40.

WANG, MARGARET C.; HAERTEL, GENEVA D.; and WALBERG, HERBERT J. "Toward a Knowledge Base for School Learning." *Review of Educational Research* 63 (1993):249–304.

WEST, J. FREDERICK, and IDOL, LORNA. "Collaborative Consultation in the Education of Mildly Handicapped and at-Risk Students." *Remedial and Special Education* 11 (1990):22–31.

WILL, MADELINE. *Educating Students with Learning Problems: A Shared Responsibility.* Washington, DC, 1986.

WRIGHT, GEORGE N. *Total Rehabilitation.* Boston, 1980.

EDNA MORA SZYMANSKI
SARAH JOHNSTON-RODRIGUEZ
DEBRA ADRIAN HEISS
MARY HEINRICHS

SPEECH

See COMMUNICATION DISABILITIES

SPINA BIFIDA

See CHILDHOOD DISABILITIES; GENETIC DISORDERS; MENTAL RETARDATION

SPINAL CORD INJURY

Spinal cord injury (SCI) results in a catastrophic and usually permanent disability that requires comprehensive treatment and rehabilitation. It presents life-long challenges in all realms of a person's life. Spinal cord injury is defined as an injury to the spinal cord as a result of trauma or disease. It includes injuries with some degree of neurological impairment, such as muscular weakness, paralysis, loss of sensation, or loss of bladder control, and does not include those with back injuries or spinal fractures without neurologic deficits.

The spinal cord is composed of nerves that carry motor (voluntary movement), sensory, and autonomic (unconscious functions such as sweating, blood pressure regulation, and bladder control) information between the brain and the rest of the body. The spinal cord has thirty segments—eight cervical, twelve thoracic, five lumbar, and five sacral (Figure 1). Injury to any of the cervical segments results in tetraplegia (also termed quadriplegia), meaning paralysis involving, to some degree, all four extremities. Injury to the thoracic, lumbar, or sacral segments is termed paraplegia, meaning paralysis involving the legs. The lowest intact segment of the spinal cord, as determined by examination of sensory and motor function, is defined as the neurologic level. It is abbreviated using the letter and number of that segment. For example, "C6 tetraplegia" means that cervical segment six and everything above it is intact. The spinal level, defined as the vertebra that is most severely fractured, may not correspond to the neurologic level. It is possible to sustain an SCI without a spinal fracture.

Estimates suggest that in the United States 8,000 to 10,000 persons sustain traumatic spinal cord injuries every year, and approximately 200,000 people are currently living with SCI in the United States. Traumatic SCI is most commonly due to motor vehicle crashes, followed by falls, acts of interpersonal violence, and recreational sporting activities. Other causes of SCI include vascular injuries, tumors, and inflammatory diseases. Traumatic SCI primarily affects young adults. Although SCI can occur at any age, the majority of injuries occur between the ages of 16 and 30 years. Men are four times more likely to sustain an SCI than are women.

The economic impact of SCI is great. Average yearly health care and living expenses that are directly attributable to SCI vary greatly according to severity of injury. In one report, first year expenses (in 1992 dollars) averaged nearly $200,000. This

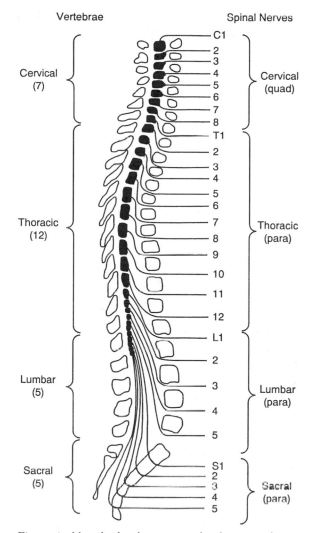

Figure 1. Vertebral column, spinal column, and nerves

ranged from $122,900 for persons with incomplete motor function to $417,000 for persons with high tetraplegia. Costs related to SCI in each subsequent year ranged from $8,600 to $74,700. The price of lost wages, fringe benefits and productivity could average nearly $38,000 but varies widely based on education, severity of injury, and pre-injury employment history.

Acute SCI Management

Because of the devastating nature of SCI, early efforts are directed toward preventing further injury and preserving as much neurologic function as possible. Initial medical care for acute SCI starts at the scene of the injury. Immobilizing the neck or back, supporting respiration and other vital functions, and transporting the injured person to a trauma center are the first priorities. Improved emergency medical services have decreased the severity of many spinal cord injuries and have saved the lives of many people with severe SCI who may have otherwise died at the scene of injury.

Initial hospital management consists of evaluating and treating spinal fractures and other injuries and preventing early complications. Persons with tetraplegia and high paraplegia are at great risk for respiratory complications, including pneumonia and respiratory failure. Initially some will require mechanical ventilation. Depending on the type of injury, overall medical condition, and severity of SCI, spinal stabilization in the form of traction, surgical fusion, or immobilization in a brace may be necessary. Providing early nutritional support and preventing medical complications such as deep venous thrombosis (blood clot forming in the veins of the legs) are important for a successful outcome.

Special attention to bladder, bowel, and skin care is crucial in the early management of SCI. Because the bladder is unable to empty voluntarily, early bladder management is usually accomplished with an indwelling catheter. Once the person is medically stable, other methods of bladder management may be started. Urologic evaluation is beneficial in determining the best method of management. The bowels function sluggishly after SCI. Early bowel care, usually facilitated by the use of rectal suppositories and laxatives, is important to prevent severe constipation and bowel obstruction. When sitting or lying down, the skin and underlying tissues are vulnerable to damage from pressure because of the loss of sensation and movement. A person with SCI must be turned in bed regularly to prevent the development of pressure ulcers, also called decubitus ulcers or bed sores. Special beds and mattresses can decrease the risk but do not eliminate the need for turning. Once sitting begins, frequent relief of pressure from the buttocks, accomplished by lifting or leaning, and a wheelchair cushion designed to distribute sitting pressures evenly is necessary. If a sore develops, rehabilitation efforts are slowed and the medical costs increase.

Psychological issues are important to address early in acute care. Recognition of the consequences of SCI and reactions to it vary greatly. Many have a fear of dying and of what the future may hold. Denial is very common. The individual is often in a state of confusion caused by a combination of medications, pain, psychological shock, sleep deprivation, or concomitant traumatic brain injury. Loss of sensation and immobilization may cause sensory deprivation leading to, in some persons, panic due to a distortion of body image and bizarre sensations such as a feeling of floating, tingling, or numbness. Confusion may also be the result of being in an environment with unfamiliar people, sights, sounds, smells, and sensations.

Family members also experience a variety of reactions, including anger, guilt, fear, anxiety, and feelings of helplessness. Persons with SCI and their families need information about their condition and possible consequences very early in the hospital stay. It is important to instill confidence in the treatment team and provide hope for the future.

Rehabilitation

After SCI even simple activities can be difficult to perform and may need to be relearned. The major emphasis in SCI rehabilitation is to teach the injured person to become as independent as possible in managing the medical, physical, psychological, social, emotional, and environmental changes that occur. This is accomplished through a program of specialized medical and nursing care; physical, occupational, and recreational therapies; counseling; and education. Recognition of the priorities of the individual, knowledge of potential levels of function, and an understanding of potential medical complications are important components of successful SCI rehabilitation.

The following paragraphs describe a potential degree of independence for persons at various levels with complete SCI (no function below the neurologic level). These are generalizations. Individual outcomes may vary because of general health, associated medical complications, psychological state, and degree of completeness of SCI.

Persons with C3 tetraplegia and above will require some form of mechanical ventilation due to the loss of respiratory function. They require total assistance in activities of daily living (ADLs), such as feeding, grooming, dressing, bathing, and toileting, and require total assistance for transfers from bed to a wheelchair. They can operate an electric wheelchair using specialized adaptations controlled with the mouth or chin. Persons with C4 tetraplegia will usually be able to wean from the ventilator, but remain dependent in most ADLs.

Persons with C5 injuries have control of their shoulders and elbow flexion. This allows them to feed themselves and perform facial hygiene tasks with use of adaptive equipment. They typically remain dependent in bathing, dressing, toileting, and transfers. An electric wheelchair with a joystick control is needed, although some are able to use a manual wheelchair for short distances. Many are able to drive a specially modified van.

Persons with C6 tetraplegia can become independent with use of adaptive equipment in most ADLs, although they may require some assistance for bathing, toileting, dressing, and transfers. Most are independent with a manual wheelchair indoors, but may need an electric wheelchair for long distances or hilly terrain. They are able to drive a modified van.

Those with C7 tetraplegia and levels below can become independent in all activities of daily living, transfers, and manual wheelchair propulsion. They are able to drive a car with hand controls or a modified van.

Persons with a low thoracic or high lumbar paraplegia (T10 to L2) are usually able to walk indoors with braces and crutches; however, the energy required for walking is so great that many do not continue. Those who walk usually do so only for exercise. Persons with level L3 and below often are able to walk with use of ankle braces and either crutches or canes.

There are vast differences in emotional responses to disability and rehabilitation. These reactions may include denial, depression, anger, acceptance, mourning, anxiety, shock, fear, aggression, rebellion, withdrawal, hostility, regression, repression, use of humor, and fantasy. Often the type of severity of response changes from moment to moment and through the initial rehabilitation period. Regaining a sense of control over one's life is extremely important. Persons with SCI should be encouraged to make decisions about their health care and personal affairs. Although they may be physically dependent, they can maintain control over their lives by directing others verbally. Rehabilitation team members, such as social workers, psychologists, vocational counselors, and other specialists, provide counseling to help the individual and family members adapt psychologically to the new situation. They also provide training in the skills necessary for independent living, such as hiring and managing persons who provide personal assistance services, finding accessible housing, and securing new sources of income.

Medical Complications

Persons with SCI are at risk for developing a number of unique, SCI-related medical complications during rehabilitation and later throughout their life. These complications are important to recognize early because some can be life threatening, while others will significantly limit a person's function and independence if not adequately treated.

Autonomic dysreflexia is a syndrome of dangerously high blood pressure associated with slow heart rate, pounding headache, facial flushing, and nasal congestion. This condition occurs only in persons with SCI above T6 and is due to noxious stimulation below the neurologic level. Prompt management of the underlying cause (often a distended bladder or bowel impaction) will lead to a rapid decrease in blood pressure. Medications to lower the blood pressure are often needed until the source of the problem is identified and treated. Untreated, this syndrome can lead to a stroke or death.

Heterotopic ossification is the appearance of bone in the soft tissue around a joint. This most often occurs at the hips and knees and is estimated to occur in 10 to 60 percent of people with SCI. The most common signs and symptoms are swelling and loss of flexibility of the joints affected. If not treated, the joint may become fused, resulting in loss of sitting ability and diminished function.

Spasticity, the presence of increased tone and involuntary movement in weak or paralyzed muscles, can also limit function or lead to complications such as pressure ulcers or falls. Stretching tight muscles is the first treatment for spasticity. Medications or surgery may be needed if the spasticity interferes with function. An increase in spasticity may indicate other medical problems, such as a urinary tract infection, an ingrown toenail, or deep venous thrombosis. Any change in spasticity should be evaluated thoroughly to exclude these and other possible complications.

Urinary tract infections (UTIs) are common because of altered bladder function. However, the usual signs and symptoms of pain and burning with urination are often absent due to loss of sensation. Many times UTIs have only vague symptoms, such as sweating, increased spasticity, and low-grade fever. Recurrent UTIs require urologic evaluation and prompt treatment to minimize risk for further complications, including kidney stones and renal failure.

Community Integration

Once a person completes the initial inpatient rehabilitation program, there are many challenges to face in order to live successfully with an SCI. One barrier to successful community reintegration is the development of medical complications that may lead to rehospitalization. The most common potentially preventable complications include pressure sores and urinary tract infections. Because of the physiologic changes that take place after injury, a person with SCI is at increased risk for developing these complications and must take an active role in their prevention. Prevention includes good hygiene, careful inspection of the skin regularly, frequent position changes and pressure relief, and careful attention to the bladder management prescribed by the physician. Medical complications are very costly, both in terms of direct medical costs for treatment, and in the loss of productivity associated with illness and hospitalization. Therefore, every effort should be made to educate the individual and family about special care needs and the importance of accepting responsibility for maintaining a healthy body. Other complications that can arise include kidney and bladder stones, chronic pain, syringomyelia (cyst formation in the spinal cord at the site of trauma), pneumonia and other respiratory conditions, osteoporosis, and fractures. Careful, routine monitoring in association with a physician trained in SCI care is important to maintaining good health.

Even though there are many changes that occur with SCI that affect sexual function, persons with SCI are capable of full participation in sexual relationships. However, changes in physical abilities, body image, bladder catheters, bowel accidents, and other problems may make sexual activities difficult and frightening. Understanding the physical and emotional changes that occur with SCI and a willingness to try new options can lead to exciting and fulfilling relationships. Many men with SCI are able to achieve erections, often adequate for intercourse. Methods to improve erections are available for those with difficulty. Most men can produce sperm capable of fertilizing an egg. However, ejaculation is generally impaired, and special methods, such as vibratory stimulation or electroejaculation (electrical stimulation of the rectum that leads to ejaculation), may be needed to collect the sperm. A woman will usually resume menstruation a few months after injury. Fertility is generally unimpaired, although she may require additional lubrication during intercourse. Women with SCI are able to become pregnant and carry the pregnancy to term.

During the first month after discharge much attention centers on the basic, practical aspects of daily life, such as getting around in the home, using the bathroom, coping with stairs, using new equipment, and arranging for necessary physical assistance and home modifications. Relearning activities that were once routine, such as cooking, housekeeping, banking, and shopping, can sometimes be overwhelming. The transition from rehabilitation to home can be eased by having the individual with SCI return home on day and weekend passes during the latter phase of inpatient rehabilitation. As a result of these visits home, the individual, the family, and the rehabilitation team are able to assess the need for further training, assistive equipment, home modifications, and paid personal assistance services.

After discharge from the hospital, emotional and social adaptation continues to be a challenge. Individuals with recent SCI must first become reintegrated into the immediate family, then into the extended family and circle of close friends, and finally into the community at large. Roles and routines are often disrupted, and new ones must be established. A period of readjustment is necessary, and the support and understanding of family and friends are essential.

Some people are able eventually to resume lives that closely resemble their preinjury situation. Many others fall short of this ideal because of barriers to community integration, such as lack of transportation, inadequate personal assistance, architectural barriers, lack of social support, society's attitude toward persons with disabilities, poor economic status, and poor physical or mental health.

It has been estimated that only about 27 percent of persons with SCI who are of working age are gainfully employed. The proportion is lower for recently injured persons and improves with increased duration of injury. People are more likely to be employed who have higher educational levels, worked in white-collar jobs before injury, are less disabled, are male, and are white. State vocational rehabilitation agencies provide economic assistance for vocational evaluation, counseling, training, education, and job placement. With appropriate training, adaptive equipment, and workplace modifications, most people with SCI can be employed in many different occupations. However, much remains to be done to eliminate barriers and promote employment opportunities.

There is hope that many of the barriers to community living and employment will be eliminated because of the Americans with Disabilities Act (ADA). Four aspects of the act are particularly relevant to the lives of persons with SCI. Employers may not refuse to hire a qualified person because of the person's disability and must provide reasonable accommodations for the person to perform the essential functions of the job. Public accommodations such as hotels, restaurants, and theaters may not refuse to serve a person with a disability, and physical barriers must be removed. Public and private transportation systems must be accessible to persons with disabilities. State and local governments may not discriminate against qualified individuals with disabilities.

Long-Term Issues

As people with SCI age, a number of changes may occur. These changes also occur in people without SCI but seem to develop earlier and, in some cases, more severely in those with SCI. Thinning skin makes it easier to develop pressure ulcers. Painful shoulder muscles due to years of use make it more difficult to push a wheelchair, transfer, or walk with crutches. Osteoporosis leads to fragile bones that are prone to fracture. A sedentary lifestyle leads to cardiovascular deconditioning and increases the risk of atherosclerosis and heart disease. Hands that take the brunt of much activity may develop numbness due to compression of nerves in the wrist (carpal tunnel syndrome). Whether these problems are due to premature aging, overuse of muscles, or biochemical changes after SCI is an area of further research.

Some individuals with SCI become better adjusted and are more satisfied with life as they age. Others have increasing difficulty with depression, substance abuse, and decreased mental abilities. Some are frightened by what the future may bring. These problems may be the result of declining physical health or environmental changes.

Weakness, fatigue, or pain may decrease a person's ability to cope with daily challenges, necessitating changes such as early retirement, more assistive equipment, or more personal assistance services. These changes can create significant problems for those on fixed and/or limited incomes. Finally, caregivers may also experience declines in physical and psychological well-being that may limit their abilities to continue to perform their caregiving roles adequately. Paid personal assistance services and respite care are possible alternatives that will allow older persons with SCI to continue to live in their own homes.

The key to the success of many "survivors"—individuals who have lived with SCI for many years—seems to be a combination of assertiveness and the ability to adapt to change. They are people who can find meaning and enjoyment in their lives despite the limitations imposed by SCI.

Prevention Efforts

Preventing SCI is much easier than curing it. Methods used to prevent SCI are grouped into three categories: educational, legislative, and environmental. Educational efforts are designed to persuade people to reduce risk-taking behavior and enhance safety. These include the "Think First Program," aimed primarily at adolescents, and a similar program designed for elementary school children. There is also a program to prevent diving-related SCI called "Feet First First Time." Legislative and enforcement efforts are also designed to restrict risky behaviors and require safety behaviors. Examples include stringent laws regarding driving under the influence of alcohol or drugs, and laws requiring use of seat belts and child restraint devices. Environmental changes designed to prevent injury do not require behavioral change by the people being protected. These measures include safer highway design, better lighting on roadways, headrests integrated into vehicle seats, air bags, and passive-restraint seat belts. These prevention strategies seem to be paying off. Trends show the proportions of injuries due to motor vehicle crashes and sporting activities have declined steadily since 1973. However, the proportions of injuries from falls and acts of violence (primarily gunshot wounds) have increased over the same period.

Future Developments

There are two main thrusts in SCI research. These can be thought of as "cure" and "care" research. The "cure" research is being done with the specific goal of finding a way to cure SCI. This may include basic science research on regeneration of the spinal cord, developing new medications and surgical techniques to minimize spinal cord damage or repair it, and developments in engineering that will allow a person to walk again using electrical stimulation. "Care" research is often in the area of finding ways to help people with SCI live full and productive lives despite their limitations. This area includes improving the care received from the time of injury through community reintegration, developing better therapy methods to facilitate recovery and strengthen weakened muscles, and preventing secondary medical complications such as UTIs, pressure ulcers, and problems related to aging. Both kinds of research are important and necessary. Both attempt to improve the lives of people with SCI but approach that goal differently.

(*See also*: FUNCTIONAL ELECTRICAL STIMULATION; HOSPITAL, REHABILITATION; PHYSICIAN; PSYCHOSOCIAL ADJUSTMENT; REHABILITATION CENTER; SEXUALITY AND DISABILITY; TECHNOLOGY; WHEELCHAIRS)

RESOURCES

SCI Organizations

Professional

American Association of Spinal Cord Injury Nurses, 75–20 Astoria Blvd., Jackson Heights, NY 11370–1177

American Association of Spinal Cord Injury Psychologists and Social Workers, 75–20 Astoria Blvd., Jackson Heights, NY 11370–1177

American Paraplegia Society, 75–20 Astoria Blvd., Jackson Heights, NY 11370–1177

American Spinal Injury Association, 345 East Superior St., Room 1436, Chicago, IL 60611

International Medical Society of Paraplegia, National Spinal Injuries Centre, Stroke Mandeville Hospital, Aylesbury, Bucks HP21 8AL, United Kingdom. U.S.A. Corresponding Secretary, R. Edward Carter, M.D., 1333 Moursund Ave., Suite E103, Houston, TX 77030

Nonprofit and Consumer

American Paralysis Association, 500 Morris Ave., Springfield, NJ 07081

California Spinal Injury Network, 3911 Princeton Drive, Santa Rosa, CA 95405

Eastern Paralyzed Veterans Association, 75–20 Astoria Blvd., Jackson Heights, NY 11370–1179

Foundation for Spinal Cord Injury Prevention, 1546 Penobscot Building, Detroit, MI 48226

National Paraplegia Foundation, 333 North Michigan Ave., Chicago, IL 60601

National Spinal Cord Injury Association, 545 Concord Ave., Cambridge, MA 02138

Paralyzed Veterans of America, 801 Eighteenth St., NW, Washington, DC 20006

Spinal Cord Society, Wendell Road, Fergus Falls, MN 56537

Governmental

U.S. Department of Education, National Institute on Disability and Rehabilitation Research-sponsored Model Regional Spinal Cord Injury Care Systems:
Georgia Regional SCI System, Atlanta, GA
Midwest Regional SCI Care System, Chicago, IL
Mount Sinai SCI Model System, New York, NY
Northern California SCI System, San Jose, CA
Northern New Jersey SCI System, West Orange, NJ
Northwest Regional SCI System, Seattle, WA
Regional SCI Care System of Southern California, Downey, CA

Regional SCI System of Delaware Valley, Philadelphia, PA

Rocky Mountain Regional SCI System, Englewood, CO

Southeast Michigan Regional SCI System, Detroit, MI

Texas Regional SCI System, Houston, TX

University of Alabama at Birmingham SCI Care System, Birmingham, AL

University of Michigan Model SCI System, Ann Arbor, MI

Department of Veterans Affairs, Regional Spinal Cord Injury Centers:

Albuquerque, NM	Miami, FL
Augusta, GA	Milwaukee, WI
Brockton/West Roxbury, MA	Palo Alto, CA
Bronx, NY	Richmond, VA
Castle Point, NY	St. Louis, MO
Cleveland, OH	San Antonio, TX
East Orange, NJ	San Diego, CA
Hampton, VA	San Juan, PR
Hines, IL	Seattle, WA
Houston, TX	Sepulveda, CA
Long Beach, CA	Tampa, FL
Memphis, TN	

BIBLIOGRAPHY

APPLE, DAVID F., and HUDSON, LESLEY, eds. *Spinal Cord Injury: The Model.* Atlanta, 1990.

BERKOWITZ, MONROE; HARVEY, CAROL; GREENE, CAROLYN G.; and WILSON, SVEN E. *The Economic Consequences of Traumatic Spinal Cord Injury.* NY, 1992.

BLOCH, RALPH F., and BASBAUM, MEL, eds. *Management of Spinal Cord Injuries.* Baltimore, 1986.

CENTERS FOR DISEASE CONTROL. *Proceeding of the First Colloquium on Preventing Secondary Disabilities Among People with Spinal Cord Injuries.* Atlanta, 1990.

EISENBERG, MYRON E.; SUTKIN, LaFAYE C.; and JANSEN, MARY A. *Chronic Illness and Disability Through the Life Span: Effects on Self and Family.* New York, 1984.

EYSTER, E. FLETCHER, and WATTS, CLARK. "An Update of the National Head and Spinal Cord Injury Prevention Program of the American Association of Neurological Surgeons and the Congress of Neurological Surgeons: Think First." *Clinical Neurosurgery* 38 (1992):252–260.

FUHRER, MARCUS J. *Rehabilitation Outcomes: Analysis and Measurement.* Baltimore, 1987.

KENNEDY, E. J., ed. *Spinal Cord Injury: The Facts and Figures.* Birmingham, AL, 1986.

MARINELLI, ROBERT P., and DELL ORTO, ARTHUR E. *The Psychological and Social Impact of Physical Disability,* 3rd ed. New York, 1991.

NATIONAL RESEARCH COUNCIL. *Injury in America: A Continuing Public Health Problem.* Washington, DC, 1985.

NATIONAL SCI STATISTICAL. *Spinal Cord Injury Model Systems: Two Decades of Managed Care.* Washington, DC, 1994.

OZER, MARK N. *The Management of Persons with Spinal Cord Injury.* NY, 1988.

RICHARDS, J. SCOTT. *Resources: A National Directory of Spinal Cord Injury Prevention Programs.* Birmingham, AL, 1990.

RICHARDS, J. SCOTT; HENDRICKS, CHARLOTTE; and ROBERTS, MICHAEL. "Prevention of Spinal Cord Injury. An Elementary Education Approach." *Journal of Pediatric Psychology* 16 (1991):595–609.

TRIESCHMANN, ROBERTA B. *Aging with a Disability.* NY, 1987.

———. *Spinal Cord Injuries: Psychological, Social, and Vocational Rehabilitation,* 2nd ed. NY, 1988.

U.S. INSTITUTE OF MEDICINE. COMMITTEE ON A NATIONAL AGENDA FOR THE PREVENTION OF DISABILITIES. *Disability in America: Toward a National Agenda for Prevention.* Washington, DC, 1991.

U.S. NATIONAL COMMITTEE FOR INJURY PREVENTION AND CONTROL. "Injury Prevention: Meeting the Challenge." Supplement to *American Journal of Preventive Medicine* 5 (1989).

WHITENECK, GALE G.; ADLER, CAROLE; CARTER, R. EDWARD; LAMMERTSE, DANIEL P.; MANLEY, SCOTT; MENTER, ROBERT R.; WAGNER, KAREN A.; and WILMOT, CONAL, eds. *The Management of High Quadriplegia.* Demos, NY, 1989.

WHITENECK, GALE G.; CHARLIFUE, SUSAN W.; GERHART, KENNETH A.; LAMMERTSE, DANIEL P.; MANLEY, SCOTT; MENTER, ROBERT R.; and SEEDROFF, KATHIE R., eds. *Aging with Spinal Cord Injury.* NY, 1993.

YOUNG, JOHN S.; BURNS, PETER E.; BOWEN A. M.; and McCUTCHEN, ROBERTA. *Spinal Cord Injury Statistics: Experience of the Regional Spinal Cord Injury Systems.* Phoenix, 1982.

MICHAEL M. PRIEBE
DIANA H. RINTALA

SPORTS

See MUSCULOSKELETAL DISORDERS; RECREATION; WELLNESS

STATE–FEDERAL REHABILITATION PROGRAM

The state–federal rehabilitation program is a joint effort by the federal and state governments to assist people with physical and/or mental disabilities to work and become self-sufficient. Established at the federal level by the Smith-Fess Act of 1920, this program is one of the oldest federal grant programs in the United States. It grew out of workers' compensation and vocational education and recognized that people who were injured in industrial accidents could be retrained for other jobs. After considerable debate about how the origin of the disability should be a basis for eligibility, Congress opened the program to disability without regard to its origin. For example, the disability could be from industrial accidents (which were common in this period) or other accidents, or by birth or disease. Early program data indicate that people with orthopedic disabilities were most commonly served by the program.

The Smith-Fess Act required the states to develop a plan for how they were going to use the grant money for returning people with disabilities to work. These state plans are still required as the instrument for defining the program. States were also required to match the federal money with state funds. State agencies actually provide the services needed to return the persons with disabilities to work, through field counselors.

Although the rehabilitation process is not a clear-cut, one-step-at-a-time sequence, there are certain logical phases through which rehabilitation counselors assist persons with disabilities. Since the underlying theory of rehabilitation is that a disability causes the problem of unemployment, the first phase is one of diagnostic services—that is, determining the specific problem the disability causes to prevent functioning on a job. This is not a simple task. In fact, a specialty in the field of rehabilitation often provides information for the counselor. That specialist is known as a vocational evaluator, and uses sophisticated tests to determine levels of physical, mental, and social functioning as well as vocational interests. This information is used by the counselor and person with a disability to understand what is needed to reach a vocational goal.

Individualized written rehabilitation programs are prepared jointly by the counselor and the program participant and may require medical, psychological, social, educational, or other services. This "plan" is common in many programs serving persons with disabilities (e.g., education, corrections, mental health, and developmental disability programs). Rehabilitation services are based on economic need except for diagnostic, counseling, and placement services. Other services—for instance, medical therapies and educational services—require some cost sharing by the person.

The state–federal rehabilitation program can be viewed as an employment program because of its goal of job placement; it can be viewed as an educational program because many of its participants receive college training or vocational training; it can be viewed as a social program because medical and psychological services are often provided. This multiple program identity has benefited the program over the years from a political perspective, since it contained conservative and liberal political elements. The multiple identities of the program are further reflected in its organizational location. In the federal code of laws, it is in the labor (employment) section; but the U.S. Department of Education, and within it, the Rehabilitation Services Administration, carries out the funding and oversight of the rehabilitation program. At the state level, the program is located variously in state departments of labor, departments of social services, or departments of education; moreover, some states have an independent organizational unit to implement the program.

Larger Policy Context of the State–Federal Rehabilitation Program

Although this entry is not devoted to the history of the state–federal rehabilitation program, a quick walk through the past is important to present and understand the larger context of the program. At its inception, the Civilian Vocational Rehabilitation Program dominated the field of disability policy. Over the years there were periods of expansion, particularly in 1954, when not only the counseling profession got a boost, but also the creation of the Social Security Disability Program affected on the state–

federal program. Many state rehabilitation agencies contracted with the Social Security Administration to make permanent disability awards through a separate program that operated in tandem with the vocational rehabilitation program. Paradoxically, upon being determined "permanently and totally disabled," a person was referred to the state–federal program, a rehabilitation counselor, and was evaluated for work potential. So one part of the state–federal program declared a person unable to work, while the other part of the agency made every effort to "rehabilitate" or return that person to work.

Severity of disability became an issue in the state-federal program, culminating in a mandate in 1973 that persons with severe disabilities be served first. The issue of whether employment should be the only goal for programs for people with disabilities gave exemption to programs for persons with developmental disabilities and independent living programs. The developmental disability programs are not usually administered by state–federal rehabilitation agencies; however, independent living became part of the state–federal program, allowing that some persons with disabilities are not able to work, or need certain services before a vocational objective could be considered.

Further, people with disabilities were given rights to education, rather than the historically special schools for such children with disabilities. Parents of children with disabilities began to sue school districts for equal educational opportunities.

In sum, since the early period of vocationally dominated disability policy, as in the state–federal program, there has been a proliferation of disability agendas and policies. Most of these policies and programs have had an impact on the state–federal rehabilitation program, and ultimately the rehabilitation professional's job. The most significant of all these is the Americans with Disabilities Act.

The Americans with Disabilities Act and the State–Federal Rehabilitation Program. The Americans with Disabilities Act (ADA) is a landmark in the history of disability policy. It provides overarching civil rights protections that have affected all other disability programs and policies. The impact of the ADA on the rehabilitation program and its counselors is of concern here. The single most important

impact of the ADA on the state–federal program is the prohibition of employment discrimination based on disability. Previous protections under Section 504 (the Rehabilitation Act of 1973, as amended) were limited in coverage. But the ADA covers private as well as public employers. The goal of the state–federal program is job placement for people with disabilities. Past discrimination made the rehabilitation counselor's job difficult, and subjected the person with a disability to unjust treatment in the job market. The ADA also has an impact on the state–federal program by prohibiting discrimination in transportation, housing, education, and public services. Many of these protections facilitate employment and independent living, while others provide a reason for working—full participation in all walks of life.

Modern Technology and the State–Federal Rehabilitation Program. In 1986, the state–federal rehabilitation program made official what it had been doing for decades—reengineering and applying technology to assist functioning by people with disabilities. Rehabilitation engineering and technology were codified in federal law and mandated to be used in every phase of the rehabilitation process when appropriate. The technology had outrun the rehabilitation program; the mandate required the state–federal program to catch up with the accelerated rate of technological growth. It established pilot projects in most states to promote the use of technology for people with disabilities.

Ironically, the advance in computerization, remote controls, telecommunications, voice recognition, and speech synthesizers on many occasions was initially pursued to increase the ease of functioning of the persons without disabilities, and as a side effect or extension in use of the device, to increase functional capabilities of people with disabilities. Moreover, the space program required development of technology that has applications in assisting persons with disabilities.

What Difference Does It Make? From the beginning of the state–federal program, public funds spent on persons with disabilities were considered an investment in human potential. Economists (e.g., Berkowitz et al., 1988; Conley, 1969) have devised cost-benefit models to show the return on the dollar through taxes collected and public assistance reduced. However, the theory of investments has been under considerable scrutiny for several years. In actuality, tremendous resources have been spent to determine the quality of the state–federal program (e.g., see Abt Associates, 1974; Jones et. al., 1990).

Casework review and compliance have been major parts of determining the success of the state-federal program (Hanks & Dean, 1990). Problems of severity of disability, eligibility, and retention of benefits have been of concern in the seemingly endless search to evaluate the performance of the programs. Dale Hanks and David Dean (1990) may have developed a unique method for determining the success of the program. By unobtrusively cross-matching closed cases with records of employment (without breaching confidentiality laws), one can determine whether pre- and postclientele are (1) still employed and (2) making more money. Using a cohort group, one could further determine aggregate tax paid over time and further public assistance benefits paid. This method allows an inference about quality of services by retention of benefits—if the client is still working, services were sufficient. On the other hand, in a case review, adequacy of services must be made by clinical judgment, which is time-consuming and not always reliable.

The Future of the State–Federal Rehabilitation Program

The state–federal rehabilitation program is one of the most politically popular programs ever enacted by Congress. The future of the program lies with how well it meets the challenge of interrelationships with other disability policies, particularly regarding information, telecommunication, and technological advances, and with the Americans with Disabilities Act. The ADA could open employment and other opportunities to such an extent that the rehabilitation program would be hard pressed to keep up with the demand.

Some difficulties in the state–federal program may come from multiple interests of specific disability groups competing for services under the act. As these groups exert more pressure on state and federal rehabilitation agencies, those agencies will have to balance the demands and resources.

(*See also:* AMERICANS WITH DISABILITIES ACT; ASSISTIVE TECHNOLOGY; DISABILITY LAW AND SOCIAL POLICY; ECONOMICS; HISTORY OF REHABILITATION; JOB PLACEMENT; EVALUATION OF REHABILITATION PROGRAMS; REHABILITATION COUNSELING; TECHNOLOGY AND DISABILITY; VOCATIONAL EVALUATION; WORK)

BIBLIOGRAPHY

ABT ASSOCIATES, INC. "Cost-Benefit Analysis." In *The Program Services and Support System of the Rehabilitation Services Administration: Final Report.* Cambridge, MA, 1974.

BERKELEY PLANNING ASSOCIATES. *Review of Design Options and Recommendations for the Impact Evaluation of the Federal-State Vocational Rehabilitation Program.* Washington, DC, 1988.

BERKOWITZ, MONROE, et al. *Analysis of Costs and Benefits in Rehabilitation.* Philadelphia, 1988.

BUREAU OF NATIONAL AFFAIRS. *The Americans with Disabilities Act: A Practical and Legal Guide to Impact, Enforcement and Compliance.* Washington, DC, 1990.

CONLEY, RONALD. "A Benefit-Cost Analysis of the Vocational Rehabilitation Program." *Journal of Human Resources* 4 (1969):226–252.

GALVIN, DONALD. "Disability and Rehabilitation Policy: Then, Now, and in the Future." In *If: The Future of VR.* Dunbar, WV, 1986.

HANKS, DALE, and DEAN, DAVID. *The State-Federal Vocational Rehabilitation Program.* Washington, DC, 1990.

JONES, ANTONIO, et al. *Accountability: Enhancing Public Confidence.* Dunbar, WV, 1990.

ANTONIO E. JONES

STATISTICS

Statistics are simply numbers that describe some aspect of reality. They depend ultimately on the ability to classify units of reality into categories. Once classified, the units can be counted, and the counts can be combined by various mathematical operations, such as addition, subtraction, multiplication, and division. The resulting combined numbers include many types of statistics, such as aggregates, percents, proportions, rates, differences, correlation coefficients, and regression coefficients. Such statistics can themselves be combined by mathematical operations, creating even more complex statistics, which are sometimes said to be models of reality.

The reality described by simple statistics, such as percents, is easily understood by most persons with a good general education; however, the reality described by complex statistics can be understood only by those with special training in statistics. The difficulty in understanding complex statistics is a serious problem for their use in the disability and rehabilitation professions: some professionals reject complex statistics as too far removed from reality to be useful, while others accept them uncritically. The purpose of this entry is to introduce key concepts in statistics that many professionals in disability and rehabilitation need to understand. While many of the concepts apply to a variety of statistical applications, the focus is on statistics from sample surveys. (For a thorough general introduction to statistics, see Snedcor & Cochran, 1989).

A population is the set of real units that is described by a statistic. In general, statistics describe populations of persons or events. In disability and rehabilitation, the population may consist of persons such as patients or personal assistants, or events such as injuries or office visits. In a population of persons, statistics may describe the number, percent, or proportion of persons who have a characteristic of interest, such as a loss of motor function. By convention, such statistics are said to describe the prevalence of the characteristic in the population. In a population of events, statistics may describe the number of events, such as head injuries, occurring in a period of time. By convention, such statistics are said to describe the incidence of events. Epidemiology is the scientific discipline that studies the prevalence and incidence of disease, and applies the results of its study to the prevention and control of disease. Professionals in disability and rehabilitation sometimes use the terminology and methodology of epidemiology in studies and applications related to the consequences of disease. (For a thorough introduction to epidemiology, see Rothman, 1986.)

A complete count of a population is an enumeration or census, and statistics derived from them are known as descriptive statistics. In many applications, it is possible to count the whole population of persons or events. This is usually the case, for instance, where medical or administrative procedures generate records with information on whole populations of persons or events. While not created to produce descriptive statistics on the population, medical and administrative records make it possible to do so at relatively low cost. National censuses of population that are undertaken for political and administrative purposes also make it possible to produce descriptive statistics for the whole population.

In many cases, however, there is no census or enumeration of the whole population for which statistics are needed. In such cases it may be possible to select a sample of the population, calculate statistics for the sample, and infer statistics for the population. The method of selecting sample cases from a population is crucial. If cases are selected because they are easily available, the resulting sample of convenience is likely to be biased, and statistics inferred from it will not describe the population correctly. In a scientific sample, also known as a probability sample, cases are selected at random and with known probability.

The simplest probability sample is the simple random sample, in which, for instance, a sample of 100 cases is randomly selected from a population of 1,000 units, each population unit having an equal probability of selection, namely 10 in 1,000 (or 1 in 100, or 1 percent). Most scientific samples of large populations of people are multistage area probability samples, in which small geographic areas are selected at random, the selected areas are visited and their housing units listed, and then housing units are selected at random. In these complex samples, the sample persons have different probabilities of selection, but they are selected at random and their probability of selection is known.

Because probabilities of selection vary among sampled units, estimates from these complex samples are adjusted by counting each sample person (or event) as if they were the number of persons they represent in the population. For instance, if a sample person's probability of selection is known to be 1 in 2,000, then that person counts as 2,000 persons, whereas a sample person whose probability of selection is 1 in 500 would count as 500 persons. This adjustment procedure is known as weighting the data, and is a necessary part of the estimation procedure that infers population statistics from a sample.

From statistical theory it is known that if many

probability samples are taken from the same population and a population statistic inferred or estimated from each sample, the estimated statistics will differ from one another, but they will tend to group around the true value of the statistic in the population. Furthermore, the estimates from different samples will vary around the true value in a predictable way. Using this statistical theory, it is possible to select one probability sample, infer or estimate a statistic for the population, and know how likely it is that the estimated value is close to the true value, without knowing what the true value is. Thus reports of statistics based on a probability sample should include statements such as "14 percent of people in the United States have a functional limitation, with a margin of error of 1 percent." More explicitly, that statement means that if many samples of the U.S. population were selected, nearly all of those samples would yield estimates of the percent with a limitation in the range of 13 percent to 15 percent, so the true population value is probably in that range and is estimated to be 14 percent. The range or "margin of error" is the sampling error of the statistic estimated from the sample. Users of statistics from samples should always ask: Was it a probability sample (random selection, known probability)? What is the sampling error (range of probable true values)?

With scientific samples, whether simple or complex, the sampling error of an estimated population statistic can be measured by a statistic called the standard error. For simple random samples, the standard error is computed using a simple algebraic formula. For complex samples there usually is no formula for computing sampling errors, and they must be approximated by iterative (repetitious) computations. Analysts of statistics from complex samples use special computer programs that estimate population statistics and their standard errors. One such program, widely used in the United States, is named Software for Survey Data Analysis, and is known by the acronym SUDAAN. SUDAAN (Research Triangle Institute, 1993) is based on a widely used analysis software package, SAS (SAS Institute, 1989). Both SUDAAN and SAS are available in personal computer versions.

Another important aspect of statistics is the collection of the information that is used to classify persons and events. There are many modes of data collection, such as telephone interview, personal interview, and self-administered interview. All use sets of actual or implicit questions, questionnaires, which may be on paper or on a computer. To meet the standards of statistics, the questions must elicit answers that have high levels of validity and reliability. Valid responses mean what they seem to mean (face validity), are consistent with responses to other questions (internal validity), and agree with information from independent sources (external validity). Reliable responses to questions about the same person or event do not change simply because they are asked by different persons (interrater reliability) or at different times (test-retest reliability). To achieve validity and reliability, questionnaires for statistical purposes are extensively tested before use and carefully monitored during use. The goal of these efforts is to standardize questionnaires and their administration so that insofar as possible any differences in responses reflect real differences in persons or events, not differences in the way the responses were elicited.

The use of standardized questionnaires to collect information from a scientific sample of persons or events is the hallmark of the modern sample survey. While there are some disability and rehabilitation statistics systems based on administrative or medical record systems, they tend to be focused narrowly or not nationally representative. Sample surveys are the source of most national, general purpose statistics on disability and rehabilitation. Although many sample surveys collect some data on disability, the focus in this entry is on those national surveys (mostly U.S.) in which disability is a major focus. (For a listing of major surveys in the United States and many excellent illustrations of the statistics they produce, see Thompson-Hoffman & Storck, 1991.)

There have been some ad hoc national sample surveys on disability that have been very influential, such as a 1986 Louis Harris poll, *Disabled Americans' Self-Perceptions* (Louis Harris and Associates, 1986). Its sample was small (about 1,000 persons with disabilities), and its estimates of statistics had relatively large sampling errors, but it focused on important policy issues and its results were disseminated effectively among policymakers. Consequently it is credited by some authors with helping to shape the policy debate that resulted in the Americans with Disabilities Act.

Among large national surveys that produce disability statistics on a regular basis are the Current Population Survey (CPS), the Survey on Income and Program Participation (SIPP), and the National Health Interview Survey (NHIS). All of these surveys are sponsored by U.S. federal agencies, and the data collection for each is conducted by the U.S. Bureau of the Census. The CPS is sponsored by the U.S. Bureau of Labor Statistics, and its principal purpose is to produce monthly labor force statistics, but it is used periodically as a vehicle for producing statistics on other topics, including work disability. The SIPP is sponsored by the Census Bureau, and was designed to plan and evaluate federal social welfare programs, including programs for persons with disabilities, and it has periodically produced statistics on disability.

The NHIS is sponsored by the National Center for Health Statistics and ad hoc cosponsors from other federal agencies (Benson & Marano, 1994). Because it has been in continuous operation since 1957 and has produced annual statistics on disability throughout its history, it is the single most important source of U.S. national disability statistics. The information used to classify a person's disability status is obtained in a series of standard questions that ask if, because of a chronic impairment or health problem, a sample person is unable to perform, or is limited in his or her performance of the major activity usually performed by persons of his or her age. The usual major activities are play for preschool children, regular school for school-age children and youth, working for pay or housekeeping for persons of working age (eighteen to sixty-four years), and unassisted personal care and home management for older persons. If persons are not limited in their performance of the usual major activity, questions are asked about limitations in their performance of other (unspecified) activities. Using the responses to these questions, persons are classified as unable to perform the major activity, limited in performance of the major activity, limited in performance of other activities, or not limited in the performance of

any activity (by reason of a chronic impairment or health problem). This general approach to measuring disability—questions about health-related limitations in performance of selected standard activities—has been widely adopted in sample surveys, although the specific questions about performance and the selected standard activities vary.

In 1993, the most recent year for which NHIS statistics were available for this entry, 4.5 percent of the U.S. population were estimated to be unable to perform the major activity of persons in their age group, another 6.1 percent were limited in performance of the major activity, and another 4.9 percent were limited in other activities, for a total of 15.5 percent who had a disability, as estimated by the NHIS. The NHIS estimate remained rather stable over time: In the ten years ending in 1993, the lowest percent with a disability was 13.7 (1990) and the highest was the 15.5 reported for 1993.

In 1993 the NHIS estimated the number of persons in the United States with a disability as 39,331,000. That estimate will seem low to readers familiar with the 43,000,000 estimate often cited during the public debate preceding passage of the Americans with Disabilities Act in 1990, and the even higher estimates that have been seen since. The ADA and later estimates were based on different surveys that used different questions and definitions. The discrepancies point to the fact that there are no widely accepted "official" standards for measuring and defining disability in sample surveys, although the long history and wide use of the NHIS make it the closest thing to a standard now available. Users should be aware of differences in sample surveys and examine closely the questions and definitions on which disability statistics are based.

Outside the United States, national sample surveys on disability have been done in a number of nations, including the United Kingdom, the Netherlands, Spain, Italy, Australia, and Canada. A Canadian disability survey, the 1991 Health and Activity Limitation Survey (HALS), is noteworthy: It used national census data (which enumerated all Canadians) to identify persons reported to have a disability, selected a scientific sample of those persons, and interviewed them in person. This efficient design made it possible to survey a large sample at a relatively low cost.

As part of its disability statistics program, the Statistical Division of the United Nations identifies national disability surveys, acquires their documentation and reports, abstracts national estimates of disability statistics, and compiles those statistics in a compendium available both on paper and in electronic media. This program goes under the name DISTAT, for Disability Statistics. The resulting DISTAT compendium makes it possible to compare disability statistics across nations. However, the Statistical Division warns that different countries use different questions and definitions, making comparisons difficult and even misleading. These problems are similar to those mentioned earlier in comparing statistics from different U.S. surveys, but they are far more difficult in international comparisons. The Statistical Division is engaged in a long-range program to improve international comparability by offering training workshops, technical assistance, and written guidelines to nations planning disability statistics systems.

As part of its effort to improve international comparability of disability statistics, the U.N. Statistical Division has adopted as its standard the International Classification of Impairments, Disabilities, and Handicaps (ICIDH). The ICIDH is one of a family of health classifications promulgated under the auspices of the World Health Organization (WHO). The ICIDH was published in 1980 and is being revised. It has been translated into fourteen languages and is used in many nations for statistical and other purposes.

The ICIDH identifies three levels or manifestations of the consequences of disease, disorder, or injury: consequences for the body, or impairments; consequences for the person, or disabilities; and consequences for the community, or handicaps. For each level the ICIDH offers a separate classification system: impairments, disabilities, and handicaps. According to one author, Jerome Bickenbach, each of these classifications is underlain by an implicit model of "disablement" (the term he uses to identify all three taken together)—the "medical model" for impairments; the "economic model" for disabilities; and the "social/political model" for handicaps; while each separate model has inherent biases, including

all three models within the ICIDH, the standard provides a balanced, overall system of classification for disablement. While Bickenbach is generally supportive of the ICIDH as a basis for statistical classification, he has many criticisms of its particulars, some of which are being addressed by the WHO in its revision of the manual.

Another international statistical group that has adopted the ICIDH as its standard is the Network on Health Expectancy and the Disability Process, better known by its French acronym, REVES, for Réseau Espérance de Vie en Santé (Bone, 1992). REVES is a group of statisticians who use an adaptation of the life table technique to study disability. In the classical life table, a hypothetical birth cohort of 100,000 babies is exposed throughout their life to a set of death rates at each age derived from the actual deaths of a real population in a one-year period. The population that "survives" to each age is exposed to a risk of dying at that age that is equal to the actual death rate in the real population, until all of the population has "died." By totaling the number of years "lived" by the hypothetical cohort over its lifetime, an average expectation of life can be calculated. Such calculations are widely used by insurance companies to set insurance payments that are equitable and profitable. The health expectancy technique used by REVES and others exposes a hypothetical cohort not only to death rates, but also to disability rates at each age, so the resulting calculations yield an estimate of disability-free life expectancy, the number of years, on average, a newborn can expect to live without a disability. Some related measures, which differ somewhat in approach, are quality-adjusted life years and disability-adjusted life years.

Like life expectancy, these health expectancy measures provide a single statistic that describes a complex reality of mortality and disability conditions in a whole population. For persons trained in these statistical techniques, those statistics are convenient summaries, rich in meaning. For those not so trained, they are (1) rejected as too far removed from the lives of persons with disabilities to have practical meaning; or (2) accepted uncritically and used inappropriately, confusing and possibly undermining the interests of persons with disabilities. And that comes around to the point with which this entry began: Statistics are simply numbers that describe some aspect of reality; as such, they can be a useful tool for understanding disability, but not without thought and care in their use.

(*See also:* DISABILITY; EVALUATION OF REHABILITATION PROGRAMS; RESEARCH)

RESOURCES

Disability Statistics Rehabilitation Research and Training Center, Institute for Health and Aging, UCSF, Box 0646, Laurel Heights, San Francisco, CA 94143–0646

U.S. Department of Health and Human Services, Public Health Service, Centers for Disease Control and Prevention, National Center for Health Statistics, 6525 Belcrest Rd, Hyattsville, MD 20782

BIBLIOGRAPHY

BENSON, VERONICA, and MARANO, MARIE. "Current Estimates from the National Health Interview Survey, 1993, National Center for Health Statistics." *Vital and Health Statistics* 10 (1994):190.

BICKENBACH, JEROME E. *Physical Disability and Social Policy.* Toronto, 1993.

BONE, MARGARET R. "International Efforts to Measure Health Expectancy." *Journal of Epidemiology and Community Health* 46 (1992):555–558.

HARRIS, LOUIS, and ASSOCIATES. *Disabled Americans' Self-Perceptions: Bringing Disabled Americans into the Mainstream.* New York, 1986.

RESEARCH TRIANGLE INSTITUTE. *SUDAAN: Professional Software for Survey Data Analysis, Version 6.34.* Research Triangle Park, NC, 1993.

ROTHMAN, KENNETH J. *Modern Epidemiology.* Boston, 1986.

SAS INSTITUTE. *SAS Language and Procedures: Usage, Version 6.* Cary, NC, 1989.

SNEDCOR, GEORGE W., and COCHRAN, WILLIAM G. *Statistical Methods.* Ames, IA, 1989.

THOMPSON-HOFFMAN, SUSAN, and STORCK, INEZ F. *Disability in the United States: A Portrait from National Data.* New York, 1991.

UNITED NATIONS. *Disability Statistics Compendium.* New York, 1990.

WORLD HEALTH ORGANIZATION. *International Classification of Impairments, Disabilities, and Handicaps: A Manual of Classification Relating to the Consequences of Disability.* Geneva, 1980.

GERRY HENDERSHOT

STROKE

Stroke is a major cause of death and the largest single cause of neurologically based disability in the United States. The term refers to the acute onset of nervous system dysfunction. The most obvious symptom is weakness on one side of the body or problems in balance. There may be visual loss as well as disturbance in sensation, such as feelings of numbness or loss of awareness of body position in space. Other symptoms can include slurring of speech and/or difficulties in finding the proper words to express one's thoughts. Other findings that are less obvious are difficulties in swallowing safely and in controlling one's bladder.

Causes

These losses of neural control are due to something going wrong in the blood vessels feeding the brain. The brain uses a major part of the entire body's blood supply to provide it with the sugar and oxygen needed for its high level of ongoing activity. Disturbance of nervous system activities can come about because blockage of the blood supply leads to what is called "ischemia," or lack of blood supply to brain tissue. The blockage can be in the blood vessels feeding the brain itself or from small clots that come from the heart and lodge in the blood vessels of the brain. The blockage can thus be caused by clots within the vessels themselves called "thrombi," or by clots from elsewhere that lodge in the vessels of the brain. These are called "emboli." Most strokes are due to thrombo-embolic disease, which thus produces blockage without hemorrhage. Less commonly, disturbance can also come about because of hemorrhage from blood vessels into brain tissue. These hemorrhages can be due to bleeding from smaller blood vessels within the brain itself or from larger blood vessels that lie in spaces alongside the brain.

The early disturbance in function due to blockage or hemorrhage can end in death of neural tissue. "Infarction" is the term used to describe this stage. The degree to which such permanent injury occurs depends on several different factors. For those with nonhemorrhagic stroke, the larger the vessel that has been blocked, the greater the degree of injury.

The degree to which other blood vessels can provide alternative sources of supply could lead to reducing the amount of permanent damage to brain tissue. Thus death of neural tissue tends to occur in areas deep in the brain where such collateral circulation is less available. The ability of other blood vessels to compensate is also compromised by the effects of aging, which limits the rapidity with which collateral circulation can respond to needs. Other chemical factors are now under investigation; their treatment could lead to reducing the amount of permanent damage to brain tissue. These treatments must take place early. Increasing attention is therefore now being addressed to more rapid treatment of persons with nonhemorrhagic stroke. For those with hemorrhagic stroke, the extent of neural injury depends on the size of the blood clot and where it occurs in the brain. The blood disrupts the metabolism of the brain tissue and can cause death of the affected area. There is eventual removal of the blood by scavenger cells, leaving an area that has now been destroyed.

There are two major systems of blood vessels feeding the brain by the major arteries from the heart. All the arteries feeding the brain are ultimately connected within the brain itself. The circulation feeding the lower part of the brain, or brainstem, is called the vertebral basilar system. The larger remainder of the brain is fed from the two carotid arteries, which are the major arteries on each side of the neck and that one can feel pulsating close to the surface. These vessels in the neck are accessible to surgery with replacement of the blocked portion as one important treatment now available for persons with stroke. Particularly important is recognition of sometimes transient episodes of neurological dysfunction. These episodes can reflect an increased likelihood of subsequent, more lasting difficulties and should occasion seeking medical attention. Surgical replacement of the affected portions of the carotid artery can be particularly useful in these circumstances.

Symptoms

The most common finding is for the weakness and disturbance in sensation to be results of abnormality in carotid artery circulation, with findings on the side of the body opposite to the side of the brain affected. For example, blockage of the vessels fed by the right carotid can lead to weakness and/or sensory disturbance in the left arm and leg. Persons with left-side brain injury are far more likely to have difficulties with language. These problems can include difficulties with expression as well as understanding of language. Persons with injury to the brainstem are more likely to have difficulties with balance as well as swallowing and slurring of speech. Those who have had several strokes affecting both sides of the brain may simulate the effects of a brainstem stroke. They will have difficulties with speech and swallowing but also greater evidence of loss of memory and confusion. This latter difficulty can ultimately have the greatest effect on the degree of recovery one can ultimately achieve. Problems in learning new ways of doing things can limit the person's ability to compensate for the effects of the stroke.

Risk Factors

Strokes most commonly occur in older persons. The sudden onset of the stroke obscures the long-term development of the conditions that have brought it about. Disease in the vascular system may be present not only in the vessels serving the brain but also in those serving the heart and the muscles of the limbs. For example, atherosclerosis, or "hardening of the arteries," is one of the major causes of stroke. Plaques due to fatty deposits in the walls of the larger arteries feeding the brain are frequently associated with similar problems in the coronary vessels feeding the heart. These plaques are associated with increased fat intake and can be alleviated even in persons who are elderly by lowering one's intake of fat from animal sources and by reducing one's use of saturated fats. Disease of the heart due to various causes additional to that of atherosclerosis can also be associated with abnormal heart rhythms, with a tendency to form clots within the heart; these clots then break off to interfere with blood supply to the brain. Heart disease is the most common cause of eventual death in those who have experienced a stroke.

The other major risk factor associated with stroke is high blood pressure. Hypertension can lead to a worsening of the atherosclerosis affecting the larger arteries feeding the brain. Hypertension also can lead to specific disease of the heart. Hypertension is also associated with worsening in the degree to which the smaller blood vessels within the brain itself, called "arterioles," are prone to blockage as well as the degree to which these same arterial walls are weakened with tendency to hemorrhage. These problems in the smaller blood vessels are compounded by the concomitant presence of diabetes. Like atherosclerosis, hypertension is treatable. There is considerable evidence that maintenance of blood pressure within given limits can reduce the frequency of stroke. One must attend to both the systolic blood pressure as well as the diastolic. In persons who are elderly, for example, control of isolated systolic hypertension has recently been found to be associated with significant reduction in incidence of stroke. Other major risk factors that can be reduced are smoking and excessive use of alcohol as well as drugs, such as cocaine. Although more evident in persons who are elderly, strokes can also occur in persons below age sixty due to the same risk factors described above but more commonly due also to abnormalities in the blood clotting process. Primary avoidance of stroke should be the focus of treatment. When a stroke does occur and risk factors remain, the likelihood of another stroke is high, particularly in the younger age group. Therefore, reducing treatable risk factors is an important task to prevent subsequent stroke with resultant worsening of the degree of brain injury.

After the Stroke

The life of the person after the onset of a stroke is naturally divided into three phases. The first, acute phase, lasting days to several weeks, takes place in an acute care setting such as a general hospital. The primary goal during this phase is to prevent death. The likelihood of death is related to the extent of the brain injury and its character. The existence of hemorrhage is of particular concern. The likelihood of death is far greater with hemorrhage than with thrombo-embolic disease. It may be necessary to remove the blood clot that contributes to dangerously increased pressure within the skull. Other issues during the acute phase are illness due to pneumonia from aspiration of food subsequent to swallowing

problems, and urinary tract infections when catheterization is done because of inability to empty the bladder. Other problems include the formation of clots in the legs; such clots can then enter the lungs and cause serious problems with breathing. This problem is attributed not only to immobilization of the limbs due to paralysis but also to a degree of increased coagulability associated with stroke. Another major emphasis of the acute phase during the days immediately after the stroke is to determine the possible cause of stroke as described above and to institute treatment to reduce recurrence. For example, there will be tests to determine the existence of clots in the heart and blockage of the carotid arteries in the neck. Long-term treatment for those with thrombo-embolic disease can include the use of several different kinds of drugs to reduce the clotting of blood to help to deal with these problems.

The other major goal is to minimize the degree to which the effects of the stroke interfere with the person's ability to carry out his or her life. This goal becomes primary during the longer-term rehabilitation phase, which may last several weeks to months and which takes place in a rehabilitation setting either as an inpatient or while living at home. The decision to enter into this phase requires an ability to participate in what may be for some a relatively strenuous exercise program. Thus entry into an intensive rehabilitation program requires the achievements of an appropriate level of physical endurance, an absence of illness, and an adequate ability to learn new ways to accomplish life goals.

The term "impairment" is useful to describe the disturbance of function that has occurred with the death of neural tissue. The effects of the injury will vary in relation to its initial severity but also in the degree to which recovery of function occurs. The pattern of recovery relates to time since onset and to the areas that are more likely to recover. The effects of the stroke are generally greatest two to three days after onset. The injured areas display increased swelling, associated with worsening. Once the swelling begins to recede there may be improvement in function. Improvement in this early acute phase is also attributed to reorganization of areas distant from the area of injury that were temporarily affected.

There is frequently ongoing improvement in function over the weeks after onset of stroke. This improvement is attributed to reorganization of the neural pathways that remain uninjured. The character of the improvement reflects the kind of alternative pathways available. The weakness and sensory loss on the side opposite the area of injury reflect the crossing over of brain fibers of the most highly developed tracts, which deal with the most versatile activities. For example, the hand requires the greatest degree of versatility in its actions. It is most sensitive to injury; is most highly controlled by neural cells on the opposite side of the brain; and is the last to recover. In the upper extremity, greater recovery occurs generally in control of the shoulder and trunk. This occurrence is attributed to the more widespread nature of neural cells controlling the actions of those parts of the body closer to the midline. The control of these areas is more frequently associated with both sides of the brain. Thus the uninjured side of the brain can take over. The pattern of recovery will also vary between the arm and the leg of the affected side. There is generally a greater degree of recovery in the leg, again more frequently at the hip than in the foot itself. There tends to be particular recovery in the leg of those actions that permit the person to hold the leg stiff at the hip and knee. Those elements that help maintain the upright posture of the body are controlled by the less highly developed motor pathways, which can remain intact even when the more advanced areas have been injured.

This pattern of recovery has significant implications for later function. The tendency for recovery at the trunk and those actions in the limbs closest to the trunk, particularly in the affected leg, enable many persons to stand upright once again. Being able to stand upright can then, in most instances, lead to being able to transfer oneself from a bed to a wheelchair, and from a wheelchair to a toilet. For example, recent experience has demonstrated that generally within four to six weeks after onset of stroke those enrolled in a rehabilitation program who were initially unable to do so are once again able to transfer to a toilet from a bed or a wheelchair completely on their own in 50 percent of cases. An additional 30 percent are able to transfer safely requiring only supervision and no physical assistance. Thus the overwhelming majority are no longer bedfast even when the only caregiver is an elderly spouse.

Given a particular degree of ongoing impairment, planning for a return to one's life activities requires a further definition of the functional consequences of those impairments in the life of the person. These "disabilities" are a result not only of the specific impairments and the pattern of recovery; they also reflect the goals of the person and the character of the resources available to the person experiencing those impairments. For example, the significance of the degree of ongoing impairment of the right hand will be greater for a person who is right-handed and for whom fine coordination is crucial to his or her life goals; the degree of coordination required is far greater and crucial to his livelihood for a man whose work is as a dental technician; a musician would be particularly distressed about the effects of the loss of hand coordination on her life as a pianist. Still another man with ongoing right hand dysfunction could show less concern about his impairment, being able to use his left hand to write his name. What is disabling to him is the lack of control he experienced in using the power tools he used in the past for his carpentry work.

The resources available also help determine the priorities of any rehabilitation plan. As an example, the goal for mobility in the case of a rather obese woman with left-side weakness is for her to be able to transfer from her bed to a wheelchair, with her husband not required to lift her up. Still another person with problems in ambulation lived in a house where there were a large number of steep front steps. He will not return to that house but could as an alternative go home to his daughter's ranch-style home.

Training during the rehabilitation phase deals with alleviation of disabilities. Such training involves use of functional capacities that remain unimpaired. One may enhance those functional capacities by training. This is the basis for work by various professional staff members. For example, disability resulting from visual loss on one side may include a lack of awareness of that side when propelling a wheelchair. One may bump into objects on the affected side. Treatment includes application of various compensatory strategies, such as learning to scan one's environment more consciously. For example, one woman with difficulty seeing on her left side found it helpful to block out vision on the right and have on the left a picture of her grandchildren. The efforts also extend to training in the use of assistive devices that may permit the person to regain mobility. These include wheelchairs as well as other devices to permit stabilization of the limb. Still another aspect must deal with the training of persons who will serve as caregivers. Modification of the physical environment is yet another alternative.

These rehabilitation efforts differ considerably from the sort of activities carried out in an acute care facility. An interdisciplinary team works with various aspects of the person. In addition to the physician and nurse, there are speech therapists, physical therapists, and occupational therapists. A psychologist and a social worker contribute their skills to deal with emotional and placement issues. The relationship between the person with stroke and the professional staff is more collaborative than usually found in the acute care setting. The rehabilitation phase is a transition between convalescence and independence in managing one's own life. Ultimately one must be able to make one's own life plans.

The goals may remain the same: to be able to get around, to care for oneself, to earn one's living. The means, however, may need to change. The way one could get around may no longer be walking but rather using a wheelchair. Life plans after the stroke require identifying goals and then considering alternative means of achieving them. Participating in the process of development of the rehabilitation plan is crucial to the necessary participation in its implementation. It is desirable for patients to learn to plan increasingly for themselves. The planning process involves the person with the problem being asked to define his or her concerns and the appropriate goals. The person is then asked to monitor the outcomes and the means by which those outcomes were achieved. Awareness of goals helps to identify them when results occur. Awareness of results helps one to have hope for the future. Awareness of what means were successful helps one to consider that alternatives exist and are worth trying.

The third and most lasting phase are those years when a person with a stroke once again enters into family and community life. During this continuing care phase the priorities are once again somewhat different from those during the earlier phases. Preventing stroke recurrence becomes even more paramount. Such prevention requires in most instances a degree of self-management of treatable risk factors. Use of medication and other techniques for control of hypertension is one example. Such control is likely to be enhanced if the person with stroke has been trained during the rehabilitation phase to be aware of the goal being sought, and to monitor the degree to which the goal has been achieved with the use of a blood pressure monitor. Another example of self-management can extend to reducing fat intake to guard against atherosclerosis.

The family life issues include dealing with the effects of role change and the relationship with spouses. One wife described her concern about now having to take responsibility for the finances and her husband's general lack of initiative. Another wife has found her husband much easier to get along with and is not disturbed about now having to make more of the family's decisions. There are increased burdens for a frequently elderly mate in providing physical assistance. Psychological issues are of greater importance and are expressed in depression and withdrawal from leisure activities and other aspects of what made life meaningful.

The reentry into community life also requires that one address stairs that block entrances to public buildings, or transportation systems that preclude accessibility to work or leisure activities. Other factors can include reimbursement systems that discourage return to work. The term "handicap" is defined here as those factors in the environment that can interfere with full participation in the wider social arena of persons with disabilities. Failure to achieve such participation depends not only on the degree of impairment and the retraining carried out to alleviate the resultant disabilities; it also depends on the response of the larger social system. The passage in 1990 of the Americans with Disabilities Act (ADA) can lead to a greater degree of integration. Support in these areas is provided by a variety of groups, including the Stroke Council of the American Heart Association and the National Stroke Association. Technical assistance is available in the application of technology to alleviate disability through government agencies in each state.

The cycle is an ongoing one. One must be aware of the warning signs of stroke and seek help to deal with the possibility of stroke recurrence. Having had a stroke and having been trained to manage one's own life during the rehabilitation phase have included the ability to use compensatory strategies to accomplish life goals. As one continues to live with the effects of the stroke it may be necessary to develop new ways of dealing with problems that arise in family life and living in the community unforeseen during the rehabilitation phase. What is sought is not only reintegration in active community life but also the ability to approach one's problems with an ongoing willingness to solve difficulties as they arise, derived from having overcome the devastation inherent in the very word "stroke."

(See also: HEAD INJURY; HOSPITAL, REHABILITATION; INDEPENDENT LIVING; LOSS AND GRIEF; NEUROLOGICAL DISORDERS; REHABILITATION CENTER)

RESOURCES

The American Heart Association, 7272 Greenville Ave., Dallas, TX 75321

National Stroke Association, 8480 East Orchard Rd, Suite 1000, Englewood, CO 80110–5015

Stroke Club of America, 805 12th St., Galveston, TX 77550

BIBLIOGRAPHY

CAPLAN, LEWIS R.; DWIKEN, MARK; and ESTON, DONALD J. Family Guide to Stroke. New York, 1994.

FRYE-PIERSON, JAMES, and TOOLE, JAMES F. Stroke: A Guide for Patients and Family. New York, 1987.

OZER, MARK N.; MATERSON, RICHARD S.; and CAPLAN, LEWIS R. Management of Persons with Stroke. St. Louis, 1994.

MARK N. OZER

SUBSTANCE ABUSE

See ALCOHOL REHABILITATION; CORRECTIONAL REHABILITATION; DRUG REHABILITATION

SUPPORTED EMPLOYMENT

Supported employment originated with federal- and state-funded demonstration projects in the late 1970s and early 1980s that showed that persons with significant mental retardation could work competitively if given the opportunity and support (Rusch & Mithaug, 1980; Wehman, Hill, and Koehler, 1979). Early pioneers of supported employment, including Dr. Frank Rusch with the University of Il-

linois at Champaign-Urbana and Dr. Paul Wehman with Virginia Commonwealth University, rejected the prevailing vocational service models based on "readiness," which required that individuals progress through a continuum of service settings leading to more independent, more normalized, and more integrated work as they acquired skills. The endeavors of these doctors laid the groundwork for a program that has improved the lives of thousands of persons with severe disabilities and inalterably changed the direction of disability services.

The origins of supported employment must be viewed within the context of the time period. During the 1970s employers' attitudes about persons with mental retardation were becoming more tolerant as training technologies improved, community presence increased, and work competencies were enhanced and demonstrated. Yet few persons with severe mental retardation crossed the bridge from training or other nonwork activities to paid employment in real jobs. Instead, they were relegated to day activity or habilitation programs or, at best, low-paying sheltered work from which they never progressed. For these individuals, success in competitive employment would require fundamental changes in job preparation and placement services, from expectations of vocational independence to employment with ongoing assistance, and from a "train, then place" approach to "place, then train." Thus supported employment participants are placed directly into jobs, with "job coaches" providing whether work or social skills training, job accommodations, community mobility assistance, case management, advocacy, or other support services are needed to maintain employment.

The supported employment model has since been modified for use with individuals with mental illness, brain injury, autism, cerebral palsy, other forms of physical impairments, and other severe disabling conditions. Moreover, this new paradigm of support has quickly spread to education, housing, recreation, family services, and other disability-related arenas.

Legislative Foundations

Although a number of state vocational rehabilitation (VR) agencies had encouraged and funded programs that were similar in concept, supported employment did not become a formal service option in the federal/

state VR program until the Rehabilitation Act Amendments of 1986. The regulations that followed (*Federal Register*, 1987) defined the components of supported employment as (1) time-limited employment services (up to eighteen months) funded by the VR agency; and (2) extended services, including periodic job skills reinforcement and ongoing support, funded by non-VR sources. The VR agency is required to develop collaborative agreements with public and nonprofit agencies to fund or provide ongoing support services after the supported employment client achieves job stabilization.

The regulations further define appropriate candidates for supported employment as individuals for whom competitive employment has not traditionally occurred or has been interrupted or intermittent due to disability, and for whom ongoing support services are essential to perform competitive work. Supported employment represented a significant policy shift for the VR program, from providing services exclusively for individuals capable of independent employment, to providing services to all persons with severe disabilities regardless of the need for long-term vocational support.

The Rehabilitation Services Administration of the U.S. Department of Education has stimulated tremendous growth in the supported employment program in a few short years, primarily through statewide systems-change grants to state VR agencies authorized by Title III (West, Revell, and Wehman, 1992). In 1985 and 1986, five-year Title III grants were awarded to twenty-seven state VR agencies, and three-year grants to an additional seventeen VR agencies in 1991, to promote conversion from segregated day services to supported employment. These grants have been used by VR agencies to build service capacity through interagency linkages, program start-up grants, vendor agreements, counselor and provider training, information system development and coordination, and similar activities.

In addition, Title VI, Part C of the act authorized VR funds specifically for supported employment clients and time-limited services. Funding from non-VR sources, primarily mental retardation and mental health funding systems for extended services, has steadily increased over the years, and in 1990 accounted for two-thirds of known supported employment funding (Sale et al., 1992).

Program Models

A number of supported employment program models have emerged that use either individual job placements with job coaching (Wehman & Kregel, 1985) or small group placements, such as enclaves, mobile work crews, and small enterprises (Moon & Griffin, 1988). The supported employment regulations limit the number of supported employees in group models to no more than eight. Typically, group-supported employment consumers are supervised and employed by the supported employment provider agency rather than by the host business. Also, group model participants are paid according to their productivity, with subminimum wages common (Wolfe, 1992).

The use of group models has been a controversial issue in supported employment. During the early years of the program, group placements were very common, largely because many rehabilitation facilities that started supported employment programs had experience with the "work stations in industry" program, albeit with individuals with less severe disabilities. By using their own work supervisors and payroll system, facilities could offer supported employment to clients with more severe disabilities without requiring major concessions from the businesses with whom they had routinely contracted for goods or services. However, as the program and the research base have advanced, all evidence indicates that those served in group models experience inferior outcomes compared to those in individual placement, and many persons believe that group placements are overly restrictive and unnecessary (Brown et al., 1991). Coincidentally, the use of group models has declined sharply in recent years (see Figure 1).

The Impact of Supported Employment on Service Participants

From its inception, supported employment has been promoted as a means of improving the vocational outlook of persons with severe disabilities. This section will summarize research on four key consumer outcomes: earnings, social integration, job retention, and quality of life.

Earnings. Early research on supported employment outcomes found that service participants typically earned higher hourly and weekly wages than

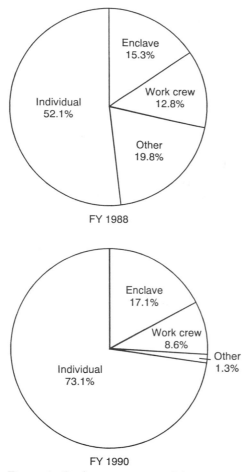

Figure 1. Decline in group models

their counterparts in segregated employment options such as sheltered workshops (Kiernan, McGaughey, and Schalock, 1986; Wehman, 1986). Moreover, individuals entering supported employment from alternative programs have substantially increased their earnings, sufficient to offset any reductions of government assistance from programs such as Social Security, public housing, and food stamps (Hill et al., 1987; Hill & Wehman, 1983; Noble & Conley, 1987).

Other investigations have examined consumer earnings across placement models and disability groups. These studies show that consumers in individual placement have experienced greater hourly and weekly wages than persons in group models (Helms, Moore, and McSweyn, 1991). In addition, Michael West, John Kregel, and P. David Banks (1990) found that participants in individual placement also received key fringe benefits, such as med-

ical coverage, more often. Individuals with severe or profound mental retardation have been found to earn significantly lower wages than persons from other disability groups (Kregel, Wehman, and Banks, 1989; Thompson, Powers, and Houchard, 1992), largely because they are more likely to be in a group program (Kregel & Wehman, 1989).

Although supported employment participants fare better than their cohorts in sheltered employment and other segregated programs, supported employment wages are generally low. Michael West, W. Grant Revell, and Paul Wehman (1992) reported that the national average hourly wage of supported employment participants in both 1988 and 1990 was just cents above the minimum wage in effect in those years ($3.38 and $3.87, respectively). However, for some supported-employment populations, such as persons with physical impairments and mental illness, wages appear to be higher (Kregel, Wehman, and Banks, 1989; West, Revell, and Wehman, 1992).

Social Integration. Promoting opportunities for positive social and work-related interaction with co-workers and the general public is a primary goal of supported employment. As with earnings, integration is typically greater for participants in individual placement models than for those in group placements. For example, Frank R. Rusch, John R. Johnson, and Carolyn Hughes (1990) found more frequent coworker interactions for individual placement consumers with mental retardation than for those in group models. These authors also found that coworkers interacted more with supported employees with mild retardation as opposed to those with severe retardation. Barbara L. Helms, Stephen C. Moore, and Cary Ann McSweyn (1991) found that supported employment participants in individual placements had greater levels of general community presence and participation than did persons in group models or in sheltered employment.

Job Retention. While many individuals with severe disabilities achieve long-term employment success in their first supported employment placement, perhaps half will not retain their first job for a year, with most leaving their first job during the initial six months (Lagomarcino, 1990; Sale et al., 1991; West, 1992). Many supported employment job changes are positive as individuals move to jobs offering greater responsibility, better pay or working conditions, or that better match their interests. The reasons for negative job loss are many and varied, including problems with the supported employee's productivity or work quality, social skills, mental or physical health status, and commitment to the job. Economic layoffs, failure of the business, and other external factors also contribute to unnecessary job loss. There is also some evidence that an individual's primary reason for job loss is related to disability group status (Lagomarcino, 1990; West, 1992), although the utility of this research for direct services is limited (Sale et al., 1991).

Considering the competitive employment histories of the supported employment target population, it is not surprising that many participants fail to achieve long-term job retention in their first placement. The larger issue is the response of supported employment provider agencies and the VR system to job loss. While some supported-employment participants will choose not to continue with the program, for many more the promise of long-term support lasts only as long as the first job. Many individuals who leave their first supported employment position, whether due to resignation, termination, or layoff, are never placed in a second position (West, 1992).

Quality of Life. The study of the relationships between quality of life (QOL) and employment has a long history, and generally confirms that increased QOL and life satisfaction are related to employment, wages, job stability, and participation in the work culture (Moseley, 1989). A growing body of evidence indicates that supported-employment consumers score higher on self-reports of QOL and life satisfaction than individuals in segregated programs, and that persons with disabilities can experience increased QOL and life satisfaction from participation in supported employment (Fabian, 1992; McCaughrin et al., 1993; Test et al., 1993).

In summary, this brief review confirms that individuals who are placed in supported employment fare better economically and socially than those who are not, and that movement to supported employment generally increases an individual's quality of life. Moreover, placement in individual jobs rather than group work typically produces the greater benefit to the individual.

Issues in Supported Employment Policy and Implementation

Supported employment as a VR service option is still very much in its infancy, and many second- and third-generation policy and implementation issues continue to emerge as state programs expand and mature. Three major issues will be discussed in this section: (1) the characteristics of supported employment consumers, particularly in regard to unserved and underserved populations; (2) facility conversion from segregated services to supported employment; and (3) the use of natural supports as time-limited and extended services.

Consumer Characteristics. As mentioned previously, the supported-employment model was originally developed for persons with mental retardation, and this group constitutes the majority of supported-employment participants. However, the participation rate of individuals with mental illness in supported employment has increased dramatically in recent years (see Table 1). It is evident that persons with mental illness are entering supported employment at a rate exceeding that of any other disability group (West, Revell, and Wehman, 1992).

Table 1. Primary disability of supported employment participants, 1988 and 1990

Disability Classification	1988	1990
Mental retardation	70.5%	65.0%
Mental illness	16.7%	24.4%
Sensory impairments	2.5%	2.2%
Cerebral palsy	1.8%	1.9%
Other	8.5%	6.6%

SOURCE: West, Revell, and Wehman, 1992

Because the supported employment regulations stipulate that prospective clients must have an identified source of extended services funding before the initiation of time-limited services, access to supported employment is determined to a large extent by the types of disability services funding that are available within a state. In most cases, mental retardation and mental health systems are the primary (and in many states the only) sources of extended services funding through fee-for-service agreements with provider agencies. Consequently, persons with mental retardation and mental illness constitute the overwhelming majority of service consumers. Many states have no extended service funding sources for persons with cerebral palsy, brain injury, hearing or visual impairments, autism, or other disabilities, and thus their participation rates have declined nationally (West, Revell, and Wehman, 1992). This problem is particularly acute for individuals who have acquired their disabilities as adults and would therefore be ineligible for services funded through their state mental retardation/developmental disabilities service system. To serve these individuals, provider agencies have had to assemble a patchwork of formal and informal supports (Rheinheimer et al., 1993).

Individuals with severe disabilities are the target population for supported employment. Yet considerable evidence indicates that individuals with the most severe disabilities are underserved in supported employment programs. For example, of participants with mental retardation, only about 12 percent are in the severe or profound range, while almost half are mildly retarded (West, Revell and Wehman, 1992). In addition, John Kregel and Paul Wehman (1989), examining service histories and functional characteristics of more than 1,500 supported employment consumers in eight states, found that although the majority had little or no competitive employment experience, few had significant physical, sensory, behavioral, or communicative problems that interfered with employment. They also found high levels of work-related skills, such as math, reading, endurance, attending to task, and other skills and behaviors. They concluded that supported employment is only partially fulfilling its mission to serve individuals with truly severe disabilities.

The Rehabilitation Act Amendments of 1992 include a number of changes to promote inclusion of individuals with significant challenges. First, the act articulates a "presumption of ability" of all potential VR clients to engage in employment, regardless of the types or severity of their disabilities. Title VI, Part C of the act now specifically defines the target population for supported employment as those with "the most severe disabilities." In addition, many state VR agencies have taken the initiative in encouraging provider agencies to serve clients with very severe disabilities through individualized fee schedules, incentive grants, and state policies that are more stringent than the federal regulations.

Facility Conversion. Since supported employment became a VR service option, there has been rapid growth in the number of organizations vendored to provide time-limited and extended services. As Michael West, W. Grant Revell, and Paul Wehman (1992) report, in 1986 there were 324 known supported-employment provider agencies, but in 1990 there were 2,647, most of which were rehabilitation facilities, sheltered workshops, or other segregated day programs. Only about 21 percent of provider agencies had downsized or terminated segregated services to provide supported employment, with the majority maintaining their primary focus and resources for segregated services. Thus, while VR agencies are increasing statewide capacity through provider agreements, few providers are converting from segregated services to supported employment to any appreciable degree. Many states have instituted policy initiatives to promote facility conversion, such as limits on funds or service slots in segregated day programs, adjusted fee scales, incentive grants, or waivers for burdensome regulatory requirements that discourage community-based placements.

Natural Supports. A major movement in the field is the use of "natural supports" in the workplace in lieu of or in addition to formal supports provided by rehabilitation professionals. Natural supports can include employer resources such as employee assistance programs, training programs, coworkers, and supervisors; natural supports may also include friends, family members, personal care attendants, generic community services, and other existing resources that may be used to provide off-site assistance (Albin & Slovic, 1992). Natural supports have been advanced as a cost-effective means of achieving maximum social integration at work and in other integrated environments (Anderson & Andrews, 1990; Nisbet, 1992; Nisbet & Hagner, 1988). The use of natural supports has been endorsed by the Rehabilitation Act Amendments of 1992, which allow natural supports as a source of extended services. This policy change should improve access to services for many individuals who have no source of extended services funding, such as persons who acquire disabilities as adults.

As natural support research and demonstration activities unfold, it will become clearer what natural-support strategies are effective and feasible. Yet some persons in the field have expressed concerns regarding the directions and empirical support for the natural-supports movement in supported employment (West, 1992; Wehman, 1993). There is as yet no evidence for a reasonable expectation that coworkers and supervisors can provide effective and responsive interventions for individuals with severe intellectual, physical, or behavioral challenges. Also, given that individuals with the most severe disabilities are now underserved in supported employment programs, the natural-supports movement may result in the further exclusion of individuals who require more intervention and support than would be found in the typical workplace, in favor of those whose support needs are fewer and more easily accommodated.

The Future of Supported Employment

The Rehabilitation Act Amendments of 1992 instituted policy changes that reinforce the value of integrated, competitive employment for all persons with severe disabilities. Many of those changes came about because of insufficient progress in fulfilling the mission of the supported-employment program to enable persons with the most severe disabilities to achieve gainful employment in the workforce. The future of the supported-employment initiative will depend to a large degree on how rigorously state VR agencies incorporate those changes into their programs, through vendor contracts, interagency agreements, and procedural standards that emphasize (1) inclusion of persons with the most severe disabilities; (2) job placements based on individualized goals, needs, and interests; (3) optimum consumer outcomes such as earnings, integration, and long-term job retention; (4) rapid replacement following job loss; and (5) consumer satisfaction with supported employment services and outcomes.

In the era of the Americans with Disabilities Act and its mandates for nondiscrimination, equal access, and reasonable accommodation, group models will increasingly be viewed as anachronisms and fewer individuals will enter supported employment in groups. The use of natural supports will continue to gain momentum and adherents, driven by the desire to integrate supported employment clients fully into work cultures, and by ever more strained funding from VR and extended-services agencies. Natural-supports research and demonstration projects of the 1990s will help supported-employment programs identify and effectively access employer and community supports and resources. Supported-employment rehabilitation professionals will be less providers of services and more facilitators of supports. Significant issues of debate will be (1) the effectiveness and durability of natural supports in relation to consumer outcomes; (2) the impact of the natural-supports movement on the participation rates of individuals with extensive support needs; and (3) the extent to which natural supports can be utilized and still retain the legislative intent of the program to provide intensive, ongoing rehabilitation services.

The trump card in the natural-supports debate will be consumers' right to choice and self-determination. The Rehabilitation Act Amendments of 1992 also empowered VR clients as never before to determine their own employment goals, services, service providers, and training and support methods. Thus supported-employment consumers will be given increased opportunities to choose the types and sources of training, accommodation, and support that they feel are desirable, effective, and appropriate for their own situation.

(See also: FACILITIES; JOB PLACEMENT; QUALITY OF LIFE; TRANSITION FROM SCHOOL TO WORK; WORK)

RESOURCES

The Association for Persons in Supported Employment (APSE), 5001 West Broad St., Suite 34, Richmond, VA 23230

Rehabilitation Research and Training Center on Supported Employment, Virginia Commonwealth University, Richmond, VA 23284–2011

BIBLIOGRAPHY

ALBIN, JOYCE, and SLOVIC, ROZ. Resources for Long-Term Support in Supported Employment. Eugene, OR, 1992.

Americans with Disabilities Act, PL 101-336 (July 26, 1990). 42 U.S.C. 12101 et seq.

ANDERSON, B., and ANDREWS, M. *Creating Diversity: Organizing and Sustaining Workplaces That Support Employees with Disabilities.* Juneau, AK, 1990.

BROWN, LOU; UDVARI-SOLNER, ALICE; FRATTURA-KAMPSHROER, ELISE; DAVIS, LOUANNE; AHLGREN, CHARLOTTE; VAN DEVENTER, PATRICIA; and JORGENSEN, JACK. "Integrated Work: A Rejection of Segregated Enclaves and Mobile Work Crews." In *Critical Issues in the Lives of People with Severe Disabilities,* eds. Luanna H. Meyer, Charles A. Peck, and Lou Brown. Baltimore, 1991.

FABIAN, ELLEN S. "Supported Employment and the Quality of Life: Does a Job Make a Difference?" *Rehabilitation Counseling Bulletin* 36 (1992):84–97.

Federal Register (August 14, 1987). 52(157), 30546-30552. 34 CFR 363.

Federal Register (June 24, 1992). 57(122), 28432-28442. 34 CFR 363.

HELMS, BARBARA L.; MOORE, STEPHEN C.; and McSWEYN, CARY ANN. "Supported Employment in Connecticut: An Examination of Integration and Wage Outcomes." *Career Development for Exceptional Individuals* 14 (1991):159–166.

HILL, MARK, and WEHMAN, PAUL. "Cost Benefit Analysis of Placing Moderately and Severely Handicapped Individuals into Competitive Employment." *Journal of the Association for the Severely Handicapped* 8 (1983):30–38.

HILL, MARK L.; BANKS, P. DAVID; HANDRICH, RITA R.; WEHMAN, PAUL H.; HILL, JANET W.; and SHAFER, MICHAEL S. "Benefit-Cost Analysis of Supported Competitive Employment for Persons with Mental Retardation." *Research in Developmental Disabilities* 8 (1987):71–89.

KIERNAN, WILLIAM E.; McGAUGHEY, MARTHA J.; and SCHALOCK, ROBERT C. *National Employment Survey for Adults with Developmental Disabilities.* Boston, 1986.

KREGEL, JOHN, and WEHMAN, PAUL. "Supported Employment: Promises Deferred for Persons with Severe Disabilities." *Journal of the Association for Persons with Severe Handicaps* 14 (1989):293–303.

KREGEL, JOHN; WEHMAN, PAUL; and BANKS, P. DAVID. "The Effects of Consumer Characteristics and Type of Employment Model on Individual Outcomes in Supported Employment." *Journal of Applied Behavior Analysis* 22 (1989):407–415.

LAGOMARCINO, THOMAS R. "Job Separation Issues in Supported Employment." In *Supported Employment:*

Models, Methods, and Issues, ed. Frank R. Rusch. Sycamore, IL, 1990.

McCAUGHRIN, WENDY B.; ELLIS, WARREN K.; RUSCH, FRANK R.; and HEAL, LAIRD W. "Cost-Effectiveness of Supported Employment." *Mental Retardation* 31 (1993):41–48.

MOON, M. SHERRIL, and GRIFFIN, SUSAN L. "Supported Employment Service Delivery Models." In *Vocational Rehabilitation and Supported Employment,* eds. Paul Wehman and M. Sherril Moon. Baltimore, 1988.

MOSELEY, CHARLES R. "Job Satisfaction Research: Implications for Supported Employment." *Journal of the Association for Persons with Severe Handicaps* 13 (1989):211–219.

NISBET, JAN, ed. *Natural Supports in School, at Work, and in the Community for People with Severe Disabilities.* Baltimore, 1992.

NISBET, JAN, and HAGNER, DAVID. "Natural Supports in the Workplace: A Reexamination of Supported Employment." *Journal of the Association for Persons with Severe Handicaps* 13 (1988):260–267.

NOBLE, JOHN, and CONLEY, RONALD. "Accumulating Evidence on the Benefits and Costs of Supported and Transitional Employment for Persons with Severe Disabilities." *Journal of the Association for Persons with Severe Handicaps* 12 (1987):163–174.

Rehabilitation Act Amendments of 1986, PL 99-506 (1986). 29 U.S.C. 701 et seq.

Rehabilitation Act Amendments of 1992, PL 102-569 (1992). 29 U.S.C. 701 et seq.

RHEINHEIMER, GAIL B.; VANCOVERN, DEBBY; GREEN, HOWARD; REVELL, GRANT; and INGE, KATHERINE J. *Finding the Common Denominator: A Supported Employment Guide to Long-Term Funding Supports and Services for People with Disabilities.* Richmond, VA, 1993.

RUSCH, FRANK R.; JOHNSON, JOHN R.; and HUGHES, CAROLYN. "Analysis of Co-worker Involvement in Relation to Level of Disability versus Placement Approach Among Supported Employees." *Journal of the Association for Persons with Severe Handicaps* 15 (1990):32–39.

RUSCH, FRANK R., and MITHAUG, DENNIS E. *Vocational Training for Mentally Retarded Adults: A Behavioral Analytic Approach.* Champaign, IL, 1980.

SALE, PAUL; REVELL, W. GRANT; WEST, MICHAEL; and KREGEL, JOHN. "Achievements and Challenges II: An Analysis of 1990 Supported Employment Expenditures." *Journal of the Association for Persons with Severe Handicaps* 17 (1992):236–246.

SALE, PAUL; WEST, MICHAEL; SHERRON, PAM; and

WEHMAN, PAUL. "An Exploratory Analysis of Job Separations from Supported Employment for Persons with Traumatic Brain Injury." *Journal of Head Trauma Rehabilitation* 6 (1991):1–11.

TEST, DAVID W.; HINSON, KAREN B.; SOLOW, JILL; and KEUL, PATRICIA. "Job Satisfaction of Persons in Supported Employment." *Education and Training in Mental Retardation* 28 (1993):38–46.

THOMPSON, LYKE; POWERS, GREG; and HOUCHARD, BERENICE. "The Wage Effects of Supported Employment." *Journal of the Association for Persons with Severe Handicaps* 17 (1992):87–94.

WEHMAN, PAUL. "Competitive Employment in Virginia." In *Competitive Employment Issues and Strategies*, ed. Frank Rusch. Baltimore, 1986.

———. "Natural Supports: More Questions Than Answers?" *Journal of Vocational Rehabilitation* 3 (1993):1–3.

WEHMAN, PAUL; HILL, JANET W.; and KOEHLER, FRANCIS. "Helping Severely Handicapped Persons Enter Competitive Employment." *AAESPH Review* 4 (1979):274–290.

WEHMAN, PAUL, and KREGEL, JOHN. "A Supported Work Approach to Competitive Employment of Individuals with Moderate and Severe Handicaps." *Journal of the Association for Persons with Severe Handicaps* 10 (1985):3–11.

WEHMAN, PAUL, and SHAFER, MICHAEL S., eds. *Emerging Trends in the National Supported Employment Initiative: A Preliminary Analysis of 27 States.* Richmond, VA, 1989.

WEST, MICHAEL. "Job Retention: Toward Vocational Competence, Self-Management, and Natural Supports." In *Supported Employment: Strategies for Integration of Workers with Disabilities*, ed. Paul Wehman, Paul Sale, and Wendy Parent. Boston, 1992.

WEST, MICHAEL; KREGEL, JOHN; and BANKS, P. DAVID. "Fringe Benefits Available to Supported Employment Participants." *Rehabilitation Counseling Bulletin* 34 (1990):126–138.

WEST, MICHAEL; REVELL, W. GRANT; and WEHMAN, PAUL. "Achievements and Challenges I: A Five-Year Report on Consumer and System Outcomes from the Supported Employment Initiative." *Journal of the Association for Persons with Severe Handicaps* 17 (1992):227–235.

WOLFE, PAMELA S. "Supported Employment: A Review of Group Models." In *Supported Employment: Strategies for Integration of Workers with Disabilities*, eds. Paul Wehman, Paul Sale, and Wendy Parent. Boston, 1992.

MICHAEL D. WEST

SURGERY

Persons disabled by trauma or disease are frequently transferred to the rehabilitation setting before reconstruction of their impairment is complete, either in anticipation of further stages of care, or to be followed for the possibility of further surgical care. The patient with burns whose rehabilitation begins before his or her eyebrows are reconstructed because of the need to let tissues soften is an example of the first type of patient. The patient with burns who slowly develops an axillary contracture after grafting and physical therapy, requiring secondary release or graft, is an example of the second type of patient. Therefore, surgeons continue to follow patients with rehabilitation specialists or are available to the rehabilitation team for consultation.

There are few surgical specialties uninvolved with improving the level of function of persons with disabilities. Neurosurgeons observe patients for improvement of their sensorium (Steward & Jane, 1989) or the development of sequelae of neurologic injury, including hydrocephalus and syrinxes. Urologists deal with problems in sexuality (Nanninga, 1989), including penile implants, urinary incontinence, bladder calculi (stones) related to chronic infection and drainage devices, and upper urinary tract calculi caused by immobility and loss of bony mass. General and vascular surgeons deal respectively with persistent problems of gastrointestinal integrity, when to internalize colostomies and problems created by short bowel syndromes, and the problems created by ongoing arteriosclerotic peripheral vascular disease, which are often hard to diagnose in the individual who is immobilized or neurologically impaired.

The plastic surgeon deals with both soft tissue and bony problems of the face, including scar revision to improve appearance of the bones of the facial skeleton, and to shape the jaws and orbits (eye sockets) to restore function such as binocular vision or effective chewing (Cohen & Kawamoto, 1992). Many of these procedures are performed in partnership with oral and maxillofacial surgeons as well as orthodontic or dental specialists.

The facial features of many patients with burns are restored in stages over relatively long periods of time. Eyelids may require release and skin graft, or reconstruction by the movement of soft tissue available in the region (Huang, Blackwell, & Lewis, 1978). Eyebrows are rebuilt either by the movement of strips of hair with their own blood supply through tunnels under the skin to the rim above the eyelid, or by taking small bunches of hair (punch grafts) from the remaining hair on the back of the head and placing them in rows on the skin of the forehead in the shape of the eyebrow arch (Tessier, Hervouet, Lekieffre, et al., 1981).

The burned or damaged nose is rebuilt using skin grafts and remaining nasal tissue, flaps from the forehead moved on their own blood supply, or expanded just by a tissue expander placed under the skin (Feldman, 1988). Missing bone and cartilage are replaced from the hip or skull, ear or rib, when adequate skin to cover has been created (Burget, 1985). The mouth can be widened and lips restored using tongue and mouth lining tissue, and local tissue rearrangements (Feldman, 1987). Soft, sometimes expressive facial skin can be provided over time by expanding unburned skin remaining in the neck or face. Occasionally tissue is moved by free tissue transfer, using a microscope to attach a blood supply (Angrigiani, 1994). Ears can be rebuilt using rib cartilage, lining tissue from the temple, and skin grafts (Brent, 1992).

Soft tissue losses of the trunk and extremities are replaced with limited or extensive procedures depending on the volume of tissue required. Webs of scar tissue around the joints of patients with burns may be released by rearranging the tissue in the area using a procedure called Z-plasty, or by the addition of skin grafts. Large ulcers caused by compression of soft tissue between bone and an underlying unyielding surface called pressure sores may require the composite movement of blocks of tissue containing skin, lining, and muscle called musculocutaneous flaps to provide durable seated surfaces (Lewis, 1990).

The function of the hand damaged by accident or burn or defunctionalized by paralysis may be improved by plastic or orthopedic surgeons. Available procedures range from releasing webbed scars and contracted joints with Z-plasties or skin grafts (Covey, Dutcher, Heimbach, et al., 1987), to transfer-

ring a big toe from the foot to the hand to create a thumb (Lister, Kalisman, and Tsai, 1983). Intermediate procedures include replacing lost tendons to let muscles move fingers, shifting the tendon of a still functioning muscle to the tendon of a paralyzed one to improve hand usefulness, and releasing of tendons trapped in scar to glide more smoothly (Earle & Fratianne, 1983).

Advances in orthopedic surgery now enable surgeons to preserve lengths of limbs damaged by trauma, or lengthen shortened limbs (Illizarov procedure). The lengthening is frequently done with the addition of bone from the hip (ilium) as a free graft (Taylor, 1977), or with the movement of a piece of the small bone of the lower leg (fibula) with its blood supply, and sometimes with attached soft tissue (Cierny & Nahai). Joints such as the knee and hip, the function of which have been lost by trauma or arthritis, can be replaced with joints of stainless steel and plastic (Effekar).

The appropriateness of an available operative procedure for an individual patient is determined by the medical team and patient together. Certain procedures may be possible but give little benefit, such as a joint replacement in a paralyzed limb. Some procedures may require long periods of retraining, which the patient may not be equipped to undergo, such as tendon transfer in the hand of a patient with brain damage. Some patients with burns may decide they have had enough feature restoration, even when more is available. The surgeon's role is to decide the preferred therapies with the disabled patient, rather than to do to the patient what is available.

(See also: AMPUTATION; BACK DISORDERS; BURNS; CORONARY ARTERY DISEASE; GASTROINTESTINAL DISORDERS; HOSPITAL, REHABILITATION; PEDIATRIC REHABILITATION; PHYSICIAN; PROSTHETICS AND ORTHOTICS; SPINAL CORD INJURY; STROKE)

RESOURCES

American Academy of Physical Medicine and Rehabilitation, 78 East Adams St., Suite 310, Chicago, IL 60603–6103

Ranchos Los Amigos, 7601 East Imperial Highway, Downey, CA 90242

Texas Institute of Rehabilitation and Research, 1333 Moursund Ave., Houston, TX 77030

BIBLIOGRAPHY

ANGRIGIANI, CLAUDIO. "Aesthetic Microsurgical Reconstruction of Anterior Neck Burn Deformities." *Plastic Reconstructive Surgery* 93 (1994): 507–518.

BRENT, BURT. "Auricular Repair with Autogenous Rib Cartilage Grafts: Two Decades of Experience with 600 Cases." *Plastic Reconstructive Surgery* 90 (1992): 355–374.

BURGET, GARY. "Aesthetic Restoration of the Nose." *Clinical Plastic Surgery* 12 (1985):463–480.

CIERNY, GEORGE, and NAHAI, FOAD. "Dialogue: Lower Extremity Reconstruction, Part II." *Perspectives in Plastic Surgery* 2 (1988): 109–121.

COHEN, STEVEN R., and KAWAMOTO, HENRY K. "The Use of Rigid Fixation in Post-traumatic Maxillary and Mandibular Reconstruction." In *Rigid Fixation of the Craniomaxillofacial Skeleton*, eds. Michael J. Yaremchuk; Joseph S. Gruss; and Paul N. Mason. Stoneham, MA, 1992.

COVEY, MARK; DUTCHER, KRISTI; HEIMBACH, DAVID M.; MARRIN, JANET A.; ENGRAV, LOREN H.; DE LATEUR, BARBARA. "Return of Hand Function Following Major Burns." *Journal of Burn Care Rehabilitation* 8 (1987): 224–226.

EARLE, SCOTT A., and FRATIANNE, RICHARD B. "Delayed Definitive Reconstruction of the Burned Hand: Evolution of a Program of Care." *Journal of Trauma* 19 (1979): 145–152.

EFTEKAR, NAS S. *Total Hip Arthroplasty.* St. Louis, MO, 1993.

FELDMAN, JOEL J. "Burn Reconstruction." *Perspectives in Plastic Surgery* 2 (1988): 146–154.

———. "Secondary Repair of the Burned Upper Lip." *Perspectives in Plastic Surgery* 1 (1987): 31–67.

HUANG, TED T.; BLACKWELL, STEVEN J.; and LEWIS, STEPHEN R. "Burn Injuries of the Eyelids." *Clinical Plastic Surgery* 5 (1978):571–581.

LEWIS JR., VICTOR L. "Pressure Ulcers." In *Medical Management of Long-term Disability*, ed. David Green. Rockville, MD, 1990.

LISTER, GRAHAM D.; KALISMAN, MICHAEL; and TSAI, TSU-MIN. "Reconstruction of the Hand with Free Microvascular Toe-to-Hand Transfer: Experience with 54 Toe Transfers." *Plastic Reconstructive Surgery* 71 (1983): 372–384.

NANNINGA, JOHN B. "Anticipated Urologic-Sexual Dysfunction." In *Surgery of Spine Trauma*, ed. Paul R. Meyer, New York, 1989.

STEWARD, OSWALD, and JANE, JOHN A. "Repair and Reorganization of Neuronal Connections Following CNS Trauma." In *Textbook of Head Injury*, eds. Donald P. Becker, and Steven K. Gudeman. Philadelphia, 1989.

TAYLOR, IAN. "Microvascular Free Bone Transfer: A Clinical Technique." *Orthopedic Clinics of North America* 8 (1977): 425–477.

TESSIER, PAUL; HERVOUET, FRANÇOIS; LEKIEFFRE, MICHEL; ROUGIER, JACQUES; WOILLEZ, MARCEL; and DEROME, PATRICK. *Plastic Surgery of the Orbit and Eyelids.* Chicago, 1981.

VICTOR L. LEWIS, JR.

SWITZER, MARY E.

Mary E. Switzer was born in 1900 and died in 1971. She completed her federal service as the first administrator of the Social and Rehabilitative Services Administration of the U.S. Department of Health, Education, and Welfare. She went on to serve as vice president of the World Rehabilitation Fund until her death.

The name Mary E. Switzer is synonymous with the federal-state partnership in the rehabilitation of persons with disabilities. After more than twenty years of federal service in Washington, DC, she was appointed Commissioner of the Office of Vocational Rehabilitation (OVR), later known as the Rehabilitation Services Administration (RSA). She was fifty years old when she took the helm of OVR and brought to the position a superior intellect and a thorough knowledge of the bureaucracy, along with experience in economics, the legislative process, health, welfare, and public education, to name some of her assets.

Miss Switzer entered the vocational rehabilitation movement at a critical juncture during this period. It was a time when this relatively new human service specialty was in its formative years and facing many challenges and obstacles. What was necessary was a leader with vision and a solid understanding of how to tame the bureaucracy and make it move in a positive direction, to make vocational rehabilitation a viable force throughout the United States.

Miss Switzer could seize any platform to advocate for persons with disabilities. As noted by Martha Lentz Walker (1985), she had a tenacity of purpose taught her by her maternal uncle, Michael J. Moore, "who coached her in speech and delivery, pointers which served her purpose all of her life. . . ." These teachings were evident as she carried the message of persons with disabilities to the U.S. Congress and the executive branch of the federal government, where she learned to deal with secretaries of health and of labor, as well as with presidents from Franklin D. Roosevelt through Richard Nixon.

In her quest for excellence she surrounded herself with the best and the brightest talent representing a broad cross section of disciplines, including physical medicine, psychology, social work, and economics. Armed with the facts and the most current research information available at the time, she proceeded to make the case for vocational rehabilitation and its myriad of needs for persons with numerous types of disabilities. "Innovation" and "persistence" were her watchwords, and she set forth on a journey that was to establish her as a legend in the field.

During her tenure she fought for new and more effective approaches to rehabilitation and introduced new concepts to be developed on a national scale in areas such as mental illness, mental retardation, independent living issues for the most severely disabled persons, facilities construction, mobility, and sensation training for blind persons. In addition, she developed education and training programs at the university level for persons to work in the field of vocational rehabilitation. Known as "Switzer traineeships," more than 100 universities offered the programs that were to provide a cadre of rehabilitation counselors, psychologists, and other rehabilitation professionals to work in state–federal programs and other rehabilitative settings in communities throughout the nation. Many of the novel programs and concepts that continue to operate today are the direct result of the seeds planted by Mary Switzer and her national team of experts in the 1950s and 1960s.

Following a life pattern in support of increased services to people and a more responsive and humanitarian government to changing human needs, Miss Switzer committed herself to the less certain but more hopefully expanded future for the field of rehabilitation. The breadth and humanity of Mary Switzer are emblazoned forever in the passage of the Vocational Rehabilitation Act Amendments of 1954, with its research and demonstration features,

its concern for rehabilitation education, its mandate to construct rehabilitation facilities, its new international efforts and cooperation regarding rehabilitation, and its expanded funding base for more personnel and programs for those needing a wide array of rehabilitative services.

Miss Switzer won numerous national and international awards and was leader of many organizations, including the National Rehabilitation Association (NRA), that have kept her name alive through the Switzer Memorial Committee and its Annual Switzer Memorial Seminar and Monograph. Monograph No. 6 (1981) contained a number of quotes of and about Mary Switzer, the person, the administrator, and the humanitarian. Excerpts of these quotes sum up her life and contributions in a concise manner, as follows: James F. Garrett, former assistant commissioner of the RSA, noted, ". . . she was a remarkable person whose daily life was a Renaissance recital. She had the broad interests of the liberal arts major, yet she was able to balance [them] with utmost pragmatism. She was "soft" in dealing with those under her and "hard" with peers and superiors. She was most skillful in her use of information, rarely making rash promises. She was superb in her capacity to delegate authority and yet knew when to draw in the reins."

Another colleague of Miss Switzer, Joseph Hunt, former commissioner of the RSA, stated, "Her leadership was not of the scientific management genre, with its jargon, charts, processes, and machinery, for which she had little taste. It was instead a unique art form—a leadership into which she put the total person, a woman of good instincts, imagination, and intelligence, with untiring interest in the social problems of her country and the world, especially the problems of poor persons, the sick, and persons with disabilities." He went on to state that in her policy-making she thought and talked from a wide reading of history, biography, literature, political philosophy, and significant years of government experience gained in high places. She was adroit, and in planning strategy and tactics was not above political maneuvers when indicated, but these moves and ploys were always directed toward good ends. She was a captivating public speaker with a good stage presence, and she liked to write and wrote well. Hunt noted that she was honored by her country and was the first woman to have a government building in Washington, DC, named in her honor.

Josephine Coe, secretary to Miss Switzer, stated that Mary Switzer believed that public servants should have the attitude of commitment and caring for each individual and a true belief in the inner capability and hope that each person has within him or her qualities that can be enhanced. She was a "bureaucrat," as government employees are often called, but in her was a mission, vision, faith, hope, and joy in obtaining the results of dedicated work. She believed that government could make a difference, inspire, and lead the way.

(*See also:* HISTORY OF REHABILITATION; STATE–FEDERAL REHABILITATION PROGRAM)

BIBLIOGRAPHY

NATIONAL REHABILITATION ASSOCIATION. "Annual Switzer Memorial Seminar and Monograph No. 6." Alexandria, VA, 1981.

PERLMAN, LEONARD G., and ARNESON, KATHALEEN, C. *Women and Rehabilitation of Disabled Persons.* Alexandria, VA, 1982.

WALKER, MARTHA LENTZ. *Beyond Bureaucracy: Mary Elizabeth Switzer and Rehabilitation.* Lanham, MD, 1985.

LEONARD G. PERLMAN
JAMES R. BURRESS

T–U

TECHNOLOGY AND DISABILITY

The landmark legislation regarding the provision of assistive technologies was the Technology-Related Assistance of Individuals with Disabilities Act of 1988 (P.L. 100-407), which was reauthorized in 1994. The original legislation defined assistive technology (AT) as: "any item, piece of equipment, or product system, whether acquired commercially off the shelf, modified, or customized, that is used to increase, maintain, or improve functional capabilities of individuals with disabilities."

ATs help individuals with disabilities live more independent lives in their communities and replace or reduce the amount of assistance required of other persons by enhancing independent functioning and minimizing "disability." An AT may be low-tech (mechanical) or high-tech (electromechanical or computerized), and the term includes products that compensate for sensory and functional losses by providing the means to move (e.g., wheelchairs, lifts, braces, quad canes), speak (e.g., manual communication boards, computerized voice synthesizers), read (e.g., magnifying devices for persons who are blind), hear (e.g., hearing aids, personal FM systems, vibrotactile pagers), and manage self-care tasks (e.g., built-up eating utensils, automatic feeders, environmental control systems).

Assistive Technologies May be Used, Avoided, or Abandoned

Data from the 1990 U.S. Census Bureau's National Health Interview Survey on Assistive Devices show that more than 13.1 million people in the United States (more than 5% of the total U.S. population) used assistive technologies in 1990. In 1969, 6.2 million people used a total of 7.2 million assistive devices. Between 1970 and 1990 the number of persons using assistive technologies doubled because of three key factors: (1) People with disabilities surviving severe trauma and disease and living longer; (2) advances in microelectronics and the availability of microcomputers; and (3) each new law regarding persons with disabilities passed since P.L. 100-407 in 1988 has mandated the consideration of assistive technology. There are no data on how these figures compare to the total number of devices prescribed or purchased during this time span, nor are there comparable indicators of this population's predisposition to technology use in general. We do know that people with disabilities differ in the degrees to which they use assistive technologies, and they have differing views of the extent to which they believe ATs improve the quality of their lives. Many individuals with disabilities avoid technologies outright, and others try them only to abandon them to the closet or bedside table. While unused and abandoned technologies represent wasted resources, so do people not performing at their functional best.

Depending on the type of AT, nonuse or abandonment can be as low as 8 percent or as high as 75 percent; on average, one-third of more optional ATs are abandoned, most within the first three months (Scherer & Galvin, 1994). One type of device with a high rate of abandonment is hearing aids. According to the results of a study conducted by Marcia J. Scherer and D. Robert Frisina (1994), factors associated with the nonuse of hearing aids include the nature and extent of hearing loss, discomfort with ear molds, the expense and visibility of the aids, and disappointment that "perfect hearing" is not restored. Additionally, users of hearing aids often comment on difficulties in discriminating a speaker's voice from background noise.

All assistive technologies are designed to improve functioning, enable a person to live at home and in the community successfully, and enhance independence. But as in the case of hearing aids, improved functioning by itself will not ensure AT use. Individuals have psychological and psychosocial needs that ATs need to accommodate. The provision of an AT is not an end. An AT is only a means to help individuals achieve their personal goals as they function in different environments. The personal aspects of a functional need must drive AT selection, not an AT's functions or features.

Regardless of the type of AT under construction, people will differ in their use, as reactions to assistive technologies are individual and complex. They emerge from varying needs, abilities, preferences, and experiences. Use may be full-time and done willingly, or partial and done reluctantly (this most frequently occurs with persons whose AT use is not optional or where a person will use an AT in one environment but not another). Nonuse may be due to the avoidance of an AT altogether (e.g., a person will not show up for an evaluation or fitting or will not purchase it) or to its abandonment. As noted in Marcia J. Scherer and Jan C. Galvin (1994), a better understanding of how and why technology users decide to accept or reject different types of ATs is critical to improving the effectiveness of assistive technology interventions and enhancing individuals' quality of life.

The Need for a Model When Matching a Person and a Technology

Successful AT use requires adapting the AT to the person's capabilities and temperament and adapting the person, family, coworkers, and others to the realities and situations of AT use. One method that has been found useful in organizing the myriad influences on a person's predisposition to the use of a more optional technology is the Matching Person and Technology (MPT) model (Scherer, 1993a), which advocates separately addressing:

1. characteristics of the **M**ilieu (environment and psychosocial setting) in which the assistive technology is used;
2. pertinent features of the individual's **P**ersonality and temperament;
3. salient characteristics of the assistive **T**echnology itself.

The MPT model promotes development of a broad as well as in-depth profile of a person's predisposition to use a particular AT. For example, a person may look like a partial or reluctant AT user as far as milieu variables but appear to be an optimal user according to the characteristics listed for personality and technology. The milieu influences on use may need some intervention or modification for the person to gain maximum satisfaction and functional gain from use of the AT. Table 1 provides examples of broad characteristics associated with AT use, avoidance, or abandonment in these areas, and Table 2 lists important questions for consumers to answer regarding their potential match with a particular AT. More detailed descriptions of factors to consider follow.

Table 1. Assessing the match of person and technology: Examples of factors associated with AT use, avoidance, and abandonment in three domains

	Milieu	Person	Technology
Use	Essential modifications and accommodations exist	Self-esteem and self-efficacy enhanced	The AT is affordable and easily obtained
	Support and assistance from family, friends, etc.	Desired level of independence achieved	The AT is safe, reliable, and comfortable
Avoidance	The environment/culture does not support use	The person does not want a technical alternative	The AT appears complex and overwhelming
	Family encourages dependence and helplessness	Person believes aptitude for success with AT is lacking	The AT is too expensive or complicated to get
Abandonment	Environment makes use awkward and otherwise unappealing	AT believed to restrict freedom and/or privacy	The gain from use is not worth resources required for use
	AT use forced on the person by others	The person finds other, easier, and preferred options	The AT becomes incompatible with need, interests, etc.

SOURCE: Marcia J. Scherer (1993a)

Influences on AT Use, Avoidance, and Abandonment in Three Areas

Milieu. An all too common occurrence is that the AT that worked so well in the rehabilitation facility is not working out in the home. The walker that made getting around easy on linoleum is useless on the shag carpeting in the living room. The wheelchair won't fit in the car, and the magnifying device is never in the same room as the current visual need. The failure of ATs to fit well with the environments of home, work, or school is a major reason for technology being abandoned.

In addition to the stress associated with the need for an AT, there may be stress from changes made to the home or workplace and anxiety/insecurity and depression at the loss of familiar routines and surroundings. There may be resistance to change and resentment from others in the work, home, or school environment toward the individual with a disability. It is important to try out ATs in the settings in which they will be used and involve all affected by them so that (1) the best AT can be recommended that requires the minimal amount of modifications to the settings themselves; and (2) everyone feels they are involved in making choices around accommodations for the AT.

Self-concept, self-efficacy, motivation, personal aspirations, and other influences on predispositions to AT use are shaped by social interactions and cultural expectations. The attitudes and expectations of others can have a profound influence on the kinds of support given for AT use. Another common reason for abandonment is that AT use was forced on the individual as a condition for being discharged to home, and the AT immediately became a focal point for resentment. Other factors, such as environmental accommodations, available resources (e.g., private insurance for specialized treatment, availability of personal assistance), and special opportunities (e.g., placement in a rehabilitation center with the newest equipment and proper training for use) are also important milieu characteristics.

Personality. People are dynamic, with changing needs and goals. ATs often must be thought of as relatively long-term solutions to functional limitations due to AT expense and funding requirements. The challenge is to meet the individual's current needs with future needs in mind.

Many people with disabilities have an aversion to replacing a natural function, however limited, with a technical device. They may believe that use of ATs will lead to a loss of functional abilities and

Table 2. Questions for consumers to answer about assistive technologies

Characteristics of the Psychosocial Arena/Milieu

- Where will I use the AT? At home, work, community, all of these?
- Will my environment or environments support the AT?
- Will I have the training and support I need to use the AT?
- Could the environment disrupt AT performance, that is, electronic interference?
- How may the AT affect other people in my environment?

Characteristics of the Person's Temperament, Abilities, and Preferences

- Are my capabilities stable or changing?
- How do I currently manage my daily activities?
- How will the AT fit my routines?
- Can I change my activities so I can do them without an AT?
- Is it important to me to do things as independently as possible?
- Am I comfortable using technology?
- Do I have the necessary capabilities to use the AT?
- Will this AT contribute significantly to my quality of life?

Characteristics of the Assistive Technology

- Does the AT reflect my lifestyle, age, personality, values?
- Have I considered all the options available?
- How well does the AT work?
- How much will it cost to buy and maintain?
- Will it be easy to use and maintain?
- How long is it likely to last?
- Will I be able to try it before I buy it?
- How does this AT fit with other equipment or technologies I use?

increasing dependence on ATs. Additionally, persons without knowledge of or exposure to technologies can exhibit anxiety when faced with them. Being anxious makes it more difficult for them to learn the skills to operate them. As well as feeling anxious around technologies, people often have a distrust of them.

The article "Technophiles and Technophobes" in *American Demographics* (Mitchell, 1994) noted that technophobes outnumber technophiles by more than two to one. The technophile embraces technology, whereas the technophobe avoids it. It is challenging to get technophobes to use new technical products; it is as much of a challenge to keep technophiles from grabbing each new product that comes along. The technophobic person avoids, even fears, such technologies as VCRs and computers.

Individuals who are technophobic typically have not been exposed to technologies. For them, the potentials achieved through use of an AT are not worth the anxiety or discomfort involved in its use.

Gender is one influence on the appeal and use of many sophisticated ATs (Scherer, 1993b and c). Women have traditionally received little exposure to technical perspectives and tend to be uninformed about and disinterested in complex high-tech products. Nontechnically oriented males, on the other hand, can feel even more threatened by technological products in that they may feel an additional assault to their egos because they lack skills that are traditionally male objects of interest.

The use of an AT is more acceptable when both low- and high-tech options are available and the person can exercise choice. While a wheelchair is not usually an optional piece of equipment for a person, the type and number of wheelchairs a person has *are* under more individual control.

ATs that require a lot of cognitive energy for the user are frequently abandoned in favor of other, easier alternatives. Other obstacles to optimal AT use include giving a person an AT that requires development of unusual or new skills and changes in accustomed patterns of doing things, having the AT eclipse the person and call undue attention to itself, and having AT use result in loss of privacy. Feelings of being conspicuous are compounded when assistive technologies leave many users feeling deviant and stigmatized.

Technology. Assistive technologies have a high rate of use when they are lightweight and portable, easy to use and set up, are cost-effective to obtain and maintain, and are the same as or similar to devices used by the general population. The flexibility of devices and the degree to which they can accommodate the addition of other devices are also important. The increased practice of integrating multiple devices controlled by a single input device often results in a more streamlined appearance but also in situations of "cognitive overload."

Devices are unlikely to be used if they "never seem to be there when needed," are seen as "not worth all the effort," do not have enough practical applications, and create discomfort or inconvenience. Adequate training in operating and maintaining the AT is very important, as is the availability of a backup system.

Assistive technology use is interactive among the above categories. An alteration in one will have an effect on the others. For example, optimal use of one assistive technology likely leads to improved functioning, improved self-esteem, wider social contacts, and enthusiasm for trying another AT. Also, at a particular time a person can be in one category with one AT and in another with a second AT. The introduction of a new technology can make use of an existing one more complicated or cumbersome. It is probable that as time goes on, AT compatibility/incompatibility will be a growing area of concern. We have become aware that a "fatal threshold" can be reached when a system composed of one or more technologies has an additive effect, resulting in a situation of frustration and "overload" for a person and even such difficulties as fatigue and musculoskeletal and cardiopulmonary stress.

Consumer Involvement in AT Selection Is Crucial

Laws regarding persons with disabilities recognize the importance of consumer involvement in rehabilitation services, including AT selection. This emphasis on consumerism advocates consumer choice, self-determination, and independent living. It leaves the person and family more in charge and with more responsibilities than ever before.

As noted in Marcia J. Scherer and Jan C. Galvin (1994), one key to achieving better person and technology matches is adopting a collaborative approach to AT selection, training, and support where consumer and professional cooperate equally in the matching process. While both consumer and professional are trying to achieve the same thing, each has particular strengths to bring to the relationship. Consumers know the goals, interests, dislikes, priorities, and practical aspects of their living situation. Professionals know about different ATs, have access to a variety of resources, and have experience evaluating technologies and people's functioning.

When consumer and professional form a partnership, each partner is responsible for completing certain tasks, gathering information, and making certain decisions. Professionals can stimulate discussion of the consumer's current capabilities and functioning and personal aspects related to technology use such as lifestyle, motivation, adjustment to disability, attitude toward technology, and values. Together, consumers and professionals can explore how these issues relate to technology use. One means developed to support such a collaborative approach is the MPT model, which consists of checklist-type assessment instruments to record consumer goals and preferences, views of the benefits to be gained from a technology, and changes in self-perceived functioning and outcome achievement over time. The items emerged from the actual experiences of technology users and nonusers, so they have "content validity." Additional psychometric evidence exists that they are quality assessments (Crewe & Dijkers, 1995). For the assistive technology version, there is a consumer and professional form so that crisscross comparisons of professional and consumer views can be made.

Regardless of the means employed to assess the potential quality of the match of person and AT, it is crucial for professionals to ensure the following:

1. Consumer needs drive the matching process, not what the AT can do or its availability.
2. Professionals have the support they need to become knowledgeable about a variety of technologies and relevant resources.
3. Different perspectives of professional and consumer become evident so they can be addressed.
4. No tech, low-tech, and high-tech interventions are all considered.
5. Trial periods with the interventions in situations of actual use are arranged.
6. Desirable interventions are selected, with the necessary support systems established to ensure their success.
7. Specific objective criteria by which to judge the intervention's usefulness to the consumer are identified, along with a timeline.

Individuals with disabilities involved in AT selection in a meaningful way will generally be more cooperative, more active and independent in using the AT, and more satisfied with rehabilitation services overall. Additionally, shared responsibility for the outcome brings personal investment in achieving that outcome.

(*See also:* COMPUTER APPLICATIONS FOR VISUAL DISABILITIES; COMPUTERS; WHEELCHAIRS)

RESOURCES

RESNA Technical Assistance Project, 1700 N. Moore St., Suite 1540, Arlington, VA 22209–1903

Trace Research and Development Center, S-151 Waisman Center, 1500 Highland Ave., Madison, WI 53705–2280

BIBLIOGRAPHY

CREWE, NANCY M., and DIJKERS, MARCEL P. "Functional Assessment." In *Psychological Assessment in Medical Rehabilitation Settings*, eds. Laura A. Cushman and Marcia J. Scherer, Washington, DC, 1995.

MITCHELL, SUSAN. "Technophiles and Technophobes." *American Demographics* 16 (1994):35–42.

SCHERER, MARCIA J. *Living in the State of Stuck: How Technology Impacts the Lives of People with Disabilities.* Cambridge, MA, 1993a.

———. "What We Know About Women's Technology Use, Avoidance, and Abandonment." *Women and Therapy* 14 (1993b):117–132; also in *Women with Disabilities: Found Voices*, eds. Mary E. Willmuth and Lillian Holcomb. New York, 1993c.

SCHERER, MARCIA J., and FRISINA, D. ROBERT. "Applying the Matching People with Technologies Model to Individuals with Hearing Loss: What People Say They Want—and Need—from Assistive Technologies." In *Technology and Disability: Deafness and Hearing Impairments*, ed. Marcia J. Scherer, Stoneham, MA, 1994.

SCHERER, MARCIA J., and GALVIN, JAN C. "Matching People with Technology." *Rehab Management* 9 (1994):128–130.

MARCIA J. SCHERER

TESTING

See ASSESSMENT; PSYCHOLOGY; VOCATIONAL EVALUATION

TRANSFERABILITY OF SKILLS

See JOB PLACEMENT

TRANSITION FROM SCHOOL TO WORK

In 1984, Madeline Will, assistant secretary in the Office of Special Education and Rehabilitation Services (OSERS), brought to the nation's attention the need for students with disabilities who were exiting the educational system to be better prepared for the world of work and independent living. She began a policy initiative for transition services, referring to transition as three bridges from the world of education to the world of work, postsecondary training, and adult living. The three bridges of transition that a student with a disability could use represented: (1) no special support services, (2) time-limited support services, and (3) ongoing special services. Each of these three bridges would lead from the school system to various types of employment: (1) regular competitive employment, (2) supported employment, and (3) sheltered employment. Will believed that most students with mild or moderate disabilities would use the bridge that required no additional support services outside the family or employers in the community, while students with more involved disabilities would require at least some time-limited services, such as those provided through vocational rehabilitation. The most severely involved population would require more constant ongoing support services. Various other models of transition were developed from that point, but all of the transition models had similar components—vocational training; assistance in the development of employability skills, independent living skills, and social skills; support services; job coaching; interagency collaboration; and parental involvement.

Legislation

Transition services for young adults with disabilities leaving school to enter the world of work were legislatively mandated in 1990. The 1990 amendments to the Individuals with Disabilities Education Act (IDEA) defined transition services as follows:

> A coordinated set of activities for a student, designed within an outcome-oriented process, which promotes movement from school to post-school activities, including: post-secondary education, vocational training, integrated employment (including supported employment), continuing and adult education, adult services, independent living, and community participation. The coordinated set of activities shall be based upon the individual student's needs, taking into account student preferences and interest, and shall include: instruction, community experiences, development of employment and other post-school adult living objectives and when appropriate, daily living skills and functional vocational evaluation [Section 602 (A), 20 U.S.C. 1401 (A)].

The law mandates that by no later than age sixteen (beginning at age fourteen or younger) each student's individualized education plan (IEP) include transition services. The IEP team (as defined by IDEA) would be responsible for integrating transition into the IEP. For transition planning to be effective, a partnership among the school, the family, and the community is necessary. In cases where an agency other than the educational agency is involved in providing agreed-upon services but does not carry them out, the educational agency must reconvene the IEP team to identify alternative strategies to meet the transition objectives.

Other pieces of legislation also contribute to the transition movement. Section 118 of the Carl D. Perkins Vocational and Applied Technology Education Act provides the following assurances:

1. To assist students in their recruitment, enrollment, and applications to enter vocational education programs and in fulfilling their transitional services requirements under IDEA.
2. To assess the special needs of students with respect to their successful completion of vocational education programs in the most integrated setting possible.
3. To provide supplementary services—such as curriculum modification, equipment modification, classroom modification, supportive personnel, and instructional aids and devices—to students who are members of special populations, including students with disabilities.
4. To provide guidance, counseling, and career development activities by professionally trained counselors and teachers who are associated with the provisions of such special services.
5. To provide counseling and instructional services designed to facilitate the transition from school to employment and career opportunities.

The Americans with Disabilities Act (1990) also supported the transition movement by guaranteeing equal access for individuals with disabilities in the following areas: employment, public accommodations, state and government agencies, transportation, and telecommunications. The Job Training and Partnership Act and the Vocational Rehabilitation Act include support for transition mandates as well.

Transition Planning. The transition planning process has been driven by the IEP since the implementation of IDEA legislation. The anticipated adult environments are targeted as transition outcomes based on assessment data, IEP team input, family input, resources, and student preferences. Adult outcomes most frequently considered in transition planning are postsecondary training, learning, occupational training, home living, civic and community participation, and recreation and leisure activities. The critical factor in transition planning is that the comprehensive needs of the student be matched to the curriculum and learning experiences that are likely to lead to the desired adult outcomes. The IEP team is responsible for planning the curriculum that will assist the student in mastering skills needed in the targeted adult environments. Skills may include the following: job-seeking and job-retention skills, specific occupational skills, generalizable skills (such as reading, computation, and writing), social skills, self-advocacy skills, community functioning skills (such as transportation), and home living skills (such as cooking).

The IEP team is responsible for the instructional planning of each student with a disability by identifying annual goals and short-term objectives for IEPs leading to the mastery of skills and competencies that increase the student's chances for success in making the transition from school to the postschool environment. The curriculum becomes an important vehicle for teaching transition skills. One approach to curriculum associated with transition is that of functional curriculum.

Functional curriculum is an approach to selecting instructional skills, activities, and experiences that will assist students in adjusting to adult life. One functional curriculum that is closely identified with the transition movement is the Life Centered Career Education (LCCE) Competency-Based Curriculum, published by the Council for Exceptional Children (CEC). The LCCE curriculum includes three domains: (1) daily living skills, (2) personal-social skills, and (3) occupational guidance and preparation skills. The LCCE curriculum was researched, developed, and refined between 1973 and 1993 by Donn E. Brolin at the University of Missouri at Columbia. The curriculum contains twenty-two competencies and ninety-seven subcompetencies that are used by IEP teams to focus on transition. The LCCE curriculum is based on the philosophy of normalization and independent living. The theory is

that through a coordinated effort by teams (schools, parents, and the community), students can better achieve transition if they master a common core of competencies designed for that outcome.

Support Services

To facilitate the acquisition of skills, the IEP team considers a wide continuum of services, such as regular education, vocational education, special education, vocational rehabilitation, community experiences, and home experiences. Services and supports can come from community organizations, agencies, guidance and career counselors, educators, job placement specialists, job coaches, peers, and family members. The stronger the cooperation and networking among the various agencies and individuals, the better chance the student has for success.

Support services are an integral part of transition from school to work. It is the emphasis on support services that most schools focus on when they are involved in transition planning. Support services for transition can include peer tutoring, transportation, residential options, medical care, child care, vocational training alternatives, job search and placement assistance, mental health services, financial assistance, assistive devices, equipment adaptations, social services, legal counseling, leisure-time support groups, attendant care, and any other services that an individual may need to achieve independent living status. Support services can be provided by educators (teachers, administrators, related service personnel, counselors), government agencies, or individuals within the community. Frequently, collaboration and coordination are required for the effective and efficient delivery of transition support services. The coordination can be either formal or informal. The formal arrangement of this type of collaboration is generally referred to as an interagency agreement.

Interagency agreements are usually articulated by educational institutions, job training programs, rehabilitative agencies, and other agencies such as organizations serving persons with developmental disabilities. Michelle Sarkees and John Scott (1985) define an interagency agreement as a written agreement between public and private agencies whose objective is to provide instruction and services to learners with special needs. The ultimate goal is to provide efficient and effective delivery of vocational assessment, vocational instruction, support services, and other related transition services depending on the resources available. There are several reasons why interagency agreements are needed: to avoid duplication of services, to provide efficient and effective services, to save valuable resources, to facilitate the delivery of services based on individual case needs, to avoid administrative problems, and to coordinate the efforts of professionals from various agencies.

The issues that are usually addressed in interagency agreements include administrative relationships, operating policies, services to be provided, specific referral procedures, eligibility requirements, provisions for exchanging appropriate information, financial costs, roles and responsibilities of personnel involved in providing services, and any other strategies useful in providing the jointly sponsored services needed to assist individuals in the transition process.

Supported Employment

Curriculum and support services are intended to bring about self-sufficiency, employment, and independent living to the maximum extent possible. The desired outcomes of carefully designed curricula and support services may be achieved through interagency agreements. However, competitive employment may not be the outcome. Supported employment is a vocational opportunity for persons with severe disabilities. Since the late 1970s it has provided an alternative to the traditional sheltered workshop service delivery model. Supported employment has been successfully implemented with individuals who have previously not had occupational choices or personal autonomy, including those who previously were considered unemployable in the competitive labor market. Paul Wehman at Virginia Commonwealth University has researched and published extensively in the field of supported employment. He has identified employment alternatives for individuals with severe disabilities such as the individual placement model, enclaves in industry, and mobile work crews. The foundations of

supported employment are paid employment, integration into the community, ongoing support, and the presence of severe disabilities. The ongoing support services closely associated with supported employment can include job coaches, natural supports, job sharing, alternating work schedules, and a variety of accommodations.

Supported employment is defined as competitive work performed in an integrated work setting by individuals with severe disabilities who have not previously been employed in the competitive market or whose competitive employment has been interrupted or intermittent. Supported employment has three distinguishing characteristics: (1) services are targeted for individuals who traditionally have not succeeded in competitive employment, (2) services are provided in integrated community settings, and (3) services include the provision of long-term support from a variety of agencies and sources (U.S. Department of Education, Office of Special Education and Rehabilitation Services, 1987).

Assessment

One of the cornerstones in transition planning is the identification of needs and the assessment process. The assessment of students with disabilities begins early and continues throughout the student's school experience. Usually by the time a student reaches junior high school or middle school, assessment will become more systematized and focused on transition to adult roles. The results of the assessment should be evident in the student's IEP. Even in the primary years the IEP should contain career awareness goals and objectives. As the student gets older, the IEP goals and objectives become more future-oriented. Typically, teachers and counselors conduct assessment. They administer assessment instruments, review portfolio records, interview students and parents, and collect as much data as possible to assist them in the transition planning efforts. Sarkees and Scott (1985) provided a list of areas that assessment should cover, including basic skills, communication skills, following directions, physical coordination, self-confidence, personal grooming, ability to work with others, work habits, and learning styles. Together, this collection of data is referred to as a vocational profile or a vocational assessment. Vocational assessment generally refers to activities that yield useful information about the employability skills and vocational needs of students with disabilities. Vocational evaluation refers to the collection of data by a team of professionals for the express purpose of making a professional judgment about program placement and instructional needs after the vocational assessment data have been collected. Pam Leconte (personal communication, 1993) identifies the following types of vocational assessment for persons with disabilities: (1) ability- and interest-matching, (2) community-based assessment, (3) behavioral observations, and (4) curriculum-based vocational assessment. Research has reported that assessment data are most frequently used to make decisions regarding service eligibility, to assist in program planning, to enhance communication among professionals, and to enhance communication between parents and professionals. Vocational assessment is used in supported employment as well as in competitive employment.

Job Placement

Job placement is a critical factor in the transition process. Gary Clark and Oliver Kolstoe (1990) identified three factors that affect the employment base in any community: (1) population trends, (2) social trends, and (3) occupational trends. In most school districts there is a job development specialist who is generally asked to assist educators in locating appropriate job sites for individuals with disabilities. The specialist visits employers and identifies vacancies and new positions that will generate a pool of alternatives for placing individuals on the job. In addition to contacting employers in the community, the job specialist also conducts community surveys to gather occupational data to assist in the effort. If it is needed, he or she also conducts a job analysis, which is a systematic way of determining the exact skills and demands that a job may require. The job analysis information is then given to vocational instructors, job coaches, and others who are able to provide the necessary training. Educators need to be familiar with community resources and job placement services so they can access transition support for their students successfully.

Student Follow-up and Program Evaluation

Student follow-up is an important part of any school district's transition program. It is important to determine how successful the school district is in preparing students for their transition into the world of work. Educators must track their students after high school to determine if they are working, if their education prepared them for what they are experiencing, and what the school district could have done differently to prepare them better for independence. The information collected by the school district is then used by the administration and teaching staff to revise curriculum, improve support services, and develop new services to aid students in the transition process. "Follow-up" should not be confused with "follow-along." "Follow-along" is a term used to describe the process used to track students who have left the education system but who still need support services for transition.

Program evaluation is also necessary for any district trying to determine the quality and effectiveness of the transition program. Lynda West (1987) identified the following issues for examination in transition program evaluations: administration of the program; adequacy of staffing to meet program design; coordination among vocational education, special education, vocational rehabilitation, and adult services providers; identification of the program's target population; curriculum content; appropriate course offerings; resource and support services available; comprehensiveness of support services; and assurances that legislative mandates are met. Data for program evaluation can be collected through internal staff reviews and by external consultants. The results are then used to improve current services, design new services, and improve overall program quality. Program evaluation determines whether the components of the transition program, either together or separately, have been effective.

The outcomes of the transition process depend on programs, services, individuals, and the community. Clark and Kolstoe (1990) make the following distinction between programs and services. Transition programs require all the formal elements that characterize a formal operation (funding, personnel, policies, procedures, etc.) and therefore demand a certain level of energy and commitment to be planned and implemented. Services, on the other hand, focus on the delivery of a needed response to problems and can occur inside or outside the formal structure of a program. Parents, advocates, school officials, and adult service providers must cooperate and coordinate in both formal and informal transition efforts.

Transition from school to work is the focus of educators, parents, advocates, and makers of public policy. The ultimate goal of transition is not a matter of debate, but opinions differ widely on the best way to achieve it successfully. School districts, employers, and adult service providers are searching for strategies that meet not only the letter but also the spirit of the law.

(See also: ADOLESCENTS; ASSESSMENT IN REHABILITATION; CAREER COUNSELING; EVALUATION OF REHABILITATION PROGRAMS; INDEPENDENT LIVING; JOB PLACEMENT; SPECIAL EDUCATION; SUPPORTED EMPLOYMENT; VOCATIONAL EVALUATION; WORK)

BIBLIOGRAPHY

BROLIN, DONN. Life Centered Career Education: A Competency Based Approach. Reston, VA, 1993.

CLARK, GARY M., and KOLSTOE, OLIVER P. Career Development and Transition Education for Adolescents with Disabilities. Needham Heights, MA, 1990.

SARKEES, MICHELLE D., and SCOTT, JOHN L. Vocational Special Needs. Alsip, IL, 1985.

U.S. DEPARTMENT OF EDUCATION, OFFICE OF SPECIAL EDUCATION AND REHABILITATION SERVICES. Federal Register Rules and Regulations. Washington, DC, 1987.

WEST, LYNDA L.; "Designing Vocational Programs for Special Needs Individuals." In Handbook of Vocational Special Needs Education, ed. Gary D. Meers. Rockville, MD, 1987.

WEST, LYNDA L.; CORBEY, STEPHANIE; BOYER-STEPHENS, ARDEN; JONES, BONNIE; MILLER, ROBERT J.; and SARKEES-WIRCENSKI, MICKEY. Integrating Transition Planning into the IEP Process. Reston, VA, 1992.

WEHMAN, PAUL. Life Beyond the Classroom: Transition Strategies for Young People with Disabilities. Baltimore, 1992.

WILL, MADELINE. Bridges from School to Working Life: Programs for Handicapped. Washington, DC, 1984.

LYNDA L. WEST

TRANSPORTATION ACCESSIBILITY

Access to transportation is critical to promoting independence and meaningful community integration for persons with disabilities. Without access to transportation, persons with disabilities are not able to participate fully in community life or take advantage of education and employment opportunities. The transportation barriers are not insurmountable. However, persons with disabilities are unlikely to be able to participate fully in society until they have greater access to such services.

A national survey conducted by the Department of Transportation (DOT) in 1978 estimated that there were 7.4 million persons with transportation handicaps (i.e., persons whose disability restricts their ability to use public transit) in the urban United States; this represents 5 percent of the urban population. Today there are an estimated 49 million persons in the nation with varying disabling conditions, not all of which prevent public transit use. In a 1986 Louis Harris poll, Bringing Disabled Americans into the Mainstream, a majority of people with disabilities indicated that their disabilities prevent them from getting around, socializing, or going to cultural events as much as they would like. A 1988 report by the National Council on the Handicapped, On the Threshold of Independence, stated that 49 percent of respondents believe that their mobility is limited because they "are not able to use public transportation or because [they] can't get special transportation or someone to give [them] a ride when [they] need one." The Harris poll also found that 24 million people with disabilities (51%) are unemployed. Approximately three of ten people said that the lack of accessible or affordable transportation is an important reason why they are not working.

Since the early 1970s, public policies have promoted mainstreaming in education, employment opportunities in integrated settings, deinstitutionalization in housing and health care, and expanded access to a range of social and recreational activities for persons with disabilities. The success of these policies has meant that growing numbers of people with disabilities, including those with severe and/or multiple impairments, are seeking to live and work within the community. Demographic changes in the American population and ongoing activities in society promise to emphasize further the need for accessible transportation. Also, persons with disabilities depend on transportation at a higher rate than people without disabilities, since the former tend to have higher unemployment rates and often are unable to drive. For many people, the lack of appropriate accessible transportation represents one of the last obstacles to their meaningful integration and independence.

Public Transportation

Legislative, regulatory, judicial, and community conflicts have characterized public transportation for persons with disabilities since the early 1970s. Federal transit policies have vacillated from requiring a bare amount of special efforts to full access. The result of these conflicting policies is that transit agencies have been confused about what they are required to provide, and people with disabilities have been frustrated at the level of transit services they have received.

As early as 1968, with the Architectural Barriers Act, Congress affirmed the right of access to federally assisted buildings and facilities, including train and subway stations. However, prior to the Urban Mass Transit Act of 1970, there was no federal pronouncement on how transportation vehicle service should be provided to people with disabilities. This law stated for the first time that it is the "national policy that elderly and handicapped persons have the same right as other persons to utilize mass transportation facilities and services . . . and that special efforts shall be made in the planning and design of such facilities and services."

The Federal Aid to Highways Act of 1973 required projects receiving federal funds to be planned, designed, constructed, and operated to allow effective utilization by older persons and people with disabilities. Many of the curb cuts and accessible roadside rest stops can be traced to this law. Also in

1973, Congress passed the Rehabilitation Act. Section 504 of this law requires that "no otherwise qualified handicapped individual shall . . . be excluded from participation in, be denied the benefits of, or be subjected to discrimination in any program or activity that receives federal financial assistance." Section 504 is viewed as the core of civil rights for persons with disabilities. After the passage of this important legislation, DOT began a long process of regulatory activity to interpret the requirements of these federal laws. The greatest source of conflict has been DOT's regulations.

The benchmark for all activity began with the regulations issued in 1976, which left provision of transit service for people with disabilities to local initiatives. These special-effort regulations required that good-faith efforts be made to provide transportation to individuals with disabilities that is reasonable in comparison to persons without disabilities and that, in a reasonable time period, meets a significant fraction of the needs of persons with disabilities. Nevertheless, most public transit providers continued to regard persons with disabilities as social service clients rather than as members of the general public. Many public transit providers assumed that the transportation needs of such persons were the exclusive duty of charitable and human service agencies. In fact, most public transit special-efforts programs relied heavily on identifying transportation services provided by social service groups as meeting the requirements of special-efforts planning. Even years after the adoption of later, more explicit regulations, many public transit agencies did not acknowledge that they had any affirmative duty to provide accessible or paratransit service.

In 1979, after a change in administration, DOT replaced the special-efforts regulations with more rigorous rules that required all new transit vehicles and train stations to be accessible; required a retrofitting of existing vehicles and stations so that within ten years 50 percent of a bus fleet must be accessible; and required "key" rail stations to be accessible in three to thirty years, depending on the type of station. These full-access regulations were met with strenuous objection from the public transit community.

From this stage, the conflict moved to the courts. The 1979 regulations were challenged by the American Public Transit Association (APTA). Two years after DOT's final regulation, the U.S. Court of Appeals for the District of Columbia ruled that there was insufficient legislative justification for the regulation. As a result of APTA v. *Lewis,* which struck down these regulations, in 1981 DOT issued interim local option regulations that reverted to the earlier concept of permitting local transit agencies again to decide how to serve people with disabilities. This could be done through accessible fixed-route service, paratransit service using lift-equipped vans, or some combination of these approaches.

A 1982 U.S. General Accounting Office report stated that despite the regulatory requirements, significant mobility barriers remained and little tangible had been done to meet the real transportation needs of persons with disabilities. Only thirty of the eighty-three bus systems that were studied intended to reach full accessibility. The report also concluded that paratransit services were not providing sufficient access. In response, Congress passed the Surface Transportation Assistance Act of 1983, which required that DOT promulgate new regulations establishing minimum criteria for accessible transportation services by recipients of federal funds.

In 1986 DOT issued final comparable-service regulations, implementing Section 504 and the Surface Transportation Assistance Act. These regulations offered transit agencies three choices: purchase only buses with lifts; provide paratransit that meets certain service criteria, subject to a cost cap; or provide a combination of both forms of service. The cost cap permitted transit agencies to disregard the service criteria if 3 percent of operating funds were spent on paratransit services. Given the chain of events focused in Washington since 1970 in the legislative, regulatory, and judicial spheres, it is no wonder that considerable discord has plagued communities across the country. Many transit agencies believed they were adequately meeting needs with combinations of paratransit and fixed-route service, while others provided the bare minimum of paratransit service.

People with disabilities argued strongly that paratransit by itself can never meet their diverse transit needs. They found support for their arguments from transit agencies that recognized that providing paratransit was very expensive. All communities that relied solely on paratransit services reported that

they could not meet the demand for these services. Because of this they placed severe limitations on paratransit services: having to call days in advance for a ride; having a limited number of rides per month; serving small geographic boundaries; and limiting hours of service. Many paratransit systems had waiting lists in the hundreds—people who received no transit at all. Cumbersome registration procedures meant that visitors with disabilities generally did not get a ride. These limitations made paratransit a poor system for regular commutes to work and school and did little to affect the unemployment rate among people with disabilities.

The legacy of this history has been the building of an adversarial relationship in many places across the country between local transit authorities and people with disabilities and their advocates. Those who preferred paratransit service were strongly disinclined to use lifts on buses. And people with disabilities who preferred fixed-route service did not want to be limited by paratransit service.

In the mid-1980s the scene began to change. First, federal financial support for public transit began to shrink. Public transit operators were faced with the reality that paratransit services were enormously expensive if more than minimal needs were to be satisfied and if the primarily operational cost must be met year after year. On the other hand, fixed-route accessible service involved largely one-time capital costs. Moreover, despite difficulties with early lift models, several transit agencies had proven that lift-equipped bus service could be provided reliably with newer technology. Articles began to appear in transportation trade publications about entities that had begun the switch with much success. It was reported that not only was fixed-route service working but also the paratransit service, now acting as a supplement instead of a substitute, was operating with more efficiency and serving more persons with severe disabilities.

Second, the disability rights movement had taken on a much more assertive role. Americans Disabled for Accessible Public Transportation (ADAPT) was regularly demonstrating and engaging in civil disobedience at APTA meetings. Local chapters of ADAPT and other organizations also targeted individual transit agencies, often blocking buses.

National attention helped revitalize the disability

rights movement and played a significant role in later regulations and laws, including, in 1990, the Americans with Disabilities Act (ADA). ADAPT also challenged the 3 percent cost cap in the 1986 DOT regulation. In *ADAPT v. Burnley*, the U.S. Court of Appeals for the Third Circuit ruled that the cost cap was arbitrary and that transit systems must purchase accessible buses.

In 1990 the ADA settled the policy debate about how to provide transportation to people with disabilities. The result is a shift in emphasis from having a local option of how to provide transportation services to giving people with disabilities in local communities a choice of which accessible transportation service they wish to use. This shift in emphasis is the cornerstone of the ADA.

The effects of each of these policy changes on the purchases of fixed-route buses can be seen in the following table:

Policy Era	Non-accessible	Accessible	Per-centage
No policy	3,218	146	4.36
Special efforts	2,249	311	12.15
Full access	3,368	5,380	61.50
Local option	9,043	6,898	43.27
Comparability	4,863	8,203	62.78
ADA	8	4,964	99.84
Total	22,749	25,902	53.24

SOURCE: Adapted from the American Public Transit Association (APTA) fleet survey (1993)

According to the 1993 American Public Transit Association fleet survey, there were a total of 48,651 fixed-route buses, of which 25,902 were lift-equipped. This represents 53 percent accessible buses (Figure 1).

The law now provides a clear federal mandate that all new vehicles used in fixed-route transportation be accessible to people with disabilities. In addition, for those individuals who cannot use the fixed-route accessible services, complementary paratransit must be provided with respect to the fixed-route system so it is comparable to the level of services provided to people without disabilities.

People eligible for paratransit services include: (1) any individual who is unable, as a result of a physical or mental disability, to use an accessible vehicle; (2) any individual who needs the assistance of a wheelchair lift to ride but no accessible vehicles are available on the route the person wants to travel; and (3) any individual with a disability who has an impairment-related condition that prevents him or her from traveling to or from a transit stop.

Public entities operating demand-response systems open to everyone in a given area and that plan to purchase or lease new vehicles must also purchase accessible vehicles unless it can be shown that the existing system provides a level of service to individuals with disabilities equivalent to that provided to people without disabilities. New and altered transit facilities must also be accessible.

One area of particular controversy in the ADA was access to over-the-road buses (i.e., buses with high floors and baggage compartments below). The ADA directed the Office of Technology Assessment (OTA) to study accessibility issues concerning access to over-the-road buses and services operated by the private sector (e.g., tour buses). This study was submitted to the president and Congress in May 1993. The OTA study examined the access needs of individuals with disabilities to over-the-road buses and service and the most cost-effective methods of providing access.

By July 26, 1994, DOT, in conjunction with the Architectural and Transportation Barriers Compliance Board, had to issue regulations to inform private transportation operators using over-the-road buses of their compliance obligations under the ADA. The final regulations are to take effect for large operators in July 1996 and for small operators in July 1997.

The OTA report identified about 340 over-the-road buses equipped with vehicle-based lifts operated by or under contract to public transportation systems. In most cases government funds were used to purchase the accessibility technologies. As of October 1992 only one operator had purchased an accessible over-the-road bus without government funding. OTA estimated that if over-the-road buses were accessible, "roughly 910,000 trips might be taken annually by persons with sensory or mobility impairments."

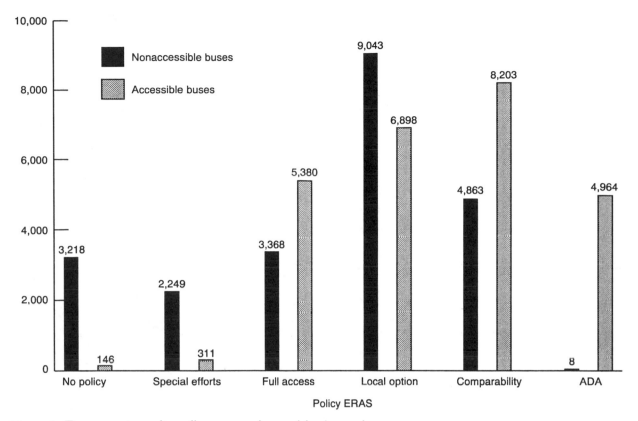

Figure 1. Transportation policy effects on purchases of fixed-route buses

SOURCE: American Public Transit Association (APTA) fleet survey (1993)

The report recommended that over-the-road buses should provide boarding assistance devices such as lifts and ramps that allow persons to remain in their wheelchairs; at least two accessible securement locations for wheelchairs; aisle seats with movable armrests; and information systems that make provisions for persons who cannot see, hear, or comprehend certain information.

Air Transportation

Problems associated with air travel for people with disabilities predate World War II. The Civil Aeronautics Board adopted a rule in 1937 limiting air travel for "ill, deformed, or disabled" people. Since then, air travel for people with disabilities has been an adventure. Different airlines had varying policies that impeded travel in one way or another. For instance, airline policies differed as to when a passenger must arrive to be assured service. Other restrictions existed as well. Some airlines required

people with disabilities to sit on blankets. Others required a medical certificate before allowing a person with a disability to board the aircraft. The lack of airline policy uniformity was also apparent within a single airline. Treatment of passengers with disabilities differed from one airline to the next and often depended on whether airline personnel were familiar with the policies that existed.

Prior to 1986, two federal laws were available to protect individuals with disabilities from discrimination when they traveled by air: Section 504 of the Rehabilitation Act of 1973, and the Federal Aviation Act of 1958. Section 504 specifically prohibits discrimination on the basis of disability in federally assisted programs. If an airline received federal funds to help pay for an airplane, for example, then it could not discriminate against people with disabilities. The Federal Aviation Act addressed discrimination in a general way, only requiring that "safe and adequate" service be provided.

The Civil Aeronautics Board wrote regulations in

1982 to enforce both Section 504 and the Federal Aviation Act. However, these regulations prohibited discrimination against people with disabilities only if an airline received federal funds. These regulations were challenged by the Paralyzed Veterans of America (PVA) in the U.S. Court of Appeals for the District of Columbia, and ultimately before the U.S. Supreme Court. PVA argued that even though airlines did not receive direct federal funds, they benefited in other ways from federal assistance by operating air traffic controls systems and maintaining runways. The Supreme Court did not agree. And since most commercial and commuter airlines do not receive direct funds from the federal government, they did not have to comply with these regulations. In ninety-three days Congress swiftly passed the Air Carrier Access Act (ACAA) to overturn the Supreme Court decision and declared that airlines should treat passengers with disabilities the same as other passengers regardless of whether federal funds were involved.

The legislation called for regulations by April 1987. Final regulations were not issued until March 6, 1990. These regulations require access to aircraft, prohibit discriminatory policies and practices, and mandate training for airline personnel and a new compliance program.

The requirements for aircraft access depend on the size of the airplane and whether it is new or existing. New aircraft must include movable aisle armrests; stowage space for a folding wheelchair; one accessible lavatory; and an on-board wheelchair. Existing aircraft require access only if there is a replacement scheduled for the cabin interior, seats, or lavatory. Airports owned, leased, or operated by one or more airlines must meet accessibility requirements within three years.

The regulations also address issues such as refusal of transportation; advance notice requirements; attendants; seat assignments; provision of services and equipment; stowage and treatment of personal equipment; accommodations for persons with hearing impairments; security screening; communicable diseases; medical certificates; and charges for accommodations.

Since the regulations were issued in March 1990, more than 590 complaints have been filed. The following chart provides information in nine categories

about complaints that were filed against various airlines (Figure 2).

Parking

In 1988 Congress passed a law establishing a uniform system of parking for persons with disabilities and encouraged the states to adopt it. The law required the DOT to write regulations that adopt the International Symbol of Accessibility as the only recognized symbol for the identification of vehicles used for transporting individuals with disabilities; provide for the issuance of license plates or windshield placards displaying the international symbol; prohibit fees charged for the licensing or registration of vehicles used to transport individuals with disabilities from exceeding fees charged for other similar vehicles; and recognize license plates and placards displaying the international symbol that have been issued by other states or countries. The 1992 Transportation Appropriations Act required a two-year study of progress by the states in adopting and implementing the uniform system for parking for persons with disabilities.

Conclusion

Excluding the millions of people with disabilities who want to work from the employment ranks costs society billions of dollars annually in support payments and lost income-tax revenues. Spending in 1990 on disability benefits and programs exceeded $60 billion. When people with disabilities are able to depend on an accessible transportation system and use it to join the workforce, society as a whole benefits. Public benefit rolls can be reduced and income-tax revenues enhanced.

In the end, all barriers to the participation of persons with disabilities in society are attitudinal. If there were no attitudinal barriers, most physical barriers would not exist. Others would simply be viewed as interesting engineering problems, and the search for a solution would be launched immediately. The ADA declared access to transportation vehicles and facilities a civil right, but attitudes change slowly. This landmark legislation has more national public awareness than any similar act and has raised expectations in the community of persons with disabili-

	American	America West	Continental	Delta	Northwest	Southwest	TWA	United	USAir	Other	Total
Refusal to board	13	4	5	5	6	3	2	6	3	13	**60**
Required attendant	1	—	1	—	—	1	—	4	2	2	**11**
Nonaccessible aircraft	2	—	1	2	4	—	1	—	2	4	**16**
Seat assignment restriction	4	4	6	7	—	—	4	8	7	10	**50**
Failure to provide assistance	39	6	23	14	23	2	13	37	24	27	**208**
Assistive device problem	26	2	10	12	14	2	11	12	9	18	**116**
Service animal problem	1	—	—	1	—	—	—	—	—	1	**3**
Unsatisfactory information	2	—	1	—	1	—	—	2	2	1	**9**
Other	17	4	9	6	8	2	10	19	11	32	**118**
Total	**105**	**20**	**56**	**47**	**56**	**10**	**41**	**88**	**60**	**108**	**591**

Figure 2. Complaints filed against various airlines

SOURCE: David Capozzi and Dennis Cannon

ties. Nevertheless, its impact on society will not be fully felt for many years.

(*See also:* ACCESSIBILITY; ADVOCACY; AMERICANS WITH DISABILITIES ACT; ARCHITECTURAL ACCESSIBILITY; CIVIL RIGHTS; HOUSING; QUALITY OF LIFE; WHEELCHAIRS; WORK)

BIBLIOGRAPHY

Air Carrier Access Act, 49 U.S.C. 1374(c) (1986).

American Public Transit Association v. *Lewis*, 556 F.2d 1271 (DC Cir. 1981).

AMERICAN PUBLIC TRANSIT ASSOCIATION. *Transit Passenger Vehicle Fleet Inventory* (1993).

Americans with Disabilities Act, P.L. 101-336, 42 U.S.C. 12101 et seq. (1990).

Americans Disabled for Accessible Public Transportation v. *Skinner*, 881 F.2d 1184 (3rd Cir. 1989).

Architectural Barriers Act, P.L. 90-489, 42 U.S.C. 4151 et seq. (1968).

Federal Aid Highway Act, 23 U.S.C. 142 et seq. (1973).

Federal Aviation Act, 49 U.S.C. 1374 et seq. (1958).

GREY ADVERTISING, INC. *Technical Report of the National Survey of Transportation Handicapped People*, Washington, DC, 1978.

HARRIS, LOUIS, and ASSOCIATES. *Bringing Disabled Americans into the Mainstream.* 1986.

NATIONAL COUNCIL ON THE HANDICAPPED. *On the Threshold of Independence.* 1988.

Paralyzed Veterans of America v. *U.S. Civil Aeronautics Board*, 752 F.2d 694 (DC Cir. 1982).

Surface Transportation Assistance Act, 49 U.S.C. 1612(d) (1982).

Uniform System of Handicapped Parking, 102 Stat. 3335.

Rehabilitation Act, P.L. 93-112, 29 U.S.C 790 et seq. (1973).

Urban Mass Transportation Act, Sec. 16, 49 U.S.C. 1601 et seq. (1970).

U.S. CIVIL AERONAUTICS BOARD. *Nondiscrimination on the Basis of Handicap*, 14 CFR Part 382 (1982).

U.S. DEPARTMENT OF TRANSPORTATION. *Nondiscrimination on the Basis of Handicap in Air Travel*, 14 CFR Part 382 (1990).

———. *Nondiscrimination on the Basis of Handicap in Federally Assisted Programs and Activities Receiving or*

Benefiting from Federal Financial Assistance, 49 CFR Part 27 (1979).

———. *Nondiscrimination on the Basis of Handicap; Interim Final Rule and Request for Comments,* 49 CFR Part 27 (1981).

U.S. Department of Transportation v. Paralyzed Veterans of America, 477 U.S. 597 (1986).

U.S. GENERAL ACCOUNTING OFFICE. *Status of Special Efforts to Meet Transportation Needs of the Elderly and Handicapped.* Washington, DC, 1982.

U.S. OFFICE OF TECHNOLOGY ASSESSMENT. *Access to Over-the-Road Buses for Persons with Disabilities.* Washington, DC, 1993.

U.S. URBAN MASS TRANSPORTATION ADMINISTRATION. *Transportation for Elderly and Handicapped Persons,* 49 CFR Part 609; 49 CFR §613.204 and the appendix to that section (1976).

DAVID M. CAPOZZI
DENNIS M. CANNON

TRAUMATIC BRAIN INJURY

See HEAD INJURY

UNIONS

See LABOR UNIONS

UNIVERSAL DESIGN

See ARCHITECTURAL ACCESSIBILITY; HOUSING

V

VETERANS' MEDICAL REHABILITATION IN THE U.S. DEPARTMENT OF VETERANS AFFAIRS

The rehabilitation programs in Veterans Health Administration (VHA) had their beginnings in the immediate post-World War II era. In 1946, the then Veterans Administration (VA) initiated an improved, formal program designed to return those wounded service members with physical disabilities to an active and productive life. Physicians who were experienced in dealing with these problems, along with the allied health specialists of the day—"physiotherapists" (PT), occupational therapists (OT), and corrective therapists (CT)—were recruited, frequently coming directly from the military as well as from the civilian population. Donald A. Covalt, M.D., was appointed assistant medical director for rehabilitation to direct the program nationally.

The new medical specialty of physical medicine and rehabilitation (PM&R) was in a fledgling state in those days, and qualified physiatrists were few and far between. Therapy personnel were an expanding entity, yet their educational qualifications were of relatively poor quality. In fact, few physiotherapists employed prior to World War II had attained a bachelor's degree level of education.

Prosthetic devices were primitive at best. Many such devices were fabricated by the disabled veterans themselves, who, knowing their own weaknesses and strengths, could design the proper assistive device to meet their specific needs.

A rapid growth of interest in this area of medicine followed this period, not only in the VA but in the private sector as well. The VA assumed national, even international, leadership in the field of prosthetics research and became an important educator of rehabilitation professionals. By the early 1960s, federal grant dollars for rehabilitation research and training centers were flowing; the VA's rehabilitation programs were flourishing; and all was well within the world of rehabilitation.

Medical rehabilitation in the VA pioneered the concept of an interdisciplinary treatment team approach to regaining functional independence. In addition to PT, OT, and CT, the disciplines of manual arts therapy (MAT), educational therapy (ET), and recreation therapy (RT) rounded out the ability of the PM&R service to provide a comprehensive rehabilitation program for veterans with disabilities.

Medical rehabilitation has continually been thrust into those more challenging programs for veterans—spinal cord injury, traumatic brain injury, stroke, amputations, and other neurological conditions—that have placed the PM&R staff and their outreach efforts into the mainstream of inpatient and outpatient areas of care.

The rehabilitation disciplines played an important role in the treatment programs related to mental health as well. Medical rehabilitation personnel participated actively in the function of psychiatric treatment teams, providing the physical, occupational, psychosocial, and life skills components of mental health treatment programs. This was true not only for general psychiatry but also for special programs in substance abuse, stress disorders, and homelessness, as well as for people with long-term schizophrenia.

As the importance of rehabilitation became more and more obvious during the late 1970s and 1980s, the VHA experienced marked shortages of rehabilitation therapists, as did the private sector. Some blamed university programs for limiting access to the therapy's curricula; others believed that salary levels were too low to make therapy a lucrative profession. A number of recruitment and retention incentive programs were implemented, among which was the health professional's scholarship program. As a result, the VHA became even more important nationally as a sponsor of rehabilitation education. The previously established postgraduate education programs for physicians in the specialty of PM&R were also continued, with the VHA consistently supporting 15 percent to 20 percent of all the PM&R residency positions in the country.

Research and development in rehabilitation have been priorities in the VHA for many years. VHA accomplishments in, for example, computer-assisted design and manufacture of prosthetic limbs, development of robotics for patients with paralysis, low-vision-enhancement systems, and cochlear implants have put VHA rehabilitation research and development on the cutting edge of new technology in this field worldwide.

As medical care in general has become more and more expensive, the need for maximum efficiency has become obvious. A standardized outcome evaluation system—the UDSMR (Uniform Data System for Medical Rehabilitation)—has been implemented throughout VHA rehabilitation services, giving local and national program officials information needed to compare their performances with their peers both within and outside the VA system. Now that outcomes of care can be quantified, a research effort is being initiated to identify those conditions necessary to produce optimal outcomes as effectively and efficiently as possible. Such factors as intensity, frequency, timing of interventions, staffing mix, therapy procedures, and sites of care will be studied.

As would seem obvious, the future of rehabilitation in the VA should be exciting. If past progress is any indicator, the future should be challenging, productive, and rewarding.

(*See also:* ASSISTIVE TECHNOLOGY; HOSPITAL, REHABILITATION; PHYSICIAN; PROSTHETICS AND ORTHOTICS; PSYCHIATRIC REHABILITATION; TECHNOLOGY AND DISABILITY; VETERAN VOCATIONAL REHABILITATION IN THE U.S. DEPARTMENT OF VETERANS AFFAIRS)

RESOURCES

American Veterans of World War II, Korea, and Vietnam (AMVETS), 4647 Forbes Blvd., Lanham, MD 20706.

Blinded Veterans Association (BVA), 477 H St., NW, Washington, DC 20006

Department of Veterans Affairs, 810 Vermont Ave., NW, Washington, DC 20420

Disabled American Veterans (DAV), P.O. Box 14301, Cincinnati, OH 45250–0301

Paralyzed Veterans of America (PVA), 801 Eighteenth St., NW, Washington, DC 20006

JAMES L. GREEN

VETERAN VOCATIONAL REHABILITATION IN THE U.S. DEPARTMENT OF VETERANS AFFAIRS

The vocational rehabilitation of America's veterans with service-connected disabilities began during World War I in 1917 (James, 1987). During and following that war, vocational rehabilitation of veterans with service-connected disabilities consisted of medical services provided by the military branches and the U.S. Public Health Service, and vocational training provided by the military branches and, upon discharge, in government-run as well as civilian vocational schools. After a year's experience, military schools and other government schools were closed, and vocational rehabilitation assumed the model it would follow off and on until 1981. Vocational rehabilitation was defined as training for suitable employment, and employment services were coordinated with the U.S. Department of Labor (Obermann, 1965). Since vocational psychology was in its infancy, trained rehabilitation professionals did not exist. It would be stated later, in congressional testimony, that the central weakness of the World War I veterans' vocational rehabilitation program was the lack of professional staff who could conduct vocational evaluations and help veterans determine "suitable" vocational goals. The World War I vocational rehabilitation program was operational from April 6, 1917, to July 2, 1928. During that time about 675,000 veterans applied for vocational rehabilitation: 330,000 were found eligible, 180,000 entered training, and almost 130,000 were declared rehabilitated (Obermann, 1965). Vocational rehabilitation for veterans with service-connected disabilities was administered during this time first by the Veterans Rehabilitation Division of the Federal Board for Vocational Education and later by the newly created Veterans Bureau.

The Veterans Bureau became the Veterans Administration (VA) in 1930, but vocational rehabilitation was not an authorized benefit for the peacetime veteran. Nor were such services available to the war-injured of World War I or to peacetime service-connected disabled veterans after 1928. While the state–federal vocational rehabilitation program was available to these veterans as civilians, the VA would not provide these services again until March 1943.

In March 1943, the vocational rehabilitation program for veterans with service-connected disabilities was reestablished fifteen months after the bombing of Pearl Harbor. By this time, large numbers of veterans with service-connected disabilities were waiting for vocational rehabilitation services in hospitals for veterans and at home. The law provided vocational training for veterans with service-connected disabilities to restore employability lost by reason of service-connected conditions. Essentially, the World War I vocational rehabilitation program was unchanged. However, efforts were made to staff the program with better-qualified rehabilitation personnel, and the VA became a leader in applying the knowledge of vocational psychology to veterans with service-connected disabilities to help them determine and pursue suitable vocational goals. Of major significance to the advances in the vocational rehabilitation program for veterans with service-connected disabilities was the knowledge gained from evaluating civilians for military service during World War II and assigning them to training for suitable military occupations. About 621,000 veterans with service-connected disabilities received vocational rehabilitation training as a result of World War II (James, 1987). The numbers would undoubtedly have been much higher if the educational benefits program, popularly known as the "G.I. Bill," had not been passed. Both programs offered approximately equal benefits, but veterans with service-connected disabilities could elect to use the G.I. Bill and select the schools and courses they wanted without personal evaluations, determinations of need, and individual approval, as was required by the vocational rehabilitation program. Many veterans with service-connected disabilities preferred the independence of attending school under the G.I. Bill.

In December 1950, the vocational rehabilitation benefits that had been available to war-injured veterans of World War II were extended to war-injured veterans of the Korean conflict. The vocational rehabilitation program was unchanged with the notable exception of professional qualification standards for program staffing. In 1952 the VA, working with the U.S. Civil Service Commission, established the position of counseling psychologist and set educational requirements at the masters and doctoral levels for the position. The agency funded the education of its program staff to obtain their degrees and continued the noncounseling psychologist staff as "vocational advisers." The maturing of the field of vocational psychology and improved standards for staffing by the creation of the counseling psychologist position contributed to the effectiveness of the vocational rehabilitation program for veterans with service-connected disabilities. The result, for the first time, was a high degree of quality in vocational rehabilitation and counseling services for veterans with service-connected disabilities. Some 77,000 disabled veterans received vocational rehabilitation training as a result of the Korean conflict (James, 1987).

In October 1962, a vocational rehabilitation law for veterans with service-connected disabilities was passed that extended vocational rehabilitation services to service-connected disabilities of veterans of peacetime service. It was made retroactively available to veterans with service-connected disabilities who served between World War II and the Korean conflict, and after the Korean conflict who were determined to need these services. It was not made available to the peacetime period between World Wars I and II. Approximately 23,600 veterans with service-connected disabilities who served during peacetime prior to the Vietnam era received vocational rehabilitation training. This program for peacetime veterans with service-connected disabilities, while of landmark significance, was severely restrictive. Unfortunately, the vast majority of war-injured Vietnam era veterans were subject to the restrictive criteria of this program, because the law was not further amended until 1975, the year the Vietnam conflict ended (James, 1987).

In 1975 a more generous vocational rehabilitation program was established. However, its benefits were far fewer than the programs of the World War II and Korean conflict periods, perhaps due to the lack of public support for Vietnam veterans. Approximately 150,000 veterans with service-connected disabilities of the Vietnam era received vocational rehabilitation services from August 1964 to May 1975.

The Rehabilitation Act of 1973 provided far-reaching changes in programs serving persons with handicaps in all federally assisted programs. As a result, the vocational rehabilitation program for veterans with service-connected disabilities was studied and major changes were recommended.

In 1981 the law governing the vocational rehabilitation program for veterans with service-connected disabilities was changed. While its purpose had been to provide supervised training for suitable employment and referral for employment assistance, it became a program that provided all services and assistance necessary to enable entitled veterans to achieve maximum independence in daily living and, to the maximum extent feasible, to become employable and to obtain and maintain suitable employment.

The vocational rehabilitation program for veterans with service-connected disabilities can address the full range of rehabilitation needs a disabled veteran may have. The emphasis is on needed services and assistance; therefore, individual programs include all services and assistance identified through the rehabilitation evaluation process needed by a veteran with service-connected disabilities to achieve vocational or independent living rehabilitation. A rehabilitation program may consist of guided employment assistance for those veterans determined suitably trained; and, if training is an indicated need, a program may include training in a vocational school, college, on-the-job, farm, self-employment, or by independent instructor. Program participants who are homeless are also assisted in locating suitable living arrangements. In addition, for those for whom suitable employment is not feasible due to their disability, a program may consist of services and assistance to enable independence in daily living. Veterans are paid a monthly subsistence allowance. The period during which vocational rehabilitation benefits may be provided is generally limited to twelve years from a veteran's release from military active duty, but may be extended for veterans with more serious service-connected disabilities. Approximately 160,000 veterans with service-connected disabilities have received vocational rehabilitation services during the post-Vietnam conflict. More than one million veterans with service-connected disabilities received vocational rehabilitation services from 1917 to 1994 (James, 1987).

The VA became the U.S. Department of Veterans Affairs in 1989. Within the Department of Veterans Affairs medical and surgical rehabilitation services are provided by the Veterans Health Administration, and nonmedical vocational rehabilitation services are administered by the Veterans Benefits Administration, Vocational Rehabilitation and Counseling Service.

Veterans who receive services in the vocational rehabilitation program for veterans with service-connected disabilities at any given time range in age from seventeen to some senior citizens who desire to be vocationally active. They are male and female and have service-connected disabilities such as low back strains, posttraumatic stress disorders, blindness, amputations, and other disabilities common to veterans and nonveterans alike. Some veterans sustained their injuries in combat; others simply in the line of duty. Past participants in the vocational rehabilitation program for veterans with service-connected disabilities now serve in Congress as well as in significant leadership positions in business and industry. But the vast majority of those who have achieved rehabilitation success are the people we all pass on the street every day: friends and neighbors, those ordinary citizens who answered the call to serve their country and who suffered physical or mental loss and have been assisted in overcoming the stigma of dependence and unemployment through a program intended to make them as whole as possible.

(*See also:* DISABILITY LAW AND SOCIAL POLICY; HISTORY OF REHABILITATION; JOB PLACEMENT; LOSS AND GRIEF; PSYCHOSOCIAL ADJUSTMENT; RUSK, HOWARD; WORK)

RESOURCES

American Veterans of World War II, Korea, and Vietnam (AMVETS), 4647 Forbes Blvd., Lanham, MD 20706

Blinded Veterans Association (BVA), 477 H St., NW, Washington, DC 20001

Department of Veterans Affairs, 810 Vermont Ave., NW, Washington, DC 20420

Disabled American Veterans (DAV), P.O. Box 14301, Cincinnati, OH 45250–0301

BIBLIOGRAPHY

JAMES, DAVID T. "Seventy Years of U.S. Veterans' Vocational Rehabilitation (1917–1987): History and Commentary." *Vocational Rehabilitation and Counseling Professional Review.* Washington, DC, 1987.

OBERMANN, C. ESCO. "The Rehabilitation of Veterans." *A History of Vocational Rehabilitation in America.* Minneapolis, 1965.

DAVID THOMAS JAMES

VIOLENCE

Violence is the use of force or power to coerce, harm, or exploit another individual or group. Violence is a major cause of a wide variety of disabilities, and some factors that predispose to violence also increase risk for disability. In addition, people with disabilities appear to be at increased risk to suffer from future violence.

The number of disabilities caused by violence remains unknown, but estimates of various researchers suggest that at least 5 to 10 percent of all disabilities are caused by violence. Traumatic brain injury and spinal cord injuries are among the best known disabling outcomes of violence. For example, about 12 percent of all traumatic brain injuries are known to result from assaults, and that number is likely to be an underestimate, since violence-induced injury is often concealed through attribution to another cause. The majority of disabling head injuries in children are caused by child abuse. Recent research suggests that many children are disabled as a result of shaking as infants, and others sustain permanent damage as a result of smothering by caregivers. Violence toward women who are pregnant may result in direct damage to their infants or to complications of pregnancy that increase the risk for subsequent disability in their offspring (McFarlane, 1989). Children exposed to chronic physical or sexual abuse may experience long-term emotional or developmental disabilities even when no physical damage is apparent.

Violence is also linked to disabilities in more complex ways. For example, chronic use of alcohol or other disinhibiting drugs within families increases the risk for violence, and victims of violence are more likely to have drug and alcohol addictions. Alcohol and many other psychoactive drugs also increase the risk for birth defects, accidents, and other events that may cause disability. Other factors, such as family dysfunction, that increase risk for violence may also contribute to the risk for various disabilities.

Severe neglect, often associated with violence, is probably responsible for another 5 to 10 percent of disabilities. In many more cases medical, educational, emotional, and rehabilitative neglect compounds the effects of disabilities with other etiologies.

Increased Vulnerability to Violence. People with disabilities resulting from any cause also appear to experience increased risk for child abuse, assault, spousal abuse, sexual assault, and other forms of violence in contemporary society (Senn, 1988). Increased risk appears to result from a number of factors that affect many people with disabilities, including: (1) impairment of abilities that are critical for self-defense or avoidance of violence; (2) social isolation that sometimes accompanies disability; (3) increased dependency on others for care; (4) negative attitudes toward people with disabilities that disinhibit violence against them; (5) institutional care; and (6) discriminatory practices in violence prevention and law enforcement (Sobsey & Mansell, 1990). Since these and many other factors that influence risk for violence affect each individual differently, no clear or simple pattern exists differentially linking specific types of disability or relative severity of disability to risk for violence or other forms of abuse.

People with disabilities appear to have a somewhat higher risk for child abuse, spousal abuse, and other forms of violence within the family than people without disabilities, but much more of the excess risk of violence experienced by people with disabilities comes from the service system on which many of them depend.

Cultural Violence. While deeds of violence are generally viewed as individual acts that contravene the rules of society, society may be more tolerant of violence toward some of its members than others. In some cases it may even condone violence toward certain minority groups. For example, a cross-cultural study of thirty-five societies (Daly & Wilson, 1988) found diverse reasons for infanticide in various cultures, including that an infant was one of twins, born out of wedlock, female, born to a mother who dies in childbirth, conceived from a nontribal father, or conceived from incest. By far the most frequently acceptable reason for infanticide, however—reported in twenty-one of the thirty-five societies studied—was the presence of obvious disability or deformity. Such children are often considered to be ghosts or demons, and cultural beliefs demand their elimination to protect society. According to social distancing theory, such dehumanizing attitudes and beliefs are crucial factors in disinhibiting violence and rationalizing its occurrence. This theory suggests that our deeply ingrained inhibitions against hurting other people can be overcome if we view the targets of our aggression as less than human and therefore not entitled to the protections accorded to other human beings (Sobsey, 1994).

Abominations and Monstrosities. While such attitudes may seem alien to our own culture, they have been well established and continue in only slightly modified contemporary forms. Terms such as "abominations" and "monstrosities" that have been applied to people with disabilities reveal the historical attitudes that connect deformity or impairment with inhuman evil. According to *The Oxford English Dictionary*, the word "abomination," used to refer to those with visible defects, derived from its conceptual roots of "an evil omen" and "away from human." "Monstrosity," an abnormality of growth, developed from the idea that something unusual was sent as a divine warning. Thus differences were strongly connected with evil and dehumanized images of people with disabilities. Such concepts are apparent in many religious teachings, such as Martin Luther's belief that "idiots are men in whom devils have established themselves" (Judge, 1987) and his admonition that drowning was required to eliminate these devils.

With the coming of the twentieth century, science has increasingly challenged religion for the role of preeminent influence on human behavior, yet the influence of science has been more to redefine the myths that legitimate violence against people with disabilities than to eliminate them. Four major scientific myths have been used to legitimate killing of people with disabilities in the twentieth century.

First, the eugenic myth suggests that most disability is inherited and that unless individuals with disabilities can be eliminated or at least denied the right to reproduction, society will be overcome by increasing numbers of people with disabilities. Thus the supernatural spiritual threat of a more religious era of the past has been transformed into a quasi-scientific genetic threat in the twentieth century. In reality, only a small percentage of disabilities are inherited, and many of these are associated with lower rates of reproduction. Genes for most inherited causes of disability also occur much more frequently in carriers who do not have the disability. Thus elimination of people with inherited disorders without eliminating the carriers would take thousands of years to make a significant difference in incidence (Suzuki, Griffiths, and Lewontin, 1989). If carriers also were eliminated, inherited disabilities might be eradicated more quickly, but since the average person carries three or four such genes, such a program would require the elimination of every human being on the planet.

Second, the growing social burden myth suggests that since modern technology has allowed us to save the lives of many people who would have died without the benefit of technology, larger and larger numbers of persons with severe handicaps are placing a growing burden on society. People with disabilities have been cast in the role of social and economic threats to modern society. In reality, while modern medicine and technology have kept many people with disabilities alive who might have died in an earlier era, medicine and technology have been even more successful in reducing the number and severity of disabling conditions. The disabling effects of polio, whooping cough, smallpox, rubella, and many other diseases have been vastly reduced; outcomes of head injury, anoxia, and many other medical emergencies also have improved. As a result, the percentage of people with disabilities is decreasing, not increasing (Orelove & Sobsey, 1991). Furthermore, technological advances along with changing social, economic, and vocational conditions allow people with various types and severities of disability to contribute more to society.

Third, the family burden myth suggests that the dependency of people with disabilities is a source of great hardship on families. This hardship has been suggested as a cause of family dysfunction and a rationale for euthanasia, abuse, and institutionalization. While disability may increase some demands on families, research suggests that this burden may have been vastly exaggerated and that the great majority of families that include members with disabilities experience stress levels within normal limits for any family (Sobsey, 1990).

Fourth, the quality of life myth suggests that people with disabilities live miserable lives with little potential for pleasure. This myth rationalizes abuse, since the maltreatment could add little to such misery or even murder, since killing such an individual could only put an end to suffering. Research regarding how people with disabilities view the quality of their own lives, however, does not support this myth. It suggests that people with disabilities typically rate their own quality of life about the same as people without disabilities rate their lives (Sobsey, 1993).

Such contemporary myths illustrate some of our culture's negative attitudes toward people with disabilities. Much more research is needed to clarify how such attitudes may contribute to violent acts against people with disabilities, but many current experts believe that such attitudes and myths are major contributors to the problem (e.g., Sobsey & Mansell, 1990; Waxman, 1991). On a direct personal level, they allow offenders greater freedom from inhibition and guilt by providing justification for their acts. Less direct but equally negative outcomes may occur as a result of social isolation and poor family attachment resulting from such attitudes. Both social isolation and poorly developed bonds between children and their parents have been identified as major risk factors in child abuse and other forms of violence.

Holocaust. The most extreme manifestation of such beliefs in the twentieth century occurred when the Nazi regime killed about 100,000 European children and adults with physical or mental disabilities. This euthanasia program was designed to rid society of "useless eaters" and improve "racial purity." Originally, only those with severe disabilities were targeted, but individuals with milder disabilities were gradually added. The methods of extermination included starvation, shooting, poisonous gas, and lethal injection. The euthanasia program was run largely by the same health care and educational professionals who provided services to people with disabilities prior to the introduction of the extermination program. Martin Hohl, director of the Wendelhöfen mental institution at Bayreuth, was one of the few who refused to kill his patients (Kater, 1989), but the doctors and nurses who held a party to celebrate the murder of their 10,000th patient at Hadamar Hospital were much more typical.

While such a large-scale program of violence against people with disabilities never existed in North America, many endorsed the objectives of the Nazi program and advocated a similar program in the Allied countries. An official editorial of the *American Journal of Psychiatry*, for example, argued for the killing of children with severe disabilities when they reached the age of about four (*Euthanasia*, 1942). It suggests that the only impediment to the implementation of such a program would be resistance from parents of these children. The bond between parents and such children was identified as a morbid obsession, and the physician's role in inhibiting the development of that attachment was described as good mental hygiene practice. While it is unlikely that many professionals would advocate a policy of mass euthanasia today, many do persist in attacking, rather than supporting, bonds between family members with and without disabilities.

Contemporary attempts at involuntary euthanasia of people with disabilities occur primarily through medical discrimination. For example, one report followed fifty infants with spina bifida (Gross et al., 1983). Although the severity of disability appeared similar, thirty-six received vigorous treatment and twenty-four received only supportive care. By the age of six months, all thirty-six receiving comprehensive medical care still survived, but all twenty-four who were denied comprehensive care had died. Some persons have suggested that the long-term use of psychotropic drugs in apparent disregard to their health consequences with people with psychiatric and mental disabilities is another, subtler form of euthanasia. For example, the rate of people with developmental disabilities who die of airway obstruction has increased twenty-five fold since such drugs have been used widely, and the rate of such deaths in some institutionalized populations is almost 100 times higher than in the general population.

Abuse and Assault. While acts of medical discrimination against people with disabilities are potentially prosecutable offenses that result in frequent and serious harm, they are rarely viewed as crimes by contemporary society or prosecuted as such. Physical and sexual assaults committed against children and adults, however, undeniably represent acts of violence. Unfortunately, no systematic database provides comprehensive statistics on crimes against people with disabilities, and therefore available information remains fragmented. Nevertheless, available data indicate a clear pattern of criminal violence against people with disabilities.

Since the inception of the contemporary study of child abuse in the 1960s, dozens of studies have found that children with physical, mental, or behavioral disabilities are more likely to be abused, and if abused are more likely to experience severe and chronic abuse than other children (Sobsey et al., 1991). While the degree of increased risk varies from study to study depending on the definitions of abuse and disability, and measures of incidence employed by the researchers, the range of results suggests that the percentage of children with disabilities experiencing abuse is two to ten times as high as the percentage of children without disabilities. Further evidence suggests that abused children with disabilities are less likely to receive protective services or abuse recovery treatment than children without disabilities, and perpetrators of abuse against children with disabilities are less likely to be prosecuted than those offending other children.

Women with disabilities are more frequently victims of sexual violence than women without disabilities and also are more likely to be battered (Sobsey et al., 1991). Liz Stimpson and Margaret C. Best (1991), for example, found that more than 70 percent of the women with disabilities they interviewed had been victims of sexual violence. Less information is available about sexual offenses against men with disabilities, but preliminary information suggests that male children, adolescents, and adults represent a larger proportion of victims of sex crimes among disabled victims than would be expected on the basis of the gender ratio reported for able-bodied victims of sex crimes (Sobsey, 1994). Evidence suggests that sexual offenses against people with disabilities are rarely reported.

Offenders. Many of the relationships between violent offenders and victims with disabilities are similar to those between offenders and other victims. They are frequently family members, acquaintances, neighbors, dates, workmates, or schoolmates. About 10 percent are strangers. People with disabilities, however, are much more likely to be victimized by paid caregivers in disability-specific health, education, rehabilitation, or social systems that provide services to them. In addition, people with disabilities in segregated services are often victimized by other people with disabilities who are clustered with them in the same settings. This result is particularly true in psychiatric and developmental disabilities institutions. Preliminary studies suggest that almost half of those committing sexual offenses against people with disabilities come in contact with their victims through the service delivery system (Sobsey & Doe, 1991).

Violence Prevention. People with disabilities should take an active part in violence prevention programs. Personal rights, decision-making, personal safety skills, sex education, and assertiveness should be part of the basic curriculum for every child and young adult with or without disabilities. Careful screening of all caregiving staff is essential to thwart habitual offenders who enter service careers to access victims, and all human service workers must receive training both to minimize the chances that they will become abusive and to ensure that they will respond appropriately if they encounter abuse. In addition to their many other benefits, integration and full participation in the community reduce the risk of violence for people with disabilities (Sobsey, 1994).

(*See also:* ALCOHOL REHABILITATION; CHILDHOOD DISABILITY; CIVIL RIGHTS; CORRECTIONAL REHABILITATION; DRUG REHABILITATION; ETHICS; FAMILY; HEAD INJURY; LOSS AND GRIEF; PEDIATRIC REHABILITATION; QUALITY OF LIFE; RELIGION; SPINAL CORD INJURY)

RESOURCES

Abuse & Disability Project, 6-102 Education North, University of Alberta, Edmonton, Alberta T6G 2G5 Canada

Clearinghouse on Child Abuse and Neglect, P.O. Box 1182, Washington, DC 20013-1182

Disabled Victims of Violence, B-150, 151 Slater St., Ottawa, Ontario K1P 5H3 Canada

National Coalition on Abuse and Disabilities, P.O. Box T, Culver City, CA 90230

National Committee for Prevention of Child Abuse (NCPCA), 332 S. Michigan Ave., Suite 1600, Chicago, IL 60604

BIBLIOGRAPHY

AMMERMAN, ROBERT T., VAN HASLETT, VINCENT B.; HERSEN, MICHAEL; McGONIGLE, JOHN J.; and LUBETSKY, MARTIN J. "Abuse and Neglect in Psychiatrically Hospitalized Multihandicapped Children." *Child Abuse & Neglect* 13 (1989):335–343.

BLACHER, JAN, and MEYERS, C. EDWARD. "A Review of Attachment Formation and Disorder of Handicapped Children." *American Journal of Mental Deficiency* 87 (1983):359–371.

BROWN, HILARY, and CRAFT, ANN. "Thinking the Unthinkable: Papers on Sexual Abuse and People with Learning Difficulties." London, England, 1989.

COLE, SANDRA S. "Facing the Challenges of Sexual Abuse in Persons with Disabilities." *Sexuality and Disability* 7 (1986):71–88.

DALY, MARTIN., and WILSON, MARGO. *Homicide.* New York, 1988.

DOUCETTE, JOANNE. *Violent Acts Against Disabled Women.* Toronto, Canada, 1986.

EGLEY, LANCE C. "Domestic Abuse and Deaf People: One Community's Approach." *Victimology* 7 (1982):24–34.

Euthanasia: The American Journal of Psychiatry 99 (1942):141–143.

GARBARINO, JAMES; BROOKHOUSER, PATRICK E.; and AUTHIER, KAREN J., eds. *Special Children—Special Risks: The Maltreatment of Children with Disabilities.* New York, 1987.

GROSS, RICHARD H.; COX, ALAN; TATYREK, RUTH; POLLAY, MICHAEL; and BARNES, WILLIAM A. "Early Management and Decision Making for Treatment of Myelominingocele." *Pediatrics* 72 (1983):450–458.

HUGHES, HONOR M., and DIBREZZO, RIO. "Physical and Emotional Abuse and Motor Development: A Preliminary Investigation." *Perceptual and Motor Skills* 64 (1987):469–470.

JUDGE, CLIFFORD. *Civilization and Mental Retardation.* Melbourne, Australia, 1987.

KATER, MICHAEL H. *Doctors under Hitler.* Chapel Hill, NC, 1989

McARTHER, SCOTT. "Crime Risk Education Is Essential for the Disabled." *Rehabilitation Digest* 19 (1989):20–21.

McFARLANE, JUDITH. "Battering During Pregnancy: The Tip of an Iceberg Revealed." *Women & Health* 15 (1989):69–84.

MORGAN, SHARON R. *Abuse and Neglect of Handicapped Children.* Boston, 1987.

ORFLOVE, FRED P., and SOBSEY, DICK. *Educating Children with Multiple Disabilities,* 2nd ed. Baltimore, 1991.

RINDFLEISCH, NOLAN, and RABB, JOEL. "How Much of a Problem Is Resident Mistreatment in Child Welfare Institutions?" *Child Abuse and Neglect* 8 (1984):33–40.

RUSCH, RANDALL G.; HALL, JULIA C.; and GRIFFIN, HAROLD C. "Abuse-Provoking Characteristics of Institutionalized Mentally Retarded Individuals." *American Journal of Mental Deficiency* 90 (1986):618–624.

SCHILLING, ROBERT F.; KIRKHAM, MAURA A.; and SCHINKE, STEVEN P. "Do Child Protection Services Neglect Developmentally Disabled Children?" *Ed-*

ucation and Training of the Mentally Retarded 21 (1986):21–26.

SENN, CHARLENE Y. Vulnerable: Sexual Abuse and People with an Intellectual Handicap. Downsview, Canada, 1988.

SOBSEY, DICK. "Disability, Discrimination and the Law." Health Law Review 2 (1993):6–10.

———. "Too Much Stress on Stress? Abuse and the Family Stress Factor." Newsletter of the American Association on Mental Retardation 3 (1990):2, 8.

———. Violence and Abuse in the Lives of People with Disabilities: The End of Silent Acceptance? Baltimore, 1994.

SOBSEY, DICK, and DOE, TANIS. "Patterns of Sexual Abuse and Assault." Journal of Sexuality and Disability 9 (1991):243–259.

SOBSEY, DICK; GRAY, SHARMAINE; WELLS, DON; PYPER, DIANE; and REIMER-HECK, BETH. Disability, Sexuality, and Abuse: An Annotated Bibliography. Baltimore, 1991.

SOBSEY, DICK, and MANSELL, SHEILA. "The Prevention of Sexual Abuse of People with Developmental Disabilities." Developmental Disabilities Bulletin 18 (1990):51–66.

STIMPSON, LIZ, and BEST, MARGARET C. Courage Above All: Sexual Assault Against Women with Disabilities. Toronto, Canada, 1991.

SULLIVAN, PATRICIA M., and SCANLON, JOHN M. "Therapeutic Issues." In Special Children—Special Risks: The Maltreatment of Children with Disabilities, eds. James Garbarino, Patrick E. Brookhouser, and Karen J. Authier. New York, 1987.

SULLIVAN, PATRICIA M.; VERNON, MCCAY; and SCANLON, JOHN M. "Sexual Abuse of Deaf Youth." American Annals of the Deaf 132 (1987):256–262.

SUZUKI, DAVID T.; GRIFFITHS, A.J.F.; and LEWONTIN, R. C. An Introduction to Genetic Analysis, 2nd ed. San Francisco, 1989.

WAXMAN, BARBARA F. "Hatred—The Unacknowledged Dimension in Violence Against Disabled People." Journal of Sexuality and Disability 9 (1991):185–199.

DICK SOBSEY

VOCATIONAL COUNSELING

See CAREER COUNSELING

VOCATIONAL EVALUATION

One of the most critical of all rehabilitation services provided to individuals with physical or mental disabilities is vocational assessment. Evaluations play an important role in enhancing clients' self-understanding and in assisting them with personal career decisions and specific occupational selections. Vocational assessment is a comprehensive, intradisciplinary process in which the physical, mental, and emotional abilities, limitations, and tolerances of a person with disabilities are evaluated in order to identify an optimal vocational course of action for him or her (Power, 1991). It is a method of acquiring information about the individual's vocational strengths and weaknesses in the areas of personality, aptitude, interests, work habits, physical tolerance, and dexterity. Evaluation is a process, consequently, involving mainly diagnosis and prediction that eventually generates a course of action that may range from competitive employment to effective, productive activity within his or her own home.

Vocational assessment information can be obtained both formally and informally. Informal assessment includes observing the client's behavior in a variety of situations, conversing with the client, or getting information about him or her from other sources. Formal assessment comprises such processes as mental testing in the form of work samples and job analyses (Power, 1991). The choice of an approach depends, of course, on the objective of the assessment. This entry will explain briefly the different approaches used within informal and formal assessment and identify the important issues within the field of vocational evaluation that have emerged since 1980 to influence the effective practice of rehabilitation.

A dominant issue that affects the use of formal and informal assessment tools is the utilization of real work environments for providing evaluation information. Identification of the environment in which the client is expected to function is now recognized as critical to a meaningful evaluation of the person's level of functioning. The closer the evaluation method is to the real situation one is measuring, the more the assessment results will facilitate the client's occupational placement.

Other issues to be considered include the shorter evaluation periods being authorized by state and private agencies; the utilization of multifactored approaches in assessment, especially for those who have severe disabilities; updated standards for psychological testing; more functional and situational approaches to evaluation; the impact of technology on the assessment field; and legislation from federal and state governments that has resulted in a decrease of available monies for vocational assessment purposes. A particularly controversial issue that has emerged since 1990 is the decrease in the use of tests that measure aptitude, intelligence, interest, and personality traits and the increase in the use of evaluation approaches that favor behavioral models. In other words, the criteria used to evaluate potential occupational success and career satisfaction may now include such factors as emotional adjustment to the needs of the workplace, getting along with others, and adapting to the behavioral necessities of punctuality, sustained energy, flexibility, and even the creativity that many jobs demand. This issue of trait versus behavioral assessment will continue to generate both conflict and renewed approaches to evaluation practice as this question is repeatedly asked: "What instruments and procedures are sufficiently discriminating for appropriate decision-making?"

Informal Assessment

For individuals with severe disabilities, the traditional approaches to vocational assessment that have mainly embraced psychological testing methods may be inappropriate for vocational planning. The lack of appropriate norms for those with disabilities, as well as the reported lack of attention paid to validity and reliability concerns for persons with physical and mental handicaps, almost forces evaluators to select other approaches that can elicit timely information and provide some predictive value. The utilization of the interview and observational methods, as well as checklists that have not been standardized but that can retrieve information about transferable skills, client needs, values, and even interests, can all be helpful when

attempting to assist individuals in identifying achievable rehabilitation goals.

The interview is a particularly important tool, for when a client can communicate information related to educational and work history, ongoing family dynamics, personal expectations and needs for career placement, and perception of his or her own strengths and limitations, then a skilled interviewer can use this solicited information to identify a central vocational-rehabilitation problem, to determine possible outcomes, and to explore alternatives. Because the interview is a "conversation with a purpose," it can be structured to provide information related to occupational readiness. During the interview, job readiness can be further determined if the evaluator is aware of the client's general orientation toward other people, ability to face his or her own problems, goal-directedness, and energy level. The interview as an assessment tool then becomes both a directive and a nondirective exploration of vocational problems, an identification of factual data, and a consideration of possible lines of action for help in decision-making.

Another informal assessment method that can aid in occupational/career-related decisions is observation, which can be differentiated into global observations and observational systems (i.e., behavioral analysis). The former involves observations made during the entire assessment process, beginning with the initial interview and continuing throughout any psychological testing to actual job tryouts during which the client may learn specific work skills. The latter focuses on relatively discrete behaviors, such as particular job strengths and weaknesses and those behaviors that are needed for appropriate work adjustment (Vacc, 1982). Observations, an evaluation method that can constitute an integral part of situational assessment, are discussed later in this entry. Both the interview and observation methods generate information that can be collected efficiently and used to enhance client self-understanding.

Formal Assessment

Formal assessment can and often does encompass all four major areas of psychological assessment: ability, achievement, personality, and interest assessment

(Solly, 1989). General ability or aptitude assessment includes the measurement of current skills or capabilities to perform a particular task, to function, or to learn. A widely used instrument in vocational evaluation that minimizes the use of written or spoken language when measuring motoric and spatial abilities is the General Aptitude Test Battery (GATB). This performance test is developed and distributed by the United States Employment Service (Capps, Heinlein, & Sautter, 1990). Other ability tests utilized frequently in assessment are the Differential Aptitude Test (DAT), a paper-and-pencil measure that can be used economically when evaluating a large number of individuals over a relatively short period of time, and the APTICOM Aptitude Test Battery, developed similarly to the GATB and now computerized.

Achievement assessment, though not as widely used in vocational assessment as the measurement of client interests and behaviors, refers to an evaluation of educational attainment or the level of accomplishment in one's prior or current occupation (Hohenshil & Solly, 1990). For the evaluator it can be particularly important in determining whether persons with disabilities have the basic academic skills necessary to enter an educational or training program. Frequently used instruments are the Wide Range Achievement Test-Revised (WRAT-R), an individually administered test of reading, spelling, and arithmetic skills, that is particularly helpful in assessing school achievement when the client has not had recent education experience; the Adult Basic Learning Examination (ABLE), second edition, which measures vocabulary, reading, spelling, computation, and problem-solving skills and is used to determine the general educational level of adults who have not completed formal education to the eighth-grade level; the Pennsylvania Bi-Manual Worksample, a test that measures a combination of finger dexterity of both hands, gross movements of both arms, eye-hand coordination, bimanual coordination, and the ability to use both hands in coordination; and the Non-Reading Aptitude Test Battery (NATB), an adaptation of the GATB for nonreaders (Power, 1991). Other tests are used to measure intellectual ability, such as the Wechsler Adult Intelligence Scale-Revised (WAIS-R), and neuropsychological functions that have implications

for daily living. Data from newer psychological tests may also be useful to help clients better understand their specific learning needs and the types of training and adaptation needed for a specific job (Capps, Heinlein, and Sautter, 1990).

Formal personality assessment has been a controversial area within the practice of vocational evaluation. The lack of extensive training for vocational evaluators in the identification of complex personality dynamics and the infrequent attention given to the impact of emotional characteristics on vocational adjustment have resulted in minimal utilization of formal personality assessment tools in evaluation practice. But the purpose of any personality assessment performed in rehabilitation is to identify (1) those strengths or deficits that affect responsiveness to job demands; (2) where and how the client can function effectively; and (3) what training might be needed to enhance the behaviors needed for suitable job adjustment (Maki, Pape, and Prout, 1979). Personality traits that might be the focus of evaluation include mood/temperament needs; attitudes toward self and others; motivation, including energy levels and goal-directedness; and adjustment to the disability, which encompasses coping resources, the ability to face one's problems, and other individual strengths. Tools to measure these characteristics can include the Sixteen Personality Factor Questionnaire (16PF), Form E; the Psychological Screening Inventory (PSI); the Tennessee Self-Concept Scale; and selected tests that focus on anxiety, self-acceptance, and depression (Power, 1991). Personality tests used to develop vocational plans include not only those that measure the "normal" personality, as in the case of the 16PF and the Tennessee Self-Concept Scale, but also those designed to detect patterns of maladjustment or characteristics impairing job performance, as in the case of the Minnesota Multiphasic Personality Inventory (MMPI) and many other scales identifying depression or severe anxiety (Brown, 1990).

Assessment of the client's interests is an integral component of an individual's vocational/career development needs and should be a major focus of evaluators providing services. Several popular interest inventories are used frequently in vocational assessment. For those with low reading skills, the Wide Range Interest-Opinion Test (WRIOT), containing items that represent jobs ranging from unskilled through the highest professional level, was developed to measure interests that appeal to a wide variety of groups. Another measure for this low reading population is the Geist Picture Interest Inventory (Revised), a self-administering tool that can facilitate interest exploration with people with verbal handicaps. For those clients with a higher reading ability, the Strong Vocational Interest Blank for Men and Women, the Career Assessment Inventory, the Kuder Occupational Interest Survey (Form DD), and Holland's Self-Directed Search and Vocational Preference Inventory can identify a broad range of interests for persons who have different occupational goals and who also may wish to explore alternative courses of action. The Self-Directed Search is also available in Form E, primarily intended for those with low reading ability.

Serious concerns arise about all of these formal assessment tools, however, when attempts are made to use them with persons with severe disabilities. These groups usually have been excluded from norm populations, and specific physical and mental limitations may affect standardized administration procedures. Also, people who have limited proficiency in English will have difficulties when taking most formal assessment measures. However, all of these special groups often need the most assistance to be integrated effectively into the job market (Maddy-Bernstein, 1990). Alternative assessment methods have been developed to provide appropriate evaluation resources that may generate findings leading to meaningful occupational decisions. Three such approaches are situational assessment, work samples, and functional assessment. These three methods satisfy the needs of many clients and professional evaluators.

Situational Assessment. This method essentially consists of the observation of people in work situations. It has been one of the most commonly used techniques in vocational evaluation (Power, 1991). A client is placed in a real work situation where, under close supervision by trained evaluators, he or she works with other employees for real wages. The evaluator focuses on the client's work behaviors, and the assessment provides the evaluator with a valuable opportunity to relate to the client within an environment with normal work behavior expecta-

tions. Situational assessment is a process of observing, evaluating, and reporting that extends over a period of time. The client usually can choose to participate in the process, and the information the client can provide during the assessment is important in predicting future work potential. Consequently, assessment performance is considered to be a function of situational variables or the interaction of situational and personal variables and to be a sample of a person's repertoire in a specific situation (Galassi & Perot, 1992).

Though the client interview may be used as one information-gathering procedure in situational assessment, the direct observation of target behaviors; behavior self-report measures; and, when possible, client self-motivation are the methods most frequently used to obtain evaluation data (Galassi & Perot, 1992). Whatever information-gathering approach is used, evaluators have to be aware of the extended time period needed for a situational assessment to be productive. The motivation of both the employer and the client will also determine the productiveness of the assessment. Supportive management can be a key factor in determining the success of this vocational evaluation method.

Work Samples. A work sample is either a simulated task or a work activity of an actual industrial operation (Power, 1991). Actual work samples are taken directly from business or industry and reproduce the processes actually conducted there; simulated work samples are developed by evaluators to simulate jobs. There are many advantages to using this assessment approach, including (1) the approximation to real-life jobs; (2) the opportunity to assess many personal characteristics in a controlled setting; (3) the appropriateness for the evaluation of many groups of people with disabilities, such as those who are brain-injured, mentally ill, or blind; and (4) the fact that during the assessment process clients can perceive themselves as involved in a work task rather than a test (Power, 1991). Work sampling has been reported to have a positive effect on clients' motivation to perform (Capps, Heinlein, and Sautter, 1990). But there are some limitations to the use of work samples. The verbal nature of the instructions usually requires a higher language capability than individuals with severe mental retardation commonly display. Also, a lack of standardization of work samples often exists, and there is no assurance that performance on work samples always predicts performance in actual jobs.

Even with these limitations, work samples can be quite useful in vocational assessment, and many commercial work sample systems are frequently offered by different rehabilitation agencies. Examples of these systems are the Jewish Evaluation Vocational Service (JEVS) work samples, Vocational Information and Evaluation Samples (VIEWS), Singer Vocational Evaluation, Micro-Tower, and VALPAR. When using these systems or other work samples, the evaluator should attempt to individualize these measures for each client.

Functional Assessment. This assessment method is a series of evaluation activities designed to measure a person's existing capabilities and/or limitations, and since 1985 has been used most often following injury or illness (Miller, 1991). Functional assessment includes measures to assess general work demands such as lifting, carrying, reaching, sitting, standing, walking, hand strength and coordination, as well as behaviors relevant to impairment and disability. This approach also focuses on the client's motor and sensory functions and on social, biographical, and environmental information and psychological and intellectual capabilities (Crewe & Athelstan, 1981). The emphasis is on the needs and functional status of individual clients. By helping establish worker readiness to return to a worksite, this evaluation benefits physicians, rehabilitation professionals, employers, insurers, attorneys, and the injured workers themselves (Miller, 1991). It also enables the classification of clients, regardless of diagnostic labels, according to type of disability and severity, for research or program evaluation.

A further advantage of this assessment is that it attempts to pinpoint the obstacles that need to be taken into account in developing a rehabilitation plan. Identifying the obstacles to rehabilitation can be helpful in determining what services are needed, and the information obtained in this diagnostic process can be used to help develop unique measurable goals for the client. Functional assessment is conducted early in the evaluation process and is comprehensive in scope. Either the Functional Assessment Inventory (Crewe & Athelstan, 1981) or related tools developed by agencies for their own use may be used to collect the necessary information.

What distinguishes this form of vocational evaluation from others is that client behaviors, including both limitations and capabilities, are placed on a hierarchical continuum. The assessment of impairments usually requires both a very fine-grained level of measurement and a consideration of the relevant environmental circumstances (Alexander & Fuhrer, 1984). Another unique characteristic is the important use of functional assessment in research. Functional assessment data have been used to quantify individual differences among rehabilitation clients in predictive studies of their functioning after they are discharged from rehabilitation hospitals (Alexander & Fuhrer, 1984).

Providers

The individuals whose main responsibility involves the vocational evaluation process usually have had in-depth training in vocational evaluation/assessment. Other professionals who provide evaluation services include instructors in elementary and secondary schools and postsecondary programs; rehabilitation counselors; occupational and physical therapists; supported employment specialists; and work adjustment specialists (Lombard et al., 1993). The roles of each type of professional require different certification and preparation. The Commission on Certification of Work Adjustment and Vocational Evaluation Specialists (CCWAVES) offers credentialing for both work evaluators and work adjustment specialists. Created as an independent commission in 1981, CCWAVES exists primarily to provide assurance that professionals engaged in vocational evaluation meet acceptable standards of quality. There are many options for the applicant seeking to be eligible to take the certified vocational evaluator exam, though all options involve academic course work and/or acceptable employment experience. The certification process is intended to assure that all individuals involved in vocational evaluation demonstrate competency or successful completion of training in competencies that include the following abilities:

1. To select, adopt, and/or develop methods and approaches that are useful in determining an individual's attributes, abilities, and needs.
2. To utilize alternative methods and approaches

that can serve to cross-validate information generated from other assessment sources.

3. To collect and interpret data in a manner that contributes to the total service delivery system and to integrate assessment approaches that are current, valid, and reliable and grounded in career, vocational, and work contexts (Lombard et al., 1993).

Conclusion

The proper and effective application of vocational evaluation information plays a prominent role in the client's attainment of rehabilitation goals. Appropriately used assessment results can make a difference in how people with disabilities make optimal use of their remaining strengths and resources.

(*See also:* ASSESSMENT; CAREER COUNSELING; CREDENTIALS; DISABILITY MANAGEMENT; FORENSIC REHABILITATION; JOB PLACEMENT; LIFE CARE PLANNING; OCCUPATIONAL INFORMATION; REHABILITATION COUNSELING; WORK)

RESOURCES

Materials Development Center, Stout Vocational Institute, School of Education and Human Services, University of Wisconsin–Stout, Menomonie, WI 54751

Vocational Evaluation and Work Adjustment Association, National Rehabilitation Association, 1910 Association Drive, Suite 205, Reston, VA 22901

BIBLIOGRAPHY

ALEXANDER, JAMES and FUHRER, MARCUS J., eds. *Functional Assessment in Rehabilitation.* Baltimore, 1984.

BROWN, MICHAEL B. "Personality Assessment in Career Counseling." *Career Planning and Adult Development Journal* 6 (1990):22–26.

CAPPS, FREDERICK C.; HEINLEIN, WILLIAM E.; and SAUTTER, SCOTT W. "Aptitude Testing in Career Assessment." *Career Planning and Adult Development Journal* 6 (1990):16–21.

CREWE, NANCY M., and ATHELSTAN, GARY T. "Functional Assessment in Vocational Rehabilitation: A Systematic Approach to Diagnosis and Goal Setting." *Archives of Physical Medicine and Rehabilitation* 62 (1981):299–305.

GALASSI, JOHN P., and PEROT, ANNETTE R. "What You Should Know About Behavioral Assessment." *Journal of Counseling and Development* 70 (1992):624–631.

HOHENSHIL, THOMAS H., and SOLLY, DAVID C. "An Overview of Career Assessment Methods and Models." *Career Planning and Adult Development Journal* 6 (1990):4–8.

LOMBARD, RICHARD; NEUBERT, DEBORAH; ROTHENBACHER, CAROL; SITLINGTON, PATRICIA; SMITH, FRAN; and LECONTE, P. *The Interdisciplinary Council on Vocational Evaluation/Assessment: A Position Paper.* Stout, WI, 1993.

MADDY-BERNSTEIN, CAROLYN. "Considerations Regarding Career Assessment for Special Groups." *Career Planning and Adult Development Journal* 6 (1990):37–40.

MAKI, DENNIS; PAPE, DEBORAH; and PROUT, H. THOMPSON. "Personality Evaluations: A Tool of the Rehabilitation Counselor." *Journal of Applied Rehabilitation Counseling* 10 (1979):119–123.

MILLER, MARGOT. "Functional Assessments." *Work* 1 (1991):6–10.

POWER, PAUL. *A Guide to Vocational Assessment,* 2nd ed. Austin, TX, 1991.

SOLLY, DAVID C. *Functional Assessment of Students with Handicaps.* Topeka, KS, 1989.

VACC, NICHOLAS A. "A Conceptual Framework for Continuous Assessment of Clients." *Measurement and Evaluation in Guidance* 15 (1982):40–47.

PAUL W. POWER

VOCATIONAL REHABILITATION

See CAREER COUNSELING; REHABILITATION COUNSELING; WORK

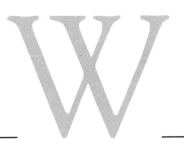

WELFARE

See DISABILITY LAW AND SOCIAL POLICY

WELLNESS

The National Institute of Wellness defines wellness as having six dimensions: social, physical, emotional, intellectual, occupational, and spiritual. The concept of "physical wellness" is essential in the prevention of illness and disability as well as during the treatment and rehabilitation process. If persons with disabilities are to meet the demands, rigors, and challenges of rehabilitation effectively and efficiently and attain a level of optimal independence in living and/or working, they should understand that the notion of wellness is an attitude about thought and behaviors regarding fitness and nutrition. This attitude is often the difference between limited options and expanded choices that can improve the quality of life and facilitate the attainment of health care and rehabilitation goals.

In the general population the beneficial effects of regular physical exercise or activity, coupled with prudent dietary practices, are well documented (American College of Sports Medicine, 1990). There is an overall improvement in cardiovascular and muscular fitness, reduction in body weight and body fat, and an increase in the sense of emotional well-being. Clinical evidence proposes that improvements in physical fitness may reduce the likelihood of premature death (Blair et al., 1989) and suggests that those persons exhibiting moderate compared to low cardiovascular fitness levels are at much lower risk for all causes of mortality. While cause and effect have yet to be determined, other literature (Erikssen, 1986; Peters et al., 1983; and Sobolski et al., 1987) has also implied that lack of activity contributes to poor physical health. The American College of Sports Medicine (ACSM) has synthesized much of the significant literature in this area and published a position statement that recommends appropriate amounts of exercise needed to provide the minimal levels of physical fitness for all adults (American College of Sports Medicine, 1990).

Beginning in the 1980s, the advantages of participating in regular exercise and improving nutrition for people living with various illnesses and disabilities became an increasingly important area of study. Recognizing that the literature is meager compared to that available for able-bodied people, in the early 1990s the American College of Sports Medicine began to encourage research and dissemination of information in the general area of chronic disease and disability. The mission of ACSM is to "promote and integrate scientific research, education and practical application of sports medicine and exercise science to maintain and enhance physical performance, fitness, health, and quality of life" (American College of Sports Medicine, 1990). This mission encompasses the potential role of exercise and nutrition professionals who strive to make life more enjoyable and healthier for people with physical and emotional disabilities.

General Guidelines for Fitness

Many people with disabilities do not generally have active lifestyles. The lack of exercise may be a result of the disease or disability itself or consequent to the nature of the disability (i.e., an individual with quadriplegia is more limited in the amount of exercise he or she can engage in than a person with a lower limb amputation). In addition, the inability to exercise or engage in active leisure may be secondary to substance abuse and depression about the disability. Because research shows an association between a lack of exercise and health problems, however, the incorporation of some form of exercise into one's lifestyle, no matter how little, is being increasingly accepted and encouraged.

It is very apparent that the body seems to suffer from inactivity. Affected are the cardiovascular system and the general body musculature, which undergoes a decrease in muscular strength, endurance, and range of motion and increases in body weight and body fat. To counteract these deleterious effects, some large muscle movement is advisable (walking, swimming, cycling, etc.). For those people unable to engage in large muscle activity (e.g., because of confinement to a wheelchair or similar restriction), alternatives include arm cranking or ergometry and wheelchair ambulation and any other large body activity. In each case the objective is to sustain the activity for a period of time, preferably

fifteen to twenty minutes initially and progressively extend to thirty minutes, for a minimum frequency of three times a week. During this time the heart rate should increase, an indication that the cardiovascular system is being stimulated. Depending on a person's disability and age, the increase should range from approximately 60 to 90 percent of the maximal achievable heart rate (maximal achievable heart rate = 220 − age). However, the amount of increase in heart rate that is advisable may be more limited in the case of some disabilities. A health professional trained in exercise evaluation and prescription should be consulted to determine the appropriate stimulus. Appropriate exercise of the musculoskeletal system includes the lifting, pulling, or pushing of various amounts of weight for a series of repetitions. Consideration should be given to the amount of weight, the number of sessions per week, and the specific area of the body being exercised. Guidelines for both the cardiovascular and musculoskeletal areas can be found in a publication by the American College of Sports Medicine (1990).

Wellness: Research, Rehabilitation, Exercise, and Sport

For more than thirty years, many health professionals have concentrated their efforts in the rehabilitation of patients with coronary heart disease. Fitness training, reduction of risk factors (such as smoking), and nutrition and exercise education have been the backbone of a comprehensive rehabilitation effort to reduce the debilitating effects of our nation's leading cause of death. These efforts have made an impact. The success of cardiac rehabilitation programs has led to an increased interest in research on the use of exercise rehabilitation for people with various disabilities. For example, exercise science researchers have studied the effects of exercise and lack of exercise in a variety of disabling conditions, such as spinal cord injury (both paraplegia and quadriplegia); mental retardation; muscular dystrophy; multiple sclerosis; cerebral palsy; diabetes; mental illness; amputation; blindness; deafness; and others. The available literature in each area has increased dramatically since the early 1980s. These findings have heightened the awareness of health professionals of the possible benefits that can be derived from exercise rehabilitation. It is now generally accepted that some form of habitual activity, regular exercise, or participation in sports improves psychomotor skills, increases motivation for other tasks of living, and reduces anxiety and tension (Sherrill, 1986). This realization has led to the establishment of research laboratories and exercise programs specializing in the study and rehabilitation of persons with disabilities.

In addition to the research and associated exercise rehabilitation programs, there are major efforts across the country to involve people with disabilities in organized forms of sports activities and competition. While recreation programs for people with disabilities in general began early in the twentieth century, contemporary competitive sports programs are reflective of the various advocacy groups associated with the many specific disabilities (Shephard, 1990). See the Resources list at the end of this entry for a list of various associations supportive of leisure activities for people with disabilities.

Diet and Chronic Disease Prevention

Among the ten leading causes of death in the United States, four (coronary heart disease, certain cancers, diabetes mellitus, and stroke) have been associated with dietary excess and imbalances. Three others (unintentional injury, suicide, and chronic liver disease) are associated with excessive alcohol consumption. Together these conditions account for nearly two-thirds of the 12 million deaths in this country each year. Other diet-related conditions, such as obesity, high blood pressure, osteoporosis, and dental caries, also inflict a substantial burden of illness on society. In response to increased recognition that nutrition problems among Americans are due to imbalances in dietary intake, numerous scientific and federal organizations have established dietary guidelines for disease prevention (McGinnis & Nestle, 1989). The implementation of sound dietary practices has notable health benefits with regard to prevention of certain diseases, and it contributes significantly to one's ability to engage in various daily activities. It is also an important factor in the successful rehabilitation of persons with physical as well as emotional disabilities. Many organizations, including the American Heart Association and the American Cancer Institute as well as scientific branches of the federal government, have generated dietary guidelines to reduce the risk of diet-related chronic diseases in Americans (National Research Council, 1989). The dietary guidelines issued by the National Research Council in 1985 are as follows:

1. Maintain ideal body weight through an appropriate balance of caloric intake and exercise.
2. Limit or reduce total fat intake to less than 30 percent of total calorie intake.
3. Reduce saturated fat to less than 10 percent of total calorie intake.
4. Limit cholesterol intake to less than 300 milligrams per day.
5. Increase intake of complex carbohydrate to at least 55 percent of total calories by consuming increased amounts of complex carbohydrates such as cereals, breads, and legumes.
6. Increase fiber intake through increased consumption of vegetables, fruits, and cereals.
7. If you drink alcohol, do so in moderation.

The Food Pyramid

To improve dietary habits and ultimately the nutrition profile of Americans, food consumption patterns that mirror these dietary recommendations must be developed (Mason & McGinnis, 1990; McGinnis & Nestle, 1989). The food pyramid is an educational tool developed in the early 1990s to inform the public about healthful choices that follow the dietary guidelines. Selection of a variety of items within each food group and consumption of fresh, wholesome foods should prevent most nutrient deficiencies in the general population. Grains make up the base of the food pyramid. Thus bread, cereals, pasta, and other grains, which are rich sources of fiber, B vitamins, and some trace elements, should be the staple of the diet. This follows the dietary recommendation to increase complex carbohydrate and fiber consumption. The second widest level of the food pyramid consists of fruits and vegetables, which are rich sources of fiber, vitamins C and A, and folic acid. This follows the dietary guidelines, which encourage increased consumption of fiber, complex carbohydrates, and a liberal intake of vitamins, minerals, and trace elements. The next level of the food pyramid includes the meat, fish, and protein group, which is rich in protein, iron, and zinc, and the dairy group, which is rich in calcium, phosphorus, and vitamins A and D. This follows the recommendation to decrease intake of fat and cholesterol, which are found in these animal food products. Decreased consumption of these may reduce the incidence of heart disease, certain cancers and obesity. The smallest food group on the pyramid, to be ingested sparingly, includes calorie-rich, nutrient-poor items such as fats, oils, and sweets. Thus the food pyramid should encourage eating habits that are more healthful, reduce the incidence of illness, and maximize the rehabilitation potential of people with disabilities.

Nutrition Problems Specific to Persons with Disabilities

Assessment of nutritional status evaluates an individual for normal growth and development, checks for the presence of dietary risk factors that may contribute to disease, and enables early detection of nutrient deficiencies and excesses (Gibson, 1990). Comparison of an individual to established norms provides a basis for nutritional intervention and evaluation of therapy. A combination of physical body measurements and biochemical, clinical, and dietary assessment parameters forms the basis of the evaluation (Gibson, 1990). Persons with physical and psychological disabilities may be at increased risk of nutritional deficiencies and dietary imbalances due to significant alterations in metabolic and physical activity status as a direct result of the disability itself or as a consequence of the lifestyle associated with it. As with the general population, nutritional assessment should focus on prevention, early detection, and treatment of nutrition-related problems.

Nutritional deficiencies and diet-related chronic diseases may be more prevalent in persons with disabilities because of problems related to abnormalities in appetite, feeding, energy expenditure, growth, or drug-nutrient interactions. Behavioral difficulties related to feeding on the part of either caregiver or client may lead to nutritional problems. Specific diet-related risk factors such as unusual eating habits, inability to purchase and prepare food, and inadequate nutritional knowledge may be present more frequently in persons with certain disabilities (American Dietetic Association, 1987).

For people with certain disabilities, problems related to feeding and the ability to consume adequate nutrients may be severe. Malnutrition, a pathologic state of varying severity, results from a deficiency or imbalance of calories or individual essential nutrients. The cause may be primary (inadequate intake) or secondary (increased requirements). Both calorie and protein deprivation results in impaired immune function, placing malnourished persons at risk for increased infections. An interdisciplinary feeding team focusing on optimal nutrient intake through improved feeding skills and eating behavior can help improve food intake.

Conversely, physical impairment may modify physical activity levels and thus place individuals with disabilities at increased risk for obesity. "Healthy People 2000" estimated obesity prevalence to be 36 percent in people with disabilities (American Dietetic Association, 1991). Obesity is often resistant to treatment; thus prevention is important. If obesity develops, treatment should include a combination of diet, exercise, and behavior modification. Lack of knowledge or motivation may be intrinsic or caregiver-related. The focus should be on educating both client and caregiver as to the goals of all dietary recommendations. Attitudes and food practices are more difficult to change; however, behavior modification techniques may be useful. Specific dietary risk factors such as increased intake of caffeine, sucrose, and alcohol, as well as disordered eating patterns, should be evaluated. Additional problems may include diarrhea or constipation, which may require dietary modification.

The increased incidence of diet-related chronic diseases has led to a strong effort for prevention through dietary intervention. The dietary guidelines listed above were developed for the general population, but they apply to persons with disabilities as well. Persons with disabilities are classified in an "at risk" group by the "Healthy People 2000" (American Dietetic Association, 1991) objectives for the nation; thus nutritional assessment should target this population for early intervention and prevention.

Summary

Although there is increasing consensus regarding dietary and exercise guidelines for wellness or the prevention of chronic disease in the general population, scientific recommendations for various populations with disabilities are lacking. More research is needed in this critical area so that precise interventions targeted at optimal lifestyle and rehabilitation possibilities may be designed. The emphasis must be on prevention of lifestyle-related chronic diseases, which may complicate disabilities and impair the rehabilitation process. Regular exercise and healthy eating habits are not a panacea for a particular disability, disease, or illness. However, the stresses of the twenty-first century and the challenges of living and working with a disability will be minimized if the basic tenets of physical wellness are practiced.

(*See also:* CORONARY ARTERY DISEASE; INDEPENDENT LIVING; QUALITY OF LIFE; RECREATION; SELF-CONCEPT; WORK)

RESOURCES

American Athletic Association of the Deaf, 1052 Darling St., Ogden, UT 84403

American Blind Bowling Association, 411 Sherriff St., Mercer, PA 16137

American Blind Skiing Foundation, 610 South William St., Mt. Prospect, IL 60056

American Water Ski Association Committee on Water Skiing for the Disabled, c/o Camp Association, P.O. Box 21, Jackson Gap, AL 36861

American Wheelchair Bowling Association, N54 W15858 Lakespur Lane, Menomonee Falls, WI 53051

National Amputee Golf Association (NAGA), P.O. Box 1228, Amherst, NH 03031

National Foundation for Happy Horsemanship for the Handicapped, Inc., P.O. Box 462, Malvern, PA 19355

National Handicap Motorcyclist Association (NHMA), 35-34 84th St., #F-8, Jackson Heights, NY 11372

National Handicapped Sports and Recreation Association, 1145 19th St., NW, Suite 717, Washington, DC 20036

National Wheelchair Athletic Association, 3595 E. Fountain Blvd., Suite L1, Colorado Springs, CO 80910

National Wheelchair Basketball Association (NWBA), 110 Seaton Center, University of Kentucky, Lexington, KY 40506

National Wheelchair Shooting Federation, P.O. Box 18251, San Antonio, TX 78218

National Wheelchair Softball Association (NWSA), P.O. Box 22478, Minneapolis, MN 55422

North American Riding for the Handicapped Association, Box 33150, Denver, CO 80233

Physically Challenged Swimmers of America, 22 William St., #225, South Glastonbury, CT 06073

BIBLIOGRAPHY

AMERICAN COLLEGE OF SPORTS MEDICINE. "Position Stand on the Recommended Quantity and Quality of Exercise for Developing and Maintaining Cardiorespiratory and Muscular Fitness in Healthy Adults." *Medicine and Science in Sports and Exercise* 22 (1990):265–274.

AMERICAN DIETETIC ASSOCIATION. "Nutrition in Comprehensive Program Planning for Persons with Disabilities: Technical Support Paper." *Journal of the American Dietetic Association* 87 (1987):1069–1074.

———. "Healthy People 2000: Nutrition Objectives." *Journal of the American Dietetic Association* 91 (1991):1515–1516.

BLAIR, STEVEN N.; KOHL, HAROLD W. III; PAFFENBARGER, RALPH S.; CLARK, DEBRA G.; COOPER, KENNETH H.; and GIBBONS, LARRY W. "Physical Fitness and All-Cause Mortality: A Prospective Study of Healthy Men and Women." *Journal of the American Medical Association* 262 (1989):2395–2401.

ERIKSSEN, JAN. "Physical Fitness and Coronary Heart Disease Morbidity and Mortality: A Prospective Study in Apparently Healthy, Middle-Aged Men." *Acta Medica Scandinavia Supplement* 711 (1986): 189–192.

GIBSON, ROSALIND S. *Principles of Nutritional Assessment.* New York, 1990.

MASON, JAMES O., and McGINNIS, J. MICHAEL. "Healthy People 2000: An Overview of the National Health Promotion and Disease Prevention Objectives." *Public Health Reports* 105 (1990):441–447.

McGINNIS, J. MICHAEL, and NESTLE, MARION. "The Surgeon General's Report on Nutrition and Health: Policy Implications and Implementation Strategies." *American Journal of Clinical Nutrition* 49 (1989):23–28.

NATIONAL RESEARCH COUNCIL. *Diet and Health: Implications for Reducing Chronic Disease Risk,* 3rd ed. Washington, DC, 1989.

———. *Recommended Dietary Allowances.* Washington, DC, 1989.

PETERS, RUTH K.; CADY, LEE D., JR.; BISCHOFF, DAVID P.; BERNSTEIN, LESLIE; and PIKE, MALCOLM C. "Physical Fitness and Subsequent Myocardial Infarction in Healthy Workers." *Journal of the American Medical Association* 249 (1983):3052–3056.

SHEPHARD, ROY, J. *Fitness in Special Populations.* Champaign, IL, 1990.

SHERRILL, CLAUDINE. *Adapted Physical Education and Recreation.* Dubuque, IA 1986.

SOBOLSKI, JOHN C.; KOMITZER, MARCEL; DEBACKER, GUY; DRAMAIX, MICHÈLE; ABRAMOWICZ, MICHEL; DEGRE, SERGE; and DENOLIN, HENRI. "Protection Against Ischemic Heart Disease in the Belgian Physical Fitness Study: Physical Fitness Rather than Physical Activity?" *American Journal of Epidemiology* 125 (1987):601–610.

WILHELMSEN, LARS; BJURE, JAN; EKSTROM-JODAL, BARBRO; AURELL, MATTIAS; GRIMBY, GUNNAR; SVARDSUDD, KURT; TIBBLIN, GOSTA; and WEDEL, HANS. "Nine Years' Follow-up of a Maximal Exercise Test in a Random Population Sample of Middle-Aged Men." *Cardiology* 68 (supp. 2, 1981): 1–8.

GARY S. SKRINAR
KRISTY M. HENDRICKS

WHEELCHAIRS

It is estimated that 1.2 million people in the United States use wheelchairs as their primary means of locomotion (Todd, 1990). For some, the wheelchair is a temporary mobility aid, but for persons with chronic physical disability that prevents safe and effective walking, the wheelchair is a permanent device and a key to independence, vocation, and recreation. While the majority of wheelchair users are persons who have impaired lower-limb motor and/or sensory function due to a neurological disorder and live in the community, a large number of wheelchair users have a more generalized disability due to aging or different medical conditions and are institutionally confined for a longer or shorter period of time.

Although most wheelchairs may look similar, numerous designs exist. Fundamentally, there are two main categories of wheelchairs: manual and externally powered. Within each category, hundreds of different designs are available worldwide, with multiple options to meet individual needs of users. Selecting an appropriate wheelchair has therefore become a complex task wherein the prescriber must evaluate the latest technological trends in wheelchair design and receive input from users and their families as well as from nurses, therapists, and suppliers. Table 1 summarizes the different factors that must be considered when a wheelchair is prescribed (Todd, 1990). When the wheelchair is prescribed, a wheelchair seat cushion must also be selected, one that improves comfort and sitting posture.

Table 1. Considerations for a wheelchair prescription

1. User's age, size, weight, etc.
2. User's disability and prognosis
3. User's functional skills and preferences
4. Indoor/outdoor use
5. Portability/accessibility
6. Reliability/durability
7. Cosmetic features
8. Options available
9. Service
10. Cost
11. Level of acceptance (total environment)

SOURCE: Wilson, 1992

History

There is little documentation available on wheelchairs until the time of the Civil War, when wooden chairs with wooden wheels were used (Wilson, 1992). Photographs and drawings exist from the latter part of the nineteenth century that show specific wheelchair designs with many features currently used. During the 1930s the first folding wheelchairs were designed and manufactured (Wilson, 1992). The folding design was further refined to decrease weight, ease operation, and secure stability of the wheelchair, and became the standard. In 1967 a stainless steel model was introduced and was referred to as a lightweight wheelchair because it reduced the average weight of the wheelchair from approximately 50 pounds to 40 pounds. During the 1970s numerous improvements in manual wheelchair designs occurred to improve performance and the comfort of users, many of whom were actively participating in different wheelchair sports and other high-level activities. Drawing on available technology in the bicycle and automobile industries, independent wheelchair makers developed sports chairs, lighter in weight, easier to maneuver, and more durable than previous designs. Many of the new features were incorporated into the standard wheelchair design to create a new generation of wheelchairs, sometimes referred to as "ultralight" wheelchairs.

During World War I, electrically powered wheelchairs were first made by crudely adding a motor, battery and on/off switch to a manual chair (Wilson, 1992). As medical care improved following World War II, and as more persons with severe disabilities, such as those with tetraplegia, survived, demand for powered wheelchairs increased along with designs improved to meet the different needs of users.

The basic or standard wheelchair (Figure 1) consists of a chrome-plated steel frame with cross bars to permit folding and with short tipping levers in the back. It weighs 30 to 50 pounds. There are two large rear wheels and two small front caster wheels. The wheels usually have solid tires when used indoors, but the rear wheels may have pneumatic tires when used primarily outdoors. Handrims for propulsion and control are attached to the large wheels, sometimes with additionally mounted projecting lugs to ease operation by users with hand impairment. The

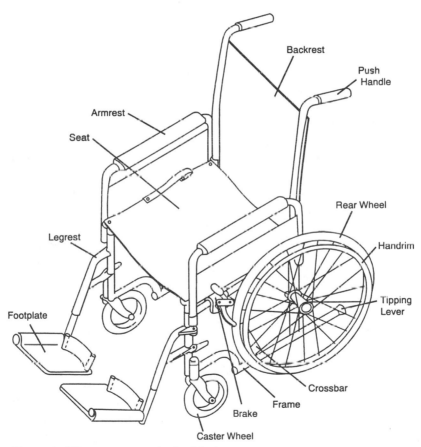

Figure 1. The conventional wheelchair

SOURCE: Ragnarsson, Kristjan T. "Prescription Considerations." *Journal of Rehabilitation Research and Development, Clinical Supplement 2* (1990):11

seat and backrest are usually fabricated in standard dimensions, with numerous modifications possible. Push handles are present in the back, armrests may be full-length or desk-type, fixed or removable, and adjustable in height. Foot- and legrests may be detachable and adjustable. For safety, the basic wheelchair has a pair of toggle or lever brakes for the rear wheels, and an antitipping extension may be added to the tipping lever. Multiple variations of the basic wheelchair can be made available, such as placing the rear wheel farther behind the seat to increase stability for the user with bilateral leg amputations, providing one hand drive, placing the large wheels in front and the casters in the rear, lowering the seat for easier propulsion with the feet, providing different sizes of frames for different body sizes, extended and reclining backrests, seat belts, thigh supports, stand-up features, and so forth.

The lightweight (sports) wheelchair in general has a sportier look than the basic type, weighs considerably less, and permits higher performance due to special design features. The wheelchair frame, which may be solid or permit folding, is made of lightweight metals, available in different colors. The rear wheels are often detachable and their axle position adjustable in different directions for better maneuverability, propulsion, power, and stability. The front caster wheels usually are made of solid polyurethane, smaller in diameter and adjustable for position. The height of the backrest is variable but tends to be lower than on the basic wheelchair. Elite wheelchair athletes often have their wheelchairs specifically built for added advantage during sports competition, such as racing.

Powered wheelchairs have in common a battery-powered source, electric motors, and user-operated control systems, but vary otherwise greatly in design. The power systems may occasionally be added on a basic wheelchair, but more often they are integral to the wheelchair itself. Such powered wheelchairs often are expensive and highly sophisticated mobility devices that may have specially mounted electronic control and communication systems, respirators, powered reclining extended backrests, and elevating footrests. While such wheelchairs are provided for people with severe physical disability, a person who is marginally able to walk may better benefit by using a different powered wheelchair, such

as the three-wheeled, scooterlike cart for long distance and outdoor mobility.

(*See also:* ARCHITECTURAL ACCESSIBILITY; ASSISTIVE TECHNOLOGY; HOUSING; INDEPENDENT LIVING; MUSCULOSKELETAL DISORDERS; REHABILITATION CENTER; SPINAL CORD INJURY; TECHNOLOGY; TRANSPORTATOPN ACCESSIBILITY)

BIBLIOGRAPHY

TODD, SELDON P., ed. *"Choosing a Wheelchair System."* *Journal of Rehabilitation Research and Development 2* (1990).
WILSON, A. BENNETT, JR. *Wheelchairs: A Prescription Guide,* 2nd ed. New York, 1992.

KRISTJAN T. RAGNARSSON

WOMEN IN REHABILITATION

Since the inception of federally mandated vocational rehabilitation services in the aftermath of World War I, many changes have occurred in the field of rehabilitation. Most notably, revisions in the underlying philosophy of rehabilitation reflect a shift both in gender balance and in assigned responsibility among providers and consumers of rehabilitation services.

Once, successful rehabilitation outcomes were believed to result from counselors' assumption of responsibility and control in the counselor-client relationship. Now, successful outcomes are believed to result from client empowerment—that is, clients' participation in the formulation of their individualized rehabilitation programs and acceptance of responsibility in bringing such programs to fruition.

Consequently, rehabilitation and health care professionals who once evaluated clients narrowly, on the basis of their functional limitations, now tend to assess them holistically, in terms of their unique patterns of strengths and weaknesses. No longer do competent rehabilitators view clients as disabled persons but as persons with disabilities—with a disability being only one of a multitude of meaningful personal characteristics.

Along with altered roles in general of clients in rehabilitation, the role of women both as consumers and as providers of rehabilitation services has also changed. Early rehabilitation legislation was designed to provide vocational rehabilitation services to men—that is, World War I veterans with service-connected disabilities. Subsequent legislation, during an era when few women were in competitive employment, specified homemaker as a feasible occupational goal, thereby expanding the focus of state-federal services.

Moreover, since most women were not employed outside their homes, the fledgling profession of rehabilitation consisted primarily of males. Today, more than sixty years later, within rehabilitation women outnumber males in junior but not in senior positions.

Whether the relationship between philosophical changes and the movement of women into the rehabilitation profession is causal or coincidental is impossible to determine. What is incontrovertible is that the status of women in rehabilitation—those who pursue a career in the profession as well as those who receive services from the profession—reflects the status of women in American society in general: overrepresentation in service occupations, underrepresentation in administrative and managerial positions, and inequities in promotions and salary levels (Murray & Keenan, 1992).

Moreover, within rehabilitation or without, women continue to be ignored as a population worthy of interest in basic research, as well as in research specifically related to rehabilitation outcomes. For example, although women historically have been excluded from employment-related research on work stressors and family stressors, the results of such research have been presumed to apply equally well to women as to men (Baruch, Beiner, and Barnett, 1987). This failure to investigate women, or often even to include them in rehabilitation-related research, has resulted in an inability to understand or address their rehabilitation needs and potential adequately (Danek, 1992).

In addition to the gender-based bias they share with their peers without disabilities, women with disabilities experience the additional consequence of being perceived as functionally limited—socially, economically, and psychologically—because of their disabilities. The resultant social position of women with disabilities has been described as "sexism without the pedestal," for in the eyes of many, they are deemed incapable of fulfilling the occupational, the reproductive, or the nurturant roles traditionally assigned to and reserved for women in American society (Fine & Asch, 1981). Moreover, the cumulative and diffusive effects of multiple devalued social statuses—gender, disability, and ethnicity or race—can have a negative impact on one's ability to adjust socially, vocationally, and psychologically. As one young woman explains, "I don't mind being Indian, and I don't mind being blind, and I don't mind being a girl, but to be a blind Indian girl is more than I can bear" (Dunham & Dunham, 1978).

Two major issues, therefore, fall within the overall topic of women in rehabilitation. One concerns the role and position of women who are themselves rehabilitation professionals. The other involves the role and position of women who are or have been consumers of rehabilitation services.

Women as Rehabilitators

"Old soldiers never die, they go into rehabilitation" encapsulates characteristics of many early rehabilitators—retired military personnel who entered the field as their second career. Others who were attracted into rehabilitation early were male clergy—ex-priests or ministers who needed to supplement incomes provided by small, sometimes impoverished, congregations.

Those few women who entered the profession often began their careers as support staff or secretaries. For example, Louise Blankenship, who was a regional director when she retired in the late 1980s, entered the field as a rehabilitation secretary. Similarly, Mary E. Switzer, who became one of the most well-known and nationally influential figures in rehabilitation, began in 1922 as a Grade 2 clerk in the Treasury Department.

Therefore, "old soldiers" with their authoritarian worldview had the greatest impact on early rehabilitation. Moreover, their influence, although somewhat diminished since the passage of consumer-oriented legislation stemming back to the Rehabilitation Act of 1973, continues to affect the implementation of rehabilitation policy today. Four discernible effects of that influence continue: (1) the persistence of the more "male" authority-based medical model as a phenotype for client-counselor roles—despite inroads made by proponents of the more "female" collaboration-based compensatory model (Cottone & Cottone, 1992); (2) the persistence of attitudinal barriers that impede full acceptance of persons with disabilities as qualified fellow professionals (Harris, 1992); (3) the persistence of rehabilitation as an undercompensated human services area in which earnings are inadequate in light of the preparation and practical experience required to provide quality services; and (4) the persistence of gender bias and resultant gender imbalance at different stages of the career ladder in both the public and the private sectors of rehabilitation (Murray & Keenan, 1992; *Rehab Brief*, 1988).

Not surprisingly, ex-military rehabilitators adapted easily to the medical model of helping, which holds that successful outcomes are dependent on a person's unquestioning acceptance of the authority of the helping professional. The medical model, unlike the compensatory model, promotes learned helplessness, not autonomy and independence, in adults with permanent disabilities.

Second, the medical model, with its distinct and rigid boundaries between service provider and service receiver, contributes to the difficulties persons with disabilities experience in being perceived as qualified service providers themselves. Oftentimes, professionals with visible disabilities find they are cast in the role of client until circumstances prove otherwise. As an example, Nancy Kerr, a rehabilitation psychologist who uses a wheelchair, recounts her experiences as a rehabilitation professional within medical rehabilitation settings:

> On countless occasions, I have been wheeling along in treatment settings in various parts of the country, tending to my business, when an attendant or nurse would hustle alongside and challengingly or sarcastically say, "Hey, where do you think you're going?" or sometimes "You're not supposed to be out here—go to your room." On one occasion, solely on the basis of my occupancy of a wheelchair, a nurse tried physically to put me to bed! More than once my wheelchair has been hijacked by an attendant who, without comment, wheeled me to the dining room of his institution [Kerr, 1970].

Although more than twenty years have passed since the incidents Kerr described, nonacceptance of persons with disabilities as colleagues, *especially in*

positions of authority within the rehabilitation field, continue, albeit more subtly than in years past. Richard Harris (1992) reports reactions "ranging from discomfort to resentment on the part of able-bodied colleagues not happy with the juxtaposition of the new roles."

Third, although the academic, credentialing, and job requirements of rehabilitation counseling closely resemble those of psychology or social work, salary or fee schedules for many rehabilitation counselors have been far below those of other related fields. This situation was especially true for state agency counselor positions until the burgeoning of private for-profit rehabilitation, supported through insurance companies and state-by-state workmen's compensation insurance, resulted in salary increases and career opportunities. In the 1990s, those with master's degrees in social work could expect a salary ranging from $25,000 to $38,000 (*Occupational Outlook Handbook, 1994–1995*; U.S. Department of Labor, Bureau of Labor Statistics); persons with a master's degree in rehabilitation counseling could expect a salary ranging from $31,000 to $49,000 (*Occupational Outlook Handbook, 1994–1995*; Department of Labor, Bureau of Labor Statistics. But, more specifically, the bottom 10 percent of rehabilitation counselors earned less than $17,000 in positions in public or private non-profit agencies (Savage & Palmisano, 1994).

Gender bias may play a major role in these compensation inequities among related professions. Despite more stringent standards within rehabilitation, the increasing prevalence of women counselors may contribute to the continuing low levels of compensation. Under similar circumstances, as women continue to outnumber male graduates of psychology programs, the American Psychological Association fears that a corresponding decrease in the level of compensation for psychological services will occur in the future.

Finally, recent surveys of the role status of women employed in rehabilitation indicate that gender imbalance and bias persist. For example, within state agencies more women are employed than men, but men far outnumber women in administrative, as opposed to counselor, positions. Within rehabilitation education programs men predominate overall. A larger percentage of men occupy faculty positions, are directors of training programs, and publish in rehabilitation journals (Datoff, 1983; Murray & Keenan, 1992; Myers & Wedl, 1985; Perlman & Arneson, 1982).

While the ratio of four male administrators to one female administrator, contrasted with a ratio of one male to two females at the counselor level, might be explained by the historical predominance of men within the profession, the discrepancy appears to be stable from the earliest surveys to the latest. According to Susan E. Murray and Deborah Keenan (1992), "Men move on to higher positions, women often do not."

Similarly, in rehabilitation education programs, "Women have failed to keep pace with men in terms of salaries, opportunities for advancement, and responsibilities for budgets and decision-making" (Murray & Keenan, 1992). For example, although from 1984 to 1992 the number of women faculty increased from 23 to 32 percent, a 1992 survey of women revealed that 53 percent of the respondents said they did not receive equal salaries, and 72 percent felt they had not received equal treatment compared to their male counterparts. Moreover, in 1992, 79 percent of the program directors or coordinators in rehabilitation training settings were men (Murray & Keenan, 1992).

Women with Disabilities

Although a few women with disabilities have attained positions of power and prominence within the field of rehabilitation, they are exceptions. As compared to other women in this society, women with disabilities are more often unemployed, receive lower salaries, and are less likely to marry than persons of either gender who do not have disabilities, or men who do. Among those who marry, the percentage of divorces or separations is greater for women with disabilities than for women without disabilities and for men with or without disabilities (Hanna & Rogovsky, 1991).

The gender bias that women with disabilities experience extends to the provision and outcomes of rehabilitation services. An internal study conducted by state vocational rehabilitation agencies in Illinois, Indiana, Michigan, Ohio, and Wisconsin (Region V) revealed the effect of this bias in the delivery of rehabilitation services:

> Whereas women constitute approximately 53 percent of the U.S. population and 40 percent of the full-time workforce, their per capita earnings are only 64 percent of men's. After being served by the VR (vocational rehabilitation) system, women find that this income differential is *not* eliminated or even reduced. Moreover, unlike closed male clients, their postclosure income does not, on the average, put them above the defined poverty level [*Rehab Brief,* 1988].

There has been much speculation as to the source of this gender-specific bias as it affects women in rehabilitation. Harlan Hahn (1988) has pointed out that disability as a distinguishing characteristic has a greater overall negative—that is, stigmatizing—effect than have racial, religious, ethnic, or gender group membership. He contends that the continued greater oppression experienced by persons with disabilities, compared to the overt gains in social acceptance and status by members of other minority groups, stems from the

> prevalent assumptions of their biological inferiority. Whereas a major thrust of social science research on other minorities during the last century has been to refute such assumptions and to demonstrate that their unequal status stems primarily from prejudicial attitudes, many . . . popular images of disabled individuals continue to harbor presuppositions of inferiority based on their functional incapacities.

In the mind of the general public the term "disability" is synonymous with "the inability to perform any adult social function." Therefore, in contrast to, for example, an African American who, when successful, is perceived as successful and black, when a person with a disability is perceived as successful, he or she is no longer perceived as disabled. The interaction of disability and gender, which appears to result in a greater degree of stigma or devaluation for women than for men, may result in women being perceived as less functionally capable than men, regardless of men's specific physical, emotional, or cognitive limitations. The degree of devaluation that women experience may stem primarily from the actual or perceived effect of their disability on their ascribed social roles—that is, the reproductive, the nurturant, and secondarily, the economic role women are still assigned in society today (Fine & Asch, 1981).

Despite the fact that men and women appear to be treated equitably during the rehabilitation process, there is a marked discrepancy in rehabilitation outcomes, depending on gender. In the longitudinal study conducted in Region V (Danek, 1992; *Rehab Brief*, 1988), no significant differences were found between the genders in regard to the total number of services provided or resources used, the amount of case monies spent, or time spent completing the rehabilitation process.

There were, however, significant differences in rehabilitation outcomes. Although overall more women were considered successful rehabilitants than men (67% to 63%), fewer women were in competitive employment (45% to 53%) and far more had their cases successfully closed as homemakers (15% to 3%) "even when in half those cases . . . the original employment objective was not homemaking" (Danek, 1992). Among those in competitive employment, approximately twice as many women as men (15% to 7%) were employed in clerical-sales occupations, and more women than men in service occupations (15% to 10%).

This apparent funneling of women into traditional occupations may account for the gender disparity in reported earnings at the time of job placement. Women earned an average of $4,814 and men $7,212 at the time their cases were determined to be closed successfully (*Rehab Brief*, 1988).

Are these discrepant rehabilitation outcomes primarily the result of gender bias by those who provide rehabilitation services, or are these outcomes largely due to conscious client choices? For women the perceived inability to perform sanctioned social roles may enhance the value of social roles that other women may be trying to avoid or redefine. Michelle Fine and Adrienne Asch (1981) suggest that women with disabilities more often subscribe to traditional roles than other women because these roles, even with their constraints, are seen as potentially more satisfying than the rolelessness or sense of neglect, invisibility, and pow-

erlessness these women experience in the absence of sanctioned social roles.

For those who reject the rolelessness ascribed them and choose options other than those offered by the traditional stereotype of what it means to be a woman in our society—weak, passive, and dependent—their disability will impact on the attribution of those nonstereotypic behaviors. In the judgment of others, the choice and the effort to become a successful professional or to live independently may be viewed not as a choice but merely as a consequence of having a disabling condition, that is, being unable to assume one's "proper" social role.

It is important to realize, however, that disability can be freeing as well as limiting. When one is deemed incapable of fulfilling social expectations, one can more easily shed the shackles of social demands. On the one hand, rolelessness can contribute to unemployment or underemployment, to low-status occupations, and to low levels of income. On the other hand, however, rolelessness can present an opportunity to define oneself, to make self-generated rather than other-generated choices. When one is already deemed a social misfit, one no longer risks becoming a social outcast by making those same decisions. By defining the situation, the disability has provided the option. The choice then becomes that of the woman with the disability, whether hindered or abetted by those who could provide her with the chance to attain maximum benefits from rehabilitation services.

Conclusion

Despite the women's movement with its attempts to demolish gender stereotyping and with its success in fostering women's entrance into men's former vocational bastions, women who are deemed capable still are assigned the role of nurturing caregiver and concierge within the family unit.

Perhaps it's time to move beyond gender-assigned or gender-assumed roles to roles determined by preference. Does one prefer and have the requisite ability and psychological stamina to direct the bulk of one's energies to career growth and development in competitive employment? Or does one prefer and have the requisite ability and psychological stamina to direct the bulk of one's energies into a supportive role that underwrites someone else's career path in the competitive arena? Individual choice and career preference, not gender or disability status, should be the factors that determine one's status, not only in rehabilitation but in every facet of our multifaceted lives as well.

(*See also:* ATTITUDES; CAREGIVING; CONSUMERS; FAMILY; HISTORY OF REHABILITATION; KELLER, HELEN; SOCIOLOGY; SWITZER, MARY E.; WORK)

BIBLIOGRAPHY

BARUCH, GRACE; BEINER, LOIS; and BARNETT, ROSALIND. "Women and Gender in Research on Work and Family Stress." *American Psychologist* 42 (1987):130–136.

COTTONE, LAURA P., and COTTONE, R. ROCCO. "Women with Disabilities: On the Paradox of Empowerment and the Need for a Trans-systemic and Feminist Perspective." *Journal of Applied Rehabilitation Counseling* 23 (1992):20–25.

DANEK, MARITA M. "The Status of Women with Disabilities Revisited." *Journal of Applied Rehabilitation Counseling* 23 (1992):7–13.

DATOFF, VILIA. "Women in Rehabilitation Management," unpublished manuscript. Washington, DC, 1983.

DUNHAM, JEROME R., and DUNHAM, CHARLIS S. "Psychosocial Aspects of Disability." In *Disability and Rehabilitation Handbook*, eds. R. M. Goldenson, J. Dunham, and C. Dunham. New York, 1978.

FINE, MICHELLE, and ASCH, ADRIENNE. "Disabled Women: Sexism Without the Pedestal." *Journal of Sociology and Social Welfare* 8 (1981):233–248.

HAHN, HARLAN. "The Politics of Physical Differences: Disability and Discrimination." *Journal of Social Issues* 44 (1988):39–47.

HANNA, WILLIAM J., and ROGOVSKY, BETSY. "Women with Disabilities: Two Handicaps Plus." *Disability, Handicap, and Society* 6 (1991):49–62.

HARRIS, RICHARD. "Musings from 20 Years of Hard-Earned Experience." *Rehabilitation Education* 6 (1992):207–212.

KERR, NANCY. "Staff Expectations for Disabled Persons: Helpful or Harmful?" *Rehabilitation Counseling Bulletin* 14 (1970):85–94.

MURRAY, SUSAN E., and KEENAN, DEBORAH. "The Role of Women as Leaders in Rehabilitation: Changing to Meet the Times." *Journal of Applied Rehabilitation Counseling* 23 (1992):34–38.

MYERS, JANE E., and WEDL, LOIS C. "Women in Rehabilitation: Publication Track Records." *Journal of Rehabilitation* 51 (1985):63–66.

PERLMAN, LEONARD, and ARNESON, KATHERYNE. *Women and Rehabilitation of Disabled Persons*. Washington, DC, 1982.

REGION V WOMEN'S STUDY GROUP. *Region V Study: Access, Services, and Benefits in Rehabilitation*. Menomonie, WI, 1987.

Rehab Brief. "Gender Bias in Vocational Rehabilitation Services." Washington, DC, 1988.

SAVAGE, KAREN M., and PALMISANO, JAMES M., eds. *Professional Careers Sourcebook*, 3rd ed. Detroit, MI, 1994.

CHARLENE POCH DELOACH

WORK

Much has been written about the importance of work to the psychological and economic health of the individual. Work is defined as "activity in which one exerts strength or faculties to do or perform something; sustained physical or mental effort to overcome obstacles and achieve an objective or a result; the labor, task, or duty that is one's accustomed means of livelihood" (Merriam-Webster, 1993). George N. Wright (1980) defines work as "goal-directed activity for social, economic, or other desired accomplishment or outcome." According to Wright (p. 343), the most important thing about work "is not remuneration but its activity and product." Different facets of these definitions are worthy of discussion. Work is designed to use one's "strengths or faculties," it is designed to have an outcome to achieve an objective or result, and one is accustomed to remuneration for that activity. All three facets of this definition are important to a study of the value of work to humans and its implications for rehabilitation.

Recognition of the Importance of Work to Health. A recognition of the intrinsic value of work to human health and life satisfaction has been growing. Kathleen J. Pottick (1989) traces references to the importance of work to human health by major psychological theorists since the 1890s. Sigmund Freud is cited as recognizing love and work as the basic requirements of human existence. Alfred Adler is noted to have been a theorist who contended that every human being has three main ties that constitute reality: the social, the sexual, and the occupational. Eric Erikson stressed the importance of work in conveying a primary sense of selfhood. Robert L. Kahn (1981) further illustrates the existence of intrinsic rewards to work by citing studies conducted by the Institute for Social Research. These studies have shown that work provides individuals with social relationships and life direction that cause the majority of workers sampled to respond that they would work even if they did not have the financial need to do so.

An expanded understanding of how work has meaning to the greater whole of people, and how people relate to their work environment, was provided by Frederick Herzberg (1966). Herzberg identified hygiene factors and motivation factors that affect people's overall satisfaction or dissatisfaction with their workplace. Level and quality of supervision, personnel policies and administrative procedures, overall working conditions, and interpersonal relationships with peers were identified as hygiene factors that can influence people's sense of dissatisfaction with their workplace. The factors identified by Herzberg as motivators for workers were achievement, the nature of the work itself, level of responsibility, the possibility for advancement and growth afforded the person, and recognition of the value of the work. Herzberg also discussed the relationship of these factors to the person's level of mental health as well as overall job satisfaction.

Recognition of Work as Therapy. In the field of rehabilitation, work itself has been used as a form of therapy or treatment that "uses the work experience to change the work personality so that the rehabilitant can function appropriately in a normal work situation" (Wright, 1980, p. 343). Thus work has been seen as having intrinsic value in and of itself, and also as a means to prepare an individual for return to the workplace subsequent to disability. Various forms of "work therapy" have been used for these purposes. Vocational rehabilitation and occupational therapy have both used work as a form of therapy to restore a person to full vocational functioning. What has been integrally important in the use of work as a therapeutic medium is a recognition of the importance of treating the whole person, looking at the skills and interests of the individual and also at the interface between the person and the

work environment. For example, Janette Schkade and Sally Schultz (1992) provide a model of occupation that presents adaptation as a change that occurs within the person's developmental structure as a result of their occupation or relationship to the world of work; these authors then apply this concept to the effective professional functioning of occupational therapists.

Clinical mental health-related disciplines also have recognized the importance of work-related feelings, thoughts, and behaviors to an individual's global mental health. Thus increasingly attention has been given to the preparation of mental health professionals to enhance understanding of the influence of work on psychological well-being and therefore on the practice of psychotherapy. The importance of the application of mental health professional functioning in the world of work has been discussed in the field of social work, for example (Mudrick, 1991; Pottick, 1989).

The Rehabilitation Act of 1973 mandated the serving of people with severe disabilities. Work adjustment services have been seen as one strategy to facilitate either the initial integration or the reintegration of individuals with severe disabilities into the workplace (Glynn et al., 1992). In the 1970s, a curriculum of training and a certification process for the professionals who provide work adjustment services were created in recognition of the importance of this function (Coffey & Ellien, 1979). The Commission on Accreditation of Rehabilitation Facilities (1991, p. 80), in its *Standard Manual*, defines work adjustment as "a transitional, time-limited, systematic training program which assists persons toward their optimal level of vocational development." This kind of therapeutic approach uses either real or simulated work to help the individual with a disability in understanding the meaning, value, and demands of the work environment. Some of the structured activities of work adjustment programs have been to learn or reestablish skills, attitudes, personal characteristics, work behaviors, and functional capacities that the individual with disability would need in the work environment. The work adjustment program is not necessarily designed to provide specific skill building for placement in a particular job title or job family, but rather the characteristics and attitudes that will enable the worker to be successful in the overall work environment. That such a separate program exists as a form of treatment is a statement about the recognition of the behaviors and attitudes of people as key elements for a successful vocational outcome, and also of the creation of a contextual work environment that can be therapeutic in and of itself.

Another therapeutic use of the work environment can be seen in work hardening programs. These programs are interdisciplinary and use the services of a variety of different professionals, such as occupational therapists, physical therapists, physiatrists, rehabilitation psychologists, and vocational rehabilitation counselors to provide an integrated service. Such programs use conditioning tasks that are graded progressively to "improve the biomechanical, neuromuscular, cardiovascular/metabolic, psychosocial functioning of the person served, in conjunction with real or simulated work activities" (Commission on Accreditation of Rehabilitation Facilities, 1991, p. 71). Work hardening programs are in either real or simulated work environments and provide a transition between acute care and return to work. They seek to address issues of productivity, safety, physical tolerances, and worker behaviors in a highly structured, goal-oriented, individualized treatment program designed to maximize the person's ability to return to work.

Several evolving concepts in the world of work have implications for the functioning of professionals in vocational rehabilitation: increasing awareness of the importance of examining work satisfaction and career development for people with disabilities, the importance of appropriate job-person match and an appreciation of skills in a diverse workforce, appropriate and expanded use of vocational evaluation, and factors in assessing quality of employment and quality of life.

Work Satisfaction and Career Development for People with Disabilities. A number of conceptualizations of job satisfaction are based on the notion that the match between the individual's needs, goals, and/or values and the rewards provided by the work environment determines, in large part, the job satisfaction expressed by the individual. However, the results of a study conducted by Vida Scarpello and John P. Campbell (1983) indicate that individual differences in aspiration level and different views of

career progression may also contribute to job satisfaction levels. This factor is most significant to the field of rehabilitation. Historically, a focus on job placement approaches for people with disabilities has often been put on fitting the person into the existing workplace, rather than starting the vocational rehabilitation process from a career development perspective. "A coming frontier for innovation in employment practices for people with disabilities is career advancement. . . . Interventions and access to mainstream training and services that provide the worker with a disability with the knowledge and skills to advance into managerial and higher-level jobs could well be the next area for advocacy and service delivery" (Greenwood, 1990, p. 14).

The sequence of employment throughout one's working life is called a "career." According to *Merriam-Webster's Collegiate Dictionary*, 10th ed., a career is "a profession for which one trains and which is undertaken as a permanent calling." George N. Wright (1980) defines career as the total pattern of vocational events over a person's lifetime, including the sequence of jobs engaged in while progressing in an occupational structure or changing from one position, job, or occupation to another. The concept of career has utility in rehabilitation both in understanding where the worker has come from in his or her work-related history, and in putting together a plan for vocational preparation and job placement in the context of the vocational rehabilitation process.

Supported employment programs were funded under the 1986 amendments for the 1973 Rehabilitation Act, providing long-term services to help moderately and severely disabled individuals to find a job, learn the job, and sustain employment. Under this program, large numbers of individuals who historically were not considered eligible for employment are now able to access integrated work sites for the first time (Brodsky, 1990). A more recent extension of this legislated protection for persons with disabilities in the workplace is the Americans with Disabilities Act of 1990 (ADA). The ADA extends civil rights protections, similar to those previously offered to persons on the basis of sex, race, or religion, to persons with disabilities. Even though the ADA has been cited as the most significant piece of nondiscrimination legislation since the Civil Rights

Act of 1964, some of the most significant barriers, both to initial employment for persons with severe disabilities and to ongoing career enhancement opportunities, remain. These are the perceptions of employers, coworkers, and perhaps even the rehabilitation specialists themselves who support these individuals in employment settings.

Research by James W. Black and Luanna H. Meyer (1992) to test for differences in judgments about the value of employment training for persons with different levels of disability by a variety of respondent groups found significant differences in the perceptions of the desirability of providing employment training to a person based on his or her disability. The researchers studied the different ratings of managers, rehabilitation counselors, teachers, parents, coworkers, and policymakers. In this study, ratings of future teachers of students with disabilities were significantly more positive about the value of employment training for persons with severe disabilities than those of potential coworkers and business managers, and to a somewhat lesser extent, those of rehabilitation counselors and policymakers. The implications of this social valuing for the training of rehabilitation professionals are significant. If we are to pursue the concepts of job satisfaction and career development for persons with severe disabilities, we must understand more about the perceptions of different groups toward persons with disabilities, and how social valuation may affect opportunities for initial employment for persons with severe disabilities and later career enhancement possibilities. The expectations of rehabilitation professionals on job placement and career development opportunities for people with severe disabilities may have the initial impact on successful vocational outcomes.

Job-Person Match and Cultural Diversity. Change has begun to occur in how people are matched to jobs. Dissatisfaction in the workplace and its incumbent problems of increased health care costs, turnover, and absences have encouraged leaders in business and industry to look for alternative ways to get the right workers in the appropriate positions. Traditionally, a job has been defined by using a job description, the policies and procedures of an organization, and the goals and objectives of the positions to identify specific tasks that actually must be performed daily or weekly. The job has more or less

been treated as somewhat "fixed" and the person treated as "variable" to match his or her respective skills, education, and experience to do the job sought (Dortch, 1989). In general, the field of rehabilitation has over the years followed suit in this job-person match approach. Persons with disabilities were slotted into existing openings in a given community, often in entry-level jobs with little opportunity to maximize use of their own interests and skills or in building options for long-term career ladders. Protection against segregation of persons with disabilities into entry-level jobs and nondiscrimination in all facets of employment are afforded by the Americans with Disabilities Act. The act also presents the concept of reasonable accommodation to all private employers, requiring them, on a case-by-case basis, to assess the accommodation needs of a particular qualified employee with a disability for a job where he or she can perform the essential functions. The provisions of the ADA again affirm the importance of looking at the individual skills, characteristics, and accommodation needs of a person with a disability, and matching those to the requirements of a particular position.

Just as each job has a what and a how, so all employees bring a set of skills, abilities, and aptitudes that they want to apply to their new position. Their personal preferences and interests influence how they design the priorities of the position and therefore the effectiveness of their work behavior. Awareness of the importance of making maximum use of the skills and abilities of each individual in the workplace has been further expanded with an awareness by companies of the importance of working effectively with a culturally diverse workforce. More and more companies are trying to attract women returners, employees from ethnic minorities, older workers, and people with disabilities to help offset the effects of the demographic downturn. In this increasingly diverse work culture, greater emphasis is placed on changing personnel practices and recruitment strategies to acknowledge a wider array of skills, and a broader perspective of assets of individuals for given positions (Paddison, 1990). In their effort to place persons with severe disabilities in integrated employment settings, rehabilitation professionals can build on this emerging new ethic by seeking out potential employers whose personnel recruitment and career development policies foster appreciation of diversity in the workplace, therefore providing expanded opportunities for people with disabilities.

Appropriate and Expanded Use of Vocational Evaluation. Historically, vocational evaluation has been used to determine the potential of an individual for specific occupations or groups of occupations in competitive employment. The process of vocational evaluation grew up in the rehabilitation facility movement in this country in the 1950s and 1960s (Corthell & Griswold, 1987). Various pieces of legislation provided funding for the establishment of rehabilitation facilities and greatly enhanced the growth of vocational evaluation. Subsequent legislation provided funding for rehabilitation training, vocational evaluation, and work adjustment services. Since the mid-1970s, changes in philosophy toward vocational exploration for people with disabilities, empowerment of persons with disabilities, and advanced medical and assistive device technologies have influenced thinking about the usefulness of vocational evaluation. Critics of vocational evaluation express concern that in traditional vocational rehabilitation processes each person with a disability receives the same standard evaluation regardless of his or her disability or particular situation. Another concern is that traditional evaluation relies too heavily on simulated rather than real work as a means of predicting job success (Corthell & Griswold, 1987). This concern is also evident in occupational therapy, where some authors critique work evaluations for their lack of attention to the meaning of work to persons (Velozo, 1993).

Such increased sensitivity to a needed expansion of factors for consideration in vocational assessment has provided a necessary broadening of the concept of vocational evaluation. For persons with more severe disabilities, standardized testing may not provide sufficient information for designing an effective assessment of what training and long-term supports are needed. Expanded methods of evaluation may be required that focus on direct observation in job settings, employing greater use of situational assessments and careful job analysis of specific jobs to create a good job match. The focus of situational assessments is similar to that in more traditional vocational evaluations—that is, helping to develop useful information to assist individuals in determining long-range career goals.

Factors in Assessing Quality of Employment and Quality of Life. As previously discussed, contemporary thinking recognizes that job satisfaction is an interplay between factors in the work environment and the needs and motivations of individual workers. Historically, theorists such as Frederick Herzberg have contributed to an understanding of some of these factors. A more recent, journalistic rather than scientific approach has been heralded by Robert Levering and Milton Moskowitz, who periodically list the hundred best companies in America to work for. Ratings for the companies are based on the following criteria: pay and benefits, promotional opportunities, job security, pride in work and company, openness and fairness, and camaraderie and friendship (Levering & Moskowitz, 1993). Levering and Moskowitz believe that workplaces improve with genuine employee participation; greater sensitivity to work and family issues; increased sharing of company wealth through profit-sharing, gain-sharing, and employee stock ownership programs; incorporation of fun into the corporate mission; and development of trust between employees and management that requires treating employees as meaningful contributors to the company.

This expanded concept of job satisfaction and related quality-of-work life variables that are valued by workers today need to be addressed in the rehabilitation service delivery system. An example of a study that reflects this needed attention is one conducted by Ellen S. Fabian (1992), investigating the quality of life for 110 individuals with severe mental illness participating in a supported employment experience. Results of this study showed that subjective quality-of-life indices for persons with disabilities increased as a result of job placement; however, social or leisure activities that were also measured did not increase. This may suggest that for persons with disabilities to make use of all of the above-mentioned factors in quality of employment, supports in addition to traditional ones found now in supported employment may need to be put in place to maximize the ability of individuals with disability to take advantage of the many elements that constitute work satisfaction as we understand it.

Implications for Rehabilitation Practice. Too often, job placement has occurred expediently, where the job-person match occurs because of a job vacancy, rather than the best application of the skills and interests of the individual. Both job satisfaction and opportunities for career enhancement will be maximized with better vocational assessments and with enhanced attention to long-term career development for persons with disabilities. The likelihood of a successful job-person match will be heightened with the application of expanded vocational evaluation strategies, including situational assessment.

Education and Training of Rehabilitation Professionals. Some of the contemporary thinking on work both philosophically and operationally has implications for current curricula and the preparation of rehabilitation counselors, vocational evaluators, and other rehabilitation specialists. Expanded concepts of vocational evaluation, including situational assessment, are important to build into preparation for rehabilitation professionals taking courses in vocational evaluation and work assessment. In addition, increased emphasis must be placed on career enhancement and opportunities for persons with severe disabilities in vocational assessment, job placement, and supported employment-related courses. One noted issue that has implications for the training of rehabilitation professionals is attitudinal barriers in the workplace, and perhaps even in the professional rehabilitationists themselves; these continue to be obstacles to the full realization of the vocational potential of persons with disabilities. It is therefore imperative that rehabilitation educators and trainers address this issue when providing training, alerting professionals to the limitations that they themselves may place on the range of opportunities for persons with disabilities, and to attitudinal barriers that may be encountered in the workplace by the worker with a disability.

Implications for Research. Several contemporary issues in the world of work and persons with disabilities are worthy of further study. Some of these are: the quality of current placements and their contribution to both the psychological and economic health of individuals; the impact of discriminatory attitudes toward persons with disabilities of supervisors and employees in the workplace; and job satisfaction factors and their implications for job placement and career enhancement for persons with disabilities. Research is needed to look at outcome data from vocational rehabilitation placements that assess the quality of the job match for the particular skills and interests of the person with the disability, job satisfaction in terms of a tangible outcome in the work being done, and the appropriateness of the remuneration the individual is being paid for the work done.

(*See also:* AMERICANS WITH DISABILITIES ACT; CAREER COUNSELING; DISABILITY MANAGEMENT; EMPLOYEE ASSISTANCE PROGRAM; JOB PLACEMENT; LABOR UNIONS; OCCUPATIONAL INFORMATION; QUALITY OF LIFE; SUPPORTED EMPLOYMENT; VOCATIONAL EVALUATION; WELLNESS)

BIBLIOGRAPHY

BLACK, JAMES W., and MEYER, LUANNA H. "But . . . Is It Really Work? Social Validity of Employment Training for Persons with Severe Disabilities." *American Journal on Mental Retardation* 96 (1992):463–474.

BRODSKY, MELVIN. "Employment Programs for Disabled Youth: An International View." *Monthly Labour Review* 113 (1990):50–52.

COFFEY, DARRELL D., and ELLIEN, VALERIE J. *Work Adjustment Curriculum Development Project: A Summary.* Menomonie, WI, 1979.

COMMISSION ON ACCREDITATION OF REHABILITATION FACILITIES. *Standard Manual for Organizations Serving People with Disabilities.* Tucson, AZ, 1991.

CORTHELL, DAVID W., and GRISWOLD, PETER P. *The Use of Vocational Evaluation in VR: The Fourteenth Institute on Rehabilitation Issues.* Menomonie, WI, 1987.

DORTCH, C. THOMAS. "Job-Person Match." *Personnel Journal* 68 (1989):49–61.

FABIAN, ELLEN S. "Supported Employment and the Quality of Life: Does a Job Make a Difference?" *Rehabilitation Counseling Bulletin* 36 (1992):84–97.

GLYNN, SHIRLEY M.; RANDOLPH, EUGENIA T.; ETH, SPENCER; PAZ, GEORGE G.; LEONG, GREGORY B.; SHANER, ANDREW L.; and VAN VORT, WALTER. "Schizophrenic Symptoms, Work Adjustment, and Behavioral Family Therapy." *Rehabilitation Psychology* 37 (1992):323–338.

GREENWOOD, REED. "Employment and Disability: Emerging Issues for the 1990s." In *Employment and Disability: Trends and Issues for the 1990s: A Report on the Fourteenth Mary E. Switzer Memorial Seminar,* eds. Leonard Pearlman and Carl E. Hansen. Alexandria, VA, 1990.

HERZBERG, FREDERICK. *Work and the Nature of Man.* New York, 1966.

KAHN, ROBERT L. *Work and Health.* New York, 1981.

LEVERING, ROBERT, and MOSKOWITZ, MILTON. *The One Hundred Best Companies to Work for in America.* New York, 1993.

MUDRICK, NANCY R. "An Underdeveloped Role for Occupational Social Work: Facilitating the Employment of People with Disabilities." *Social Work* 36 (1991):490–495.

PADDISON, LORRAINE. "The Targeted Approach to Recruitment." *Personnel Mangement* 22 (1990):54–58.

POTTICK, KATHLEEN J. "The Work Role as a Major Life Role." *Social Casework: The Journal of Contemporary Social Work,* Oct. 1989, pp. 488–494.

SCARPELLO, VIDA, and CAMPBELL, JOHN P. "Job Satisfaction and the Fit Between Individual Needs and Organizational Rewards." *Journal of Occupational Psychology* 56 (1983):315–328.

SCHKADE, JANETTE P., and SCHULTZ, SALLY. "Occupational Adaptation: Toward a Holistic Approach for Contemporary Practice," Part 1. *The Journal of Occupational Therapy* 46 (1992):829–837.

VELOZO, CRAIG A. "Work Evaluations: Critique of the State of the Art of Functional Assessment of Work." *The American Journal of Occupational Therapy* 47 (1993):203–209.

WRIGHT, GEORGE N. *Total Rehabilitation.* Boston, 1980.

SUSANNE M. BRUYÈRE
JOYCE A. HOYING

List of Resources

AARP Disability Initiative
601 E Street NW
Washington, DC 20049

ABLEDATA Database Program
Macro International
8455 Colesville Road, Suite 935
Silver Spring, MD 20910-3319

ACCESS: The Foundation for Accessibility by the
Disabled
P.O. Box 356
Malverne, NY 11565

Access to Respite Care and Help (ARCH)
800 Eastowne Drive
Suite 105
Chapel Hill, NC 27514

ADA Materials Development Project Relating to
Employment
Cornell University
106 ILR Extension
Ithaca, NY 14853-3901

Adaptive Environments Center
374 Congress Street
Suite 301
Boston, MA 02110

Al-Anon Family Group Headquarters, Inc.
P.O. Box 862, Midtown Station
New York, NY 10018

Alcoholism and Drug Treatment Addiction Center
The McDonald Center for Alcoholism and Drug Addiction
Department of Behavioral Medicine
Scripps Memorial Hospital
9888 Genesee Avenue
La Jolla, CA 92037

Alexander Graham Bell Association for the Deaf
3417 Volta Place NW
Washington, DC 20007

Alliance of Genetic Support Groups
35 Wisconsin Circle, Suite 440
Chevy Chase, MD 20815

Alzheimer's Association
919 North Michigan Avenue
Suite 1000
Chicago, IL 60611

Alzheimer's Disease Education and Referral (ADEAR)
Center
P.O. Box 8250
Silver Spring, MD 20907-8250

American Academy of Orthotists and Prosthetists
1650 King Street
Alexandria, VA 22314

American Academy of Physical Medicine and
Rehabilitation (AAPM&R)
122 South Michigan Avenue
Suite 1300
Chicago, IL 60603-6107

American Alliance for Health, Physical Education,
Recreation and Dance (AAHPERD)
1900 Association Drive
Reston, VA 22091

American Amputee Foundation, Inc. (AAF)
P.O. Box 250218
Little Rock, AR 72225

American Anorexia/Bulimia Association, Inc.
418 East 76th Street
New York, NY 10021

American Art Therapy Association (AATA)
1202 Allanson Road
Mundelein, IL 60060

American Association for Music Therapy (AAMT)
P.O. Box 80012
Valley Forge, PA 19484

American Association for Respiratory Care (AARC)
11030 Ables Lane
Dallas, TX 75229

American Association of Kidney Patients (AAKP)
111 South Parker Street

Suite 405
Tampa, FL 33606

American Association of Pastoral Counselors (AAPC)
9504A Lee Highway
Fairfax, VA 22031

American Association of People with Disabilities (AAPD)
4401 Connecticut Avenue
Suite 223
Washington, DC 20008

American Association of Spinal Cord Injury Nurses
(AASCIN)
75-20 Astoria Boulevard
Jackson Heights, NY 11370-1177

American Association of the Deaf-Blind
814 Thayer Avenue
Suite 302
Silver Spring, MD 20910

American Athletic Association of the Deaf (AAAD)
3607 Washington Boulevard
Ogden, UT 84403-1731

American Bar Association (ABA)
1800 M Street NW
Washington, DC 20036

American Blind Bowling Association
411 Sheriff Street
Mercer, PA 16137

American Blind Skiing Foundation
610 South William Street
Mt. Prospect, IL 60056

American Board for Certification in Orthotics
and Prosthetics (ABC)
1650 King Street
Suite 500
Alexandria, VA 22314

American Burn Association
New York Hospital Cornell Medical Center
525 East 68th Street, Room L-706
New York, NY 10021

American Camping Association (ACA)
Bradford Woods
5000 State Road 67 North
Martinsville, IN 46151-7902

American Cancer Society (ACS)
National Office
1599 Clifton Road NE
Atlanta, GA 30329

American Chronic Pain Association (ACPA)
P.O. Box 850
Rocklin, CA 95677

American Congress of Rehabilitation Medicine (ACRM)
Association Management Center

5700 Old Orchard Road
Skokie, IL 60077-1057

American Council of the Blind (ACB)
1155 15th Street NW
Suite 720
Washington, DC 20005

American Council on Rural Special Education (ACRES)
221 Milton Bennion Hall
Department of Special Education
University of Utah
Salt Lake City, UT 84112

American Counseling Association (ACA)
5999 Stevenson Avenue
Alexandria, VA 22304

American Dance Therapy Association (ADTA)
2000 Century Plaza
Suite 108
Columbia, MD 21044

American Deafness and Rehabilitation Association
(ADARA)
P.O. Box 251554
Little Rock, AR 72225

American Diabetes Association, Inc. (ADA)
National Center
1660 Duke Street
Alexandria, VA 22314

American Disability Prevention and Wellness Association
18113 Town Center Drive
Olney, MD 20832

American Disabled for Attendant Programs Today
(ADAPT)
12 Broadway
Denver, CO 80203

American Epilepsy Society (AES)
638 Prospect Avenue
Hartford, CT 06105

American Foundation for the Blind (AFB)
15 West 16th Street
New York, NY 10011

American Geriatrics Society (AGS)
770 Lexington Avenue
Suite 300
New York, NY 10021

American Heart Association (AHA)
7272 Greenville Avenue
Dallas, TX 75231

American Kidney Fund, Inc.
6110 Executive Boulevard
Suite 1010
Rockville, MD 20852

The American Liver Foundation
1425 Pompton Avenue
Cedar Grove, NJ 07009

American Lung Association (ALA)
1740 Broadway
New York, NY 10019

The American Lupus Society (TALS)
3914 Del Amo Boulevard, Suite 922
Torrance, CA 90503

American Occupational Therapy Association (AOTA)
1383 Piccard Drive
P.O. Box 1725
Rockville, MD 20849

American Orthotic and Prosthetic Association (AOPA)
1650 King Street
Suite 500
Alexandria, VA 22314

American Pain Society (APS)
5700 Old Orchard Road
First Floor
Skokie, IL 60077-1057

American Paralysis Association (APA)
500 Morris Avenue
Springfield, NJ 07081

American Parkinson Disease Association (APDA)
60 Bay Street
Staten Island, NY 10301

American Physical Therapy Association (APTA)
1111 North Fairfax Street
Alexandria, VA 22314

American Printing House for the Blind (APH)
1839 Frankfort Avenue
P.O. Box 6085
Louisville, KY 40206

American Psychiatric Association (APA)
Division of Public Affairs
1400 K Street NW
Washington, DC 20005

American Red Cross
National Headquarters
17th & D Streets NW
Washington, DC 20006

American Rehabilitation Association (ARA)
P.O. Box 17675
Washington, DC 20041

American Rehabilitation Counseling Association (ARCA)
5999 Stevenson Avenue
Alexandria, VA 22304

American Self-Help Clearinghouse
St. Clares-Riverside Medical Center
Denville, NJ 07834

American Sickle Cell Anemia Association (ASCAA)
10300 Carnegie Avenue
Cleveland, OH 44106

American Sledge Hockey Association (ASHA)
10933 Johnson Avenue South
Bloomington, MN 55437

American Society of Plastic and Reconstructive Surgeons
(ASPRS)
444 East Algonquin Road
Arlington Heights, IL 60005

American Speech-Language-Hearing Association (ASHA)
10801 Rockville Pike
Rockville, MD 20852

American Spinal Injury Association (ASIA)
345 East Superior Street
Room 1436
Chicago, IL 60611

Americans with Disabilities Act: Implementation
and Evaluation
Suffolk University
Department of Public Management
Eight Ashburton Place
Boston, MA 02108-2770

American Tinnitus Association (ATA)
P.O. Box 5
Portland, OR 97207

American Trauma Society (ATS)
8903 Presidential Parkway
Suite 512
Upper Marlboro, MD 20772-2656

American Veterans of World War II, Korea, and Vietnam
(AMVETS)
4647 Forbes Boulevard
Lanham, MD 20706-4380

American Wheelchair Archers (AWA)
5318 Northport Drive
Brooklyn Center, MN 55429

American Wheelchair Bowling Association
3620 Tamarack Drive
Redding, CA 96003

The American Wheelchair Table Tennis Association
(AWTTA)
23 Parker Street
Port Chester, NY 10573

Amyotrophic Lateral Sclerosis Association (ALSA)
21021 Ventura Boulevard
Suite 321
Woodland Hills, CA 91364

Apple Computer, Inc.
Worldwide Disability Solutions Group
Mail Stop 38DS
1 Infinite Loop
Cupertino, CA 95014

Applications of Technology to the Rehabilitation of
Children with Orthopedic Disabilities

Rancho Los Amigos Medical Center
Los Amigos Research and Education Institute, Inc.
(LAREI)
7503 Bonita Street, Bonita Hall
Downey, CA 90242

The Arc
500 East Border Street
Arlington, TX 76010

The Arc/Baker International Resource Center for Down
Syndrome
The Keith Building
1621 Euclid Avenue
Suite 514
Cleveland, OH 44115

Architectural and Transportation Barriers Compliance
Board (ATBCB)
1331 F Street NW
Suite 1000
Washington, DC 20004

Arthritis Foundation
1314 Spring Street NW
Atlanta, GA 30309

Artificial Language Laboratory (ALL)
405 Computer Center
Michigan State University
East Lansing, MI 48824

Assessing Independent Living Center Capabilities to
Deliver ADA-Related Services
The Institute for Rehabilitation and Research
Independent Living Research Utilization
2323 South Shepherd
Suite 1000
Houston, TX 77019

Assistance Dog Institute
P.O. Box 2334
Rohnert Park, CA 94927-2334

Assisting Community-Based Rural Independent Living
Programs
The Institute for Rehabilitation and Research
Independent Living Research Utilization
2323 South Shepherd Street, Suite 1000
Houston, TX 77019

Associated Services for the Blind (ASB)
919 Walnut Street
Philadelphia, PA 19107

Association for Children with Down Syndrome, Inc.
(ACDS)
2616 Martin Avenue
Bellmore, NY 11710

Association for Habilitation and Employment of the
Developmentally Disabled (AHEDD)
3300 Trindle Road
Camp Hill, PA 17011-4432

Association for Macular Diseases, Inc. (AMD)
210 East 64th Street
New York, NY 10021

Association for Persons in Supported Employment (APSE)
5001 West Broad Street
Suite 34
Richmond, VA 23230

Association for the Care of Children's Health (ACCH)
7910 Woodmont Avenue
Suite 300
Bethesda, MD 20814

Association of Birth Defect Children, Inc. (ABDC)
5400 Diplomat Circle
Suite 270
Orlando, FL 32810

Association of Rehabilitation Nurses (ARN)
5700 Old Orchard Road
First Floor
Skokie, IL 60077-1057

Association of Sudden Infant Death Syndrome Program
Professionals (ASPP)
c/o Massachusetts Center for SIDS
Boston City Hospital
818 Harrison Avenue
Boston, MA 02118

Asthma and Allergy Foundation of America (AAFA)
1125 15th Street NW
Suite 502
Washington, DC 20005

AT&T Accessible Communications Products Center
(ACPC)
5 Woodhollow Road
Room 1119
Parsippany, NJ 07054

Autism National Committee
7 Teresa Circle
Arlington, MA 02174

Barrier Free Environments (BFE)
P.O. Box 30634
Water Garden
Highway 70 West
Raleigh, NC 27622

Beach Center on Families and Disability
The University of Kansas
Institute for Life Span Studies
3111 Haworth Hall
Lawrence, KS 66045

Blind Childrens Center (BCC)
4120 Marathon Street
P.O. Box 29159
Los Angeles, CA 90029

Blinded Veterans Association (BVA)
477 H Street NW
Washington, DC 20001

The Candlelighters Childhood Cancer Foundation
(CCCF)
7910 Woodmont Avenue
Suite 460
Bethesda, MD 20814-3015

The Caption Center
125 Western Avenue
Boston, MA 02134

Catholics United for Spiritual Action (CUSA)
176 West 8th Street
Bayonne, NJ 07002

CDC National AIDS Clearinghouse
P.O. Box 6003
Rockville, MD 20850

CDC National AIDS Hotline
American Social Health Association
P.O. Box 13827
Research Triangle Park, NC 27709

Center for Accessible Housing
North Carolina State University
Box 8613
Raleigh, NC 27695-8613

Center for Children with Chronic Illness and Disability
Division of General Pediatrics and Adolescent Health
University of Minnesota
420 Delaware Street
Minneapolis, MN 55455

Center for Recreation and Disability Studies in the
Curriculum in Leisure Studies and Recreation
Administration
CB #8145
730 Airport Road
Suite 204
The University of North Carolina at Chapel Hill
Chapel Hill, NC 27599-8145

Center for Rehabilitation Technology (CRT)
490-10th Street NW
Atlanta, GA 30332-0156

Center on Human Policy
Syracuse University
200 Huntington Hall
Syracuse, NY 13244

Charcot-Marie-Tooth Association (CMTA)
601 Upland Avenue
Upland, PA 19015

Children and Adults with Attention Deficit Disorders
(CHADD)
499 Northwest 70th Avenue
Suite 109
Plantation, FL 33317

Children's Hospice International (CHI)
700 Princess Street

Suite LL
Alexandria, VA 22314

Children's PKU Network (CPN)
10515 Vista Sorrento Parkway
San Diego, CA 92121

Clearinghouse on Child Abuse and Neglect Information
P.O. Box 1182
Washington, DC 20013-1182

Cleft Palate Foundation
1218 Grandview Avenue
Pittsburgh, PA 15211

Commission on Accreditation of Rehabilitation Facilities
(CARF)
101 North Wilmot Road
Suite 500
Tucson, AZ 85711

Cooley's Anemia Foundation, Inc.
129-09 26th Avenue
Flushing, NY 11354

Cooperative Wilderness Handicapped Outdoor Group
(CWHOG)
Idaho State University
Box 8118
Pond Student Union
Pocatello, ID 83209

Cornelia de Lange Syndrome Foundation
(CdLS Foundation)
60 Dyer Avenue
Collinsville, CT 06022-1273

The Council for Exceptional Children (CEC)
1920 Association Drive
Reston, VA 22091

Council of Citizens with Low Vision International
(CCLVI)
5707 Brockton Drive, Suite 302
Indianapolis, IN 46220-5481

Council of State Administrators of Vocational
Rehabilitation (CSAVR)
1055 Thomas Jefferson Street NW
P.O. Box 3776
Suite 401
Washington, DC 20007

Council on Rehabilitation Education, Inc. (CORE)
P.O. Box 1788
Champaign, IL 61824-1788

Courage Center
3915 Golden Valley Road
Golden Valley, MN 55422

Crohn's & Colitis Foundation of America, Inc. (CCFA)
386 Park Avenue South
New York, NY 10016

Cystic Fibrosis Foundation (CFF)
6931 Arlington Road
Bethesda, MD 20814

Deaf and Hard of Hearing Entrepreneurs Council
(DHHEC)
817 Silver Spring Avenue
Suite 305-F
Silver Spring, MD 20910-4617

The Deafness Research Foundation
9 East 38th Street
New York, NY 10016

Deafpride, Inc.
1350 Potomac Avenue SE
Washington, DC 20003

Delta Society
Service Dog Center
P.O. Box 1080
321 Burnett Avenue South, 3rd Floor
Renton, WA 98057-9906

Department of Veterans Affairs (VA)
810 Vermont Avenue NW
Washington, DC 20420

Disability Statistics Rehabilitation Research and Training
Center Institute for Health and Aging, UCSF
Box 0646, Laurel Heights
San Francisco, CA 94143-0646

Disabled American Veterans (DAV)
P.O. Box 14301
Cincinnati, OH 45250

Division of Birth Defects and Developmental Disabilities
Center for Environmental Health and Injury Control
Centers for Disease Control
1600 Clifton Road
Atlanta, GA 30333

Dogs for the Deaf, Inc.
10175 Wheeler Road
Central Point, OR 97502

Dysautonomia Foundation, Inc.
20 East 46 Street
Room 302
New York, NY 10017

Epilepsy Foundation of America (EFA)
4351 Garden City Drive
Landover, MD 20785

ERIC Clearinghouse on Disabilities and Gifted Education
(ERIC/EC)
Council for Exceptional Children (CEC)
1920 Association Drive
Reston, VA 22091

Eye Bank Association of America, Inc. (EBAA)
1001 Connecticut Avenue NW

Suite 601
Washington, DC 20036-5504

FacioScapuloHumeral Society, Inc. (FSH Society, Inc.)
c/o Carol A. Perez
3 Westwood Road
Lexington, MA 02173

Families of Spinal Muscular Atrophy (SMA)
P.O. Box 1465
Highland Park, IL 60035

The Family Caregiver Alliance (FCA)
425 Bush Street
Suite 500
San Francisco, CA 94108

Fanconi Anemia Research Fund, Inc. (FA)
66 Club Road
Suite 390
Eugene, OR 97401

Federal Transit Administration (FTA)
400 7th Street SW
Room 9400
Washington, DC 20590

FES Information Center
11000 Cedar Avenue
Suite 322
Cleveland, OH 44106

Foundation for Hospice and Homecare
513 C Street NE
Stanton Park
Washington, DC 20002

Gallaudet University
800 Florida Avenue NE
Washington, DC 20002

Gazette International Networking Institute (GINI)
5100 Oakland Avenue
Suite 206
St. Louis, MO 63110

General Rare Disorder Network
Vanderbilt University
AA3223, Medical Center North
Nashville, TN 37232-2195

Glaucoma Research Foundation
490 Post Street #830
San Francisco, CA 94102

Guide Dog Foundation for the Blind, Inc.
371 East Jericho Turnpike
Smithtown, NY 11787

Hearing Information Center
Swarthmore Medical Center
300 South Chester Road
Swarthmore, PA 19081

Helen Keller International, Inc. (HKI)
909 Washington Street, 15th Floor
New York, NY 10006

Housing for Elderly and Handicapped People Division
451 7th Street SW
Room 6116
Washington, DC 20410

Huntington's Disease Society of America (HDSA)
140 West 22nd Street
6th Floor
New York, NY 10011

Institute for Child Health Policy (ICHP)
5700 Southwest 34th Street
Suite 323
Gainsville, FL 32608-5367

The Institute for Rehabilitation and Research (TIRR)
1333 Moursund
Houston, TX 77030

Institute on Alcohol, Drugs, and Disability (IADD)
1801 East Cotati Avenue
Rohnert Park, CA 94928

International Association of Laryngectomees (IAL)
c/o American Cancer Society (ACS)
1599 Clifton Road NE
Atlanta, GA 30329

International Association of Psychosocial Rehabilitation
Services (IAPSRS)
10025 Governor Warfield Pkwy, #301
Columbia, MD 21044

International Center for the Disabled (ICD)
340 East 24th Street
New York, NY 10010

The International Council for Learning Disabilities (CLD)
National Office
P.O. Box 40303
Overland Park, KS 66204

International Federation of Physical Medicine and
Rehabilitation (IFPMR)
600 University Avenue
Suite 1160
Toronto, Ontario M5G 1X5

International Hearing Dog, Inc. (IHDI)
8901 East 89th Avenue
Henderson, CO 80640

International Hearing Society
20361 Middlebelt Road
Livonia, MI 48152

International Lutheran Deaf Association (ILDA)
1333 South Kirkwood Road
St. Louis, MO 63122

International Polio Network (IPN)
5100 Oakland Avenue
Suite #206
Saint Louis, MO 63110

International Rehabilitation Medicine Association
(IRMA)
1333 Moursund Avenue
Suite A-221
Houston, TX 77030

International Ventilator Users Network (I.V.U.N.)
5100 Oakland Avenue, Suite 206
Saint Louis, MO 63110

International Wheelchair Aviators
1117 Rising Hill
Escondido, CA 92029

Job Accommodation Network (JAN)
918 Chestnut Ridge Road
Suite 1
P.O. Box 6080
Morgantown, WV 26506-6080

Job Opportunities for the Blind (JOB)
1800 Johnson Street
Baltimore, MD 21230

Judge David L. Bazelon Center for Mental Health Law
1101 15th Street NW
Suite 1212
Washington, DC 20005-5002

Juvenile Diabetes Foundation International
(JDF International)
432 Park Avenue South
New York, NY 10016

Klinefelter Syndrome and Associates (KS and Associates)
P.O. Box 119
Roseville, CA 95678-0119

Leukemia Society of America
600 Third Avenue, 4th Floor
New York, NY 10016-1901

The Lighthouse, Inc.
111 East 59th Street
New York, NY 10022

Little People of America (LPA)
P.O. Box 9897
Washington, DC 20016

Lowe's Syndrome Association (LSA)
222 Lincoln Street
West Lafayette, IN 47906

Lupus Foundation of America, Inc.
4 Research Place
Suite 180
Rockville, MD 20850

March of Dimes Birth Defects Foundation (MOD)
1275 Mamaroneck Avenue
White Plains, NY 10605

Materials Development Center (MDC)
Stout Vocational Rehabilitation Institute

School of Education and Human Services
University of Wisconsin-Stout
Menomonie, WI 54751

Model Spinal Cord Injury System
Thomas Jefferson University
Jefferson Medical College
11th and Walnut Streets
Philadelphia, PA 19107

Model System of Comprehensive Rehabilitation for
Persons with TBI
Virginia Commonwealth University
Medical College of Virginia
Department of Physical Medicine and Rehabilitation MCV
Station, Box 542
Richmond, VA 23298-0542

Muscular Dystrophy Association (MDA)
3300 East Sunrise Drive
Tucson, AZ 85718

Myasthenia Gravis Foundation (MGF)
222 South Riverside Plaza
Suite 1540
Chicago, IL 60606-6001

Narcotics Anonymous (NA)
P.O. Box 9999
Van Nuys, CA 91409

National Adrenal Disease Foundation (NADF)
505 Northern Boulevard
Suite 200
Great Neck, NY 11021

National Alliance for the Mentally Ill (NAMI)
2101 Wilson Boulevard
Suite 302
Arlington, VA 22201

National Alliance of Blind Students (NABS)
1155 15th Street NW
Suite 720
Washington, DC 20005

National Amputation Foundation (NAF)
73 Church Street
Malverne, NY 11565

National Amputee Golf Association (NAGA)
P.O. Box 1228
Amhearst, NH 03031-1228

National Arthritis and Musculoskeletal and Skin Diseases
Information Clearinghouse
Box AMS
9000 Rockville Pike
Bethesda, MD 20892

National Association for Children of Alcoholics
(NACoA)
11426 Rockville Pike, Suite 100
Rockville, MD 20852

National Association for Hearing and Speech Action
(NAHSA)
10801 Rockville Pike
Rockville, MD 20852

National Association for Home Care (NAHC)
519 C Street NE
Stanton Park
Washington, DC 20002

National Association for Music Therapy (NAMT)
8455 Colesville Road
Suite 930
Silver Spring, MD 20910

National Association for Parents of the Visually Impaired
(NAPVI)
P.O. Box 317
Watertown, MA 02272

National Association for Rights, Protection, and Advocacy
(NARPA)
587 Marshall Avenue
St. Paul, Minnesota 55102

National Association for the Craniofacially Handicapped
(FACES)
P.O. Box 11082
Chattanooga, TN 37401

National Association for Visually Handicapped (NAVH)
22 West 21st Street
New York, NY 10010

National Association of Anorexia Nervosa and Associated
Disorders (ANAD)
P.O. Box 7
Highland Park, IL 60035

National Association of Protection and Advocacy Systems,
Inc. (NAPAS)
900 Second Street NE
Suite 211
Washington, DC 20002

National Autism Hotline
Prichard Building
605 9th Street
P.O. Box 507
Huntington, WV 25710

National Braille Association, Inc. (NBA)
3 Townline Circle
Rochester, NY 14623-2513

National Brain Tumor Foundation
785 Market Street
Suite 1600
San Francisco, CA 94103

National Burn Victim Foundation (NBVF)
32 Scotland Road
Orange, NJ 07050

National Cancer Institute (NCI)
National Institutes of Health
U.S. Department of Health and Human Services
Bethesda, MD 20892

National Captioning Institute, Inc. (NCI)
5203 Leesburg Pike
Suite 1500
Falls Church, VA 22041

National Catholic Office for Persons with Disabilities
(NCPD)
P.O. Box 29113
Washington, DC 20017

National Catholic Office for the Deaf
814 Thayer Avenue
Silver Spring, MD 20910

National Center for Education in Maternal and Child
Health (NCEMCH)
2000 Fifteenth Street North
Suite 701
Arlington, VA 22201-2617
Internet: ncemch01@gumedlib.dml.georgetown.edu

National Center for Medical Rehabilitation Research
(NCMRR)
6100 Executive Boulevard
Room 2A03
Rockville, MD 20852

National Christian Resource Center on Mental
Retardation
Bethesda Lutheran Homes and Services, Inc.
700 Hoffman Drive
Watertown, WI 53094

The National Clearinghouse for Alcohol and Drug
Information (NCADI)
Center for Substance Abuse Prevention (CSAP)
Substance Abuse and Mental Health Services
Administration (SAMHSA)
U.S. Department of Health and Human Services
P.O. Box 2345
Rockville, MD 20847-2345

National Clearinghouse for Professions in
Special Education
The Council for Exceptional Children
1920 Association Drive
Reston, VA 22091

National Clearinghouse on Family Support and
Children's Mental Health
Portland State University
P.O. Box 751
Portland, OR 97207-0751

National Consumers League (NCL)
815 15th Street NW
Suite 928
Washington, DC 20005

The National Council of the Churches of Christ
in the USA
Committee on Disabilities
A Program of Ministries in Christian Education
475 Riverside Drive, Room 848
New York, NY 10115

National Council on Communicative Disorders (NCCD)
Attention: Mary Schreder
10801 Rockville Pike
Rockville, MD 20852

National Council on Disability
1331 F Street NW
Suite 1050
Washington, DC 20004-1107

National Council on Family Relations (NCFR)
3989 Central Avenue NE
Suite 550
Minneapolis, MN 55421

National Council on Independent Living (NCIL)
2111 Wilson Boulevard, Suite 405
Arlington, VA 22201

National Council on the Aging, Inc. (NCOA)
409 3rd Street SW
Washington, DC 20024

National Data Bank for Disability Support Services
Room 0126
Shoemaker Building
University of Maryland
College Park, MD 20742

National Diabetes Information Clearinghouse (NDIC)
P.O. Box NDIC9000
Rockville Pike
Bethesda, MD 20892

National Digestive Diseases Information Clearinghouse
(NDDIC)
9000 Rockville Pike
Box NDDIC
Bethesda, MD 20892

National Down Syndrome Congress (NDSC)
1605 Chantilly Drive
Suite 250
Atlanta, GA 30324

National Down Syndrome Society (NDSS)
666 Broadway
New York, NY 10012

National Easter Seal Society (NESS)
230 West Monroe Street
Suite 1800
Chicago, IL 60606

National Eating Disorders Organization (NEDO)
Ashlawn Building/Harding Hospital
445 E. Granville Road
Worthington, OH 43085

National Eldercare Institute on Health Promotion
American Association of Retired Persons (AARP)
601 E Street NW, 5th Floor-B
Washington, DC 20049

National Eye Care Project (NECP)
P.O. Box 429098
San Francisco, CA 94102-9098

National Eye Research Foundation (NERF)
910 Skokie Boulevard
Suite 207
Northbrook, IL 60062

National Federation of Interfaith Volunteer
Caregivers, Inc.
368 Broadway
Suite 103
P.O. Box 1939
Kingston, NY 12401

National Federation of the Blind (NFB)
1800 Johnson Street
Baltimore, MD 21230

National Foundation for Facial Reconstruction (NFFR)
317 East 34th Street
New York, NY 10016

National Foundation of Wheelchair Tennis
940 Calle Amanecer
Suite B
San Clemente, CA 92673

National Fragile X Foundation
1441 York Street
Suite 215
Denver, CO 80206

National Fraternal Society of the Deaf (NFSD)
1300 West Northwest Highway
Mt. Prospect, IL 60056

National Handicap Housing Institute, Inc. (NHHI)
4556 Lake Drive
Robbinsdale, MN 55422

National Head Injury Foundation, Inc. (NHIF)
1776 Massachusetts Avenue NW
Suite 100
Washington, DC 20036

National Heart, Lung, and Blood Institute (NHLBI)
Information Center
P.O. Box 30105
Bethesda, MD 20824-0105

The National Hemophilia Foundation (NHF)
The Soho Building
110 Greene Street
Suite 303
New York, NY 10012

National Hospice Organization (NHO)
1901 North Moore Street

Suite 901
Arlington, VA 22209

National Information Center for Children and Youth
with Disabilities (NICHCY)
P.O. Box 1492
Washington, DC 20013

National Information Clearinghouse for Infants with
Disabilities & Life-Threatening Conditions
Center for Developmental Disabilities
Benson Building, 1st Floor
University of South Carolina
Columbia, SC 29208

National Institute for Burn Medicine (NIBM)
909 East Ann Street
Ann Arbor, MI 48104

National Institute of Allergy and Infectious Diseases
(NIAID)
National Institutes of Health
U.S. Department of Health and Human Services
Building 31, Room 7A50
9000 Rockville Pike
Bethesda, MD 20892

National Institute of Art and Disabilities (NIAD)
551 23rd Street
Richmond, CA 94804

National Institute of Diabetes and Digestive and Kidney
Diseases (NIDDK)
U.S. Department of Health and Human Services
Building 31
Room 9A04
9000 Rockville Pike
Bethesda, MD 20892

National Institute of Neurological Disorders and Stroke
(NINDS)
National Institutes of Health
U.S. Department of Health and Human Services
Building 31, Room 8A 06
9000 Rockville Pike
Bethesda, MA 20892

National Institute on Deafness and Other Communication
Disorders (NIDCD)
National Information Clearinghouse
Program Planning and Health Reports Branch
Building 31, Room 3C 35
9000 Rockville Pike
Bethesda, MD 20892

National Jewish Center for Immunology and Respiratory
Medicine
1400 Jackson Street
Denver, CO 80206

National Kidney and Urologic Diseases Information
Clearinghouse (NKUDIC)
Box NKUDIC

3 Information Way
Bethesda, MD 20892-3580

National Kidney Foundation (NKF)
30 East 33rd Street
New York, NY 10016

National Legal Center for the Medically Dependent
and Disabled, Inc.
50 South Meridian
Suite 605
Indianapolis, IN 46204-3541

National Library Service for the Blind and Physically
Handicapped (NLS)
Library of Congress
1291 Taylor Street NW
Washington, DC 20542

National Mental Health Association (NMHA)
1021 Prince Street
Alexandria, VA 22314

National Multiple Sclerosis Society
733 Third Avenue
6th Floor
New York, NY 10017

National Network of Learning Disabled Adults (NNLDA)
P.O. Box 32611
Phoenix, AZ 85064-2611

National Neurofibromatosis Foundation (NNFF)
141 Fifth Avenue
Suite 7-S
New York, NY 10010-7105

The National Odd Shoe Exchange (NOSE)
7102 North 35th Avenue
Suite 2
Phoenix, AZ 85051

National Oral Health Information Clearinghouse
(NOHIC)
One NOHIC Way
Bethesda, MD 20892-3500

The National Organization for Rare Disorders (NORD)
P.O. Box 8923
New Fairfield, CT 06812

National Organization on Fetal Alcohol Syndrome
(NOFAS)
1815 H Street NW
Suite 710
Washington, DC 20006

National Osteoporosis Foundation (NOF)
1150 17th Street NW
Suite 500
Washington, DC 20036-4603

National Parent Network on Disabilities (NPND)
1600 Prince Street

Suite 115
Alexandria, VA 22314

National Parkinson Foundation
1501 NW Ninth Avenue
Miami, FL 33136

National Rehabilitation Association (NRA)
633 South Washington Street
Alexandria, VA 22314-4193

National Rehabilitation Information Center (NARIC)
8455 Colesville Road
Suite 935
Silver Spring, MD 20910-3319

National Rehabilitation Research and Training Center on
Blindness and Low Vision
Mississippi State University
P.O. Drawer 6189
Mississippi State, MS 39762

National Retinitis Pigmentosa Foundation (RP Foundation
Fighting Blindness)
1401 Mt. Royal Avenue
Fourth Floor
Baltimore, MD 21217

The National Scoliosis Foundation
72 Mount Auburn Street
Watertown, MA 02172

National Skeet Shooting Association (NSSA)
P.O. Box 680007
San Antonio, TX 78268-0007

National Spinal Cord Injury Association (NSCIA)
545 Concord Avenue
Cambridge, MA 02138

National Stroke Association (NSA)
8480 East Orchard Road
Suite 1000
Englewood, CO 80111-5015

National Stuttering Project (NSP)
4601 Irving Street
San Francisco, CA 94122

National Tay-Sachs and Allied Diseases Association, Inc.
(NTSAD)
2001 Beacon Street
Suite 204
Brookline, MA 02146

National Technical Information Service (NTIS)
U.S. Department of Commerce
5285 Port Royal Road
Springfield, VA 22161

National Therapeutic Recreation Society (NTRS)
National Recreation and Park Association
2775 South Quincy Street
Suite 300
Alexandria, VA 22206

National Wheelchair Softball Association (NWSA)
1616 Todd Court
Hastings, MN 55033

Neurofibromatosis, Inc. (NF, Inc.)
8855 Annapolis Road
Suite 110
Lanham, MD 20706-2924

North American Riding for the Handicapped Association
(NARHA)
Box 33150
Denver, CO 80233

NRH International Polio Institute National Rehabilitation
Hospital
102 Irving Street NW
Washington, DC 20010

Obsessive Compulsive Foundation, Inc. (OCF)
P.O. Box 70
New Haven, CT 06535

Office of Technology Transfer (OTT)
Department of Veterans Affairs Prosthetics Research
& Development Center
103 South Gay Street
Baltimore, MD 21202

Osteogenesis Imperfecta Foundation, Inc. (OIF)
5005 Laurel Street
Tampa, FL 33607-3836

Paralyzed Veterans of America (PVA)
801 Eighteenth Street NW
Washington, DC 20006

Parkinson's Disease Foundation, Inc. (PDF)
William Black Medical Research Building
Columbia-Presbyterian Medical Center
650 West 168th Street
New York, NY 10032

Partners of the Americas PATH (Partners Appropriate
Technology for the Handicapped)
Americas Program
1424 K Street NW
Suite 700
Washington, DC 20005

Perkins School for the Blind
175 North Beacon Street
Watertown, MA 02172

The Phoenix Society for Burn Survivors, Inc.
11 Rust Hill Road
Levittown, PA 19056

Polycystic Kidney Research Foundation (PKRF)
922 Walnut Street
Suite 411
Kansas City, MO 64106

Prader-Willi Syndrome Association
1821 University Avenue West
St. Paul, MN 55104-2801

President's Committee on Employment of People with
Disabilities (PCEPD)
1331 F Street NW
Washington, DC 20004-1107

PRIDE Foundation (Promote Real Independence for the
Disabled and Elderly)
391 Long Hill Road
Box 1293
Groton, CT 06340-1293

Recovery, Inc.
The Association of Nervous and Former Mental Patients
802 North Dearborn Street
Chicago, IL 60610

Registry of Interpreters for the Deaf, Inc. (RID)
8719 Colesville Road
Suite 310
Silver Spring, MD 20910

Rehabilitation Engineering Research Center in
Augmentative Communication
University of Delaware
E.I. duPont Institute
1600 Rockland Road
P.O. Box 269
Wilmington, DE 19899

Rehabilitation Engineering Research Center on Hearing
Enhancement and Assistive Devices
The Lexington Center, Inc.
Research Division
30th Avenue and 75th Street
Jackson Heights, NY 11370

Rehabilitation Engineering Research Center on Prosthetics
and Orthotics
Northwestern University
Rehabilitation Institute of Chicago
345 East Superior Street, Room 1441
Chicago, IL 60611

Rehabilitation Engineering Research Center on
Technology to Improve Wheelchair Mobility
University of Pittsburgh
Rehabilitation Technology Program (RTP)
915 William Pitt Way
Pittsburgh, PA 15238

Rehabilitation International (RI)
25 East 21st Street
New York, NY 10010

Rehabilitation Research and Training Center for Substance
Abuse and People with Disabilities
Wright State University
Projects on Drugs and Disability
School of Medicine
3640 Colonel Glenn Highway
Dayton, OH 45435

Rehabilitation Research and Training Center on Aging
with a Disability

Rancho Los Amigos Research and Education Institute
Rancho Los Amigos Medical Center
7601 East Imperial Highway
Downey, CA 90242

Rehabilitation Research and Training Center on Aging
with Mental Retardation
University of Illinois/Chicago
Institute on Disability and Human Development
A University Affiliated Program
College of Associated Health Professions
1640 W. Roosevelt Road
Chicago, IL 60608-6904

Rehabilitation Research and Training Center on Aging
with Spinal Cord Injury
Craig Hospital
University of Colorado Health Science Center
Research Department
3425 South Clarkson
Englewood, CO 80110

Rehabilitation Research and Training Center on Personal
Assistance Services
World Institute on Disability
510 16th Street
Oakland, CA 94612

Rehabilitation Robotics to Enhance the Functioning of
Individuals with Disabilities
University of Delaware
Center for Applied Sciences and Engineering
E.I. duPont Institute
1600 Rockland Road
P.O. Box 269
Wilmington, DE 19899

Rehabilitation Services Administration (RSA)
Office of Special Education and Rehabilitative Services
(OSERS)
U.S. Department of Education
Switzer Building, Room 3028
330 C Street SW
Washington, DC 20202-2531

Research and Training Center in Management of
Information and Information Systems in State Vocational
Rehabilitation Agencies, West Virginia University
HRE/Research and Training Center
806 Allen Hall
P.O. Box 6122
Morgantown, WV 26506-6122

Research and Training Center in Rehabilitation and
Childhood Trauma Tufts University
New England Medical Center
Department of Rehabilitation Medicine
750 Washington Street, 75K-R
Boston, MA 02111

Research and Training Center on Functional Assessment
and Evaluation of Rehabilitation Outcomes

State University of New York (SUNY/Buffalo)
Department of Rehabilitation Medicine
232 Parker Hall
SUNY South Campus
Buffalo, NY 14214

Resource Center on Substance Abuse Prevention and
Disability
VSA Educational Services
1331 F Street NW
Suite 800
Washington, DC 20004

Resource Unit for Information and Education (RU)
Northwestern University REC
345 East Superior Street
Room 1441
Chicago, IL 60611

Respiratory Nursing Society (RNS)
5700 Old Orchard Road
First Floor
Skokie, IL 60077-1057

Rubinstein-Taybi (RTS) Parent Group
RR1, Box 2
Cedar, KS 67628

Scleroderma Federation
Peabody Office Building
One Newbury Street
Peabody, MA 01960

Self Help for Hard of Hearing People (SHHH)
7910 Woodmont Avenue
Suite 1200
Bethesda, MD 20814

Sickle Cell Disease Association of America, Inc.
(SCDAA)
3345 Wilshire Boulevard
Suite 1106
Los Angeles, CA 90010

The Simon Foundation for Continence
P.O. Box 835
Wilmette, IL 60091

Skating Association for the Blind and Handicapped
(SABAH)
c/o Kaufmann's
1255 Niagara Falls Boulevard
Buffalo, NY 14226

Ski for Light, Inc. (SFL)
5 McAuliffe Drive
North Brunswick, NJ 08902

Smith-Kettlewell Eye Research Institute
Rehabilitation Engineering Research Center and
Rehabilitation Engineering Service
2232 Webster Street
San Francisco, CA 94115

Social Security Administration (SSA)
6401 Security Boulevard
Baltimore, MD 21235

Society for Cognitive Rehabilitation, Inc. (SCR)
P.O. Box 53067
Albuquerque, NM 87153-3067

Society for Disability Studies (SDS)
c/o Department of Sociology
Gallaudet University
Washington, DC 20005

Society for Muscular Dystrophy Information International
(SMDI International)
P.O. Box 479
Bridgewater, Nova Scotia
Canada, B4V 2X6

Society for the Advancement of Travel for the
Handicapped (SATH)
347 Fifth Avenue
Suite 610
New York, NY 10016

Special Olympics International (SOI)
1350 New York Avenue NW
Suite 500
Washington, DC 20005

Spina Bifida Association of America (SBAA)
4590 MacArthur Boulevard NW
Suite 250
Washington, DC 20007-4226

Spinal Cord Injury Network International (SCINI)
3911 Princeton Drive
Santa Rosa, CA 95405-7013

Spinal Cord Society (SCS)
Route 5, Wendell Road
Fergus Falls, MN 56537

Spinal Network
23815 Stuart Ranch Road
Malibu, CA 90265

Stuttering Foundation of America (SFA)
3100 Walnut Grove Road, #603
P.O. Box 11749
Memphis, TN 38111-0749

TASH
11201 Greenwood Avenue North
Seattle, WA 98133

TBI INFO
Rehabilitation Research and Training Center on
Traumatic Brain Injury
State University of New York (SUNY)/Buffalo
194 Farber Hall
3435 Main Street
Buffalo, NY 14214

Telecommunications for the Deaf, Inc. (TDI)
8719 Colesville Road, Suite 300
Silver Spring, MD 20910

Tourette Syndrome Association (TSA)
42-40 Bell Boulevard
Bayside, NY 11361

Trace Research and Development Center on
Communication, Control and Computer Access for
Handicapped Individuals
S-151 Waisman Center
1500 Highland Avenue
Madison, WI 53705

United Cerebral Palsy Associations, Inc. (UCPA)
1522 K Street NW
Suite 1112
Washington, DC 20005

United States Association of Blind Athletes (USABA)
33 North Institute Street
Colorado Springs, CO 80903

United States Blind Golfers Association
3094 Shamrock Street N
Tallahassee, FL 32308

United States Cerebral Palsy Athletic Association
3810 W. Northwest Highway
Suite 205
Dallas, TX 75220

United States Deaf Skiers Association, Inc. (USDSA)
0400 SW Palatine Hill Road
Portland, OR 97219-6551

United States Wheelchair Swimming
229 Miller Street
Middleboro, MA 02346

University of Washington Burn Injury Rehabilitation
Model System
University of Washington Burn Center
Harborview Medical Center
325 Ninth Avenue
Seattle, WA 98104

U.S. Department of Labor
Employment Standard Administration
Office of Federal Contract Compliance Programs (OFCCP)
200 Constitution Avenue NW
Washington, DC 20210

U.S. Disabled Ski Team
P.O. Box 100
Park City, UT 84060

U.S. Equal Employment Opportunity Commission
(EEOC)
ADA Services Office
1801 L Street NW
Washington, DC 20507

Vermont Rehabilitation Engineering Research Center
in Low-Back Pain
University of Vermont
Department of Orthopedics and Rehabilitation

One South Prospect Street
Burlington, VT 05401

Vestibular Disorders Association (VEDA)
P.O. Box 4467
Portland, OR 97208-4467

Visiting Nurse Associations of America (VNAA)
3801 East Florida Avenue
Suite 900
Denver, CO 80210

Vocational Evaluation and Work Adjustment Association
(VEWAA)
202 East Cheyenne Mountain Boulevard
Colorado Springs, CO 80906

Von Hippel-Lindau Family Alliance
171 Clinton Road
Brookline, MA 02146

Voyageur Outward Bound School
111 Third Avenue South
Suite 120
Minneapolis, MN 55401-2551

Well Spouse Federation (WSF)
P.O. Box 801
New York, NY 10023

Wheelchair Motorcycle Association, Inc. (WMA)
101 Torrey Street
Brockton, MA 02401

Wheelchair Sports, U.S.A.
3595 East Fountain Boulevard
Suite L1
Colorado Springs, CO 80910

Wilderness Inquiry
1313 5th Street SE
Box 84
Minneapolis, MN 55414-1546

Williams Syndrome Association
P.O. Box 297
Clawson, MI 48017

Wilson's Disease Association
P.O. Box 75324
Washington, DC 20013

World Institute on Disability (WID)
510 16th Street
Suite 100
Oakland, CA 94612

World Recreation Association of the Deaf/USA (WRAD)
P.O. Box 3211
Quartz Hill, CA 93586

Young Adult Institute (YAI)
460 West 34th Street
New York, NY 10001

Zain Hansen MPS Foundation
1200 Fernwood Drive
Arcata, CA 95521

Index

Numbers in **boldface** refer to the main entry on the subject

A

Abdominal injury, 152
Ability, **1–3**, 31, 236
ABLEDATA database, 408
Abortion, 348, 349, 459
Abuse. *See* Violence; *specific type*, e.g.,
   Child abuse
Academy of Physical Medicine and
   Rehabilitation, 267
Accessibility, **3–7**
   ADA requirements, 50, 52
   affirmative action requirements, 25–
      26
   architectural, **69–74**
   assistance animals to aid, 63
   assistive technology, **89–93**
   civil rights legislation for, 177
   housing, **384–387**
   international rehabilitation, 411, 412
   reasonable accommodation, **611–613**
   self-concept affected by, 661
   self-help to attain, 665
   transportation, **731–737**
Accessible society, 3–4, 7
Accidental injury
   of aged, 29
   childhood disabilities caused by,
      153
   communication disabilities caused
      by, 194
   forensic rehabilitation, 326
   head, **361–366**
   HIV/AIDS and, 388
   pediatric rehabilitation following,
      535–536
   prevention of, 40
   of spinal cord, 689

surgery for, 716
violence as cause, 743
in workplace, 206–207, 270–274
see also specific type, e.g., Highway
   accidents
Accommodation. *See* Job placement;
   Public accommodation; Reason-
   able accommodation
Accreditation, 223–226, 563
Achievement assessment, 750
Achondroplasia, 357
Acknowledgment stage, 600
Acquired disabilities, 257
Acquired immunodeficiency syndrome.
   See Human immunodeficiency vi-
   rus disease and acquired immuno-
   deficiency syndrome
ADA. *See* Americans with Disabilities
   Act of 1990
Adaptation stage, 600
Adaptive technology. *See* Assistive
   technology
ADAPT. *See* Americans Disabled for
   Attendant Programs Today
ADAPT v. Burnley (1986), 734
ADA Standards for Accessible Design,
   386
Addiction. *See* Alcohol abuse; Alcohol
   rehabilitation; Drug abuse; Drug
   rehabilitation; Gambling rehabili-
   tation; Smoking
Addison's disease, 294
ADHD. *See* Attention-deficit hyperac-
   tivity disorder
Adjustment to Blindness program, 9
Adjustment services, **8–12**, 143
Adler, Alfred, 767–768

Adolescents, rehabilitation of, **12–16**,
   537
   adjustment services, 8–9, 11
   career counseling, 144
   for communication disabilities, 192–
      193
   for developmental disabilities, 250,
      254
   for drug abuse, 276
   for eating disorders, 279
   for eye disease, 235
   for growth disorders, 357
   for hemophilia, 123, 125
   for learning disabilities, 435
   massage therapy, 455
   for psychiatric disorders, 156, 164–
      165
   psychological issues affecting, 155
   sexuality issues, 670
   see also Childhood disabilities; Family
Adrenal disorders, 294–295
Adult Basic Learning Examination, 750
Advocacy, **17–21**, 259, 324, 337
   ADA and, 48–49
   for architectural accessibility, 72
   for children with disabilities, 248, 259
   for deaf and hearing impaired, 242–
      243
   deinstitutionalization and, 248
   for developmentally disabled, 255
   disability law and social policy sup-
      porting, 248, 267, 268
   for genetic disorders, 354
   for growth disorders, 358
   for hospice, 379
   for housing, 385
   for independent living, 402

Advocacy (*cont.*)
  in international rehabilitation, 409
  for kidney patients, 427
  for mentally retarded, 18, 248, 461
  for minorities, 465–466
  for organic mental syndromes, 529
  for personal assistance services, 544–545
  by physicians, 565
  for private sector rehabilitation, 572
  by psychologists, 595, 598
  for rehabilitation assessment, 83–84
  by rehabilitation center professionals, 617
  by religious professionals, 631
  self-help groups for, 665–666
  by social workers, 677
Affective disorders. *See* Mood disorders; Psychiatric rehabilitation; Psychology, rehabilitation; *specific disorders*
Affirmative action, **22–26**, 48; *see also* Advocacy; Americans with Disabilities Act of 1990; Civil rights
AFL-CIO, 431
African Americans, 462, 463, 465, 466
  blindness and visual impairment of, 118
  endocrine disorders in, 290, 292
  homelessness, 372
  income levels, 464
  lupus in, 79
  sickle cell disease and, 351, 673–675
African ancestry, 344, 351, 673
Aggression, 162, 165
Aging, **27–33**
  accessibility issues, 5
  Alzheimer's disease, **42–46**
  amputation and, 55, 576
  animals for companionship, 64
  architectural accessibility needs, 74
  arthritis and, 76–77
  art therapy for elders, 75
  attitudes toward, 97
  back disorders due to, 105
  burn risk and, 126, 128
  caregiving for aged, **146–148**
  civil rights issues, 177
  coronary artery disease risk and, 212
  dance/movement therapy, 233
  deaf-blindness and, 234
  effect on workforce, 333–334
  genetic disorders due to maternal, 348
  housing issues, 384, 385, 386, 387
  independent living and, 401, 621
  kidney disorders and, 424
  medication dosage affected by, 470

  neurological disorders and, 504
  occupational therapy and, 527
  organic mental syndromes and, 529
  personal assistants for aged, 543
  prosthetics and, 576
  Rusk's programs for, 652
  spinal cord injury and, 693
  stroke and, 704, 705, 707
  veterans' vocational needs, 743
  vision loss and, 118–119
Agoraphobia, 66
Aid to Families with Dependent Children, 375
AIDS. *See* Human immunodeficiency virus disease and acquired immunodeficiency syndrome
Air bags, 365
Air Carrier Access Act of 1986, 5, 48, 736
Air transportation, 735–736
Albee, Fred, 367
Alcohol abuse
  adolescent, 535
  alcoholism definition, 34–35
  attitudes toward, 97
  death caused by, 757
  drunk-driving and, 36, 365
  eating disorders and, 279
  fetal alcohol syndrome as result, 458
  highway accidents due to, 535
  homelessness and, 372, 374, 375
  medications with, 553
  mood disorders and, 469, 470
  schizophrenia and, 655
  as stroke risk, 705
  veterans, 740
  as violence risk, 743
Alcoholics Anonymous (AA), 37, 39, 207, 219–220, 277
Alcohol rehabilitation, **34–39**, 275
  art therapy, 75
  centers for, 617
  future of, 333, 334
  for prisoners, 218, 219–220
  see also Drug rehabilitation; Psychiatric rehabilitation
Alexander v. Choate (1985), 176
Alliance of Genetic Support Groups, 355
Allied health professionals, **40–42**
  alcoholism treatment by, 38–39
  clinical supervision, **178–187**
  decrease in students for, 617
  disability management, 271
  for employee assistance programs, 288
  head injury and, 364–365

  hospice, **378–381**
  international rehabilitation, 409
  mood disorders and, 474
  for neurology, 509
  for physical therapy, **561–562**
  in psychiatry, 590
  recreation programs by, 615
  in rehabilitation hospital, 383
  for respiratory disease, 637
  social workers and, 677
  for veterans' rehabilitation, 739
Alzheimer's disease, **42–46**, 503, 504, 529
  communication disabilities caused by, 195
  consumer groups for, 210
  family and, 324
  hospice and, 380
Alzheimer's Disease and Related Disorders Association, 46
American Academy of Neurology, 508
American Academy of Orthotists and Prosthetists, 578
American Art Therapy Association, 75–76
American Association for Music Therapy, 498
American Association of Kidney Patients, 427
American Association of Mental Retardation, 459, 460
American Board for Certification in Orthotics and Prosthetics, 578
American Braille Press, 421–422
American Cancer Society, 136, 137, 138, 664, 757
American Chronic Pain Association, 533
American Coalition of Citizens with Disabilities, 209, 267
American College of Rheumatology, 81
American College of Sports Medicine, 755–756
American Congress of Rehabilitation Medicine, 508
American Counseling Association, 144
American Dance Therapy Association, 231
American Federation of State, County, and Municipal Employees, 432
American Foundation for Overseas Blind, 422
American Foundation for the Blind, 421, 422
American Heart Association, 707, 757
American Lung Association, 664

American Massage Therapy Association, 456

American National Standards Institute, 72

American Occupational Therapy Association, 528

American Orthotic and Prosthetic Association, 579

American Osteopathic Association, 318

American Pain Society, 533

American Psychiatric Association, 35

American Psychological Association (APA), 307, 593, 598–599, 622

American Public Transit Association, 733

American Rehabilitation Association, 566

American Rehabilitation Counseling Association, 621, 622

American School for the Deaf, 244

Americans with Disabilities Act of 1990 (ADA), **47–53**, 175, 176, 177, 178, 191, 258, 268–269
  ability evaluation for employment under, 2
  accessibility issues addressed by, 5
  adjustment services supported by, 10
  advocacy procedures under, 19
  affirmative action under, **22–26**
  assistance dogs' rights under, 63
  assistive technology and, 91
  blindness/vision loss under, 119, 238
  cancer patients covered by, 139
  communication disabled protected by, 193
  computers and, 201, 202
  deaf/hearing impaired under, 245
  developmentally disabled under, 250
  diabetes under, 294
  disability surveys and, 701
  drafting and signing of, 568, 569
  education programs and, 447
  effect on career development, 145
  ergonomics and, 304
  future of rehabilitation, 333, 335
  history, 210–211, 370
  HIV/AIDS under, 390
  housing issues, 384, 386
  independent living and, 405
  information resource centers under, 408
  job placement under, 414, 415
  labor unions and, 431–432
  mentally retarded under, 248, 461–462
  Native American exclusion, 648
  philosophy of rehabilitation and, 557
  prisoner coverage, 221
  rehabilitation assessment and, 86, 87
  rehabilitation counseling, 621
  rehabilitation education, 627
  rehabilitation psychology and, 598
  religious community affected by, 629
  research affected by, 633
  self-help groups and, 664, 667
  small firms under, 333
  spinal cord injury victims and, 693
  state-federal rehabilitation program and, 697, 698
  transition movement supported by, 727
  transportation accessibility under, 732, 734
  work issues and, 273, 540–541, 568, 584, 769–770

Americans Disabled for Attendant Programs Today (ADAPT), 210, 665, 733

American Sign Language (ASL), 3, 41, 102, 195, 196, 239, 241, 340, 341

American Society of Neurorehabilitation, 508

American Speech-Language-Hearing Association, 69, 99, 195, 196

Amnesia. *See* Memory impairment

Amniocentesis, 459

Amphetamine, 552

Amputation, **54–61**, 564
  animals to assist amputee, 62–63
  childhood injury as cause, 152, 153
  diabetes as cause, 291, 292, 293
  prosthetics for, 574, 576
  rehabilitation engineering, 297, 299
  wheelchairs for, 762

Amyotrophic lateral sclerosis (Lou Gehrig's disease), 194, 512, 514, 640

Analgesics, 173, 533, 552

Anatomy, 303

Androgen excess, 294, 295

Anemia. *See* Sickle cell anemia and thalassemia

Angina pectoris, 213, 214

Angleman syndrome, 353

Animals, **62–64**

Ankylosing spondylitis, 80

Anorexia nervosa. *See* Eating disorders

Anthony, William, 370

Anticoagulant drugs, 550, 551

Anticonvulsant drugs, 471, 552

Antidepressants
  for children, 165, 166–167
  for chronic fatigue syndrome, 173
  for eating disorders, 280
  for HIV/AIDS patients, 390
  for mood disorders, 468–469, 470–471
  for pain, 532
  pharmacology of, 553
  see also specific drug

Anti-inflammatory drugs, 173

Antioxidents, 215

Antipsychotic drugs, 552, 553, 656

Antisocial personality disorder, 547

Anxiety disorders, **65–67**, 471
  behavior therapy for, 112
  in children, 166, 168
  coronary artery disease as cause, 216
  eating disorders and, 279, 280
  of HIV/AIDS patients, 390
  following loss-related grief, 445
  massage therapy for, 455
  neurological disorders as cause, 503
  organic mental syndromes and, 529–530
  pharmacology for, 552–553
  of prisoners, 221
  psychiatry for, 579, 590, 591
  psychological approaches to, 598
  respiratory disease and, 636, 637

Anxiolytic drugs, 553

Aphasia, **68–69**, 195, 196

Appearance. *See* Attitudes; Clothing; Self-concept

Apprenticeship programs, 433

Apraxia, 194

APTA v. Lewis (1981), 733

Architectural accessibility, 3–7, **69–74**
  ADA requirements, 50, 52–53
  affirmative action requirements, 24, 25–26
  for amputees, 59
  for children, 155
  as civil right, 175, 208
  housing, **384–87**
  international, 412
  life care planning and, 441–442
  for musculoskeletal disorders, 496
  self-help advocacy for, 666, 667
  for stroke victims, 707
  see also Public accommodation

Architectural and Transportation Barriers Compliance Board, 73

Architectural Barriers Act of 1968, 4, 5, 6, 47, 72, 73, 208, 386, 732

Arline v. School Board of Nassau County (1987), 20

Arteriosclerosis, 54, 502

Arthritis, **76–81**, 177
    bursitis and, 484
    gastrointestinal disorders link, 342
    hemophilia as cause, 122, 124, 125
    of homeless, 374
    occupational therapy for, 527
    surgery for, 716
    see also specific type, e. g., Osteoar-
        thritis
Arthritis Foundation, 81
Articulation disabilities, 193–194
Artificial Limb Program, 297, 298
Art therapy, **74–76**, 221, 379, 739;
    see also Music therapy
Asian Americans, 463, 464, 465, 466
Asian ancestry, 344
ASL. See American Sign Language
Aspirin, 215, 342
Assembly of Specialized Accrediting
    Bodies, 226
Assertive community treatment, 585
Assessment in rehabilitation, **82–88**
    for behavior therapy, 111
    for cancer treatment, 135, 138
    for childhood disabilities, 153–155
    of clinical supervisors, 181–182
    for hemophiliacs, 123
    for mentally retarded, 457
    philosophy of rehabilitation, 555–
        559
    by physical therapist, 561
    for prosthetics/orthotics, 575, 576
    psychological, 597–598
    for transition from school to work,
        729–730
    for vision loss, 119
    vocational evaluation, **748–753**
Assistive technology, **89–93**, 371,
    564, 721–726
    for accessibility, 3, 5, 6
    for aged, 32
    allied professionals and, 41
    for Alzheimer's patients, 46
    architectural accessibility and, 70, 71
    for cancer patients, 136–137, 138
    clothing adaptations for, 191
    computers for visual impairments,
        197–201
    for deaf/hearing impaired, 240–241
    future of, 334
    housing as, 385–386
    for international rehabilitation, 411
    for job placement, 414
    for kidney disorders, 423–424
    life-care planning and, 439, 441
    for neurological disorders, 505

    for neuromuscular disorders, 513–514
    for pediatric rehabilitation, 539
    for rehabilitation assessment, 83
    rehabilitation education, 627
    rehabilitation engineering, **296–302**
    for rehabilitation psychology, 598
    in rural areas, 647–648
    self-concept affected by, 661
    as sexual aid, 671
    for spinal cord injury, 690–691, 692
    for stroke victims, 706–707
    for veterans, 739
    wheelchairs, **760–762**
Association for Children with Learning
    Disabilities, 685
Association for Retarded Children/
    Citizens (ARC), 248, 255, 267,
    459, 664
Association for the Advancement of
    Behavior Therapy, 109
Association of Children's Prosthetic-
    Orthotic Clinics, 579
Association of Machinists Center for
    Administering Rehabilitation and
    Employment Services (IAM
    CARES), 432
Association of Persons with Severe
    Handicaps, 685
Association of Rehabilitation Nurses,
    521, 523–524
Asthma, 374, 636
Atherosclerosis. See Coronary artery
    disease
Attendant care. See Personal assistance
    services
Attention-deficit hyperactivity disorder
    (ADHD), 75, 151, 160–162, 195
Attitudes, **94–99**, 568, 570
    about aging, 30
    about blindness, 207
    about burn victims, 133
    about cancer patients, 139
    about communication disabilities, 192
    about deaf-blind, 236, 421
    about deinstitutionalization, 249
    about disabled, 178, 259, 268, 269,
        396–397
    about HIV/AIDS, 392–393
    about kidney disorders, 425–426
    about psychology, 598
    about wellness, 755
    about women with disabilities, 765–
        766
    ADA and, 50
    civil rights issues, 175
    clothing as influence on, **190–192**

    Helen Keller's role in altering, 421
    violence resulting from, 744
    see also Emotions; Normalization and
        social role valorization; Self-
        concept
Attribution, 604
Audiogram, 100
Audiology, 42, **99–101**, 193
Audiotape for training, 180
Australian Disability Technology Asso-
    ciation, 300
Autism, **101–102**, 249, 253
    communication affected by, 195
    as genetic condition, 352
    mental retardation and, 460
    multiple disabilities and, 477
    respite care, 642
    supported employment for, 708
Autoimmune disorders, 77
Automobiles
    belts and seats, 365, 366, 535, 536,
        538, 694
    parking accessibility, 736
    see also Highway accidents
Autonomic dysreflexia, 691
Autonomy, 305
Avoidant personality disorder, 547

B
Baby-boom generation, 334
"Baby Doe" case regulations, 156, 176
Back disorders, **105–107**
    behavior therapy for, 111
    lower, 479–480
    occupational therapy for, 527
    pain from, 531
    in workplace, 283
Back Pain Association of America, 107
Balloon coronary angioplasty, 212
Bank-Mikkelsen, Niels Eric, 515, 516
Barden-LaFollette Act of 1943, 368, 581
Barrier-free design, 70, 71
Beach Center on Family and Disabil-
    ity, 325
Becker's dystrophy, 506
Behavior
    childhood psychiatric disorders and,
        159, 161, 163
    drug abuse effects on, 276
    emotional impairment and, 253
    following head injury, 363, 364
    HIV/AIDS and, 392–393
    learning disabilities and, 435
    multiple disabilities and, 476
    neurological disorders and, 503
    nutrition affected by, 758

organic mental syndromes and, 528, 530

following pediatric rehabilitation, 539

Behavioral medicine, 109

Behavioral technology, 598

Behavior therapy, **108–113**
  for addicted prisoners, 220
  for adjustment problems, 10
  for aged, 27, 33
  for Alzheimer's patients, 45
  art used for, 75
  for autism, 101, 102
  for back pain, 106
  by caregivers, 147
  following head injury, 363
  as loss-related grief aid, 446
  for mentally retarded, 459, 460
  for mood disorders, 473–474
  for personality disorders, 548

Be Head-Smart Campaign, 365

Beneficence, 257, 305

Benzodiazepine agents, 552, 553

Bereavement. *See* Loss and grief

Berkeley Center for Independent Living, 208, 399, 667

Beta blockers, 215

Bicycle safety, 365, 366

Bioengineering. *See* Engineering; Rehabilitation

Biofeedback, 598, 637

Biopsychosocial model, 112, 220

Bipolar disorder, 372, 469–470, 471–473, 552, 590

Birth defects. *See* Developmental disabilities; Genetic disorders

Bladder stimulators, 331

Blankenship, Louise, 763

Blatt, Burton, 248

Bleuler, Eugen, 653

Blindness and vision disorders, **115–119**
  accessibility needs, 3, 6
  adjustment services, 9
  affirmative action, 24
  attitudes toward, 94, 95, 207
  childhood screening for, 149, 150, 151–152
  computer applications for, 6, **197–201**, 205
  definition, 116–117
  diabetes as cause, 294
  disability law and social policy, 266
  government jobs for people with, 209
  guide dogs for, 62–63
  housing issues, 385
  Keller, Helen, **421–423**

management of care, 451

multiple disabilities and, 477

rehabilitation education for, 625

rehabilitation engineering, 297

societal allowances for, 207

stroke as cause, 703, 706

student rights, 370

in veterans, 740

work ability and, 207

Blocking/inhibition medication, 550

Blood clots, 705

Blood disorders, **120–125**
  hemophilia, 121–123, 352, 353
  HIV/AIDS, **388–393**
  sickle cell anemia/thalassemia, 351, 352, **673–676**

Blood oxygenation impairment, 635–638

Blood transfusion, 388, 675–676

Board of Education of the Hendrick Hudson School District v. *Rowley* (1982), 19

Body image. *See* Self-concept

Bone cancer, 138

Bone disorders, 486–489

Bone fractures, 152

Bone marrow transplant, 676

Borderline personality disorder, 547

Braces. *See* Prosthetics and orthotics

Braille, Louis, 367

Braille technology, 199–200, 205, 421, 422

Brain cancer, 138, 139

Brain chemicals, 532

Brain death, 258

Brain function, 636

Brain injury. *See* Head injury

Brain malformations, 150, 151

Brainstem auditory evoked response, 100

Brain tumors, 68

Breaking New Ground program, 648

Breast cancer, 137–138

Breast implants, 138

Bridgewater State Hospital (Massachusetts), 248

Bronchodysplasia, 635

Brown v. *Board of Education* (1954), 681

Bulimia nervosa. *See* Eating disorders

Bupropion (Wellbutrin), 470

Bureau of Labor Statistics, 701

Burgdorf, Robert, 49

Burns, **126–133**, 152, 715–716

Bursae, 484

Bursitis, 484

Bush, George, 49, 50

Buspirone (Buspar), 470–471

Bus transportation, 732, 733, 734, 735

C

Caffeine, 342

Calcium antagonists, 472

Calcium disorders, 295–296

Campanella, Roy, 652

Canada, 258, 516, 701–702

Canadian Association for Community Living, 516

Canadian Association for Music Therapy, 498

Cancer
  arthritis link, 79
  communication disabilities caused by, 194
  hospice care, 380
  ostomy following, 345
  pain from, 531, 532
  survival rates, 146
  see also specific type, e.g., Breast cancer

Cancer rehabilitation, **135–139**

Caption services, 241

Carbamazepine (Tegretol), 472

Cardiac pacemakers, 330

Cardiomyopathy, 511

Cardiomyoplasty, 331

Cardiovascular disorders. *See* Coronary artery disease; Stroke

Career counseling, **140–145**, 769–771
  ability evaluation for, **1–3**
  for developmentally disabled, 254
  following head injury, 365
  international, 409
  job placement, **413–419**
  occupational information for, **525–527**
  rehabilitation, **618–623**
  see also Vocational evaluation

Caregiving, **146–148**
  abuse by caregiver, 743, 746
  for Alzheimer's patients, 44–46
  for cancer patients, 135
  family and, 324
  for HIV/AIDS patients, 392
  hospice, **378–381**
  life care planning and, 441
  management, **449–454**
  for mood disorders, 474
  nutrition issues, 758
  personal assistance services, **542–545**
  respite, **641–642**
  sexuality issues, 670

Caregiving (*cont.*)
  social workers' help in, 677
  for spinal cord injury victims, 693
  by women, 766
CARF. *See* Commission on Accreditation of Rehabilitation Facilities
Carl D. Perkins Vocational and Applied Technology Education Act, 727
Carpal tunnel syndrome, 88, 293, 294, 489–490
Cartilage disorders, 484–486
Case management movement, 438
Case review, 180
Case Review System, 312
Catalogs, 191
Catapres. *See* Clonidine
Cataract, 118
Catastrophic disabilities, 437
CD-ROM information systems, 200
Center for Disability and Socioeconomic Policy Studies, 466
Center for Independent Living, 466
Center for Substance Abuse Prevention, 276, 277
Center, hemodialysis, 425
Central nervous system, 152, 153
Cerebral palsy, 249, 250, 252–254
  advocacy project for, 18
  animals to aid, 62, 63
  attitudes toward, 95
  communication disabilities and, 193
  definition, 152
  multiple disabilities and, 477
  occupational therapy for, 527
  rehabilitation engineering, 299
  sexuality and, 671
  speech/language professionals for, 41
  supported employment for, 708
Cerebrovascular disease, 529
Certification, 223, 226–227
Chace, Marian, 232
Character disorders. *See* Personality disorders
Charcot-Marie-Tooth disease, 511–512, 514
Charter of Rights and Freedoms (Canada), 258
Chelation therapy, 675
Chemical burns, 130
Chemical dependence, 275, 552; *see also specific dependence, e.g.* Drug abuse; Drug rehabilitation
Chemotherapy, 135, 136, 139
Child abuse, 130, 535, 538, 547, 743, 744, 746

Childbirth. *See* Pregnancy and childbirth
Childhood disabilities, **148–156**
  abuse/neglect as cause, 130, 458
  advocacy groups, 18, 248
  amputation as result, 55, 59–60
  animals to assist, 63
  arthritis, 78–79
  assistive technology for, 91–92
  attitudes toward, 97
  burns causing, 126, 128, 130, 133
  civil rights issues, 175
  communication, **192–197**
  computers to aid, 205–206
  dance/movement therapy, 233
  deaf-blindness, 234, 235, 247
  deafness/hearing impairment, 239, 244–245
  developmental, **249–255**
  disability law/social policy, 266–267
  euthanasia programs for, 745–746
  gastrointestinal disorders, 344
  genetic disorders, **347–355**
  growth disorders, **355–358**
  head injury prevention, 365–366
  hemophilia, 122, 123, 124–125
  learning disabilities, **434–436**
  loss-related grief and, 447–48
  massage for, 455
  mental retardation, 18, 248, **457–462**
  neurological, 503, 506, 507
  occupational therapy for, 527
  organic mental syndromes, 529
  pain from, 531
  pediatric rehabilitation, 59–60, 153–156, **534–541**
  physician for, 565
  psychosocial adjustment to, 601
  quality of life and, 609
  respite care for, 642
  self-concept and, 661
  sexuality and, 669–670
  sickle cell anemia, 674–675
  social worker to aid family with, 676–677
  thalassemia, 675
  thalidomide causing, 297
  see also Adolescents, rehabilitation of; Special education
Childhood psychiatric disorders, **158–168**
  art therapy, 75
  autism, **101–102**
  mood, 470
  sexual abuse as cause, 547

Chloropromazine, 582
Cholesterol, 212
Cholinomimetics, 472
Christmas in Purgatory (Blatt and Kaplan), 248
Chromosome disorders. *See* Genetic disorders
Chronic disease/disability
  aging and, 29, 30, 32
  alcoholism as, 35
  amputation as result of, 54
  arthritis as, 177
  back pain as, 105, 106, 111
  behavior therapy for, 110, 111, 112–113
  blood disorders as, 120, 121–123
  burns and, 130
  cancer as, **135–139**
  caregiving for, **146–148**
  childhood disability caused by, 153
  coronary artery disease, **212–217**
  developmental disabilities as, **249–255**
  diabetes as, 291
  gastrointestinal disorders, **341–346**
  HIV/AIDS as, 390–391
  homelessness and, 374
  pain and, 531, 532
  prevention of, 40
  psychosocial adjustment to, 601
  rehabilitation assessment and, 83
  rehabilitation psychology for, 597
  respiratory, 637
  in rural areas, 645
  self-help groups for, 664
  sociological views, 679
  visual impairment as, 118
  wellness programs for, 757
Chronic fatigue syndrome, **172–174**
Chronic obstructive pulmonary disease. *See* Respiratory disease
Chronic sorrow, 13–14
City of Cleburne v. Cleburne Living Center (1985), 177
Civil Aeronautics Board, 735–736
Civilian Rehabilitation Act of 1920, 261
Civilian Vocational Rehabilitation Program, 696
Civil rights, **174–178**
  accessibility as, **3–7**
  ADA and, **47–53**
  affirmative action for, **22–26**
  assistive technology as, 91
  disability law/social policy, 268–269
  influence on disability consumer groups, 208, 210

legal advocacy for, 19–20
normalization and, 15
reasonable accommodation as, 612–613
see also Disability rights movement; Discrimination
Civil Rights Act of 1964, 22, 47, 50, 51
Civil Rights Restoration Act of 1988, 48, 175, 176
Civil War, U.S., 206, 573
Class action suits, 19, 20
Clearinghouse on Disability Information, 408
Cleft palate and lip, 193
Client-centered approach, 548
Clinical supervision, **178–187**
Clonidine (Catapres), 472, 553
Clothing, **190–192**
Clotting factors, 121, 122, 123, 124, 125
Clozapine, 587, 657
Clubhouse model, 583, 584–585
Cocaine abuse, 275
Cocaine Anonymous, 277
Cochlear implants, 100, 740
Code of Professional Ethics for Rehabilitation Counselors, 308
Coehlo, Tony, 49
Cognitive/developmental impairment, 44
autism and, 101
behavior therapy for, 109–110, 112
caregiving for, 147
of children, 151, 155, 164
head injury as cause, 363
multiple disabilities and, 476
neurological disorders as cause, 503
personal assistance services for, 542
physician for, 564
psychological assessment of, 593, 598
Colleges and universities
accreditation for, 223–226
affirmative action requirements, 24
architectural accessibility at, 71–72
assistive technology programs at, 93
courses for prisoners, 219
for deaf/hearing impaired, 243
disabled students accepted by, 208
disabled students denied entrance by, 207–208
Gallaudet University, **339–341**
information resources, 407
physical therapy research at, 562
for prosthetics/orthotics professionals, 578

psychiatric rehabilitation and, 583–584
rehabilitation counseling training at, 618
rehabilitation credentials from, 223–226
rehabilitation education, 623–625, 626, 627
rehabilitation engineering, 299
rehabilitation training shortages at, 740
Rusk's contribution to, 652
Switzer traineeships at, 718
see also Credentials; Students with disabilities
Colon cancer, 136
Colostomy, 344
Commission on Accreditation of Rehabilitation Facilities (CARF), 9, 314, 318, 383, 563
Commission on Certification of Work Adjustment and Vocational Evaluation Specialists, 752
Commission on Recognition of Postsecondary Accreditation, 226
Commission on Rehabilitation Counselor Certification, 226–227
Committee on Prosthetics Research and Development, 297, 298
Communication barriers, 50, 52–53, 269
Communication disabilities, **192–197**
allied health professionals aids, 40, 41–42
Alzheimer's disease as cause, 43
animal aids, 61
aphasia, **68–69**, 195, 196
architectural accessibility for, 74
art therapy, 75
audiology, **99–101**
autism and, 102
cancer-caused, 136–137
in children, 152, 154
deaf-blindness, **233–238**
deafness/hearing impairment, **239–247**
future of rehabilitation, 335
music therapy, 497
physician for, 563
rehabilitation assessment, 87
rehabilitation engineering, 299
rehabilitation hospital, 383
stroke-caused, 703, 704
technology aids, 6, 90–91
Community care
for aged, 30

attitudes toward, 97
for developmentally disabled, 254
early management of, 450–451
hospice, 379
international rehabilitation, 409–410
for pediatric rehabilitation, 537–539
for psychiatric rehabilitation, 583
respite, 641
following spinal cord injury, 692–693
Community living. *See* Deinstitutionalization; Housing; Independent living
Community Mental Health Center Act of 1963, 582
Community rehabilitation, 320–321, 364–365
Community Rehabilitation Programs, 319
Community Supported Living Arrangements Act, 544
Comorbidity. *See* Multiple disabilities
Compensatory devices. *See* Assistive technology
Competitive placement, 414
Comprehensive outpatient rehabilitation facilities, 319
Computer application for persons with visual impairments, 6, **197–201**
Computer-controlled appliances, 205
Computers, **201–206**
for ability and job matching, 1
for allied health professionals' tasks, 41–42
for autistics, 102
for back disorders' registry, 107
for career counseling, 143–144
for deaf/hearing impaired, 241, 246, 740
for homebound work, 414
for improved communication accessibility, 6, 41
for information resources, 408
for music therapy, 498–499
for neurological disorders, 505
for occupational information, 526
for occupational therapy, 527
for prosthetics design, 577, 740
for rehabilitation assessment, 83
for rehabilitation education, 627
for rehabilitation professionals, 335
for rehabilitation program evaluation, 315
for research, 634
speech activated, 90–91
for statistics, 700, 702
talking, 6

Computers (*cont.*)
  for veterans' rehabilitation, 740
  for visual impairments, 6, **197–201**
Conduct disorders, 162–165, 547
Confidentiality, 307, 393
Congenital disorders. *See* Developmental disorders; Genetic disorders
Conn's syndrome, 294
Consortium for Citizens with Disabilities, 49
Constipation, 456
Consumers, **206–211**
  addiction groups, 277
  architectural accessibility and, 73–74
  arthritis groups, 81
  for assistive technology, 725–726
  clothing, **192–194**
  communication disabilities groups, 196
  deaf-blind groups, 238
  deaf/hearing impaired groups, 243, 245
  developmentally disabled groups, 255
  disability law/social policy, 267
  disabled groups, 259
  family groups, 325
  future of rehabilitation, 336, 337
  head injury groups, 366
  hemophilia centers, 125
  independent living, 400, 404
  information resources, 406
  international rehabilitation, 410
  job placement, 413–414, 418
  kidney disorder groups, 426–427, 428
  mental retardation groups, 248
  multiple disabilities groups, 478
  neuromuscular disorders groups, 514
  pain groups, 533
  personal assistance services, 544–545
  of physical therapy, 561
  for psychiatric rehabilitation, 584, 586–587
  of rehabilitation counseling, 620
  rehabilitation engineering, 299, 301
  rehabilitation program evaluation and, 313
  for respiratory disease, 640
  self-help groups for, 664
  of supported employment, 711–712, 713
  women in rehabilitation as, 762–763
Contagious diseases, 20
Contingency management, 161
Convalescent Assistance to Recovering Employees, 272
Cooley's Anemia Foundations, 676

Coping
  adolescent rehabilitation for, 13, 16
  for burn victims, 133
  by child/family, 155
  by disabled, 155, 259
  in family, 322
  with loss and grief, 444, 446
  with pediatric rehabilitation, 537
  psychiatric rehabilitation for, 580
  psychosocial adjustment and, 604
  self-help groups for, 664
  see also Psychiatric rehabilitation; Psychology, rehabilitation; Psychosocial adjustment
Copp, Tracy, 368
Coronary angiography, 214
Coronary artery disease, **212–217**
  bypass grafting for, 215
  death rates from, 146
  diabetes and, 292, 293
  functional electrical stimulation for, 330, 331
  hospice and, 380
  pharmacology for, 550, 551
  respiratory disease symptoms and, 636
  stroke caused by, 704–705, 707
  study of children with, 13
  wellness programs to prevent, 755, 756
Corporate rehabilitation counseling, 621
Correctional rehabilitation, **217–222**, 621
Corticosteroids, 494
Cortisol excess, 295
Cost-benefit analysis, 313
Coulter, John Stanley, 368
Council for Exceptional Children, 459, 685
Council of Rehabilitation Counselor Education, 625
Council on Postsecondary Accreditation, 226
Council on Rehabilitation Education (CORE), 225–226, 619, 622, 626
Counseling. *See* Adjustment services; Allied health professionals; Career counseling; Psychology; Rehabilitation counseling; Social work
Counselor-facilitator roles, 183
Covalt, Donald, 369
Credentials, **222–229**
  for allied health professionals, 42
  for career counselors, 148
  for counselors of deaf/hearing impaired, 242
  for dance/movement therapist, 233

  for life care planning, 438
  for massage therapists, 456
  for music therapists, 498
  neurology, 507–508
  for occupational therapists, 528
  for physical therapy, 652
  for physicians, 563
  for private sector rehabilitation professionals, 571–572
  for prosthetics/orthotics professionals, 578
  psychiatry, 588–589
  psychologist, 592–593
  for recreation professionals, 615
  for rehabilitation centers, 617
  for rehabilitation counseling, 619, 621–622
  for rehabilitation education, 626–627
  rehabilitation engineering, 300–301
  rehabilitation nurse, 521–522
  for rehabilitation psychology, 598
  for social worker, 678
  for sociologists, 680
  for special educators, 684–685
  for speech-language pathologists, 195
  of vocational evaluators, 752–753
  see also Colleges and universities; Education, professional
Crime. *See* Correctional rehabilitation; Violence
Crohn's disease, 343–344, 346
Cryotherapy, 495
Current Population Survey, 701
Cushing's syndrome, 294
Cybernetics (Weiner), 301
Cystic fibrosis, 351, 352, 635

D
Dance/movement therapy, **231–233**
Danish Mental Retardation Service, 515
Dart, Justin, 48–49, 568, 569
Data collection, 700
Deaf-blindness, **233–238**, 266, 421
Deaf Education Initiative, 247
Deafness and hearing impairment, **239–247**
  accessibility needs, 3, 5, 6
  ADA and, 53
  affirmative action, 24
  allied health professionals to aid, 41–42
  audiology for, **99–101**
  autism as cause, 101
  in children, 149, 150, 151–152, 154, 340
  civil rights legislation for, 176

commmunication affected by, 192, 193
computers for, 205
disability law/social policy, 266
future of rehabilitation, 335
Gallaudet University, **339–341**
hearing dogs for, 62
housing issues, 385
Keller, Helen, **421–423**
management of care, 451
mental retardation and, 460
rehabilitation education, 625
special education, 683
student protests about, 210
technology for, 722
in veterans, 740
Death
alcoholism as cause, 36
Alzheimer's disease as cause, 43
arthritis as factor, 78, 79
attitudes toward, 97
burns as cause, 126
coronary artery disease rates, 212
of hemophiliacs, 121
hospice, **378–381**
lifestyles as cause of, 112
loss and grief, **443–48**
from neurological disorders, 505, 506
rates, 146
right to, 176
see also Euthanasia; Suicide
Debridement, 130
Degenerative joint disease, 76–77
Deinstitutionalization, **247–249**
architectural accessibility and, 72, 74
history, 370
homelessness and, 373
housing issues, 386
of injured worker, 271
international rehabilitation, 410
psychiatric rehabilitation and, 581–583
rehabilitation counseling following, 620–621
residential/community rehabilitation following, 320
respite care following, 641
DeJong, Gerben, 402–403, 405
Delirium, 529
Dementia, 42, 43, 44, 126
caregiving for, 147
in HIV/AIDS patients, 391, 393
Rusk's programs for, 652
see also Alzheimer's disease
Dental care, 122, 123
Deontology, 305

Department of. See name of department, e.g., Education, U.S. Department of
Dependent personality disorder, 547
Depression, economic (1930s), 207
Depressive disorders, 469, 470–471, 473, 532
in aged, 30
alcoholism combined with, 35, 37
aphasia as cause, 69
arthritis as cause, 80–81
behavior therapy for, 111
in children, 166–168
communication disabilities and, 193
following coronary artery disease, 216
in deaf-blind, 236
eating disorders and, 279, 280
HIV/AIDS and, 390
homelessness and, 374
kidney disorders as cause, 425–426
following loss-related grief, 443–444, 445
massage for, 455
neurological disorders and, 503
neuromuscular disorders and, 514
pharmacology for, 550, 552
of prisoners, 220, 221
psychiatry for, 590
psychosocial adjustment to, 601
rehabilitation psychology for, 598
religious professionals as aid, 629
respiratory disease and, 636
following stroke, 530, 707
see also Antidepressants
Dermatomyositis, 79
Desyrel, 470, 553
Devaluation. See Normalization and social role valorization
Developmental disabilities, **249–255**, 257
adjustment services for, 9
animals to assist, 63
architectural accessibility and, 74
autism, **101–102**
of children, 149, 150, 151–152
communication affected by, 195
definition, 150
deinstitutionalization, **247–249**
euthanasia for, 746
hearing deficit as cause, 152
legislation protecting people with, 48
psychosocial adjustment to, 600, 601
quality of life and, 609
respite care for, 642
sexuality and, 669
speech/language professionals for, 41

state-federal rehabilitation program for, 697
thalidomide as cause, 297
violence as cause, 743
vision deficit as cause, 152
see also Autism; Cerebral palsy; Epilepsy; Mental retardation
Developmental Disabilities Assistance and Bill of Rights Act of 1975, 48, 175, 248, 250, 461
Developmental Disabilities Service and Construction Act of 1970, 249
Development of sexuality, 669–670
Deviancy, 366–367
Diabetes mellitus, 126, 290–294
amputation as result of, 54, 55
gastrointestinal disorders and, 343
of homeless, 374
kidney disorders and, 424
sexuality and, 671
as stroke risk, 502
vision loss and, 118–119
Diagnosis and screening
alcoholism, 36
Alzheimer's disease, 43–44
arthritis, 77
art therapy for, 74
autism, 101
blindness/vision impairment, 117–118, 149, 150, 151–152
breast cancer, 137
childhood disabilities, 149, 150, 151–152
childhood psychiatric disorders, 158–160
coronary artery disease, 212, 213–214
deaf-blindness, 235
disabled, 257–258
drug abuse, 275–276
gastrointestinal disorders, 343, 344
genetic disorders, 351, 354
growth disorders, 356–357
hemophilia, 124
learning disabilities, 434
life care planning and, 439
mental retardation, 157, 160
multiple disabilities, 477
neurological disorders, 506, 508
neuromuscular disorders, 510–511
psychiatric, 589–590
psychological, 593–594
rehabilitation, 83–84
respiratory disease, 636, 638–639
schizophrenia, 654
sickle cell anemia, 674
Dialysis. See Kidney disorders

Dictionary of Occupational Titles, The,
525, 526
Diet. *See* Food and nutrition
Differential Aptitude Test, 750
Diffuse connective tissue disorders,
77–79
Digestive diseases. *See* Gastrointestinal
disorders
Dilantin, 554
Disability, **257–260**, 270, 303, 327;
see also Disability law and social
policy; Disability management;
specific disabilities
Disability and Business Technical Assistance Centers, 407–408
Disability and Family Support Act
(model), 325
Disability insurance. *See* Social Security Disability Insurance; Workers'
compensation
Disability law and social policy, 258–
259, **260–269**
accessibility issues, 4–5, 6, 7
ADA, **47–53**
advocacy views, 18, 19–20
affirmative action, **22–26**
alcoholics and, 35–36
for assistive technology, 91
attitudes affected by, 98
for cancer patients, 139
for career counseling, 140–141
for childhood psychiatric disorders,
165
for children, 149, 151, 155–156
civil rights, **174–176**
consumers groups, **206–211**
for deaf-blind, 236
for developmental disability, 249, 250
forensic rehabilitation, **326–330**
gender issues, 762–763
history, 367–371
housing issues, 386–387
international, 410–411
life care planning, 437, 438
for mentally retarded, 461
personal assistance services, 543–544
to prevent spinal cord injury, 694
reasonable accommodation, **611–613**
rehabilitation assessment and, 87
research affected by, 633
self-concept affected by, 661
for special education, 684
for supported employment, 708–709
for technology and disability, 721
for transition from school to work,
727–728

for transportation accessibility, 732–
735
see also specific legislation
Disability management, 2, **270–274**
cancer rehabilitation, **135–139**
career counseling to aid, 141, 143–
144
family role in, 321
rehabilitation counseling for, 621
Disability rights movement, 268, 369–
370, 410, 568, 733–734
Disabled Americans' Self-Perceptions
(poll), 700–701
Disabled American Veterans, 4, 55
Discrimination
ADA prohibition, **47–53**, 86
affirmative action and, 22, 24
against aged, 30
against cancer patients, 139
civil rights issues, **174–178**, 268
against disabled children, 155
against HIV/AIDS patients, 392
see also Attitudes; Disability law and
social policy; Minorities
Disease. *See* Chronic disease/disability;
specific diseases
Disfluent speech, 194
DISTAT (Disability Statistics), 702
Distraction therapy, 130
Divalproex sodium (Depakote), 472
Dix, Dorothea, 367
DNA, 347, 357
Dogs, assistance, 62–63, 64
Dominant genetic conditions, 352
Dopamine, 552, 656
Douglas, Rick, 569
Douglas, William O., 652
Down syndrome, 151, 348, 458
Draper, Warren, 369
Drowning/near-drowning, 36, 152
Drug abuse
adolescent, 168, 535
affirmative action exclusion, 23
alcoholism and, 35
attitudes toward, 97
eating disorders and, 280
highway accidents due to, 535
HIV/AIDS and, 388, 392, 393
homelessness and, 372, 374
medications with, 553
mood disorders and, 470
organic mental syndromes caused by,
530
prenatal effects, 150, 458, 477
schizophrenia and, 655
as stroke risk, 705

veterans, 740
as violence risk, 743
Drug Enforcement Administration, 554
Drug rehabilitation, **275–277**
art therapy, 75
centers, 617
future of, 333, 334
for prisoners, 218, 219–220
Drugs, therapeutic. *See* Pharmacology;
specific drug
Duchenne muscular dystrophy, 506,
512–513
Du Pont survey (1990), 2
Dybwad, Gunnar, 248, 516
Dysarthria, 194
Dysfunctional behavior. *See* Behavior
therapy
Dyslexia, 434
Dysphagia, 647
Dyspnea, 637
Dysthymia, 166, 469

E
EAP. *See* Employee assistance programs
Ear infections, 193
Early Intervention Program for Infants
and Toddlers with Disabilities, 537
Earnings capacity, 328–329
Ears. *See* Deafness and hearing impairment; Ear infections
Eating disorders, **279–281**, 333; *see
also* Feeding disorders
Economics, **281–286**
of ability management, 2
of accidents, 271–272
of aging, 30
of Alzheimer's disease, 44
of back disorders, 105, 106
of cancer care, 139
of caregiving, 147
of coronary artery disease, 212
of disability management, 2
of drug rehabilitation, 275
of eating disorders, 280–281
of endocrine disorders, 290
of hemophiliac care, 122, 124, 125
of hospice care, 380, 381
of illegal drug use, 219
of independent living, 399–400
job market effects, 145
of job placement, 418
of kidney disorders, 425
minorities and, 462–464, 466–467
of pain, 531
of personal assistance services, 543
of psychiatric rehabilitation, 582

of rehabilitation centers, 617–618
rural, 643–645
of spinal cord injury, 689
of state-federal rehabilitation program, 697–698
of supported employment, 710
of workplace accessibility, 6–7
Education. See Colleges and universities; Learning disabilities; Rehabilitation education; Special education; Students with disabilities
Education, professional
allied health professionals, 42
career counselors, 144
caregivers, 147
clinical supervision, **178–187**
counselors for deaf/hearing impaired, 242
credentials, **222–229**
for disabled, 207–208, 387
ethics, 308
federal funding, 267
for independent living, 404, 405
physical therapy, 562
physicians, 563
post-employment, 186
private sector rehabilitation specialists, 571–572
psychiatric rehabilitation, 581
rehabilitation counseling, 618–619, 772
rehabilitation education, **623–627**
rehabilitation engineering, 299
religious leaders, 629
sexuality counseling, 672–673
Switzer traineeships, 718
for veterans' rehabilitation, 739, 740
see also Colleges and universities
Education, U.S. Department of, 197, 210, 267, 682
Education for All Handicapped Children Act of 1975, 48, 149, 151, 155, 209, 267, 268
architectural accessibility, 73
future of rehabilitation, 336
housing, 386
learning disabilities, 434
mentally retarded, 461
pediatric rehabilitation, 537
special education, 681
E. E. Black, Ltd. v. Marshall (1980), 24
EEOC. See Equal Employment Opportunity Commission
Effleurage, 454
Eisenhower, Dwight D., 369
Elderly. See Aging

Electrical burns, 127, 130
Electrical stimulation. See Functional electrical stimulation
Electroconvulsive therapy (ECT), 471, 472
Electroejaculation, 331, 692
Electronic mail (e-mail), 200–201
Elementary and Secondary Education Act of 1965 (ESEA), 209, 236
Elizabethan Poor Law of 1601, 396
Emergency medical services, 129, 690
Emotions
art therapy to express, 75
behavior impairment and, 253
childhood disabilities affecting, 152, 155
childhood psychiatric disorders and, 159
dance/music therapy for, 233
about disabled, 178, 396
drug abuse affected by, 276
in family, 322
learning disabilities and, 435
loss and grief, **443–448**
neuromuscular disorders and, 514
during pediatric rehabilitation, 536
religious support for, 629
self-help groups for, 664
about sexuality, 670
see also Attitudes; Psychology, rehabilitation
Employee assistance programs (EAP), **287–289**, 433
Employment. See Affirmative action; Career counseling; Job placement; Labor unions; Occupational therapy; Supported employment; Unemployment; Vocational evaluation; Work
Empowerment
of alcoholic, 39
assistive technology and, 725
consumer groups for, 210–211
of deaf/hearing impaired, 245
of disabled, 258
family and, 324, 325, 326
history, 371
international rehabilitation, 410
for learning disabled, 435
management team and, 453
President's Committee on Employment of People with Disabilities, **568–570**
psychiatric rehabilitation and, 584
rehabilitation assessment and, 84–85

rehabilitation program evaluation and, 313
self-concept and, 661
self-help groups for, 664
see also Advocacy; Civil rights
ENCOR regional service system (Omaha, Nebraska), 516
Endocrine disorders, **290–296**; see also Growth disorders
Endogenous chemicals, 532
End stage renal disease. See Kidney disorders
Engineering, rehabilitation, 89, 91, **296–302**
centers for, 298
for childhood disabilities, 154–155
computers for, **197–206**
information resources, 407
state-federal rehabilitation program and, 697
see also Assistive technology
Environmental adaptations
allied health professionals to aid, 40
for Alzheimer's patients, 44–45
assistive technology for, 91, 723
behavior therapy for, 110
as civil right, 175, 177
for neurological disorders, 506
to prevent spinal cord injury, 694
for stroke victims, 707
Environmental barriers. See Architectural accessibility
Environmental control units, 71
Environmental influences
on alcoholism, 36
on arthritis, 77, 80
autism and, 102
on childhood psychiatric disorders, 159
on coronary artery disease, 212
on eating disorders, 280
genetic disorders, 347
mental retardation, 458
for multiple disabilities, 477
on neurological disorders, 504
on psychosocial adjustment, 600, 603
rehabilitation assessment and, 83
on respiratory disease, 635–636, 637
sensitivity to, 74, 102
Environmental safety, 20, 193
Epidemiology, 699
Epilepsy, 64, 126, 249, 502–503
functional electrical stimulation to prevent, 331
pharmacology for, 551

Epilepsy Foundation of America, 255, 267
Epstein-Barr virus, 172
Equal Employment Opportunity Commission (EEOC)
    ADA enforcement by, 51, 53
    affirmative action, 23, 24, 26
    brain cancer/workplace discrimination case, 139
    legal advocacy procedures, 19
    workplace accommodation study, 6–7
Ergonomics, 302–304
    assessment for rehabilitation, 86, 87
    for back disorders, 107
Erikson, Erik, 768
Esophageal speech, 136
ESRD. See Kidney disorders
Ethics, 305–308
    HIV/AIDS information, 393
    of personal assistants, 543
    of private sector rehabilitation, 572
    for rehabilitation centers, 618
    of rehabilitation research, 634–635
Ethnic issues. See Minorities
Ethnography, 679
Eugenic myth, 744–745
European Conference for the Advancement of Rehabilitation Technology, 300
Euthanasia, 176, 258, 307
    medically assisted, 258, 543
    Nazi programs, 745–746
Evaluation of rehabilitation programs, 309–315
Executive Order 11246, 22
Exercise. See Dance/movement therapy; Physical exercise; Physical therapy; Recreation; Sports
Exercise testing, 636
Expert witness. See Forensic rehabilitation
Externalizing disorders, 167, 168
Eyegaze computer system, 204
Eyes. See Blindness and vision disorders

F
Facial disfigurement, study of children with, 13
Facilities, 317–321
    affirmative action requirements, 25–26
    architectural accessibility, 71, 74
    life care planning and, 441
    management, 452–453
    for supported employment, 712
Fair Housing Act of 1988, 5, 73, 384, 386

Families of Children with Spinal Muscular Atrophy, 640
Family, 321–326
    accessibility issues for, 6
    adolescent rehabilitation and, 13–14
    allied health professionals and, 40
    Alzheimer's disease and, 44
    animals to assist disabled and, 63
    aphasia and, 69
    arthritis and, 81
    attitudes toward disabled, 96
    autism in, 102
    of burn victims, 130, 132, 133
    caregiving by and for, 146–148, 544
    childhood psychiatric disorders and, 159, 161–162, 164–165, 166
    communication disabilities and, 192, 193
    coronary artery disease and, 216
    of deaf-blind person, 236
    developmentally disabled in, 254, 255
    of disabled children, 153, 155
    drug rehabilitation role, 277
    dysfunction as violence risk, 743
    genetic disorders and, 354
    head injury and, 362
    of hemophiliacs, 122, 124–125, 365
    of HIV/AIDS patients, 393
    international rehabilitation, 411–412
    life care planning, 437, 438–439
    loss-related grief and, 447
    minority, 462
    neurological disorders and, 507, 509
    pediatric rehabilitation and, 535–536, 537, 538, 539
    psychiatric rehabilitation and, 580, 584, 587
    psychological support for, 595
    rehabilitation center to assist, 617
    religious support for, 630
    respite care, 641–642
    of schizophrenics, 656, 657
    self-help groups, 664, 666
    siblings in, 677
    social workers to aid, 676–677
    of spinal cord injury victims, 690, 691
    of stroke victims, 707, 708
    see also Genetic disorders
Family burden myth, 745
Fascio-scapulo-humeral syndrome, 513, 514
Fat, dietary, 212
Faulkes, William F., 368
Federal agencies
    affirmative action requirements, 24
    see also specific agencies

Federal Aid to Highways Act of 1973, 732
Federal Aviation Act of 1958, 735
Federal programs. See specific program or legislation
Federal Security Agency, 368
Federal-state. See State-federal benefits; State-federal rehabilitation program
Feeding disorders, 154, 758
Feet First First Time program, 694
Felty's syndrome, 78
Female sexuality, 671–672
FES. See Functional electrical stimulation
Fetal alcohol syndrome (FAS), 458
Fidelity, 306
Fires, alcoholism as cause, 36
First aid, for burns, 127–129
Fitness guidelines, 756
Fluency disabilities, 194
Fluoxetine (Prozac), 470, 471, 552, 553
Folic acid, 347, 353–354
Follow-along, 730
Food and Drug Administration, 138, 301, 331
Food and nutrition
    additives affecting children, 160
    for Alzheimer's patients, 45, 46
    for burn victims, 132
    gastrointestinal disorders and, 342, 343, 344, 345, 346
    for hemophiliacs, 122
    for hospice, 379
    for kidney disorders, 423, 425
    mental retardation and, 458, 459
    for PKU disorder, 351, 458
    to prevent coronary artery disease, 212
    to prevent multiple disabilities, 477
    to prevent stroke, 704, 707
    respiratory disease and, 637
    for wellness, 755–756, 757–759
    see also Eating disorders; Feeding disorders
Food pyramid, 757–758
Forensic rehabilitation, 326–330
    education for, 625
    psychologist role, 595
Fragile X syndrome, 352–353, 458
Freud, Sigmund, 767
Friction stroke, 454
Frieden, Lex, 49
Friendly Societies, 663
Friendship, attitudes toward disabled and, 96
Full Inclusion Movement, 683

Functional assessment, 330, 567, 752
Functional curriculum, 728
Functional electrical stimulation, **330–332**
Future of rehabilitation, **333–337**

G

Gallaudet, Thomas Hopkins, 244, 367, 451
Gallaudet University, 210, **339–341**
Gallstones, 343
Gambling rehabilitation, for prisoners, 218
Gastrointestinal disorders, **341–346**, 715
Gazette International Network Inc., 640
Geist Picture Interest Inventory, 751
Gender
    assistive technology use and, 724
    attitudes toward, 98
    blood disorders linked with, 121
    deafness/hearing impairment differences, 239
    endocrine disorders and, 294
    genetic disorders linked with, 349–350, 352–353
    neuromuscular disorders linked with, 512–513
    as psychosocial adjustment factor, 602
    sexuality and, 669, 671–672
    Social Security payments and, 266
    see also Women in rehabilitation
Gene disorders, 350
General Aptitude Test Battery, 750
General Electric Company (GE), 272
Genetic disorders, 257, **347–355**
    alcoholism as, 36, 39
    amputation as result of, 54, 55
    arthritis as, 77, 80
    autism and, 101
    of the blood, 121, 125
    childhood disabilities caused by, 151
    childhood psychiatric disorders caused by, 160–161, 166
    communication disabilities caused by, 196
    coronary artery disease risk and, 212
    deaf-blindness as, 235, 237
    drug abuse link, 275
    learning disabilities, 434, 436
    mental retardation, 458–459, 460, 461
    multiple disabilities, 477
    neurological, 503, 504, 505, 507
    neuromuscular, 511–513

psychosocial adjustment to, 600, 601
schizophrenia as, 655
speech/language professionals for, 41
    see also specific type, e.g., Huntington's disease
Genetic engineering, 123, 125
German measles. See Rubella
Germany
    adolescent rehabilitation in, 14
    gastrointestinal disorders in, 345
G.I. Bill, 741
Glasgow Coma Scale, 364
Glaucoma, 118
Glossopharyngeal breathing, 639
Goffman, Erving, 248
Grant recipients, affirmative action requirements, 24
Gray, Boyden, 49
Greve, Bell, 367
Grief. See Loss and grief
Group homes. See Supported living
Group therapy, 277, 661
Grove City College v. Bell (1984), 25, 176
Growth disorders, 349, **355–358**
Growth hormone, 357
Grumman, Inc., 24
Grunewald, Karl, 248
Guide dogs. See Dogs, assistance
Guide to Occupational Exploration, 525–526
Gynecological cancers, 136

H

Hahn, Harlan, 259–260
Halderman v. Pennhurst State School and Hospital, 248
Halfway houses, 219, 376
Halstead-Reitan test, 87, 593
Handicap, 270, see also Disability
Hard of hearing. See Deafness and hearing impairment
Harkin, Tom, 49
Headaches, 531
Head cancers, 136–137
Head injury, **361–366**
    adjustment services for, 9
    alcohol as cause, 36
    aphasia caused by, **68–69**
    behavior therapy following, 111
    childhood disability caused by, 152–153
    child psychiatric disorders caused by, 160
    communication disabilities caused by, 195

developmental disabilities following, 250
future of rehabilitation, 334
loss-related grief following, 445
mental retardation as result, 458
multiple disabilities and, 477
pediatric rehabilitation following, 535, 537, 538
pharmacology for, 550, 551
physician for, 564
psychological testing following, 593
rehabilitation assessment following, 83, 86, 87
self-help for students, 665–666
sexuality and, 671
speech/language professionals for, 41
supported employment for, 708
violence as cause, 743
Health. See Wellness
Health and Activity Limitation Survey, 701–702
Health and Human Services, U.S. Department of, 196, 255
Health care
    for aging population, 29
    for Alzheimer's patients, 45–46
    behavior therapy used in, 110–113
    independent living and, 404
    in rural areas, 646–647
Health Care Financing Administration, 267, 268, 427, 428
Health Care for the Homeless, 374
Health care workers
    attitudes toward disabled, 97
    back disorders of, 106
    for developmentally disabled, 254
Health, Education, and Welfare, U.S. Department of, 297, 298
Health expectancy, 702
Health insurance. See Medical insurance
Health psychology, 109, 110
Healthy People 2000, 196, 758
Hearing. See Audiology; Communication disabilities; Deafness and hearing impairment
Heart disease. See Coronary artery disease
Heart disorders, 249, 513
Helen Keller International, 422–423
Helen Keller National Center Act of 1967, 236
Helms, Edgar James, 367
Hemodialysis, 423–424
Hemoglobinopathies. See Sickle cell anemia and thalassemia

Hemophilia, 121–123, 352, 353
Hemorrhage, 703, 705
Hepatitis, 122, 123
Heredity. *See* Genetic disorders
Heroin, 553
Herpes simplex, 390, 529
Heterocyclic antidepressants, 470, 471
Heterotopic ossification, 691
Heumann, Judith, 209, 370
High blood pressure. *See* Hypertension
Highway accidents, 4
    alcoholism as cause, 36, 365
    childhood disabilities caused by, 153
    head injury, 361, 362, 365, 366
    pediatric rehabilitation following, 535–536, 538
    safety devices to prevent, 365, 366, 535, 536, 538, 694
Hippocratic oath, 307
Hispanic Americans, 462, 463, 464, 465, 466
    endocrine disorders, 290, 292
    homelessness, 372
History of rehabilitation, **366–371**
    ADA and, 210–211, 370
    consumer groups, **206–211**
    dance/movement therapy, 231
    disability law/social policy, 261, 265–266
    Gallaudet University, 339
    hospice, 379
    international, 409–410
    kidney disorders, 424–425
    prosthetics/orthotics, 573
    psychiatric, 581–582
    rehabilitation engineering, 297–299
    Rusk, Howard A., **651–652**
    self-help groups, 663–664
    special education, 681–682
    state-federal program, 696–697
    Switzer, Mary E., **718–719**
    wheelchairs, 760–762
HIV. *See* Human immunodeficiency virus disease and acquired immunodeficiency syndrome
Holocaust, 745–746
Homebound employment, 202, 414
Home care. *See* Caregiving; Independent living; Personal assistance services
Home hemodialysis, 424, 425
Homelessness, **372–376**
    effect on childhood disabilities, 150
    of mentally ill, 580
    of veterans, 740
Homophobia, 392

Hormones
    arthritis link, 77, 78
    burns and, 129
    cancer treatment manipulation of, 135
    organic mental syndromes caused by, 530
Horseback riding, 63–64
Hospice, 147, **378–381**
Hospital, mental. *See* Deinstitutionalization
Hospital, rehabilitation, 318–319, **382–383**
    assessment for, 83
    for burn victims, 126, 129–130, 133
    caregivers at, 147
    for children, 153, 536–537
    for diabetics, 293
    ethics committees, 307–308
    nurses, 523
    physical therapy programs, 562
    physicians, 565–566
    psychiatric, 373, 374, 548, 580, 581, 590
    psychological approaches, 597
    rural, 644
    for spinal cord injury, 690
    for stroke, 706–707
    see also Nursing, rehabilitation; Rehabilitation center
Housing, **384–387**
    accessibility issues, 5
    for aged, 31
    architectural accessibility, 70–71, 73
    attitudes toward disabled, 94
    disability law and social policy, 266
    for disabled prisoners, 221
    laws against discrimination, 48
    for mentally ill, 580
    in rural areas, 648
    see also Homelessness; Independent living; Institutional living; Supported living
Housing and Community Development Amendments of 1974, 266
Howard A. Rusk Institute of Rehabilitation Medicine, 651, 652
Howe, Samuel Gridley, 367
Hudson Institute Report, 466
Human factors. *See* Ergonomics
Human Genome Project, 354–355, 460
Human immunodeficiency virus disease and acquired immunodeficiency syndrome, **388–393**
    consumer groups, 210
    endocrine disorders and, 294

    family and, 324
    future of rehabilitation, 333, 334–345
    hemophiliacs infected with, 123, 353
    homelessness and, 374
    hospice and, 380
    legislation, 48, 49
    massage therapy for, 454
    mental retardation and, 461
    psychiatry for, 591
    psychological support, 596
    rehabilitation assessment, 83
    research about, 635
    vocational rehabilitation, 320
Human resource development, **394–395**
Human Resources Development Institute Handicapped Placement Program, 432
Human services, **395–397**; *see also* Caregiving; Personal assistance services
Huntington's disease, 352
Hydrocephaly, 151, 458
Hyperactivity. *See* Attention-deficit hyperactivity disorder
Hypercalcemia, 295
Hypercapnia, 637
Hypertension, 51, 212, 215, 292, 374
    massage therapy for, 456
    as stroke risk, 502, 704–705, 707
Hyperthyroidism, 294
Hypoglycemia, 291
Hypothyroidism, 294

I

IDEA. *See* Individuals with Disabilities Education Act of 1990
Ileostomy, 344
Imipramine, 552, 553
Immune therapy, 135
Immunizations, 234
Impairment, 270, 303, 705
Imprinting, 353
Independent living, 324, **399–405**
    ability for, 1
    for aged, 31, 32
    allied health professionals to aid, 40, 41
    architectural accessibility, **69–74**
    computers to aid, 202, 205, 206
    for disabled veterans, 742
    future of, 336
    history, 369–370, 371
    housing for, 386–387
    international, 410
    legislation, 210
    for mentally retarded, 461

for minorities, 465–466
movement for, 48, 208, 211, 410
personal assistance services for, 542
rehabilitation education for professionals, 623
in rural areas, 646, 647
self-concept and, 661
self-help for, 208, 666–667
state-federal rehabilitation program for, 697
transition from school to work for, 728
Independent Living Research Utilization program, 403
Individual/client advocacy, 18, 21
Individualized education plan (IEP), 84, 91, 155, 209, 681
for mentally retarded, 459
for transition from school to work, 727–728
Individualized Family Service Plan, 155, 538
Individualized Service Plans, 84
Individuals with Disabilities Education Act of 1990 (IDEA), 48
assistive technology, 92
developmental disabilities, 250
future of rehabilitation, 336
pediatric rehabilitation, 537, 538, 540
rehabilitation engineering, 299
special education, 681, 682, 685
transition from school to work, 727, 729
Individual written adjustment plan, 8
Individual written rehabilitation plan, 84, 91, 557, 696
Industrial ergonomics, 303
Industrial rehabilitation. See Occupational therapy
Industrial Revolution (U.S.), 261, 367
Infanticide, 367, 744
Infarction, 703
Infection, 33, 194, 195
Inflammatory bowel disease, 343–345
Information-processing approach, 142
Information resources, 406–408
for back disorders, 107
for independent living, 401
to influence attitudes toward disabled, 95–96
privacy of, 25
Injury. See Accidental injury; Head injury; Occupational injury
Input devices, 202 204
Input evaluation, 310
Institute on Rehabilitation Issues, 32

Institutionalization. See Institutional living
Institutional living
for aged, 29–30, 31
correctional rehabilitation, 217–222
psychiatric rehabilitation, 581–582
see also Deinstitutionalization
Insulin, 290–291, 292
Insurance. See Medical insurance; Social Security Disability Insurance; Workers' compensation
Integrated employment, 558
Intelligence
ability as, 1
developmental disability and, 251, 253
infant testing, 150
learning disabilities and, 434
of mentally retarded, 457, 460
neuromuscular disorders and, 514
following pediatric rehabilitation, 539
psychological tests, 593
Interagency agreements, 728–729
Interest groups. See Consumers
Internalizing disorders, 165 167, 168
Internal programs, 288
International Association for the Study of Pain, 533
International Association of Psychological Rehabilitation Services, 586
International Center on Deafness, 340
International Classification of Impairments, Disabilities, and Handicaps, 702
International Council on Disability, 410
International rehabilitation, 409–412, 421–423
International Rehabilitation Associates, 327
International Society for Prosthetics and Orthotics, 579
International symbols, 412
Interpersonal relationships. See Personality disorders
Interpreters for deaf, 240–241
Irritation medication, 550
Ischemia, 502, 674, 703

J
Japanese vocational training, 14
Jewish ancestry, 344
Job accommodation. See Job placement; President's Committee on Employment of People with Disabilities; Reasonable accommodation
Job Accommodation Network, 570

Job counseling. See Career counseling
Job placement, 413–419
ability factors for, 1–3
adjustment services for, 9, 11–12
affirmative action, 23–24, 25
allied health professionals for, 41
career counseling for, 140–145
for developmentally disabled, 254
information resources for, 408
for injured worker, 273
occupational information for, 525–527
rehabilitation counseling for, 618–623
rehabilitation education for, 623
state-federal rehabilitation program for, 696
supported employment, 708–713
transition from school to work, 730
see also President's Committee on Employment of People with Disabilities; Reasonable accommodation; Vocational evaluation
Job titles, 328–329
Job Training and Partnership Act, 727
Joint Commission for the Accreditation of Health Organizations (JCAHO), 563
Joint Commission of Healthcare Organizations, 383
Joint Commission on Accreditation of Healthcare Organizations, 318
Joint disorders. See Arthritis; Musculoskeletal disorders
Journal of Learning Disabilities, The, 685
Joysticks, computer, 204
Justice, 305
Justice, U.S. Department of, 51, 52, 53, 197
Juvenile rheumatoid arthritis, 78–79

K
Kahn, Robert L., 768
Kanner, Leo, 101
Kant, Immanuel, 305
Kaplan, Fred, 248
Keller, Helen, 234, 235, 421–423
Kemp, Evan, 49
Kennedy, Joseph P., 652
Kennedy, Robert, 248
Kessler, Howard, 368–369
Keyboard, computer, 202–203
Kidney disorders, 293, 357, 380, 423–428, 549
Killing or inactivating organisms, 550

Kim Manufacturing v. Superior Metal Treating (1976), 327
Kinney v. Pennsylvania Transportation Department (1993), 19
Koop, C. Everett, 663
Korean War, 72, 741–742
Korsakoff's syndrome, 529
Kraepelin, Emil, 653
Kratz, John A., 368
Kropotkin, Peter, 663, 667
Krusen, Frank, 368–369, 382

L
Labor, U.S. Department of, 24
Labor Market Access, 328–329
Labor Statistics, U.S. Bureau of, 701
Labor unions, 207, 261, 288, **431–433**
Language disabilities. *See* Aphasia; Communication disabilities
Larynx cancer, 136, 194
Law. *See* Disability law and social policy; *specific legislation*
Learning disabilities, **434–436**
   art therapy, 75
   communication effects, 195
   consumer groups, 210
   genetic disorders as cause, 349
   pediatric injury as cause, 538
   premature birth as cause, 151
   rehabilitation of adolescents with, 13
   rehabilitation assessment for, 87
Least restrictive environment, 209, 245, 682
Legal advocacy, 18, 19–20
Legal blindness, 117
Legal issues. *See* Disability law and social policy
Legal Nurses Association, 327
Leisure. *See* Recreation
Leukemias, 120
Levering, Robert, 771
Libraries, public, 24; *see also* Information resources
Licensure. *See* Credentials
Life care planning, 327–328, **436–442**
Life Centered Career Education curriculum, 728
Life expectancy, 125, 146, 151
Life stages, 27
Lifestyle patterns, 112, 630
Limb girdle syndrome, 513, 514
Literacy programs, 218–219
Lithium, 165, 471–472, 549, 552, 553, 554
Liver disorders, 346, 549
Local area networks, 200–201

Lopez, Vincent, 652
Loss and grief, **443–448**
   aphasia and, 69
   burn victims and, 132
   disabled adolescents and, 13–14
   disabled child and, 155
   during pediatric rehabilitation, 537
   psychiatry for, 591
   religious professionals for, 630
   self-concept process and, 660–661
   sexual adjustments and, 670
Lou Gehrig's disease. *See* Amyotrophic lateral sclerosis
L-P-E method, 329
Lung cancer, 136, 138
Lung disease. *See* Respiratory disease
Lupus erythematosus, 79
Lupus Foundation, 81
Luria-Nebraska test, 87
Luther, Martin, 744
Lymphedema, 138
Lymph nodes, 137

M
Macular degeneration, 118
Magnification software/hardware, 199
Mail-order catalogs, 191
Mainstreaming
   attitudes toward, 97
   childhood disabilities and, 155
   computers to aid, 202
   consumers for, 209
   for deaf and hearing impaired, 245
   for disability management, 271
   future of rehabilitation, 336
   human services and, 397
   international rehabilitation, 410
   social worker to aid, 677
   see also Deinstitutionalization; Normalization and social role valorization; Transition from school to work
Malaria, 673
Male sexuality, 671
Malnutrition, 758
Managed care. *See under* Medical insurance
Management, **449–454**
   of ability, 2–3
   of neurological disorders, 502
   of neuromuscular disorders, 513–514
   private sector rehabilitation, **570–572**
   of respite care, 648–649
   of spinal cord injury, 689–690
Management by objective (MBO), 313

Mania, 470, 472
Manic-depressive illness. *See* Bipolar disorder
Manually Coded English (MCE), 240, 241
Marchand, Paul, 49
March of Dimes, 207, 355
Marfan syndrome, 357
Marijuana abuse, 275
Marriage and relationships
   abuse in, 744
   burn injury effect on, 133
   mental illness and, 590–591
   mental retardation and, 461
Mary E. Switzer Memorial Seminar, 32
Massage therapy, **454–456**
Matching Person and Technology model, 722, 725
McCarron-Dial Work Evaluation System, 87
McKinney Homeless Assistance Act of 1987, 376
Medicaid, 267, 396
   for childhood disabilities, 156
   as civil right, 176
   creation of, 582
   for developmental disabilities, 255
   for the homeless, 375
   hospice and, 379, 380
   medical rehabilitation coverage, 563
   for personal assistance services, 543, 544
   for psychiatric rehabilitation, 586
Medicaid waiver, 248
Medical assessment. *See* Diagnosis and screening
Medical insurance
   aphasia coverage, 69
   behavior therapy coverage, 113
   cancer coverage, 139
   disability management, 272
   effect on caregiving, 146
   ethical considerations, 306–307
   for hemophiliacs, 124, 125
   for independent living, 404
   for kidney disorders, 427
   managed care, 113, 289, 586
   medical rehabilitation coverage, 563
   for private sector rehabilitation, 570–571
Medical model
   for childhood disabilities, 149
   for older adult, 32
   for personal assistance services, 542
   for rehabilitators, 764
Medical rehabilitation. *See* Physician

Medicare, 318, 319, 379, 380, 396
  creation of, 582
  for kidney disorders, 424, 425, 427–428
  medical rehabilitation coverage, 563
  rural areas, 644
Medicare Hospice Benefit Program Evaluation, 381
Medication. *See* Pharmacology
Melanocytes, 129
Memory impairment, 43, 45, 594
Mendelian inheritance, 350
Mental health, 590–591
Mental hospitals
  historical trends, 581
  population, 248, 249
  see also Deinstitutionalization; Psychiatric rehabilitation
Mental illness
  of adolescents, 14
  of alcoholics, 35
  anxiety disorders, **65–67**
  art therapy, 74
  attitudes toward, 95
  behavior therapy, 109
  burn risk and, 126
  caregiving for, 147
  childhood psychiatric, **158–168**
  computers to aid, 205
  dance/movement therapy, 233
  deinstitutionalization, **247–249**
  disability law/social policy, 49, 51, 266
  euthanasia for, 746
  family and, 324
  future of rehabilitation, 333
  historical views of, 367, 368
  homelessness and, 372, 374, 375
  management, 449
  mental retardation and, 253, 460
  mood disorders, **468–475**
  as multiple disability, 476
  music therapy, 497
  neurological disorders and, 503
  occupational therapy, 527
  pharmacology, 552–553
  psychiatric rehabilitation, **579–587**
  psychiatric therapy, **588–591**
  psychological therapy, **592–596**
  psychology, rehabilitative, **597–599**
  quality of life, 607, 609
  rehabilitation assessment, 84
  rehabilitation counseling, 620–621
  rehabilitation of labor union members, 431
  rehabilitation of prisoners, 218, 219–220, 221

schizophrenia, **653–658**
self-help groups, 664
supported employment, 708, 710, 711–712
  in veterans, 740
  work issues, 771
  see also specific illness, e.g., Bipolar disorder
Mental retardation, 249, 250, 251, 258, **457–462**
  adjustment services, 9
  of adolescents, 14
  advocacy project, 18
  art therapy, 75
  attitudes toward, 95, 97
  autism and, 101
  blindness/deafness and, 152, 236
  burn risk and, 126
  civil rights legislation, 177
  communication effects, 195
  definition, 151
  deinstitutionalization, **247–249**
  disability law/social policy, 48, 209, 266
  as Down Syndrome component, 151
  future of rehabilitation, 333
  genetic aspects, 352
  historical views of, 368
  mental illness and, 253
  multiple disabilities and, 477
  normalization/social role valorization, 248, **515–520**
  PKU disorder as cause, 351
  of prisoners, 221
  respite care, 642
  rubella syndrome as cause, 234
  special education, 681
  supported employment, **708–713**
Mental Retardation Facilities and Community Mental Health Centers Construction Act, 266
Mentor. *See* Clinical supervision
Metabolic disorders. *See* Developmental disability; Endocrine disorders; Genetic disorders; Mental retardation
Migraine headaches, 531
Milbank, Jeremiah, 367
Mills v. Board of Education of the District of Columbia (1971–1972), 209, 268
Minnesota Multiphasic Personality Inventory, 750
Minorities, **462–467**
  ADA applied to, 50
  affirmative action, 22
  civil rights, **174–178**
  deaf/hearing impaired, 239

disabled as, 268
disabled compared with, 601–602
drug abuse link, 276
endocrine disorders, 290
history of disabled, 370
mental retardation, 457
quality of life for, 609
in special education, 685
violence against, 744
vocational rehabilitation, 320
in workforce, 145, 334
Miracle Worker, The (play/film), 421
Mitochrondrial inheritance, 353
Mobility impairments. *See* Musculoskeletal disorders; Prosthetics and orthotics; Spinal cord injury; Transportation accessibility; Wheelchairs
Model State Plan for Deaf-Blind Persons, 242, 246
Monkeys, assistance, 63
Monoamine Oxidase Inhibitors (MAOIs), 470, 471
Mononucleosis, 172
Mood disorders, 253, **468–475**
  Alzheimer's disease as cause, 43, 44
  homelessness and, 372
  organic mental syndromes and, 529–530
  pharmacology for, 552
  psychiatric rehabilitation, 579
  see also specific disorders, e.g., Depressive disorders
Moskowitz, Milton, 771
Motoneuron diseases, 503–504
Motor development, 152
Motor impairment, 505–506
Motor neurons, 510
Mouse, computer, 203–204
Mouth cancer, 136
Movement therapy. *See* Dance/movement therapy
Multicultural issues. *See* Minorities
Multiple disabilities, 167–168, **476–478**
  deaf-blindness, **233–238**
  Keller, Helen, **421–423**
  kidney disorders and, 424–425
  sexuality and, 671
Multiple sclerosis, 445, 505–506, 551, 672
Murder. *See* Violence
Muscle disorders, 482–484
Muscular dystrophies, 506–507, 513, 550, 671
Muscular Dystrophy Association, 514, 640

Musculoskeletal disorders, **478–496**
  assistive technology for, 90
  back disorders, **105–107**
  cancer, 138–139
  of children, 150, 151, 154
  pain and, 532
  prosthetics/orthotics for, 573
  surgery for, 716
  wellness programs for, 756
Music therapy, 379, **497–499**
Myasthenia gravis, 513
Myelomeningocele, 151
Myoblast transfer, 514
Myocardial infarction, 212, 214–215, 283
Myocardial ischemia, 212, 213–214, 215
Myofascial disorders, 490
Myotonic muscular dystrophy, 513

N
NARC. *See* National Association for
  Retarded Children
Narcissistic personality disorder, 547
Narcotic Addict Rehabilitation Act of
  1966, 219
Narcotic drugs, 533, 551–552, 674; *see
  also* Drug abuse
Narcotics Anonymous (NA), 219–220,
  277
National Alliance for the Mentally Ill,
  584, 590, 664
National Association for Music Ther-
  apy, 498
National Association for Retarded
  Children, 18, 248
National Association for Ventilator
  Dependent Individuals, 640
National Association of Alcoholism
  and Drug Abuse, 39
National Association of Rehabilitation
  Professionals in the Private Sec-
  tor, 623
National Cancer Institute, 135
National Center for Law and Deafness,
  340
National Center for Law and the
  Handicapped, 18
National Chronic Pain Outreach Asso-
  ciation, 107
National Council on Disability, 49,
  210, 370
National Council on Rehabilitation
  Education, 625
National Defense Act of 1916, 367
National Head Injury Foundation, 255,
  366
National Health Interview Survey, 701

National Hemophilia Foundation, 125,
  664
National Hospice Organization, 379
National Hospice Study, 381
National Institute for Drug Abuse, 39,
  277
National Institute for Disability and
  Rehabilitation Research, 210
National Institute for Handicapped
  Research, 210
National Institute of Alcohol Abuse
  and Alcoholism, 39
National Institute of Child Health and
  Human Development, 459
National Institute of Handicapped Re-
  search, 33, 298
National Institute of Mental Health, 583
National Institute on Deafness and
  Other Communication Disabili-
  ties, 196
National Institute on Disability and
  Research, 53, 514, 632
National Institute on Mental Retarda-
  tion (Canada), 516
National Institutes of Health, 514,
  632–633
National Joint Committee for Learning
  Disabilities, 434
National Kidney Foundation, 427
National Mental Health Consumers'
  Association, 584
National Rehabilitation Association,
  144, 267, 465, 718
National Rehabilitation Counseling
  Association, 621, 622
National Rehabilitation Information
  Center, 634
National Stroke Association, 707
National Transition Study, 685
Native Americans, 462, 464–465, 466
  arthritis in, 78
  disability rates, 463
  endocrine disorders in, 290
  gastrointestinal disorders in, 343
  rehabilitation programs for, 648
Natural supports, 712–713
Neck cancers, 136–137
Needs assessment, 311–312
Neglect, 743
Nerve blocks, 533
Nerve disorders, 489–490
Network on Health Expectancy and
  the Disability Process, 701
Neural prosthesis, 331
Neural tube defects, 151, 347, 353–
  354, 458

Neurodegenerative disorders, 503–505,
  550
Neurofibromatosis, 352
Neuroleptic drugs, 165, 656
Neurological disorders, **501–507**
  assessment for, 87
  autism, **101–102**
  multiple disabilities, 476
  physician for, 565
  psychological testing for, 594
  respiratory disease and, 638
  special education for, 681
  speech/language professionals for, 41
  following spinal cord injury, 689
  wheelchairs for, 760
Neurology, **507–509**
  Alzheimer's disease, **42–46**
  autism, **101–102**
  blood disorders and, 120, 124
  childhood disorders, 150, 151, 347
  communication disabilities and, 193
  developmental disabilities, **249–255**
  diabetes and, 293
  head injury, **361–366**
  learning disabilities, **434–436**
  loss-related grief following injury, 445
  mood disorders, **468–475**
  organic mental syndromes, **528–530**
  of pain, 532
  pediatric rehabilitation, 539
  schizophrenia and, 655–656
  of stroke, 703
  surgeons for, 715
  see also specific disorders, e.g., Epilepsy
Neuromuscular disorders, **509–514**
  animals to aid, 62, 63
  architectural accessibility for, 71
  functional electrical stimulation for,
  331
  physician for, 564
  prosthetics/orthotics for, 573, 574
  psychiatry for, 591
  psychological testing for, 594
  respiratory disease and, 638
Neuropsychology, 111, 539, 592–593,
  598
Neurotransmitters, 552, 553
*New York State Association for Retarded
  Children, Benevolent Society for
  Retarded Children, et al. v. Mario
  Cuomo, et. al.* (1975, 1993), 20
New York State Human Rights Law, 19
New York State mental institutions,
  248
Nicotine. *See* Smoking
Nirje, Bengt, 248, 515, 516

Nondiscrimination. *See* Affirmative action; Disability law and social policy
Nonmaleficence, 257–258, 305
Non-Reading Aptitude Test Battery, 750
Nonsteroidal anti-inflammatory drugs (NSAIDs), 494, 551
Noradrenergic agents, 472
Norfluoxetine, 471
Normalization and social role valorization, 397, **515–520**
  advocacy programs for, 17–18
  aging and, 28, 31
  allied health professionals to aid, 40
  Alzheimer's patients and, 45
  architectural accessibility and, 72
  attitudes toward disabled, **94–99**
  for autistics, 102
  for mentally retarded, 248, 461
  rehabilitation program evaluation and, 313
  transition from school to work for, 728
  see also Deinstitutionalization; Mainstreaming
Norpramin, 553
Not-for-profit institutions, 449, 450, 451
NSAIDS. *See* Nonsteroidal anti-inflammatory drugs
Nursing, rehabilitation, 383, **521–524**, 563, 564
  for children and families, 154
  clinical supervision of, 184
  education for, 624
  forensic issues, 326–327
  hospice, 378, 380
  private sector, 571
  psychiatric, 184
Nursing homes, 210, 293, 318, 365, 401
Nutrition. *See* Food and nutrition

O
Obesity, 111–112, 216, 343, 758
Observation methods, 180–181, 749, 751
Obsessive-compulsive disorder, 66, 67, 111, 279, 547–548
Occupational Access Systems, 526
Occupational bonding, 273
Occupational information, **525–527**
Occupational injury, 4, 206–207, 261, 266, 367, 415, 431, 591; *see also* Social Security Disability Insurance; Veterans; Workers' compensation

Occupational medicine, 288
Occupational Outlet Handbook, 525, 526
Occupational Safety and Health Act of 1970, 571
Occupational therapy, 40, 41, **527–528**, 564
  adjustment services of, 11
  architectural accessibility and, 73
  assistive technology for, 89
  for back disorders, 106
  for burn victims, 132
  for childhood disabilities, 153, 154
  clinical supervision of, 184–185
  clothing as aid to, 191
  disability management, **270–274**
  education for, 624
  future of, 333–334
  for hospice care, 380
  international rehabilitation, 409
  for neurological disorders, 504–505
  occupational therapy for, 527
  physician for, 563
  rehabilitation assessment for, 87
  in rehabilitation hospital, 383
  for respiratory disease, 636–637
  see also Employee assistance programs; Private sector rehabilitation
O'Connor v. Donaldson (1975), 248
Office of Civil Rights, 612–613
Office of Personnel Management, 24
Office of Special Education Programs, 246
Office of Special Education and Rehabilitation Services, 682
Office of Technology Assessment, 734
Office of Vocational Rehabilitation, 368, 717
Office workers, 106
Older adulthood. *See* Aging
Older Americans Act, 27, 543
On-line services, 201
On-the-job training, 419
Ophthalmologist. *See* Blindness and vision disorders
Oppositional defiant disorders, 162
Optical character recognition systems, 200, 204
Organic mental syndromes, **528–530**; *see also* Alzheimer's disease; Dementia
Organ transplants, 346, 424, 425
Orthopedics. *See* Musculoskeletal disorders
Orthotics. *See* Prosthesis and orthotics
Osteoarthritis, 76–77, 479–480
Ostomies, 345

Outcome evaluation, 311, 312–313
Output devices, computer, 204–205
Oxygen therapy, 637

P
Pacemakers, 330, 331
Pacific Islanders, 463
Pain, **531–534**
  arthritis, 81
  back disorder, 105, 106
  behavior therapy for, 110–111
  burn, 130, 132
  hemophilia-related, 124
  musculoskeletal disorder, 492, 494
  neurological disorder, 506
  pharmacology for, 551–552
  physical therapy for, 561
  prosthetics/orthotics for, 573, 574
  sickle cell anemia, 674
  spinal cord injury, 693
Palliative care, 379
Pancreatitis, 532
Panic disorder, 66, 67, 471, 590
Paralysis. *See* Neurological disorders; Neuromuscular disorders; Spinal cord injury; Stroke
Paralyzed Veterans of America, 4, 72, 736
Paranoid personality disorder, 546–547
Paraplegia, 331
Paratransit services, 733, 734
Parents. *See* Family
Parking accessibility, 736
Parkinson's disease, 194, 454, 455, 503–504
Paroxetine (Paxil), 470, 552, 553
Parrino, Sandra, 49
Parsons, Frank, 141–142
Patient-controlled drugs, 552
Paxil. *See* Paroxetine
Pediatric rehabilitation, 59–60, 153–156, **534–541**
Peer counseling, 401–402
Peer pressure, 276
Peer supervision, 181
Pennsylvania Association for Retarded Children (PARC) v. Commonwealth of Pennsylvania (1971–72), 209, 268
Pennsylvania Attendant Care Program, 542
Pennsylvania Bi-Manual Worksample, 750
People First, 248, 255
Peptic ulcer, 342–343, 346
Performance appraisal, 182, 453

Peritoneal dialysis, 424, 425
Perkins Institute for the Blind, 451
Perrin, Burt, 516
Personal assistance services, 94, 210, **542–545**
  for independent living, 402, 404
  respite care, **641–642**
  for spinal cord injury victims, 693
Personal computers. *See* Computers
Personality disorders, 9, **546–548**, 552
Personality evaluation, 750
Petrissage, 454
Pets. *See* Animals
Pharmacodynamics, 549, 552
Pharmacokinetics, 549
Pharmacology, **548–554**
  for Alzheimer's disease, 44
  for anxiety disorders, 66
  for arthritis, 77, 78, 79
  for autism, 102
  for back disorders, 106
  for burns, 130
  for childhood psychiatric disorders, 161, 162, 164, 165, 166
  for chronic fatigue syndrome, 173
  for coronary artery disease, 214–215
  deinstitutionalization and, 373
  depression as result of, 469
  for eating disorders, 280
  for endocrine disorders, 290–291, 294
  for euthanasia, 764
  for gastrointestinal disorders, 342, 344, 346
  for genetic disorders, 349
  for growth disorders, 357
  for HIV/AIDS, 389, 390, 391
  for hospice care, 380
  for kidney disorders, 423, 424
  life care planning and, 441
  following loss-related grief, 445
  massage therapy effect on, 455
  for mood disorders, 468, 470–473
  for musculoskeletal disorders, 494
  for neurological disorders, 505, 506
  for neuromuscular disorders, 513
  for pain, 532, 533
  psychiatric, 581, 589, 590, 591
  for respiratory disease, 637
  for schizophrenia, 656–657
  for sickle cell anemia, 674, 675
  following spinal cord injury, 691–692
  for stroke prevention, 707
Pharmacotherapeutics, 549
Phenylketonuria (PKU), 351, 352, 458
Philosophy of rehabilitation, **555–559**
  international, 409

rehabilitation education, 624–625
special education, 682–683, 684
women's role in, **762–767**
Phobias, 66, 67, 579–580, 590
Phrenic nerve pacers, 331
Physiatrist, 86, 153, 369, 563, 564, 565
Physical disabilities, 252
  affirmative action, 24
  of aged, 28, 31
  alcoholism as cause, 35
  allied health professionals for, 40, 41
  art therapy, 75
  attitudes toward, 97
  computers for, 202, 205
  coronary artery disease as cause, 216
  dance/movement therapy, 233
  drug abusers with, 275, 276, 277
  historical view, 367
  homelessness and, 372
  legislation, 51
  management of, 449
  multiple, 476
  music therapy, 497
  physical therapy, 561
  psychiatry for, 589, 591
  rehabilitation center, 617
  rehabilitation of labor union members, 431
  rehabilitation of prisoners, 221
  in rural areas, 646
  self-help groups, 664
  state-federal rehabilitation program, 696
  supported employment, 708, 710, 712
Physical exercise
  for Alzheimer's patients, 45
  for arthritis, 77, 79
  for back disorders, 107
  for chronic fatigue syndrome patients, 173
  coronary artery disease and, 213–214, 215–216, 217
  for hemophiliacs, 124
  for musculoskeletal disorders, 495–496
  for neuromuscular disorders, 513–514
  for wellness, 755–757
  see also Sports
Physically Disabled Students Program, 208
Physical medicine and rehabilitation specialty, 739
Physical therapy, 40, 41, **561–562**
  for amputees, 55–56
  for arthritis, 81
  for burn victims, 132

for cancer patients, 138
for children, 153, 154
clinical supervision of, 180, 184–185
clothing as aid to, 191
for diabetics, 293
education for, 624
federal funds for, 267
following head injury, 364
for hemophiliacs, 121–122, 123, 124
horseback riding as, 63–64
for hospice care, 380
international rehabilitation, 409
for musculoskeletal disorders, 495–496
for neurological disorders, 504, 507
physician for, 563
in rehabilitation hospital, 383
for respiratory disease, 636–637, 638
Physician, 317–319, **562–567**
  for childhood disabilities, 153–154
  for hospice care, 380
  for management of care, 450–451
  for neurology, **507–509**
  pharmacology and, 554
  psychiatry and, **588–591**
  rehabilitation counseling role, 619
  rehabilitation education for, 624
  in rehabilitation hospital, 383
  rural, 644
  Rusk, Howard A., **651–652**
  for surgery, **715–716**
Physiology, 303, 363
Physiotherapists, 739
Pinel, Philippe, 581
Pituitary disorders, 295, 357
PKU. *See* Phenylketonuria
Placement specialist, 413–415
Plastic surgeon, 715–716
Playground safety, 365
Play therapy, 158
Policy. *See* Disability law and social policy; State-federal rehabilitation program
Polio, 512
  architectural accessibility and, 72
  consumers groups, 207
  pharmacology, 551
  prosthetics/orthotics, 573
Polymyositis, 79, 512
Population. *See* Statistics
Poststroke depression, 530
Post-traumatic stress disorder, 66
  of burn victims, 133
  future of rehabilitation and, 333
  loss-related grief and, 445

Poverty, 175, 372, 458, 643; *see also* Homelessness
Prader Willi syndrome, 353
Pregnancy and childbirth
  alcohol use during, 458, 477
  childhood disabilities following, 150–151, 152
  electroejaculation to conceive, 331, 692
  genetic disorders, 347–348, 349, 351, 353–354
  in vitro fertilization, 671
  learning disabilities-prenatal conditions link, 434–435
  lupus during, 79
  massage therapy during, 455
  maternal prenatal drug use effects, 150, 458, 477
  maternal rubella effects, 234
  mental retardation and, 458
  multiple disabilities following, 477
  premature birth, 151, 455, 527
  prenatal testing, 348, 459, 477
  protective effect for maternal neurological disorders, 505
  sickle cell anemia and, 673, 675
  following spinal cord injury, 692
  termination of pregnancy, 348, 349, 459
  thalassemia and, 675
  thalidomide use during, 297
  violence against mother effects, 743
Prejudice. *See* Attitudes; Discrimination
Premature births, 151, 455, 527
Prenatal testing, 348, 459, 477
President's Committee for the Employment of People with Disabilities, **568–570**
President's Committee on Mental Retardation, 459
Prevention programs
  alcoholism, 37, 39
  Alzheimer's disease, 44–45
  amputation, 55
  back disorders, 107
  behavior therapy as, 112
  communication disabilities, 196
  coronary artery disease, 214–216
  drug abuse, 276
  employee assistance programs, 288
  endocrine disorders, 292–293
  ergonomics as, 87–88, 107
  head injury, 365–366
  hearing loss, 100
  hemophilia, 122
  immunization programs, 234

international programs, 411
kidney disorders, 423
loss-related grief, 447
mental retardation, 458–459
mood disorders, 471
multiple disabilities, 477
neurological, 509
occupational therapy as, 527
for prisoners, 220
spinal cord injury, 693–694
stroke, 704–705, 707
violence, 747
vision loss, 118
for wellness, **755–759**
see also Safety
Principle of Normalization in Human Services, The (Wolfensberger), 515, 516
Printers, computer, 205
Prisons. *See* Correctional rehabilitation
Private sector rehabilitation, **570–572**
  ethics and, 306–307
  forensic issues, 327
  job placement and, 415
  research in, 633
Probability samples, 699–700
Process evaluation, 310–311, 312
Professional organizations. *See specific organizations*
Professional training. *See* Education, professional
Program evaluation. *See* Evaluation of rehabilitation programs
Progression, 35
Progressive Era, 206
Project Enable, 408
Projects with Industry, 414
Prophylaxis. *See* Prevention programs
Prostate cancer, 136
Prosthetics and orthotics, **573–579**
  following amputation, 56–59
  for cancer patients, 136, 137–138
  for children, 154
  Civil War (U.S.) role in development of, 206, 573
  for developmentally disabled, 255
  for eye replacement, 118
  functional electrical stimulation for, **330–332**
  international rehabilitation, 409–410
  life care planning and, 439, 441
  for musculoskeletal disorders, 495
  for neurological disorders, 506
  physician for, 564
  rehabilitation engineering, 297, 301
  technological changes, 90
  for veterans, 740

Prozac. *See* Fluoxetine
Psychiatric disorders. *See* Mental illness; Mood disorders; Psychiatric rehabilitation; *specific disorders*
Psychiatric rehabilitation, **579–587**
  for anxiety disorders, 66–67
  art therapy, 75
  assessment for, 83, 86
  for burn victims, 133
  centers for, 617
  for children, 159–160
  coronary artery disease and, 216
  dance/movement therapy, 232
  deinstitutionalization and, 247–249, 373, 374
  for drug abuse, 277
  federal funds for professionals, 267
  for mood disorders, 468–469, 473–474
  for neurological disorders, 503
  personal assistance services for, 542
  for personality disorders, 548
  pharmacology and, 550, 552–554
  rehabilitation counseling and, 621
  of schizophrenics, 657–658
  for veterans, 740
Psychiatry, **588–591**
Psychology, 563, **592–596**
  of career counseling, 140, 142
  of coronary artery disease, 216
  deficits following head injury, 363–364
  for disabled, 257
  ergonomics and, 303
  ethical principles of, 307
  of neurological disorders, 503
  of organic mental syndromes, 528
  psychiatry and, 589
  for rehabilitation hospital patients, 383
  support by religious professionals, 629
  for vocational evaluation, 749–750
Psychology, rehabilitation, **597–599**
  for alcoholics, 37, 38–39
  for Alzheimer's patients, 44
  assessment for, 84, 86, 87
  for back disorders, 106
  behavior therapy for, **108–113**
  for burn victims, 133
  for childhood disabilities, 155
  dance/movement therapy, 232
  for deaf-blind, 237
  for developmentally disabled, 254
  forensic issues, 330
  for growth disorders, 358
  for hemophiliacs, 121–122
  for HIV/AIDS patients, 389–390

Psychology, rehabilitation (*cont.*)
  horseback riding advantages, 63–64
  following loss-related grief, 445
  for neurological disorders, 506
  for prisoners, 218
  prosthetics/orthotics and, 574
  rehabilitation counseling and, 619
  for self-concept, 661
  self-help groups for, 664
  sexuality issues, 670
  for spinal cord injury, 690, 691
  state-federal rehabilitation program,
    696
  for stroke victims, 707
  for veterans, 741
  work's role in, 768
Psychopharmacology, 552, 553
Psychosis, 470, 471, 503, 654, 656
Psychosocial adjustment, 8–9, 564,
    599–604
  adolescent rehabilitation for, 13,
    14–16
  advocacy programs for, 17
  of aged, 28, 31
  of alcoholics, 35
  animal assistants, 63
  aphasia and, 69
  of arthritics, 80–81
  for autistics, 102
  behavior therapy for, 112–113
  for burn victims, 132–133
  for cancer patients, 135
  caregivers to aid, 147
  chronic fatigue syndrome and, 172–
    173
  clothing and, **190–192**
  for communication disabilities, 192–
    193, 194
  for deaf-blind, 235, 236–237
  for disabled, 259
  for eating disorders, 280–281
  for hemophiliacs, 124–125
  history of specialty, 207
  for mentally retarded, 460
  for mood disorders, 473–474
  to pain, 532–533
  for respiratory disease, 637
  for schizophrenics, 657
  self-concept, **660–662**
  self-help for, **663–668**
  sexuality and, 670–671
  sociological views, 679
  transportation accessibility to aid,
    731
  to vision loss, 119
  for women in rehabilitation, 763

Psychosocioecological approach, 597
Psychotherapy. *See* Mood disorders;
    Pharmacology; Psychiatric rehabil-
    itation; Psychiatry; Psychology;
    Psychology, rehabilitation
Public accommodation
  ADA requirements and, 52–53
  affirmative action, 24
  architectural accessibility, 71, 208
  assistance animals and, 63
  disability law/social policy, 269
  for spinal cord injury victims, 693
  see also Reasonable accommodation
Public Health Service, U.S., 741
Public rehabilitation system. *See* State-
    federal rehabilitation program
Public sector rehabilitation, 306, 327,
    415, 633
Public transportation, 732–735
Pulmonary disorders. *See* Respiratory
    disease

Q
Quality of life, **607–609**
  for Alzheimer's patients, 44–46
  aphasia and, 69
  art therapy for, 75
  computers to aid, 206
  for disabled, 258
  ergonomics, **303–304**
  functional electrical stimulation for,
    331
  gastrointestinal disorders and, 342,
    344, 346
  for hemophiliacs, 124
  for hospice patients, 381
  job placement and, 415
  myth of, 745
  normalization and, 17
  personal assistants/patients and, 543
  philosophy of rehabilitation and,
    558–559
  psychological issues, 594–596
  rehabilitation center for, **616–618**
  respiratory disease and, 636
  respite care, **641–642**
  of schizophrenics, 658
  social workers to aid, 676
  supported employment for, 711
  work issues, 771
Quinlan, Karen, 307

R
Radiation therapy, 135, 136, 137, 139
Rain Man (film), 101
Rancho scale, 364

Randolph-Sheppard Act, 266
Randomization, 284–285
Random sample, 699
Rare disorders. *See* Developmental dis-
    abilities; Endocrine disorders; Ge-
    netic disorders
Rate dependency, 161
Rational Recovery, 39
Reach to Recovery Program, 138
Reading evaluation, 750–751
Reading machines, 199, 200, 204
Realization stage, 600
Reasonable accommodation, **611–613**
  for accessibility, 6
  ADA and, 51, 52–53
  adjustment specialist as aid to, 10
  affirmative action for, 22, 23–24, 25
  allied health professionals for, 41
  architectural accessibility and, 73
  assistive technology for, 91
  civil rights legislation and, 177
  disability law/social policy, 268, 269
  psychiatric rehabilitation and, 584
  at work, 770
Recessive genetic conditions, 350–352
Recreation, **614–615**
  attitudes toward disabled in, 94
  clinical supervision of professionals,
    185
  communication disabilities and, 193
  computers to aid, 202
  life care planning and, 442
  in rehabilitation hospital, 383
  for veterans' rehabilitation, 740
  for wellness, 757
  see also Sports
Rectal cancer, 136
Registration, 223, 228–229
Regular Education Initiative, 683
REHABDATA database, 408
Rehabilitation Act of 1920, 624
Rehabilitation Act of 1954, 394
Rehabilitation Act of 1973, 47–48, 50,
    175–176, 268
  accessibility issues, 4–5, 6
  affirmative action, 23, 24
  aged and, 31, 33
  architectural accessibility, 73
  assistive technology, 91
  cancer patients covered by, 139
  children and, 155
  family services, 298, 324
  history, 208–209, 370
  housing issues, 386
  information resource centers under,
    407, 408

for mentally retarded, 248
professional credentials and, 228
for psychiatric rehabilitation, 581
rehabilitation counseling, 619
rehabilitation engineering, 298
rehabilitation program evaluation, 309, 314
research affected by, 633
for self-help groups, 666
transportation accessibility under, 735
veteran rehabilitation under, 742
work adjustment services under, 768
Rehabilitation Act Amendments of 1973, 399, 611
Rehabilitation Act Amendments of 1986, 709
Rehabilitation Act Amendments of 1987, 583
Rehabilitation Act Amendments of 1992, 228
affirmative action, 24
aging, 31, 33
assistive technology, 91
consumers and, 209–210
developmental disabilities, 250
future of rehabilitation, 335–336
independent living, 403, 404
job placement, 415
minorities, 465
rehabilitation counseling, 619, 620
rehabilitation education, 626
rehabilitation engineering, 298
research affected by, 633
for supported employment, 712, 713
Rehabilitation center, 564, **616–618**
architectural accessibility, 71
for burn victims, 130–132
for deaf-blind, 236
for hemophiliacs, 125
for independent living, 399–400
psychological approaches at, 597
religious support at, 628–629
self-help groups at, 664, 666
sexuality issues at, 672–673
Rehabilitation, Comprehensive Services, and Developmental Disabilities Act of 1978, 209–210, 666
Rehabilitation counseling, 319–320, 371, 563, **618–623**, 769
adjustment services of, 9, 11
for adolescents, **12–16**
advocacy role in, 17
for aged, 27, 30–33
by allied health professionals, **40–42**
for Alzheimer's patients, 45–46
for amputees, 55–56, 58–60

architectural accessibility and, 73
assessment by, 87
career counseling and, 144
clinical supervision of, **178–187**
credentials, **222–229**
for deaf/hearing impaired, 242
disability law/social policy on, 267
education for, **623–627**
ethics education for, 308
historical views of, 207
for HIV/AIDS patients, 391–393
kidney disorders and, 425, 426, 427, 428
life care planning and, 442
Medicaid denial of coverage for, 586
for minorities, 464–465
for pain, 533
philosophy of rehabilitation and, **555–559**
private sector, 571
in rural areas, 647
special education and, 681–682
for spinal cord injury, 691
state-federal rehabilitation program and, 697
supported employment and, **708–713**
Switzer, Mary E., **717–719**
for veterans, **740–743**
for vision loss, 119
women's role in, **762–767**
see also Assessment in rehabilitation; Career counseling
Rehabilitation education, **623–627**
accessibility needs of students, 3
adjustment services for, 10, 11
for adolescents, 14, 15
for aged, 32, 33
for arthritics, 81
assessment for, 83, 84, 86, 87
assistive technology for, 93
for back disorders, 106
for blind, 207
computers for, 202
for deaf-blind, 235
for deaf/hearing impaired, 244–245, 246–247
for hemophiliacs, 121–122
human resources development, **394–395**
international, 411
for kidney disorders, 425, 426
normalization/social role valorization and, 518
for prisoners, 218
for supported employment, 708
for veterans, 739–740

see also Students with disabilities
Rehabilitation engineering. See Engineering, rehabilitation
Rehabilitation Engineering Society of Japan, 300
Rehabilitation Engineering Society of North America, 298, 300
Rehabilitation hospital. See Hospital, rehabilitation
Rehabilitation International, 409
Rehabilitation psychology. See Psychology, rehabilitation
Rehabilitation research. See Research
Rehabilitation Services Administration (RSA), 267, 312, 314
for adjustment services, 11
for aging, 32
consumers and, 209
for deaf/hearing impaired, 245
for kidney disorders, 426, 427, 428
for psychiatric rehabilitation, 585–586
rehabilitation education and, 625, 626
state-federal rehabilitation program, 696
supported employment under, 709
Switzer, Mary E., **717–719**
Rehabilitation team, 563
Reiter's syndrome, 80
Relaxation training, 112
for burn victims, 130
for childhood psychiatric disorders, 166
for respiratory disease, 637
Religion, **628–631**
ADA coverage of workplace holidays, 50
alcohol rehabilitation and, 39
attitudes about, 98
deviancy views, 367
hospice counselors, 378
international rehabilitation, 412
role in coping with loss-related grief, 446
role in early care management, 450–451
views linking disabilities with evil, 744
Remote control systems, 90
Renal disease. See Kidney disorders
Replacement medication, 550
Research, **632–635**
on aged rehabilitation, 33
on back disorders, 107
on behavior therapy, 110–111

Research (*cont.*)
on caregiving effects, 147
deafness-related, 340
first national institute devoted to disability, 210
on gastrointestinal disorders, 343
on hemophilia-caused arthritis, 125
on independent living, 402–403
information resources, 406–407
on learning disabilities, 436
on mental retardation, 461
on minorities with disabilities, 464
on mood disorders, 474–475
on neuromuscular disorders, 514
on personal assistance services, 545
on physical therapy, 562
on psychiatric rehabilitation, 586
on quality of life, **607–609**
on serotonin levels, 553
sociological, 680
on spinal cord injury, 694
on stroke, 502
on vocational assessment, 730
on wellness issues, 756–757
on work issues, 772
Research and Training Center on Independent Living, 407
Research and Training Centers on Psychiatric Rehabilitation, 586
Residential rehabilitation, 320–321
Respirators, 564
Respiratory disease, **635–640**
architectural accessibility and, 74
neuromuscular disorders and, 511, 512
sickle cell anemia and, 674
Respite care, 46, 147, **641–642**, 693
Retinal degeneration, 118–119
Retinitis pigmentosa (tunnel vision), 235
REVES statistical group, 702
Revolutionary War, 261
Rheumatoid arthritis, 77–78, 479–480, 550, 551
Right-to-die, 176, 307; *see also* Euthanasia
Rimland, Bernard, 101
Risperidone, 657
Ritalin, 161
Rivera, Geraldo, 248
Roberts, Edward, 208, 209, 370, 399
Roeher, G. Allan, 516
Role modeling. *See* Normalization and social role valorization
Role-playing, 180
Roosevelt, Franklin D., 207

RSA. *See* Rehabilitation Services Administration
Rubella (German measles), 234, 236
Rural rehabilitation, **643–649**
Rusch, Frank, 708
Rusk, Howard A., 369, 382, **651–652**
Rusk Institute, 652
Russell, Harold, 568

S
Safe Kids Campaign, 366
Safety
auto belts and seats, 365, 535, 536, 538, 694
bicycle, 365, 366
environmental, 20, 193
playground, 365
San Antonio Independent School District v. Rodriguez (1973), 176
SAS software, 700
Saunders, Cecily, 379
Savage, Liz, 49
Savant, 101
Scandinavian formulations of normalization, 248, 515, 516
Scars, 132
Schizoid personality disorder, 547
Schizophrenia, **653–658**
adolescent, 14
alcoholism and, 38
caregiving for, 147
homelessness and, 372
pharmacology for, 552
psychiatric rehabilitation for, 579, 580, 582, 587
psychiatry for, 589–590
psychological support for families, 596
of veterans, 740
School for the Deaf, 451
Schools. *See* Colleges and universities; Learning disabilities; Special education; Students with disabilities
Scleroderma, 79, 80
Scleroderma Federation, 81
Screen displays, computer, 198–199, 204–205
Seizure drugs, 165
Self-advocacy. *See* Advocacy; Consumers
Self-care. *See* Independent living; Self-help in disability
Self-concept, **660–662**
aging and, 30
of alcoholic, 37
assistive technology and, 723
of breast cancer patients, 137

of burn victims, 133
career counseling and, 143
clothing and, **190–192**
dance/movement therapy for, 233
growth disorders and, 357
kidney disorders and, 425
following loss-related grief, 445
personality disorders and, 547
prosthetics/orthotics and, 574
psychosocial adjustment and, 601, 602
rehabilitation engineering and, 299
social workers to aid, 676
survey about, 700–701
see also Attitudes; Self-esteem
Self-Directed Search, 142
Self-employment, 647
Self-empowerment. *See* Empowerment
Self-esteem, 175
anxiety disorders and, 67
child and adolescent, 155, 192, 448
communication disabilities and, 192, 193, 194
dance/movement therapy for, 233
gastrointestinal disorders and, 345
growth disorders and, 357
following head injury, 363–364
learning disabilities and, 435
mental hospital effect on, 248
mood disorders affecting, 468
neuromuscular disorders and, 514
following pediatric rehabilitation, 539
personality disorders and, 547
programs for, 661
psychiatric rehabilitation and, 584
psychiatry for, 591
religious professionals to aid, 629–630
see also Self-concept
Self-help in disability, **663–668**
for addiction, 277
for adjustment problems, 10
for alcoholics, 39, 207
for arthritics, 81
for breast cancer survivors, 138
for burn victims, 133
for cancer survivors, 137
for caregivers, 147
for communication disabilities, 196
dance/movement therapy, 232
for families of schizophrenics, 657
hypnosis for burn victims, 130
inception of movement, 207
for independent living, 208
for pain sufferers, 533
prosthetics/orthotics and, 574

for psychiatric rehabilitation, 586–587

rehabilitation assessment for, 84–85

rural rehabilitation and, 646

for sexual disorders, 672

for stroke victims, 707

see also Advocacy; Consumers; *specific groups*, e.g., Alcoholics Anonymous

Sensory/neurological impairment. *See* Neurological disorders

Separation anxiety, 168

Serotonin levels, 455, 532, 552, 553

Serotonin Reuptake Inhibitors (SRIs), 470

Sertraline (Zoloft), 470, 552, 553

Service center programs, 288

Sex-linked conditions, 349–350, 352–353, 512–513

Sex offender rehabilitation, 220–221

Sexual abuse, 221, 547, 743, 746

Sexuality and disability, **668–673**

adolescent rehabilitation and, 15–16

arthritis effect on, 81

behavior therapy for problems with, 111

cancer effect on, 136

functional electrical stimulation for, 331

HIV/AIDS and, 388, 392, 393

neurological disorders and, 506

self-help for, 666

following spinal cord injury, 692

Sheltered employment. *See* Supported employment

Shingles, 390

Shock phase, 600

Shontz's model, 600

Sickle cell anemia and thalassemia (hemoglobinopathies), 120, 351, 352, **673–676**

Sign language. *See* American Sign Language

Silicone-filled breast implants, 138

Silverstein, Bob, 49

Sinus cancer, 136

Site-of-lesion testing, 100

Situational assessment, 751

Skilled nursing facilities (SNF), 318

Skin, 129, 131–132

Skin graft, 131, 132

Sleep disorders, 390, 455, 532, 553

Smith-Fess Act of 1920, 4, 367, 696

Smith-Hughes Act of 1917, 367

Smoking, 275

as cancer cause, 135

as coronary artery disease risk, 212, 215

effect on medication, 554

gastrointestinal disorders from, 342

nicotine addiction from, 35

respiratory disease and, 637

as stroke risk, 502, 705

Snellen System, 116, 117

Social and Rehabilitative Services Administration, 717

Social burden myth, 745

Social policy. *See* Disability law and social policy

Social role theory, 518–519

Social role valorization. *See* Normalization and social role valorization

Social Security Act of 1935, 27, 368, 369, 396

Social Security Administration (SSA), 267, 268, 327, 425, 427, 428, 697

Social Security Disability Insurance (SSDI), 84, 267, 572

for developmental disabilities, 255

ethical issues, 306

gender-related benefits differences, 266

homeless and, 375, 376

job placement and, 415

kidney disorders and, 425

state-federal rehabilitation program and, 696 697

see also Workers' compensation

Social Security international programs, 411

Social Security Supplemental Security Income (SSI), 84, 156, 255, 375, 376, 396, 425

Social service agencies, 288

Social Service block grants, 543

Social situations. *See* Psychosocial adjustment

Social work practice in rehabilitation, 563, **676–678**

for developmentally disabled, 254

for hospice, 378

for rehabilitation hospital patients, 383

salary for, 764

for spinal cord injury, 691

Society of Disability Studies, 210

Sociology, **678–680**

Software programs, 205

Software for Survey Data Analysis, 700

Soldier Rehabilitation Act of 1918, 261, 367

Somatopsychology, 597

Souder v. Brennan (1973), 581

Southeastern Community v. Davis (1979), 176

Spasticity, 691–692

Special education, 153, **681–686**

adjustment services, 11

adolescent rehabilitation programs, 13

assistive technology for, 93

computers for, 202

international rehabilitation, 409

for learning disabilities, 435

for mentally retarded, 459

following pediatric rehabilitation, 538–540

Speech and language disorders. *See* Aphasia; Communication disabilities

Speech synthesis systems, 198

Spina bifida, 151, 347, 458, 746

Spinal cord cancer, 138

Spinal cord injury, 105, **688–694**

adjustment services for, 9

assistance animals for, 63

assistive technology for, 90

functional electrical stimulation for, 331

orthotics for, 574

pediatric rehabilitation and, 537

pharmacology for, 550

physician for, 564

rehabilitation assessment for, 86

rehabilitation engineering for, 297–298

sexuality following, 671, 672

violence as cause, 743

Spinal muscular atrophy, 512, 640

Spirituality. *See* Religion

Spondyloarthropathies, 80

Sports

musculoskeletal disorders and, 491, 495–496

pediatric injuries caused by, 535

prostheses/orthoses used for, 574

psychologists and sports medicine, 593

psychotherapy following injury, 591

therapeutic recreation using, 615

for wellness, 755–757

using wheelchairs, 574, 615, 761, 762

SRV. *See* Normalization and social role valorization

SSDI. *See* Social Security Disability Insurance

SSI. *See* Social Security Supplemental Security Income

Stage theory, 600

Stanford-Binet scale, 457
State-federal benefits
  for the blind, 117
  statistics, 6, 175
State-federal rehabilitation program,
  11, **696–698**
  for career counseling, 140–141
  counseling for, 619
  for deaf/hearing impaired, 241–244,
    246
  for disabled, 6
  economics of, 282
  for hemophiliacs, 125
  history of, 368
  for minorities, 463
  psychiatric, 581
  Switzer, Mary E., **717–719**
  vocational, 334
  welfare programs, 6, 175, 261, 265–
    268
State mental hospitals, 248, 249
State Plan Assurance Review, 312
Statewide Independent Living Coun-
    cils, 404
Statistics, **698–703**
  accidental injury, 363
  amputation, 54, 574
  aphasia, 68
  back injury, 105
  blindness/vision impairment, 117,
    118
  burns, 126
  cancer, 135, 136, 137, 139
  causes of death, 112
  communication disabilities, 192,
    193
  coronary artery disease, 146, 212, 217
  deaf-blindness, 234
  deafness/hearing impairment, 239,
    242
  disability, 4, 6, 301, 334, 385, 409,
    569, 632
  disability payments, 217
  drug abusers in prison, 219
  drug rehabilitation, 275
  eating disorders, 279
  Employee Assistance Programs, 287
  endocrine disorders, 290
  head injury, 361, 362
  hemophilia, 121
  homelessness, 372, 374
  hospice, 380
  international rehabilitation, 409
  mentally ill, 248, 249, 582
  mental retardation, 457
  musculoskeletal disorders, 479, 480

neurological disorders, 501, 504,
    505, 506
nursing homes, 318
occupational therapy, 528
pain, 531
pediatric rehabilitation, 535
respiratory disease, 636
respite care, 642
rural rehabilitation, 643
schizophrenia, 654–655
spinal cord injury, 689
sports for disabled, 574
technology and disability, 721
transportation accessibility, 731
unemployment, 6, 22–23, 175
violence, 743
welfare benefits, 6, 175
wheelchairs, 760
women in prison, 221
work, 334
workplace accidents, 272
Sterilization, 461
Steroid abuse, 275
Steroidal medication, 551
Stimulation medication, 161, 550
Strategic planning, 452
Stress
  of assistive technology use, 723
  behavior therapy for, 112
  of burn victims, 132
  career development as cause of, 141
  in clinical supervisor/trainee rela-
    tionship, 184–185
  effect on Alzheimer's disease, 44
  endocrine disorders and, 290
  in family, 322
  gastrointestinal disorders from, 342
  hemophilia as cause of, 122
  loss and grief following, 444, 446
  management for back disorders, 106
  massage therapy for, 455
  occupational therapy for, 527
  psychiatric rehabilitation for, 580
  psychological approaches to, 595, 598
  recreation services for, 614
  respite care to relieve, **641–642**
  on veterans, 740
Stroke, 501–502, **703–708**
  aphasia caused by, 68
  blood disorders as cause of, 120
  communication disabilities following,
    192, 194, 195
  depression following, 530
  diabetes as cause of, 292
  loss-related grief following, 445
  occupational therapy for, 527

pharmacology for, 550, 551
physician for, 563, 564
sickle cell anemia and, 674
speech/language professionals for, 41
following spinal cord injury, 691
Students with disabilities, 271
  adjustment services for, 11
  adolescent rehabilitation programs, 13
  art therapy for, 75
  attitudes toward, 94, 95, 97
  blindness, 422
  career counseling for, 144
  clothing for, 190
  college acceptances, 208
  computers for, 202, 206
  deaf/hearing impaired, 243, 247
  denied acceptance into professional
    programs, 207–208
  developmentally disabled, 254, 255
  disability law/social policy for, 266–
    267, 269
  future of, 336
  gastrointestinal problems, 345
  history of, 370
  learning disabilities, **434–436**
  legislation protecting, 155, 209
  pediatric rehabilitation and, 539, 540
  rehabilitation assessment for, 84, 87
  self-concept of, 660
  self-help advocacy for, 665–666, 667
  sickle cell anemia, 674–675
  social worker to aid, 677
  special education, **681–686**
  state-federal rehabilitation program
    for, 697
  teachers of, 96, 154, 155
  thalassemia, 675–676
  transition from school to work,
    726–731
  see also Mainstreaming; Rehabilita-
    tion education
Stuttering, 194
Substance abuse. See specific type, e.g.,
    Drug abuse
Suction sockets, 297
Suicide
  alcoholism-related, 36
  following loss-related grief, 445
  medically assisted, 258, 543
  mood disorders as cause, 468, 469, 471
  prevention of, 591
  schizophrenia as cause, 655
Sullivan, Anne Mansfield, 421
Sullivan, Oscar, 368
Sullivan v. Zebley (1990), 156
Supervision. See Clinical supervision

Supported education, 583–584
Supported employment, 371, **708–713**, 769, 771
  for adolescents, 14
  career counseling for, 144
  facilities for, 319
  future of rehabilitation, 336–337
  following head injury, 365
  job placement and, 414, 417
  for psychiatric rehabilitation, 581–582
  rehabilitation education and, 623
  for transition from school to work, 727, 729
Supported living, 320, 401
  for aged, 32
  for alcoholics, 37
  for Alzheimer's patients, 46
  for autistics, 102
  following head injury, 365
  rehabilitation assessment for, 86
  respite care and, 642
Support groups. See Self-help in disability
Support services for transition, 728–729
Surface Transportation Assistance Act of 1983, 733
Surgery, **715–716**
  amputation, **53–61**
  for burns, 127, 130–131, 132
  for cancer, 136, 137–138, 139
  for childhood disabilities, 151, 153
  communication disabilities caused by, 194
  for coronary artery disease, 212
  for deafness, 100
  for endocrine disorders, 294, 295
  for gastrointestinal disorders, 341, 342, 343, 344, 345, 346
  for genetic disorders, 347
  joint replacement for arthritis, 77, 124
  for kidney disorders, 424, 425
  massage therapy following, 454
  mental retardation and, 459
  for neurological disorders, 506
  for neuromuscular disorders, 513
  organ transplants, 346, 424, 425
  pain and, 531, 532, 533
  for pediatric injuries, 536
  prenatal, 459
  reconstructive, 130–131, 136, 137–138
  for spinal cord anomalies, 151, 458
  following spinal cord injury, 691–692
  following stroke, 704, 705
  for thalassemia, 676
Survey on Income and Program Participation, 701
Surveys. See Statistics; specific surveys

Swedish Association for Retarded Children, 515
Switzer, Mary E., 369, **717–719**, 763
Systems advocacy, 18, 20–21
Systems evaluation, 311

T
Talking books, 422
Tapotement, 454–455
Tardive dyskinesia, 656
Target joint, 123–124
Tax Equity and Fiscal Responsibility Act of 1982, 563
TDD. See Telecommunication device for the deaf
Technology and disability, 258, 371, 564, **721–726**
  for amputees, 60–61
  architectural accessibility and, 71, 72, 74
  assistive technology, **89–93**
  for burn victims, 131–132
  computers for visual impairments, **197–201**
  for deaf-blindness, 235
  effect on caregivers, 146
  future of, 334, 335
  at Gallaudet University, 340
  for growth disorders, 357–358
  for head injury prevention, 365
  for hemophiliacs, 124
  legislation, 5, 89, 91, 298, 647–648, 721
  minorities and, 467
  occupational therapy and, 527
  prenatal screening, 348, 459, 477
  for psychiatric rehabilitation, 587
  quality of life affected by, 608
  rehabilitation assessment and, 83
  rehabilitation education and, 627
  rehabilitation program evaluation, 315
  in rural areas, 647–648
  state-federal rehabilitation program, 697
  for stroke victims, 707
  for veterans, 740
Technology Related Assistance for Persons with Disabilities Act of 1988, 5, 89, 91, 298, 647–648, 721
Teenagers. See Adolescents, rehabilitation of
Telecommunication device for the deaf (TDD), 241
  ADA requirements, 53, 91, 269
  future of, 335
  to provide accessibility, 3, 5, 6

Television systems, closed-circuit, 199
Tendon and ligament disorders, 479–482
Testing. See Assessment in rehabilitation; Psychology; Vocational evaluation
Thalassemia. See Sickle cell anemia and thalassemia (hemoglobinopathies)
Thalidomide, 297
Therapeutic recreation. See Recreation
Think First Program, 693–694
Thorazine, 552
Throat cancer, 136
Thrombocytosis, 120
Thrombo-embolic disease, 703, 705
Thrombolytic agents, 551
Thyroid disorders, 294
Thyroid hormone, 471
Tissue inflammation, 490–491
Titticut Follies (documentary), 248
Tobacco. See Smoking
Tongue cancer, 137
Toxicology, 549
Toxins. See Environmental influences
Trace Center, 407
Traffic accidents. See Highway accidents
Training in Community Living program, 658
Train transportation, 732
Tranquilizer abuse, 275
Transferability of skills. See Job placement
Transitional employment, 584–585
Transitionalism, 582–583
Transition from school to work, 336–337, **726–731**
  for adolescents, 14
  career counseling for, 144
  for deaf-blind, 238
  for deaf/hearing impaired, 243
  for developmentally disabled, 255
  rehabilitation assessment for, 87
  special education for, 681, 685–686
Transplantation. See Organ transplants
Transportation, U.S. Department of, 52, 732–735, 736
Transportation accessibility, 4, **731–737**
  ADA requirements, 50, 52
  for aged, 32
  for Alzheimer's patients, 46
  civil rights legislation, 176
  life care planning and, 441
  for minorities, 463
  in rural areas, 645–646
  for spinal cord injury victims, 693
  for stroke victims, 707
  for wheelchairs, 6

Trauma
  abuse of women as, 221
  amputation as result of, 54–55
  back disorders caused by, 106
  behavior therapy following, 111
  burns, **126–133**
  childhood disability caused by, 152–153
  communication disabilities caused by, 194, 195
  developmental disabilities following, 250
  ergonomics to control, 304
  family reaction to, 322
  future of rehabilitation, 334
  head injury, **361–366**
  among homeless, 374–375
  housing issues following, 385
  loss and grief following, 444–445, 446
  management of, 449
  massage therapy for, 454
  musculoskeletal disorders caused by, 480, 492
  pediatric rehabilitation, **534–541**
  personality disorders following, 547
  physiatrist's role, 564, 565
  psychologist's role, 595, 597
  rehabilitation psychology following, 597
  sexuality following, 670, 671
  social worker's role, 677
  spinal cord injury as result, 689, 690
  see also Violence
Trazone (Desyrel), 470, 553
Treatment Alternatives to Street Crime, 220
Trisomy 21. See Down syndrome
Tuberculosis, 374
Tuke, William, 515, 581
Tullman, Steve, 517
Tumors, 68, 194, 195
  bone, 489
  endocrine, 294, 295
  genetic, 352
  see also specific cancers
Turner syndrome, 349, 357

U
Ulcerative colitis, 344
Unemployment
  adjustment services for, 10–11
  aging and, 29
  eating disorders and, 280
  kidney disorders and, 424–425, 426
  minority rates of, 463, 464, 466
  neuromuscular disorders and, 514

statistics, 6, 22–23, 175, 569
transportation accessibility as factor, 733
Unions. See Labor unions
United Cerebral Palsy Association, 18, 255
United Mine Workers, 369
United Nations, 258–259, 411–412, 702
United Nations Year of Disabled Persons, 409, 410
United Ostomy Association, 136, 664
United States. See Statistics; specific government agencies and legislation
Universal Declaration of Human Rights, 258–259
Universal design. See Architectural accessibility; Housing
Universities. See Colleges and universities
Unparental disomy, 353
Urban Mass Transportation Act of 1970, 73, 732
Urinary tract infections, 692, 705, 715
Urologists, 715
U.S. Department of. See key word, e.g., Justice, U.S. Department of
Usher's syndrome, 235, 237
Utilitarianism, 305

V
VALPAR system, 526
Vascular surgeon, 715
Venlafaxine, 553
Ventilatory impairment, 638–640
Verapamil (Calan), 472
Vermont Rehabilitation Engineering Research Center for Low Back Pain, 107
Veterans
  accessibility needs, 4–5
  amputation and, 55
  architectural accessibility needs, 71–72
  attitudes toward, 98
  Civil War, 206, 573
  disability law/social policy, 261
  homelessness of, 375
  Korean War, 72, 741–742
  rehabilitation engineering, 298
  Revolutionary War, 261
  Rusk's work with, 651–652
  self-help groups for, 664, 666–667
  Vietnam War, 4, 72, 742
  vocational rehabilitation for, 319, 740–741

World War I, 4, 207, 333, 367, 409, 421, 528, 740–741
World War II, 4, 71, 207, 297, 318, 528, 568, 651–652, 664, 666–667
  see also Paralyzed Veterans of America
Veterans Administration, 298, 739, 741, 742
Veterans Affairs, U.S. Department of. See Veterans' medical rehabilitation in the U.S. Department of Veterans Affairs; Veteran vocational rehabilitation in the U.S. Department of Veterans Affairs
Veterans Benefits Administration, Vocational Rehabilitation and Counseling Service, 742
Veterans Health Administration, 739, 740, 742
Veterans' medical rehabilitation in the U.S. Department of Veterans Affairs, **739–740**
Veteran vocational rehabilitation in the U.S. Department of Veterans Affairs, **740–743**
Vibration stroke, 455
Vibrotactile aid, 100
Videotape for training, 180
Vietnam War, 4, 72, 742
Violence, **743–747**
  against aged, 543
  alcoholism-related, 36
  by caregiver, 543
  against children, 130, 535, 538, 547
  loss and grief following, 444
  personality disorders following, 547
  prevention programs, 362, 366
  against schizophrenics, 653
  spinal cord injury as result of, 694
  against women, 221
  see also Child abuse; Sexual abuse; Trauma
Viral infection, 172
Vision disorders. See Blindness and vision disorders
Visual functions, 116–117
Visual-motor integration, 151
Visual system, 115–116
Vitamins, 102, 129, 215
Vocal cord cancer, 136
Vocational counseling. See Career counseling
Vocational evaluation, **748–753**, 771
  ability factors for, **1–3**
  adjustment services following, 8
  by career counselors, 144

computers to aid, 206
education for, 623
occupational information for, **525–527**
rehabilitation counseling and, 622
state-federal rehabilitation program for, 696
for transition from school to work, 729–730
Vocational Evaluation and Work Adjustment Association, 623
Vocational expert, 327
Vocational Rehabilitation Act of 1943, 624
Vocational Rehabilitation Act of 1973, 155, 297, 727
Vocational Rehabilitation Amendments of 1954, 369, 624, 718
Vocational Rehabilitation program, 282, 283, 284, 286, 314
Vocational rehabilitation. *See* Career counseling; Rehabilitation counseling
Vocational training
  for adolescents, 14, 15, 125
  affirmative action, 25
  for aged, 30–32, 33
  allied health professionals and, 41
  assessment for, 84, 86
  assistive technology for, 92, 93
  for blind, 422
  for cancer patients, 135, 139
  career counseling and, 140, 141, 142
  clinical supervision of personnel, 183–184
  computers for, 202, 206
  for deaf-blind, 235, 237
  disability law/social policy concerning, 266
  for hemophiliacs, 125
  legislation, 211
  for prisoners, 218–219
  state-federal rehabilitation program, 696
  for transition from school to work, **726–731**
  outside United States, 14
Voice-activated appliances, 90
Voice disabilities, 194
Voice output devices, 205
Voice recognition computers, 204
Voice synthesizers, 136–137, 154, 204, 205
Von Willebrand's disease, 121
Voting Accessibility for the Elderly and Handicapped of 1984, 5, 48

W
Wagner-Peyser Act Amendments of 1954, 266
Walker, Sylvia, 370
Walkers, 723
War veterans. *See* Veterans
Wechsler intelligence scales, 457, 750
Wehman, Paul, 708
Weicker, Lowell, 49
Welfare. *See* State-federal rehabilitation programs
Wellness, **755–759**
  employee assistance programs, 288
  mental, 590–591
  psychology and, 593
  quality of life, **607–609**
  recreation, **614–615**
  work and, 767–768
  workplace programs, 334
  see also Prevention programs
Wheelchairs, 564, 723, 724–725, **760–762**
  accessibility needs, 3, 6, 70, 71, 177, 665, 734, 735, 736
  ADA requirements, 50
  adjustment services for users, 9
  for amputees, 59
  animals to assist with, 63
  for cancer patients, 138
  for children, 154
  clothing and, 191
  for hemophiliacs, 124
  housing issues, 385, 386
  life care planning and, 439
  for neuromuscular disorders, 512, 513
  occupational therapy and, 527
  rehabilitation engineering, 298, 299
  self-help for accessibility, 665
  for spinal cord injury, 691
  sports competition using, 574, 615, 761, 762
  for stroke victims, 706, 707
  student rights, 370
  technological changes, 71, 90–91
  transportation accessibility and, 734, 735, 736
  wellness programs for users of, 756
Wide Range Achievement Test, 750
Wide Range Interest-Opinion Test, 750–751
Wiener, Norbert, 301
Wilbur, Harvey, 367
Will, Madeline, 683, 726
Willowbrook State School (New York), 20, 248
Wiseman, Frederick, 248

Witchcraft, 367
Wolfensberger, Wolf, 17, 248, 515–518
Women in rehabilitation, **762–767**
  assistive technology, 724
  cancer patients, 136, 137–138
  endocrine disorder patients, 295–296
  prison inmates, 221
Women's sexuality, 671–672
Work, **767–772**
  ability for, **1–3**
  accessibility, 4, 6
  ADA application to, 50, 51
  adjustment services for, 9, 10–11
  for adolescents, 14, 540–541
  advocacy programs, 20, 540–541
  affirmative action, **22–26**
  aging and, 29, 30, 32, 33
  alcoholism and, 36, 38
  architectural accessibility, 70, 71, 73
  arthritis disability and, 81
  attitudes about disabled workers, 94, 95, 97
  back disorders and, 106–107, 284
  behavior therapy for stress from, 112
  for blind/visually disabled, 207
  burn victims and, 133
  cancer patients and, 137, 139
  career counseling for, **140–145**
  civil rights issues, 174, 177, 178
  clothing for, 190, 191
  communication disabilities and, 193, 194
  compensation legislation. *See* Workers' compensation
  computers for, 202, 206
  following coronary artery disease, 216–217
  for deaf/hearing impaired, 244
  diabetics and, 293
  disability management, **270–274**
  education for, 208
  employee assistance programs, **287–289**
  ergonomics, **302–304**
  forensic rehabilitation, 327, 328–329
  future of rehabilitation, 333–334
  Gallaudet alumni, 341
  gastrointestinal disorders and, 344, 345
  following head injury, 365
  for hemophiliacs, 124
  history for life planning, 438
  history of rehabilitation, 371
  for HIV/AIDS patients, 391, 392
  at home, 202, 414

Work (*cont.*)

human resource development, **394–395**

injury from. *See* Occupational injury

international rehabilitation, 409

kidney disorders and, 425, 426, 427

labor unions, **431–433**

mental illness and, 590–591

for minorities, 464, 467

musculoskeletal disorders and, 479–480, 491

occupational information, **525–527**

occupational therapy, 527

pain effect on workers, 531, 533

President's Committee on Employment of People with Disabilities, **568–570**

private sector rehabilitation, **570–572**

psychiatric rehabilitation and, 581–583, 584–585

reasonable accommodation, **611–613**

rehabilitation assessment for, 83, 84, 86, 87

rehabilitation counseling for, **618–623**

rehabilitation economics for, 283, 284

rehabilitation psychology and, 598

rehabilitation research about, 635

respiratory disease and, 640

in rural areas, 647

special education to aid, 685

spinal cord injury and, 693

state-federal rehabilitation program, **696–698**

for stroke victims, 707

supported employment, **708–713**

termination of/adverse action, 1–2, 26, 711

vision loss and, 119

vocational evaluation, **748–753**

vocational rehabilitation, 319–320

see also Career counseling; Job placement; Labor unions; Transition from school to work; Unemployment; Vocational training

Work acclimation model, 9

Work design. *See* Ergonomics

Workers' compensation, 84, 261, 266, 272, 415, 571

first legislation, 207

forensic rehabilitation and, 327

psychologist role in, 595

rehabilitation programs, 625

Work hardening programs, 9, 106, 533, 769

Work readiness, 418

Work samples, 751–752

World Crusade for the Blind, 422

World Disability Fund, 640

World Federation of Occupational Therapy, 528

World Health Organization, 702

World Rehabilitation Fund, 652, 717

World War I, 4, 207, 333, 367, 409, 421, 528, 740–741

World War II, 4, 71, 207, 297, 318, 528, 568, 651–652, 664, 666–667

Wright, Pat, 49

Wyatt v. *Stickney*, 248

Y

Yeast infection, 172

Youngberg v. *Romeo* (1982), 20

Young people. *See* Adolescents, rehabilitation of; Childhood disabilities

Z

Zoloft. *See* Sertraline